S0-AIQ-633

BEHAVIORAL NEUROLOGY AND NEUROPSYCHOLOGY

NOTICE

BEHAVIORAL NEUROLOGY AND NEUROPSYCHOLOGY

SECOND EDITION

EDITORS

Todd E. Feinberg, M.D.

Chief
Betty and Morton Yarmon Division of Neurobehavior and Alzheimer's Disease
Associate Attending, Psychiatry and Neurology
Beth Israel Medical Center
New York, New York
Associate Professor, Neurology and Psychiatry
Albert Einstein College of Medicine
Bronx, New York

Martha J. Farah, Ph.D.

Professor of Psychology and Director
Center for Cognitive Neuroscience
University of Pennsylvania
Philadelphia, Pennsylvania

McGraw-Hill
MEDICAL PUBLISHING DIVISION

New York Chicago San Francisco Lisbon London Madrid
Mexico City Milan New Delhi San Juan Seoul Singapore Sydney Toronto

The McGraw·Hill Companies

BEHAVIORAL NEUROLOGY AND NEUROPSYCHOLOGY, Second Edition

1 2 3 4 5 6 7 8 9 0 DOC DOC 0 9 8 7 6 5 4 3

ISBN 0-07-137432-9

This book was set in Times Roman by The GTS Companies/York, PA Campus.
The editors were Marc Strauss, Lisa Silverman, and Lester A. Sheinis.
The production supervisor was Richard C. Ruzycka.
The cover designer was Aimée Nordin.
The indexer was Alexandra Nickerson.
RR Donnelley was printer and binder.

This book is printed on acid-free paper.

Cataloging-in-publication data for this title is on file at the Library of Congress.

In memory of Eleanor M. Saffran,
beloved colleague and friend to so many of us.

CONTENTS

Contributors xiii

Preface xxi

PART 1 GENERAL PRINCIPLES 1

1 The Development of Modern Behavioral Neurology and Neuropsychology 3
Todd E. Feinberg
Martha J. Farah

2 The Mental Status Exam 23
Susan K. Guy
Jeffrey L. Cummings

3 Principles of Neuropsychological Assessment 33
Muriel D. Lezak

4 Some Anatomic Principles Related to Behavioral Neurology and Neuropsychology 45
M.-Marsel Mesulam

5 Mechanisms of Plasticity and Behavior 57
Albert M. Galaburda
Alvaro Pascual-Leone

6 The Lesion Method in Behavioral Neurology and Neuropsychology 71
Hanna Damasio
Antonio R. Damasio

7 Functional Imaging in Behavioral Neurology and Neuropsychology 85
Geoffrey Karl Aguirre

8 Functional Neuroimaging Studies of Neuropsychological Patients 97
Cathy J. Price
Karl J. Friston

9 Electrophysiological Methods and Transcranial Magnetic Stimulation in Behavioral Neurology and Neuropsychology 105
Leon Y. Deouell
Richard B. Ivry
Robert T. Knight

10 Computational Modeling in Behavioral Neurology and Neuropsychology 135
Martha J. Farah

PART 2 APHASIA AND OTHER DOMINANT HEMISPHERE SYNDROMES 145

11 Aphasia: Clinical and Anatomic Issues 147
Michael P. Alexander
12 Aphasia: Cognitive Neuropsychological Issues 165
Eleanor M. Saffran
13 Rehabilitation of Aphasia 179
Myrna F. Schwartz
Ruth B. Fink
14 Acquired Disorders of Reading 195
H. Branch Coslett
15 Acalculia and Number Processing Disorders 207
Stanislas Dehaene
16 Disorders of Skilled Movements: Limb Apraxia 217
Kenneth M. Heilman
Robert T. Watson
Leslie J. Gonzalez Rothi

PART 3 AGNOSIA AND DISORDERS OF PERCEPTION 225

17 Visual Perception and Visual Imagery 227
Martha J. Farah
18 Visual Object Agnosia 233
Martha J. Farah
Todd E. Feinberg
19 Prosopagnosia 239
Martha J. Farah
20 Disorders of Color Processing 243
Daniel Tranel
21 Auditory Agnosia and Amusia 257
Russell M. Bauer
Carrie R. McDonald
22 Tactile Agnosia and Disorders of Tactile Perception 271
Richard J. Caselli
23 Disorders of Body Perception and Representation 285
Georg Goldenberg
24 Visuospatial Function 295
Martha J. Farah

PART 4 DISORDERS OF ATTENTION AND AWARENESS 301

25 Neglect: Clinical and Anatomic Issues 303
Kenneth M. Heilman
Robert T. Watson
Edward Valenstein

26 Neglect: Cognitive Neuropsychological Issues 313
Anjan Chatterjee
H. Branch Coslett

27 Balint's Syndrome and Related Disorders 325
H. Branch Coslett
Anjan Chatterjee

28 Disorders of Consciousness in Coma, Stupor, and Minimally Responsive States 337
Joseph T. Giacino

29 Anosognosia 345
Todd E. Feinberg
David M. Roane

30 Confabulation 363
Todd E. Feinberg
Joseph T. Giacino

31 Misidentification Syndromes 373
Todd E. Feinberg
David M. Roane

PART 5 FRONTAL, CALLOSAL, AND SUBCORTICAL SYNDROMES 383

32 Frontal Lobes: Clinical and Anatomic Issues 385
Bruce L. Miller
D. Frank Benson
Julene K. Johnson

33 Frontal Lobes: Cognitive Neuropsychological Issues 393
Martha J. Farah

34 Callosal Disconnection 401
Kathleen Baynes
Michael S. Gazzaniga

35 Syndromes due to Acquired Basal Ganglia Damage 411
Bruce Crosson
Anna Bacon Moore
Christina E. Wierenga

36 Syndromes due to Acquired Thalamic Damage 419
Neill R. Graff-Radford

PART 6 MEMORY AND AMNESIA 429

37 Amnesia: Neuroanatomic and Clinical Issues 431
Matthias Brand
Hans J. Markowitsch

38 Amnesia: Cognitive Neuropsychological Issues 445
Margaret M. Keane
Mieke Verfaellie

39 Semantic Memory Impairment 457
Martha J. Farah
Murray Grossman
40 Learning and Memory Dysfunction Following Traumatic Brain Injury 463
Frank G. Hillary
John DeLuca
41 Memory Impairment Following Anterior Communicating Artery Aneurysm 477
John DeLuca
Deborah Bryant
Catherine E. Myers
42 Rehabilitation of Memory Dysfunction 487
Elizabeth L. Glisky

PART 7 DELIRIUM, DEMENTIA, AND EPILEPSY 493

43 Delirium and Dementia: an Overview 495
Daniel I. Kaufer
Jeffrey L. Cummings
44 Alzheimer's Disease: Clinical and Anatomic Issues 515
François Boller
Charles Duyckaerts
45 Alzheimer's Disease: Biochemical and Pharmacologic Issues 545
Gang Tong
Leon J. Thal
46 Alzheimer's Disease: Cognitive Neuropsychological Issues 573
William Milberg
Regina McGlinchey-Berroth
47 Frontotemporal Dementia and Variants 582
Mario F. Mendez
48 Dementia in Parkinson's Disease, Huntington's Disease, and Related Disorders 593
Diane M. Jacobs
Gilberto Levy
Karen Marder
49 Vascular Dementia 609
John V. Bowler
Vladimir Hachinski
50 Infective Causes of Dementia Including Human Immunodeficiency Virus 629
Clement T. Loy
Bruce J. Brew
51 Wernicke-Korsakoff and Related Nutritional Disorders of the Nervous System 639
Mieke Verfaellie
52 Neurobehavioral Aspects of Vasculitis and Collagen Vascular Syndromes 651
Nancy N. Futrell
Clark H. Millikan
53 Normal Pressure Hydrocephalus 659
Thomas A. Krefft
Neill R. Graff-Radford

54 Cognitive and Behavioral Aspects of Epilepsy 675
Melanie Shulman
Orrin Devinsky
55 Neuropsychological Aspects of Temporal Lobe Epilepsy Surgery 695
David W. Loring
Kimford J. Meador

PART 8 EMOTIONAL DISORDERS 709

56 Emotion and the Brain: An Overview 711
Kevin S. LaBar
Joseph E. LeDoux
57 Emotional Disorders in Relation to Unilateral Brain Damage 725
Guido Gainotti
58 Emotional Disorders in Relation to Nonfocal Brain Dysfunction 735
Elizabeth S. Ochoa
Hulya M. Erhan
Todd E. Feinberg
59 The Aprosodias 743
Elliott D. Ross
60 Violence and the Brain 755
Jonathan M. Silver
Karen E. Anderson
Stuart C. Yudofsky

PART 9 NEUROBEHAVIORAL DISORDERS IN CHILDREN 763

61 The Neurobehavioral Examination for Children 765
Martha Bridge Denckla
62 Pediatric Neuropsychological Assessment 773
Jane Holmes Bernstein
Deborah P. Waber
63 Acquired Disorders of Language in Children 783
Maureen Dennis
64 Developmental Reading Disorders 801
Maureen W. Lovett
Roderick W. Barron
65 Nonverbal, Social, and Emotional Learning Disabilities 821
Kytja K.S. Voeller
66 Attention Deficit Hyperactivity Disorder 831
Bruce F. Pennington
Nomita Chhabildas
67 Mental Retardation 843
Kytja K.S. Voeller

68 The Pervasive Developmental Disorders: Autism and Related Conditions 853
Nancy J. Minshew
Jessica A. Meyer

69 Molecular Genetics of Cognitive Developmental Disorders 867
James Swanson
John Fosella
Deborah Grady
Robert Moyzis
Pam Flodman
Anne Spence
Michael Posner

COLOR PLATES FALL BETWEEN PAGES 72 AND 73

Glossary of Linguistic Terms **881**

Index **883**

CONTRIBUTORS

Geoffrey Karl Aguirre, M.D., Ph.D.
University of Pennsylvania
Center for Cognitive Neuroscience
Philadelphia, Pennsylvania
(Chapter 7)

Michael P. Alexander, M.D.
Departments of Neurology
Beth Israel Deaconess Medical Center
and Harvard Medical School
Boston, Massachusetts
Stroke Rehabilitation, Youville Lifecare Hospital
Cambridge, Massachusetts
Memory Disorders Research Center
Boston University School of Medicine
Rotman Research Institute
Baycrest Geriatric Centre
Toronto, Canada
(Chapter 11)

Karen E. Anderson, M.D., M.S.
Functional Neuroimaging Laboratory
University of Maryland School of Medicine
Baltimore, Maryland
(Chapter 60)

Roderick W. Barron, Ph.D.
Professor, Department of Psychology
University of Guelph
Guelph, Ontario, Canada
(Chapter 64)

Russell M. Bauer, Ph.D.
Professor, Associate Chair for Academic Affairs
Department of Clinical and Health Psychology
University of Florida
Gainesville, Florida
(Chapter 21)

Kathleen Baynes, Ph.D.
Associate Professor of Neurology
University of California at Davis
Davis, California
(Chapter 34)

D. Frank Benson, M.D.
Augustus S. Rose Professor Emeritus of Neurology
University of California at Los Angeles
Los Angeles, California
(Chapter 32)

Jane Holmes Bernstein, Ph.D.
Assistant Clinical Professor of Psychology
Department of Psychiatry
Harvard Medical School
Children's Hospital
Boston, Massachusetts
(Chapter 62)

François Boller, M.D., Ph.D.
Director, Department of Neuropsychology and Neurobiology
INSERM (The French Institute of Health and Medical Research)
Paris, France
(Chapter 44)

John V. Bowler, M.D.
Department of Neurology
Royal Free Hospital
London, England
(Chapter 49)

Matthias Brand, Ph.D.
University of Bielefeld
Department of Physiological Psychology
Bielefeld, Germany
(Chapter 37)

Bruce J. Brew, M.B.B.S., M.D., F.R.A.C.P.
Professor of Medicine (Neurology)
University of New South Wales
Consultant Physician and Neurologist
Head of Department of Neurology and Neurosciences
St. Vincent's Hospital, Darlinghurst
Sydney, Australia
(Chapter 50)

Deborah Bryant, Ph.D.
Kessler Medical Rehabilitation Research
and Education Corporation
West Orange, New Jersey
(Chapter 41)

Richard J. Caselli, M.D.
Department of Neurology
Mayo Clinic Scottsdale
Scottsdale, Arizona
(Chapter 22)

Anjan Chatterjee, M.D.
Department of Neurology
and the Center for Cognitive Neuroscience
University of Pennsylvania
Philadelphia, Pennsylvania
(Chapters 26, 27)

Nomita Chhabildas
Department of Psychology
University of Denver
Denver, Colorado
(Chapter 66)

H. Branch Coslett, M.D.
Department of Neurology
and the Center for Cognitive Neuroscience
University of Pennsylvania
Philadelphia, Pennsylvania
(Chapters 14, 26, 27)

Bruce Crosson, Ph.D.
Department of Clinical and Health Psychology
University of Florida Health Science Center
Gainesville, Florida
(Chapter 35)

Jeffrey L. Cummings, M.D.
Director, UCLA Alzheimer's Disease Center
Los Angeles, California
(Chapters 2, 43)

Antonio R. Damasio, M.D.
M.W. Van Allen Professor and Head of Neurology
University of Iowa Hospitals and Clinics
Iowa City, Iowa
(Chapter 6)

Hanna Damasio, M.D.
Professor of Neurology
University of Iowa Hospitals and Clinics
Iowa City, Iowa
(Chapter 6)

Stanislas Dehaene, Ph.D.
Director, Cognitive Neuroimaging Unit
INSERM (The French Institute of Health and Medical Research)
Service Hospitalier Frédéric Joliot
Orsay, France
(Chapter 15)

John DeLuca, Ph.D.
Professor of Physical Medicine and Rehabilitation
University of Medicine and Dentistry–New Jersey Medical School
Newark, New Jersey
Director of Neuroscience Research
Kessler Medical Rehabilitation Research and Education Corporation
West Orange, New Jersey
(Chapters 40, 41)

Martha Bridge Denckla, M.D.
Director of the Developmental Cognitive Neurology Clinic
Kennedy Krieger Institute
Baltimore, Maryland
(Chapter 61)

Maureen Dennis, Ph.D.
Institute of Medical Science, Department of Psychology
University of Toronto
Hospital for Sick Children
Toronto, Ontario, Canada
(Chapter 63)

Leon Y. Deouell, M.D., Ph.D.
Helen Willis Neuroscience Institute
University of California, Berkeley
Berkeley, California
(Chapter 9)

Orrin Devinsky, M.D.
Director
NYU/Mount Sinai Comprehensive Epilepsy Center
New York, New York
(Chapter 54)

Charles Duyckaerts, M.D., Ph.D.
Hospital of the Pitiè-Salpêtrière
Paris, France
(Chapter 44)

Hulya M. Erhan, Ph.D.
Assistant Professor
Department of Psychiatry and Behavioral Sciences
Albert Einstein College of Medicine
Beth Israel Medical Center
New York, New York
(Chapter 58)

Martha J. Farah, Ph.D.
Professor of Psychology
and Director, Center for Cognitive Neuroscience
University of Pennsylvania
Philadelphia, Pennsylvania
(Chapters 1, 10, 17, 18, 19, 24, 33, 39)

Todd E. Feinberg, M.D.
Chief
Betty and Morton Yarmon Division of
Neurobehavior and Alzheimer's Disease
Associate Attending, Psychiatry and Neurology
Beth Israel Medical Center
New York, New York
Associate Professor, Neurology and Psychiatry
Albert Einstein College of Medicine
Bronx, New York
(Chapters 1, 18, 29, 30, 31, 58)

Ruth B. Fink, M.A.
Moss Rehabilitation Research Institute
Philadelphia, Pennsylvania
(Chapter 13)

Pam Flodman, M.S., M.Sc.
Department of Human Genetics and Birth Defects
University of California, Irvine
Irvine, California
(Chapter 69)

John Fosella, Ph.D.
Sackler Institute for Developmental Psychobiology
Department of Psychiatry
Weill Medical College of Cornell University
New York, New York
(Chapter 69)

Karl J. Friston, M.D.
Head, Functional Imaging Laboratory
Institute of Neurology
University College London
London, England
(Chapter 8)

Nancy N. Futrell, M.D.
Intermountain Stroke Center
Salt Lake City, Utah
(Chapter 52)

Guido Gainotti, M.D.
Universita Cattolica del Sacro Cuore (Cuore-Heart)
Facolta di Medicince e Chirurgia
Instituto di Clinica Delle
Malattie Nervose e Mentali
Rome, Italy
(Chapter 57)

Albert M. Galaburda, M.D.
Emily Fisher Landau Professor of Neurology and Neuroscience
Harvard Medical School
Chief, Division of Behavioral Neurology
Beth Israel-Deaconess Medical Center
Boston, Massachusetts
(Chapter 5)

Michael S. Gazzaniga, Ph.D.
Director, Center for Cognitive Neuroscience
Dartmouth College
Hanover, New Hampshire
(Chapter 34)

Joseph T. Giacino, Ph.D.
Associate Director, Neuropsychology
JFK Medical Center
Edison, New Jersey
Assistant Professor
Seton Hall University
Department of Neuroscience
South Orange, New Jersey
Clinical Assistant Professor
Department of Physical Medicine and Rehabilitation
University of Medicine and Dentistry of New Jersey
Robert Wood Johnson Medical School
New Brunswick, New Jersey
(Chapters 28, 30)

Elizabeth I. Glisky, Ph.D.
Professor of Psychology
University of Arizona
Tucson, Arizona
(Chapter 42)

Georg Goldenberg, M.D.
Neuropsychologische Abteilung
Krankenhaus Munchen-Bogenhausen
Munich, Germany
(Chapter 23)

Deborah Grady, Ph.D.
Department of Biological Chemistry
University of California, Irvine
Irvine, California
(Chapter 69)

Neill R. Graff-Radford, M.D.
Professor of Neurology
Mayo Clinic Jacksonville
Jacksonville, Florida
(Chapters 36, 53)

Murray Grossman, M.D.
Associate Professor
Department of Neurology
Hospital of the University of Pennsylvania
Philadelphia, Pennsylvania
(Chapter 39)

Susan K. Guy, M.D.
Dementia and Neurobehavior Fellow
UCLA Alzheimer's Disease Center
Los Angeles, California
(Chapter 2)

Vladimir Hachinski, M.D., F.R.C.P.C., M.Sc., D.Sc.
Director, Southwestern Ontario Stroke Programme
Professor of Neurology
Department of Clinical Neurological Sciences
University of Western Ontario
London, Ontario, Canada
(Chapter 49)

Kenneth M. Heilman, M.D.
The James D. Rooks Jr. Distinguished Professor of Neurology and Health Psychology
University of Florida
Program Director and Chief, NF/SG VAMC
Gainesville, Florida
(Chapters 16, 25)

Frank G. Hillary, Ph.D.
Clinical Research Associate
Neuropsychology and Neuroscience Laboratory
Kessler Medical Rehabilitation Research and Education Corporation
West Orange, New Jersey
(Chapter 40)

Richard B. Ivry, Ph.D.
Department of Psychology
University of California, Berkeley
Berkeley, California
(Chapter 9)

Diane M. Jacobs, Ph.D.
Assistant Professor of Clinical Neuropsychology
Department of Neurology
Columbia University College of Physicians and Surgeons
New York, New York
(Chapter 48)

Julene K. Johnson, Ph.D.
Institute for Brain Aging and Dementia
University of California at Irvine
Irvine, California
(Chapter 32)

Daniel I. Kaufer, M.D.
Assistant Professor of Psychiatry and Neurology
University of Pittsburgh School of Medicine
Pittsburgh, Pennsylvania
(Chapter 43)

Margaret M. Keane, Ph.D.
Associate Professor
Department of Psychology
Wellesley College
Wellesley, Massachusetts
(Chapter 38)

Robert T. Knight, M.D.
Department of Psychology and the Helen Willis Neuroscience Institute
University of California, Berkeley
Berkeley, California
(Chapter 9)

Thomas A. Krefft, M.D.
Behavioral Neurology Fellow
Mayo Clinic Jacksonville
Jacksonville, Florida
(Chapter 53)

Kevin S. LaBar, Ph.D.
Assistant Professor of Psychological and Brain Science
Center for Cognitive Neuroscience
Duke University
Durham, North Caroina
(Chapter 56)

Joseph E. LeDoux, Ph.D.
Henry and Lucy Moses Professor of Science
Professor of Neural Science and Psychology
New York University
New York, New York
(Chapter 56)

Gilberto Levy, M.D.
Associate Research Scientist
Gertrude H. Sergievsky Center
Columbia University
New York, New York
(Chapter 48)

Muriel D. Lezak, Ph.D.
Department of Neurology
Oregon Health and Sciences University
Portland, Oregon
(Chapter 3)

David W. Loring, Ph.D.
Department of Neurology
Medical College of Georgia
Augusta, Georgia
(Chapter 55)

Maureen W. Lovett, Ph.D.
Senior Scientist, Brain and Behavior Program
Director, Learning Disabilities Research Program
Hospital for Sick Children
Professor of Pediatrics and Psychology
University of Toronto
Toronto, Ontario, Canada
(Chapter 64)

Clement T. Loy, B.A., M.B.B.S., Mmed. (Clin Epi)
Department of Neurology
St. Vincent's Hospital
Sydney, Australia
(Chapter 50)

Karen Marder, M.D., M.P.H.
Associate Professor of Neurology
Gertrude H. Sergievsky Center
Columbia University College of Physicians and Surgeons
New York, New York
(Chapter 48)

Hans J. Markowitsch, Ph.D.
Department of Physiological Psychology
University of Bielefeld
Bielefeld, Germany
(Chapter 37)

Carrie R. McDonald, Ph.D.
University of Florida
Gainesville, Florida
(Chapter 21)

Regina McGlinchey-Berroth, Ph.D.
Department of Veterans Affairs Medical Center
West Roxbury, Massachusetts
(Chapter 46)

Kimford J. Meador, M.D.
Professor, Department of Neurology
Medical College of Georgia
Augusta, Georgia
(Chapter 55)

Mario F. Mendez, M.D., Ph.D.
Professor of Neurology and Psychiatry
and Biobehavioral Sciences
UCLA School of Medicine
Los Angeles, California
(Chapter 47)

M.-Marsel Mesulam, M.D.
Professor of Neurology and Psychiatry
Cognitive Neurology and Alzheimer's Disease Center
Northwestern University Medical School
Chicago, Illinois
(Chapter 4)

Jessica A. Meyer
University of Miami
Miami, Florida
(Chapter 68)

William Milberg, Ph.D.
Department of Veterans Affairs Medical Center
West Roxbury, Massachusetts
(Chapter 46)

Bruce L. Miller, M.D.
A.W. & Mary Margaret Clausen Distinguished Chair
Professor of Neurology
Clinical Director, Memory and Aging Center
University of California at San Francisco
San Francisco, California
(Chapter 32)

Clark H. Millikan, M.D.
Salt Lake City, Utah
(Chapter 52)

Nancy J. Minshew, M.D.
Associate Professor
Department of Psychiatry and Neurology
University of Pittsburgh School of Medicine
Pittsburgh, Pennsylvania
(Chapter 68)

Anna Bacon Moore, Ph.D.
Assistant Professor, Department of Clinical
and Health Psychology
University of Florida
Research Investigator
Division of Research/Brain Rehabilitation Research Center
Malcom Randall VA Medical Center
Gainesville, Florida
(Chapter 35)

Robert Moyzis, Ph.D.
Professor
Department of Biological Chemistry
University of California, Irvine
Irvine, California
(Chapter 69)

Catherine E. Myers, Ph.D.
Department of Psychology
Rutgers University
Newark, New Jersey
(Chapter 41)

Elizabeth S. Ochoa, Ph.D.
Assistant Professor
Department of Psychiatry and Behavioral Sciences
Albert Einstein College of Medicine
Beth Israel Medical Center
New York, New York
(Chapter 58)

Alvaro Pascual-Leone, M.D., Ph.D.
Associate Professor of Neurology
Harvard Medical School
Director of Research at the Behavioral Neurology Unit
Beth Israel Deaconess Medical Center
Boston, Massachusetts
(Chapter 5)

Bruce F. Pennington, Ph.D.
Department of Psychology
University of Denver
Denver, Colorado
(Chapter 66)

Michael Posner, Ph.D.
Professor, Department of Psychology
Institute of Cognitive and Decision Sciences
University of Oregon Institute of Neuroscience
Eugene, Oregon
(Chapter 69)

Cathy J. Price
Wellcome Department of Imaging Neuroscience
Institute of Neurology
University College London
London, England
(Chapter 8)

David M. Roane, M.D.
Department of Geropsychiatry
Beth Israel Medical Center
New York, New York
(Chapters 29, 31)

Elliott D. Ross, M.D.
VA Medical Center
Oklahoma City, Oklahoma
(Chapter 59)

Leslie J. Gonzalez Rothi, Ph.D.
Professor, Departments of Neurology, Clinical and Health Psychology and Communicative Processes and Disorders
Program Director, VA Brain Rehabilitation Research Center
University of Florida
Gainesville, Florida
(Chapter 16)

Eleanor M. Saffran, Ph.D.*
Department of Communication Sciences
Weiss Hall
Temple University
Philadelphia, Pennsylvania
(Chapter 12)

Myrna F. Schwartz, Ph.D.
Moss Rehabilitation Research Institute
Philadelphia, Pennsylvania
(Chapter 13)

Melanie Shulman, M.D., M.Phil.
Director, Cognitive and Behavioral Neurology Program
NYU/Mount Sinai Comprehensive Epilepsy Center
New York, New York
(Chapter 54)

Jonathan M. Silver, M.D.
Clinical Professor of Psychiatry
New York University School of Medicine
Assistant Director of Clinical Services and Research
Chief of Ambulatory Services in the Department of Psychiatry
Lenox Hill Hospital
New York, New York
(Chapter 60)

Anne Spence, Ph.D.
Department of Human Genetics and Birth Defects
University of California, Irvine
Irvine, California
(Chapter 69)

James Swanson, Ph.D.
Professor of Pediatrics
Executive Director, Child Development Center
University of California, Irvine
Irvine, California
(Chapter 69)

*Deceased

Leon J. Thal, M.D.
Professor and Chairman
Department of Neurosciences, University of California, San Diego
La Jolla, California
(Chapter 45)

Gang Tong, M.D., Ph.D.
Adjunct Assistant Professor and Staff Attending Physician
Department of Neurosciences
University of California, San Diego
La Jolla, California
(Chapter 45)

Daniel Tranel, Ph.D.
Department of Neurology
University of Iowa Hospital and Clinic
Iowa City, Iowa
(Chapter 20)

Edward Valenstein, M.D.
Chair, Department of Neurology
The William L. and Janice M. Neely
Professor of Neurology and Clinical and Health Psychology
University of Florida
Gainesville, Florida
(Chapter 25)

Mieke Verfaellie, Ph.D.
Associate Professor
Department of Psychiatry and Psychology
Boston University School of Medicine
Boston, Massachusetts
(Chapters 38, 51)

Kytja K.S. Voeller, M.D.
Research Neurologist
Greenwood Genetics Center
JC Self Research Center
Center for Molecular Studies
Greenwood, South Carolina
(Chapters 65, 67)

Deborah P. Waber, M.D.
Clinical Assistant Professor, Pediatrics
University of Maryland Hospital for Children
Mercy Medical Center
Baltimore, Maryland
(Chapter 62)

Robert T. Watson, M.D.
Jules B. Chapman Professor in Clinical Care and Humaneness
Professor of Neurology and Clinical and Health Psychology
Senior Associate Dean for Educational Affairs
Vice-Chair, Department of Neurology
University of Florida
Gainesville, Florida
(Chapters 16, 25)

Christina E. Wierenga, M.S.
Department of Clinical and Health Psychology
University of Florida Health Science Center
Gainesville, Florida
(Chapter 35)

Stuart C. Yudofsky, M.D.
Professor
D.C. and Irene Ellwood Chair of Psychiatry
Baylor College of Medicine
Houston, Texas
(Chapter 60)

PREFACE

The difference between editing the first and second edition of a textbook is a little like the difference between parenting and grandparenting. The first edition is a huge investment of time and effort, and one has to accept the sleepless nights, worries, and disappointments along with the pleasure and pride. The second edition involves work too, of course, but mostly of a purely enjoyable nature. Our main task was to step back, take a broad look at our field and ask "what is new and significant?" In the six years since the first edition was published, there have been a number of exciting developments.

Among the important methodological developments we felt compelled to feature in this new edition is the growing use of functional neuroimaging. This family of methods, and functional Magnetic Resonance Imaging in particular, has become an essential tool in behavioral neurology and cognitive neuropsychology. Anyone working in our field must now be familiar with the basic principles and techniques, if only to be an informed consumer of the functional neuroimaging literature. Our new coverage of imaging includes an expanded chapter on the acquisition and interpretation of fMRI data from normal humans and a new chapter on the use of functional imaging with neurological patients. The growing use of transcranial magnetic stimulation and the burgeoning of genetic approaches to neurodevelopmental disorders are two other methodological developments that have come to the fore in recent years and are included in this second edition.

Theoretical progress is harder to measure than methodological progress, perhaps because a change in theoretical approach is not as easy to identify as a change of laboratory equipment. Regardless, there is no mistaking the growth in this aspect of our field as well. Many chapters have been extensively revised to accommodate new knowledge, and all reflect the steady and vigorous growth of understanding since the first edition was written. We are therefore filled with grandparently pride as this second edition goes to press, not just for the outstanding contributions of the book's many authors, but also for the ongoing progress in behavioral neurology and cognitive neuropsychology embodied here.

In closing, we should like to thank our new editors at McGraw Hill, Marc Strauss and Lisa Silverman, the ever-presiding editing supervisor, Lester Sheinis, and our colleagues, families, and friends for their continuing support.

BEHAVIORAL NEUROLOGY AND NEUROPSYCHOLOGY

Part 1

GENERAL PRINCIPLES

Chapter 1

THE DEVELOPMENT OF MODERN BEHAVIORAL NEUROLOGY AND NEUROPSYCHOLOGY

Todd E. Feinberg
Martha J. Farah

HISTORICAL ROOTS OF BEHAVIORAL NEUROLOGY AND NEUROPSYCHOLOGY

The history of the study of brain function could be said to start with a different organ, the heart. The ancient Egyptians held that the heart and diaphragm were the seats of mental life. They held this belief despite their observations of the behavioral effects of head injury, including descriptions of aphasia dating back as far as 3500 B.C.[1–6] In ancient Greece, we see the first statements of and debate over a cerebrocentric view of the mind. Alcmaeon of Croton,[6] a Greek of the fifth-century B.C. who may have been a pupil of Pythagoras,[2,7] could well be considered the first neurologist or neuropsychologist. On the basis of his clinical and pathologic investigations, he proposed that the brain was the organ responsible for sensation and thought. He also taught that the various sensations each had a particular localization in the brain,[2,3,6,8] thus articulating for the first time a localist view of brain function. Starting in the eighteenth century, localism would become such a controversial hypothesis that it would polarize the field and become the driving motivation for almost 300 years of research.

A century after Alcmaeon, the writings of Hippocrates constitute another major turning point. Hippocrates believed that the brain was responsible for the intellect, senses, knowledge, emotions, and even mental illness.[9] A particularly revolutionary idea, recorded in the Hippocratic tract entitled "On the Sacred Disease," was that epilepsy is a medical condition and not the result of demonic possession.[2] However, even at this point the issue of cerebrocentrism versus cardiocentrism was not yet settled for all time. Plato, a contemporary of Hippocrates, accepted a cerebrocentric view of the mind, but a century later Aristotle rejected it in favor of the more traditional cardiocentric view.[2,3,8] Furthermore, even in the cerebrocentric camp, more than a few details concerning mind-brain relations remained to be worked out. Herophilus of Chalcedon, a follower of Hippocrates in the third century B.C. and a pioneer in the practice of human dissection, believed that the brain's ventricles, particularly the fourth ventricle, were the seat of human intelligence.[3,6,7,10]

The Greek natural philosophers taught an influential "doctrine of the spirits."[7] They proposed that a *spiritus naturalis* originated in the liver and was transported to the heart and lungs. Here it was mixed with air and thereby transformed into the *spiritus vitalis,* which was identified with the essential principle of life. Finally it is transported to the brain where it is converted into the *spiritus animalis,* the essence of the soul and mind. The doctrine of the spirits was to appear in various forms over the centuries and was frequently incorporated into later theories that were based on more objective knowledge of the brain.

One of the great physicians of the classical period was Galen of Pergamus (A.D. 131–201).[2,3] Galen firmly rejected the cardiocentric position of Aristotle and reaffirmed the position of the brain as the seat of the psyche. His thinking on brain physiology reflected the continuing belief in the spirit doctrine and the importance of the ventricular system in brain functioning. He taught that the *vital spirits,* produced by the left ventricle of the heart, were transferred via the vessels to the brain where, in the *rete mirabile,* they were transformed into *animal spirits.* The *rete mirabile,* previously described by Herophilus, is a vascular network that surrounds the pituitary gland and is prominently present in the ox but absent in humans. This error is testament to the degree to which the ancients relied upon animal dissection for the knowledge of anatomy. After transformation in the *rete mirabile,* the animal spirits could be stored in the ventricles and, when needed, sent through the nerves to the rest of the body for use in action or sensation.[10] While Galen taught that the ventricles were crucial to action and sensation, he also believed that brain tissue itself played a role in mental life.[11]

For the entire period of the middle ages in Europe (approximately the fourth to fourteenth centuries), the ventricles continued to be the focus of theories relating mind and brain.[11] For example, according to fourth-century church fathers, the anterior ventricles were associated with perception (later to be known as the *sensorium commune*), the middle with reason, and the posterior with memory.[10] It has been suggested that this focus on the ventricles accorded better with the dualism of Christian theology, as the hollow cavities could be said to contain the soul without hypothesizing an identity between mind and the physical substrate of brain tissue.[11] Figure 1-1 shows an early illustration of the ventricular system.

During the Renaissance, the ventricular doctrine and the role of the *rete mirabile* began to lose their influence on theories of mind-brain relations.[4,10,12] The seventeenth-century writings of René Descartes mark a transitional phase, in which the interaction between fluid in the ventricles and brain tissue itself was hypothesized to explain intelligent action, as shown in Fig. 1-2. For reflexive action, Descartes proposed a simple loop, in which stimulated nerves caused the release of animal spirits in the ventricles, which, in turn, caused efferent nerves and muscles to act. For intelligent human action, this loop was modulated by the soul via its effects on the pineal gland. The pineal gland was chosen in part because it is unpaired and centrally located and also because it is surrounded by cerebrospinal fluid. It was also mistakenly thought to be uniquely human. Of course, the pineal gland was just the vehicle for the mind's influence on the body; Descartes' theory still denied any form of identity between the mind and neural tissue.[4,13–16]

Descartes' theory was formulated at a time when neuroanatomic knowledge was quite primitive. This situation began to change with the work of such figures as Thomas Willis later in the seventeenth century[4,17]

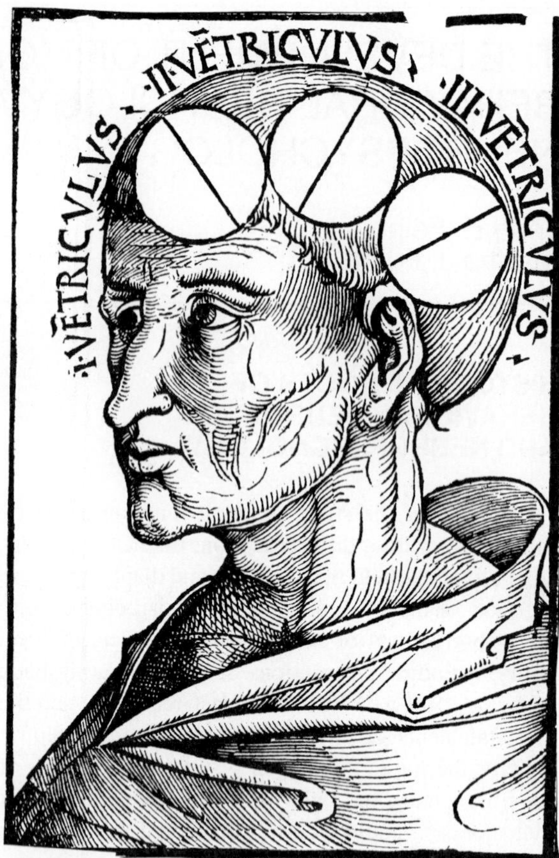

Figure 1-1
The ventricular system according to Albertus Magnus from his Philosophia naturalis *(1506).*[10]

and Malpighi Pacchioni and Albrecht von Haller in the eighteenth.[8,18] For example, Von Haller stimulated the nerves of live animals in an effort to discover the pathways for perception and motor action, thus establishing the experimental method in neurophysiology. This work set the stage for the explosion of experimental and clinical research of the nineteenth century, in which the brain organization underlying perception, action, language, and many other cognitive functions was revealed.

Some of the earliest inroads into meaningful localization in the nervous system began not with the brain but the peripheral nervous system. Von Haller had suggested that the same nerves subserved motor and sensory functions.[2] Sir Charles Bell and François Magendie, independently, discovered the segregation

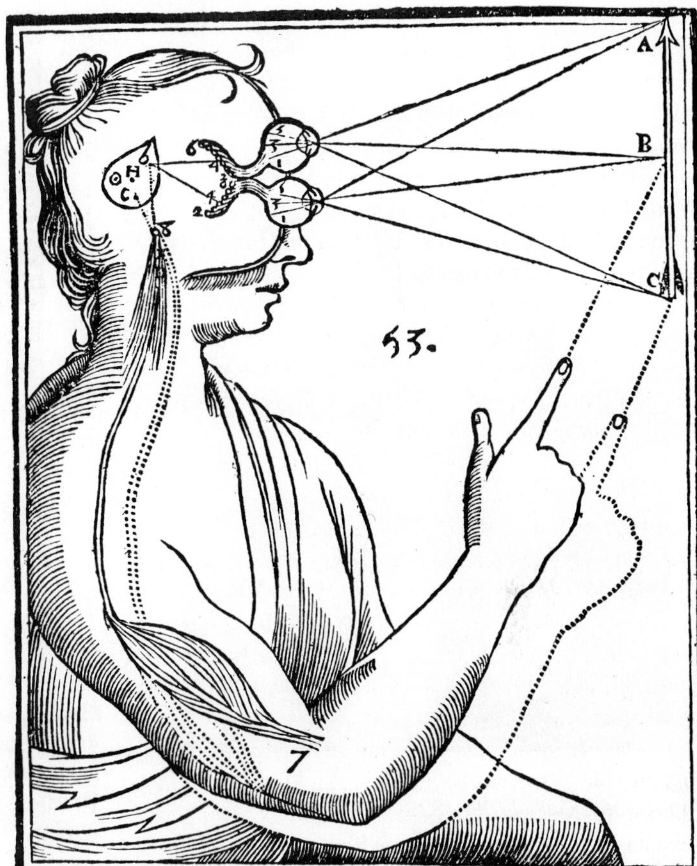

Figure 1-2
Descartes' conception of sensation and action as conceived in his De homine *(1662). Light was transferred from the retina to the ventricles, causing the release of animal spirits. The pineal gland modulated this mechanism for voluntary action.*[3]

of sensory functions to the posterior spinal roots and motor functions to the anterior spinal roots, which has come to be known as the Bell-Magendie law. The clear-cut division of function provided by these observations, coupled with a straightforward anatomic basis and its proof by experiment, was both a model for localization of function within the nervous system and a triumph for the experimental method.[2,4,8,18–20]

THE LOCALISM/HOLISM DEBATE OF THE NINETEENTH CENTURY

One of the more notorious figures in the history of behavioral neurology is Franz Josef Gall, shown in Fig. 1-3. In the late eighteenth and early nineteenth centuries, he and his collaborator Johann Spurzheim made a number of important contributions to functional neuroanatomy, including proving by dissection the crossing of the pyramids and establishing the distinction between gray and white matter.[21–23] Gall is also credited with one of the earliest descriptions of aphasia linked to a lesion of the frontal lobes.[24] He is most famous, however, for his general theory of cerebral localization, known today as phrenology. At the age of 9, Gall had noted that his schoolmates who excelled at rote memory tasks had quite prominent eyes, *"les yeux à fleur de tête"* (cow's eyes). He reasoned that this was the result of the overdevelopment of the subjacent regions of the brain, and speculated that these regions of the brain might be particularly involved in language functions and especially verbal memory.

Gall identified 27 basic human faculties and associated them with particular brain centers that could affect the shape of the skull, as shown in Fig. 1-4. These included memory of things and facts, sense of spatial

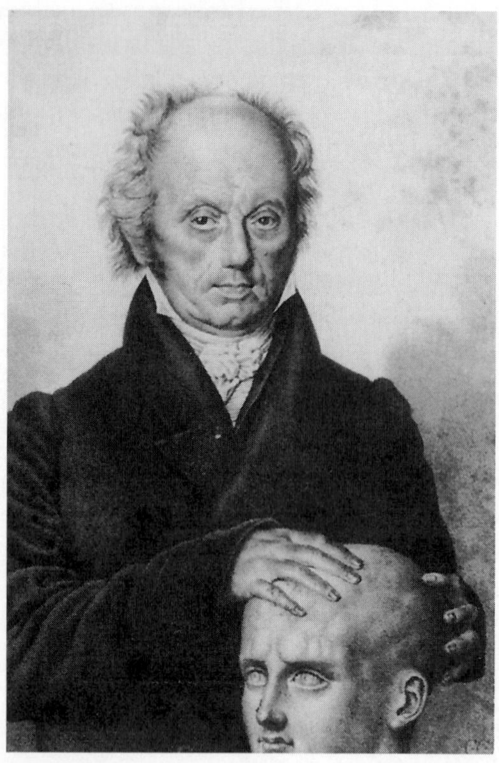

Figure 1-3
Franz Josef Gall (1758–1828).

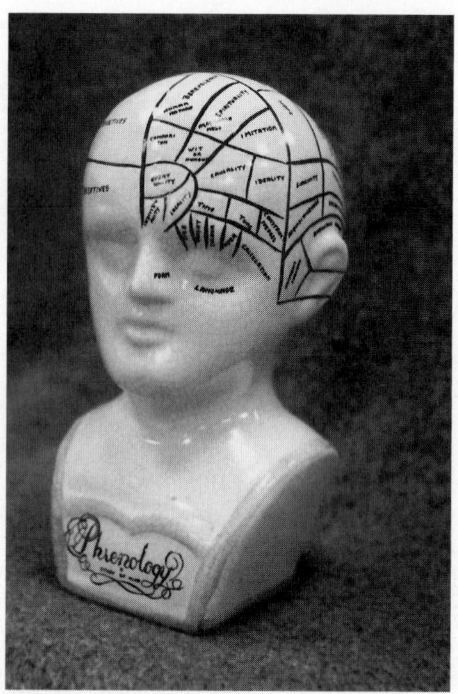

Figure 1-4
An example of a porcelain phrenology bust with demarcations that demonstrate the reflection of the human faculties on the skull. (Photograph courtesy of Joseph A. Hefta.)

relations, vanity, God and religion, and love for one's offspring.[23] His theory was based on hundreds of skulls and casts of humans and beasts. For instance, the disposition to murder and cruelty was based on a bump above the ear possessed by carnivorous animals. He located the same feature in sadistic persons whom he had examined personally,[4] skulls of famous criminals, and the busts and paintings of famous murderers.[18] Gall taught and practiced medicine in Vienna from 1781 to around 1802, until Emperor Francis I banned Gall's public lectures because they were materialistic and thus opposed to morality and religion.[18] Gall then took to the road, lecturing across Europe to enthusiastic popular audiences. By the time he settled in Paris in 1807, he was hugely popular and internationally known. However, phrenology continued to create controversy in scientific circles.

The best-known critic of Gall was Marie-Jean-Pierre Flourens. Flourens mounted a scientific research program to disprove Gall's theory, but it appears to have been motivated at least as much by religious discomfort with the implications of Gall's straightforward mind-brain equivalences as by scientific considerations. Flourens viewed Gall's theory as tantamount to denying the existence of the soul, because it divided the mind and brain into functionally distinct parts and Flourens believed the soul to be unitary.[18,25–27] He carried out extensive lesion experiments on a variety of animal species to demonstrate the equipotentiality of cortex.

Gall's status as a popularizer, and Flourens's empirical attacks, helped to push localism out of the mainstream of contemporary scientific thought in the early nineteenth century. When, in 1825, Jean-Baptiste Bouillaud, shown in Fig. 1-5, presented a large series of clinical cases of loss of speech following frontal lesions,[21,27,28] his work was largely ignored. This landmark work, in which speech per se was distinguished from nonspeech movements of the mouth and tongue, is still relatively unknown.

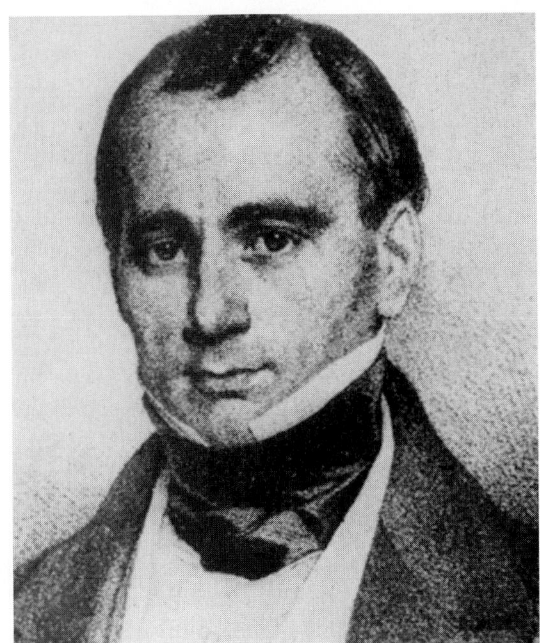

Figure 1-5
Jean-Baptiste Bouillaud (1796–1881).

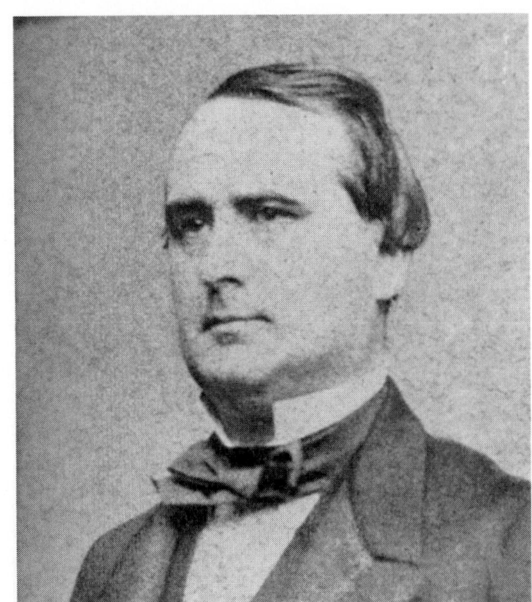

Figure 1-6
Ernest Aubertin (1825–1865).

Bouillaud was not the only one to suggest a frontal location for language functions. During this period and lasting up to the 1860s, numerous clinical reports of patients with frontal lobe damage and loss of speech were recorded in Europe and America. Indeed, this idea had considerable historical precedence throughout antiquity.[5,29,30] However, intense interest in localization of brain functions, particularly language, was now developing. It was during this time that Marc Dax noted the association between left-hemispheric damage, right hemiplegia, and aphasia, based upon his examination of 40 patients over a 20-year period. This paper was handwritten in 1836 and not published at the time,[31] but copies may have been distributed to friends and colleagues.[4]

It was not until 1861 that the field reconsidered localism with a more open mind. That year the Société d'Anthropologie in Paris held a series of debates between Pierre Gratiolet, arguing in favor of holism or equipotentiality, and Ernest Auburtin, the son-in-law of Bouillaud, arguing in favor of localism.[21,32,33] Auburtin, shown in Fig. 1-6, reported his clinical observations of a patient whose frontal bone was removed following a suicide attempt. He reported that when the blade of a spatula was applied to the "anterior lobes," there was complete cessation of speech without loss of consciousness.[4,21,33] Auburtin went on to describe a patient of Bouillaud's who had a speech disturbance and was near death. Auburtin boldly vowed if this patient lacked a frontal lesion he would renounce his views.[21,32–35]

The 1861 debate is best known not for the presentations of Gratiolet and Auburtin but for the eventual participation of the society's founder and secretary, Paul Broca, shown in Fig. 1-7. Although Broca did not initially take a strong position, his observations of a patient then under his care led him to play a pivotal role in the debate. His patient, Leborgne, suffered from epilepsy, right hemiplegia, and loss of speech, the last for a period of over 20 years. Leborgne had been institutionalized for some 31 years and throughout the hospital was known by the name "Tan," as this was his only utterance along with a few obscenities.[3,4] In light of Auburtin's declaration, Broca invited him to examine Tan, which Auburtin did and afterward concluded that indeed the patient met the criteria of his prior challenge. Six days later Leborgne died; the following day, April 18, 1961, Broca presented the brain to the society along

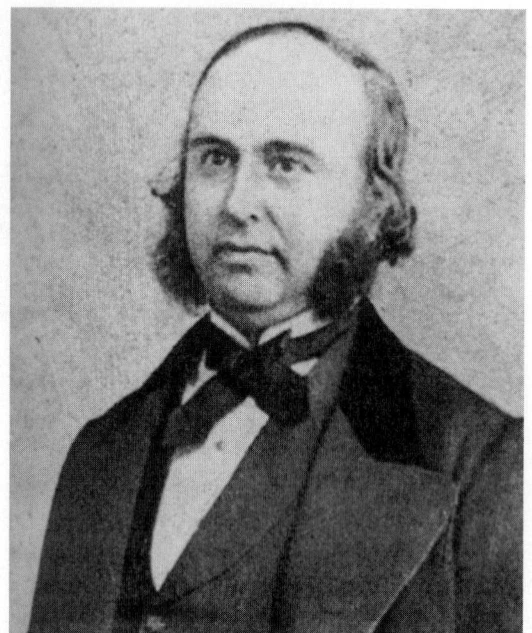

Figure 1-7
Paul Broca (1824–1880).

with a brief statement but without firm conclusions.[33] Figure 1-8 shows the brain of Leborgne.

Four months later, at a meeting of the Société Anatomique de Paris in August, Broca made a more extensive report. The brain of Leborgne had demonstrated an egg-sized fluid-filled cavity located in the posterior second and third frontal convolutions, with involvement of adjacent structures as well, including the corpus striatum.[36] In this report, Broca claimed that his findings would "support the ideas of M. Bouillaud on the seat of the faculty for language";[33,36] he later suggested a possible localization of speech functions to the second or more probably third frontal convolution. Later the same year, Broca presented another patient with speech disturbance, an 84-year-old laborer whose lesion also involved the left second and third frontal convolutions. The lesion was more circumscribed than that found in Leborgne and strengthened the association of those structures with speech localization.

In the mid-1860s the issue of hemispheric asymmetry entered the debate on localization. The previous cases strongly suggested that speech is localized to the left hemisphere, and an additional series of eight cases published by Broca in 1863 were exclusively left-sided.[4,31,37] In spite of the strong lateralization of lesion locus in these cases, Broca made note of this "remarkable" observation but made no further claims.[31] In this same year and shortly before Broca's paper was presented,[4] Gustave Dax, son of Marc Dax, sent a handwritten copy of his father's manuscript to the Académie de Médecine in Paris. In this document, Marc Dax had previously described his view on the relation between speech and the left hemisphere. The

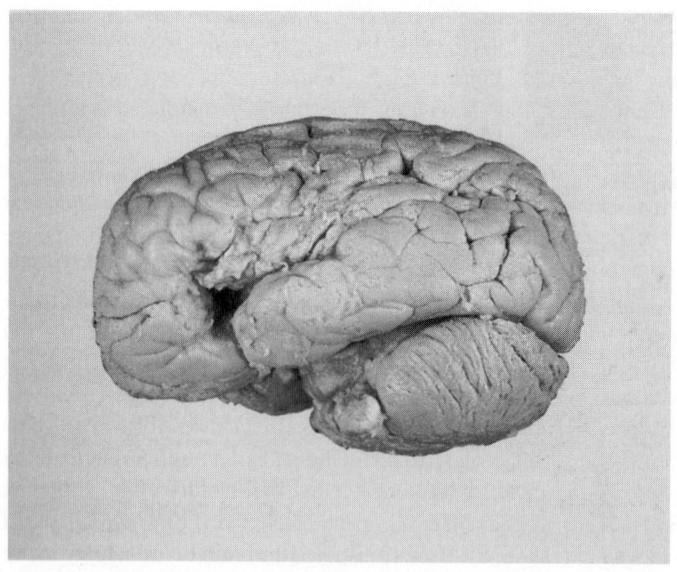

Figure 1-8
Photograph of the brain of Broca's first patient, Leborgne ("Tan"). It is now housed in the Musée Dupuytren.

paper was read before the Académie in December 1864 and published in 1865.[38,39] By 1865, Broca clearly expressed the opinion that the left hemisphere played a dominant role in speech production.[40,41] As far as the issue of priority of discovery is concerned (a matter of controversy among historians), most writers agree that the Dax paper in its original form in 1836 had no influence on Broca or the scientific community when first written. This paper did, however, make clear the association of language functions and the left hemisphere. While Broca alone clarified the role of the second and third frontal convolutions, he apparently did not take a firm position on the specific role of the left hemisphere until after the Dax paper was read before the Académie de Médecine in Paris in December 1964.[4] It appears that the reemergence of the Dax manuscript and Broca's discovery were nearly simultaneous events.

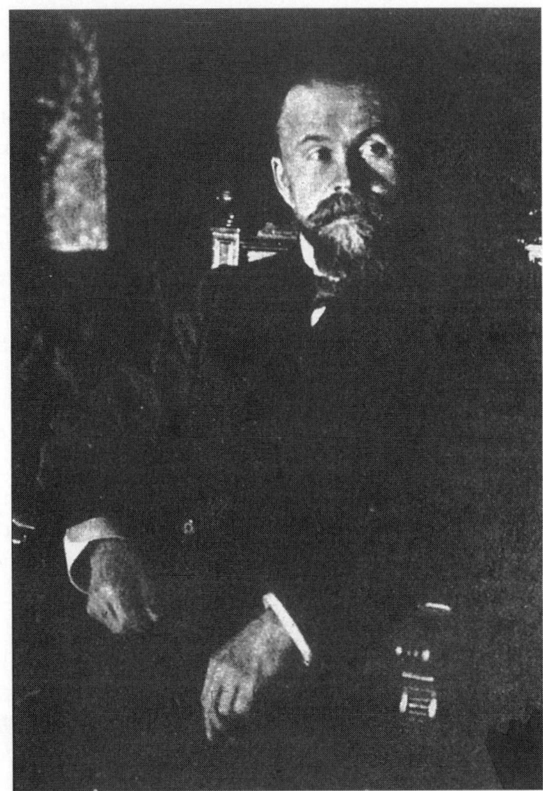

Figure 1-9
Carl Wernicke (1848–1904).

THE AFTERMATH OF 1861: THE EMERGENCE OF MODERN BEHAVIORAL NEUROLOGY AND NEUROPSYCHOLOGY

The events in Paris in the 1860s constituted a turning point in the history of ideas regarding brain function. The concepts and methods developed in the course of debating the localization of speech were extended to a variety of different higher functions, and experimental work on animals also developed apace. From this period onward, it is impossible to trace a single line of scientific development. Here we simply present a summary of some of the major advances seen in the behavioral neurology and neuropsychology of the late nineteenth and early twentieth centuries.

In the decade following Broca's contributions, two important developments took place in Germany. First, Edward Hitzig and Gustav Fritsch performed a series of experiments in which the cortex of a dog was stimulated while the dog lay on a dressing table in Hitzig's Berlin home.[3,4,42] These experiments established that motor functions are localized to anterior cortex and demonstrated experimentally the somatotopic organization of motor cortex inferred indirectly from previous clinical-anatomic correlations in humans. In their report, the investigators specifically noted that their results refuted the holism of Flourens. Following their work, Sir David Ferrier in England confirmed the findings of Hitzig and Fritsch and improved upon their method of stimulation to discover more detailed structure-function relationships.[18]

About the same time, the German neurologist Carl Wernicke began to investigate language functions other than speech. Wernicke, shown in Fig. 1-9, documented a form of aphasia different from the nonfluent variety that followed frontal damage. In what he called sensory aphasia, a posterior lesion in the region of the first temporal gyrus caused a disturbance in auditory comprehension, inappropriate word selection in spontaneous speech, and impaired naming and writing. In his landmark monograph *Der aphasische Symptomencomplex,* Wernicke reasoned that Broca's area was the center for the motor representation of speech, and the posterior first temporal gyrus was the center for "sound images." Wernicke also described global aphasia and explained it as a result of destruction of both anterior and posterior language areas. He also made a prediction that a disturbance of the pathways between these two areas would produce another variety of aphasia he called "conduction aphasia," in which comprehension would be preserved but output would be as impaired as in sensory aphasia.[43–46] Wernicke had, in effect, proposed a model that could explain a number of different aphasic syndromes by lesions to different combinations of centers and connections between centers. This type of theorizing came to be known as "associationism," because language use was viewed in terms of associating representations in different brain centers, or as "connectionism," because of the emphasis that view put on the connections between centers, as shown in Fig. 1-10.

The connectionist paradigm was quickly extended to explain other disorders. Ludwig Lichtheim placed pure word deafness in this framework, predicting the critical lesion site as well as noting that, given the connectionist explanation for this syndrome, a disturbance in repetition should accompany conduction aphasia.[46,47] Hugo Liepmann described the apraxias, including ideomotor apraxia,[48] and, with Maas, callosal apraxia,[49] explaining them in terms of connectionist principles. Joseph Jules Déjerine, shown in Fig. 1-11, also used the framework of centers and connections in his explanation of alexia without agraphia.[50]

Figure 1-10
Wernicke's model of the speech mechanism.[44] The auditory areas (a) project to centers subserving vocal output (b) and areas which contain tactile (c) and visual (d) images.

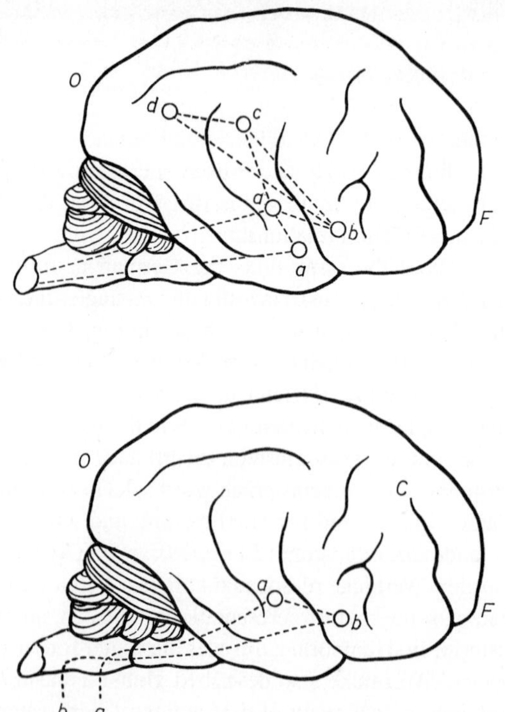

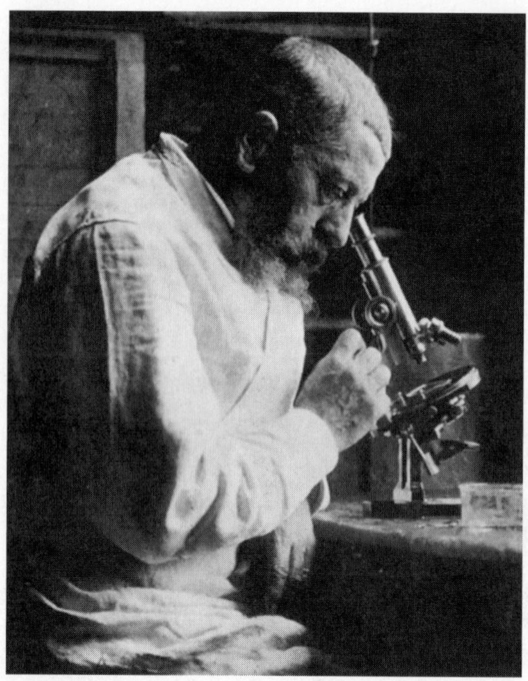

Figure 1-11
Joseph Jules Déjerine (1849–1917).

The nineteenth-century connectionist framework proved to have both parsimony and explanatory power. Rather than hypothesizing a new center for every ability or every observed deficit, after the fashion of Gall, a relatively small number of basic centers (vision, sound images, motor outputs) could be combined through connections to explain a wide variety of higher functions and their deficits. Connectionist explanations of aphasia, apraxia, alexia, and other disorders survived well into the twentieth century; indeed, Norman Geschwind, one of the most influential behavioral neurologists of our time, championed them throughout his career.[51] Despite the current proliferation of theories and approaches in our field, the theories of Déjerine,

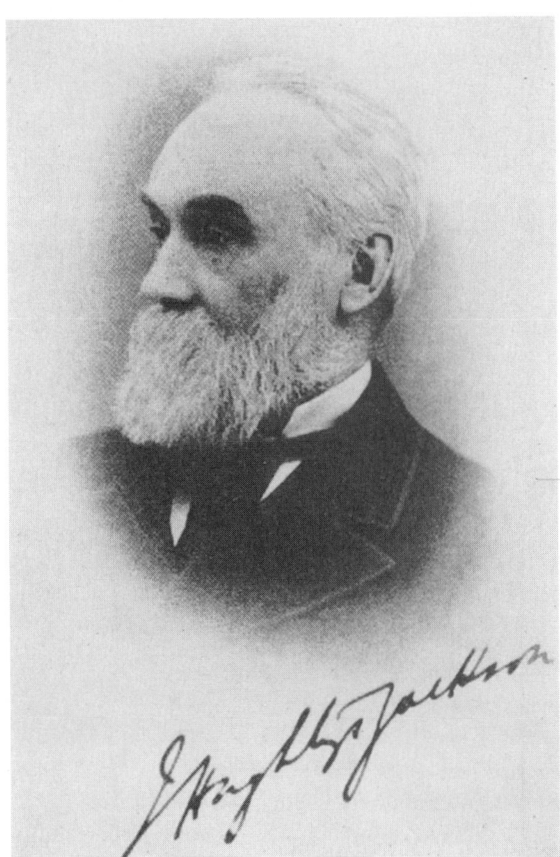

Figure 1-12
John Hughlings Jackson (1835–1911).

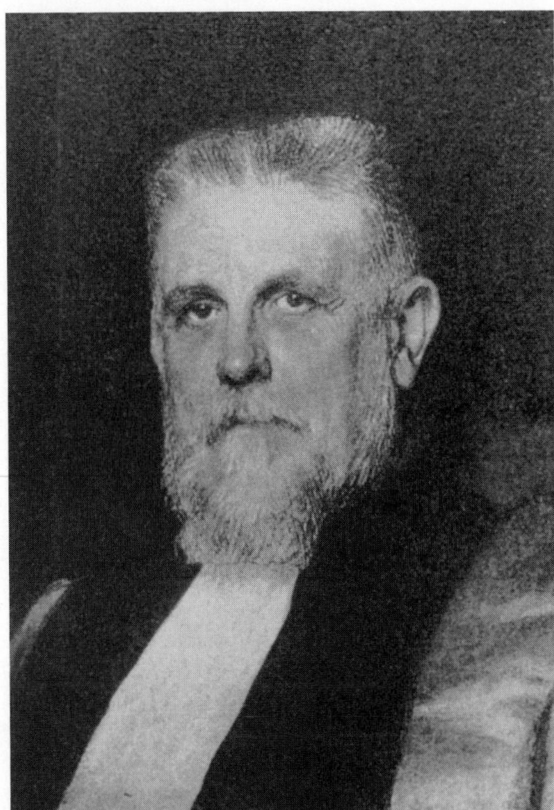

Figure 1-13
Pierre Marie (1853–1940).

Liepmann, Lichtheim, and Wernicke are still held to be correct by many.

Nevertheless, as successful as the connectionist framework was in late nineteenth century in explaining a variety of disorders, skeptics continued to reject the localism implicit in it. One of the most influential of these was the English neurologist John Hughlings Jackson, shown in Fig. 1-12. He viewed the nervous system not as a series of centers connected by pathways but rather as a hierarchically organized and highly interactive whole that could not be understood piecemeal.[32] Figure 1-13 shows Pierre Marie, a Parisian student of Broca and Charcot, who also took issue with the connectionist theorizing of the late nineteenth century. His style was direct, to say the least. One of his articles was so offensive to Déjerine that it provoked the latter to challenge Marie to a duel. His article questioning the empirical basis of the early claims concerning speech localization was entitled *"La troisiéme circonvolution frontale gauche ne joue aucun rôle spécial dans la fonction du langage"* ("The third frontal convolution plays no special role at all in the function of language").[52] Marie believed that there was just one basic form of aphasia, a posterior aphasia, which was a type of general intellectual loss not specific to language per se. He held that the speech problems of anterior aphasics were motoric in nature. When aphasia is viewed this way, a network of specialized centers is superfluous. A movement toward holism continued into the early twentieth century, with Jackson and Marie followed by a number of influential neurologists and psychologists, including Henry Head in England,[32] shown in Fig. 1-14, Kurt Goldstein in Germany,[53–55] shown in Fig. 1-15, and Karl Lashley in the United States.[56–59] This swing of the pendulum back toward holism has

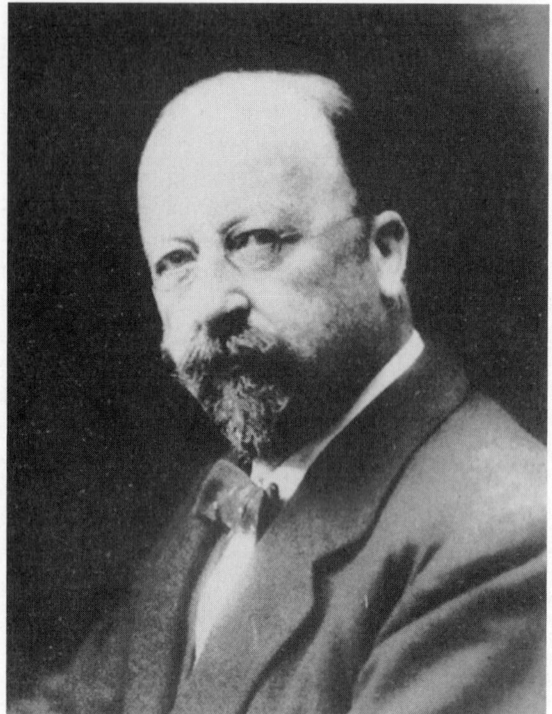

Figure 1-14
Henry Head (1861–1940).

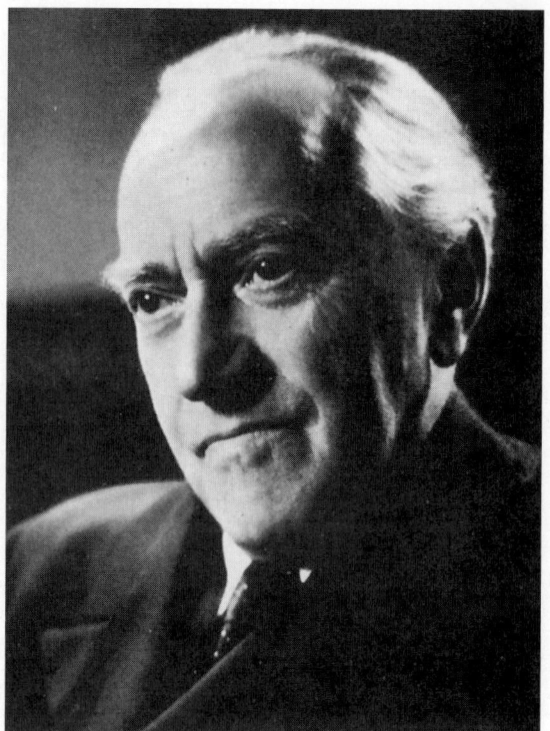

Figure 1-15
Kurt Goldstein (1878–1965).

been explained by the waning of German influence following World War I[60] and the growing influence of Gestalt psychology.[61]

While these workers emphasized the brain's unity, other researchers had pointed out the difference between brain regions in cellular morphology, cell densities, and lamination and produced the first cytoarchitectonic maps. Oskar and Cécile Vogt[62,63] and Alfred W. Campbell[64,65] produced some of the earliest examples of these architectonic maps, followed by many others, including those of Korbinian Brodmann,[66] whose cortical maps of the human brain have had the most widespread application. While these workers did not agree on the number and location of cortical areas (the Vogts counted over 200, Brodmann only 52[4]) it could not be contested that there were clear regional neuroanatomic differences.

The late nineteenth century also saw the beginnings of the modern study of memory and vision. Theodule Ribot introduced the distinction between anterograde and retrograde memory impairments and observed what is now known as "Ribot's law," that the most recently laid down memories were the most vulnerable to brain damage.[67–69] Ribot can also be credited with describing preserved learning in amnesia, thus anticipating the distinction between declarative and nondeclarative forms of memory that has been so intensively investigated in our own recent times. An additional contribution to memory research in the latter nineteenth century was the description by Wernicke and Korsakoff (shown in Fig. 1-16) of the syndrome that bears their names, including Korsakoff's observations of what he called "pseudo-reminiscence," now known as confabulation.[70,71]

In 1881, Hermann Munk reported that when he ablated the occipital lobes of dogs, they seemed unable to recognize objects despite seeing well enough to navigate the visual environment.[72] Shortly thereafter, Lissauer presented one of the earliest clinical descriptions of visual recognition impairment in a human and suggested the distinction between apperceptive and

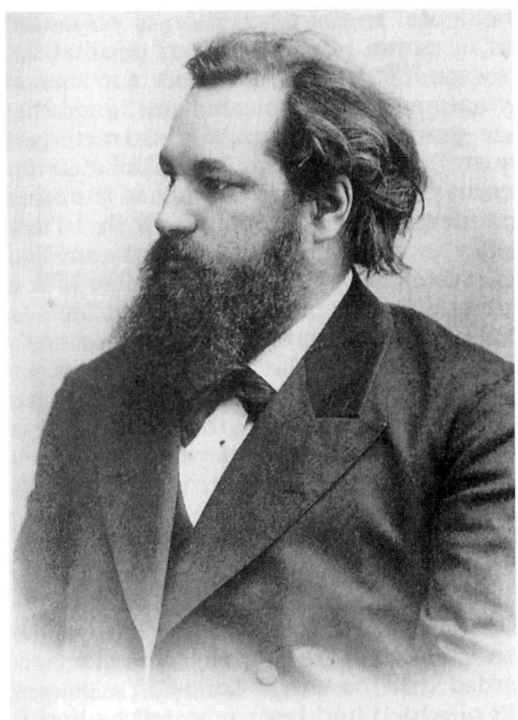

Figure 1-16
Sergei S. Korsakoff (1853–1900).

associative impairment—a clinical dichotomy still in use today.[73] Freud would later introduce the term *agnosia* to describe these conditions.[74] In the decades that followed, the visuospatial functions of the right hemisphere finally attracted the attention of neurologists and neuropsychologists.[75–77] The relatively delayed entry of this realm of functioning into the research arena is probably a result of the field's original focus on language and the left hemisphere, reflected in the nineteenth-century terminology of *major* and *minor hemisphere.*

THE RISE OF EXPERIMENTAL NEUROPSYCHOLOGY

Most of the advances described so far in this chapter were made by studying individual patients, or at most a small series of patients with similar disorders. In many instances, particularly before the middle of this century, patients' behavior was studied relatively naturalistically, without planned protocols or quantitative measurements. In the nineteen sixties and seventies, a different approach to the study of brain-behavior relations took hold. Neurologists and neuropsychologists began to design experiments patterned on research methods in experimental psychology.

Typical research designs in experimental psychology involved groups of normal subjects given different experimental treatments (for example, different training or different stimulus materials), and the effects of the treatments were measured in standardized protocols and compared using statistical methods such as analysis of variance. In neuropsychology, the "treatments" were, as a rule, naturally occurring brain lesions. Groups of patients with different lesion sites or behavioral syndromes were tested with standard protocols, yielding quantitative measures of performance, and these performances were compared across patient groups and with non-brain-damaged control groups. Unlike the impairments studied previously in single-case designs, which were so striking that control subjects would generally have been superfluous, experimental neuropsychology often focused on group differences of a rather subtle nature, which required statistical analysis to substantiate.

The most common question addressed by these studies concerned localization of function. Often the localization sought was no more precise than left versus right hemisphere or one quadrant of the brain (which, in the days before computed tomography, often amounted to left versus right hemisphere with presence or absence of visual field defects and/or hemiplegia). Given the huge amount of research done during this period on language, memory, perception, attention, emotion, praxis, and so-called executive functions, it would be hopeless even to attempt a summary. For those interested in some examples of this approach, we cite here some classic papers from a variety of the active laboratories of the period, addressing the question "Is the right hemisphere specialized for spatial perception of properties such as location,[78–80] orientation,[81,82] and large-scale topography?[83,84]"

The influential research program of the Montreal Neurological Institute also began during this period. In the wake of William Scoville's discovery that the bilateral medial temporal resection he performed on epileptic patient H.M. resulted in permanent and dense amnesia, Brenda Milner and her colleagues investigated this patient and groups of other operated epileptic patients. This enabled them to address questions of functional localization with the anatomic precision of known surgical lesions (e.g., see Refs. 85 and 86 for reviews of research from that period on frontal lobe function and temporal lobe function, respectively). At the same time, another surgical intervention for epilepsy, callosotomy, also spawned a productive and influential research program. Roger Sperry and his students and collaborators were able to address a wide variety of questions about hemispheric specialization by studying the isolated functioning of the human cerebral hemispheres.[87]

In addition to answering questions about localization, the experimental neuropsychology of the sixties and seventies also uncovered aspects of the functional organization of behavior. By examining patterns of association and dissociation among abilities over groups of subjects, researchers tried to determine which abilities depend on the same underlying functional systems and which are functionally independent. For example, the frequent association of aphasia and apraxia had been taken by some to support the notion that aphasia was not language-specific but was just one manifestation of a more pervasive loss of the ability to symbolize or represent ("asymbolia"). A classic group study by Goodglass and Kaplan[88] undermined this position by showing that severity of apraxia and aphasia were uncorrelated in a large sample of left-hemisphere-damaged subjects. A second example of the use of dissociations between groups of patients from this period is the demonstration of the functional distinction, by Newcombe and Russell, within vision between pattern recognition and spatial orientation.[89]

By the end of the seventies, experimental neuropsychology had matured to the point where many perceptual, cognitive, and motor abilities had been associated with particular brain regions, and certain features of the functional organization of these abilities had been delineated. Accordingly, it was at this time that first editions of some of the best-known neuropsychology texts appeared, such as those by Hécaen and Albert,[90] Heilman and Valenstein,[91] Kolb and Whishaw,[92] Springer and Deutsch,[93] and Walsh.[94]

Despite the tremendous progress of this period, experimental neuropsychology remained distinct from and relatively unknown within academic psychology. Particularly in the United States, but also to a large extent in Canada and Europe (the three largest contributors to the world's psychology literature), experimental neuropsychologists tended to work in medical centers rather than university psychology departments and to publish their work in journals separate from mainstream experimental psychology. An important turning point in the histories of both neuropsychology and the psychology of normal human function came when researchers in each area became aware of the other.

THE MARRIAGE OF EXPERIMENTAL NEUROPSYCHOLOGY AND COGNITIVE PSYCHOLOGY

The predominant approach to human experimental psychology in the 1970s was cognitive psychology. The hallmark of this approach was the assumption that all of cognition (broadly construed to include perception and motor control) could be viewed as information processing. Although the effects of damage to an information-processing mechanism might seem to be a good source of clues as to its normal operation, cognitive psychologists of the seventies were generally quite ignorant of contemporary neuropsychology.

The reason that most cognitive psychologists of the 1970s ignored neuropsychology stemmed from an overly narrow conception of information processing, based on the digital computer. A basic tenet of cognitive psychology was the computer analogy for the mind: the mind is to the brain as software is to hardware in a computer. Given that the same computer can run different programs and the same program can be run on different computers, this analogy suggests that hardware and software are independent and that the brain is therefore irrelevant to cognitive psychology. If you want to understand the nature of the program that is the human mind, studying neuropsychology is as pointless as trying to understand how a computer is programmed by looking at the circuit boards.

The problem with the computer analogy is that hardware and software are independent only for very special types of computational systems: those systems that have been engineered, through great effort and ingenuity, to make the hardware and software independent, enabling one computer to run many programs and enabling those programs to be portable to other computers. The brain was "designed" by very different pressures, and there is no reason to believe that, in general, information-processing functions and the physical subtrate of those functions will be independent. In fact, as cognitive psychologists finally began to learn about neuropsychology, it became apparent that cognitive functions break down in characteristic and highly informative ways after brain damage. By the early 1980s, cognitive psychology and neuropsychology were finally in communication with one another. Since then, we have seen an explosion of meetings, books, and new journals devoted to so-called cognitive neuropsychology. Perhaps more important, existing cognitive psychology journals have begun to publish neuropsychological studies, and articles in existing neuropsychology and neurology journals frequently include discussions of the cognitive psychology literature.

Let us take a closer look at the scientific forces that drove this change in disciplinary boundaries. By 1980, both cognitive psychology and neuropsychology had reached stages of development that were, if not exactly impasses, points of diminishing returns for the concepts and methods of their own isolated disciplines. In cognitive psychology, the problem concerned methodologic limitations. By varying stimuli and instructions and measuring responses and response latencies, cognitive psychologists made inferences about the information processing that intervened between stimulus and response. But such inferences were indirect, and in some cases they were incapable of distinguishing between rival theories. In 1978 the cognitive psychologist John Anderson published an influential paper[95] in which he called this the "identifiability" problem and took as his example the debate over whether mental images were more like perceptual representations or linguistic representations. He argued that the field's inability to resolve this issue, despite many years of research, was due to the impossibility of uniquely identifying internal cognitive processes from stimulus-response relations. He suggested that the direct study of brain function could, in principle, make a unique identification possible, but he indicated that such a solution probably lay in the distant future.

That distant future came to pass within the next 10 years, as cognitive psychologists working on a variety of different topics found that the study of neurologic patients provided a powerful new source of evidence for testing their theories. In the case of mental imagery, taken by Anderson to be emblematic of the identifiability problem, the finding that perceptual impairments after brain damage were frequently accompanied by parallel imagery impairments strongly favored the perceptual hypothesis.[96] The study of learning and memory within cognitive psychology was revolutionized by the influx of ideas and findings on preserved learning in amnesia, leading to the hypothesis of multiple memory systems.[97–99] In the study of attention, cognitive psychologists had for years focused on the issue of early versus late attentional selection without achieving a resolution, and here too neurologic disorders were crucial in moving the field forward. The phenomena of neglect provided dramatic evidence of selection from spatially formatted perceptual representations, and the variability in neglect's manifestations from case to case helped to establish the possibility of multiple loci for attentional selection as opposed to a single early or late locus. The idea of separate visual feature maps, supported by cases of acquired color, motion, and depth blindness, provided the inspiration for the most novel development in recent cognitive theories of attention—namely, feature integration theory.[100]

What did neuropsychology gain from the rapprochement with cognitive psychology? The main benefits were theoretical rather than methodologic. Traditionally, neuropsychologists studied the localization and functional organization of *abilities,* such as speech, reading, memory, object recognition, and so forth. But few would doubt that each of these abilities depends upon an orchestrated set of *component cognitive processes,* and it seems far more likely that the underlying cognitive components, rather than the task-defined abilities, are what is implemented in localized neural tissue. The theories of cognitive psychology therefore allowed neuropsychologists to pose questions about the localization and functional organization of the components of the cognitive architecture, a level of theoretical analysis that was more likely to yield clear and generalizable findings.

Among patients with reading disorders, for example, some are impaired at reading nonwords (e.g, *plif*) while others are impaired at reading irregular words (e.g., *yacht*). Rather than attempt to localize nonword reading or irregular word reading per se and delineate them as independent abilities, neuropsychologists have been able to use a theory of reading developed in cognitive psychology to interpret these disorders

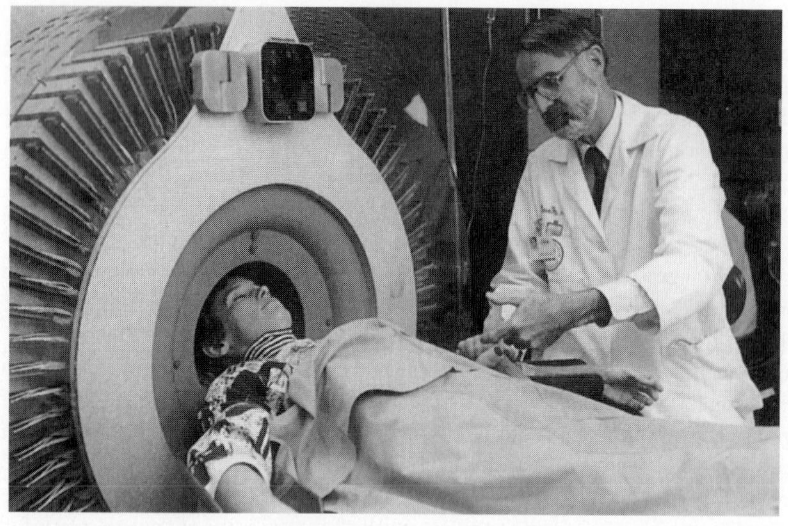

Figure 1-17
A subject about to undergo positron emission tomography. (From Marcus E. Raichle, M.D., Washington University, St. Louis, Missouri, with permission.)

in terms of damage to a whole-word recognition system and a grapheme-to-phoneme translation system, respectively.[101] This interpretation has the advantage of correctly predicting additional features of patient behavior, such as the tendency to misread nonwords as words of overall similar appearance when operating with only the whole-word system.

In recent years the neurology and neuropsychology of every major cognitive system has adopted the theoretical framework of cognitive psychology in a general way, and in some cases specific theories have been incorporated. This is reflected in the content and organization of the present book. For the most intensively studied areas of behavioral neurology and neuropsychology—namely, visual attention, memory, language, frontal lobe function, and Alzheimer disease—integrated pairs of chapters review the clinical and anatomic aspects of the relevant disorders and their cognitive theoretical interpretations. Chapters on other topics will cover both the clinical and theoretical aspects together.

NEW TOOLS FOR THE STUDY OF MIND AND BRAIN

In the past two decades, behavioral neurology and neuropsychology have been transformed not only by the influx of theoretical ideas from cognitive psychology but also by the advent of powerful new methods for studying brain activity during cognition. The first of these methods to find wide use was functional neuroimaging.

Functional Neuroimaging

Following its introduction in the 1970s, positron emission tomography (PET) was quickly embraced by researchers interested in brain-behavior relations. This technique provides images of regional glucose utilization, blood flow, oxygen consumption, or receptor density in the brains of live humans. Resting studies, in which subjects are scanned while resting passively, have provided a window on differences between normal and pathologic brain function in a number of neurologic and psychiatric conditions. With the use of radioactive ligands, abnormalities can be localized to specific neurotransmitter systems as well as specific anatomic regions. Activation studies, in which separate images are collected while normal subjects perform different tasks (typically one or more active tasks and one resting baseline), yielded new insights on the localization of cognitive processes. These localizations were not studied region by region, as necessitated by the lesion technique, but could be apprehended simultaneously in a whole intact brain. Figure 1-17 shows a subject in a PET scanner.

Positron emission tomography was soon joined by other techniques for measuring regional brain activity, each of which has its own strengths and weaknesses.

Single photon emission computed tomography (SPECT) was quickly adapted for some of the same applications as PET, providing a less expensive but also less quantifiable and spatially less accurate method for obtaining images of regional cerebral blood flow. With new developments in the measurement and analysis of electromagnetic signals, the relatively old techniques of electroencephalography (EEG) and event-related potentials (ERPs), as well as magnetoencephalography (MEG), joined the ranks of functional imaging techniques allowing some degree of anatomic localization of brain activity, with temporal resolution that is superior to the blood flow and metabolic techniques.

Most recently, functional magnetic resonance imaging (fMRI) has become the dominant functional neuroimaging method in cognitive neuroscience. This can be understood in view of its many advantages for the study of human cognition. It is noninvasive, using the magnetic properties of blood in lieu of an exogenous tracer or contrast medium. It can be implemented with equipment available for clinical purposes in many hospitals. Its spatial resolution allows localization to within millimeters, and its temporal resolution is sufficient to detect changes on the second-by-second time scale of most cognitive processes. Figure 1-18 shows an example of an fMRI signal as it varies in time over the different conditions of an experiment. Correlations between the signal change and the timing of changes among experimental conditions are computed throughout the brain, revealing those regions in which cognitive and brain activity are correlated. This and other methods of functional brain imaging are discussed in detail in Chaps. 7–9.

Much of the early work with functional neuroimaging could be considered a form of "calibration," in that researchers sought to confirm well-established principles of functional neuroanatomy using the new techniques—for example, demonstrating that visual stimulation activates visual cortex. As functional neuroimaging matured, researchers began to address new questions, to which the answers were not already known in advance. An important development in this second wave of research was the introduction of theories and methods from cognitive psychology, which specified the component cognitive processes involved in performing complex tasks and provided a means of isolating them experimentally. In neuroimaging studies of normal subjects, as with the purely behavioral studies of patients, the entities most likely to yield clear and consistent localizations are these component cognitive processes and not the tasks themselves. Starting in the mid-1980s, a collaboration between cognitive psychologist Michael Posner and neurologist Marcus Raichle at Washington University led to a series of pioneering studies in which the neural circuits underlying language, reading, and attention were studied by functional neuroimaging.[102] This approach is now widely used with normal subjects (see Chap. 7) and patient populations (see Chap. 8), and recent examples are to be found throughout this book.

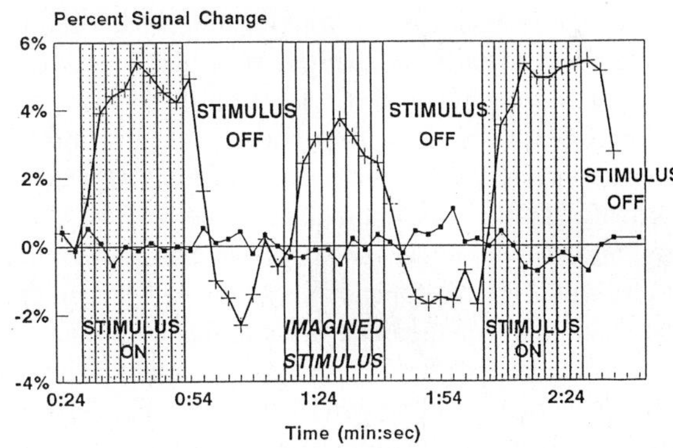

Figure 1-18
An example of the times series data that underlie fMRI, showing the percent signal change over time superimposed in the temporal onsets and offsets of the three different conditions of the experiment (stimulus on, stimulus off, and stimulus imagined). Both the perceptual processing of a stimulus and the imagining of a stimulus are correlated in time with signal changes in visual cortex but not in a nonvisual control region.

Computational Modeling of Higher Brain Function

A second and even more recent methodologic development is computational modeling of higher brain function. Computational models enable us to test hypotheses about the functioning of complex, interactive systems and about the effects of lesions to individual parts of such a system by building, running, and "lesioning" the models.

The roots of the computational approach can be traced back to earlier thinking in both behavioral neurology and cognitive psychology. Within behavioral neurology, the perennial critiques of localizationism can be viewed as an early expression of the need to consider the brain as "more than the sum of its parts" for purposes of understanding cognition. Aleksandr Luria's concept of "functional systems"[103] placed explicit emphasis on the importance of the system or circuit as the correct level of analysis for understanding brain function, and this point has been reemphasized more recently by such writers as Marcel Mesulam,[104] Kenneth Heilman and others,[105] and Patricia Goldman-Rakic.[106] The most radical reconceptualization of brain function in terms of global system properties as opposed to local centers can be attributed to Marcel Kinsbourne,[107,108] who has argued that local phenomena such as spreading activation or competition between reciprocally connected areas can lead the system as a whole to become "captured" in certain global states of attention, awareness, or asymmetrical hemispheric control of behavior.

Within cognitive psychology, a parallel evolution has taken place, from discrete-state models of human information processing, in which cognition unfolds through a series of functionally and temporally isolable stages, to models in which information is processed simultaneously and interactively over a network of processors. The latter type of model, similar in spirit to behavioral neurology's system-level theorizing, often takes the form of a running computer simulation in cognitive psychology. Such models have been termed "parallel distributed processing" (PDP) models, calling attention to the parallel or simultaneous nature of processing at multiple loci within the model and the distributed as opposed to localist nature of representation and processing within the model.[109] They have also been called "artificial neural networks," calling attention to the analogy between the units in the network and neurons in the brain. Like neurons, PDP units are highly interconnected; they process information by summing inputs received from other units across excitatory and inhibitory connections and sending outputs to a large number of other units in the same way.

By embodying the general ideas of distributedness, parallelism, and interactivity in concrete computer simulations, the specific predictions of hypotheses could be derived and tested. This is valuable because predictions about the effects local lesions in a highly interactive network on the behavior of the network as a whole can be difficult to derive by intuition alone and can sometimes be quite counterintuitive. The nature of these models, and their use in behavioral neurology and neuropsychology, is discussed further in Chap. 10.

CONCLUSIONS

It is impossible to revise a textbook and not reflect on the growth of the field since the last edition. The subject matter of some chapters has changed little, and these chapters needed only a little "freshening up" with some more recent literature citations. But in other areas, 6 years has brought substantial change in what we know about the brain and in how we study it. This is reflected in the complete rewriting of some chapters and the addition of new chapters on topics that were not covered in the first edition. In the context of the field's long history, we are in a period of explosive growth. The chapters that follow summarize our current understanding of the brain bases of higher mental functions, an understanding that surely ranks among humanity's most impressive achievements.

REFERENCES

1. Breasted JH: *The Edwin Smith Surgical Papyrus.* Chicago: University of Chicago Press, 1930.
2. McHenry LC Jr: *Garrison's History of Neurology.* Springfield, IL: Charles C Thomas, 1969.
3. Clarke E, O'Malley CE: *The Human Brain and Spinal Cord.* Berkeley, CA: University California Press, 1968.
4. Finger S: *Origins of Neuroscience. A History of Explorations into Brain Function.* New York: Oxford University Press, 1994.
5. Sondhaus E, Finger S: Aphasia and the CNS from Imhotep to Broca. *Neuropsychology* 2:87–110, 1988.
6. Woollam DHM: Concepts of the brain and its functions in classical antiquity, in Poynter FNL (ed): *The Brain and Its Functions.* Oxford, England: Blackwell, 1958, pp 5–18.

7. Bruyn GW: The seat of the soul, in Rose FC, Byrum WF (eds): *Historical Aspects of the Neurosciences.* New York: Raven Press, 1981, pp 55–81.
8. Mazzolini RG: Schemes and models of the thinking machine. In Corsi P (ed): *The Enchanted Loom: Chapters in the History of Neuroscience.* New York: Oxford University Press, 1991, pp 68–143.
9. Hippocrates: The sacred disease, in Adams F (trans): *The Genuine Works of Hippocrates.* New York: William Wood, 1932.
10. Clarke E, Dewhurst K: *An Illustrated History of Brain Function.* Berkeley, CA: University of California Press, 1972.
11. Pagel W: Medieval and Renaissance contributions to knowledge of the brain and its functions, in Poynter FNL (ed): *The Brain and Its Functions.* Oxford, England: Blackwell, 1958, pp 95–114.
12. Bakay L: *An Early History of Craniotomy.* Springfield, IL: Charles C Thomas, 1985.
13. Wozniak RH: *Mind and Body: René Descartes to William James.* National Library of Medicine, Bethesda, MD, and the American Psychological Association, Washington, DC, 1992.
14. Riese W: Descartes' ideas of brain function, in Poynter FNL (ed): *The Brain and Its Functions.* Oxford, England: Blackwell, 1958, pp 115–134.
15. Descartes R: *De homine figuris et latinitate donatus a Florentio Schuyl.* Leyden: Franciscum Moyardum and Petrum Leffen, 1662.
16. Descartes R: *Les passions de l'âme. Paris:* Henry Le Gras, 1649.
17. Willis T: *Cerebri anatome: Cui accessit nervorum descriptio et usus.* London: Martyn and Allestry, 1664.
18. Young RM: *Mind, Brain and Adaptation in the Nineteenth Century.* New York: Oxford University Press, 1990.
19. Bell C: *Idea of a New Anatomy of the Brain: Submitted for the Observations of His Friends.* London: Strahan and Preston, 1811.
20. Magendie F: Expériences sur les fonctions des racines des nerts rachidiens. *J Physiol Exp Pathol* 2:276–279, 1822.
21. Stookey B: A note on the early history of cerebral localization. *Bull NY Acad Med* 30:559–578, 1954.
22. Ackerknecht EH: Contribution of Gall and the phrenologist to knowledge of brain function, in Poynter FNL (ed): *The Brain and Its Functions.* Oxford: Blackwell, 1958, pp 149–153.
23. Pogliano C: Between form and function: A new science of man, in Corsi P (ed): *The Enchanted Loom: Chapters in the History of Neurosciences.* New York: Oxford University Press, 1991, pp 144–203.
24. Brown JW, Chobor KL: Phrenological studies of aphasia before Broca: Broca's aphasia or Gall's aphasia? *Brain Lang* 43:475–486, 1992.
25. Flourens P: *Phrenology Examined* (Charles De Lucena Meigs, trans). Philadelphia: Hogan and Thompson, 1846.
26. Flourens P: *Recherches Expérimentales sur les Propriétés et les Fonctions du Système Nerveux dans les Animaux Vertèbras* (1824), 2d ed. Paris: Baillière, 1842.
27. Harrington A: Beyond phrenology: Localization theory in the modern era, in Corsi P (ed): *The Enchanted Loom. Chapters in the History of Neuroscience.* New York: Oxford University Press, 1991, pp 207–239.
28. Bouillaud JB: *Traité clinique et physiologiquede l'encephalite ou inflammation du cerveau.* Paris: Baillière, 1825.
29. Benton AL, Joynt RJ: Early descriptions of aphasia. *Arch Neurol* 3:205–221, 1960.
30. Benton AL, Joynt RJ: Three pioneers in the study of aphasia. *J His Med Sci* 18:381–383, 1963.
31. Joynt RJ, Benton AL: The memoir of Marc Dax on aphasia. *Neurology* 14:851–854, 1964.
32. Head H: *Aphasia and Kindred Disorders of Speech.* New York: Macmillan, 1926.
33. Stookey BL: Jean-Baptiste Bouillaud and Ernest Aubertin: Early studies on cerebral localization and the speech center. *JAMA* 184:1024–1029, 1963.
34. Critchley M: The Broca-Dax controversy, in Critchley M (ed): *The Divine Banquet of the Brain and Other Essays.* New York: Raven Press, 1979.
35. Joynt RJ: Centenary of patient "Tan": His contribution to the problem of aphasia. *Arch Intern Med* 108:953–956, 1961.
36. Broca P: Remarques sur le siège de la faculté du langage articulé: Suivies d'une observation d'aphemie. *Bull Soc Anat (Paris)* 6:330–357, 1861.
37. Broca P: Localisation des fonctions cérébrales: Siège du langage articulé. *Bull Soc Anthropol (Paris)* 4:200–203, 1863.
38. Dax M: Lesions de la moitié gauche de l'encéphale coincident avec l'oublie des signes de la pensée. *Gaz hbd Méd Chir (Paris)* 2:259–262, 1865.
39. Dax G: Notes sur la mème sujet. *Gaz hbd Méd Chir (Paris)* 2:262, 1865.
40. Broca P: Sur le siège de la faculté du langage articulé. *Bull Soc Anthropol* 6:337–393, 1865.

41. Berker EA, Berker AH, Smith A: Translation of Broca's 1865 report: Localization of speech in the third left frontal convolution. *Arch Neurol* 43:1065–1072, 1986.
42. Fritsch G, Hitzig E: On the electrical excitability of the cerebrum (1870), in von Bonin G (ed): *Some Papers on the Cerebral Cortex.* Springfield, IL: Charles C Thomas, 1960, pp 73–96.
43. Geschwind N: Wernicke's contribution to the study of aphasia. *Cortex* 3:449–463, 1967.
44. Wernicke C: *Der aphasische Symptomemkomplex: Eine psychologische Studie auf anatomischer Basis.* Breslau: Cohn und Weigert, 1874.
45. Lecours AR, Lhermitte F: From Franz Gall to Pierre Marie, in Lecours AR, Lhermitte F, Bryans B (eds): *Aphasiology.* London: Baillière Tindall, 1983.
46. Geschwind N: Carl Wernicke, the Breslau School and the history of aphasia, in Carterette EC (ed): *Brain Function:* Vol III. *Speech, Language, and Communication.* Berkeley, CA: University of California Press, 1963, pp 1–16.
47. Lichtheim L: On aphasia. *Brain* 7:433–484, 1885.
48. Liepmann H: Das Krankheitsbild der Apraxie ("motorische Asymbolie") auf Grund eines Falles von einseitiger Apraxie. *Monatschr Psychiatr Neurol* 8:15–44, 102–132, 182–197, 1900.
49. Liepmann H, Maas O: Fall von linksseitiger Agraphie und Apraxie bei rechtsseitiger Lähmung. *J Psychol Neurol* 10:214–227, 1907.
50. Déjerine J: Contribution à l'étude anatomopathologique et clinique des différentes variétés de cécité verbale. *CRH Séances Mem Soc Biol* 44:61–90, 1892.
51. Geschwind N: Disconnexion syndromes in animals and man. *Brain* 88:237–294, 585–644, 1965.
52. Brais B: The third left frontal convolution plays no role in language: Pierre Marie and the Paris debate on aphasia (1906–1908). *Neurology* 42:690–695, 1992.
53. Goldstein K: *The Organism.* New York: American Book, 1939.
54. Goldstein K: *Language and Language Disturbances.* New York: Grune & Stratton, 1948.
55. Lecours AR, Cronk C, Sébahoun-Balsamo M: From Pierre Marie to Norman Geschwind, in Lecours AR, Lhermitte F, Bryans B (eds): *Aphasiology.* London: Baillière Tindall, 1983.
56. Franz SI, Lashley KS: The retention of habits by the rat after destruction of the frontal portion of the cerebrum. *Psychobiology* 1:3–18, 1917.
57. Lashley KS, Franz SI: The effects of cerebral destruction upon habit-formation and retention in the albino rat. *Psychobiology* 1:71–139, 1917.
58. Lashley KS: *Brain Mechanisms and Intelligence: A Quantitative Study of Injuries to the Brain.* Chicago: University of Chicago Press, 1929.
59. Lashley KS: In search of the engram. *Symp Soc Exp Biol* 4:454–482,1950.
60. Geschwind N: The paradoxical position of Kurt Goldstein in the history of aphasia. *Cortex* 1:214–224, 1964.
61. Harrington A: A feeling for the "whole": The holistic reaction in neurology from the fin de siècle to the interwar years, in Teich M, Porter R (eds): *Fin de Siècle and Its Legacy.* Cambridge, England: Cambridge University Press, 1990.
62. Vogt O, Vogt C: Zur anatomischen Gliederung des cortex cerebri. *J Psychol Neurol* 2:160–180, 1903.
63. Haymaker WE: Cecile and Oskar Vogt, on the occasion of her 75th and his 80th birthday. *Neurology* 1:179–204, 1951.
64. Campbell AW: Histological studies on cerebral localization. *Proc R Soc Lond B Biol Sci* 72:488–492, 1903.
65. Campbell AW: *Histological Studies on the Localization of Cerebral Function.* Cambridge, England: Cambridge University Press, 1905.
66. Brodmann K: *Vergleichende Lokalisationslehre der Grosshirnrinde in ihren Prinzipien dargestellt auf Grund des Zellenbaues.* Leipzig: Barth, 1909.
67. Levin HS, Peters BH, Hulkonen DA: Early concepts of anterograde and retrograde amnesia. *Cortex* 19:427–440, 1983.
68. Ribot T: *Diseases of Memory.* London: Kegan Paul, Trench, 1882.
69. Squire LR, Slater PC: Anterograde and retrograde memory impairment in chronic amnesia. *Neuropsychologia* 16:313–322, 1978.
70. Victor M, Adams RD, Collins GH: *The Wernicke-Korsakoff Syndrome and Related Neurologic Disorders due to Alcoholism and Malnutrition,* 2d ed. Philadelphia: Davis, 1989.
71. Victor M, Yakovlev PI: SS Korsakoff's psychic disorder in conjunction with peripheral neuritis: A translation of Korsakoff's original article with brief comments on the author and his contribution to clinical medicine. *Neurology* 5:394–406, 1955.
72. Munk H: Über die Functionen der Grosshirnrinde: Gesammelte Mitteilungen aus den Jahren. Berlin: Hirschwald, 1877–1880.
73. Lissauer H: Ein fall von seelenblindheit nebst einem Beitrage zur Theori derselben. *Arch Psychiatr Nervenkrankh* 21:222–270, 1980.
74. Freud S: *Zur Auffassung der Aphasien.* Leipzig and Vienna: Deuticke, 1891.

75. Paterson A, Zangwill OL: Disorders of visual space perception associated with lesions of the right cerebral hemisphere. *Brain* 40:122–179, 1944.
76. Hécaen H, Ajuriaguerra J, Massonet J: Les troubles visuoconstructives par lésion pariéto-occipitale droite. *Encéphale* 40:122–179, 1951.
77. Benton A: Neuropsychology: Past, present and future, in Boller F, Grafman J (eds): *Handbook of Neuropsychology*. New York: Elsevier, 1988, vol 1, pp 3–27.
78. Hannay HJ, Varney NR, Benton AL: Visual localization in patients with unilateral brain disease. *J Neurol Neurosurg Psychiatry* 39:307–313, 1976.
79. Ratcliff G, Davies-Jones GAB: Defective visual localization in focal brain wounds. *Brain* 95:46–60, 1972.
80. Warrington EK, Rabin P: Perceptual matching in patients with cerebral lesions. *Neuropsychologia* 8:475–487, 1970.
81. De Renzi E, Faglioni P, Scotti G: Judgement of spatial orientation in patients with focal brain damage. *J Neurol Neurosurg Psychiatry* 34:489–495, 1971.
82. Carmon A, Benton AL: Tactile perception of direction and number in patients with unilateral cerebral disease. *Neurology* 19:525–532, 1969.
83. Hécaen H, Tzortzis C, Masure MC: Troubles de l'orientation spatiale dans une épreuve de recherche d'itinéraire lors des lesions corticales unilaterales. *Perception* 1:325–330, 1972.
84. Semmes J, Weinstein S, Ghent L, Teuber HL: Correlates of impaired orientation in personal and extrapersonal space. *Brain* 86:747–772, 1963.
85. Milner B: Some effects of frontal lobectomy in man, in Warren JM, Akert K (eds): *The Frontal Granular Cortex and Behavior.* New York: McGraw-Hill, 1964.
86. Milner B: Memory and the medical temporal regions of the brain, in Pribram KH, Broadbent DE (eds): *Biological Bases of Memory.* New York: Academic Press, 1970.
87. Trevarthen C, Roger W: Sperry's lifework and our tribute, in Trevarthen C (ed): *Brain Circuits and Functions of the Mind: Essays in Honor of Roger W. Sperry.* Cambridge, England: Cambridge University Press, 1990.
88. Goodglass H, Kaplan E: Disturbance of gesture and patomime in aphasia. *Brain* 86:703–720, 1963.
89. Newcombe F, Russell W: Dissociated visual perceptual and spatial deficits in focal lesions of the right hemisphere. *J Neurol Neurosurg Psychiatry* 32:73–81, 1969.
90. Hécaen H, Albert ML: *Human Neuropsychology.* New York: Wiley, 1978.
91. Heilman KM, Valenstein E: *Clinical Neuropsychology.* New York: Oxford University Press, 1979.
92. Kolb B, Whishaw I: *Fundamentals of Human Neuropsychology.* New York: Freeman, 1980.
93. Springer SP, Deutsch G: *Left Brain/Right Brain.* San Francisco: Freeman, 1981.
94. Walsh KW: *Neuropsychology: A Clinical Approach.* New York: Churchill Livingstone, 1978.
95. Anderson JR: Arguments concerning representation for mental imagery. *Psychol Rev* 85:249–277, 1978.
96. Farah MJ: Is visual imagery really visual? Overlooked evidence from neuropsychology. *Psychol Rev* 95:307–317, 1988.
97. Schacter DL: Implicit memory: History and current status. *J Exp Psychol Learn Mem Cogn* 13:501–518, 1987.
98. Squire L: *Memory and Brain.* New York: Oxford University Press, 1987.
99. Weiskrantz L: On issues and theories of the human amnesic syndrome, in Weinberger N, McGaugh JL, Lynch G (eds): *Memory Systems of the Brain.* New York: Guilford Press, 1985.
100. Treisman A: Features and objects: The fourteenth Bartlett lecture. *Q J Exp Psychol* 40A:201–237, 1988.
101. Coltheart M: Cognitive neuropsychology and the study of reading, in Marin IP, Marin OSM (eds): *Attention and Performance XI.* London: Erlbaum, 1985.
102. Posner MI, Raichle ME: *Images of Mind.* New York: Scientific American Library, 1994.
103. Luria AR: *The Working Brain.* New York: Basic Books, 1973.
104. Mesulam M-M: A cortical network for directed attention and unilateral neglect. *Ann Neurol* 10:309–325, 1981.
105. Heilman KM, Watson RT, Valenstein E: Hemispatial neglect, in Heilman KM, Valenstein E (eds): *Clinical Neuropsychology.* New York: Oxford University Press, 1979.
106. Goldman-Rakic P: Topography of cognition: Parallel distributed networks in primate association cortex. *Annu Rev Neurosci* 11:137–156, 1988.
107. Kinsbourne M: Lateral interactions in the brain, in Kinsbourne M, Smith WL (eds): *Hemispheric Disconnection and Cerebral Function.* Springfield, IL: Charles C Thomas, 1974.
108. Kinsbourne M: Integrated field theory of consciousness, in Marcel AJ, Bisiach E (eds): *Consciousness in Contemporary Science.* Oxford, England: Clarendon Press, 1988.
109. Rumelhart DE, McClelland JL: *Parallel Distributed Processing: Explorations in the Microstructure of Cognition.* Cambridge, MA: MIT Press, 1986.

Chapter 2

THE MENTAL STATUS EXAM

Susan K. Guy
Jeffrey L. Cummings

Despite a technological revolution in diagnostic studies, the foundation of an accurate neurobehavioral diagnosis remains a careful history and examination. The neurobehavioral examination draws on the general neurologic exam and the psychiatric mental status exam and expands these to develop an understanding of function of specific brain regions and domains. To accommodate practical time constraints, it has become particularly important to be able to tailor the exam to target areas of suspected deficit.

The basis of examination is observation. The traditional psychiatric mental status examination emphasizes this and as such is in play throughout one's interaction with the patient. With the exception of issues of thought content and subjective affective state, it does not involve direct inquiry. The psychiatric mental status examination presents information on appearance, behavior, language, mood, affect, thought process, thought content, insight, and judgment. The neurobehavioral exam adds to the psychiatric examination by assessing cognition using a brain-based model. Cognitive domains assessed include attention, language, memory, visuospatial skills, and executive function. While behavioral observations are integral to language assessment, language is here discussed as one of the five cognitive domains targeted for directed examination.

Examination aids in the localization of pathology, but detection of localized lesions is only one goal of the mental status examination. Other goals include establishing an alliance with the patient and developing diagnostic hypotheses to be further explored with laboratory tests and imaging.

As discussed in the final section of Chap. 4, most cognitive functions depend on multiple brain regions. For instance, it is well recognized that mesial temporal lobe structures are important for memory formation, but the frontal cortex also plays a role in information retrieval.[1] Just as single cognitive domains depend on multiple anatomic sites for integrity, a given cognitive screening test may reflect the function of several domains. For example, while verbal fluency tests evaluate frontal function, they also assess temporal lobe integrity.[2] Conclusions regarding localization as based on mental status testing must take this into account.

BEHAVIORAL OBSERVATIONS

Appearance

The patient's grooming, any signs of systemic or neurocutaneous syndromes, or evidence of trauma should be noted. Patients with dementia may be unbathed and have misbuttoned or disheveled clothing. Scars may suggest brain injury, dyscontrol, posttraumatic stress disorder, drug abuse, or self-injurious behavior.

Behavior

Note the patient's cooperativeness with the exam as well as any motoric abnormalities. Impulsivity is characteristic of the orbitofrontal syndrome. Lack of gesturing can be seen as part of the initiation difficulties seen with medial frontal lobe lesions.[3] Bradykinesia (also known as psychomotor retardation) can occur with depression or parkinsonism. Hyperkinesias may reflect neurologic conditions, such as choreoatheotic movements in Huntington's disease. Myoclonic jerks may suggest corticobasal degeneration[4] or Creutzfeldt-Jakob disease.[5] Psychomotor activation describes general restlessness, which may be seen in a variety of circumstances including anxiety, mania, akathisia, and stimulant intoxication. Hyperorality may be seen in Klüver-Bucy syndrome[6] or in frontotemporal degeneration.[7] Tremors and observations elicited through physical exam, such as abnormalities of tone, are generally recorded in the elemental neurologic examination.

Affect

Affect refers to the patient's facial expression and other body movements. While bradykinesia and decreased facial expression may suggest depression to one observer, they may suggest parkinsonism or frontal lobe pathology to another. As such, it is generally most useful to describe observations rather than make inferences. Commonly used descriptive terms are *constricted, blunted,* and *flattened affect,* in order of increasing restriction of emotional range. A constricted affect is common in depression. A blunted affect can be seen in frontotemporal degeneration, while a flattened or mask-like affect may suggest Parkinson's disease. It is not necessary to limit oneself to these terms, however, as others may be more descriptive (i.e., the "alien stare" described with frontotemporal degeneration). Mention of tearfulness, smiling, lability, and the mood congruence of affect also is useful. Mood and affect are typically congruent but may be dissociated in neurologic conditions such as pseudobulbar palsy.[8]

Mood

In documenting mood, it is most informative to quote the patient's own report of his or her internal state. Reported mood is often influenced by factors such as the patient's rapport with you as well as his or her culture, age cohort, and recent stressors (i.e., finding a place to park). Apathy and depression should be distinguished, as they are probably discrete entities involving different anatomic substrates. Depression tends to occur acutely after insults to left frontal regions.[9] Apathy is associated with insults to structures in the medial prefrontal cortex, anterior cingulate, and amygdala. Depression may be differentiated from apathy by inquiring about sadness, tearfulness, feelings of hopelessness and helplessness, guilt, and thoughts of death. Apathetic patients generally do not present with these symptoms. Although family members are concerned that the patient is "depressed," they are distressed by his or her lack of motivation, interest, and decreased expression of emotion, opinions, and desires.[10] Apathy is more common than depression in Alzheimer's disease[11] and, in contrast to depression, has been found to be strongly correlated with impairment of independence in activities of daily living in these patients.[12] Apathy may be a presenting symptom of frontotemporal degeneration.[13]

Thought Process

The style in which patients present ideas and beliefs during an interview reflects the efficiency and organization of their thinking. It is important to remember, however, that such higher levels of communication are dependent not only on executive functioning but also on other cognitive domains such as memory and language. General descriptive terms are useful in providing an overview to suggest areas of more detailed investigation. For instance, with further testing it may be apparent that vague responses are an indicator of aphasia or that tangentiality is reflective of a memory deficit (or hearing impairment). The disjointed, stilted, echolalic speech and odd mannerisms of a hebephrenic schizophrenic are considered to reflect disorganized thoughts. Such a pattern can also be seen in frontotemporal degeneration. Thought *blocking* describes the abrupt cessation of speech in midconversation that is seen in schizophrenia; derailment also is common. Flight of ideas generally implies mania, while a loosening of associations suggests a psychotic process. Manic discourse follows an unusual but discernible path (for instance, a comment about a candy wrapper on the floor might be followed by an exaltation of a rap artist). During psychosis, the connectivity of ideas is lost to the outside observer; the schizophrenic assumes that strangers are aware of his or her personal thoughts and their details.

Thought Content

In evaluating the content of another's thoughts, both observations and direct questioning are useful. Three key areas to be addressed are psychotic symptoms as well as thoughts of harming self or others. Hesitancy and suspicious glances about the room by the patient should lead the examiner to careful questioning about the patient's perceived safety and possible paranoid delusional systems. Enquiring about personal messages from the television or radio can elucidate ideas of reference. When asked about special talents, schizophrenics may report thought reading, thought broadcasting (i.e., sending messages to others telepathically), or thought insertion (receiving thoughts from others). Delusions such as beliefs that the patient's possessions are being stolen, his or her spouse is unfaithful, and that people are not who they claim to be (misidentification) are common in dementing disorders.[14]

Perceptual Disorders and Hallucinations Auditory hallucinations are more characteristic of schizophrenia,[15] while visual hallucinations are a hallmark of dementia with Lewy bodies.[16] Olfactory, or less frequently, gustatory hallucinations may occur as epileptiform auras.[15] Tactile hallucinations commonly occur during stimulant intoxication.[17] Hallucinations can occur in a wide variety of neurologic disorders, and their presence and content is not pathognomonic of any disease. It is important to ascertain whether hallucinations occur in the context of a delusional system or as isolated symptoms that the patient can evaluate objectively. This can help diagnostically and can also give guidance as to the likelihood that command hallucinations will be acted upon. For instance, a schizophrenic patient who believes he is the messiah may more readily kill himself when he perceives God telling him to. A patient such as this may not appear depressed, underscoring the importance assessing suicidality in all patients.

Suicidal and Homicidal Ideation Suicide assessment can begin with asking whether the patient has had thoughts of giving up. Further questioning probes thoughts of going to sleep and not waking up (i.e., passive suicidal ideation) or actively harming oneself (including how and the availability of means, including guns). It is important to inquire about the chronicity of suicidal ideation, prior attempts (including medical care required), and reasons holding the person back from completing suicide (i.e., children, religious beliefs, fears, etc.). If present, suicidal ideation generally warrants psychiatric evaluation. A similar train of questioning is pursued in the evaluation of homicidal ideation. If homicidal ideation is present, this should be reported to authorities as well as to the targeted individual.[18]

Insight

The amount of understanding patients have of their current situation and illness is useful in targeting educational interventions and has implications for issues such as medication compliance. Early loss of insight has been proposed as a core diagnostic feature of frontotemporal degeneration[13] but also occurs in Alzheimer's disease.[19]

Judgment

Even if patients are aware of their condition, neurobehavioral deficits can still affect their ability to make practical decisions and plan for the provision of food, clothing, shelter, and self-care. In the psychiatric setting, this often has legal implications concerning the institution of involuntary treatment for grave disability.

DIRECTED EXAMINATION OF COGNITIVE FUNCTION

In addition to the general psychiatric mental status exam, the neurobehavioral examination evaluates specific realms of cognitive functioning. These are presented in a hierarchical fashion, as performance on the latter parts of the examination will be dependent on preservation of function in the earlier domains of testing. Domains assessed include attention, language, memory, visuospatial skills, and executive function.

Screens of Cognitive Function

There are several standardized measures of neurobehavioral functioning commonly employed by clinicians. They can be used as adjuncts to the traditional neurobehavioral exam to quantitatively monitor symptom progression over time and response to treatment. Some tools that are potentially useful to the clinical practice are listed in Table 2-1. The most widely used is the Mini-Mental State Exam (MMSE).

Table 2-1
Some commonly used mental status assessment tools

Rating scale	*How administered*	*Minutes to administer*	*Domains examined*	*Comments*
MMSE	Patient interview	5	Orientation, registration, attention and calculation, recall, language, construction	Gross measure of global cognitive functioning. Initially intended as a dementia screening tool. Limited behavioral or frontal systems information. Not sensitive to less severe disease.
CDR	Patient and caregiver interview	30	Memory, orientation, judgment/problem solving, community affairs, home and hobbies, personal care	Estimate of functional capacity. Often used in dementia research. Applicability to other populations unclear.
NPI	Caregiver interview	15	Delusions, hallucinations, agitation/aggression, depression, anxiety, elation/euphoria, apathy/indifference, disinhibition, irritability/lability, motor disturbance, nighttime behavior, appetite/eating	Focuses on behavioral symptomatology. Distinguishes apathy from depression. Also in a validated brief clinical version, the NPI-Q.
BDI	Self	10	Mood including suicidality	May be preferable to use an examiner-administered scale, such as the Ham-D, in cognitively impaired individuals, or the GDS in elderly populations.

Key: MMSE, Mini-Mental State Exam[38]; CDR, Clinical Dementia Rating Scale[25]; NPI, Neuropsychiatric Inventory[39]; NPI-Q, Neuropsychiatric Inventory, brief clinical version[40]; BDR, Beck Depression Inventory[41]; Ham-D, Hamilton Depression Scale[42]; GDS, Geriatric Depression Scale.[43]

Attention

The word *attention* is used in multiple different ways in connection with neurologic patients, sometimes referring to a specific perceptual process, whereby external stimuli enter a patient's awareness (see Chaps. 25 and 26), and sometimes referring to a more general state of cognitive awareness and focus (see Chaps. 28 and 43). A key component of the mental status exam is the assessment of attention in the latter sense. Attention is dependent on level of consciousness, which is an important determinant of the state of one's higher cognitive functioning. This is particularly relevant in the case of acute inpatient admissions, where the history preceding admission may not be clear and delirium can complicate the diagnostic picture. Consciousness is more impaired as one progresses through alertness, lethargy, obtundation, and stupor to coma.[20] Alertness is commonly considered the ability to interact meaningfully with the environment.[15] Lethargy, also known as somnolence, implies a sleepy state from which an individual can be fully aroused with verbal stimulation. The transition from lethargy to coma involves a progressive diminution of response to tactile and verbal stimuli. Obtundation implies the inability to regain full alertness and clarity of thinking even with vigorous repetitive stimulation. Coma is a state in which the patient's level of consciousness is not affected by external stimulation. Such patients may manifest posturing in response to noxious stimuli. The stages of consciousness are not discrete, and—as with much of the neurobehavioral exam—it is more useful to provide a description of behavior than use a label that may not be consistent across examiners.[20]

If a patient is not alert, subsequent testing will be unreliable. Alertness, however, does not imply intact attention. Attention requires the ability to maintain concentration on a task and may be impaired during an acute psychiatric disturbance, confusional state, or executive disorder. Attentional assessment is important in the recognition of delirium, which has a high mortality rate.[21]

One commonly used measure of attention is digit span. The patient is asked to repeat increasingly long digit sequences after one presentation of each sequence. A normal adult should be able to recite 7 digits forward. Inability to recite 5 or more numbers implies impairment.[2] Another attentional task is the "A test," during which the examiner reads a sequence of letters that includes the letter *A* at greater than random frequency. The patient is asked to raise and lower his or her index finger when the letter *A* is heard. The number of commissions and omissions is noted.[20]

Language

Language assessment involves observation of spontaneous language production as well as directed inquiry into areas potentially involved in aphasia and related syndromes. Taking note of any irregular words or errors in word usage as well as the prosody and rate of spontaneous speech can aid in the differential diagnosis of neurobehavioral syndromes. Simple direct testing is useful in the assessment of fluency, comprehension, repetition, and naming.

Language conveys meaning and is dependent on higher cognitive functions. Speech involves the mechanical production of sounds that are combined to produce spoken communication. Dysarthria is a disturbance of speech and may reflect stroke or motor neuron disease, while aphasias involve language disturbances and can occur with stroke or neurodegenerative disorders such as Alzheimer's disease and the frontotemporal dementias. In subcortical dementias, impairment of speech is more pronounced than are language deficits. Such patients may be dysarthric and hypophonic but generally are not aphasic.[22]

Paraphasic errors are common in fluent aphasias and can be classified as semantic (verbal) or phonemic (literal). An incorrect word usage (i.e., *cabbage* for *potato*) is a semantic paraphasic error. A syllable substitution (i.e., *flapper* for *trapper*) indicates a phonemic paraphasia. Neologisms involve the generation of new words. In schizophrenia, neologisms often acquire specific meaning (for instance, *fume* to mean a vehicle with the potential to cause immolation).[22]

Prosody involves altering the inflection and volume of speech to convey emotional content and meaning. Receptive aprosody, or difficulty distinguishing meaning conveyed by prosody, can occur with lesions to the area of the right hemisphere that is similar in location to Wernicke's area in the left hemisphere (posterosuperior temporal lobe). Executive aprosody, or difficulty expressing meaning using prosody, can occur with lesions of the right premotor cortex[23] or in subcortical disorders such as Parkinson's disease.[22]

Fluent speech generates at least 40 words a minute and is generally grammatically intact and not effortful. Aspontaneity of speech can occur with frontal-subcortical dysfunction, which is seen in a number of conditions, including depression, schizophrenia, and frontotemporal degeneration. Nonfluent speech suggests lesions anterior to the rolandic sulcus.[23]

In addition to listening to the patient's spontaneous speech, two verbal fluency tasks are commonly administered during the neurobehavioral exam. Both category and letter-fluency tasks have been found to activate frontal structures.[24] Asking the patient to name as many animals as possible in 1 min assesses category fluency. Scores of less than 12 are abnormal.[8] Animal naming norms for 70-, 80-, and 90-year-olds with 12 years of education are 18, 17, and 15 respectively. The FAS test is also a letter-fluency task. The patient is asked to name as many words as possible beginning with F, A, and then S (excluding proper nouns). He or she is given 1 min per letter. The total words named for all three letters should be 30 or more for people under age 60 and at least 18 for older people (with a minimum of a ninth-grade education).[2]

Comprehension is assessed by asking patients about a simple paragraph they have read or by having them perform commands that are increasingly syntactically complex. Preserved comprehension suggests sparing of posterior left-hemispheric structures.[23]

Repetition is readily tested by asking the patient to repeat a phrase. Intact repetition is characteristic of transcortical aphasias and is also seen in pure anomic aphasia. Preserved repetition in an aphasia syndrome suggests that the area of pathology lies outside the perisylvian language regions in the left hemisphere.[23]

Confrontation naming is generally impaired in aphasia and is assessed by asking the patient to name a variety of objects. One commonly used tool to facilitate this is the 15-item Abbreviated Boston Naming Test.[25] A significant decline in scores on the Boston Naming Test does not occur until nonimpaired individuals are in their seventies.[26]

Assessment of singing and reciting overlearned sequences (i.e., the alphabet, prayers, and nursery rhymes) may enhance understanding of the patient's verbal capacities.

Depending on the stage of a progressive illness, different language deficits may arise. In Alzheimer's disease, word-finding difficulties appear first, with impairment of category naming. Empty speech soon develops, followed closely by decreased confrontation naming. Next, difficulties with language comprehension arise and paraphasic errors occur. Repetition, motor speech, and reading out loud are preserved until late in the course of the illness.[22] Disturbances of language that can occur in frontotemporal degeneration (FTD) include stereotyped, sparse, or rapid speech; echolalia; and perseveration. In the later stages of FTD, patients are often mute.[13]

Memory

Memory concerns are among the most common complaints assessed by the behavioral neurologist. Bedside testing can help in the differential diagnosis of their etiology. The MMSE presents a three-word list, which is used to test recall after 1 to 2 min. More sensitive testing is achieved by longer list-learning tasks. There are a number of word lists that have established norms for recall tasks, including the California Verbal Learning Test (CVLT).[27] Generally, the patient is asked to recall as many items as possible immediately after presentation of the list over several trials. The patient's learning curve is noted. After a delay, the patient is asked to spontaneously recall as many items as possible from the list. The patient is then given a list of words that includes the original list as well as number of foils and is asked to indicate which were on the initial list. Patients with amnestic disorder or Alzheimer's disease generally demonstrate a poor learning curve, with little improvement in the number of items recalled over repeated trials; they exhibit poor delayed recall and have difficulty distinguishing targets from foils in the recognition portion of the test.[28] Patients with subcortical dementias have a retrieval-type memory deficit and may demonstrate a marked improvement in score during cued recall and recognition testing.[29] Initially, memory loss in patients with Alzheimer's disease involves predominantly recent memory. As the disease progresses, more distant memories are lost.[23] This pattern is not typical in patients with Parkinson's disease[30] or Huntington's disease,[31] in which there is relatively minimal retrograde amnesia.

While verbal memory is generally dependent on left-sided structures, visual memory performance is more dependent on right-sided structures.[23] Nonverbal memory is assessed by having the patient copy an image (such as the Rey-Osterrieth figure[32]) and then redraw it from memory. Alternatively, the examiner can present a series of visual or tactile figures and test the patient's recollection of these items after a delay. A test of visual memory, which is independent of language function or drawing ability, involves having the patient locate items which he or she has watched the examiner hide about the room earlier.

Visuospatial Function

Visuospatial functioning is assessed by asking the patient to copy figures such as the intersecting pentagons of the MMSE (Fig. 2-1). Copies of three-dimensional figures, such as a cube, and more complex two-dimensional figures, such as the Rey-Osterrieth figure, can reveal more subtle deficits. Patients with right parietal lesions often produce figure copies that appear disorganized and may also demonstrate left

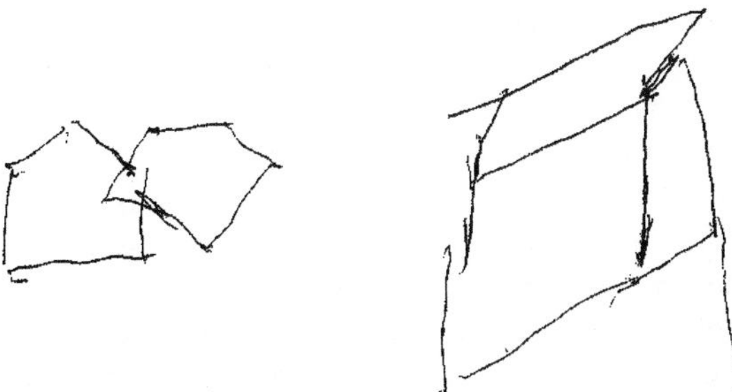

Figure 2-1
Impaired cube copy with relatively intact pentagon copy by a patient with Alzheimer's disease.

hemineglect.[23] Lesions in other brain regions can also disrupt visuospatial function. Asking the patient to give directions to his or her home can be particularly useful in visually impaired subjects or those who have a motor disturbance such as tremor that interferes with writing.

Patients with visual agnosia have difficulty recognizing a visually presented object, although they may be able to draw the item and can describe details of the object. Such disturbances are associated with left occipitotemporal damage. Prosopagnosia is a form of visual agnosia in which subjects have difficulty recognizing faces, although they can describe the details of facial characteristics, match similar faces, and recognize people by voice. Prosopagnosia may result from lesions in the right occipitotemporal region.[33] Balint's syndrome involves simultanagnosia, oculomotor apraxia, and optic ataxia and implies bilateral occipitoparietal lesions. Simultanagnosia is the inability to see multiple visual stimuli simultaneously despite preserved visual acuity. Patients often are able to identify smaller components of the image correctly. For instance, when presented with a letter *E* composed of smaller *A*'s, the patient will report seeing *A*'s but will not recognize the larger *E*. Optic ataxia refers to the inability to voluntarily control gaze to examine desired parts of the visual field. A person with oculomotor apraxia has difficulty using vision to accurately guide directed movements, such as touching a pen.[23]

Clock drawing is a task that is easy to administer and provides substantial information regarding visuospatial function. The examiner instructs the patient to draw a clock face with numbers and the time

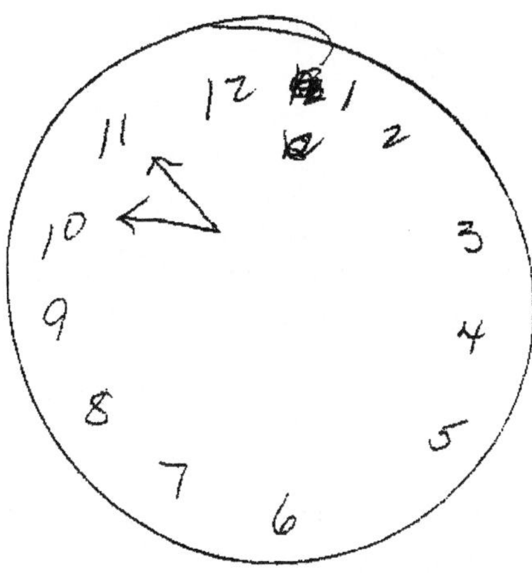

Figure 2-2
"Frontal pull" in a clock drawing by a 49-year-old patient with frontotemporal degeneration asked to set the hands to read 10 min past 11.

reading 11:10. Performance reflects not only visuospatial functioning but also executive functions, including planning. Frontal systems dysfunction is implied by "frontal pull" or stimulus-boundedness, whereby the patient places the hands on the numbers 11 and 10 rather than 11 and 2.[34] (Fig. 2-2).

Executive Function

Frontostriatal systems aid in tasks involving strategy, organization, cognitive flexibility and set shifting, and abstraction. Backwards digit span reflects cognitive flexibility and can be impaired after frontal injury.[35] In formal neuropsychological testing, the Wisconsin Card Sort Test is often used to assess set shifting. Patients are asked to sort cards according to color, shape, and other criteria. Although not formally studied, the "coin test" also attempts to assess set-shifting ability and may readily be done at the bedside. The examiner switches coins from one hand to the other behind his or her own (i.e., the examiner's) back and then asks the patient to guess which hand the coin is in. The examiner changes the pattern without warning, for instance, placing the coin in one hand twice before switching to the other hand. The average person can guess each pattern in about four trials. Set shifting also can be assessed with the Trails B test,[2] in which the patient is asked to connect alternating letters and numbers by drawing lines on

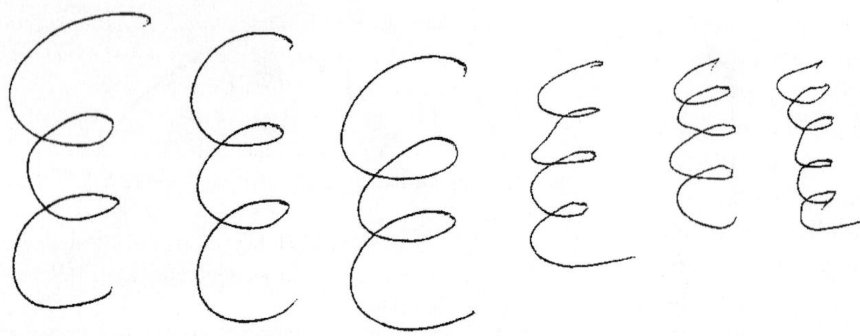

Figure 2-3
Perseveration in multiple loops and alternating programs copied by a patient with Alzheimer's disease.

paper. A similar test can be given verbally at the bedside by asking the patient to continue the set 1A, 2B, 3C, 4D, and so on.[8] Alternating program tests in combination with go, no-go tests measure set-shifting ability. In the former, the patient is asked to tap on the table once each time the examiner taps twice and to respond to one tap by the examiner with two taps. For the go, no-go task, the patient is asked to refrain from tapping when the examiner taps twice but continue to tap twice each time the examiner taps once. Difficulties with response inhibition and perseverative behavior can be elicited with tapping tasks. Patients with frontal lobe pathology may demonstrate perseverations when asked to copy multiple loops or alternating programs (such as cursive *m*'s and *n*'s)[20] (Fig. 2-3). Abstraction is tested using proverbs, idioms, similarities, and differences. Concrete proverb interpretation (i.e., stating "you might break the glass" when asked the meaning of "people in glass houses shouldn't throw stones") can be seen in a variety of processes involving frontal-subcortical dysfunction, including schizophrenia.[36] Other tests of abstraction include idioms (i.e., *hard-headed* and *level-headed*) and similarities (i.e., *table and chair*, *bike and train*, and *poem and statue*). Utilization behavior, demonstrated by a tendency to handle objects in the immediate environment, may also indicate frontal circuit dysfunction.[37]

DESCRIPTION OF A BRIEF NEUROBEHAVIOR EXAM

The core of the neurobehavioral exam includes behavioral observations, noting appearance, behavior, affect, mood, thought process (i.e., circumstantial, tangential, disorganized), thought content (including hallucinations, delusions, and suicidal and homicidal ideation), and insight and judgment.

Cognitive domains assessed directly include attention, language, memory, and visuospatial and executive function. The MMSE allows quick quantification of current cognitive function and is readily recognized by other clinicians. Assessment of attention begins with a determination of level of consciousness (alert, lethargic, obtunded, stuporous, comatose). Also noted are forward digit span (which should be at least five) and number of commissions and omissions made during the *A* test (the patient is instructed to raise and lower an index finger whenever the letter *A* appears in a series of letters read aloud by the examiner). In examining language, dysarthria, volume, paraphasic errors (semantic or phonemic), aprosody (receptive and expressive), and fluency are noted. Verbal fluency is tested by asking the patient to name as many animals as possible in 1 min and to repeat this for words beginning with the letter *F*. To test comprehension, the patient is asked to read a short passage and asked questions regarding its content. The patient is asked to repeat a simple phrase (such as "The quick brown dog jumped over the lazy fox") and to name body and clothing parts. To test verbal memory, the patient is presented with a list of 5 to 10 words and asked to repeat as many of them as possible. This is repeated twice with the same word list. The patient is then asked to try to remember the words and, after a 10- to 15-min delay, to recall as many as possible. Then a list with twice as many words is presented, including the entire original list, and the patient is asked to indicate whether a given word was on the original list. To test visual memory, the patient is asked to draw the figure from the MMSE from memory. Visuospatial function is tested with the cube copy and clock drawing (with the time as 11:10).

Measures of executive function include the following:

1. The "coin test" (the examiner moves a coin from hand to hand behind his or her back and asks the patient guess the pattern. The complexity of the patterns is increased as the patient successfully guesses the preceding one, generally after four repetitions of a given pattern).
2. Verbal "Trails B" (the patient continues the set: "1A, 2B, 3C," etc.).
3. Tapping tests ("when I tap once, you tap twice; when I tap twice, you tap once," and go, no-go: "when I tap once, you tap twice; when I tap twice, you don't tap").
4. Multiple loops (the examiner draws spirals with three loops and asks the patient continue the pattern).
5. Alternating programs (the patient copies and continues a pattern of alternating *m*'s and *n*'s).
6. The ability to abstract is tested with proverb interpretation, similarities (i.e., a bike and a train, a watch and a ruler, a poem and a statue), and idioms (i.e., *level-headed* and *hard-headed*).

REFERENCES

1. Buckner RL, Kelley WM, Petersen SE: Frontal cortex contributes to human memory formation. *Nat Neurosci* 2(4):311–314, 1999.
2. Spreen O, Strauss E: *A Compendium of Neuropsychological Tests: Administration, Norms, and Commentary*, 2d ed. New York: Oxford University Press, 1998, p 736.
3. Cummings JL: Anatomic and behavioral aspects of frontal-subcortical circuits. *Ann NY Acad Sci* 769(3): 1–13, 1995.
4. Thompson PD, Shibasaki H: Myoclonus in corticobasal degeneration and other neurodegenerations. *Adv Neurol* 82(39):69–81, 2000.
5. Poser S, Zerr I, Schroeter A, et al: Clinical and differential diagnosis of Creutzfeldt-Jakob disease. *Arch Virol Suppl* 48(16):153–159, 2000.
6. Cummings JL, Trible MR: *Concise Guide to Neuropsychiatry and Behavioral Neurology.* Washington DC: American Psychiatric Press, 1995, p 272.
7. Snowden JS, Bathgate D, Varma A, et al: Distinct behavioral profiles in frontotemporal dementia and semantic dementia. *J Neurol Neurosurg Psychiatry* 70(3):323–332, 2001.
8. Cummings JL: Neuropsychiatry: clinical assessment and approach to diagnosis, in Kaplan HI, Sadock BJ (eds): *Comprehensive Textbook of Psychiatry.* Baltimore: Williams & Wilkins, 1995, vol VI, pp 167–186.
9. Salzman D: Mood disorders, in Coffey CE, Cummings JL (eds): *Textbook of Geriatric Neuropsychiatry.* Washington, DC: American Psychiatric Press, 2000, pp 313–328.
10. Levy ML: Apathy is not depression. *J Neuropsychiatry Clin Neurosci* 10(3):314–319, 1998.
11. Marin RS, Firinciogullari S, Biedrzycki RC: Group differences in the relationship between apathy and depression. *J Nerv Ment Dis* 182(4):235–239, 1994.
12. Tekin S, Fairbanks LA, O'Conner S, et al: Activities of daily living in Alzheimer's disease: neuropsychiatric, cognitive, and medical illness influences. *Am J Geriatr Psychiatry* 9(1):81–86, 2001.
13. Neary D, Smowden JS, Gustafson L, et al: Frontotemporal lobar degeneration: A consensus on clinical diagnostic criteria. *Neurology* 51(6):1546–1554, 1998.
14. White KE, Cummings JL: Neuropsychiatric aspects of Alzheimer's disease and other dementing illnesses, in Yudofsky SC, Hales RE (eds): *The American Psychiatric Press Textbook of Neuropsychiatry.* Washington, DC: American Psychiatric Press, 1997, pp 823–854.
15. Victor M, Ropper AH, Adams RD: *Adams and Victor's Principles of Neurology,* 7th ed. New York: McGraw-Hill, 2001, p 1692.
16. Ballard CG, O'Brien JT, Swann AG, et al: The natural history of psychosis and depression in dementia with Lewy bodies and Alzheimer's disease: Persistence and

new cases over 1 year of follow-up. *J Clin Psychiatry* 62(1):46–49, 2001.
17. Koo JY: Skin disorders, in Kaplan HI, Sadock BJ (eds): *Comprehensive Textbook of Psychiatry.* Baltimore: Williams & Wilkins, 1995, vol VI, pp 1528–1538.
18. Felthous AR: The clinician's duty to protect third parties. *Psychiatr Clin North Am* 22(1):49–60, 1999.
19. Verhey FR, Ponds RW, Rozendaal N, et al: Depression, insight, and personality changes in Alzheimer's disease and vascular dementia. *J Geriatr Psychiatry Neurol* 8(1):23–27, 1995.
20. Strub RL, Black FW: *The Mental Status Examination in Neurology,* 4th ed. Philadelphia: Davis, 2000, p 208.
21. Cole MG, Primeau FJ, Elie LM: Delirium: Prevention, treatment, and outcome studies. *J Geriatr Psychiatry Neurol* 11(3):126–137, discussion 157–158, 1998.
22. Benson DF, Ardila A: *Aphasia: A Clinical Perspective.* New York: Oxford University Press, 1996, p 441.
23. Devinsky O: *Behavioral Neurology: 100 Maxims.* St Louis: Mosby–Year Book, 1992, p 348.
24. Szatowska I, Grabowska A, Szymanska O: Phonological and semantic fluencies are mediated by different regions of the prefrontal cortex. *Acta Neurobiol Exp* 60(4):503–503, 2000.
25. Morris JC, Heyman A, Mohs RC, et al: The Consortium to Establish a Registry for Alzheimer's Disease (CERAD). Part I. Clinical and neurpsychological assessment of Alzheimer's disease. *Neurology* 39(9):1159–1165, 1989.
26. Van Gorp WG, Satz P, Kiersch ME, et al: Normative data on the Boston Naming Test for a group of normal older adults. *J Clin Exp Neuropsychol* 8(6):702–705, 1986.
27. Delis DC, Freeland J, Kramer JH, et al: Integrating clinical assessment with cognitive neuroscience: Construct validation of the California Verbal Learning Test. *J Consult Clin Psychol* 56(1):123–130, 1989.
28. Masur DM, Fuld PA, Blau AD, et al: Distinguishing normal and demented elderly with the selective reminding test. *J Clin Exp Neuropsychol* 11(5):615–630, 1989.
29. Brandt J, Corwin J, Krafft L: Is verbal recognition memory really different in Huntington's and Alzheimer's disease? *J Clin Exp Neuropsychol* 14(5):773–784, 1992.
30. Freedman J, Rivoira P, Butters N, et al: Retrograde amnesia in Parkinson's disease. *Can J Neurol Sci* 11(2):297–301, 1984.
31. Beatty WW, Salmon DP, Butters N, et al: Retrograde amnesia in patients with Alzheimer's disease or Huntington's disease. *Neurobiol Aging* 9(2):181–186, 1988.
32. Osterrieth P: Le teste de copie d'une figure complexe. *Arch Psychol* 30:206–356, 1944.
33. De Renzi E: Disorders of visual recognition. *Semin Neurol* 20(4):479–485, 2000.
34. Shulman KI: Clock-drawing: Is it the ideal cognitive screening test? *Int J Geriatr Psychiatry* 15(6)548–561, 2000.
35. Leskela M, Hietanen M, Kalska H, et al: Executive functions and speed of mental processing in elderly patients with frontal or nonfrontal ischemic stroke. *Eur J Neurol* 6(6):653–661, 1999.
36. De Vries PJ, Honer WG, Kemp PM, et al: Dementia as a complication of schizophrenia. *J Neurol Neurosurg Psychiatry* 70(5): 588–596, 2001.
37. Eslinger PJ, Warner GC, Grattan LM, et al: "Frontal lobe" utilization behavior associated with paramedian thalamic infarction. *Neurology* 41(3):450–452, 1991.
38. Folstein MF, Folstein SE, McHugh PR: Mini-Mental State. A practical method for grading cognitive states of patients for the clinician. *J Psychiatr Res* 12:189–198, 1975.
39. Cummings JL: The Neuropsychiatric Inventory: Assessing psychopathology in dementia patients. *Neurology* 48(5 Suppl 6):S10–S16, 1997.
40. Kaufer DI, Cummings JL, Ketchel P, et al: Validation of the NPI-Q, a brief clinical form of the Neuropsychiatric Inventory. *J Neuropsychiatry Clin Neurosci* 12(2):233–239, 2000.
41. Beck AT: *Depression Inventory.* Philadelphia: Philadelphia Center for Cognitive Therapy, 1978.
42. Hamilton M: Development of a rating scale for primary depressive illness. *Br J Soc Clin Psychol* 6(4):278–296, 1967.
43. Yesavage JA, Brink TL, Rose TL, et al: Development and validation of a geriatric depression screening scale: A preliminary report. *J Psychiatr Res* 17(1):37–49, 1982.

Chapter 3

PRINCIPLES OF NEUROPSYCHOLOGICAL ASSESSMENT

Muriel D. Lezak

EVOLUTION AND APPLICATIONS OF NEUROPSYCHOLOGICAL ASSESSMENT

The rapid development of neuropsychological assessment procedures during the last three decades reflects the growing appreciation of its value for neurodiagnostic issues, for the care and treatment of neurologically impaired patients, and for patients needing cognitive and behavioral rehabilitation. Neuropsychological assessment also makes significant contributions to basic science research and in practical clinical knowledge in the neurologic sciences, in psychiatry, and in clinical and cognitive psychology. In practice, a neuropsychological evaluation may serve one or more purposes. For example, the same information used for diagnostic studies or in a research program may provide a patient's caregivers with the descriptive data on which they can build an individualized rehabilitation program. In other cases, data acquired for research or diagnosis may provide the necessary information for determining the behavioral impact of a cerebral lesion.[1]

The first systematic applications of neuropsychological assessment dealt with diagnosis, for before the days of sophisticated neuroimaging, the identification and—where possible—localization of a cerebral lesion was neuropsychology's most important function.[2–5] As neuropsychologists became more knowledgeable and adept, they not only became more skilled at localizing lesions on the basis of neuropsychological data but also were able to develop criteria for predicting the nature of the lesion—whether it involved damaged or absent tissue, whether the damage was due to a slow or a rapid process.[6–9]

Recent developments in neuroradiologic techniques have greatly reduced the contributions of neuropsychological assessment to diagnosis and lesion localization.[5,10–13] Yet imaging does not reveal the psychological expression—or nonexpression—of the lesion. That requires neuropsychological assessment.[14–16] Moreover, the neuropsychological examination continues to provide critical information in the differential diagnosis of the dementias,[17–19] in differentiating depression from dementia in elderly patients,[20–23] as well as in identifying behavioral problems that may presage a developing cerebral disorder.[24–26] After a mild traumatic brain injury[27–30] or exposure to toxic substances,[31–34] neuropsychological deficits may be the only residual evidence indicating the presence of cerebral damage.

Today, neuropsychological assessment is most usually called upon for the detailed behavioral descriptions necessary for intelligent patient care, for rational treatment, and for appropriate rehabilitation training and vocational/educational placement. For example, to be effective, the goals of rehabilitation as well as the procedures must be based on pertinent and detailed neurobehavioral data.[35–38] The evaluation of medical treatments or neurosurgery also requires appropriate and precise neuropsychological evaluations.[39–44] Repeated neuropsychological examinations help to predict the degree and quality of improvement in acute conditions (e.g., stroke, head trauma) or of decline in deteriorating conditions (e.g., dementias, multiple sclerosis).[39,45–50]

Descriptive neuropsychological data can provide the information needed for patients or their caregivers to make practical decisions necessitated by the patient's neurologic disorder. These decisions may concern the patient's legal status or financial options; whether the patient returns to work or when return to work is feasible; or such domestic issues as whether the patient needs help with household chores or is ready to return home from a care facility.

Contributions of neuropsychological assessment to research in the clinical neurosciences have proven invaluable. This includes treatment evaluation; development of criteria for classifying neuropsychological functions; behavioral descriptions of neurologic disorders; and the growing understanding of the functional organization of the nervous system. Moreover, the findings of neuropsychological evaluations have proven invaluable in the forensic domain. More and more, lawyers as well as judges appreciate the importance of cerebral dysfunction in contributing to criminal behavior, to mental incompetence, or to impaired ability to resume a normal life after an accident, toxic exposure, or other noxious event has resulted in brain damage.[51–53]

THE NEUROPSYCHOLOGICAL COMPONENTS OF BEHAVIOR

Traditional western epistemology has provided a three-dimensional schema for conceptualizing the psychological components of behavior. Within this framework, the intellect—i.e., the cognitive functions—is differentiated from two other, equally important categories of nonintellectual behavior: motivation and the emotions on the one hand and the executive functions—which include capacities for initiating and carrying out self-directed, goal-directed activities effectively—on the other. This conceptual organization has facilitated the identification and classification of behavioral phenomena. It has also received empirical support in that neuropsychological rsearch has shown that these concepts correspond to the major cerebral structural systems.[11,54–57]

Cognitive Functions

Information processing is the province of the cognitive functions. *Perceptual functions* select, organize, and classify stimuli received by the organism. *Memory* functions encode and store this information that *thinking* can reorganize and deal with conceptually, or which may determine a *response* in the form of a verbal or motoric activity. For most persons, the two cerebral hemispheres are each specialized for processing and storing information that is predominantly linear (the left hemisphere) or configurational (the right hemisphere) in its presentation. The bilateral organization of the hemispheres allows processing and storage of information in each perceptual modality as well as in their various combinations.[1,55,58–59] Along with the anterior/posterior dimension, functions can be roughly divided into output/input or perceptual/performance activities. Further divisions of functions characterize specific areas within anterior and posterior regions. This multidimensional organization of the brain provides for highly specialized information processing for the many subsystems of perception and memory.[60–62]

Several different and independent capacities contribute to the conceptual functions and to different kinds of responses.[1,9,63–65] The variety of mental functions and their relative independence from one another becomes apparent in comparing the many different kinds of cognitive deficits. For example, a patient who no longer can make conceptual classifications may be still able to perform fairly complex arithmetic operations; many aphasic patients are able to make known their intentions and feelings by means of facial expressions, gestures, and posture. Thus the neuropsychological evaluation must include the examination of many distinctly different cognitive functions.

Well before the relationship between specific mental activities and brain structure was known, the cognitive functions had been identified and measured with considerable accuracy.[66–68] It was only after World War II that the mental functioning of brain-damaged patients was studied in a systematic manner or that large-scale studies looking for correlations between cerebral and behavioral functions were undertaken.[56,69–70] These studies provided the first neuropsychologically grounded bases and methodologies for the behavioral evaluation of cerebral functioning.

Noncognitive Functions

It is much more difficult to characterize and measure emotional behavior and executive functions than cognitive functions. Since many cerebral disorders can alter emotional behavior, often in a quite characteristic manner,[1,71–72] we need reliable and accurate techniques to identify and quantify specific aspects of emotional behavior. However, the fact that many emotional responses are both multidetermined and multidimensional makes it difficult if not impossible to delineate precisely the differences between the effects of a lesion, of personality predispositions, and of situational reactions, particularly since most often the patient's emotional behavior results from interactions between these factors. Thus, in comparison with the cognitive functions, both the understanding and the assessment of emotional alterations accompanying cerebral damage are less precise.

The executive functions comprise capacities for volitional activity (initiation, self-awareness), planning, carrying out activities effectively, and self-regulation.[54,56] The executive functions are integral to all independently undertaken goal-directed activities. Some disorders of executive function are now known to be associated with specific focal lesions, mostly involving well-defined areas of the frontal lobes.[1,73–76] Yet despite good practical understanding of the executive functions, it has been difficult to develop satisfactory methods for demonstrating and quantifying them. The structured nature of most examinations rarely gives the patient the opportunity to exercise any independent judgment or activity—i.e., the executive functions. Moreover, executive behavior or its absence typically becomes evident in the qualitative aspects of the patient's test performances, such as abilities to identify and correct errors, to develop an effective solution strategy, or even to recognize that erasure crumbs should be swept from the page. Complicating the problem of measuring the executive functions is the tendency for the most common and obvious cognitive deficits to mask them. Too often examiners who do not understand the behavioral disorders that can accompany brain damage tend to misinterpret serious executive disorders, such as apathy or impulsivity, as emotional problems or personality aberrations.

THE ASSESSMENT OF NEUROPSYCHOLOGICAL DEFICIT

Cognitive Defects and Cognitive Deficits

Given that psychology's involvement in the identification and measurement of cognitive functions dates back more than a century,[77] it is not surprising that the neuropsychological examination has been especially focused on these functions. The evaluation of cognitive disorders concerns their severity, how they affect the patient's behavior generally, the interrelations between specific defects and deficits, as well as the correlations between specific aspects of cognitive dysfunction and underlying neuropathology.

Cognitive dysfunction can appear in the form of measurable *deficits* in skills, in knowledge, or in intellectual capacities, or it can appear as specific *defects*. Pathognomonic phenomena such as inattention to what occurs on the left of the patient's midline or characteristic behavioral symptoms such as the telegraphic speech of patients with Broca's aphasia are examples of cognitive defects. Many of the cognitive defects tend to be obvious to any observer; most of them will be identified in a careful neurologic examination. A neuropsychological examination providing a systematic review of functions may bring to light subtle defects which would not be apparent to a naive observer.

Cognitive deficits appear in the relative weakening or diminution of skills or knowledge. Fine-grained examinations are not necessary for identifying the presence of these deficits when they are obvious, as when the patient cannot tell what happened more than 5 min ago. However, in many cases, cognitive impairment may not become evident without an adequate neuropsychological examination. For example, a retired elderly person may no longer need to use highly refined visuospatial skills and thus may not appreciate that he or she has been compromised by a stroke. Also, many patients tend to avoid activities involving the affected functions and thus do not complain about losing these skills or understandings. Neuropsychological assessment may also be the best means of documenting mildly diminished cognitive capacities when they are of sufficient magnitude to affect the patient's functioning but not severe enough to be obvious. This is a not uncommon occurrence for persons whose mathematical abilities had been of *high average* or *superior* caliber but who, after sustaining brain damage may be able to solve arithmetic problems at only an *average* level. In such cases, isolated defects do not provide diagnostic information, and the patient's complaints about mental troubles may be misinterpreted until the examiner takes account of the patient's history (e.g., a software engineer; a physician) to make an objective comparison between premorbid functioning and the patient's present relatively lower level of mathematical competence.

Identifying Deficit

Finding an Appropriate Comparison Standard

The premorbid level of cognitive abilities provides a comparison standard that allows the examiner to determine whether an individual has been impaired to a significant degree.[1] The identification of cognitive impairment is easiest when there is concrete evidence of premorbid competencies, such as school or army test scores, course grades, etc. However, such information is often not available, forcing the examiner to turn to other sources to make a reasonable estimate. While some examiners have used population means as a comparison standard for this purpose, this practice is not only inappropriate but can be grossly misleading, since one-quarter of the population performs at levels above the *average* range and one-quarter fall below it.

Another method for estimating premorbid ability levels is based on the highest test scores or historical indicators of mental competence.[1] This method is applicable only to persons with known brain disorders; it should not be applied to cognitively intact persons. Underlying this practice are the assumptions that, by and large, people who perform well in one area perform well in others.[78,79] Conversely, cognitive potential can be either realized or reduced by external influences, but it is not possible to function at a higher level than biological capacity will permit. Marked discrepancies between the levels at which a person performs different cognitive functions or skills probably reflect disease, developmental anomalies, cultural training biases or deficiencies, emotional disturbances, or some other condition that has interfered with the full expression of that person's potential. For cognitively impaired persons, the least depressed abilities will likely be the best remaining behavioral representatives of the original cognitive potential. Moreover, since—within the limits of chance variations—a person's ability to perform a task is at least as high as the level of performance of that task, the patient's best performances, whether they be in the neuropsychological examination or taken from historical data (e.g., educational level, work status), are probably the best indicators of premorbid ability. Since chance variations do occur, the wise examiner who has only access to test performances will not rely on a single high score but look for a cluster of highest scores on which this estimate can be based.

Some examiners use demographic data,[80,81] residual ability to read phonetically irregular words,[82–84] or a combination of these techniques.[85] However, these methods have not proven satisfactory, overpredicting high scores and underpredicting low ones.[86–88] Johnstone and colleagues, examining postacute traumatically brain-injured patients, found that evaluations using education level as the comparison standard underestimated impairments in cognitive functioning generally and in motor skills; reading level-based comparisons were most sensitive to processing speed and mental flexibility.[89]

Deficit Measurement The presence of a cognitive impairment is most readily demonstrated when related functions show a deficit relative to other kinds of cognitive functions.[90,91] For example, when scores on tests involving visuospatial organization run significantly lower than performance levels on tests of language and verbal reasoning, a neuropsychological deficit may be hypothesized. Studies involving patients with different kinds of deficits and those suffering from the many known cerebral disorders have documented many distinctive deficit patterns that aid in diagnosing and understanding patients' disorders and cerebral functioning.[1,17,19] These known deficit patterns also help the knowledgeable clinician to distinguish organically based conditions from diminished cognitive functioning due to different sociocultural experiences or to poor education.[92–96]

TESTS IN NEUROPSYCHOLOGICAL ASSESSMENT

Test Contributions to the Neuropsychological Examination

The data of the neuropsychological examination consists of observations by the examiner and reports by others–such as caregivers or spouses, the patient's psychosocial and medical history, and findings from psychometric tests and other psychological examination techniques.[1,97] Observation of the patient's behavior during the examination provides important information about the patient's emotional status, social skills, and both cognitive and executive functioning. The patient's history and medical reports provide the context for developing hypotheses to guide the direction of the examination and for interpreting its data.

Tests can serve several purposes: They can be used to establish a comparison standard—i.e., for estimating premorbid ability. They may elicit behavioral indications of a cerebral disorder. They are indispensable for making precise comparisons between test performances on different functions or at different times (e.g., for evaluating treatments or following a patient's course). Tests may also elicit behavioral abnormalities that require special attention in a rehabilitation program, in readaptation to living at home, etc.

Many of the tests used by neuropsychologists have their origins in the tests of mental abilities, academic performance, and various aptitudes which have been used for educational placement and guidance since the early 1900s.[98,99] A well-developed psychometric technology provides the theoretical and statistical foundations for the tests and measurements used in neuropsychology. For example, it is in no small measure that the Wechsler Intelligence Scales (WIS)[100,101] owe their popularity to these technological accomplishments.

Other popular neuropsychological tests and examination techniques have come from quite different sources: Porteus's Mazes[102] and Raven's Progressive Matrices[103] were responses to the desire for culture-free measures of mental ability. The original purpose of the Bender-Gestalt Test[104] was to examine the perceptual development of children. Industry's needs for efficient employee selection led to a number of interesting tests, such as The MacQuarrie Test for Mechanical Ability[105] and the Purdue Pegboard Test.[106] Neuropsychologists have also developed tests, typically to examine specific neuropsychological functions.[90,107]

Test Selection

Hundreds of tests are available for examining different aspects of the many cognitive functions, differing from one another in presentation formats, complexity of the tasks involved, scoring criteria, and adequacy of standardization. Moreover, each year dozens of new tests appear in the literature and in test catalogues. By selecting appropriately from this profusion of tests, innovative examiners acquire the means to identify most of the organically based cognitive disorders and, often, to describe them with considerable precision. However, in order to establish the parameters of a patient's cognitive status and the severity of dysfunction, it is also necessary to have baseline data from a broad-range assessment that considers both those functions known or suspected to be impaired and those which have been relatively spared by the patient's organic condition.

Because of the need for baseline data,[79] many examiners always use the same general-purpose battery that will both measure a number of specific functions and provide a fairly global evaluation. Some of these batteries are available commercially, such as the Halstead-Reitan Battery[107,108]; others have been assembled by the individual examiner.[1,32,39] Another advantage of using a test battery is that repeated experience with a specific set of tests enhances the examiner's ability to use and interpret them. Two important technical advantages of formalized batteries are their provision of standardized assessment procedures and their reproducibility for comparisons between examinations and for research. Their chief disadvantage is that none are fully appropriate for any particular patient, resulting in both overtesting and undertesting in every case.[109] Additionally, examiners who rely on a formalized battery are less likely to explore their patients' unique strengths and deficits and less likely to have the tools or experience to make such explorations.

Most neuropsychologists compromise between a completely individualized examination and a set battery approach.[1,37,84,91,110] The usual practice consists of choosing a core set of tests that will provide a general review of cognitive functions. Based on the findings obtained from this standardized and wide-ranging assessment, the examiner can identify problem areas that need further, individualized exploration. Ideally, this exploration can be conducted with well-established tests, but the examiner may select less well known or well standardized tests when they are most appropriate for the specific issues presented by the patient.[37,90,91,111]

INTERPRETING NEUROPSYCHOLOGICAL TEST DATA

Application and Limitations of Test Scores

Test scores are essentially abstractions from observations. A score obtained from a standardized test is a mathematical calculation communicating a performance level evaluated relative to the performance of a normative group on a well-defined task. The score serves as an objective reference point on a linear scale of values. Objective tests benefit from uniformity in their items, in administration procedures, in the standardizations that determine their scores, and in their normative populations. Standard scores are powerful tools because, by using them, statistically sound comparisons can be made between an individual's performances on different tests, between different tests examining the same or similar abilities, between different persons taking the same tests, or between groups from different cultures or with different educational levels. However, in interpreting test scores achieved by an individual, it is of the utmost importance that the norms be appropriate for that person. Norms developed on subjects whose education level or cultural exposure differ from the individual can under- or overestimate performance and either create an erroneous appearance of deficit or obscure evidence of genuine deficit.

These characteristics of standardized test scores make them particularly useful in the neuropsychological evaluation. Because of their objective nature they can become comparison standards when evaluating deficits in an individual's test performances. However, even the highest among a patient's test scores do not provide appropriate comparison standards when that person has suffered global deterioration or has a psychosocial or cultural background that may have compromised their cognitive development.

By comparing a patient's test scores with one another, the examiner can identify both cognitive strengths and cognitive weaknesses. Moreover, particular cerebral disorders tend to affect cognitive functioning differently, producing score patterns characteristic for many of these disorders. For example, early in the course of Alzheimer's disease, scores on the Block Design and Digit Symbol tests of the WIS battery tend to drop significantly, as do scores on most memory tests, while many verbal abilities as well as immediate verbal memory span remain unchanged or close to premorbid levels.[17,112–114] In contrast, patients with early symptoms of another dementing disorder, progressive supranuclear palsy, tend to do everything extremely slowly[115] so that, even when most cognitive functions are still fairly well preserved and their memory performances are still intact, they may appear impaired if not properly examined.[18,115]

Nevertheless, because they are abstractions from observations, test scores offer only an artificially attenuated description of the test performance. Test scores taken in isolation from other scores and from the history and observations of the patient can easily be misinterpreted. When scores are reported without any information about the qualitative aspects of the patient's test performance, it is not possible to know, for example, whether they are valid representations of the patient's ability, whether they were based on a too restrictive test format so that a full knowledge of the patient's strengths or deficits could not become apparent, or whether improper administrative procedures affected the patient's performance.

This problem of test score limitations is well illustrated by the Arithmetic test in the WIS battery[1,101]. Since the administration instructions require the subject to solve mentally and within time limits problems that the examiner reads once, patients whose auditory-verbal span is reduced, or who have difficulty performing complex mental operations without visual supports, or whose mental processing is abnormally slow, will receive low scores regardless of their level of mathematical competence. Unless the examiner allows these patients to work out the problems on paper and/or acknowledges the validity of slow but accurate responses, these patients' actual arithmetic ability does not become apparent to the examiner, and the nature and practical implications of their actual deficits are neither documented nor appreciated.

For valid test interpretation, an appropriate reference group must be used for evaluating the patient's scores. Even though age is the most important variable affecting cognitive functioning,[116–119] a number of popular tests still lack adequate age norms. When age norms are not used, in most instances an older person's test scores are compared with those of a younger normative group, resulting in artificially lowered scores that can be misinterpreted as indicating some kind of abnormality.[120] Education is also a powerful variable for cognitive functioning. The effects of education on tests of verbal and academic abilities are obvious. Less obvious have been its significant contributions to scores on tests of nonverbal and nonacademic mental abilities[92,121–123] and memory abilities.[124–126]

Moreover, the way in which patients respond to the requirements of the examination reveals important information about the practical ramifications of their impairments as well as information about the presence and nature of these impairments. For example, observations on whether a patient introduces strategies when problem solving; or initiates, self-monitors, and self-regulates activities appropriately if at all; or how well a patient follows directions and can maintain an instructional set become invaluable information when evaluating for rehabilitation potential or for educational or vocational planning.[9,37,111,127] This kind of information may also contribute to a better understanding of the nature of the patient's dysfunction(s).[1,111]

Methods for Interpreting Test Data

Three methods have proven value in neuropsychological assessment. Since each of these methods is most suitable for different problems or different tests, all three can contribute to the interpretation of the findings of a single examination.

Cutting Scores Some tests were developed to detect organic brain damage or a particular cerebral dysfunction. These tests are based on observations that patients who have sustained certain specific conditions often show characteristic cognitive aberrations rarely seen in normal subjects. For example, most people can locate fairly accurately the middle of a horizontal line, but patients with left-sided visuospatial inattention tend to mark the middle at a point situated somewhat to the right of the line's center.[128] For diagnostic purposes, the cutting score aids in discriminating between persons who show such pathologic characteristics to a significant degree and those who do not. Although not all patients who have the condition of interest will perform below the cutting score (false-negative cases), very few—typically less than 5 percent—of normal subjects will perform at abnormal levels (false-positive cases) when age especially[129] but also education are taken into account.[130] Thus cutting scores only indicate the probability that brain damage—or a particular kind of cerebral dysfunction—is present or absent. Moreover, no diagnostic decisions can rest on the score obtained for any single test, regardless of how far below the designated level of abnormality; nor does the cutting score provide much information about the nature of the abnormality that a low score reflects.

Double Dissociation This procedure requires performances on at least three—preferably more—tests to identify the critical neuropsychological disorder underlying poor performances of complex tasks.[8,131] Most cognitive tests call upon two or more different functions. For example, to accomplish the task of copying a complex design requires at least visuoperceptual accuracy, visuospatial analyzing and synthesizing abilities, visuomotor integrity, and fine hand coordination: failure in any one of these areas would result in a poorly constructed copy. In the individual case, only one of these functions may be impaired. In order to determine which it is, the examiner can compare performances on different tests that each measure just one or two of the several functions in question. Thus, to identify the source of a problem in copying a complex design, the examiner would give the patient a visuomotor task—such as one calling for symbol substitutions that has virtually no visuospatial components, a visual recognition test that has neither visuospatial nor motor components, and a task involving visuospatial analysis and synthesis that also has no motor component. Failure on one or two of these tests when the others are performed adequately will indicate which functions involved in drawing from a copy are impaired, which preserved. By means of this kind of procedure, the functions making the critical contribution to the impaired performance may be best identified.

Pattern Analysis This approach takes into account the scores from all of the tests.[1,9,111] The examiner compares the pattern of cognitive strengths and weaknesses with the deficit patterns characteristic for particular disorders or lesion sites or evaluates the score pattern to determine whether it makes neuropsychological or neurologic sense. Competent pattern analysis requires a neuropsychologically sophisticated examiner.

Integrated Interpretation

In evaluating test performances, most neuropsychologists consider the patient's background, personality, and current situation along with the medical history. They also pay attention to neuropsychologically relevant behavioral characteristics, such as idiosyncrasies of speech, inappropriate emotional responses, carelessness or overcautiousness, distractibility, perseveration, and confabulation, characteristics which can often convey as much or more information about the patient than the test data. While recognizing that formal testing procedures constitute the basis of most neuropsychological evaluations, a valid and meaningful interpretation of test findings requires the integration of all available data. The neuropsychological examination is not a psychometric exercise but rather an opportunity for understanding the behavioral functioning of the patient in the broadest sense as appropriate for the needs and circumstances that led to the examination.

REFERENCES

1. Lezak MD: *Neuropsychological Assessment,* 3d ed. New York: Oxford University Press, 1995.
2. Teuber HL: Neuropsychology, in Harrower MR (ed): *Recent Advances in Diagnostic Psychological Testing.* Springfield, IL: Charles C Thomas, 1948, p 30.
3. Reitan RM: Problems and prospects in studying the psychological correlates of brain lesions. *Cortex* 2:177, 1966.
4. Yates AJ: The validity of some psychological tests of brain damage. *Psychol Bull* 51:359, 1954.
5. Benton AL: Clinical neuropsychology: 1960–1990. *J Clin Exp Neuropsychol* 14:407, 1992.
6. Anderson SW, Damasio AR, Tranel D: Neuropsychological impairments with lesions caused by tumor or stroke. *Arch Neurol* 47:397, 1990.
7. Crosson B: *Subcortical Functions in Language and Memory: A Working Model.* New York: Guilford, 1992.
8. Jones-Gotman M: Localization of lesions by neuropsychological testing. *Epilepsia* 32:S41, 1991.
9. Walsh KW: *Neuropsychology,* 2d ed. Edinburgh: Churchill-Livingstone, 1987.
10. Beauchamp NJ, Bryan RN: Neuroimaging of stroke, in Welch KMA, Caplan LR, Reis DJ, et al.(eds): *Primer on Cerebrovascular Diseases.* San Diego, CA: Academic Press, 1997, p 599.
11. Kertesz A (ed): *Localization and Neuroimaging in Neuropsychology.* New York: Academic Press, 1994.
12. Papanicolaou AC: *Fundamentals of Functional Brain Imaging. A Guide to the Methods and Their Applications to Psychology and Behavioral Neuroscience.* Lisse, The Netherlands: Swets and Zeitlinger, 1999.
13. Thatcher RW, Hallett M, Zeffiro T, et al (eds): *Functional Neuroimaging.* New York: Academic Press, 1994.
14. Bigler ED: Neuropsychological testing defines the neurobehavioral significance of neuroimaging-identified abnormalities. *Arch Clin Neuropsychol* 16:227, 2001.
15. Bigler ED: Quantitative magnetic resonance imaging in traumatic brain injury. *J Head Trauma Rehabil* 16:117, 2001.
16. Naugle R, Cullum CM, Bigler ED: *Introduction to Clinical Neuropsychology. A Casebook.* Austin, TX: Pro-Ed, 1998.
17. Bondi MW, Salmon DP, Kaszniak AW: The neuropsychology of dementia, in Grant I, Adams KM (eds): *Neuropsychiatric Assessment of Neuropsychiatric Disorders,* 2d ed. New York: Oxford University Press, 1996, p 164.
18. Derix MMA: *Neuropsychological Differentiation of Dementia Syndromes.* Berwyn PA: Swets & Zeitlinger, 1994.
19. Parks RW, Zec RF, Wilson RS (eds): *Neuropsychology of Alzheimer's Disease and Other Dementias.* New York: Oxford University Press, 1993.
20. King DA, Caine ED: Cognitive impairment and major depression: Beyond the pseudodementia syndrome, in Grant I, Adams KM (eds): *Neuropsychological Assessment of Neuropsychiatric Disorders,* 2d ed. New York: Oxford University Press, 1996, p 221.
21. Godwin-Austin R, Bendall J: *The Neurology of the Elderly.* New York: Springer-Verlag, 1990.
22. Kaszniak AW, Sadeh M, Stern LZ: Differentiating depression from organic brain syndromes in older age, in Chaisson-Stewart GM (ed): *Depression in the Elderly: An Interdisciplinary Approach.* New York: Wiley, 1985. p 161.
23. Marcopulos BA: Pseudodementia, dementia, and depression: test differentiation, in Hunt T, Lindley CJ (eds): *Testing Older Adults: A Reference Guide for Geropsychological Assessments.* Austin, TX: Pro-ed, 1989, p 70.
24. Albert MS, Moss MB, Tanzi R, Jones K: Preclinical prediction of AD using neuropsychological tests. *J Int Neuropsychol Soc* 7:631, 2001.
25. O'Rourke N, Tuokko H, Hayden S, Beattie BL: Early identification of dementia: Predictive validity of the clock test. *Arch Clin Neuropsychol* 12:257, 1997.
26. Zec RF: Neuropsychological functioning in Alzheimer's disease, in Parks RW, Zec RS, Wilson RL (eds): *Neuropsychology of Alzheimer's Disease and Other Dementias.* New York: Oxford University Press, 1993, p 3.

27. Mateer, CA: Assessment issues, in Raskin SA, Mateer CA (eds): *Neuropsychological Management of Mild Traumatic Brain Injury.* New York: Oxford University Press, 2000, p 39.
28. Raskin SA, Mateer CA, Tweeten R: Neuropsychological assessment of individuals with mild traumatic brain injury. *Clin Neuropsychol* 12:21, 1998.
29. Reitan RM, Wolfson D: The two faces of mild head injury. *Arch Clin Neuropsychol* 14:191, 1999.
30. Stuss DT, Ely P, Hugenholtz H, et al: Subtle neuropsychological deficits in patients with good recovery after closed head injury. *Neurosurgery* 17: 41, 1985.
31. Anger WK, Storzbach D, Amler RW, Sizemore OJ: Human behavioral neurotoxicology: Workplace and community assessments, in WN Rom (ed): *Environmental and Occupational Medicine.* 3d ed. Philadelphia: Lippincott-Raven, 1998.
32. Bowler RM, Lezak MD, Booty A, et al.: Neuropsychological dysfunction, mood disturbance, and emotional status of munitions workers. *Appl Neuropsychol* 8:74, 2001.
33. Morrow LA, Stein L, Bagovich GR, et al: Neuropsychological assessment, depression, and past exposure to organic solvents. *Appl Neuropsychol* 8:65, 2001.
34. White RF, Feldman RG, Proctor SP: Neurobehavioral effects of toxic exposures, in White RF (ed): *Clinical Syndromes in Adult Neuropsychology: The Practitioner's Handbook.* New York: Elsevier,1992, p 3.
35. Diller L: Poststroke rehabilitation practice guidelines, in Christensen A-L, Uzzell BP (eds): *International Handbook of Neuropsychological Rehabilitation.* New York: Kluwer Academic/ Plenum, 2000, p 167.
36. Johnstone, B, Frank RG: Neuropsychological assessment in rehabilitation: Current limitations and applications. *Neurorehabilitation* 5:75, 1995.
37. Sohlberg MM, Mateer CA: *Cognitive Rehabilitation. An Integrative Neuropsychological Approach.* New York: Guilford, 2001.
38. Wilson BA: Rehabilitation of memory. New York: Guilford, 1987.
39. Fischer JS, Priore RL, Jacobs LD, et al: Neuropsychological effects of interferon ß-1a in relapsing multiple sclerosis. *Ann Neurol* 48:885, 2000.
40. Meador KJ, Loring DW, Allen ME, et al: Comparative cognitive effects of carbamazepine and phenytoin in healthy adults. *Neurology* 41:1537, 1991.
41. Meyers CA: Neurocognitive dysfunction in cancer patients. *Oncology* 14:75, 2000.
42. Ryan CM, Hendrickson R: Evaluating the effects of treatment for medical disorders: Has the value of neuropsychological assessment been fully realized? *Appl Neuropsychol* 5:209, 1998.
43. Smith A: Changes in Porteus Maze scores of brain-operated schizophrenics after an eight-year interval. *J Ment Sci* 106:967, 1960.
44. Vingerhoets G, Van Nooten G, Jannes C: Effect of asymptomatic carotid artery disease on cognitive outcome after cardiopulmonary bypass. *J Int Neuropsychol Soc* 2:236, 1996.
45. Basso A, Burgio F, Paulin M, Prandoni P: Long-term follow-up of ideomotor apraxia. *Neuropsychol Rehabil* 10:1, 2000.
46. Cullum CM, Thompson LL: Neuropsychological diagnosis and outcome in mild traumatic brain injury. *Appl Neuropsychol* 4:6, 1997.
47. Rourke SB, Grant I: The interactive effects of age and length of abstinence on the recovery of neuropsychological functioning in chronic male alcoholics: A 2-year follow-up study. *J Int Neuropsychol Soc* 5:234, 1999.
48. Stern Y, Tang M-X, Jacobs DM, et al: Prospective comparative study of the evolution of probable Alzheimer's disease and Parkinson's disease demention. *J Int Neuropsychol Soc* 4:279, 1998.
49. Wild KV, Kaye JM: The rate of progression of Alzheimer's disease in the later stages: Evidence from the Severe Impairment Battery. *J Int Neuropsychol Soc* 4:512, 1998.
50. Filley CM, Heaton RK, Thompson LL, et al: Effects of disease course on neuropsychological functioning, in Rao SM (ed): *Neurobehavioral Aspects of Multiple Sclerosis.* New York: Oxford University Press, 1990, p 136.
51. Doerr HO, Carlin AS (eds): *Forensic Neuropsychology. Legal and Scientific Bases.* New York: Guilford, 1991.
52. Murrey GJ (ed): *The Forensic Evaluation of Traumatic Brain Injury. A Handbook for Clinicians and Attorneys.* Boca Raton, FL: CRC Press, 2000.
53. Titolo TR: There is nothing minor about a mild brain injury: A legal look at the medical aspects. *Neurolaw Lett* 9:2000, 37.
54. Goldberg E: *The Executive Brain. Frontal Lobes and the Civilized Mind.* New York: Oxford University Press, 2001.
55. Mesulam M-M: Behavioral neuroanatomy: large-scale networks, association cortex, frontal syndromes, the limbic system, and hemispheric specializations, in Mesulam M-M (ed): *Principles of Behavioral Neurology and Cognitive Neurology*, 2d ed. New York: Oxford University Press, 2000, p 1.
56. Luria AR: *Higher Cortical Functions in Man.* Haigh B (trans). New York: Basic Books, 1973.

57. Shepherd GM (ed): *The Synaptic Organization of the Brain,* 2d ed. New York: Oxford University Press, 1998.
58. Goldberg E: Higher cortical functions in humans: The gradiental approach, in Goldberg E (ed): *Contemporary Neuropsychology and the Legacy of Luria.* Hillsdale, NJ: Erlbaum, 1990, p 229.
59. Kolb B, Whishaw Q: *Fundamentals of Neuropsychology,* 4th ed. New York: Freeman, 1996.
60. Benton AL, Tranel D: Visuoperceptual, visuospatial, and visuoconstructive disorders, in Heilmann KM, Valenstein E (eds): *Clinical Neuropsychology,* 3d ed. New York: Oxford University Press, 1993, p 165.
61. Damasio AR, Tranel D, Rizzo M: Disorders of complex visual processing, in Mesulam M-M (ed): *Principles of Behavioral and Cognitive Neurology,* 2d ed. New York: Oxford University Press, 2000, p 332.
62. Mayes AR: *Human Organic Memory Disorders.* New York: Cambridge University Press, 1988.
63. Andreassi JL: *Psychophysiology: Human Behavior and Physiological Response,* 3d ed. Hillsdale, NJ: Erlbaum, 1995.
64. Filley CM: *Neurobehavioral Anatomy.* Niwot, CO: University Press of Colorado, 1995.
65. Heilman KM, Valenstein E (eds): *Clinical Neuropsychology,* 3d ed. New York: Oxford University Press, 1993.
66. Binet A, Simon T: Le développement de l'intelligence chez les enfants. *Année Psychol* 14:1, 1908.
67. Guilford JP: *A Revised Structure of Intellect.* Reports from the Psychological Laboratory of the University of Southern California, No.19, 1957.
68. Thurstone LL: *Primary Mental Abilities.* Chicago, University of Chicago Press, 1938.
69. Newcombe F: *Missile Wounds of the Brain.* London: Oxford University Press, 1969.
70. Teuber H-L: Effects of brain wounds implicating right or left hemisphere in man, discussion, in Mountcastle VB (ed): *Interhemispheric Relations and Cerebral Dominance.* Baltimore: Johns Hopkins Press, 1962.
71. Lishman WA: *Organic Psychiatry,* 3d ed. Oxford, UK: Blackwell, 1997.
72. Heilman KM, Bowers D, Valenstein E: Emotional disorders associated with neurological diseases, in Heilman KM, Valenstein E (eds): *Clinical Neuropsychology,* 3d ed. New York: Oxford University Press, 1993, p 461.
73. Lezak MD: The problem of assessing executive functions. *Int J Psychol* 17:281, 1982.
74. Fuster JM: *The Prefrontal Cortex,* 2d ed. New York: Raven Press, 1989.
75. Robbins TW: Dissociating executive functions of the prefrontal cortex, in Roberts AC, Robbins, TW, Weiskrantz L (eds): *The Prefrontal Cortex. Executive and Cognitive Functions.* Oxford, UK: Oxford University Press, 1998, p 117.
76. Stuss DT, Benson DF: *The Frontal Lobes.* New York: Raven Press, 1986.
77. Spearman CE: "General intelligence" objectively determined and measured. *Am J Psychol* 15:72, 1904.
78. Bell BD, Roper BL: "Myths of neuropsychology": another view. *Clin Psychol* 12:237, 1998.
79. Crawford JR: Assessment, in Beaumont JG, Sergent J (eds): *The Blackwell Dictionary of Neuropsychology.* London: Blackwell, 1996, p 108.
80. Barona A, Reynolds CR, Chastain R: A demographically based index of premorbid intelligence for the WAIS-R. *J Consult Clin Psychol* 52:885–887, 1984.
81. Wilson RS, Rosenbaum G, Brown G: The problem of premorbid intelligence in neuropsychological assessment. *J Clin Neuropsychol* 1:49–54, 1979.
82. Nelson HE: *The National Adult Reading Test (NART): Test Manual.* Windsor, Berks, UK: NFER-Nelson, 1982.
83. Crawford JR, Parker DM, Besson JAO: Estimation of premorbid intelligence in organic conditions. *Br J Psychiatry* 153:178, 1988.
84. Spreen O, Strauss E: *A Compendium of Neuropsychological Tests,* 2d ed. New York: Oxford University Press, 1998.
85. Vanderploeg RD: Estimated premorbid level of functioning, in Vanderploeg RD (ed): *Clinician's Guide to Neuropsychological Assessment.* Hillsdale, NJ: Erlbaum, 1994, p 43.
86. Goldstein FC, Gary HE, Levin HS: Assessment of the accuracy of regression equations proposed for estimating premorbid intellectual functioning on the Wechsler Adult Intelligence Scale. *Clin Neuropsychol* 8:405, 1986.
87. Karzmark P, Heaton RK, Grant I, Matthews CG: Use of demographic variables to predict full scale IQ: a replication and extension. *J Clin Exp Neuropsychol* 7:412, 1985.
88. Silverstein AB:Accuracy of estimates of premorbid intelligence based on demographic variables. *J Clin Psychol* 43:493, 1987.
89. Johnstone B, Slaughter J, Schopp L, et al: Determining neuropsychological impairment using estimates of premorbid intelligence: Comparing methods based on level of education versus reading scores. *Arch Clin Neuropsychol* 12:591, 1997.

90. McCarthy RA, Warrington EK: *Cognitive Neuropsychology: A Clinical Introduction.* San Diego, CA: Academic Press, 1990.
91. Stringer AY: *A Guide to Adult Neuropsychological Diagnosis.* Philadelphia: Davis, 1996.
92. Anger WK, Sizemore OJ, Grossmann SJ, et al: Human neurobehavioral research methods: impact of subject variables. *Environ Res* 73:18, 1997.
93. Greenfield PM: You can't take it with you: why ability assessments don't cross cultures. *Am Psychol* 52:1115, 1997.
94. Neisser U, Boodoo G, Bouchard TJ Jr, et al: Intelligence: knowns and unknowns. *Am Psychol* 51:77, 1996.
95. Pontón MO, León-Carrión J (eds): *Neuropsychology and the Hispanic Patient. A Clinical Handbook.* Mahwah, NJ: Erlbaum, 2001.
96. Suzuki LA, Valencia RR: Race-ethnicity and measured intelligence: educational implications. *Am Psychol* 52:1103, 1997.
97. Holden U: Crossing the i's and dotting the t's. *Neuropsychol Rehab* 11:197, 2001.
98. Anastasi A, Urbina S: *Psychological Testing,* 7th ed. Upper Saddle River, NJ: Prentice Hall, 1997.
99. Cronbach LJ: *Essentials of Psychological Testing,* 4th ed. New York: Harper & Row, 1984.
100. Jarvis PE, Barth JT: *The Halstead-Reitan Neuropsychology Battery. A Guide to Interpretation and Clinical Applications.* Odessa, FL: Psychological Assessment Resources, 1994.
101. Wechsler D: *WAIS-III Manual.* San Antonio, TX: Psychological Corporation, 1997.
102. Porteus SD: *The Maze Test and Clinical Psychology.* Palo Alto, CA: Pacific Books, 1959. [*Modified Manual.* Wood Dale, IL: Stoelting, no date.]
103. Raven JC: *Raven's Progressive Matrices. Examination Kit.* Los Angeles: Western Psychological Services, no date.
104. Bender L: *A Visual Motor Gestalt Test and Its Clinical Use.* New York: American Orthopsychiatric Association, 1938.
105. MacQuarrie TW: *MacQuarrie Test for Mechanical Ability.* Monterey, CA, CTB/McGraw-Hill, 1925, 1953.
106. Purdue Research Foundation: *Examiner's Manual for the Purdue Pegboard.* Chicago: Science Research Associates, 1948.
107. Benton AL, Sivan, AB, Hamsher K de S, et al: *Contributions to Neuropsychological Assessment,* 2d ed. New York: Oxford University Press, 1994.
108. Reitan RM, Wolfson D: *The Halstead-Reitan Neuropsychological Test Battery: Theory and Clinical Interpretation.* Tucson, AZ: Neuropsychology Press, 1993.
109. Benton AL: Clinical neuropsychology: 1960–1990. *J Clin Exp Neuropsychol* 14:407, 1992.
110. Lezak MD: Responsive assessment and the freedom to think for ourselves. *Rehabil Psychol.* In press, 2002.
111. Milberg WP, Hebben N, Kaplan E: The Boston Process approach to neuropsychological assessment, in Grant I, Adams KM (eds): *Neuropsychological Assessment of Neuropsychiatric Disorders,* 2d ed. New York: Oxford University Press, 1996.
112. Brandt J, Rich JB: Memory disorders in the dementias, in Baddeley AD, Wilson BA, Fraser NW (eds): *Handbook of Memory Disorders.* Chichester, UK: Wiley, 1995, p 243.
113. Huff FJ, Becker JT, Belle SH, et al.: Cognitive deficits and clinical diagnosis of Alzheimer's disease. *Neurology* 38:786, 1988.
114. Albert MS, Moss MB, Milberg W: Memory testing to improve the differential diagnosis of Alzheimer's disease, in Igbal K, Wisniewski HM, Winblad B (eds): *Alzheimer's Disease and Related Disorders.* New York: Liss, 1989.
115. Pillon B, Dubois B: Cognitive and behavioral impairments, in Litvan I, Agid Y (eds): *Progressive Supranuclear Palsy. Clinical and Research Approaches.* New York: Oxford University Press, 1992.
116. Albert MS: Age-related changes in cognitive function, in Albert ML, Knoefel LE (eds.): *Clinical Neurology of Aging,* 2d ed. New York: Oxford University Press, 1994.
117. Howieson DB, Holm LA, Kaye JA, et al: Neurologic function in the optimally healthy oldest old: Clinical neuropsychological evaluation. *Neurology* 43:1882, 1993.
118. Schaie KW: The course of adult intellectual development. *Am Psychol* 49:304, 1994.
119. Storandt M: Longitudinal studies of aging and age-associated dementias, in Boller F, Grafman J (eds): *Handbook of Neuropsychology.* Amsterdam: Elsevier, 1990, vol 4, p 349.
120. Bornstein RA: Classification rates obtained with "standard" cut-off scores on selected neuropsychological measures. *J Clin Exp Neuropsychol* 8:413, 1986.
121. Bornstein RA, Suga LJ: Educational level and neuropsychological performance in healthy elderly subjects. *Dev Neuropsychol* 4:17, 1988.

122. Heaton RK, Ryan L, Grant I, Matthews CG: Demographic influences on neuropsychological test performances, in Grant I, Adams KM (eds): *Neuropsychological Assessment of Psychiatric Disorders,* 2d ed. New York: Oxford University Press, 1996, p 100.
123. Kaufman AS, Reynolds CR, McLean JE: Age and WAIS-R intelligence in a national sample of adults in the 20 to 74-year age range: A cross-sectional analysis with educational level. *Intelligence* 13:235, 1989.
124. Craik FIM, Anderson ND, Kerr SA, Li KZH: Memory changes in normal ageing, in Baddeley AD, Wilson BA, Fraser NW (eds): *Handbook of Memory Disorders.* Chichester, UK: Wiley, 1995, p 211.
125. Rey A: *L'Examen Clinique en Psychologie.* Paris, Presses Universitaires de France, 1964.
126. Wechsler D: *Wechsler Memory Scale-III. Manual.* San Antonio, TX: Psychological Corporation, 1997.
127. Stuss DT, Eskes GA, Foster JK: Experimental neuropsychological studies of frontal lobe functions, in Boller F, Grafman J (eds): *Handbook of Neuropsychology.* Amsterdam: Elsevier, 1994, vol 9.
128. Schenkenberg T, Bradford DC, Ajax ET: Line bisection and visual neglect in patients with neurologic impairment. *Neurology* 30:509, 1980.
129. Benton AL: Basic approaches to neuropsychological assessment, in Steinhauer SR, Gruzelier JH, Zubin J (eds): *Handbook of Schizophrenia.* Amsterdam: Elsevier Science, 1991, vol V, reprinted in Benton A: *Exploring the History of Neuropsychology.* New York: Oxford University Press, 2000, p 223.
130. Stern Y, Andrews H, Pittman J, et al: Diagnosis of dementia in a heterogeneous population: Development of a neuropsychological paradigm-based diagnosis of dementia and quantified correction for the effects of education. *Arch Neurol* 40:8, 1992.
131. Milner B, Teuber HL: Alteration of perception and memory in man: Reflections on methods, in Weiskrantz L (ed): *Analysis of Behavior Change.* New York: Harper & Row, 1968, p 265.

Chapter 4

SOME ANATOMIC PRINCIPLES RELATED TO BEHAVIORAL NEUROLOGY AND NEUROPSYCHOLOGY

M.-Marsel Mesulam

The study of the human cerebral cortex can be quite challenging. Some of the difficulties arise because there are no agreements on terminology, no distinct boundaries that completely separate one region from another, and, in most instances, no one-to-one correspondence among lobar designations, traditional topographic landmarks, cytoarchitectonic boundaries, and behavioral specializations. One part of the brain can have more than one descriptive name, and cytoarchitectonic (striate cortex), eponymic (Brodmann area 17), functional (primary visual cortex), and topographic (calcarine cortex) terms can be used interchangeably to designate the same area.

Cytoarchitectonic maps, especially Brodmann's map, have introduced a useful and widely used approach to the parcelation of the cerebral hemispheres. Brodmann delineated individual architectonic areas on the basis of microscopic criteria. In contemporary usage, however, a statement such as "activation was seen in area 9" almost invariably means that the investigator estimated the area of activation to be in a part of the hemisphere analogous to the part which Brodmann designated as area 9. This usage can lead to potential inaccuracies, since the topographic fit between the imaged brain slice and Brodmann's hand-drawn brain may not be exact and there may be interindividual differences in the distribution of cytoarchitectonic areas. Brodmann's map is also quite unclear about cytoarchitectonic designations for sulcal banks, which contain a very significant proportion of the cerebral cortex.

There is no immediate solution to these difficulties, but it is important to be aware of their existence. In this chapter, descriptive neuroanatomic designations are used wherever possible. When used, cytoarchitectonic designations follow the nomenclature of Brodmann. Since the anatomic information in this chapter is highly condensed, the reader may want to consult more comprehensive treatments of this subject by Brodmann (now available in English translation),[1] Duvernoy,[2] Nieuwenhuys et al.,[3] Pandya and Yeterian,[4] and Mesulam.[5]

Neurons of the central nervous system are engaged in three major operations: (1) reception and registration of sensory stimuli from outside and from within (input), (2) planning and execution of complex motor acts (output), and (3) intermediary processing interposed between input and output. Thought, language, memory, self-awareness, and mood constitute different manifestations of intermediary processing. The neural substrates for these intermediary processes are located principally within the limbic system and cortical association areas. From a behavioral point of view, therefore, the cerebral hemispheres can be divided into four major components: primary sensory cortex, primary motor cortex, association cortex, and limbic-paralimbic cortex (Table 4-1, Fig. 4-1). The last two components, those associated with intermediary processing, are most relevant to behavioral neurology and neuropsychology and receive the most emphasis in this chapter.

CORTICAL TYPES

Regions of the cerebral cortex display a variety of architectures. The simplest type of cortex is located in the basal forebrain. Components of the basal forebrain—such as the septal nuclei, the substantia innominata, and the amygdaloid complex—are situated directly on

Table 4-1
Types of cortical areas and some of their corresponding Brodmann numbers

Primary sensory and motor cortex
Primary visual (area 17)
Primary auditory (areas 41, 42)
Primary somatosensory (areas 3, 1, 2 but mostly area 3b)
Primary motor (area 4 and caudal part of area 6)

Association cortex
Unimodal visual (areas 18, 19, 20, parts of 21 and possibly 37)
Unimodal auditory (area 22, possibly parts of superior temporal sulcus and middle temporal gyrus)
Unimodal somatosensory (area 5, rostral area 7)
Unimodal motor (rostral area 6, caudal area 8, area 44)
Heteromodal prefrontal (areas 9, 10, 11, 45, 46, 47, and possibly rostral areas 8, 12, and 32)
Heteromodal parietotemporal (areas 39, 40, caudal area 7, possibly banks of superior temporal sulcus and parts of middle temporal gyrus, area 36)

Limbic system (cortical components)
Corticoid formations (amygdala, substantia innominata, septal nuclei)
Allocortex (hippocampus, pyriform olfactory cortex)
Paralimbic cortex [insula (areas 14, 15), temporopolar cortex (area 38), caudal orbitofrontal cortex (caudal areas 11, 12, 13), cingulate complex (areas 23, 24, 33, 31, 26, 29), parolfactory region (area 25, caudal area 32), parahippocampal cortex (areas 28, 34, 35, 30)]

the ventral and medial surfaces of the hemispheres and are thus considered part of the cortical mantle. These structures contain the simplest and most undifferentiated type of cortex. The organization of the constituent neurons is rudimentary, and no consistent lamination or dendritic orientation can be discerned. These three components of the basal forebrain could be designated as having a "corticoid" or cortex-like structure. Corticoid areas (especially the amygdala) have architectonic features which are in part cortical and in part nuclear.[5]

The next stage of cortical differentiation is known as allocortex. This type of cortex contains one or two principal bands of neurons arranged into moderately well differentiated layers. The two allocortical formations of the brain are (1) the hippocampal formation, which also carries the designation of archicortex, and (2) the piriform or primary olfactory cortex, which is also known as paleocortex. Corticoid and allocortical formations collectively make up the limbic zone of cortex.

The next level of structural complexity is encountered in the paralimbic zone of the cerebral cortex. These areas provide a gradual transition from allocortex to isocortex. Allocortical cell layers often extend into the periallocortical component of paralimbic areas. Several gradual changes in the direction of increased complexity and differentiation occur from the allocortical toward the isocortical side of paralimbic regions. These changes include (1) progressively greater accumulation of small granular neurons in layer IV and then in layer II, (2) sublamination and columnarization of layer III, (3) differentiation of layer V from layer VI and of layer VI from the underlying white matter, and (4) an increase of intracortical myelin, especially along the outer layer of Baillarger (layer IV).

There are five major paralimbic formations in the primate brain: (1) the caudal orbitofrontal cortex, (2) the insula, (3) the temporal pole, (4) the parahippocampal gyrus (which includes the entorhinal, prorhinal, perirhinal, presubicular, and parasubicular areas), and (5) the cingulate complex (which includes the retrosplenial, cingulate, and parolfactory areas). These five paralimbic regions form an uninterrupted girdle surrounding the medial and basal aspects of the cerebral hemispheres.[6]

The greatest extent of the cortical surface in the human brain consists of six-layered homotypical isocortex, also known as association cortex. Association isocortex can be subdivided into two major types: modality-specific (unimodal) isocortex and high-order (heteromodal) isocortex. Unimodal association isocortex is defined by three essential characteristics: (1) The constituent neurons are almost exclusively responsive to stimulation in only a single sensory modality, (2) the predominant cortical inputs are provided by the primary sensory cortex or by other unimodal regions in that same modality, (3) damage yields modality-specific deficits confined to tasks guided by cues in that modality.

The unimodal areas for the three major sensory modalities have been determined experimentally in the

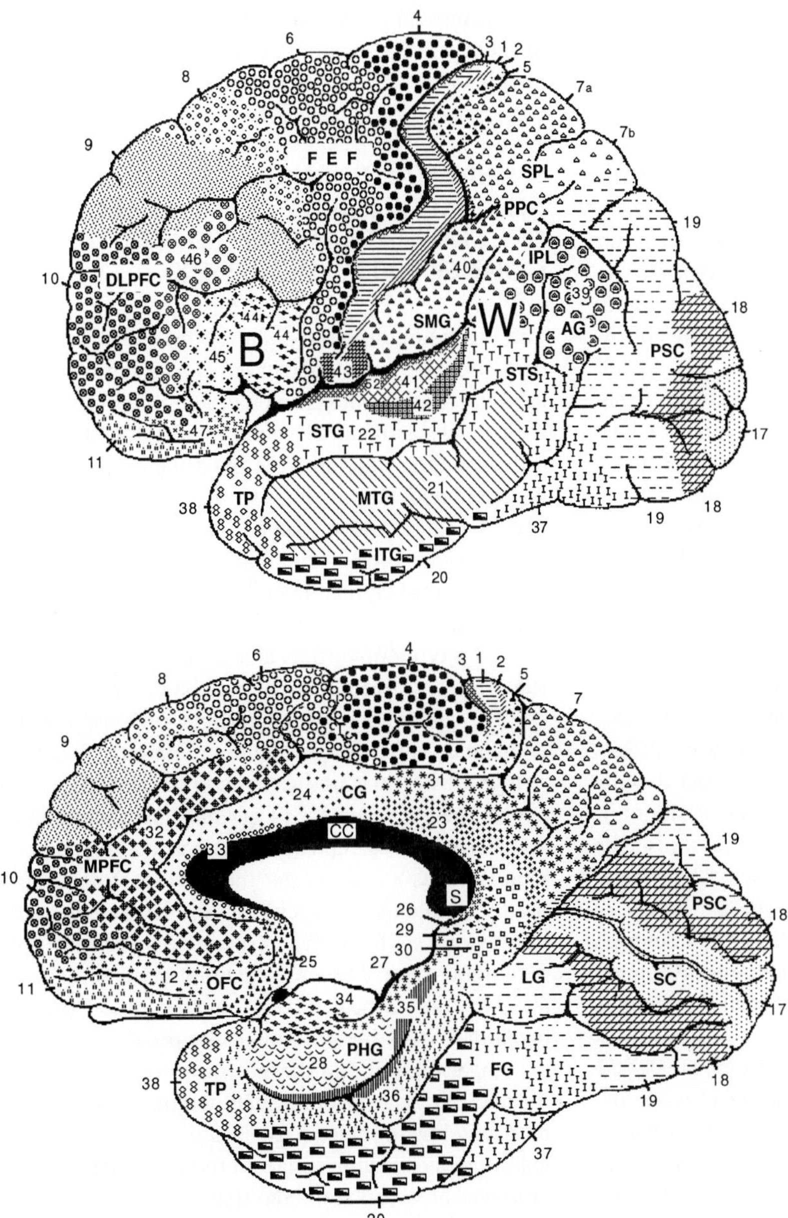

Figure 4-1
Lateral (top) *and medial* (bottom) *views of the cerebral hemispheres. The numbers refer to the Brodmann cytoarchitectonic designations. Area 17 corresponds to primary visual cortex, 41 to 42 to primary auditory cortex, 1 to 3 to primary somatosensory cortex, and 4 to primary motor cortex. The rest of the cerebral cortex contains association areas. AG, angular gyrus; B, Broca's area; CC, corpus callosum; CG, cingulate cortex; DLPFC, dorsolateral prefrontal cortex; FEF, frontal eye fields (premotor cortex); FG, fusiform gyrus; IPL, inferior parietal lobule; ITG, inferior temporal gyrus; LG, lingual gyrus; MPFC, medial prefrontal cortex; MTG, middle temporal gyrus; OFC, orbitofrontal gyrus; PHG, parahippocampal gyrus; PPC, posterior parietal cortex; PSC, peristriate cortex; SC, striate cortex; SMG, supramarginal gyrus; SPL, superior parietal lobule; STG, superior temporal gyrus; STS, superior temporal sulcus; TP, temporopolar cortex; W, Wernicke's area.*

brain of the macaque monkey. Such experiments have shown that the superior temporal gyrus contains a unimodal auditory association area, that the superior parietal lobule contains a somatosensory unimodal association area, and that the peristriate, and inferotemporal regions contain unimodal association regions in the visual modality. An analogous organization is likely to exist in the human.[5]

The heteromodal component of isocortex is identified by the following characteristics: (1) neuronal responses are not confined to any single sensory modality, (2) the cortical inputs originate from unimodal areas in more than one modality and/or from other heteromodal areas, and (3) damage to this type of cortex leads to deficits that transcend any single modality. Some neurons in heteromodal association areas respond to stimulation in more than one modality, indicating the presence of direct multimodal convergence. More commonly, however, there is an admixture of neurons with different preferred modalities. Defined in this fashion, heteromodal cortex includes the types of regions that have been designated as high-order association cortex, polymodal cortex, multimodal cortex, polysensory areas, and supramodal cortex.[5]

There are essentially two and perhaps three major heteromodal fields in the brain of the monkey. One is in the prefrontal region, including the anterior orbitofrontal surface and the dorsolateral frontal convexity. The second heteromodal field includes the inferior parietal lobule and extends into the banks of the superior temporal sulcus and parts of the midtemporal gyrus. There may be a third heteromodal region in the ventral temporal lobe.

There are some relatively subtle architectonic differences between unimodal and heteromodal areas. In general, the unimodal areas have a more differentiated organization, especially with respect to sublamination in layers III and V, columnarization in layer III, and more extensive granularization in layer IV and especially in layer II. On these architectonic grounds, it would appear that heteromodal cortex is closer in structure to paralimbic cortex and that it provides a stage in the hierarchy of architectonic differentiation intercalated between paralimbic and unimodal areas.

The koniocortex of primary sensory areas and the macropyramidal cortex of the primary motor region constitute unique and highly specialized regions that can be designated as having an idiotypic architecture. There are two divergent opinions about these primary areas. One is to consider them as the most basic and elementary components of cortex; the other is to see these areas as the most advanced and highly differentiated components of the cortical mantle. I favor the latter point of view. The location of idiotypic regions is well known: the primary visual area covers the occipital pole and the banks of the calcarine fissure, the primary auditory cortex covers Heschl's gyrus on the supratemporal plane, the primary somatosensory cortex covers the postcentral gyrus, and the primary motor area is located in the precentral gyrus.

A GENERAL PLAN OF ORGANIZATION FOR PATTERNS OF BEHAVIORAL SPECIALIZATION AND NEURAL CONNECTIVITY IN CORTEX

The preceding discussion shows that the hemispheric surface can be subdivided into five zones (limbic, paralimbic, unimodal, heteromodal, and idiotypic), which collectively provide a spectrum of cytoarchitectonic differentiation ranging from the simplest to the most differentiated. Although each cortical area is interconnected with dozens of distant cortical and subcortical structures, the relative magnitudes of these connections reflect the underlying hierarchy of architectonic differentiation.

All types of cortical areas, including association isocortex, receive direct hypothalamic projections.[7] For the great majority of cortical regions, this hypothalamic input is quite minor. The only exception is provided by the limbic structures. Thus the septal nuclei, the basal nucleus of the substantia innominata, the amygdaloid complex, the piriform cortex, and the hippocampus stand out by the presence of substantial hypothalamic connections. Another major source of connections for limbic structures is located in the paralimbic zone. The amygdala, for example, receives an extensive cortical input from the insula; the hippocampus from the entorhinal sector of the parahippocampal region; and the piriform cortex as well as the nucleus basalis from insular, temporopolar, and orbitofrontal paralimbic areas. Paralimbic areas have extensive monosynaptic connections with limbic and heteromodal areas; heteromodal areas with paralimbic and unimodal areas; and unimodal areas with primary and heteromodal areas. Primary areas derive their major cortical connections from unimodal areas and major subcortical connections from the relevant thalamic relay nuclei.[5]

These patterns are relative rather than absolute. For example, the amygdala is also known to receive direct input from association isocortex, but this does not appear to be as substantial as its connections with the hypothalamus and paralimbic regions. The primary areas in the more advanced primates receive very little limbic or paralimbic cortical input. This may ensure that the initial processing of sensory information is not influenced by drive and mood, so that emotional state does not alter the shape of an object or the pitch of a sound.

Many cortical areas have connections with other constituents of the same functional zone. These are extremely well developed within the limbic, paralimbic, and heteromodal zones. For example, of all the cortical neurons that directly projected to a subsector of prefrontal heteromodal cortex, 26 percent were located within unimodal areas, 13 percent in paralimbic regions, and 61 percent in other heteromodal cortex.[8] Furthermore, the insula as well as cingulate cortex have major interconnections with virtually each of the other paralimbic regions of the brain. The situation is different in the unimodal and primary sensory areas. Although unimodal regions may receive extensive input from other unimodal areas in the same modality, there is essentially no interconnectivity between areas belonging to different modalities. In a similar vein, except for the intimate interconnections between the primary somatosensory and motor areas, there are no neural projections among primary areas belonging to separate modalities. It appears, therefore, that there is a premium on channel width within the limbic, paralimbic, and heteromodal zones, whereas the emphasis is on fidelity within the unimodal and primary zones.

As noted above, the corticoid and allocortical areas, collectively designated as "limbic" structures, are the parts of the cerebral cortex that have the closest association with the hypothalamus. Through neural and also hormonal mechanisms, the hypothalamus is in a position to coordinate electrolyte balance, blood glucose levels, basal temperature, metabolic rate, autonomic tone, sexual phase, feeding behaviors, circadian oscillations, and even immunoregulation. In keeping with these functions of the hypothalamus, areas in the limbic zone of the cerebral cortex assume an important role in the regulation of behaviors and states related to memory, drive, emotion, hormonal balance, and autonomic tone.

At the other pole of the cytoarchitectonic hierarchy lie the most highly specialized primary sensory and motor areas. These parts of cortex are most closely related to the extrapersonal space: sensory input from the environment has its first cortical relay in primary koniocortical areas, and motor cortex coordinates actions that lead to the manipulation of the extrapersonal world. Intercalated between these two zones of limbic and primary sensorimotor cortex, the zones of association and paralimbic cortex provide neural bridges that link the internal milieu to the extrapersonal environment. The heteromodal and unimodal areas are predominantly involved in perceptual elaboration and motor planning, whereas the paralimbic zone is involved predominantly in directing drive and emotion to the appropriate extrapersonal and intrapsychic targets.[9]

Unimodal areas can be divided into *upstream* and *downstream* components. Upstream components receive their major modality-specific information directly from the corresponding primary area, whereas the downstream areas receive their major modality-specific input from the corresponding upstream unimodal areas. In the visual modality, for example, the peristriate region (areas 18 and 19) constitutes an upstream unimodal association area, whereas inferotemporal cortex (areas 20 and 21) constitutes a downstream unimodal association area.[9]

Heteromodal cortex receives convergent input from multiple unimodal areas, especially downstream unimodal areas, whereas paralimbic cortex acts as a relay between sensory association cortices and the limbic zone of the cerebral cortex.[4] Heteromodal and paralimbic formations support two major types of neural processing: (1) the associative linkage of unimodal sensory information into distributed templates that encode word meaning, face recognition, event memory, and so on and (2) the integration of this information with drive, emotion, and visceral state. In contrast to the idiotypic and unimodal belts, which are characterized by relatively more "dedicated" and homogeneous neural mechanisms confined to single modalities of information processing, the heteromodal and paralimbic areas support a more "generalized" type of processing with heterogeneous input-output relationships so that no uniform behavioral specialization can be assigned to individual components of the paralimbic and heteromodal zones.

SUBCORTICAL STRUCTURES: STRIATUM AND THALAMUS

Striatum

The striatum can be divided into three components: the caudate, the putamen, and the olfactory tubercle–nucleus accumbens complex. Each striatal component receives cortical input, but none projects back to cortex. The caudate and putamen, which are also collectively designated as the neostriatum, receive cortical input predominantly from association cortex and primary idiotypic areas. The dopaminergic input to the neostriatum originates in the pars compacta of the substantia nigra. The cortical input to the olfactory tubercle–nucleus accumbens complex originates in limbic and paralimbic parts of the brain, including the amygdala and the hippocampus. On the basis of this connectivity pattern, the nucleus accumbens–olfactory tubercle complex may be designated as the limbic striatum.[10] The dopaminergic innervation of the limbic striatum originates in the ventral tegmental area of Tsai, which is just medial to the substantia nigra, and dopamine turnover is higher in the limbic striatum than in the neostriatum.[11]

All parts of cortex project to the striatum. These corticostriatal projections display a complex topographic arrangement. Inputs from each cortical area form multiple patches of axonal terminals within the striatum. Yeterian and Van Hoesen[12] made the interesting suggestion that terminal patches from separate cortical areas are more likely to show partial overlap if the relevant cortical areas are interconnected with each other. This implies that there may be some replication of corticocortical interaction patterns within the striatum.

The caudate may have a lesser role than the putamen in motor control. For example, motor cortex projects to the putamen but not to the caudate.[13] The head of the caudate receives most of its input from dorsolateral prefrontal cortex. It is therefore interesting to note that lesions in the head of the caudate yield deficits that are essentially identical to those that emerge upon ablating prefrontal cortex.[14] This raises the possibility that each striatal region may have behavioral specializations that are similar to those of the cortical area from which it receives its major cortical input.

Globus Pallidus

The globus pallidus of the primate has four easily identifiable components: (1) the outer (lateral) segment, (2) the inner (medial) segment, (3) the ventral pallidum, and (4) the pars reticulata of the substantia nigra. The globus pallidus receives projections from the striatum and projects to the thalamus. The globus pallidus is thus an essential link in the striato-pallido-thalamo-cortical loops that are thought to have important organizing roles in a number of complex behavioral domains.

The globus pallidus plays an important role in motor control. In humans, lesions of the globus pallidus are frequently associated with severe extrapyramidal disturbances. Local cooling in the area of the globus pallidus in monkeys yields a severe and reversible breakdown of a learned flexion-extension movement, but only when the animal is blindfolded. In the presence of visual input, the deficit is no longer observed.[15]

The medial zone of the inner pallidal segment and also the ventral pallidum have close associations with limbic structures. For example, in contrast to the more dorsal parts of the pallidum that receive their striatal input from the caudate and putamen, the ventral pallidum receives its major striatal projections from the nucleus accumbens. Furthermore, a substantial number of ventral pallidal neurons respond to amygdaloid stimulation.[16]

In the monkey, the core of the internal pallidal segment projects to the motor thalamus. However, a medial crescent of this pallidal segment projects predominantly to the lateral habenula, which is generally considered as a structure closely related to the limbic regions of the brain.[17] In keeping with this anatomic pattern, some types of pallidal lesions interfere with behaviors generally associated with limbic mechanisms. For example, MacLean[18] showed that damage to the medial globus pallidus of monkeys severely disrupts species-specific sexual display patterns. Thus, the ventral pallidum and the medial portion of the inner pallidal segment could be considered as having preferential limbic affiliations.

The pars reticulata of the substantia nigra is a caudal extension of the globus pallidus. There is evidence suggesting that this portion of the pallidal complex may participate in the programming of saccadic eye movements in response to actual or remembered targets.[19]

Thalamus

One function of the thalamus is to relay sensory inputs to cortical areas. Almost all thalamic nuclei have well-developed reciprocal connections with the cortex. The one exception is the reticular nucleus, which receives subcortical and cortical input but does not project back to cortex.[20] There is very little interconnectivity among individual thalamic nuclei, so that there is very little interaction at the thalamic level among the different types of information that are being relayed to cortex. The one exception is provided by the reticular and intralaminar nuclei, which have extensive connections with other thalamic nuclei. Specifically, the reticular nucleus sends GABAergic inhibitory projections to other thalamic nuclei in a way that inhibits the thalamocortical transmission of neural signals.

The large number of thalamic nuclei can be subdivided into several functional groups on the basis of their preferred cortical and subcortical projections.[5] The primary relay nuclei are the easiest to identify (Fig. 4-2). The caudal part of the ventroposterior lateral nucleus (VPL_c) and the principal division of the ventroposterior medial nucleus (VPM) receive fibers from the medial lemniscus and trigeminothalamic tract and constitute the somatosensory relay nuclei of the thalamus. The lateral geniculate nucleus (LGN) and the part of the medial geniculate nucleus (MGN) that receives the brachium of the inferior colliculus are the primary relay nuclei for the visual and auditory modalities, respectively. Damage to the VPL_c or to the LGN gives rise to hemihypesthesia and hemianopia, respectively. Since inputs from both ears reach the MGN in each hemisphere, unilateral damage to this thalamic nucleus does not lead to contralateral ear deafness. In fact, unilateral MGN lesions may be extremely difficult to detect clinically. The major thalamic input into primary motor cortex (M1) comes from the caudal ventrolateral nucleus (VL_c) and the anterior ventroposterior lateral nucleus (VPL_a). The behavioral effect of lesions in these nuclei are poorly understood.

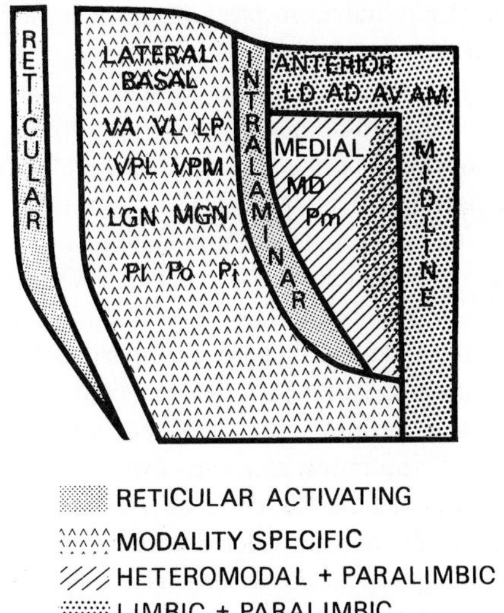

Figure 4-2
A schematic diagram of the four major groups of thalamic nuclei. AD, anterior dorsal; AM, anterior medial; AV, anterior ventral; LD, laterodorsal; LGN, lateral geniculate; LP, lateroposterior; MD, mediodorsal; MGN, medial geniculate; Pi, inferior pulvinar; Pl, lateral pulvinar; Pm, medial pulvinar; Pa, anterior pulvinar; VA, ventral anterior; VL, ventral lateral; VPL, ventroposterior lateral; VPM, ventroposterior medial.

A second group of thalamic nuclei project predominantly to unimodal association areas. In the rhesus monkey, the major thalamic projections to the somatosensory association cortex of the superior parietal lobule (area 5) come from the lateroposterior nucleus (LP) and perhaps also from the anterior subdivision of the pulvinar nucleus (P_a). In the visual modality, the nuclei which provide the major projection to visual unimodal association areas include the inferior (P_i) and lateral (Pl) subdivisions of the pulvinar nucleus. In the auditory modality, the unimodal association region receives its major thalamic input from the anterior MGN and probably also from a ventral rim of the medial pulvinar. Thus, the MGN is the source of thalamic projections not only to A1 but also to the auditory association cortex. The motor association cortex receives its major thalamic input from the anterior ventrolateral nucleus (VL_a) and from parts of the ventral anterior nucleus (VA).

A third group of thalamic nuclei have no specific modality affiliations and project predominantly to heteromodal and limbic cortex. The lateral part of the medial dorsal nucleus (MD) is the major thalamic nucleus for the prefrontal heteromodal fields, whereas the medial pulvinar nucleus (P_m) and parts of the adjacent lateral posterior nucleus (LP) are the major nuclei for the heteromodal fields in the inferior parietal lobule and within the banks of the superior temporal sulcus.

The close interaction between cortical heteromodal and paralimbic zones is also reflected in the arrangement of thalamic connectivity patterns. Thus, the MD and P_m nuclei, which are the major nuclei for heteromodal cortical areas, also have extensive paralimbic connections. For example, the medial part of MD (including the magnocellular MD_{mc} component) is the major thalamic nucleus for the orbitofrontal paralimbic region, while the P_m has reciprocal projections with all components of the paralimbic belt and is probably the major nucleus for the temporopolar paralimbic area. The MD and P_m also have direct limbic connections. Thus, the medial and magnocellular parts of MD have connections with the amygdala, piriform cortex, and the septal region, whereas the P_m has reciprocal projections with the amygdaloid complex.[21]

Another group of dorsally and medially placed nuclei are collectively known as the nuclei of the "anterior tubercle." These nuclei include the anterior thalamic nucleus [including its dorsal (AD), ventral (AV), and medial (AM) components] and the laterodorsal nucleus (LD). They provide the major thalamic connections for the posterior cingulate cortex, for the retrosplenial area, and for some of the parahippocampal paralimbic areas. The anterior thalamic nuclus receives the mammillothalamic tract and is therefore an important component of Papez's circuit.

A number of nuclei which are situated close to the thalamic midline are collectively known as midline nuclei. These include the paratenial, paraventricular, subfascicular, central, and reuniens nuclei. These nuclei have extensive connections with paralimbic areas (e.g., temporal pole and anterior cingulate gyrus) and also with the hippocampal formation.

The effects of lesions in these nuclei are consistent with their patterns of cortical connectivity. For example, in the rhesus monkey, bilateral MD lesions reproduce deficits in spatial delayed alternation similar to those associated with prefrontal ablations.[22] In humans, lesions involving MD can lead to a frontal network syndrome.[23] More medial MD lesions that also involve adjacent midline nuclei lead to visual object recognition deficits similar to those obtained after medial temporal ablations.[24] In some patients, even unilateral lesions in the more medial parts of MD and in the anterior tubercle nuclei have been associated with severe amnestic conditions.[25] In Wernicke's encephalopathy, involvement of the MD and P_m is thought to play a major role in the genesis of the amnestic state.[26] Lesions of the right pulvinar nucleus, including its medial component, have been described in conjunction with contralateral neglect for the left extrapersonal space.[27] Electrical stimulation of the left medial pulvinar has been reported to induce transient anomia.[28] These behavioral relations are consistent with the connections of the P_m with the parietotemporal parts of heteromodal cortex and with limbic-paralimbic structures.

A fourth group of thalamic nuclei are closely affiliated with the ascending reticular activating system (ARAS). The reticular nucleus of the thalamus as well as the intralaminar nuclei (e.g., the limitans, paracentralis, centralis lateralis, centromedian, and parafascicularis) have strong associations with the ascending reticular activating pathways. In contrast to other thalamic nuclei, which have somewhat restricted projection zones, the intralaminar nuclei have more widespread connections and are also known as "diffuse projection nuclei."

THE ASCENDING RETICULAR ACTIVATING SYSTEM

The cerebral cortex has three sources of afferent neural projections: cortical, thalamic, and extrathalamic. The existence of corticocortical and thalamocortical projections had been established by classical neuroanatomic methodology. During the past 20 years, the advent of more powerful methods based on axonally transported tracers helped to uncover a third set of cortical afferents with origins in the ventral tegmental area (dopaminergic), raphe nuclei (serotoninergic), nucleus locus ceruleus (noradrenergic), hypothalamus (mostly histaminergic), and basal forebrain (mostly cholinergic). These extrathalamic afferents exert a modulatory influence upon cortical activity and constitute important components of the ARAS.[29,30]

Moruzzi and Magoun[30] had introduced the concept of a brainstem-based ARAS that acted to desynchronize the cortical electroencephalogram via a relay in the thalamus. Subsequent work revealed that a most important component in this system consists of a cholinergic reticulothalamic pathway that facilitates the activation of corticopetal relay neurons in the thalamus.[31–35] These cholinergic projections arise from the pedunculopontine and laterodorsal tegmental nuclei of the upper brainstem. Although all thalamic nuclei receive these cholinergic projections, the reticular and intralaminar nuclei are traditionally considered to have the most intimate relation to the ARAS. In addition to these transthalamic pathways, the ARAS also includes direct ascending projections that reach the cerebral cortex without a thalamic relay. One group of these projections originates in the brainstem and the second in the basal forebrain.

The direct corticopetal pathways from the brainstem include dopaminergic projections from the substantia nigra–ventral tegmental area, serotoninergic projections from the raphe nuclei, and noradrenergic projections from the nucleus locus ceruleus. In the basal forebrain, the nucleus basalis and nuclei of the septal/diagonal band region provide the source of a very substantial cholinergic projection directed to the entire cerebral cortex, hippocampus, and amygdala. These projections have complex effects upon cortical neurons but generally tend to act as excitatory neuromodulators that increase the impact of behaviorally relevant sensory events upon cortical neurons.[36] The ascending corticopetal cholinergic projection originating from the basal forebrain is a crucial telencephalic component of the ARAS.

The cerebral cortex sends descending feedback projections to several components of the ARAS. Almost all parts of the cerebral cortex project to the reticular nucleus and therefore influence its inhibitory effect upon other thalamic nuclei.[20] The projection from the cerebral cortex to the reticular nucleus of the thalamus is mostly excitatory, whereas the projections to this thalamic nucleus from the brainstem cholinergic nuclei are inhibitory. The reticular nucleus is thus in a position to gate thalamocortical transmission in a way that reflects the integrated influence of the brainstem and cerebral cortex.

Although the basal forebrain projects to the entire cerebral cortex, it receives feedback projections from a very limited set of cortical areas—namely, those that belong to the limbic and paralimbic zones of the cerebral cortex.[37] This asymmetry is a feature of all the other extrathalamic ascending pathways of the ARAS: they project widely to the cerebral cortex but receive very few reciprocal connections from the cerebral cortex.[38]

NEURAL NETWORKS

The anatomic substrate of individual cognitive domains takes the form of large-scale neurocognitive networks consisting of interconnected cortical and subcortical nodes.[40] Each major node of such a network belongs to multiple intersecting networks. Consequently, the same cognitive domain may be disrupted after damage to several different regions of the brain, and damage confined to a single region may yield more than one type of cognitive deficit.

Five large-scale neurocognitive networks can be identified in the human brain: the left hemisphere language network, the right hemisphere attentional network, the temporal face- and object-recognition network, the limbic system, and the frontal network.[40,41] The major cortical nodes of the language network are located in Broca's area (areas 44 and 45) and Wernicke's area (posterior part of area 22 and parts of areas 39 and 40) of the left hemisphere. These two nodes are interconnected with several perisylvian cortical areas and with specific regions of the thalamus and striatum. Damage to components of this network leads to distinct aphasic disturbances, the clinical features of which reflect the specializations of the primary lesion site.[9] The three major cortical nodes of the attentional network are located in frontal cortex, the posterior parietal cortex, and the cingulate gyrus of the right hemisphere. Damage to cortical or subcortical components of this network leads to the various manifestations of the spatial neglect syndrome.[42] The face- and object-recognition system revolves around temporal heteromodal cortex and unimodal visual association cortex in the fusiform gyrus. Damage to this system leads to prosopagnosia and visual object agnosia.[43] The limbic system includes the limbic and paralimbic cortical areas, the limbic striatum, the limbic nuclei of the thalamus, and the hypothalamus. Damage to components of this network leads to deficits of retentive memory, emotion, motivation, and affiliative behaviors.[44] The frontal network includes the heteromodal and paralimbic cortices of the frontal lobes, the head of the caudate nucleus, and the mediodorsal nucleus of the thalamus. Damage to components of this network lead to complex deficits of the attentional matrix, personality, and comportment.[45]

Neuroanatomic investigations show that cortical nodes of individual networks are interconnected in ways that are suitable for distributed processing (see Chap. 10).[46] In resolving a cognitive problem, this sort of interconnectivity allows the execution of extremely rapid surveys of vast informational landscapes until the entire system settles into a best fit with respect to the multiple goals and constraints engendered by the problem.[40] This computational architecture is quite compatible with cognitive tasks such as deciding which words best express a thought or how to reconstruct a specific complex memory. There are no single "correct" solutions to such tasks but an entire family of possibilities, each leading to a different compromise within the relevant context of goals and constraints.

Several computational models have been proposed for understanding how the central nervous system converts experience into knowledge. One possibility is to postulate the existence of a hierarchical synaptic chain for the transfer of information from primary sensory areas first to upstream unimodal areas, then to downstream unimodal areas, and finally to multimodal areas where knowledge is encoded in convergent form. This "convergent encoding" model faces several well-known objections.[47] An alternative "selectively distributed processing" model proposes that the most realistic building blocks of experience are to be found in unimodal rather than heteromodal association cortices.[47] According to this model, heteromodal, paralimbic, and limbic areas of the cerebral cotex provide transmodal nodes for binding this modality-specific information into coherent but distributed (nonconvergent) knowledge. Lesions that interrupt the flow of information within unimodal areas or from unimodal to transmodal areas result in disconnection syndromes such as pure alexia, word deafness, prosopagnosia, and so on.[5,48] The cerebral substrate for cognition is thus both distributed and regionally specialized but neither modular nor diffuse. This model, based predominantly on the anatomic organization of the cerebral cortex, helps to generate hypotheses for probing the complex relationship between cerebral structure and cognition.

REFERENCES

1. Brodmann K: *Localisation in the Cerebral Cortex.* London: Smith-Gordon, 1994.
2. Duvernoy H: *The Human Brain.* Vienna: Springer-Verlag, 1991.
3. Nieuwenhuys R, Voogd J, van Huijzen C: *The Human Central Nervous System.* Berlin: Springer-Verlag, 1988.
4. Pandya DN, Yeterian EH: Architecture and connections of cortical association areas, in Peters A, Jones EG (eds): *Cerebral Cortex.* New York: Plenum Press, 1985, vol 4, pp 3–61.
5. Mesulam M-M: Behavioral neuroanatomy: Large-scale networks, association cortex, frontal syndromes, the limbic system and hemispheric specialization, in Mesulam M-M (ed): *Principles of Behavioral and Cognitive Neurology.* New York: Oxford University Press, 2000, pp 1–120.
6. Mesulam M-M, Mufson EJ: Insula of the old world monkey: I. Architectonics in the insulo-orbito-temporal component of the paralimbic brain. *J Comp Neurol* 212:122, 1982.
7. Mesulam M-M, Mufson EJ, Levey AI, Wainer BH: Cholinergic innervation of cortex by the basal forebrain: cytochemistry and cortical connections of the septal area, diagonal band nuclei, nucleus basalis (substantia innominata), and hypothalamus in the rhesus monkey. *J Comp Neurol* 214:170–197, 1983.
8. Barbas H, Mesulam M-M: Organization of afferent input to subdivisions of area 8 in the rhesus monkey. *J Comp Neurol* 200:407–431, 1981.
9. Mesulam M-M: From sensation to cognition. *Brain* 121:1013–1052, 1998.
10. Heimer L, Wilson RD: The subcortical projections of the allocortex: Similarities in the neural associations of the hippocampus, the piriform cortex and the neocortex, in Santini M (ed): *Golgi Centennial Symposium: Proceedings.* New York: Raven Press, 1975, pp 177–193.
11. Walsh FX, Thomas TJ, Langlais PJ, Bird ED: Dopamine and homovanillic acid concentrations in striatal and

limbic regions of the human brain. *Ann Neurol* 12:52–55, 1982.

12. Yeterian EH, Van Hoesen GW: Cortico-striate projections in the rhesus monkey: The organization of certain cortico-caudate connections. *Brain Res* 139:43–63, 1978.
13. Künzle H: Bilateral projections from precentral motor cortex to the putamen and other parts of the basal ganglia: An autoradiographic study in *Macaca fascicularis*. *Brain Res* 88:195–209, 1975.
14. Iversen SD: Behavior after neostriatal lesions in animals, in Divac I, Oberg RGE (eds): *The Neostriatum*. Oxford, UK: Pergamon Press, 1979, pp 195–210.
15. Horel J, Meyer-Lohmann J, Brooks VB: Basal ganglia cooling disables learned arm movements of monkeys in the absence of visual guidance. *Science* 195:584–586, 1977.
16. Yim CY, Mogenson GJ: Response of ventral pallidal neurons to amygdala stimulation and its modulation by dopamine projections to nucleus accumbens. *J Neurophysiol* 50:148–161, 1983.
17. Parent A, de Bellefeuille L: Organization of efferent projections from the internal segment of the globus pallidus in primate as revealed by fluorescence retrograde labeling method. *Brain Res* 245:201–213, 1982.
18. MacLean PD: Effects of lesions of globus pallidus on species-specific display behavior of squirrel monkey. *Brain Res* 149:175–196, 1978.
19. Hikosaka O, Wurtz RH: Visual and oculomotor functions of monkey substantia nigra pars reticulata: III. Memory-contingent visual and saccade responses. *J Neurophysiol* 49:1268–1284, 1983.
20. Jones EG: Some aspects of the organization of the thalamic reticular complex. *J Comp Neurol* 162:285–308, 1975.
21. Jones EG, Burton H: A projection from medial pulvinar to the amygdala in primates. *Brain Res* 104:142–147, 1976.
22. Isseroff A, Rosvold HE, Galkin TW, Goldman-Rakic PS: Spatial memory impairments following damage to the mediodorsal nucleus of the thalamus in rhesus monkeys. *Brain Res* 232:97–113, 1982.
23. Sandson TA, Daffner KR, Carvalho PA, Mesulam MM: Frontal lobe dysfunction following infarction of the left-sided medial thalamus. *Arch Neurol* 48:1300–1303, 1991.
24. Aggleton JP, Mishkin M: Visual recognition impairment following medial thalamic lesions in monkeys. *Neuropsychologia* 21:189–197, 1983.
25. Michel D, Laurent B, Foyatier N, et al: Etude de la mémoire et du langage dans une observation tomodensitométrique d'infarctus thalamique paramedian gauche. *Rev Neurol (Paris)* 138:533–550, 1982.
26. Signoret J-L: Memory and amnesias, in Mesulam M-M (ed): *Principles of Behavioral Neurology*. Philadelphia: Davis, 1985, pp 169–192.
27. Cambier J, Elghozi D, Strube E: Lésion du thalamus droit avec syndrome de l'hémisphere mineur. Discussion du concept de négligence thalamique. *Rev Neurol (Paris)* 136:105–116, 1980.
28. Ojemann GA, Fedio P, VanBuren JM: Anomia from pulvinar and subcortical parietal stimulation. *Brain* 91:99–116, 1968.
29. Mesulam M-M: Cholinergic pathways and the ascending reticular activating system of the human brain. *Ann NY Acad Sci* 757:169–179, 1995.
30. Moruzzi G, Magoun HW: Brain stem reticular formation and activation of the EEG. *Electroencephalogr Clin Neurophysiol* 1:459–473, 1949.
31. Dingledine R, Kelly JS: The brainstem stimulation and acetylcholine-invoked inhibition of neurons in the feline nucleus reticularis thalami. *J Physiol* 271:135–154, 1977.
32. Hoover DB, Jacobowitz DM: Neurochemical and histochemical studies of the effect of a lesion of the nucleus cuneiformis on the cholinergic innervation of discrete areas of the rat brain. *Brain Res* 70:113–122, 1970.
33. Hoover DB, Baisden RH: Localization of putative cholinergic neurons innervating the anteroventral thalamus. *Brain Res Bull* 5:519–524, 1980.
34. McCance I, Phillis JW, Westerman RA: Acetylcholine-sensitivity of thalamic neurons: Its relationship to synaptic transmission. *Br J Pharmacol* 32:635–651, 1986.
35. Phillis JW, Tebecis AK, York DH: A study of cholinoceptive cells in the lateral geniculate nucleus. *J Physiol* 192:695–713, 1967.
36. Mesulam M-M: The systems-level organization of cholinergic innervation in the cerebral cortex and its alterations in Alzheimer's disease. *Prog Brain Res* 109:285–298, 1996.
37. Mesulam M-M, Mufson EJ: Neural inputs into the nucleus basalis of the substantia innominata (Ch4) in the rhesus monkey. *Brain* 107:253–274, 1984.
38. Mesulam M-M: Asymmetry of neural feedback in the organization of behavioral states. *Science* 237:537–538, 1987.
39. Mesulam M-M: Attentional networks, confusional states and neglect syndromes, in Mesulam M-M (ed): *Principles of Behavioral and Cognitive Neurology*. New York: Oxford University Press, 2000, pp 174–256.

40. Mesulam M-M: Large-scale neurocognitive networks and distributed processing for attention, language, and memory. *Ann Neurol* 28:597–613, 1990.
41. Mesulam M-M: Aphasias and other focal cerebral disorders, in Braunwald E, Fauci AS, Kasper DL, et al (eds): *Harrison's Principles of Internal Medicine,* 14 ed. New York: McGraw Hill, 2001, pp 140–147.
42. Mesulam M-M: Functional anatomy of attention and neglect: from neurons to networks, in Karnath H-O, Milner D, Vallar G (eds): *The Cognitive and Neural Bases of Spatial Neglect.* New York: Oxford University Press. In press.
43. Mesulam M-M: Higher visual functions of the cerebral cortex and their disruption in clinical practice, in Albert DM, Jakobiec FA (eds): *Principles and Practice of Ophthalmology,* 2d ed. Philadelphia: Saunders, 2000, pp 4211–4224.
44. Mesulam M-M: Notes on the cerebral topography of memory and memory distortion: A neurologist's perspective, in Schacter DL, Coyle JT, Fischbach GD, et al (eds): *Memory Distortion.* Cambridge, MA: Harvard University Press, 1995, pp 379–385.
45. Mesulam M-M: The human frontal lobes: Transcending the default mode through contingent encoding, in Stuss D, Knight R, (eds): *Principles of Frontal Lobe Function.* New York: Oxford University Press, 2002.
46. Morecraft RJ, Geula C, Mesulam M-M: Architecture of connectivity within a cingulo-fronto-parietal neurocognitive network for directed attention. *Arch Neurol* 50:279–284, 1993.
47. Mesulam M-M: Neurocognitive networks and selectively distributed processing. *Rev Neurol (Paris)* 150:564–569, 1994.
48. Geschwind N: Disconnection syndromes in animals and man. *Brain* 88:237–294, 1965.

Chapter 5

MECHANISMS OF PLASTICITY AND BEHAVIOR

Albert M. Galaburda
Alvaro Pascual-Leone

PLASTICITY AS AN INTRINSIC PROPERTY OF THE BRAIN

It is not possible to understand psychological function in normal individuals or patients with cognitive or emotional deficits without invoking the concept of brain plasticity. Even though clinicians and researchers in behavioral neurology and cognitive neuroscience know better, discussions of patients with developmental, acquired, or degenerative brain injury affecting behavior often imply that the observed behaviors are the result of simple loss of function from some steady state caused by the injury. In fact, loss of function is not the only and even perhaps not the most important clinical behavioral consequence of brain damage. Injury can lead to changes in behavior by loss of function, by uncovering normally suppressed behaviors, and by the emergence of totally novel behaviors that result from brain remodeling, otherwise known as neural plasticity.

The brain is designed to be able to change in response to changes in the environment. This, in fact, is the mechanism for learning and for growth and development—changes in the anatomy of the input of a particular neural system, or in the information coming in along its afferent connections, or changes in the targets of its efferent connections can lead to system reorganization that can be demonstrable at the level of behavior, anatomy, and physiology, and down to the cellular and molecular levels. Initial damage and plasticity confer either no perceptible change in the behavioral capacity of the brain or can lead to changes that are demonstrated only under special testing conditions and not otherwise clinically significant. Otherwise, behavioral changes will bring the patient to medical attention. There may be loss of a previously acquired behavioral capacity; there may be release of behaviors normally suppressed in the uninjured brain; there may be the takeover of lost function by semiadapted neighboring systems that can complete some of the lost function (albeit perhaps via different strategies or computations); there may be the emergence of new behaviors that are adaptive or maladaptive. Reorganization does not necessarily mean recovery of function. In other words, plasticity at the neural level does not speak to the question of behavioral change and certainly does not necessarily imply functional recovery or even functional change.

It is reasonable to assume that plasticity is a characteristic of the nervous system that evolved for coping with changes in the environment associated with learning and development and that are coopted as a response to brain injury. Yet, as these mechanisms did not specifically evolve to cope with injury, they are not altogether successful in this regard. It is also safe to say, at this stage of our knowledge, that structural plasticity does not predict for behavioral plasticity, even though a fuller understanding will probably lead to such predictions.

The brain has millions of cells that are connected with each other by billions of synapses. In the course of development, very complex processes having to do with the intrinsic properties of neurons, as well as with influences arising either externally to the brain or in one brain region with respect to another, help to establish this intricate and highly specific network. Given that changes in the brain during development serve in part as a record of the history of the interaction between the brain and its environment (and among the different interconnected brain components), it is reasonable to think that the brain would, once development is completed, be resistant to change. Indeed, for many years, this notion of a rather static and unchanging postdevelopmental brain was the pervasive belief. More recently, it has become clear that this notion is wrong. The brain does not only undergo reorganization after injury, but it is in fact constantly reorganizing itself in response to change taking place around and within it.[1–3] The brain's intrinsic capacity to change persists throughout the human life span. A striking example lending support to this claim is witnessed during the acquisition of new skills. Neuroimaging studies have found decreases, increases, and shifts in regional brain activation resulting from task practice as a function of the amount of repetition and priming, level of learning proficiency, and overlearning and automatization.[4–6] Behavioral plasticity requires that structural and physiologic properties of the brain change to permit representation of new knowledge and implementation of new behaviors. As with learning, plasticity is seen in response to pathologic conditions, including injury to the central or peripheral nervous system.[7,8] As in learning, whereby input information into various brain areas changes, thus modifying plasticity, in injury structural changes also change input-output relationships in areas connectionally related to the area of damage and therefore also modify plasticity. In this setting, plasticity is likely to represent the mechanisms by which recovery of function after the injury is possible,[9] but, as already noted, could instead lead to maladaptive remodeling.

Plasticity is not an occasional state of the nervous system; instead, it is the normally ongoing state of the nervous system. A full, coherent account of any sensory or cognitive theory has to build into its framework the ongoing changes that occur as the brain continually learns from and updates its model of the world while reshaping its structure at multiple levels in response to changes in its input afferents and output targets. The need to understand the brain as an intrinsically plastic and hence changing system becomes critical not only for comprehending the effects of injury but also for the interpretation of behavioral, neurophysiologic, and functional imaging studies. Implicit in the commonly held notion of plasticity is the concept that there is a definable starting point after which it may be possible to record and measure change. In fact, there is no such beginning point, since any event, which could be exposure to a new learning situation, a seizure, or an infarct, falls upon a moving target—i.e., a brain that is undergoing constant change triggered by previous events or resulting from intrinsic remodeling activity. We should therefore not conceive of the brain as a stationary object capable of activating a cascade of changes that we shall call plasticity, nor as an orderly stream of events, driven by plasticity. We might be better served by thinking of the nervous system as a continuously changing structure of which plasticity is an integral property and the obligatory consequence of each sensory input, each motor act, association, reward signal, action plan, or awareness. In this framework, notions such as psychological processes as distinct from organic-based functions or dysfunctions cease to be informative. Behavior will lead to changes in brain circuitry (just as changes in brain circuitry will lead to behavior), hence establishing organic symbiosis between learned attitudes, dispositions, or thinking styles and functional brain circuits.

MECHANISMS OF PLASTICITY

There are a number of mechanisms for plasticity in humans that can be studied at different levels, ranging from systems physiology all the way down to cellular and molecular levels. Thus far, our understanding of these mechanisms remains incomplete. Nonetheless, it can be said that descriptions at the level of large systems of interconnected neurons more specifically characterize human psychological processes than do descriptions at molecular and cellular levels, which seem to be shared not only between human and nonhuman primates but among all vertebrate and invertebrate organisms thus far studied. There are no known molecular mechanisms of learning unique to humans. Therefore, descriptions of plasticity at the systems levels are stressed in this chapter.

Expansion of a specialized cortical area or recruitment of a remote area as a result of learning or brain disease or injury comprises the two most characteristic forms of brain plasticity. The underlying general phenomenon is that neurons in one area assume properties of neurons in an adjacent or remote area. Such remodeling might take place within the cortex but could also implicate related subcortical levels.[10,11] Such remodeling can take place across brain areas within a given modality, for example within visual, tactile, or motor distributed systems (homotypic or intramodal plasticity), or may bridge across modalities (heterotypic or cross-modal plasticity), as in the case of tactile information processing in the occipital ("visual") cortex in the blind.[12,13] The time course of plasticity is extended, with some changes appearing within seconds of the initial event and continuing many years after an intervention or injury.[14,15]

Regardless of the physiologic mechanisms underlying plasticity, a series of principles can be put together. First, changes in the balance between excitatory and inhibitory influences can take place in established connectivity.[10] Such changes can take place in a very short time, because neural connectivity is larger than functional connectivity. Thus, learning- or injury-induced loss of inhibition can quickly expand the functional reach of a neural system. This process is commonly known as "unmasking." The application of the GABA antagonist bicuculline, for demonstrating the effects of unmasking, is a now classic strategy to study mechanisms of plasticity in animal models.[16,17] In humans, magnetic resonance spectroscopy or paired-pulse transcranial magnetic stimulation (TMS) can be used to provide similar insights.

A second process underlying fast-onset plasticity is the modulation (strengthening or weakening) of existing synapses. Processes such as long-term potentiation (LTP) or long-term depression (LTD) are examples of such mechanisms. LTP or LTD occurs following specific patterns of synaptic activity and may last for long periods of time. Such processes have been shown to occur in a variety of brain regions, most notably in the hippocampus, but also in the cortex.[18,19] Thus, in many regions of the cerebral cortex, calcium ion influx through NMDA (*N*-methyl-D-aspartate)-sensitive glutamate receptors (NMDA receptors) can trigger both LTP or LTD. LTD is induced by low levels of postsynaptic NMDA-receptor activation, for instance in response to low-frequency stimulation, whereas LTP is induced by the stronger activation that occurs following high-frequency stimulation.[20]

A third mechanism playing a role in early plasticity is the change in neuronal membrane excitability.[21] There are multiple described mechanisms for changing membrane excitability; these have been shown with the use of cell and patch clamp techniques and implicate the function of calcium and sodium channels, calcium-dependent potassium channels, and other potassium channels, as well as transmitters like serotonin and genes affecting the function of membrane components.[22,23]

A fourth mechanism is anatomic change demonstrable under the microscope, with axonal and dendritic sprouting and the establishment of new synaptic connections.[24–28] Such anatomic change would take place over a longer time period and may indeed require for its induction the initial activation of one or several of the previously mentioned faster mechanisms of plasticity. Synaptic reorganization and local changes in axonal and dendritic architecture would take less time than changes involving longer corticocortical connections, and some connections acting at greater distances may not be able to regrow and remodel following injury in the mature brain, while this may still be possible in young brains in which excess connectivity, even long connections, has not as yet been pruned. Synaptic changes may take the form of increase or decrease in synaptic density, hence strengthening or weakening preexisting connections, rearrangement of synapses into novel synaptic architectures capable of new functions, or a combination of these, with unpredictable effects on function.

Finally, a fifth process is the generation and maturation of new neurons that can be incorporated into preexisting networks.[29–33] This possibility has generated a great deal of excitement lately, with both supporters and detractors of the idea that new neurons are generated in the cerebral cortex of the mature human brain, which can establish functionally relevant connectivity.

METHODS FOR THE STUDY OF PLASTICITY IN HUMANS

Information about brain plasticity in humans can be gathered using a variety of methods. The rapid development of noninvasive mapping methodologies in the past two decades has greatly accelerated progress in this area of research. The basic approach, common to all methodologies, is to identify, localize, and characterize changes in brain function (e.g., changes in glucose or oxygen utilization, blood flow, electrical activity) in relation to the performance of a specific psychological task, and to document how this brain "representation" changes according to various circumstances. The motor and visual systems have been particularly extensively studied, but the approach is also applicable to regions linked to the performance of cognitive functions, specifically the multimodal areas of the frontal, temporal, and parietal lobes.

Functional neuroimaging with positron emission tomography (PET) or functional magnetic resonance imaging (fMRI) depends on serial changes in regional blood flow, which demarcate a functionally active area or areas (PET can also be used to study specific neurotransmitter activity, including GABA and glutamate, using radioactive tracers). These techniques, discussed in greater detail in Chap. 7, are only indirect measures of synaptic activity, and depend on predictable blood-flow responses to metabolic needs. Signals obtained in optical brain imaging—e.g., near-infrared spectroscopy (NIRS)—are also indirect measures of synaptic activity, but their source is largely limited to the cortex. All of the above methods have relatively good spatial resolution, down to the millimeter or submillimeter range, but poor temporal resolution, on the order of seconds to minutes.

Magnetic resonance spectroscopy (MRS), whereby spectral signatures of brain chemical constituents and metabolites of brain function can be mapped, may eventually allow for the study of behavior as correlations of regional chemical change and specific behaviors are established. The anatomic resolution of MRS would certainly be superior to that of tracer PET, and it would have the additional advantage of not exposing the subjects to radiation.

Electroencephalography (EEG) and magnetoencephalography (MEG) represent direct measures of neuronal activity in real psychological time—that is, on the order of milliseconds. Unfortunately, as discussed in Chap. 9, the anatomic sources of the EEG/MEG signals cannot be accurately determined and thus the topographic organization of the psychological function remains underdetermined. The combined use of EEG/MEG with fMRI will certainly enhance the utility of either method alone.

Transcranial magnetic stimulation (TMS), covered in more detail in Chap. 9, has proven to be a valuable tool for studying brain plasticity.[34] Using repetitive stimulation with a variable, rapidly changing magnetic stimulus, TMS transiently deactivates a region of the brain, thus creating a virtual patient. Cortical areas seen to activate in PET or fMRI images during psychological tasks can be suppressed with TMS and the effects on the behavior noted. Thus, a causal relationship between regional brain activation and behavior can be tested and confirmed.[35] Moreover, TMS can accurately measure changes in cortical excitability, thus providing a way to assess one of the mechanisms by which plasticity takes place in the brain.[36] The technique allows for the exploration of corticocortical interactions, e.g., intracortical inhibition and facilitation, which are likely markers of glutamatergic, dopaminergic, and GABAergic effects. Lesion studies and direct cortical stimulation have hitherto been the only approaches for the study of causal interactions between brain and behavior. TMS allows for the gathering of comparable information in a relatively noninvasive manner, with the additional possibility of the serial testing of normal subjects in carefully designed experimental paradigms. In addition, when appropriately delivered in time and space, TMS can provide information regarding the exact time when activity in a brain area is critical for a given behavior. The combined use of these different methodologies enables us to inquire with exquisite anatomic and temporal resolution about the causal roles of specific brain activities in behavior and hence about the plastic changes resulting from specific circumstances, influences, or dysfunction.

PLASTICITY IS NOT NECESSARILY BENEFICIAL

An intrinsic property of brain function, plasticity during a learning situation and especially after brain damage need not lead to improvement of function. Indeed, plastic changes might result in behavioral gain or loss in normal subjects or in the development or amelioration of symptoms in disease states. The concept of "maladaptive plasticity" was introduced to capture the idea of potentially functionally undesirable consequences of plasticity (see, for instance,[37] in development and[38] in acquired disease). However, we might be better served by discarding the notion of an obligatory link between plasticity and adaptation and rather think of plasticity as a generator of change, some of which may be behaviorally adaptive and some not, much the same as what is seen in the implementation of Darwinian theory. Thus, brain change generated by plasticity is adaptive only if the environment can support and maintain the resultant behavior. For example, imagine a patient who, because of an ankle injury, requires weeks of immobilization of the distal leg and foot. This immobilization leads to diminished activity in the cortical output to the spinal segment subserving the tibialis anterior muscle, which is primarily responsible for the extension of the foot at the ankle. This reduction in efferent demand leads to a reduction in the size of the motor output map of the tibialis anterior muscle in the precentral cortex, and the extent of reduction is correlated with the duration of the immobilization and can be reversed by voluntary muscle contraction.[39] In this case, the plastic changes are adaptive only in relation to the immobilized limb, but the moment the ankle is released from restriction the plasticity is maladaptive and might result in the need for physical therapy of longer duration. Other examples of maladaptive plasticity include the possible exacerbation of cognitive deficits in Alzheimer's disease occasioned by hippocampal sprouting following cell loss[38] and the exacerbation of the distortion of the visual field in hamsters in which a collicular lesion leads to reactive cross innervation.[37]

The role played by plasticity in task-specific dystonia, for example in "pianist's cramp," is another heuristically useful example. A pianist confronted with a new composition, after understanding the task and its demands, develops a cognitive representation of the behavior and initiates an initial, centrally guided response that consists of a sensorimotor feedback and movement correction. At the beginning, the limbs move slowly, with fluctuating accuracy and speed, and success requires visual, proprioceptive, and auditory feedback. Eventually, each single movement is refined, the different movements are chained into the proper sequence with the desired timing, a high probability of stability in the ordered sequence is attained, and a fluidity of all movements is developed. Only then can the pianist shift his or her attention away from the mechanical details of the performance and focus on the emotional content of the task. We can think of the acquisition of such a skill as the conversion of declarative knowledge (facts) into procedural knowledge (actions, skills).

Normal subjects taught to perform with one hand a five-finger exercise on a piano keyboard require several days of practice to acquire proficiency.[40] Over the course of 5 days, and 2 h of practice each day, the number of sequencing errors and unevenness of the intervals separating key presses decrease significantly and accuracy improves. These behavioral gains are associated with changes in the motor output maps to the muscles involved in the task, which can be demonstrated using TMS. As the subjects' performance improve, the thresholds for TMS activation of the finger flexor and extensor muscles (a measure of cortical excitability) decrease steadily and, even taking this change in activation threshold into account, the sizes of the cortical representation for both muscle groups increase significantly (Fig. 5-1).

The plastic reorganization associated with piano practice results from increased demand for sensorimotor integration and poses the risk of unwanted plasticity. One outcome of this unwanted cortical rearrangement can be the development of overuse syndrome and focal, task-specific dystonias. The style of piano playing seems to affect the risk of developing clinical problems. Thus, forceful playing with the fingers held bent and executing hammer-like movements is more frequently associated with overuse syndrome and dystonia than softer playing with extended fingers "caressing" the keys. A guitarist experiencing dystonia during playing shows significantly greater activation of the contralateral primary sensorimotor cortices and lesser bilateral activation of premotor areas as compared with dystonia-free practice[41] (Fig. 5-2, Plate 1). Furthermore, the somatosensory homunculi of patients with focal, task-specific dystonia are abnormal.[42,43] They show distortions in the representation of adjacent fingers and excessive overlap among them, likely reflecting extensive practice of coordinated hand postures in which two or more digits function as a unit, as in arpeggios and chords. The map distortions are more striking when small repeated traumas are added, for example in forceful, "hammer-finger" piano practice. In these cases, the plasticity associated with learning to play a musical instrument can produce abnormal sensorimotor remodeling leading to the development of clinically significant motor problems.

PLASTICITY IN THE PATHOGENESIS OF DISEASE

As suggested by the example of task-specific dystonia during learning in normal subjects, plasticity can in fact be the mechanism underlying the symptomatology of clinical conditions. A case in point is illustrated by developmental dyslexia.

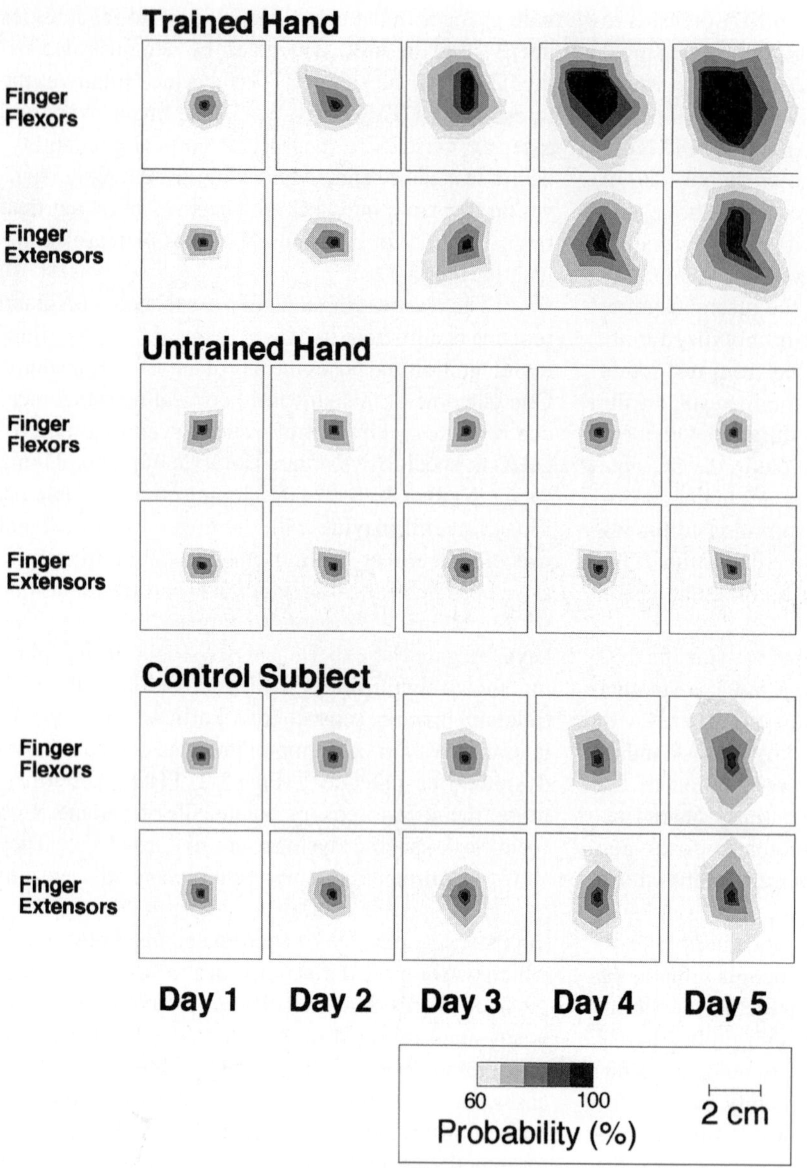

Figure 5-1
Representative examples of the cortical motor output maps for the long finger flexor and extensor muscles on days 1–5 in a test subject (trained and untrained hand) and a control subjects. The maps express the probability of evoking a motor potential with a peak-to-peak amplitude of at least 50,/u181/'b5V in the contralateral muscles with a stimulus intensity of 10% above motor threshold at the optimal scalp position. Eight stimuli were given at each scalp position. Each contour map represents 25 scalp positions (1 cm apart) arranged in a 5 × 5 grid around the optimal positions. (Modified from Pascual-Leone et al.[40] with permission.)

As reviewed in Chap. 64, most dyslexics have difficulties with phonological tasks—e.g., pseudoword reading, rhyming, phoneme deletion tasks.[44] They have also been shown to have problems with sound perception.[45] Dyslexic brains show focal cortical malformations consisting most often of nests of ectopic neurons and glia in the first cortical layer.[46,47] They also show changes in the sizes of neurons in the (auditory) medial geniculate nucleus.[48] Experiments in rats to produce cortical ectopias by early freezing damage to the incipient cortex indicate that the cortical anomalies produce the cell changes in the thalamus as part of developmental plasticity.[49] Moreover, it appears that the plastic changes in the thalamus, and not the cortical malformations themselves, are associated with the sound processing deficits. Female rats, which receive the injury and develop the same cortical malformations, but do not show cell changes in the thalamus, do not

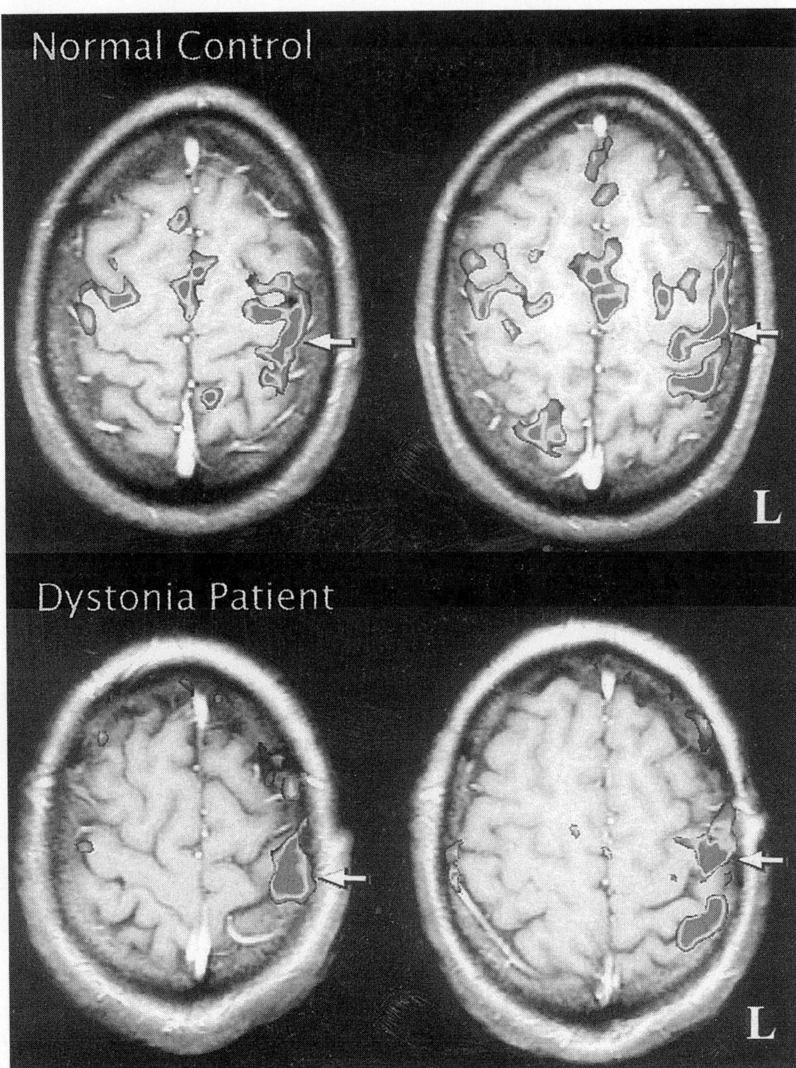

Figure 5-2 (Plate 1)
The figure displays the fMRI images of a normal and a dystonic guitar player executing right hand arpeggios in the scanner. Note the greater activation of the sensory-motor cortex (arrows) and the lack of activation of premotor and supplementary motor cortices in the dystonic patient. (Modified from Pujol et al,[41] with permission.)

exhibit sound processing problems.[50,51] In other words, developmental plasticity associated with early cortical injury, and not the cortical injury itself, leads to the abnormal behavior.

PLASTICITY IN THE ADAPTATION TO BLINDNESS

The changes in sensorimotor representation of the reading finger of proficient Braille readers and the cross-modal plasticity by which the deafferented "visual" cortex is recruited for processing auditory and tactile information provide useful illustrations of many of the principles of plasticity discussed so far. One may argue that early blindness represents a "pathologic state" resulting in substantial cross-modal brain plasticity.[12,13,52,53] A person who has suffered the total loss of a particular form of sensory input has, in reality, suffered a brain lesion. For example, with blindness, the brain is functionally deprived of approximately 2 million sensory fibers. This deprivation has a bottom-up effect and implicates multiple stages of processing, from the lateral geniculate nucleus in the thalamus,

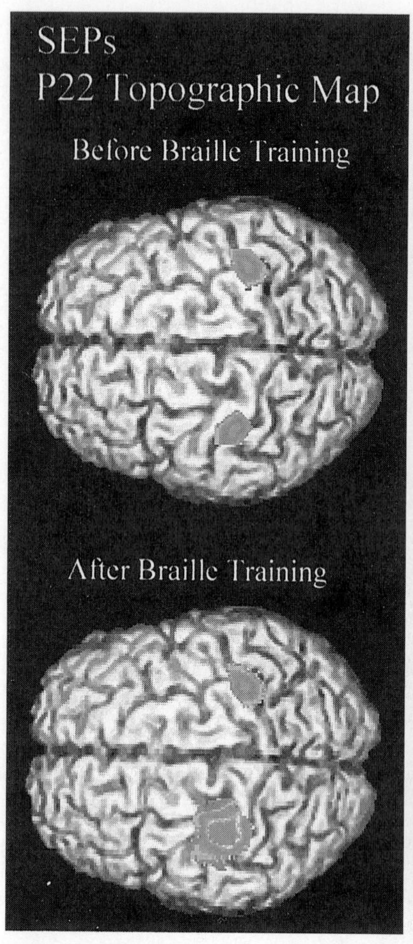

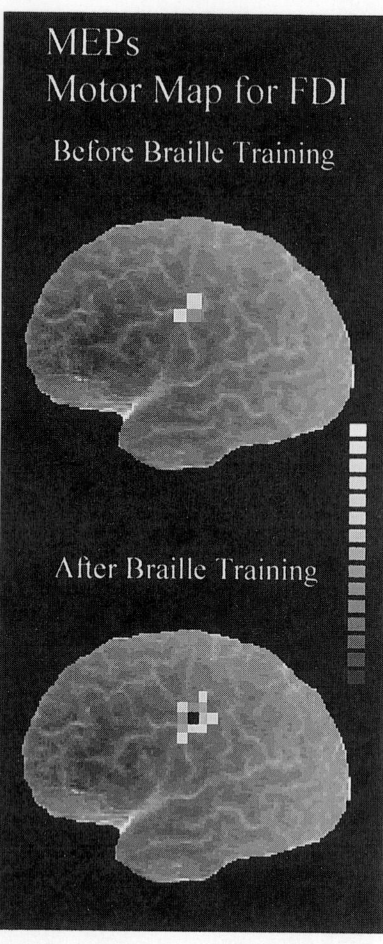

Figure 5-3 (Plate 2) *Evidence of plasticity in sensory, motor, and occipital cortex in early blind subjects after learning Braille. Representative example of the studies performed before and at the end of one year of learning Braille are shown. The different studies were conducted on different subjects using somatosensory evoked potentials (SEPs) to mechanical stimuli to the index finger pad (adapted from Pascual-Leone and Torres,[54] with permission), motor mapping with transcranial magnetic stimulation of the potentials evoked in the first dorsal interosseus muscle FDI, side-to-side mover of the index finger (adapted from Pascual-Leone et al.,[43] with permission), and functional magnetic resonance imaging (fMRI) while reading Braille characters. (Modified from Hamilton and Pascual-Leone,[12] with permission.)*

through the primary visual cortex, to subsequent stations of associative visual processing. This dramatic change in the brain's experience of the outside world is likely to lead to reorganization. Therefore, blindness provides a reasonable model for studying mechanisms underlying brain plasticity in response to sensory deprivation and loss of acquisition of modality specific skills.

Learning Braille poses a logistical challenge, because it demands a marked increase (over normal use) in functional afferent input and efferent demand from a restricted body space (the pads of Braille-reading fingers) not evolutionarily designed for this task. Blind Braille readers must first discriminate, with exquisite sensitivity and accuracy, subtle patterns of raised and depressed dots with the pads of their fingers, after which they must translate this spatial representation into associative meaning. Faced with the complex cognitive demands of Braille reading, the brain undergoes striking adaptive changes (Fig. 5-3, Plate 2). Recording somatosensory evoked potentials (SEPs) arising in the tips of the reading and nonreading index fingers of blind Braille readers, Pascual-Leone and Torres[54] demonstrated that the sensory map of the reading finger is enlarged as compared with the representation of the contralateral, homologous, nonreading finger or with the finger of a sighted or non-Braille-reading blind control subject. TMS revealed similar enlargement of the Braille-reading finger map.[55] Serial measurements of the cortical output maps of blind subjects learning Braille show that this enlargement seems to develop in two stages: (1) A rapid, dramatic, and transient enlargement that is likely the result of the unmasking of connections or upregulation of synaptic efficacy and

A

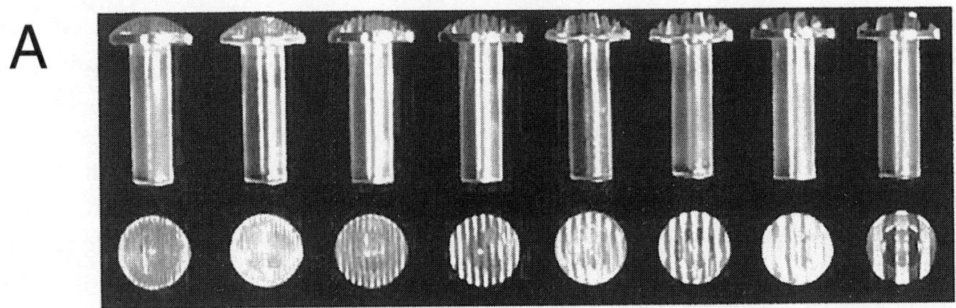

B

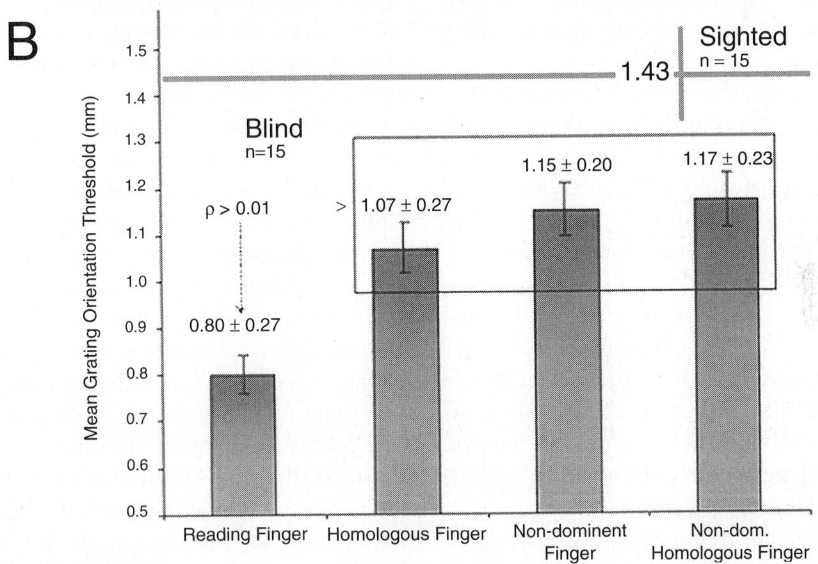

Figure 5-4 (Plate 3)

A. JVP Domes used for gratings orientations discrimination testing. B. Histogram displaying the thresholds for grating orientation discrimination in early blind and sighted control subjects. Note the marked superiority (lower thresholds) of the blind subjects in general and in paricular of their dominant Braille reading finger. (Modified from van Boven et al,[58] with permission.)

(2) a slower, less prominent, but more stable enlargement of the cortical representation of the reading finger that may represent structural plasticity.[56] If this finding can be extrapolated to other forms of skill learning, we might infer that learning involves a transient rapid change in the efficacy of existing connections, which leads the way to a more enduring structural modification in the face of continued practice.

Preceding activity affects the size of the motor output maps in Braille readers.[57] A comparison of motor output maps following a day of intensive reading to those obtained after being off for 2 days demonstrates significant differences in the cortical representation of the reading finger of proficient Braille proofreaders. Disuse, in this case by virtue of the 2 days' respite, results in a measurable decrease in the sizes of the cortical output maps. Vacation consisting of a week of minimal Braille reading leads to an even more dramatic reduction in the motor output maps. These disuse-related changes might underlie the common experience of "rustiness" upon returning to work following a break, and constitute a regressive form of neural plasticity.

In addition to the expanded cortical representation of the fingers used in Braille reading, there is enhanced fidelity in the neural transmission of spatial details of a stimulus that results in heightened tactile spatial acuity. Using the grating orientation discrimination task (Fig. 5-4, Plate 3), in which threshold performance is accounted for by the spatial resolution limits of the neural image evoked by a stimulus, van Boven et al.[58] quantified the psychophysical limits of spatial resolution at the middle and index fingers of blind Braille readers and sighted control subjects. The mean grating orientation threshold was significantly lower in the blind group compared to the sighted group. The self-reported dominant reading finger in blind subjects had the lowest grating orientation threshold in all subjects and was significantly better than other fingers tested. In this case, neural plasticity is probably causally linked to superior skill.

However, it does not appear that it is just the expansion of the sensorimotor cortical map of the reading finger that confers superior spatial skills to it, because the relative map size does not correlate with Braille reading or sensory discrimination ability. In fact, although appropriate somatosensory cortical representations expand as subjects develop sensorimotor skills, eventually they decrease in size as subjects gain mastery of those skills.[59,60] Instead, there appears to be recruitment of other cortical areas. In the case of Braille learning, the recruitment of parts of the occipital cortex, ordinarily the visual cortex (V1 and V2), for tactile information processing appears to be a critical contributor to the improved tactile acuity.

In blind, proficient Braille readers, the occipital cortex can be shown not only to be associated with tactile Braille reading[61,62] but indeed to be critical for reading accuracy[63] (Fig. 5-5, Plate 4). Peripherally blind subjects have very large areas of their cerebral cortex deafferented from visual input; hence portions of what would have been visual cortex are in principle available to be recruited for processing tactile and auditory information. Indeed, proficient Braille reading by blind subjects activates the dorsal and ventral portion of the occipital cortex.[61,62] Furthermore, there is suppression in the parietal operculum and activation in the ventral portion of the occipital cortex in blind subjects during tactile discrimination tasks, opposite to the pattern of activation and deactivation observed in sighted subjects. Studies using event-related potentials, cerebral blood flow, and magnetoencephalography (MEG) also demonstrate occipital cortex activation by tactile stimuli in persons blind from an early age.[12,13] Participation of the striate cortex in a tactile task seems related to the difficulty of the tactile discrimination regardless of whether there is a linguistic component.[61,62] These findings suggest that the pathway for tactile discrimination changes with blindness. The interpretation that occipital lobe activation is causally related to the performance of the Braille task in the congenitally blind is supported by findings from a repetitive TMS experiment that found that Braille reading was disrupted by occipital stimulation.[63] Subjects were aware of the presence of Braille characters, but during rTMS to their occipital cortex they were unable to discriminate them. Some of the subjects reported phantom tactile sensations–Braille dots that were not there—or distortions of the Braille symbols. In sighted subjects, rTMS to the visual cortex does not interfere with the ability to detect or discriminate embossed Roman letters by touch. Therefore, it would appear that Braille reading in the blind is an example of true "cross-modal sensory plasticity" by which the deafferented occipital cortex is recruited for demanding tactile tasks.

Cohen et al.[64] argued for a critical time window for the above-mentioned plasticity associated with peripheral blindness, such that beyond the age of age 14 years the striate cortex is no longer recruited for the processing of tactile information. The argument is based on the study of subjects who became blind after age 15, in whom tactile stimulation failed to reveal activation of the striate cortex on PET and rTMS to the striate cortex did not interfere with reading of embossed Roman characters.

Recruitment of occipital cortical areas for processing of auditory information in blind subjects has also been reported.[13,65] The use of transient event-related potentials (ERPs) and the oddball paradigm, which consists of a repeating stimulus (standard) that is replaced occasionally by a physically different (oddball) stimulus, allows the investigation of stimulus discrimination and change detection during passive and active conditions. No significant differences were found between early-blind and sighted individuals in the distribution of brain activity associated with the automatic detection of sound change as indexed by mismatch negativity (usually peaking at about 100 to 200 ms from stimulus change onset). However, when oddball tones had to be detected, they elicited an additional response, one with a scalp distribution that was more posterior in the blind than in the sighted subjects.[13] This effect was observed with sound

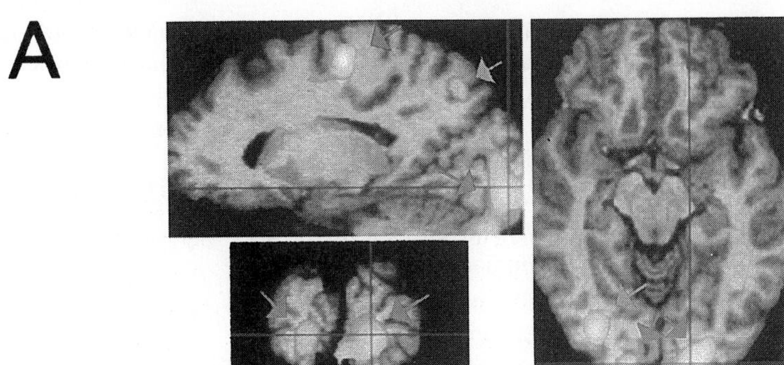

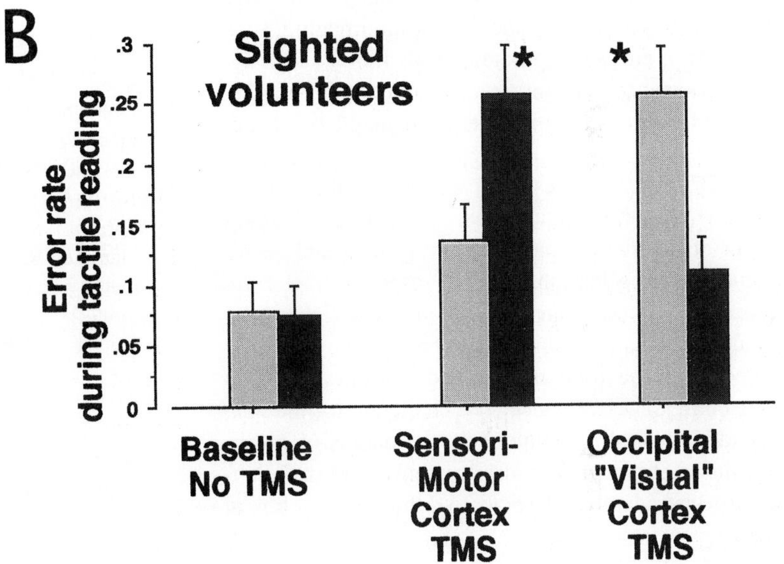

Figure 5-5 (Plate 4)
A. Activation of the occipital cortex in congenitally and early blind subjects during tactile Braille reading as demonstrated by positron emission tomography (PET). (Modified from Sadato et al,[61] with permission.) B. Effects of repetitive transcranial magnetic stimulation (TMS) to the occipital or somatosensory cortex on tactile Braille reading ability in early blind subjects and on tactile perception of embossed Roman letter in sighted controls. (Modified from Cohen et al.,[63] with permission.)

frequency, amplitude, or location change. Remarkably, and reminiscent of the findings regarding activation of the occipital cortex in tactile tasks, the results in early-blind subjects differed from those found in late-blind subjects. These results indicate that both temporal and occipital brain areas of individuals with early blindness are involved in attentive sound-change detection. Recent work using PET has demonstrated similar findings.[65] During tasks that required auditory localization both the sighted and blind subjects strongly activated posterior parietal areas. In addition, the blind subjects activated association areas in the right occipital cortex, the foci of which were similar to areas previously identified in visual location and motion detection experiments in sighted subjects. The blind subjects, therefore, demonstrated auditory to "visual" (occipital) cross-modal plasticity with auditory localization activating occipital association areas ordinarily intended for dorsal-stream visual processing. Interestingly, during auditory localization in the blind subjects, regional cerebral blood flow in the right posterior parietal cortex was positively correlated with that in the right occipital region, whereas in sighted subjects correlations were generally nonsignificant. This indicates that in congenitally blind subjects the right occipital cortex participates in a functional network for auditory localization and that this occipital activity is likely to arise from connections with posterior parietal cortex.

SUMMARY

This chapter introduces the notion that plasticity is an intrinsic property of the human nervous system. Changes in the structural and/or functional properties of neuronal circuits subserving perception and cognition occur for many different reasons throughout life and are inseparable from other properties of the brain. Plasticity can be demonstrated in the bench lab in experimental animal model, and a variety of in-vivo techniques can be used to probe brain plasticity in humans. These methods include functional brain imaging, such as positron emission tomography or functional magnetic resonance imaging, evoked potentials, magnetoencephalography, and transcranial magnetic stimulation.

Plasticity changes occur which take place in seconds, while others require years to develop. Changes occur during the normal course of growth and development, during learning, and in response to disease processes. Some changes result in beneficial behavioral consequences, while others produce no clinically detectable behavioral change, and still others lead to worsening of performance. The challenge for the next decade is to learn enough about the details of mechanisms of plasticity in order to manipulate maladaptive toward adaptive plasticity and thus gain a clinical benefit.

REFERENCES

1. Fuster JM: *Memory in the Cerebral Cortex. An Empirical Approach to Neural Networks in the Human and Nonhuman Primate.* Cambridge, MA: MIT Press, 1995.
2. Kaas JH (ed): *Functional Plasticity in Adult Cortex.* Orlando, FL Academic Press, 1997.
3. Merzenich MM: Representational plasticity in somatosensory and motor cortical fields. *Biomed Res* 10(suppl. 2):85–86, 1989.
4. Schachter DL, Buckner RL: On the relations among priming, conscious recollection, and intentional retrieval: Evidence from neuroimaging research. *Neurobiol Learn Mem* 70:284–303, 1998.
5. Poldrack RA: Imaging brain plasticity: Conceptual and methodological issues–a theoretical review. *Neuroimage* 12:1–13, 2000.
6. van Mier H: Human learning, in Mazziotta JC, Toga AW, Frackowiak RS (ed): *Brain Mapping: The Systems.* San Dieg, CAo: Academic Press, 2000, pp 605–620.
7. Kaas JH: The reorganization of somatosensory and motor cortex after peripheral nerve or spinal cord injury in primates. *Prog Brain Res* 128:173–179, 2000.
8. Chollet F: Plasticity of the adult human brain, in Mazziotta JC, Toga AW, Frackowiak RS (ed): *Brain Mapping: The Systems.* San Diego, CA: Academic Press, 2000, pp 621–638.
9. Chollet F, Weiller C: Recovery of neurological function, in Mazziotta JC, Toga AW, Frackowiak RS (ed): *Brain Mapping: The Disorders.* San Diego, CA: Academic Press, 2000, pp 587–597.
10. Donoghue JP: Plasticity of adult sensorimotor representations. *Curr Opin Neurobiol* 5:749–754, 1995.
11. Donoghue JP, Hess G, Sanes JN: Substrates and mechanisms for learning in motor cortex, in Bloedel J, Ebner T, Wise SP (ed): *Acquisition of Motor Behavior in Vertebrates.* Cambridge, MA: MIT Press, 1996, pp 363–386.
12. Hamilton R, Pascual-Leone A: Cortical plasticity associated with Braille learning. *Trends Cogn Sci* 2:168–174, 1999.
13. Kujala T, Alho K, Naatanen R: Cross-modal reorganization of human cortical functions. *Trends Neurosci* 23:115–120, 2000.
14. Gilbert CD: Rapid dynamic changes in adult cerebral cortex. *Curr Opin Neurobiol* 3:100–103, 1993.
15. Gilbert CD: Adult cortical dynamics. *Physiol Rev* 78:467–485, 1998.
16. Lane RD, Killackey HP, Rhoades RW: Blockade of GABAergic inhibition reveals reordered cortical somatotopic maps in rats that sustained neonatal forelimb removal. *J Neurophysiol* 77:2723–2735, 1997.
17. Chagnac-Amitai Y, Connors BW: Horizontal spread of synchronized activity in neocortex and its control by GABA-mediated inhibition. *J Neurophysiol* 61:747–758, 1989.
18. Debanne D: Associative synaptic plasticity in hippocampus and visual cortex: Cellular mechanisms and functional implications. *Rev Neurosci* 7:29–46, 1996.
19. Iriki A, Pavlides C, Keller A, et al: Long-term potentiation in the motor cortex. *Science* 245:1385–1387, 1989.
20. Kirkwood A, Rioult MC, Bear MF: Experience-dependent modification of synaptic plasticity in visual cortex. *Nature* 381:526–528, 1996.

21. Woody CD, Guruen E, Birt D: Changes in membrane currents during pavlovian conditioning of single cortical neurons. *Brain Res* 539:76–84, 1991.
22. Patil N, Cox DR, Bhat D, et al: A potassium channel mutation in weaver mice implicates membrane excitability in granule cell differentiation. *Nat Genet* 11:126–129, 1995.
23. Sarkisian MR, Rattan S, D'Mello SR, et al: Characterization of seizures in the flathead rat: a new genetic model of epilepsy in early postnatal development. *Epilepsia* 40:394–400, 1999.
24. Okazaki MM, Evenson DA, Nadler JV: Hippocampal mossy fiber sprouting and synapse formation after status epilepticus in rats: visualization after retrograde transport of biocytin. *J Comp Neurol* 352:515–534, 1995.
25. Cotman C, Geddes J, Kahle J: Axon sprouting in the rodent and Alzheimer's disease brain: A reactivation of developmental mechanisms? in Storm-Mathisen J, Zimmer J, Ottersen OP (ed): *Progress in Brain Research.* Amsterdam: Elsevier , 1990, pp 427–434.
26. Aigner L, Arber S, Kapfhammer JP, et al: Overexpression of the neural growth-associated protein GAP-43 induces nerve sprouting in the adult nervous system of transgenic mice. *Cell* 83:269–278, 1995.
27. Murakami F, Song WJ, Katsumaru H: Plasticity of neuronal connections in developing brains of mammals. *Neurosci Res* 15:235–253, 1992.
28. Darian-Smith C, Gilbert CD: Axonal sprouting accompanies functional reorganization in adult cat striate cortex. *Nature* 368:737–740, 1994.
29. Alvarez-Buylla A, Lois C: Neuronal stem cells in the brain of adult vertebrates. *Stem Cells* 13:263–272, 1995.
30. Bayer SA: Neurogenesis in the anterior olfactory nucleus and its associated transition areas in the rat brain. *Int J Dev Neurosci* 4:225–249, 1986.
31. Corotto FS, Henegar JA, Maruniak JA: Neurogenesis persists in the subependymal layer of the adult mouse brain. *Neurosci Lett* 149:111–114, 1993.
32. Kempermann G, Kuhn HG, Gage FH: More hippocampal neurons in adult mice living in an enriched environment. *Nature* 386:493–495, 1997.
33. Shankle WR, Landing BH, Rafii MS, et al: Evidence for a postnatal doubling of neuron number in the developing human cerebral cortex between 15 months and 6 years. *J Theor Biol* 191:115–140, 1998.
34. Pascual-Leone A, Tarazona F, Keenan JP, et al: Transcranial magnetic stimulation and neuroplasticity. *Neuropsychologia* 37:207–217, 1999.
35. Pascual-Leone A, Walsh V, Rothwell J: Transcranial magnetic stimulation in cognitive neuroscience—virtual lesion, chronometry, and functional connectivity. *Curr Opin Neurobiol* 10:232–237, 2000.
36. Pascual-Leone A, Tormos JM, Keenan J, et al: Study and modulation of human cortical excitability with transcranial magnetic stimulation. *J Clin Neurophysiol* 15:333–343, 1998.
37. Finlay BL, Wilson KG, Schneider GE: Anomalous ipsilateral retinotectal projections in Syrian hamsters with early lesions: Topography and functional capacity. *J Comp Neurol* 183:721–740, 1979.
38. Geddes JW, Cotman CW: Plasticity in Alzheimer's disease: Too much or not enough? *Neurobiol Aging* 12: 330–333, 1991.
39. Liepert J, Tegenthoff M, Malin JP: Changes of cortical motor area size during immobilization. *Electroencephalogr Clin Neurophysiol* 97:382–386, 1995.
40. Pascual-Leone A, Nguyet D, Cohen LG, et al: Modulation of muscle responses evoked by transcranial magnetic stimulation during the acquisition of new fine motor skills. *J Neurophysiol* 74:1037–1045, 1995.
41. Pujol J, Roset-Llobet J, Rosines-Cubells D, et al: Brain cortical activation during guitar-induced hand dystonia studied by functional MRI. *Neuroimage* 12:257–267, 2000.
42. Bara-Jimenez W, Catalan MJ, Hallett M, et al: Abnormal somatosensory homunculus in dystonia of the hand. *Ann Neurol* 44:828–831, 1998.
43. Pascual-Leone A: The brain that plays music and is changed by it, in Zatorre R, Peretz I (ed): *Music and the Brain.* New York: New York Academy of Sciences, 2001.
44. Liberman IY, Shankweiler D: Phonology and the problems of learning to read and write. *Remed Spec Educ* 6:8–17, 1985.
45. Tallal P: Auditory temporal perception, phonics, and reading disabilities in children. *Brain Lang* 9:182–198, 1980.
46. Galaburda AM, Kemper TL: Cytoarchitectonic abnormalities in developmental dyslexia: A case study. *Ann Neurol* 6:94–100, 1979.
47. Galaburda AM, Sherman GF, Rosen GD, et al: Developmental dyslexia: four consecutive cases with cortical anomalies. *Ann Neurol* 18:222–233, 1985.
48. Galaburda AM, Menard MT, Rosen GD: Evidence for aberrant auditory anatomy in developmental dyslexia. *Proc Natl Acad Sci U S A* 91:8010–8013, 1994.
49. Herman AE, Galaburda AM, Fitch HR, et al: Cerebral microgyria, thalamic cell size and auditory temporal processing in male and female rats. *Cereb Cortex* 7:453–464, 1997.
50. Rosen GD, Herman AE, Galaburda AM: Sex differences in the effects of early neocortical injury on neuronal

size distribution of the medial geniculate nucleus in the rat are mediated by perinatal gonadal steroids. *Cereb Cortex* 9:27–34, 1999.

51. Fitch RH, Brown CP, Tallal P, et al: Effects of sex and MK-801 on auditory-processing deficits associated with developmental microgyric lesions in rats. *Behav Neurosci* 111:404–412, 1997.
52. Rauschecker JP: Compensatory plasticity and sensory substitution in the cerebral cortex. *Trends Neurosci* 18:36–43, 1995.
53. Rauschecker JP: Mechanisms of compensatory plasticity in the cerebral cortex. *Adv Neurol* 73:137–146, 1997.
54. Pascual-Leone A, Torres F: Plasticity of the sensorimotor cortex representation of the reading finger in Braille readers. *Brain* 116:39–52, 1993.
55. Pascual-Leone A, Cammarota A, Wassermann EM, et al: Modulation of motor cortical outputs to the reading hand of Braille readers. *Ann Neurol* 34:33–37, 1993.
56. Pascual-Leone A, Hamilton R, Tormos JM, et al: Neuroplasticity in the adjustment to blindness., in Grafman J, Christen Y (ed): *Neuroplasticity: Building a Bridge from the Laboratory to the Clinic.* Munich and New York: Springer-Verlag, 1998.
57. Pascual-Leone A, Wassermann EM, Sadato N, et al: The role of reading activity on the modulation of motor cortical outputs to the reading hand in Braille readers. *Ann Neurol* 38:910–915, 1995.
58. van Boven R, Hamilton R, Kaufman T, et al: Tactile spatial resolution in blind Braille readers. *Neurology* 54:2030–2036, 2000.
59. Pascual-Leone A, Grafman J, Hallett M: Modulation of cortical motor output maps during development of implicit and explicit knowledge. *Science* 263:1287–1289, 1994.
60. Karni A, Bertini G: Learning perceptual skills: Behavioral probes into adult cortical plasticity. *Curr Opin Neurobiol* 7:530–535, 1997.
61. Sadato N, Pascual-Leone A, Grafman J, et al: Activation of the primary visual cortex by Braille reading in blind subjects. *Nature* 380:526–528, 1996.
62. Sadato N, Pascual-Leone A, Grafman J, et al: Neural networks for Braille reading by the blind. *Brain* 121:1213–1229, 1998.
63. Cohen LG, Celnik P, Pascual-Leone A, et al: Functional relevance of cross-modal plasticity in blind humans. *Nature* 389:180–183, 1997.
64. Cohen LG, Weeks RA, Sadato N, et al: Period of susceptibility for cross-modal plasticity in the blind. *Ann Neurol* 45:51–460, 1999.
65. Weeks R, Horwitz B, Aziz-Sultan A, et al: A positron emission tomography study of auditory localization in the congenitally blind. *J Neurosci* 20:2664–2672, 2000.

Chapter 6

THE LESION METHOD IN BEHAVIORAL NEUROLOGY AND NEUROPSYCHOLOGY

Hanna Damasio
Antonio R. Damasio

The lesion method aims at establishing a correlation between a circumscribed region of brain damage, a lesion and a pattern of alteration in some aspect of an experimentally controlled cognitive or behavioral performance. The brain-damaged region is conceptualized as part of a large-scale network of cortical and subcortical sites that operate in concert, by virtue of their interlocking connectivity, to produce a particular function. Given a theoretical framework for how such networks are constituted and carry out that particular function, a lesion is thus a *probe* to test a specific hypothesis. A lesion probe allows the investigator to decide whether damage to a component of the putative network, responsible for function X, alters the network behavior according to the predictions made for it. In other words, given a theory about the operations of a normal brain, lesions are a means to support or falsify the theory.

The subjects for the lesion method may be humans or animals. The lesions may have been produced by neurologic disease alone or incurred in the process of treating it (e.g., a surgical procedure). They may be small or large and may be studied in vivo or at postmortem. The indispensable requirements are that lesions be stable, well demarcated, and referable to a neuroanatomic unit. In this chapter we focus on human lesions, produced by neurologic disease or surgical ablation and studied in vivo with modern neuroimaging techniques.

The lesion approach provided the first method in what was to become neuroscience. In the very least, it dates to Morgagni's demonstration of an association between unilateral brain disease and contralateral sensory and motor disabilities. Bouillaud's and Broca's finding of a correlation between speech and focal damage to the frontal lobe are reasonable signposts to mark the modern era of lesion studies.

In the latter decades of the nineteenth century, the lesion method led to pathbreaking discoveries. But although most of the findings have stood the test of time and gained wide acceptance, the theories that were associated with them did not. The pioneering neurologists conceived of the existence of brain centers capable of performing complex psychological functions with relative independence. What little interaction there was among those few and noncontiguous centers was achieved by unidirectional pathways. These concepts were subject to deserved criticism, the best known of which came from Sigmund Freud and Hughlings Jackson. As the theoretical account lost influence, the lesion method, which was closely interwoven with the theory, lost favor as a means of valid scientific inquiry.

The lesion method began to regain some prominence in the 1960s, perhaps as a reaction to the impasses of "equipotential" antilocalizationism and "black-box" behaviorism. The revival was spearheaded by Geschwind's reflections on the work of Wernicke, Lichtheim, Liepmann, and Déjerine and by the work of notable neuropsychologists, among whom were A. R. Luria, Henri Hécaen, Brenda Milner, Arthur Benton, Hans-Lukas Teuber, and Oliver Zangwill. The full value of the lesion method, however, only began to be appreciated after the development of new neuroimaging technologies—computed tomography (CT), which had its inception in 1973, and magnetic resonance imaging (MRI), which emerged a decade later.

It has gradually become evident that the lesion method should be separated from the theoretical accounts historically connected with it. As with any other approach, this method has limitations and misapplications. Nonetheless, it is one entity, with its virtues and pitfalls, and the theoretical constructs that make use of it represent another. Nothing prevents practitioners of the lesion method from proposing the richest and most dynamic accounts of brain function.

In short, the classically discovered links between certain brain regions of the cerebral cortex and signs of neuropsychological dysfunction have been validated, remain a staple of clinical neurology, and allow for relatively accurate predictions of *localization of damage* from neurologic signs. That is, more often than not, the presence of certain neuropsychological defects indicates to the clinical expert that there is dysfunction in a specific brain area. These valid links, however, should not be taken to mean that the functions disturbed by the lesion were inscribed in the tissue that the lesion destroyed. The complex psychological functions, which usually constitute the target of neuropsychological studies in humans, are not localizable at that level.

The neural architectures revealed by neuroanatomy and neurophysiology and the cognitive architectures revealed by experimental neuropsychology suggest that single-center functions, single-purpose pathways, and unidirectional cascades of information process are unrealistic. Moreover, the residual performance that follows focal brain insults, and the ensuing patterns of recovery, suggest that knowledge must be widely distributed, at multiple neural levels, and complex psychological functions must emerge from the cooperation of multiple components of integrated networks (see Chaps. 4 and 10).

Two key developments made human lesion studies rewarding again. First, lesion studies in nonhuman primates brought major advances to the understanding of the neural basis of vision and memory, as demonstrated, among others, by Mishkin and colleagues. Second, the advent of CT and MRI began to permit human lesion studies in vivo. It is apparent now that the lesion method is indispensable to cognitive neuroscience, especially when it comes to human studies. The *new* lesion method is not concerned with "localizing functions," nor is it a contest for "localizing lesions." It is a means to test, at systems level, hypotheses regarding *both* neural structure *and* cognitive processes. What investigators from Déjerine to Geschwind gleaned from single cases can now be replicated systematically in a suitable group of subjects. Hypotheses old and new, including some advanced by the pioneer neuropsychologists, can be tested experimentally.

Beyond their intrinsic value, the results from the new lesion method in humans provide a welcome complement to results from neuroanatomic and neurophysiologic experiments in animals. Lesion work in humans has revealed characteristics of neural systems that could not have been investigated in experimental animals. The example of linguistic processes is the most obvious. Lesion results have also been the source of hypotheses that were further investigated in animals and in humans. Ungerleider and Mishkin's study of ventral and dorsal visual pathways in nonhuman primates[1] was inspired by Newcombe's work in humans.[2] Conversely, Ungerleider and Mishkin's work was followed up in humans, and the inferotemporal system has now been anatomically and functionally fractionated.[3–5] Moreover, the lesion method offers the possibility of conducting indepth experiments on some cognitive operations whose temporal characteristics are not suitable for other approaches (for instance, experiments requiring the monitoring of psychophysiologic variables).

We also see the lesion method as joining forces with two other approaches to the investigation of human brain function: electrophysiologic studies and functional imaging. The first includes the use of event-related potentials, the study of cognitive and behavioral changes induced by electrical stimulation of exposed cerebral cortex, and the direct recording of activity from cerebral cortex. The second involves the imaging of brain activity inferred from the differential emission of radio signals. It encompasses positron emission tomography (PET), single photon emission computed tomography (SPECT), and functional magnetic resonance imaging (fMRI). The combination of results from the lesion method with those from the other approaches will strengthen our conceptualization of the human brain and bring to light discrepancies that require new theorizing and experimentation. Many well-established facts from the lesion method remain the benchmark against which some results of the new dynamic methods must be measured. Moreover, the actual combination of procedures is likely to generate more powerful tools. This will become reality, for instance, with the performance of PET and fMRI studies in patients with focal lesions causing specific cognitive disorders.

COLOR PLATES

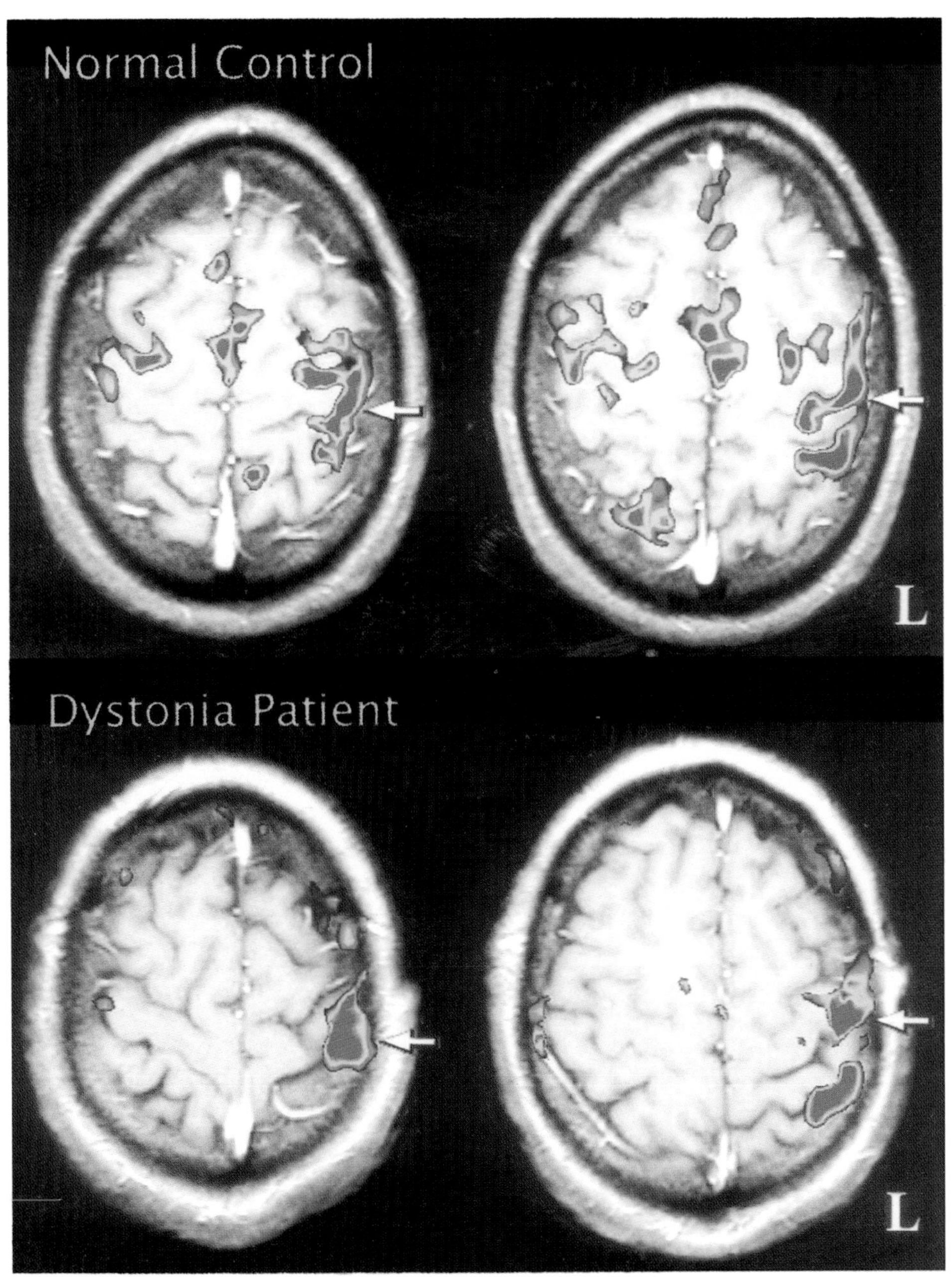

PLATE 1 (Figure 5-2)
The figure displays the fMRI images of a normal and a dystonic guitar player executing right hand arpeggios in the scanner. Note the greater activation of the sensory-motor cortex (arrows) and the lack of activation of premotor and supplementary motor cortices in the dystonic patient. (Modified from Pujol et al.,[41] with permission.)

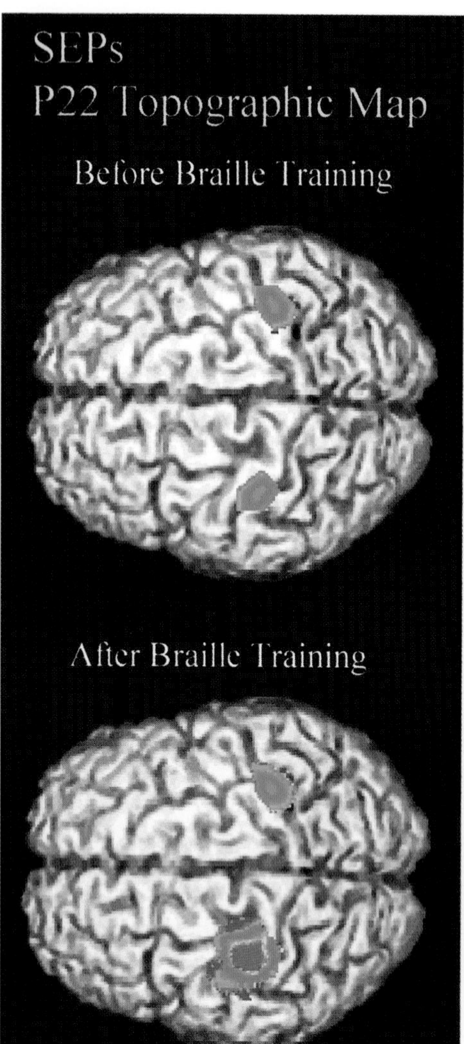

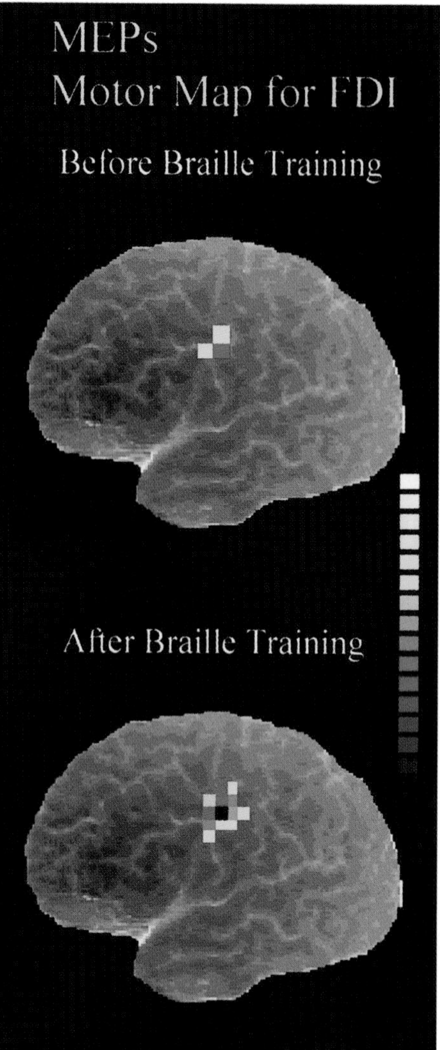

PLATE 2 (Figure 5-3)
Evidence of plasticity in sensory, motor, and occipital cortex in early blind subjects after learning Braille. Representative example of the studies performed before and at the end of one year of learning Braille are shown. The different studies were conducted on different subjects using somatosensory evoked potentials (SEPs) to mechanical stimuli to the index finger pad (adapted from Pascual-Leone and Torres,[54] with permission), motor mapping with transcranial magnetic stimulation of the potentials evoked in the first dorsal interosseus muscle FDI, side-to-side mover of the index finger (adapted from Pascual-Leone et al.,[43] with permission), and functional magnetic resonance imaging (fMRI) while reading Braille characters. (Modified from Hamilton and Pascual-Leone,[12] with permission.)

A

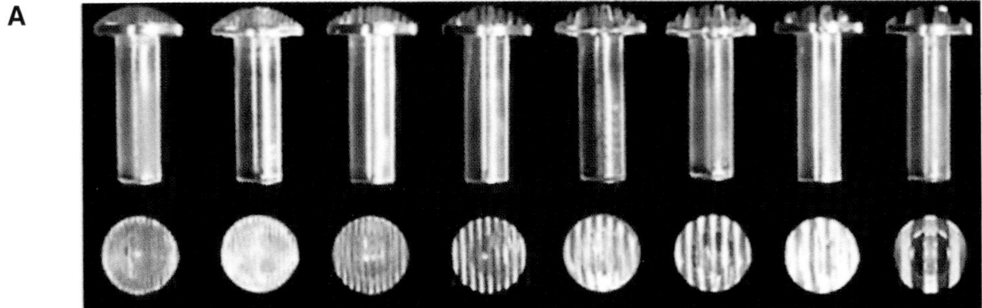

B

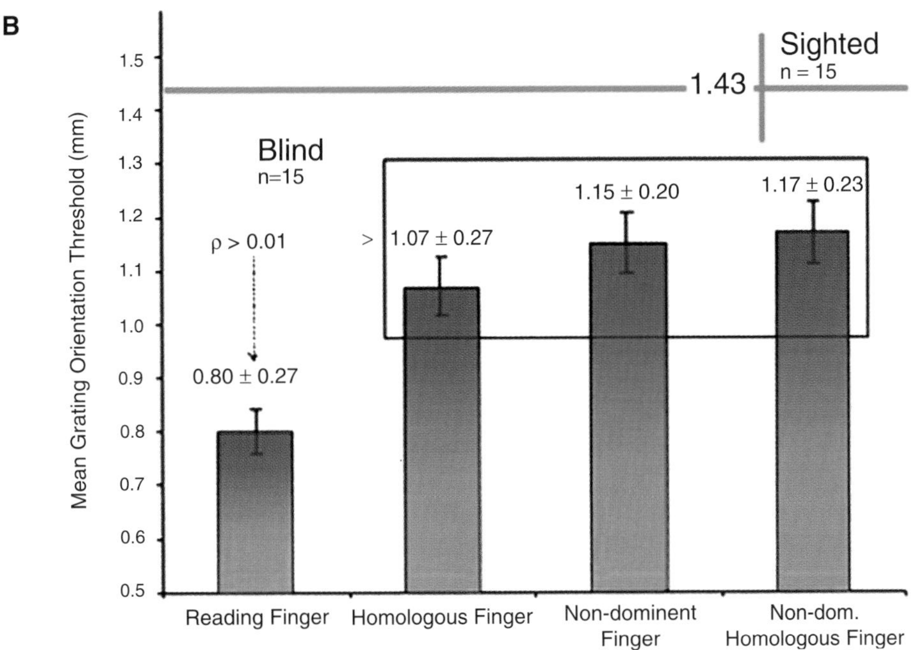

PLATE 3 (Figure 5-4)

A. JVP Domes used for gratings orientations discrimination testing. B. Histogram displaying the thresholds for grating orientation discrimination in early blind and sighted control subjects. Note the marked superiority (lower thresholds) of the blind subjects in general and in paricular of their dominant Braille reading finger. (Modified from van Boven et al.,[58] with permission.)

PLATE 4 (Figure 5-5)
A. Activation of the occipital cortex in congenitally and early blind subjects during tactile Braille reading as demonstrated by positron emission tomography (PET). (Modified from Sadato et al.,[61] with permission.) B. Effects of repetitive transcranial magnetic stimulation (TMS) to the occipital or somatosensory cortex on tactile Braille reading ability in early blind subjects and on tactile perception of embossed Roman letter in sighted controls. (Modified from Cohen et al.,[63] with permission.)

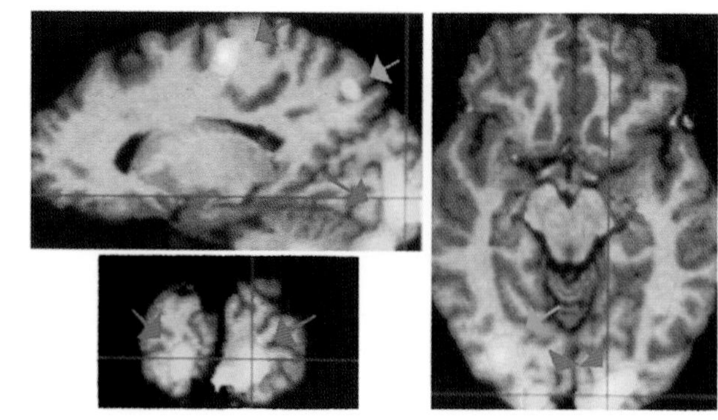

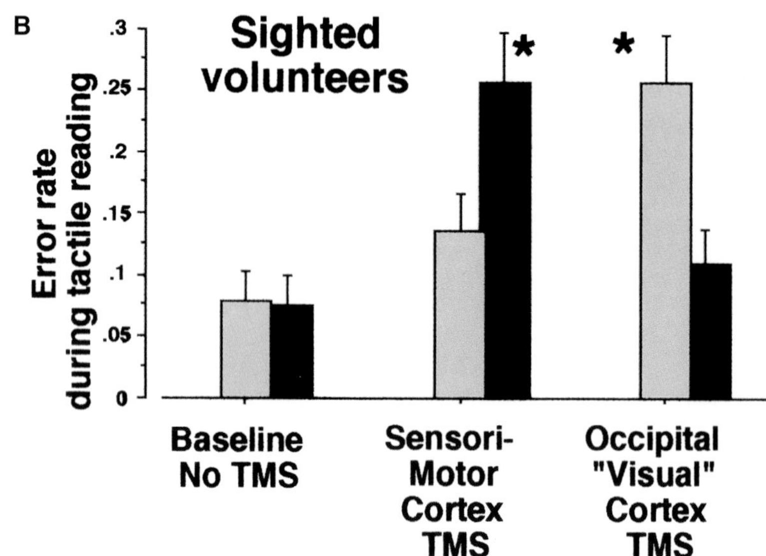

PLATE 5 (Figure 6-1) ►
Three-dimensional reconstruction (obtained from 124 contiguous thin coronal MRI slices) of the brain of a subject with an infarct in the left frontal lobe. Acutely, the subject had a nonfluent aphasia and mild paresis of the right face and arm. At the time of the MRI (1 year later), both language deficit and paresis had improved. Several sulci were identified and color-coded on the 3D reconstructed brain: central sulcus (red), precentral sulcus (green), inferior frontal sulcus (yellow), superior frontal sulcus (brown), and sylvian fissure (magenta). Inspection of the left lateral and top views of the brain shows that the area of infarct is centered on the precentral sulcus, which is clearly visible only in the top view. The most anterior sector of the precentral gyrus is damaged, as well as the posterior sector of the middle frontal and inferior frontal gyrus. The brain volume was also resectioned in axial (ax), coronal (co), and parasagittal (ps) slices (as shown in the three rows of brain slices in the lower segment of the image). Whenever any of the slices intersected a color-coded sulcus, the color automatically appeared on the slice, thus permitting an accurate identification of sulci and of gyri. Resectioning allowed us to inspect the lesion in depth and show that it extended all the way to the insula, which is compromised in its most superior sector (best seen in slice ps-3).

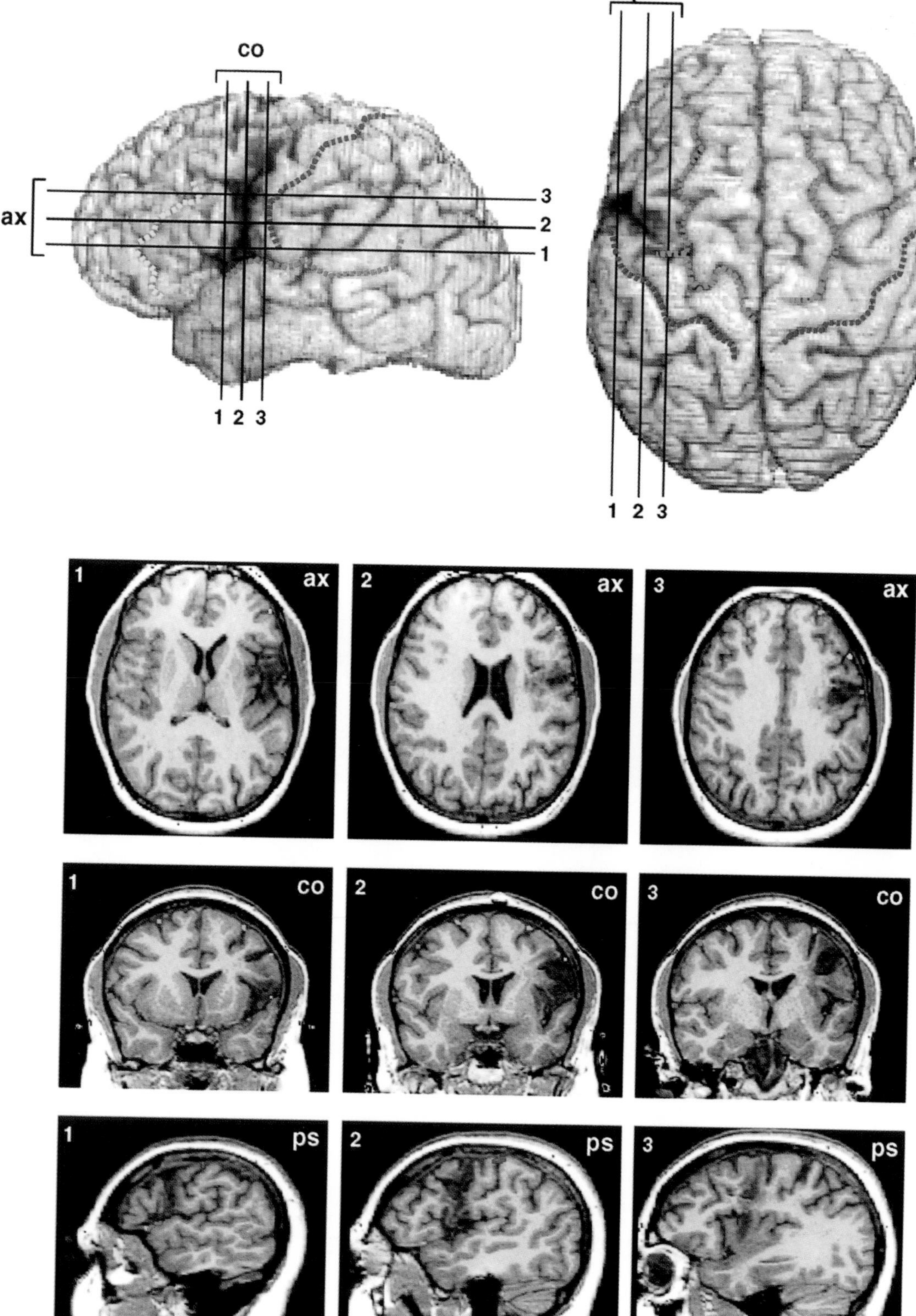

co
ax
3
2
1
1 2 3
ps
1 2 3
1 ax
2 ax
3 ax
1 co
2 co
3 co
1 ps
2 ps
3 ps

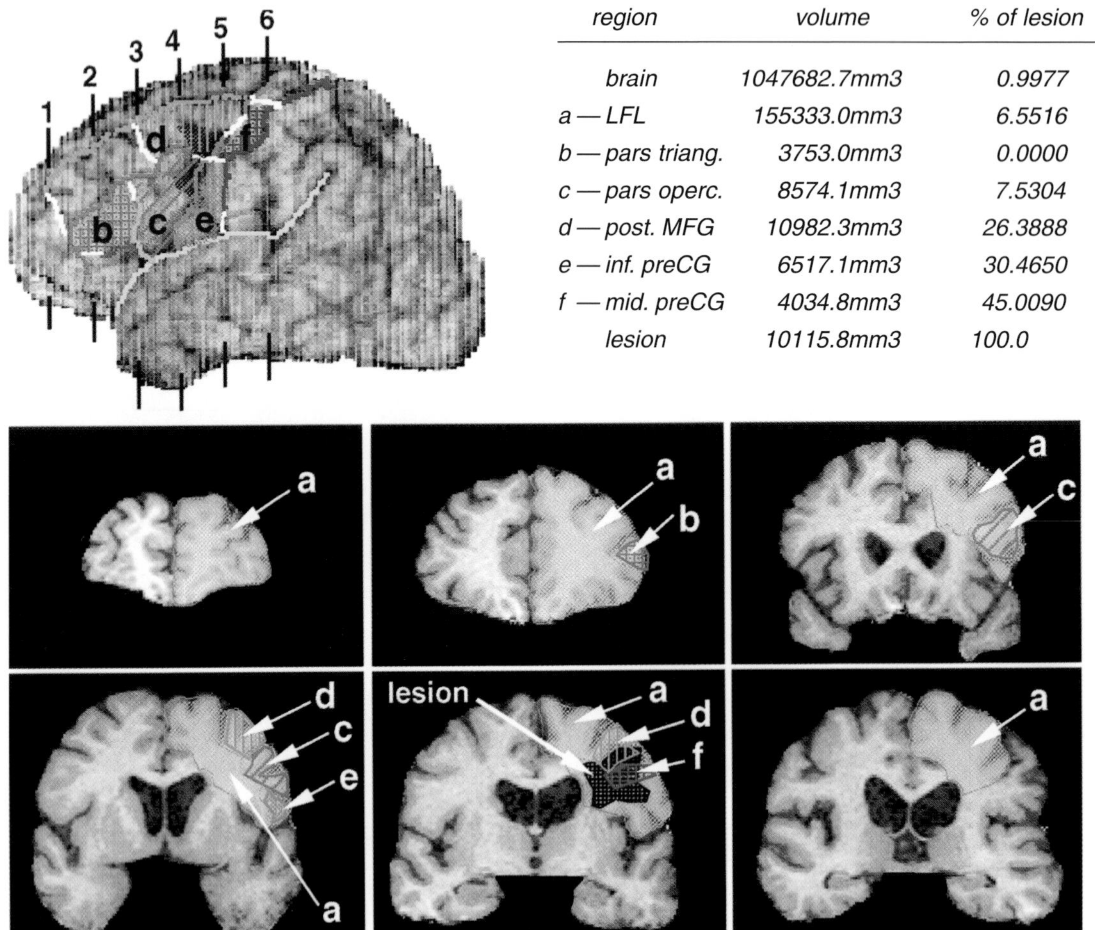

region	volume	% of lesion
brain	1047682.7mm3	0.9977
a — LFL	155333.0mm3	6.5516
b — pars triang.	3753.0mm3	0.0000
c — pars operc.	8574.1mm3	7.5304
d — post. MFG	10982.3mm3	26.3888
e — inf. preCG	6517.1mm3	30.4650
f — mid. preCG	4034.8mm3	45.0090
lesion	10115.8mm3	100.0

PLATE 6 (Figure 6-2)

Three-dimensional reconstruction of a human brain with a lesion in the left frontal lobe. The questions addressed here concerned the size of the lesion and the percentage of volume it occupied in the whole brain, in the left frontal lobe (LFL), and in some subdivisions of the frontal lobe: the pars triangularis (pars triang.) and the pars opercularis (pars operc.), the posterior half of the middle frontal gyrus (post. MFG), and the precentral gyrus in its inferior (inf. preCG) and middle thirds (mid. preCG). The limits of all of these regions of interest (ROI) were marked on the 3D reconstructed brain. On all coronal slices, the several ROIs are individually traced, as is the contour of the lesion. Six coronal slices are shown as an example. The different ROIs are color- and texture-coded. The automatically calculated absolute volumes and the percentage of damage in each of them are recorded on the top right-hand corner.

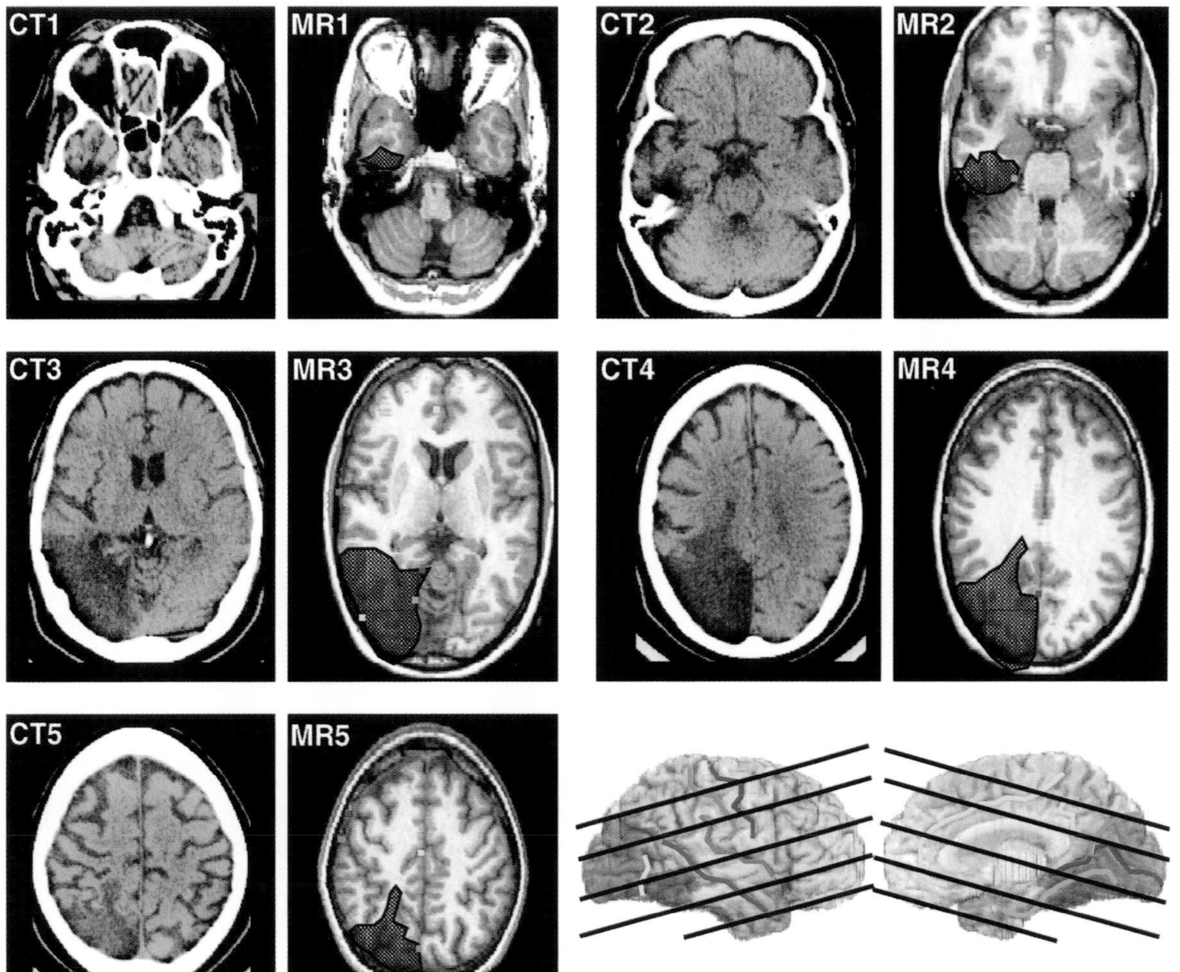

PLATE 7 (Figure 6-3)

Demonstration of the improved template method. Brain CT (CT 1–5) of a subject who could not undergo an MRI study. A normal 3D reconstructed brain was resliced so as to match the orientation and level of the CT slices (MR 1–5). The lesion seen on the CT slices was transferred onto each matched MR slice, taking into account all identifiable sulci and gyri. Once the sulci were color-coded on the 3D reconstruction, the lesion could be read off each individual slice. The object defined by the transferred traces could be fused with the normal brain to visualize the lesion's surface extent (right lower corner).

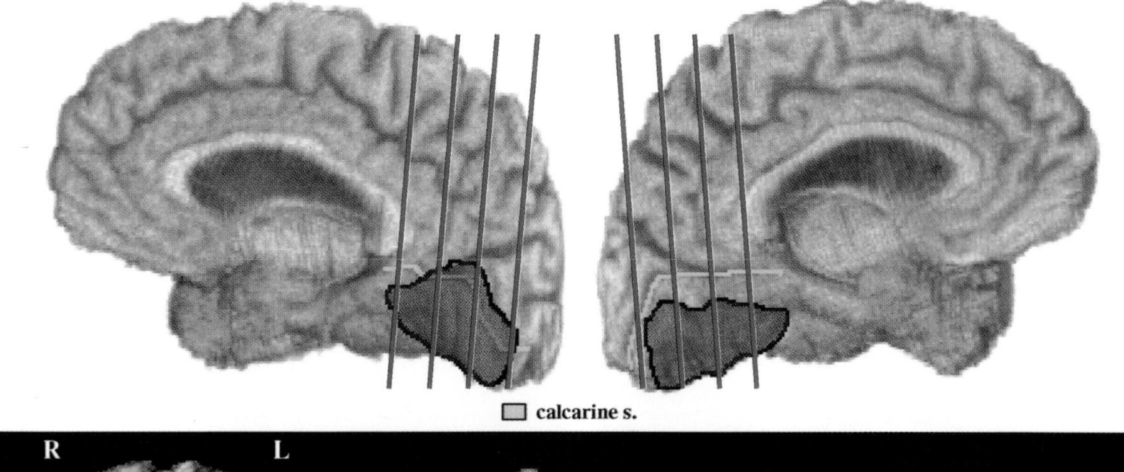

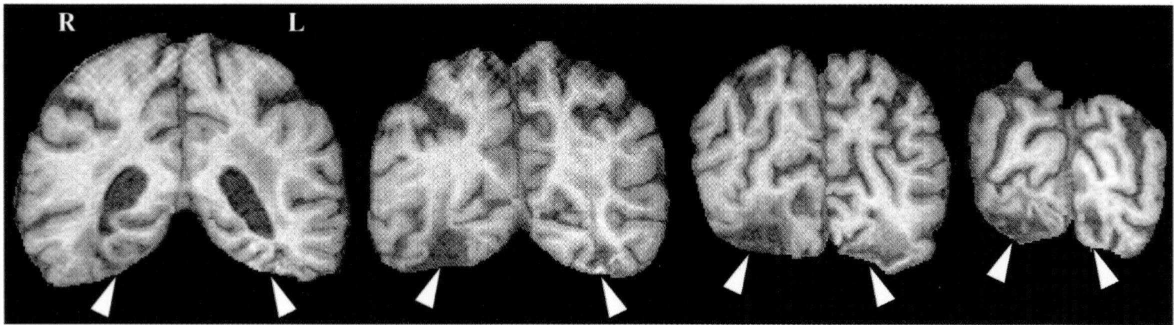

PLATE 8 (Figure 20-2)

Top: Mesial views of a three-dimensional MRI reconstruction of a patient who sustained bilateral infarcts in the infracalcarine visual association cortices (the right hemisphere is on the left, and, vice, versa). Bottom: The lesions are shown in coronal MRI sections (arrows), which correspond to the four planes marked with red lines in the mesial hemispheric views. The patient had a superior altitudinal hemianopia. In the lower fields, form vision was normal, but color perception was impaired—i.e., the patient was achromatopsic. The patient also had prosopagnosia in connection with these lesions.

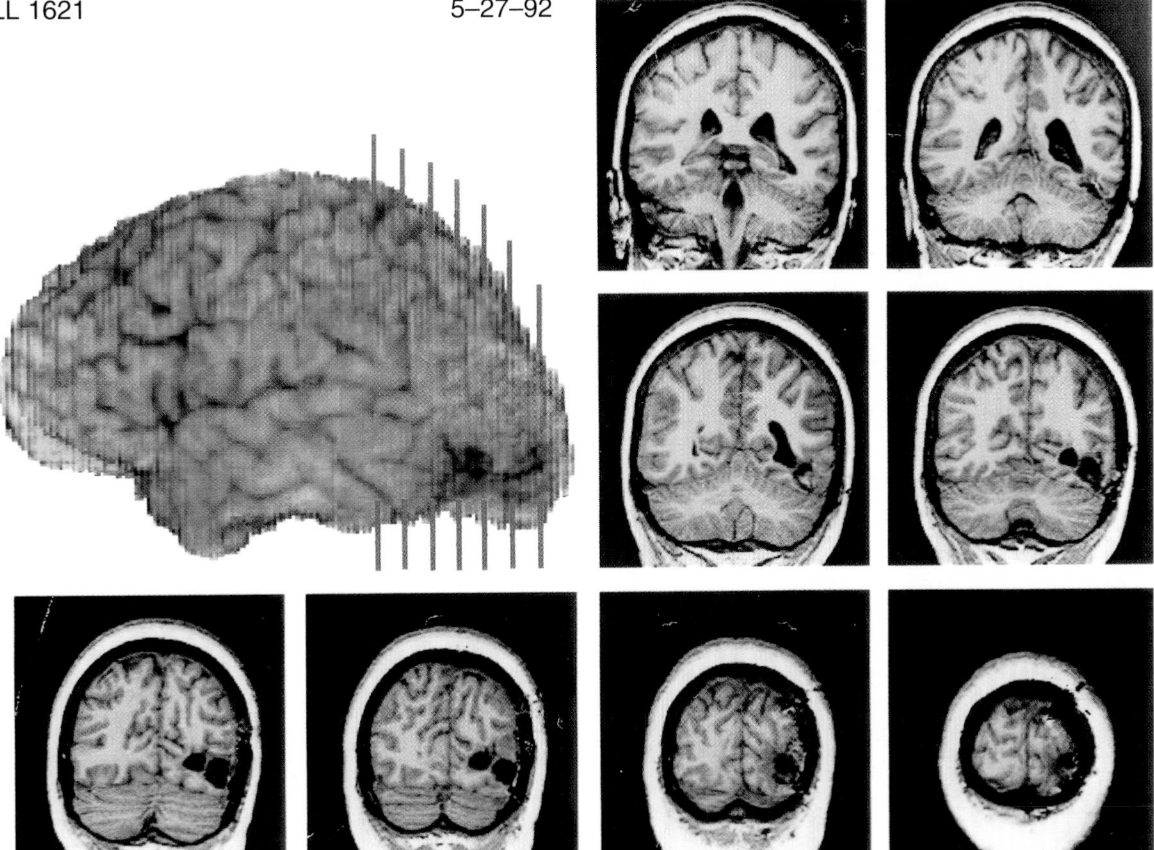

PLATE 9 (Figure 20-3)
Three-dimensional reconstruction of a T1-weighted MRI in a patient with hemiachromatopsia, pure alexia, and category-specific visual object agnosia. The lesion, centered in the left occipitotemporal region, involves parts of the lingual and fusiform gyri.

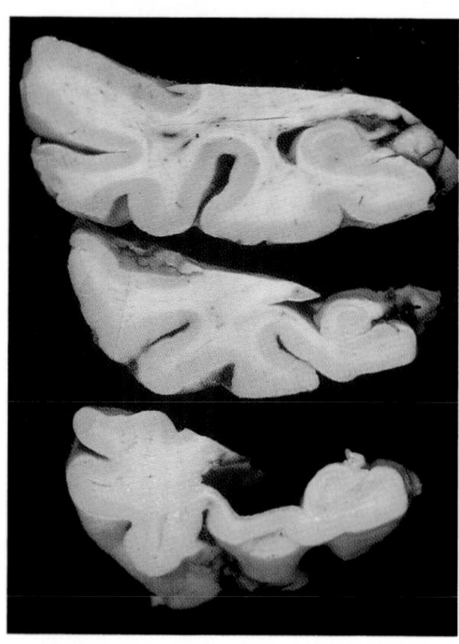

PLATE 10 (Figure 44-2)
Atrophy of the hippocampus. The upper section comes from a control without neurologic symptoms. The hippocampus has a normal volume. The two other sections come from patients with Alzheimer's disease at various stages. Maximal atrophy is seen on the lowest section.

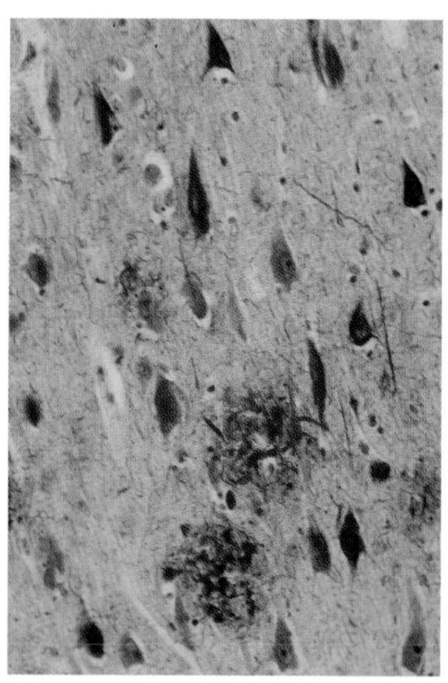

PLATE 11 (Figure 44-3)
The two main lesions of Alzheimer's disease: (1) neurofibrillary tangles (NFT) are located in the neuronal cell body and appear in black; (2) SPs are seen as spheres made of entangled neurites. Bielschowsky silver impregnation counterstained by cresyl violet. Staining performed by Dr. Joachim Kauss. Initial magnification: x750.

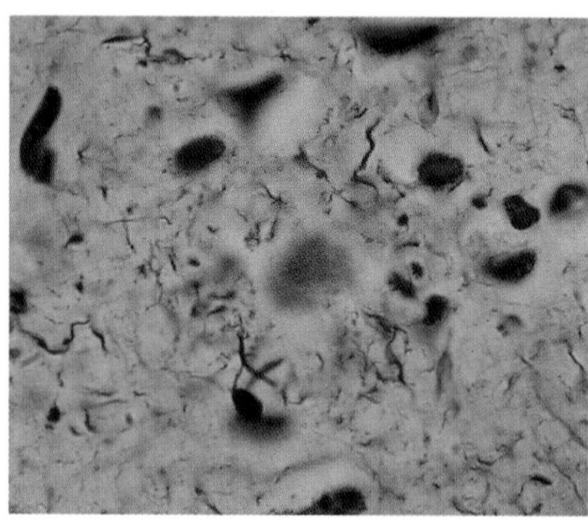

PLATE 12 (Figure 44-4)
Senile plaques. The SP, in the center of the picture, is a composite lesion. Its center, stained gray, is made of amorphous extracellular material, mainly composed of Aβ peptide. Other stains, such as Congo red, would show its "amyloid" nature. Around the amyloid center a crown of degenerating neurites is clearly seen. The nuclei that are in contact with the plaque belong for the most part to microglial cells. Initial magnification: x1200.

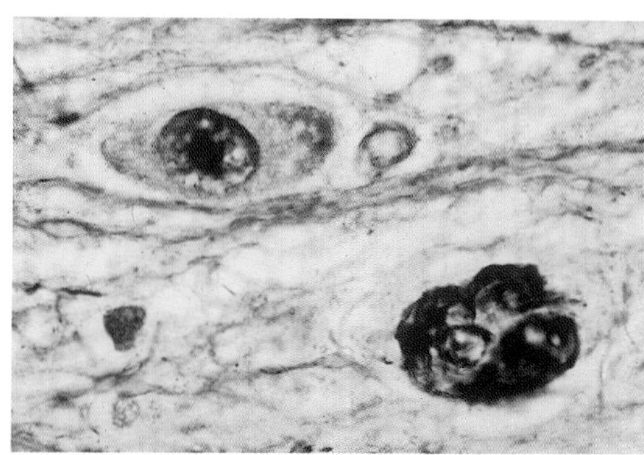

PLATE 13 (Figure 44-5)
Neurofibrillary tangle. This high-power view of the nucleus basalis of Meynert shows two neurons; the cytoplasm of the normal neuron appears light brown. The second neuron contains an NFT made of deep black fibrils surrounding and partly overlapping the nucleus. Bodian silver impregnation. Initial magnification: x2500.

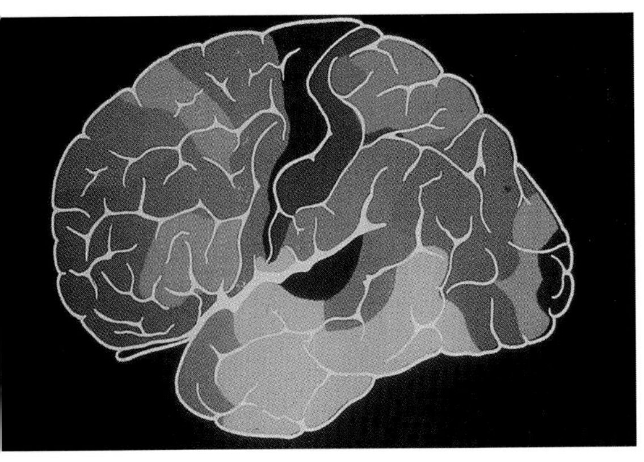

PLATE 14 (Figure 44-6A)
Comparison of the distribution of neurofibrillary tangles with the functional organization of the cortical areas. Distribution of the cortical NFTs. (From Arnold et al.,[147] with permission.) The density of the lesions is indicated by the following color scale: dark blue (no lesion); light blue, green, yellow, and orange (maximal density of lesions).

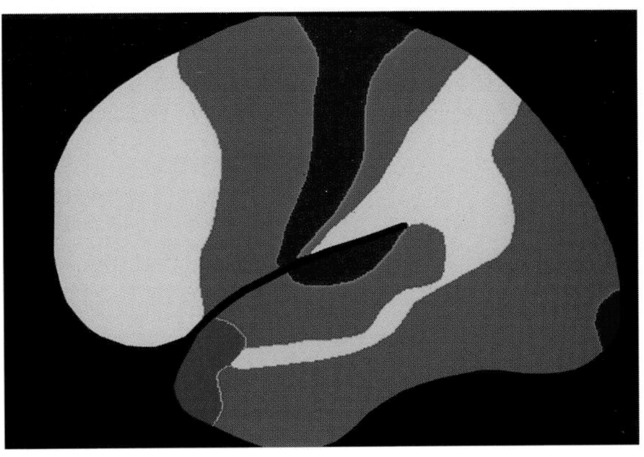

PLATE 15 (Figure 44-6B)
Classification of functional cortical zones in relation with Brodmann's map according to Mesulam.[77] Blue: primary sensory areas. Green: unimodal association cortex. Yellow: multimodal association areas. Red: paralimbic areas.

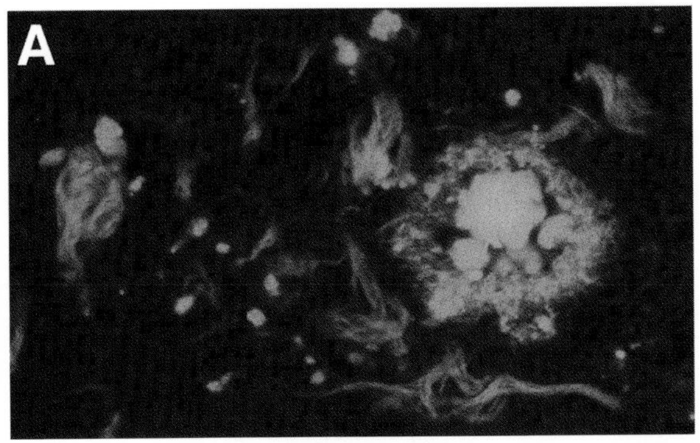

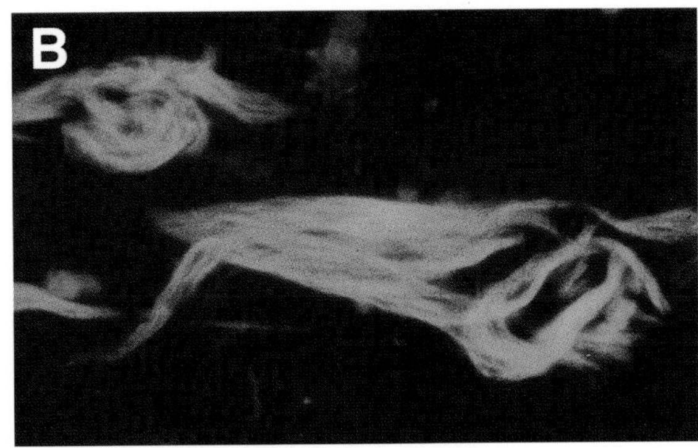

PLATE 16 (Figure 45-1)
The classic lesions of AD, as seen using thioflavin S staining and fluorescent microscopy. A. Mature plaque with dense amyloid core. B. NFTs in the entorhinal cortex. (Photographs provided by Dr. Robert D. Terry.)

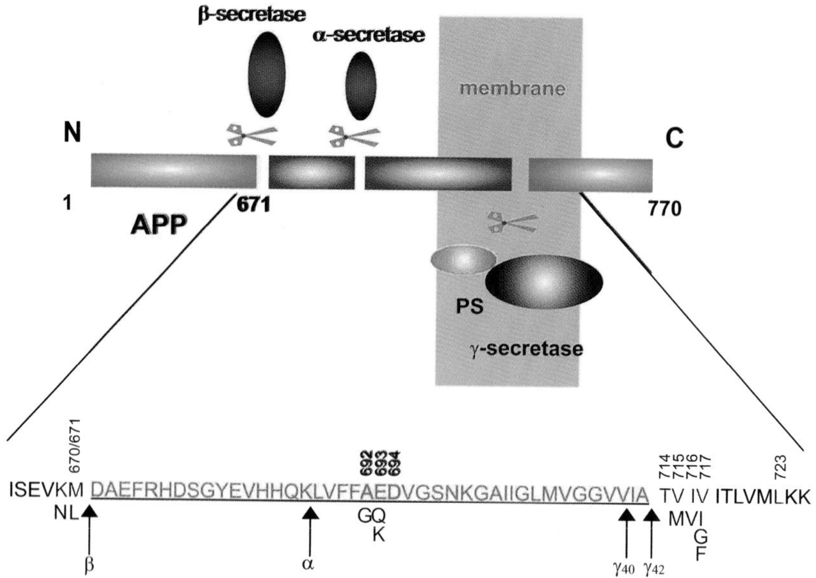

PLATE 17 (Figure 45-2)
Schematic diagram of APP and its mutations genetically linked to familial AD. The sequence in APP that contains the Aβ and the transmembrane region is expanded. The underlined residues represent $A\beta_{1-42}$. The letters below the line indicate the currently known missense mutations linked to familial AD.

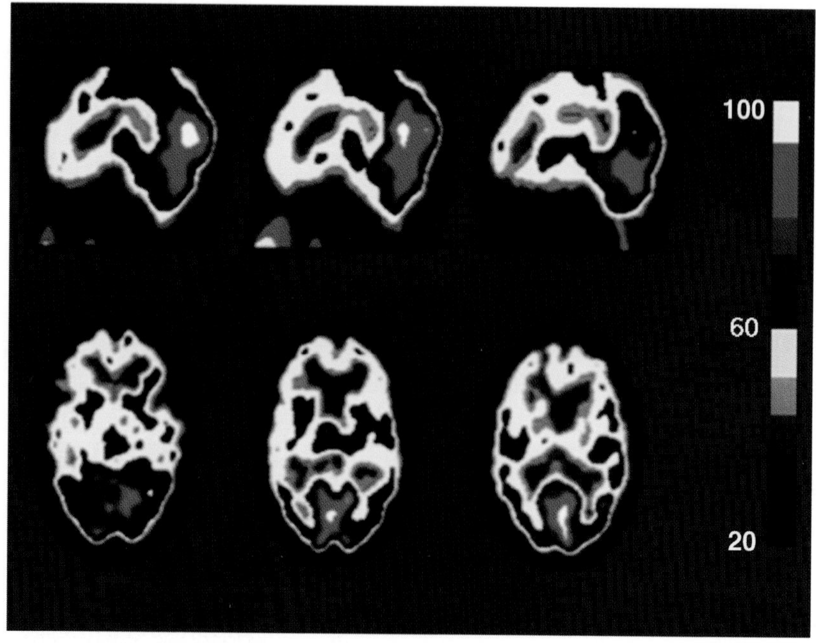

PLATE 18 (Figure 47-2)
Single photon emission computed tomography (SPECT) scans of patient with Pick's disease demonstrating frontal hypometabolism.

The lesion method does have its limitations. Not every anatomic region of the human nervous system can be properly sampled by natural lesions, and the size of the lesions provides a natural limit to the structures the method can probe with confidence. And yet, in its modern incarnation, the approach provides data currently unavailable through other means.

Only a concerted set of approaches from the molecular to the systems levels, in both humans and experimental animals, can eventually provide answers to the questions currently posed in cognitive neuroscience. The lesion method is a key partner in systems-level studies.

THE MODERN PRACTICE OF THE LESION METHOD IN HUMANS

There are at least five prerequisites for the modern practice of the lesion method: first, the availability of fine-grained structural imaging of the living human brain; second, the availability of a reliable method for the anatomic study of lesion probes; third, access to a large pool of subjects with lesions in varied brain sites, so that hypotheses regarding the operation of different systems can be experimentally tested in comparable target subjects and in appropriate controls; fourth, the availability of reliable techniques for various cognitive measurements; and fifth, the guidance of testable hypotheses concerning the neural basis of specific cognitive processes at systems level. In the following pages, we discuss some of these requisites.

Neuroanatomy from Neuroimaging

For many years, we have conceptualized the systematic neuroimaging studies pursued in our laboratory as a means to practice *human neuroanatomy from imaging data,* i.e., a means for detection and description of a lesion and consideration of its placement in the context of the anatomic systems to which it belongs. This purpose, which requires detailed knowledge of human neuroanatomy, is distinguishable from the traditional role of neuroimaging in *clinical neurologic diagnosis,* i.e., the detection of structural alterations and the prediction of its possible neuropathologic basis. The original tool for these studies was the template technique,[6] but we have since developed a new technique for individualized lesion analysis based on the three-dimensional (3D) reconstruction of the human brain from high-resolution MRI.[7] This new technique is known as BRAINVOX. It permits us to identify reliably, in vivo, every major gyrus and sulcus of the human brain; to slice and reslice the human brain in whatever incidence is necessary for anatomic analysis; and to define and measure volumes or surfaces of interest in single cases and across groups. The technique dispenses with charting onto brain templates and permits instead a customized definition of each subject. We will comment on this technique first and complete this section with a review of the template technique.

BRAINVOX

BRAINVOX is a 3D volumetric imaging and analysis system. The software was originally developed to facilitate the 3D display and mapping of acquired human brain lesions using a volume-rendering approach, but it has grown to support a wide range of advanced multimodality neuroanatomic visualization and analysis techniques. Although BRAINVOX was designed for the analysis of high-resolution volumetric MRI, it can be used with CT and PET.

BRAINVOX consists of several interconnected software components: (1) a slice/contour–based tracing module, (2) a multivolume 3D rendering system, (3) a set of general-purpose volume-manipulation tools, (4) a basic volume–data-handling system, (5) a palette editor, and (6) a volumetric object-measurement system.

BRAINVOX allows for explicit definition of volumes bounded by tracings that can be separated from the full MRI volume. The software allows users to define many such volumes simultaneously, slice by slice, taking advantage of common borders, edge tracking, and flexible trace-editing tools. Volume and intersection volume statistics can be computed for all objects defined in this manner. Histograms of volumes and individual slices can be computed.

Lesion Analysis with BRAINVOX

Using the 3D reconstructed brain to determine which anatomic sectors of each hemisphere are damaged obviates the need to adjust the angle in which the MRI sections are obtained to the angle of available template systems. The accuracy of interpretation no longer depends on the "reading" of a template with the transferred lesion but rather on the direct reading from the identified landmarks in the unique brain in question.

The new technique permits a direct identification of gyri and sulci, comparable to what can be achieved at the autopsy table in a postmortem brain after the meninges have been removed. The technique permits the accurate marking of such structures in coronal axial or parasagittal slices, with the advantage that the extension of lesions into the depths of sulci can also be determined (Fig. 6-1, Plate 5).

Other advantages of the new technique are as follows. First, the identification of anatomic structures is based on each individual brain rather than on an idealized "average" brain. The standard landmarks of each area of interest can be localized in the brain of each individual subject rather than on a template. Although templates use anatomic constants, they cannot account for individual variation and thus introduce an error of measurement, albeit small in some cases. Second, because each area of interest has been customized for each subject, it is possible to determine with considerable rigor the proportion of a given area that has been destroyed by a lesion as well as the proportion of subjacent white matter that has been involved by the lesion (Fig. 6-2, Plate 6). Again, error is reduced.

This new technique requires a T1-weighted MRI scan with contiguous thin slices (1.5 mm). For best results, the scan should be performed in the chronic stage. Regular MRI scans obtained for diagnostic purposes with thicker slices, interslice gaps, and other pulse specifications are not adequate for reconstruction. Furthermore, application of this elaborate procedure to acute lesions would be a waste of effort.

The Template Technique

Whenever MRI or CT scans are obtained with regular parameters (thick slices, and, in the case of MRI, interslice gaps), anatomic analyses must rely on the template technique.

The template technique relies on film transparencies of MRI or CT. For research purposes, it is advisable to have a technician collect all the films for a given case, mask the subject identification in all of them, and substitute a numerical entry code on the basis of which imaging data can be stored. This step ensures that the investigator performing the anatomic study is blind to the neurologic and neuropsychological data available for the same subject.

Figure 6-1 (Plate 5)

Three-dimensional reconstruction (obtained from 124 contiguous thin coronal MRI slices) of the brain of a subject with an infarct in the left frontal lobe. Acutely, the subject had a nonfluent aphasia and mild paresis of the right face and arm. At the time of the MRI (1 year later), both language deficit and paresis had improved.

Several sulci were identified and color-coded on the 3D reconstructed brain: central sulcus (red), precentral sulcus (green), inferior frontal sulcus (yellow), superior frontal sulcus (brown), and sylvian fissure (magenta).

Inspection of the left lateral and top views of the brain shows that the area of infarct is centered on the precentral sulcus, which is clearly visible only in the top view. The most anterior sector of the precentral gyrus is damaged, as well as the posterior sector of the middle frontal and inferior frontal gyrus.

The brain volume was also resectioned in axial (ax), coronal (co), and parasagittal (ps) slices (as shown in the three rows of brain slices in the lower segment of the image). Whenever any of the slices intersected a color-coded sulcus, the color automatically appeared on the slice, thus permitting an accurate identification of sulci and of gyri. Resectioning allowed us to inspect the lesion in depth and show that it extended all the way to the insula, which is compromised in its most superior sector (best seen in slice ps-3).

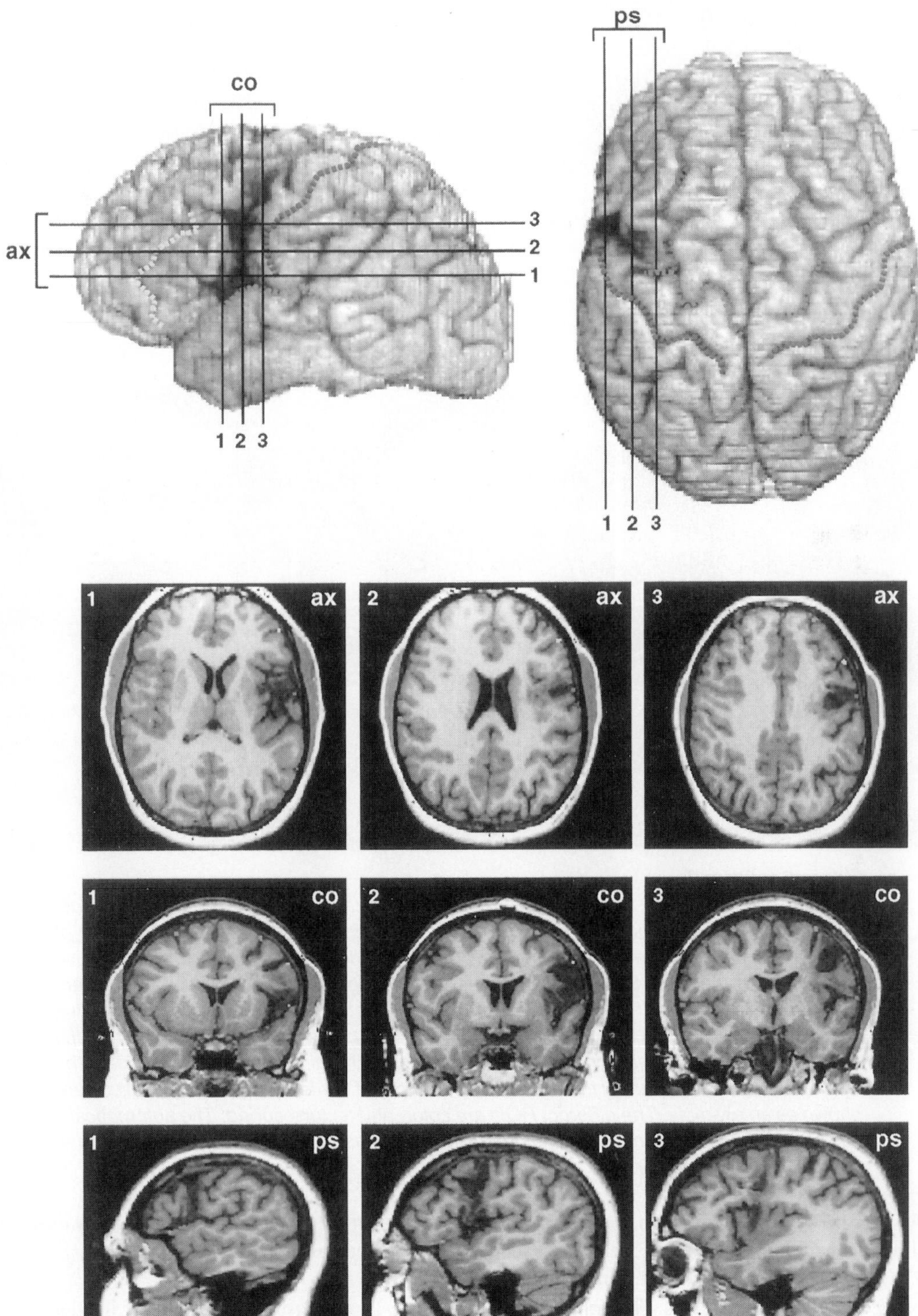
co
1 2 3
ax
3
2
1
1 2 3
ps
1 2 3
1 ax
2 ax
3 ax
1 co
2 co
3 co
1 ps
2 ps
3 ps

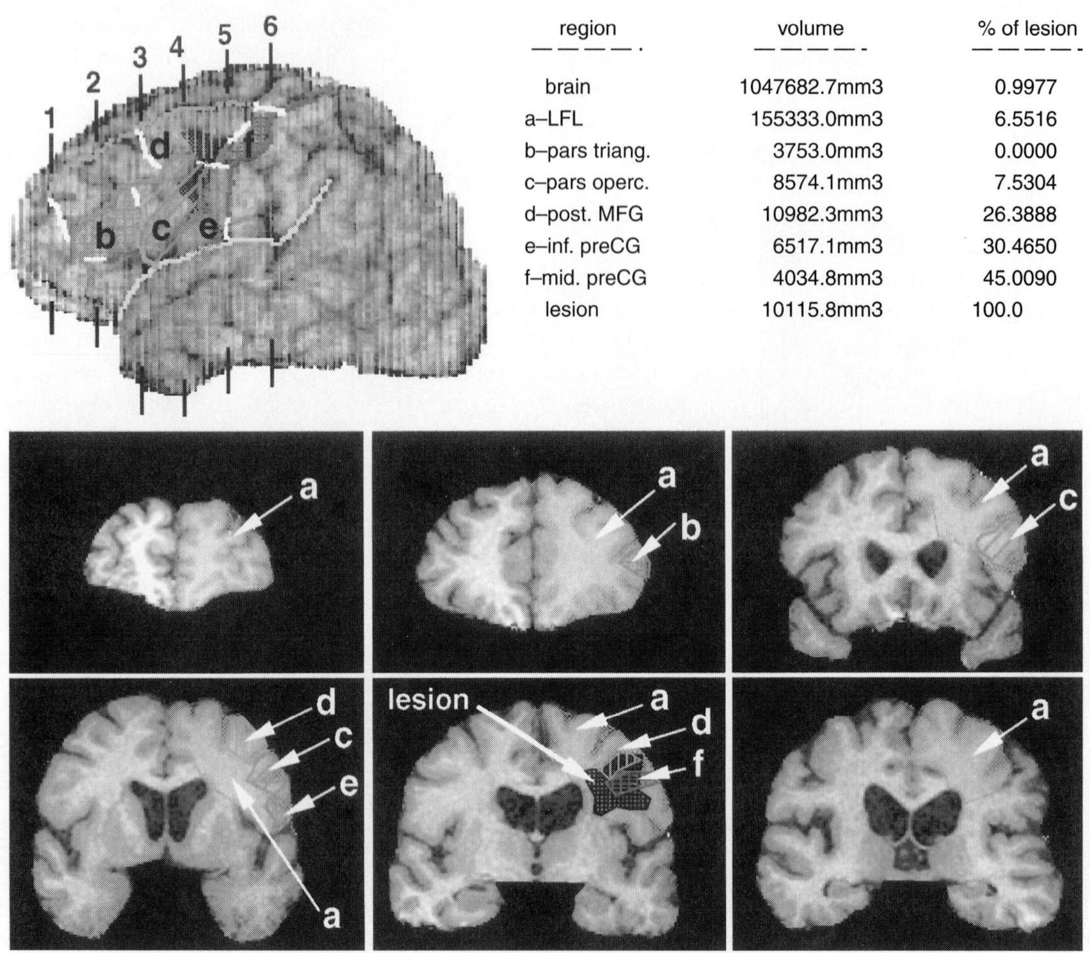

region	volume	% of lesion
brain	1047682.7mm3	0.9977
a–LFL	155333.0mm3	6.5516
b–pars triang.	3753.0mm3	0.0000
c–pars operc.	8574.1mm3	7.5304
d–post. MFG	10982.3mm3	26.3888
e–inf. preCG	6517.1mm3	30.4650
f–mid. preCG	4034.8mm3	45.0090
lesion	10115.8mm3	100.0

Figure 6-2 (Plate 6)
Three-dimensional reconstruction of a human brain with a lesion in the left frontal lobe. The questions addressed here concerned the size of the lesion and the percentage of volume it occupied in the whole brain, in the left frontal lobe (LFL), and in some subdivisions of the frontal lobe: the pars triangularis (pars triang.) and the pars opercularis (pars operc.), the posterior half of the middle frontal gyrus (post. MFG), and the precentral gyrus in its inferior (inf. preCG) and middle thirds (mid. preCG). The limits of all of these regions of interest (ROI) were marked on the 3D reconstructed brain. On all coronal slices, the several ROIs are individually traced, as is the contour of the lesion. Six coronal slices are shown as an example. The different ROIs are color- and texture-coded. The automatically calculated absolute volumes and the percentage of damage in each of them are recorded on the top right-hand corner.

As with the previous technique, detailed knowledge of human neuroanatomy is indispensable. Needless to say, the investigator must be conversant with the imaging techniques themselves. The template technique relies on the availability of brain templates of the normal brain such as those published by us in 1989 and 1995. The key steps are as follows:

1. Determine the angle of incidence in which CT or MRI were obtained. This can be achieved on the

basis of a pilot scan or by inspection of the lower axial slices in which the relative positions of structures in the three main cranial fossae can be observed.

2. On the basis of the above determination, select the set of templates that best fits the subject's films.

3. Chart the lesion on the templates at every level at which it occurs, using an *X/Y* plotting strategy.

4. Superimpose over the template an appropriate "in register" transparency that contains anatomic cells representing neural "areas of interest" in both gray and white matter structures. Each of those cells is limited by a linear boundary and has a letter and number code on the basis of which it can be anatomically identified.

5. Assign the area of damage charted in the template to the cells that encompass the abnormal images.

6. Assign the estimation of the amount of involvement within target cells. We usually code this 0 when there is less than 25 percent involvement of the total, 1 if the involvement is between 25 and 75 percent; and 2 if more than 75 percent of the total area is damaged. This step can be achieved in two ways: (a) using a transparent square grid and counting the number of units involved by the lesion at each level, then calculating the percentage in relation to the total number of units encompassed by each area of interest (which is the sum of units occupied by the region at each template level); or (b) transferring the template system into computer software, tracing the lesion's limits as marked on the template with a digitizer, and then using automated determination of the percentage of area involved.

The number of cuts in the scan and in the correctly chosen set of templates may not coincide for two reasons: varied thickness of cuts and variations in individual brain size. Therefore, the investigator must search for the most appropriate scan/template matches, on a cut-by-cut basis, using all available anatomic constants—for example, ventricular system and prominent sulci. Fortunately, current MRI resolution provides such a wealth of landmarks that finding appropriate correspondences is no longer a daunting task. Correspondences are a necessary complement to the *X/Y* plotting approach. The results of *X/Y* plotting should be counterchecked by inspection of identifiable landmarks, since "blind" plotting may produce an inaccurate chart. This is why we do not advocate the use of fully automated lesion analysis with the template technique.

The major source of error in the template technique is the choice of the wrong template set. The key to the correct choice of templates is the inspection of *all* available brain cuts, especially the lower ones, which contain crucial landmarks for the determination of the incidence of a particular scan. In practical terms, it is necessary to compare the proportion of frontal lobe, temporal lobe, and posterior fossa structures shown in the scan with those seen in the various template sets and to select the best match. It is not possible to find the right match based on the inspection of high cuts alone, because in high-lying cuts, the cues from anatomic constraints such as the ventricular system or bony landmarks are lost.

Improved Template Technique

The availability of BRAINVOX and of 3D reconstructed normal brains has allowed us to improve the template technique. It is now possible to create "customized templates" for any set of CT or MRI slices. Instead of using published templates, a 3D reconstructed normal brain can be resliced so as to match the incidence of cut and the level of slices in the CT or MR images to the analyzed (Fig. 6-3, Plate 7). The key steps are as follows:

1. All major sulci are identified and color-coded in the 3D reconstructed normal brain.

2. The normal brain is resliced on the computer screen so as to match the slice orientation and thickness of the 2D images of the brain to be analyzed, creating an equal number of brain slices (the "customized template set"). The color codes generated in (1) are automatically transferred onto the single brain slices.

3. On each matched pair of normal/abnormal brain slices, the lesion is transferred in much the same manner as described for the basic template technique.

4. The result is a 3D transfer of the lesion, which can then be "read off" the normal 3D reconstructed brain.

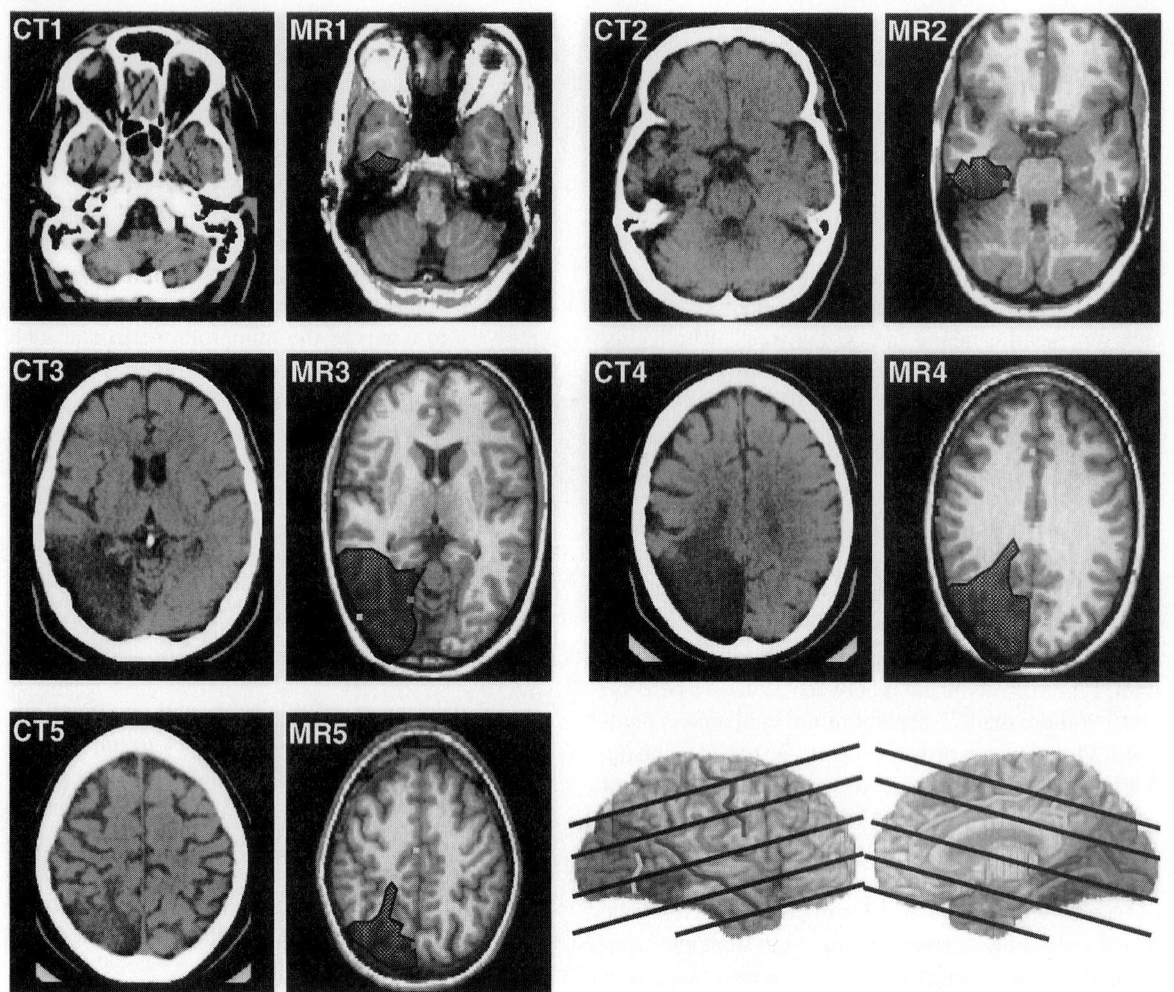

Figure 6-3 (Plate 7)
Demonstration of the improved template method. Brain CT (CT 1–5) of a subject who could not undergo an MRI study. A normal 3D reconstructed brain was resliced so as to match the orientation and level of the CT slices (MR 1–5). The lesion seen on the CT slices was transferred onto each matched MR slice, taking into account all identifiable sulci and gyri. Once the sulci were color-coded on the 3D reconstruction, the lesion could be read off each individual slice. The object defined by the transferred traces could be fused with the normal brain to visualize the lesion's surface extent (right lower corner).

Analysis of Groups of Subjects

Whenever a study involves a large number of subjects, it may be advantageous to create maps of lesion overlap. For this purpose we have developed a technique that permits the determination of the region of maximal overlap in terms of brain surface ("Map-2," a 2D map), or in volumetric terms ("Map-3," a 3D map). Each of these techniques entails the transfer of all individual lesions onto a normal reference brain.

For Map-2, the steps are as follows:

1. For each case, each view of the 3D brain showing the lesion is matched with the corresponding

view of the normal reference brain, in terms of spatial coordinates.

2. The surface contour of the lesion is transferred from the subject's brain and fitted onto the normal reference brain, taking into account its relation to sulcal and gyral landmarks.

3. The lesions are then superimposed to form a surface map. A region of maximal lesion overlap is determined on the basis of the superimpositions and assigned a numerical weight based on the number of contributing lesions.

To obtain a Map-3, we transfer and fit the limits of all the target lesions onto the normal reference brain reconstructed in 3D (by transferring the contour of each lesion as seen in each slice into the corresponding slices of the reference brain in the way described above). The sum total of lesion contours for each case constitutes a 3D object. Given the collection of such objects, we then determine the intersection of their volumes in whatever plane we prefer. This allows us to determine overlap in both cortical "surface" and white matter "depth." We refer to the area of maximal overlap as the "center of volume."

Identifying Lesions with Computed Tomography and Magnetic Resonance Imaging

The identification of neuropathologic changes using CT depends on the detection, within a given brain region, of an x-ray absorption that departs from the norm. The presence of cerebral infarction, edema, or tumor at a specified anatomic location alters the standard x-ray absorption for that region and produces an abnormal image.

In the case of MRI, the identification of neuropathologic changes depends on the production of a locally different rate of hydrogen proton spinning, within the affected brain region, after the brain is exposed to a magnetic field. In other words, after the brain is subjected to a magnetic field, with varied magnetic pulse sequence parameters, the presence of a pathologic brain region due to edema, infarction, or tumor will determine hydrogen proton spinning rates within the area that are different from what normally would be expected for the given anatomic structure subjected to the same magnetic pulse sequence. Lesion-detection sensitivity with either method varies according to the specific procedure, the nature of the pathology, the stage at which the imaging measurement is made in relation to the onset of the pathologic process, and the quality of the equipment and proficiency of the technique.

The potential for false negatives or false positives is considerable, their magnitude depending on the factors listed above. For example, CT is often negative in the first 24 h following an infarct but is usually positive in the days after. However, in the second and third weeks after an infarct, because the infarcted tissue absorbs x-rays at the same rate as normal tissue, the CT may become negative again if not performed after the injection of a contrast-enhancing substance. Contrast seeps out of damaged vessels in the damaged region and increases the density of the area.

Neuroanatomic Resolution

The limits of resolution in the lesion method are set by the state of the technology. Current-generation CT and MRI scanners detect lesions as small as 1 mm on the plane of section. From the perspective of microstructure, these seemingly astounding resolutions are actually modest, since such small areas contain so many neurons and connections. Nonetheless, from the perspective of cytoarchitecture or of cortical regions defined neurophysiologically, this resolution is quite respectable. In short, current imaging technology visualizes neural structure at a level that permits the neuroanatomic definition of most lesions resulting from acquired neurologic disease or neurosurgical ablations.

Neither CT nor MRI can detect discrete cellular pathology except when a fairly large cortical region or subcortical nucleus is affected over a sizable surface or volume that turns out to be, in the aggregate, larger than the lower limit of resolution discussed above. This is why, in the early stages of degenerative dementia of either the Alzheimer or Pick types, when neuropsychological assessment already reveals marked cerebral dysfunction, CT and MRI studies may be so deceptively normal. At the same stage, however, dynamic neuroimaging using emission tomography procedures, of either the SPECT or PET types, may show changes in cerebral blood flow or metabolism.

Decreased radio signal in posterior temporal and temporoparietal regions is quite characteristic of Alzheimer's dementia.[8–11] This is probably the consequence of both local pathologic changes and local physiologic changes brought about by anterior temporal lesions.

In moderate to advanced stages of Alzheimer's disease, CT and MRI often show fairly widespread cerebral atrophy or ventricular enlargement. In addition, MRI studies may also show a reduction in the volume of medial temporal structures, the result of accumulated damage in entorhinal and perirhinal cortices, and subsequent degeneration in hippocampus.[12,13]

In Pick's disease, autopsy studies have shown repeatedly that the characteristic pathology is especially evident in the frontal and anterior temporal cortices,[14] and in moderate to advanced cases, anatomic analysis of CT or MRI of patients with progressive dementia does reveal severe atrophy localized to those regions.[15]

The Choice of Neuropathologic Specimens

The choice of pathologic specimen is a major technical consideration in the lesion method, given that the neuropathologic characteristics of infarctions, intraparenchymal hemorrhages, or varied types of tumor are entirely different.

Nonhemorrhagic infarctions provide the best specimens for neuroanatomic investigation and correlation with neuropsychological findings, because cerebral infarctions actually destroy brain parenchyma. The infarcted area is eventually replaced by scar tissue and by cerebrospinal fluid, and CT or MRI in the chronic state provide a clear demarcation of the infarct. In CT, the damage is depicted as an area of decreased density, seen as a darker area in the gray scale that accompanies the images. In MRI, infarctions show as a dark area in T1-weighted images and a white bright signal region in T2-weighted images.

Herpes simplex encephalitis provides comparable anatomic detail. In adults, the virus has an affinity for a limited set of brain structures, mostly within the limbic system, and it destroys those areas rather completely by a mechanism that includes vascular collapse. In the chronic state, both CT and MRI produce extremely accurate images of the involved territories.

In most other varieties of neuropathologic process, the precise anatomic definition of lesions is less accurate and the functional impact of the lesion itself is less well defined. For instance, earlier in their growth, *gliomas* infiltrate brain tissue by dislocating local populations of neurons but may not destroy them immediately. Moreover, the region of low or high density seen on the CT or MRI of such tumors corresponds not just to the tumor tissue but also to edema surrounding it and to brain tissue that may still be functionally competent. In other words, in such cases it may be impossible to decide that the brain parenchyma is destroyed or that the area is functionally inoperative, or, for that matter, that an area without apparent abnormality is free of tumor. For these reasons, we do not believe that patients with glial tumors are a first choice for the lesion method. This point is made clear in a study by Anderson and coworkers,[16] who compared the neuropsychological profile of patients with confirmed gliomas to that of patients with strokes in the same regions.

Where subjects with glial tumors pose problems for the lesion method, those in whom *meningiomas* have been excised and who have had a circumscribed ablation of brain tissue are actually ideal cases. The images from such cases are entirely appropriate to establish a link between the anatomic site of the ablation and the neuropsychological profile obtained *after* the ablation has taken place.

Patients who have had ablations for seizure treatment also afford a good opportunity for behavioral and anatomic studies. In those cases, MRI obtained with T1-weighted images can help delineate the extent of brain tissue removal with extraordinary precision, although some caution is recommended in the interpretation of neuropsychological data obtained in such patients. Some patients who undergo surgical removal of brain tissue for the treatment of uncontrollable seizures may have developmental brain defects. Those whose seizures began early in life are likely to have had some degree of compensatory brain reorganization before surgery. Frequent and long-standing seizural discharges may also produce changes elsewhere in the brain. The participation of such patients in lesion studies must be evaluated on an individual basis.

The inclusion in lesion method studies of subjects with *metastatic disease, intracerebral hemorrhages,* or *severe head injury* must also be decided on an individual basis, lest it contaminate otherwise valid results. For instance, data from patients with a single brain metastasis, removed surgically and studied in the stable, postoperative state, concomitantly with a good-quality CT or MRI, are quite acceptable.

Intracerebral hemorrhages affect the brain by two different mechanisms. They destroy neural tissue, as nonhemorrhagic infarctions do, and they cause a space-occupying blood collection that displaces neurons, as tumors do. During the acute phase of a hemorrhage, neither CT nor MRI provides an accurate picture of the abnormality, because within the area of abnormal signal some neurons are truly destroyed, whereas others are simply displaced. The amount and location of tissue destruction can be estimated only after the resolution of the hematoma.

In conclusion, the specimen of choice for the purpose of establishing correlates between dysfunction and site of brain destruction are cases of nonhemorrhagic infarction and herpes encephalitis. Surgical ablations performed for the treatment of meningiomas also provide excellent material. Other material should be used on an individual basis, after careful assessment of the dynamics of lesion development.

Timing of Imaging

The timing of CT and MRI data collection is of the essence, especially in relation to subjects with stroke. Both CT and MRI may fail to show *any* abnormality when they are obtained immediately after the occurrence of a stroke. With modern-generation CT and MRI scanners, most images will be positive after 24 h. This is certainly not the case with older scanners, however. It is important to keep in mind that many CT (or even MRI) studies obtained less than 24 h after the onset of a stroke may be negative, especially when a patient with an acute stroke happens to have a CT or MRI that shows a well-demarcated area of low density with sharp margins. Such an image, early after stroke, should suggest a previous infarct, probably unrelated to the new set of symptoms.

Positive CT images obtained in the first week post-onset usually show areas of abnormality that are far larger than the region of actual structural damage because of confounding phenomena—for example, edema. This commonly occurs and means that the results of observations and experiments conducted at later epochs should not be correlated with the anatomic analysis performed in the acute images.

When CT is obtained in the second or third week after a stroke's onset without intravenous infusion of a contrast-enhancing substance, the images are negative in a good number of cases. The image can change even after a previous CT obtained earlier showed a large area of decreased density. During this period, the damaged area can show the same density as the normal tissue. On the other hand, in contrast-enhanced CT images, those normal-looking areas will appear as areas of increased density (primarily due to seepage of contrast substance through the walls of newly formed vessels in the affected region). In the chronic stage, which we define as 3 months post-onset and beyond, most CT studies of infarction are unequivocally positive. Even then, however, when strokes are small and located close to a major sulcus or to the wall of a ventricle, the chronic CT may mislead the observer, resembling images of focal "atrophy" with sulcal enlargement or images of ventricular dilatation. When no previous images are available for comparison with those obtained in the chronic stage, the correct interpretation and the establishment of an adequate behavioral/anatomic correlation may not be possible.

Similar problems befall MRI with images obtained with only one pulse sequence. T1-weighted images obtained with an inversion recovery (IR) pulse sequence provide maximal anatomic detail. With this pulse sequence, however, infarctions appear as dark areas, in precisely the same range of grays used to depict the ventricular system or any region filled with cerebrospinal fluid, such as the cerebral sulci and fissures. When infarcts are small and close to one of these structures, they may not be readily distinguishable. Images obtained with different pulse sequences on MRI (proton density or T2-weighted) show the damaged area as a region of intense bright signal, more easily distinguishable from the bright signals generated by white and even gray matter.

A meaningful relation between an anatomic image and a particular neuropsychological pattern requires reasonable temporal closeness between the epochs at which the image and the neuropsychological data were obtained. Because, during the acute period, edema and brain distortion often occur, it is not easy to define precisely the location and amount of destroyed tissue. The pairing of such images with observations made in the chronic state may lead to error. Likewise for the inverse situation—that is, pairing the results of acute neuropsychological observations obtained in the acute state with the anatomy gleaned during the chronic stage. The most reliable anatomic and neuropsychological data are obviously those obtained in the chronic stage.

Other Considerations

A traditional limitation of the lesion method in humans has been the excessive reliance on single cases. Many of the important observations made in the past were uncontrolled and went unreplicated, the significance of the results being thus diminished. Notable exceptions—for instance, Milner's collection of epileptic patients with surgical ablations in temporal and frontal lobe, Newcombe's head injury project, or Gazzaniga's group of epileptics with split brain interventions—simply confirm the rule. In our laboratory, we have obviated this limitation by creating a continuously renewed population of patients with lesions in varied neural systems who would be willing to participate in neuropsychological experiments. The goal was to conduct multiple single-subject studies in target patients and in controls with an approach as rigorous as the one used in the traditional experimental setting and to make it possible to design and carry out experiments in which certain hypotheses regarding anatomy and function could be probed comprehensively, using many individual data sets.

It goes without saying that, given optimal neuroanatomic analysis, the lesion method will be only as successful as the quality of the cognitive tasks used in the experiments and the quality of the theoretical framework and hypotheses being tested. The rapidly evolving fields of cognitive science and experimental neuropsychology have provided investigators with many useful tasks applicable to most aspects of cognition and behavior likely to be studied with the lesion method. There are also many relevant theoretical developments concerning the conceptualization of both the cognitive and neural architectures in humans. The traditional divisions between behaviorist and cognitivist views seem to have been largely overcome by theoretical positions that combine the best of both (see, for examples, Refs. 17 to 19). The conceptualization of neural structures and of their operations, insofar as mental processes and behaviors are concerned, has also changed radically, as indicated at the beginning of this chapter. Neural signaling is seen as both massively parallel and massively sequential, and, no less importantly, massively recurrent. The prevalence of feedforward and feedback loops disposed along as well as across neural streams has been duly noted, and so has the convergent/divergent nature of those neuron streams. The dependence on timing mechanisms for the normal operations of these networks is well accepted.[20–24]

REFERENCES

1. Ungerleider LG, Mishkin M: Two cortical visual systems, in Ingle DJ, Mansfield RJW, Goodale MA (eds): *The Analysis of Visual Behavior.* Cambridge, MA: MIT Press, 1982.
2. Newcombe F, Russell WR: Dissociate visual, perceptual and spatial deficits in focal lesions of the right hemisphere. *J Neurol Neurosurg Psychiatry* 332:73–81, 1969.
3. Damasio A, Tranel D, Damasio H: Face agnosia and the neural substrates of memory. *Annu Rev Neurosci* 13:89–109, 1990.
4. Damasio AR, Damasio H, Tranel D, Brandt JP: Neural regionalization of knowledge access: Preliminary evidence. *Symposia on Quantitative Biology* 55:1039–1047, 1990.
5. Tranel D, Damasio H, Damasio AR, Brandt JP: Separate concepts are retrieved from separate neural systems: Neuroanatomical and neuropsychological double dissociations (abstr). *Soc Neurosci* 21:1497, 1995.
6. Damasio H, Damasio A: *Lesion Analysis in Neuropsychology.* New York, Oxford University Press, 1989; Japanese edition, Tokyo: Igaku-Shoin, 1992.
7. Damasio H: *Human Brain Anatomy in Computerized Images.* New York: Oxford University Press, 1995.
8. Chase TN, Foster NL, Fedio P, et al: Regional cortical dysfunction in Alzheimer's disease as determined by positron emission tomography. *Ann Neurol* 15(suppl): S170–S174, 1984.
9. Foster NL, Chase TN, Mansi L, et al: Cortical abnormalities in Alzheimer's disease. *Ann Neurol* 16:649–654, 1984.
10. Friedland RP, Budinger TF, Ganz E, et al: Regional cerebral metabolic alterations in dementia of the Alzheimer

type: Positron emission tomography with (18F) fluorodeoxyglucose. *J Comp Assist Tomogr* 7:590–598, 1983.
11. Rezai K, Damasio H, Graff-Radford N, et al: Regional cerebral blood flow abnormalities in Alzheimer's disease. *J Nucl Med* 26(5):105, 1985.
12. Hyman BT, Damasio AR, Van Hoesen GW, Barnes CL: Cell specific pathology isolates the hippocampal formation in Alzheimer's disease. *Science* 225:1168–1170, 1984.
13. Van Hoesen GW, Damasio A: Neural correlates of the cognitive impairment in Alzheimer's disease, in Plum F (ed): *The Handbook of Physiology.* Bethesda, MD: American Physiological Society, 1987, pp 871–898.
14. Escourelle R, Poirier J: *Manual of Basic Neuropathology.* Philadelphia: Saunders, 1978.
15. Graff-Radford NR, Damasio AR, Hyman BT, et al: Progressive aphasia in a patient with Pick's disease: A neuropsychological, radiologic and anatomic study. *Neurology* 40:620–626, 1990.
16. Anderson SW, Damasio H, Tranel D: The use of tumor and stroke patients in neuropsychological research: A methodological critique. *J Clin Exp Neuropsychol* 10:32, 1988.
17. Kosslyn SM: *Image and Brain: The Resolution of the Imagery Debate.* Cambridge, MA: Bradford Books/MIT Press, 1994.
18. Damasio AR: *Descartes' Error: Emotion, Reason and the Human Brain.* New York: Grosset/Putnam, 1994.
19. Churchland PS, Sejnowski JF: *The Computational Brain: Models and Methods on the Frontiers of Computational Neuroscience.* Cambridge, MA: Bradford Books/MIT Press, 1992.
20. Damasio AR: The brain binds entities and events by multiregional activation from convergence zones. *Neural Comput* 1:123–132, 1989.
21. Damasio AR, Damasio H: Cortical systems for retrieval of concrete knowledge: The convergence zone framework, in Koch C (ed): *Large-Scale Neuronal Theories of the Brain.* Cambridge, MA: MIT Press, 1994, pp 61–74.
22. Crick F: *The Astonishing Hypothesis: The Scientific Search for the Soul.* New York: Scribner's, 1994.
23. Edelman G: *Neural Darwinism.* New York: Basic Books, 1987.
24. Rockland KS (ed): Special issue: Local cortical circuits. *Cerebral Cortex* 3:361–498, 1993.

Chapter 7

FUNCTIONAL IMAGING IN BEHAVIORAL NEUROLOGY AND NEUROPSYCHOLOGY

Geoffrey Karl Aguirre

The methods of behavioral neurology and neuropsychology fall into two broad categories, each of which has a long history. The first category includes manipulations of the neural substrate itself. Such an intervention might inactivate a brain area, perhaps through a lesion, with Paul Broca's 1861 observation of the link between language and left frontal lobe damage providing a prototypical example. The effects of stimulation of brain areas can also be studied, as Harvey Cushing did with the human sensory cortex in the early twentieth century. In the second category, observation techniques relate a measure of neural function to behavior. Hans Berger's work in the 1920s on the human electroencephalographic response is a good starting point.

Impressive refinements and additions to both of these categories have taken place over the last century. For example, beyond the static lesions of "nature's accidents" that have been the mainstay of cognitive neuropsychology for many years, it is now possible to reversibly inactivate areas of human cortex using transcranial magnetic stimulation (see Chap. 9 for additional details). The realm of "observational" methodology has also grown dramatically in the last few decades, with the development of functional neuroimaging.

In this chapter we concern ourselves with the theoretical and practical properties of functional neuroimaging techniques in general and with blood oxygen level–dependent (BOLD) functional magnetic resonance imaging (fMRI) in particular. We begin with a brief consideration of the nuts-and-bolts physics and physiology that underlie common imaging methods. Next, we consider several aspects of the inferential basis of neuroimaging. Our deliberations here include a "two-systems" model of neuroimaging inference and three general types of hypotheses that can be tested using these methods. We also explore the relationship between neuroimaging and lesion studies and describe different methods for behaviorally isolating cognitive processes of interest within a neuroimaging experiment. Finally, we discuss some idiosyncratic properties of BOLD fMRI as they relate to different categories of temporal organization of experiments (e.g., blocked, event-related, etc.). Except for a few glancing references, the subject of the statistical analysis of neuroimaging data in general and BOLD fMRI in particular is avoided.

PROPERTIES OF FUNCTIONAL NEUROIMAGING DATA

In general, functional neuroimaging can be defined as the class of techniques that provide volumetric, spatially localized measures of neural activity from across the brain and across time—in essence, a three-dimensional movie of the active brain. Importantly, functional imaging data have a particular order in time that cannot be changed without fundamentally altering the nature of the original data. Virtually all neuroimaging experiments vary an experimental condition over time and evaluate the relationship between the experimental manipulation and the observed time series.

Relatively noninvasive measurements of blood flow in the human brain were first accomplished in 1963 by Glass and Harper by measuring the decay of inhaled, radioactive xenon gas. This method could provide only global measurements of blood flow within the head, so it could not be used to generate images. This was to change soon after the introduction of computed tomography (CT) in the 1970s. Developed for use with x-ray images, CT methods allowed the reconstruction of a volumetric image of the body by passing x-rays through the subject from multiple directions. These ideas were soon applied to measurements of metabolic function in the human brain, with the twist that instead of directing radiation energy through the body, the source of radiation was located within the subject. In positron emission tomography (PET), the subject is injected with a radioisotope that, as it decays, produces positrons. These are immediately annihilated by joining with electrons, producing two photons that travel outward in opposite directions. An array of sensors located around the subject's head uses "coincidence detection" to determine the source of the radioactive decay in space.

Using radiolabeled water, PET was initially applied as a method of measuring local cerebral tissue perfusion. In the 1980s, functional changes in blood flow became the object of study, by comparing the distribution of cerebral perfusion during different cognitive states. In the following decades, PET techniques were used extensively in the service of research in cognitive neuropsychology. While PET provides for a spatial resolution on the order of a few millimeters, temporal resolution is limited by the half-life of the radioisotope used. Practically, PET images can be obtained only every few minutes, limiting the ability of the method to dynamically track changes in neural activity related to cognitive processes. It is this limitation in temporal resolution, coupled with the invasive and expensive need for radioisotope injection, that ultimately led fMRI methods to supplant PET as the primary tool of investigation in cognitive neuroscience.

The use of MRI to assay neural function was initiated by Belliveau and his colleagues in 1991, who used an injected contrast agent (gadolinium) to obtain perfusion MR images of the occipital cortex during visual stimulation. The widespread application of fMRI awaited the development of a noninvasive endogenous tracer method, subsequently introduced by Ogawa and colleagues in 1993 (see Ref. 26). Fortuitously, hemoglobin, the primary oxygen-carrying molecule in the blood, has different magnetic properties when bound and unbound to oxygen, and this serves as the agent of contrast in BOLD fMRI. Local changes in neural activity give rise to a chain of physiologic and imaging events, many of the details of which are still under study. In brief, increases in neural activity produce local increases in blood flow,[1] which in turn engender a delayed decrease in local deoxyhemoglobin concentration.[2] This is sometimes referred to as a paradoxical change, as increased metabolic activity leads to a decrease in deoxyhemoglobin. Because deoxyhemoglobin has stronger magnetic properties than oxyhemoglobin, a decrease in the deoxyhemoglobin concentration results in a decreased perturbation of the local magnetic field (referred to as a *susceptibility* gradient). This increases the T2*-weighted fMRI signal[3] from the area, which serves as the dependent data for fMRI. Several excellent reviews of the physics and physiology underlying BOLD fMRI are available for the interested reader (e.g., Moonen and Bandettini[4]).

Unlike PET, where the signal measured can be expressed as a physical quantity (e.g., milliliters of blood per grams of tissue per minute), the BOLD fMRI signal has no simple, absolute interpretation. This is because the particular signal value obtained is not *exactly* a measure of deoxyhemoglobin concentration but is instead a measure that is *weighted* by this concentration (i.e., is T2*-weighted) and is also influenced by a number of other factors that can vary from voxel to voxel, scan to scan, and subject to subject. As a result, experiments conducted with BOLD fMRI generally test for differences in the magnitude of the signal between different conditions within a scan. One could not, for example, directly contrast the absolute level of the BOLD fMRI signal obtained within the temporal lobe of schizophrenic patients with that from controls with much hope of obtaining a reliable or unbiased statistical test. Notably, recent developments in perfusion imaging offer the ability to obtain an fMRI signal that can be interpreted in concrete physical units.[5,6]

The spatial and temporal resolution of BOLD fMRI is limited by the neurovascular coupling that is the source of contrast. While MR images can readily be obtained every 100 ms and with spatial resolution in the tenths of a millimeter, this fine resolution has little practical advantage. Changes in neural activity give rise to a change in BOLD fMRI signal that evolves over seconds (described in detail below). As a result, BOLD fMR images are seldom acquired more frequently than once a second. Additionally, a point of neural activity engenders a change in BOLD signal that spreads over several millimeters; thus BOLD images are typically composed of voxels (the smallest-volume "pixel" of which the image is composed) no smaller than 1 mm on a side.

THE "TWO-SYSTEMS" MODEL OF FUNCTIONAL NEUROIMAGING EXPERIMENTS

Engineers frequently find it convenient to discuss an object of study as a *system.* Simply defined, a system is something that takes input and provides output. One can imagine many different examples of systems, such as a car, where the pressure upon the gas pedal is the input and the speed of the car is the output. Certain types of systems are particularly amenable to study and characterization.

What is the system under study in functional neuroimaging experiments of cognitive neuropsychology hypotheses? A profitable way of answering this question is with a *two-systems* model, in which the domain of mental operations and cognitive processes is held separate from vascular physiology and imaging physics (Fig. 7-1).

The first system is that of cognition, in which the inputs are the instructions, stimuli, and tasks presented to the subject by the experimenter and the output is the pattern of neural activity evoked within the brain. The second system is the domain of physiology

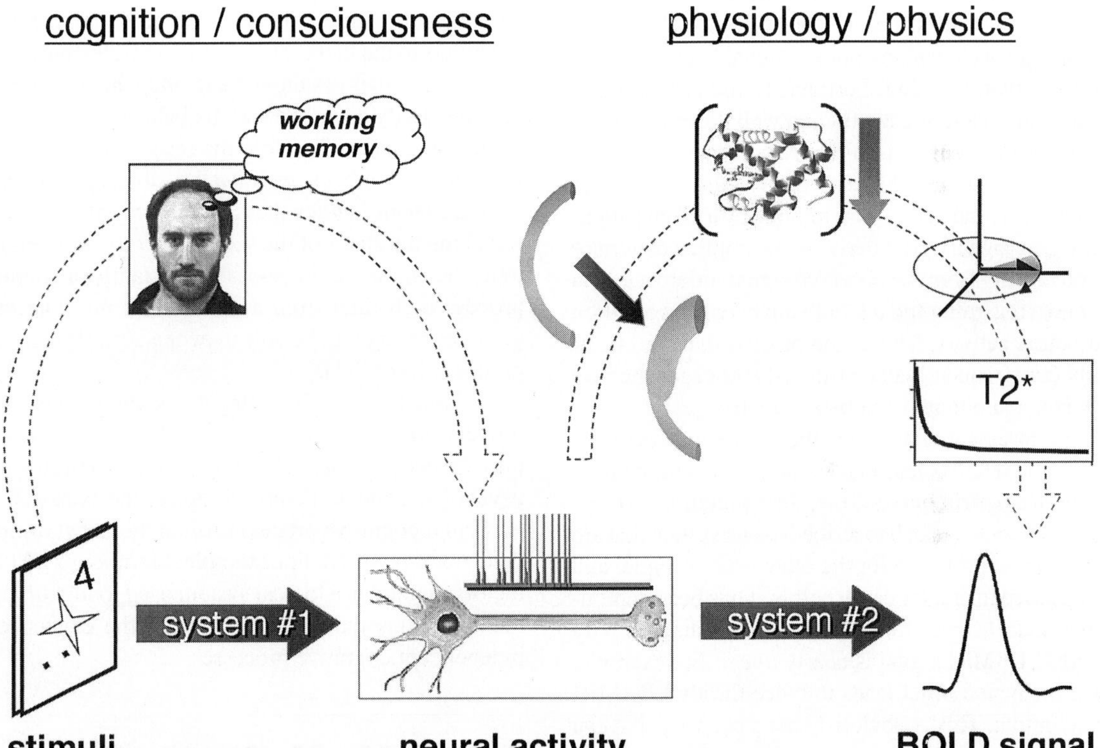

Figure 7-1
Depiction of the "two-systems" model of BOLD fMRI experiments. The left side of the figure represents the system that mediates the transformation of stimuli and instructions into neural activity. The cognitive processes that mediate this transformation are typically the subject of study of neuropsychology experiments. The right side of the figure depicts the system that transforms neural activity into BOLD fMRI signal. Following along the curved arrow on the right, the chain of events that follows an increase in neural activity includes dilatation of local vasculature, a decrease in the concentration of deoxyhemoglobin, and an alteration in local magnetic field inhomogeneity, impacting T2 signal and ultimately BOLD fMRI signal. As is described in the text, the complicated sequence of events that take place under the "system #2" label can be efficiently modeled by a linear system.*

and physics; it mediates the transformation of neural activity inputs into blood-flow responses and imaging signal. In most cognitive neuroscience experiments, the hypotheses of interest concern the patterns of neural activity that are evoked by cognitive processes and therefore chiefly concern the first of these two systems. Of course, many scientists have great interest in the exact physical mechanisms that mediate the neurovascular response; the second system is therefore a frequent target of experiments that do not strictly fall within the realm of cognitive neuroscience.

If it were the case that the properties of both systems were unknown, then it would be a daunting (if not impossible) task to study cognition using functional neuroimaging. This is because one would not be able to assign a given change in imaging signal to cognition or neurovascular coupling. Fortunately the properties of the second system are lawful and well described, even if the exact mechanisms of the transformation are still not well understood. Therefore one is able to state what changes in neural activity are implied by a given pattern of imaging signal. After deriving the implied pattern of neural activity from the observed signal, inferences can be drawn regarding the relationship between cognition and neural activity. This is the process that we effortlessly (and frequently unconsciously) engage when we look at a neuroimaging statistical map.

It is essential to keep the distinction between these two systems clear in considering functional neuroimaging experiments and their interpretation, as there are properties that can be ascribed to one system that are clearly not appropriate for the other. For example, and as discussed in greater depth below, it has been demonstrated that the system that transforms neural activity into BOLD fMRI signal is nearly *linear.* For example, twice the neural input leads to twice the BOLD fMRI signal output. This is obviously not a property that can be readily assumed to be true of the cognition system—presenting twice as many words to be remembered is not a priori assumed to produce twice as much neural activity (although this is a property of the system that might be tested).

What aspect of the first system is studied in a neuroimaging experiment? Typically, these experiments involve a subject in the scanner performing a task of the design of the experimenter. (Although there are certainly exceptions: consider studies of seizure activity or rapid-eye-movement sleep.) As depicted, it is the stimuli and instructions from the task that constitute the inputs to the first system. Ultimately, the purpose of the experiment is to state some relationship between the neural activity observed and the behavior in which the subject engaged. Therefore the researcher often seeks to control not only the *task* that the subject performs but also the *mental states* that the subject enters. The internal mental states of the subject are typically referred to as the cognitive processes. Importantly, a cognitive process is distinct from a task in that multiple tasks might be thought to be able to evoke a single cognitive process (Table 7-1).

Table 7-1
Examples of cognitive processes and tasks purported to evoke them

Task	*Cognitive process*
Determine if a stimulus is the same as one seen several seconds earlier	Working memory
Match rotated figures	Mental rotation
Generate a verb for a supplied noun	Semantic recall

Note that simply stating that something is a cognitive process does not make it so! The notion of a cognitive process has a fairly rigorous instantiation within psychology, and the demonstration of the existence of a particular cognitive process is often the target of much behavioral research. For example, Sternberg's additive factors method is a logical system used to identify task manipulations that can demonstrate the existence of independent cognitive processes.[7]

BASIC TYPES OF NEUROIMAGING INFERENCE

Although there are many neuroimaging methods and a seemingly limitless number of applications, the basic type of question being asked usually fits within one of a few categories. Each type of approach makes different assumptions and permits different inferences about the relationship between the brain and behavior. Worth noting now and developed below, an experiment that tries to fit into more than one category at once is likely on shaky logical ground.

By far the most common application of neuroimaging methodology is to *localization* questions, which ask: "what are the neural correlates of a given cognitive process?" Generally, the subject is presented with a task designed to selectively evoke a particular cognitive state of interest, and the neuroimaging method identifies whether and where bulk changes in neural activity accompany that cognitive process. The key assumption for this type of design is that a given cognitive process exists and that the task isolates only that cognitive process. Various techniques are used (such as cognitive subtraction or parametric manipulation, discussed below) to isolate the mental operation of interest from the other processes that invariably are present (e.g., button pushing, preparing responses, etc.).

It is important to understand what these types of experiments *cannot* conclude. Activity evoked by a particular cognitive process cannot be taken as evidence that the activated cortical region is necessary for the cognitive process (in the sense that a lesion of the area would impair the subject's ability to perform the task). If the assumptions of the localization framework are perfectly met, the strongest inference that can be made is that the region is *activated* by the cognitive process. Demonstration of necessity requires a lesion study (or some other method of inactivating neural structures, such as transcranial magnetic stimulation; see below).

In contrast, *implementation* studies ask about the computational mechanisms of a cognitive process within a cortical region. This type of study begins with the assumption that a cortical region is involved in a particular cognitive process. The purpose of the study is then to determine the neurocomputational parameters that mediate the area's participation in that process. For example, one might know that area MT is involved in the cognitive process of motion detection. However, what is the relationship between speed of motion and the MT response? Does motion directed toward the viewer, as opposed to motion directed across the visual field, change the magnitude of neural activity? As another example, consider a region of prefrontal cortex assumed to be involved in the cognitive process of working memory. Does this region change its bulk level of neural activity with increasing memory load (i.e., remember four items instead of two)?

Finally, an *evocation* design turns the familiar direction of neuroimaging inference on its head and asks: "What cognitive process does a given task evoke? Also termed "reverse inference," this framework is used to make inferences about cognition as opposed to neural activity; i.e., the behavior of the subject is the unknown variable. One begins by assuming that a particular cortical region is activated by a *single cognitive process.* This mapping must be unique, in that one and only one cognitive process is capable of activating a particular region. The subject performs a task that may or may not evoke the cognitive process of interest. The fMRI data are then examined to determine whether increased neural activity was present within the specified region during the task; if so, the conclusion is drawn that the subject recruited the cognitive function. In other words, the evocation paradigm may be used to test hypotheses regarding the engagement of cognitive processes during a behavioral state in which the cognitive processes need not be under experimental control.

Suppose, for example, we assume that neural activity in area MT indicates the presence of the cognitive process of motion perception. By examining the neural activity within this area, it becomes possible to learn how unrelated distractors affect motion perception.[8] In another example, we might assume that activity in the "fusiform face area" indicates the cognitive process of face perception. We can then monitor the responses of this area during a binocular-rivalry paradigm that pits face stimuli against house stimuli to learn about the time course of perceptual switching.[9]

What provides the evidence that a particular region is uniquely activated by a specific cognitive process? Logically, only an exhaustive neuroimaging examination of every possible cognitive process under every possible circumstance could provide the necessary evidence. This is obviously impractical, so a series of neuroimaging experiments that demonstrate activation of a particular region during a given cognitive process and no other usually suffices to support the assumption (a logical inference termed *enumerative induction*).

It is worth noting that a common logical error in neuroimaging studies is to try to conduct both evocation *and* localization inferences at the same time. Often, the discussion section of a paper will identify activity in one cortical area as the consequence of a cognitive process the experimenter intended to manipulate in the task and then, in the next paragraph, suggest that activity in some other location (e.g., the frontal lobe) is the result of some other behavior in which the subject engaged (e.g., working memory). This is an error, because the assumptions of each type of inferential framework contradict the other. The localization framework assumes that only a single cognitive process is being manipulated, while the evocation framework assumes that multiple, unspecified mental states are in play.

These three categories of neuroimaging inference should be taken as guidelines and do not exhaust the realm of possible designs. For example, studies of effective connectivity[10] examine the relationship of neural activity in different areas of the brain and are often used to support inferences about implementation, although other applications are certainly possible as well. The primary use of this tripartite division is to help organize one's thinking about the assumptions that underlie a particular experiment.

THE RELATIONSHIP BETWEEN LESION AND NEUROIMAGING STUDIES

Although perhaps counterintuitive, lesion and neuroimaging studies provide for very different and nonoverlapping inferences about the relationships between the brain and behavior. One way to think about these differences is in terms of the logical construct of *necessity.* A common neuropsychological hypothesis states that a particular brain region is necessary for the performance of a particular mental operation. If the region in question is removed (perhaps through a lesion) and the cognitive process is impaired, the hypothesis has been affirmed. While this seems straightforward, several inferential complications can ensue, and the interested reader is directed to Chaps. 6 and 8 for further discussion. One wrinkle discussed here is the possibility that more than one region is capable of supporting the process of interest (perhaps working in parallel, or one serving as a "backup" for the other). In this case, the region still plays an interesting role in the cognitive process, although it is not strictly *necessary* in that a lesion of only that region will not impair the cognitive process. Therefore an alternate relationship between a neural substrate and a behavior that might be sought is *involvement* (I am indebted to my colleague Eric Zarahn for this particular construct and to his general contribution to the ideas in this chapter). A region is *involved* in a cognitive process if it is necessary under some circumstance (the circumstance being that all the other potential "backup" regions have also been damaged).

Does finding activation of a cortical region in a functional neuroimaging study imply that the region is necessary (or even just involved) in the cognitive process? In short, the answer is no; not only for functional neuroimaging but for all "observation" methods mentioned at the outset (electroencephalography, depth electrode recording, etc.). The primary cause of this state of affairs is the observational, correlative nature of neuroimaging. Although we make inferences regarding cognitive processes, these processes are not themselves directly subject to experimental manipulations. Instead, the investigator controls the presentation of stimuli and instructions, with the hope that these circumstances will provoke the subject to enter a certain cognitive state and *no other.* Careful consideration reveals how this assumption might fail. Although cooperative, the subject may unwittingly engage in confounding cognitive processes in addition to that intended by the experimenter or, alternatively, may fail to differentially engage the process. For example, a subject might constantly engage in the process of declarative memory formation, even during periods of time when he or she is "supposed" to be performing some other control behavior. It is therefore not possible to know if observed changes in neural activity in a brain region are the result of the evocation of the cognitive process of interest or an unintended, confounding process. Negative results (even in the face of arbitrarily high statistical power) are also not conclusive, not only because of the failure of perfect control of evocation of cognitive processes but also because of the possibility that the neuroimaging method employed is not sensitive to the critical change in metabolic activity (e.g., pattern of neuronal firing as opposed to bulk, integrated synaptic activity).

What about the converse inference? If a region is involved in a cognitive process, may we deduce that it would be activated by that cognitive process in a neuroimaging experiment? Again, the answer is no.

Consider the situation in which two cortical regions are both involved in the same cognitive process. One is the "primary" region and the other is the "backup" region. As long as the primary region is functioning, the backup region is quiescent. Thus, a neuroimaging study might fail to demonstrate activation of the backup region even though it is involved in the cognitive process. Interestingly, one might study a patient with a lesion of the primary region and thereby demonstrate activation of the backup region by the cognitive process of interest under that circumstance (see Chap. 8).

What about the case in which a region is actually *necessary* for a cognitive process? Can we now expect that the region will be activated by the cognitive process? The answer is yes, but with a number of caveats. For example, we must be able to assume that the necessity of the region is not some side effect of the lesion method itself—for example, damaging axons that simply passed through the area ("fibers of passage"[11]) or affecting the metabolic activity of remote areas (causing, for example, diaschisis[12]). Also, we must assume that our neuroimaging method is sensitive to all possible changes in neural activity that might be induced by the cognitive process (not just bulk neural activity but synchronicity of firing). If not, then it is possible that the necessary cortical region undergoes a change in state associated with the cognitive process that our technique is unable to observe.

The upshot is that caution should be exercised in applying neuroimaging results to the clinical interpretation of the necessity of a cortical region for behavior. For example, there has been interest in using BOLD fMRI to replace the "Wada" or intracarotid amobarbital test.[13] When this test is performed to guide surgical resection of epileptic foci, each internal carotid artery is in turn catheterized and instilled with anesthetic to determine which hemisphere is dominant for language. The hope is that BOLD fMRI can be used to determine which hemisphere responds to language tasks and thus to replace this invasive procedure. While results so far have indicated a good correlation between the two methods, there is no logical requirement that this be the case. In fact, counterexamples have been presented in which neuroimaging has demonstrated activation in frontal cortical areas not subsequently found to be necessary for language function, and vice versa.[14] Further discussion of the inferences possible from the joint consideration of imaging data and neurologic patients is deferred until the next chapter.

MANIPULATION OF THE COGNITIVE PROCESS

As was discussed in the setting of inferential framework, many neuroimaging experiments depend upon the isolation of a particular cognitive process for study. Specifically, the fundamental assumption of the localization category of neuroimaging inference is that the cognitive process of interest can be isolated from other mental operations so that the neural correlates of that solitary process can be observed. Here we consider several broad classes of manipulations designed to do this. Note that any of these techniques for evoking a particular cognitive process can be coupled with different temporal structures of designs, described in the next section.

Cognitive subtraction is the prototypical neuroimaging method for putative isolation of cognitive processes, the logic of which derives from similar arguments made in the study of reaction times (e.g., Donders[15]). One condition of the experiment is designed to engage a particular cognitive process, such as face perception, episodic encoding, or semantic recall. This "experimental" condition is contrasted with a "control" condition that is designed to evoke all of the cognitive processes present in the experimental period except for the cognitive process of interest. Under the assumptions of "cognitive subtraction,"[16] differences in neural activity between the two conditions can be attributed to the cognitive process of interest.

Cognitive subtraction assumes, as do the other manipulations described below, that the particular cognitive process of interest can be evoked uniquely. This is a fundamental inferential weakness of many cognitive neuroimaging studies. As has been discussed, although we make inferences regarding cognitive processes, these processes are not themselves directly subject to experimental manipulations. Even the cooperative subject might engage other, confounding mental operations unintentionally, rendering this assumption invalid.

Cognitive subtraction (in neuroimaging) relies upon two additional assumptions: "pure insertion" and linearity. Pure insertion is the idea that a cognitive process can be *added* to a preexisting set of cognitive processes without affecting them. This assumption is difficult to prove, because one would need an independent measure of the preexisting processes in the absence and presence of the new process. If pure insertion fails as an assumption, a difference in neuroimaging signal between the two conditions might be observed not because of the simple addition of the cognitive process of interest, but because of an interaction between the added component and preexisting components. For example, the act of pressing a button to signal a semantic judgment may be different from pressing a button in response to a visual cue. Effects upon the imaging signal that result from this difference would be erroneously attributed to semantic judgment per se.

A second assumption of cognitive subtraction is that the transformation of neural activity into fMRI signal is linear. While the BOLD fMRI system has been shown to exhibit behavior close to that of a linear system, there is some evidence for systematic departures.[17] Failures of linearity can cause adjacent neural events to produce more or less signal than those events would in isolation, rendering subtraction approaches invalid. In fact, failures of cognitive subtraction along these lines have been empirically demonstrated for working memory experiments.[18]

Several other cognitive process manipulations have as their goal a reduction in the reliance upon the assumption of pure insertion. *Factorial* experiments[19] are designed to examine the interactions of two different candidate cognitive processes. The scheme of the design involves (in the simplest case) four conditions, during which two different processes are evoked individually and then jointly. The proposed advantage of the design is that interactions between the two processes can be examined. The presence of an interaction is indicated if the difference in imaging signal between the presence and absence of cognitive process A is itself different when cognitive process B is present or absent. While factorial designs do provide a compelling method for gaining greater insight into the neural implementation of cognitive processes, it is a mistake to claim that such designs obviate the need for the pure insertion assumption. Interpretation of the design requires the assumption that the two cognitive processes have indeed been isolated. The logic by which this isolation is to occur is the same as that outlined for cognitive subtraction above. That is, process A and process B must be purely inserted into the other cognitive components that allow the experiment to evoke these processes.

The *cognitive conjunction* design[20] has also been proposed to reduce reliance upon the assumption of pure insertion. The logic of the approach is that, if one wishes to discount the possibility of an interaction (i.e., a failure of pure insertion) between the cognitive component to be added and the set of preexisting processes, one should repeat the experiment with a different set of preexisting processes and replicate the result. A rigorous implementation of this notion involves conducting a series of categorical subtraction experiments that all aim to isolate the same cognitive process. The novel twist is that the subtractions need not be complete; that is, the experimental and control conditions can differ in several cognitive processes in addition to the one of interest. The imaging data are then analyzed to identify areas that have a significant, consistent response to the putatively isolated process (i.e., a significant main effect across subtractions in the absence of any significant interactions). Again, while this design reduces the plausibility of some failures of cognitive subtraction, it does not eliminate the possibility. In particular, some cognitive processes by their very nature require the evocation of an antecedent process. For example, can working memory be meaningfully present if not preceded by the presentation of a stimulus to be remembered? If not, then any cognitive conjunction design that attempts to demonstrate the presence of neural activity during a delay period will be susceptible to erroneous results due to interactions between the task manipulation and preexisting task components.

Finally, *parametric* designs offer an attractive alternative to cognitive subtraction approaches. In a parametric design, the experimenter presents a range of different levels of some parameter and seeks to identify relationships (linear or otherwise) between imaging signal and the values that the parameter assumes. This can be done to identify the neural correlates of straightforward changes in stimulus properties or manipulations of a cognitive process. Unlike cognitive subtraction methods, parametric designs do not rely as heavily upon the assumption of pure insertion, as the cognitive process is present during all conditions.

PROPERTIES OF THE BOLD fMRI SYSTEM THAT AFFECT EXPERIMENTAL DESIGN

So far we have described properties of all neuroimaging techniques and considered the inferential consequences of different ways of influencing a subject's mental state. We now turn our attention to the idiosyncratic properties of one particular neuroimaging method: BOLD fMRI. We focus here on two key properties of BOLD fMRI data that fundamentally affect the design of BOLD fMRI experiments: the hemodynamic response function and the presence of low-frequency noise.

As was mentioned earlier, the cascade of neurovascular events that ensue following changes in neural activity and produce changes in BOLD fMRI signal are still under investigation. Fortunately, the BOLD fMRI system has properties of a *linear system,* allowing us to ignore for the most part the messy details of physics and physiology. Like any other system, a linear system takes input and provides output (in this case, neural activity in, BOLD fMRI signal out). Importantly, a linear system can be completely characterized by a property called the impulse response function (IRF), which is the output of the system to an infinitely brief, infinitely intense input. In the context of BOLD fMRI, the hemodynamic response function (HRF) is taken as an estimate of the IRF of the BOLD fMRI system and is the change in BOLD fMRI signal that results from a brief (< 1 s) period of neural activity. Knowledge of the IRF can be used to predict the output of the system to any arbitrary pattern of input by a mathematical process called *convolution.* Therefore knowledge of the shape of the HRF allows one to predict the BOLD fMRI signal that will result from any pattern of neural activity.

The HRF itself can be empirically measured from human subjects by studying the BOLD fMRI signal that is evoked by experimentally induced, brief periods of neural activity in known cortical areas (e.g., neural activity in the primary motor cortex in response to a button press). The shape of the HRF reflects its vascular origins (Fig. 7-2) and rises and falls smoothly over a period of about 16 s. While the shape of the HRF varies significantly across subjects, it is very consistent within a subject, even across days to months.[21] There is some

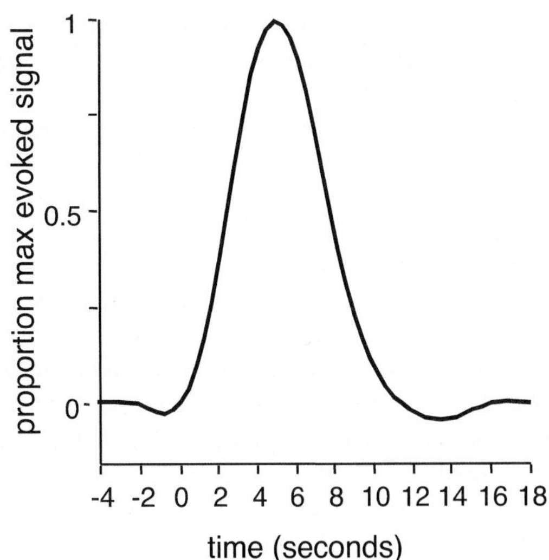

Figure 7-2
An average, across-subject hemodynamic response function. The brief period of neural activity that produced this signal change took place at time zero.

evidence that the shape of the HRF varies from one region of the brain to another (perhaps from variations in neurovascular coupling), but this is a difficult notion to test, as it is necessary to induce patterns of neural activity in disparate areas of the brain that can be guaranteed to be very similar.

The temporal dynamics of neural activity are quite rapid, on the order of milliseconds, but changes in blood flow take place over the course of seconds. One consequence of this, as demonstrated by the smooth shape of the HRF, is that rapid changes in neural activity are not well represented in the BOLD fMRI signal. The "temporal blurring" induced by the HRF leads to many limitations placed on the types of experiments that can be conducted using BOLD fMRI. Specifically, the smooth shape of the HRF makes it difficult to discriminate closely spaced neural events. Despite this, it is still possible to detect (1) brief periods of neural activity; (2) differences between neural events in a fixed order, spaced as closely as 4 s apart; (3) differences between neural events, *randomly* ordered and closely spaced (e.g., every second or less); and (4) neural onset asynchronies on the order of 100 ms. The reason that these seemingly paradoxical experimental designs can work is that some patterns of events that occur rapidly or switch rapidly create a low-frequency "envelope"—a larger structure of pattern of alternation that can pass through the hemodynamic response function. In the next section, several types of temporal structures for BOLD fMRI experiments are discussed as well as how the shape of the HRF dictates the properties of these designs.

Another important property of BOLD fMRI data is that greater power is present at some temporal frequencies than others under the null hypothesis (i.e., data collected without any experimental intervention). The power spectrum (a frequency representation) of data composed of independent observations (i.e., white noise) should be "flat," with equal power at all frequencies. When calculated for BOLD fMRI, the average power spectrum is found to contain ever-increasing power at ever lower frequencies (Fig. 7-3), often termed a 1/frequency distribution. This pattern of noise can also be called "pink," named for the color of light that would result if the corresponding amounts of red, orange, yellow, etc., of the visible light frequency spectrum were combined. The presence of noise of this type within BOLD fMRI data has two primary consequences. First, traditional parametric and nonparametric statistical tests are invalid for the analysis of BOLD fMRI data, which is why much of such analysis is conducted using Keith Worsley and Karl Friston's "modified" general linear model[22] as instantiated in SPM and other statistical packages. The second impact is upon experimental design. Because of the greater noise at lower frequencies, slow changes in neural activity are more difficult to distinguish from noise.

Figure 7-3
The power spectrum representation of the "pink," or "1/frequency" noise present in BOLD fMRI data under the null hypothesis. Data composed of independent observations over time is termed "white" noise and would have a flat line in this representation.

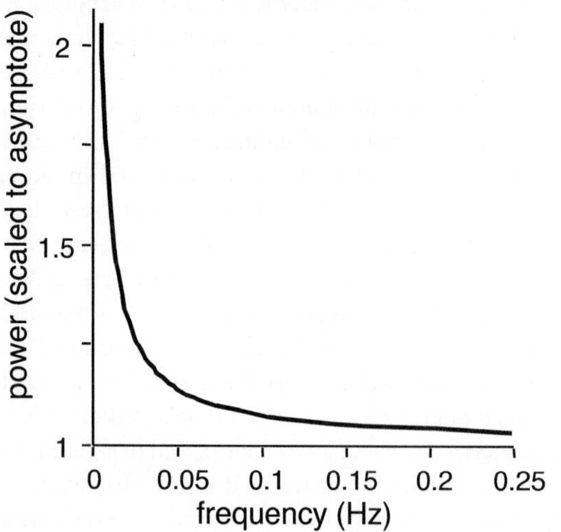

The astute reader might note that the consequences of the shape of the hemodynamic response function and the noise properties of BOLD fMRI are at odds. Specifically, the shape of the HRF would tend to favor experimental designs that induce slow changes in neural activity, while the presence of low-frequency noise would argue for experimental designs that produce more rapid alterations in neural activity. As it happens, knowledge of the shape of the HRF and the distribution of the noise is sufficient to provide a principled answer as to how best balance these two conflicting forces.

It is worth noting that other neuroimaging methods have different data characteristics, with different consequences for experimental design. For example, perfusion fMRI is a relatively new approach that provides a noninvasive, quantifiable measure of local cerebral tissue perfusion.[5] Perfusion data do not suffer from the elevated, low-frequency noise present in BOLD, and as a result, perfusion fMRI can be used to detect extremely long time-scale changes in neural activity (over minutes to hours to days) that would simply be indistinguishable from noise using BOLD fMRI.[6]

DIFFERENT TEMPORAL STRUCTURES OF BOLD fMRI EXPERIMENTS

As BOLD fMRI experiments by necessity include multiple task conditions (prototypically, an "experimental" and "control" period), several ways of ordering the presentation of these conditions exist. Different terms are used to describe the pattern of alternation between experimental conditions over time; they include such familiar labels as *blocked* or *event-related.* While these are often perceived as rather concrete categories, the distinction between blocked, event-related, and other sorts of designs is actually fairly artificial. These may be better considered as extremes along a continuum of arrangements of stimulus order. Consider every period of time during an experiment as a particular experimental condition. This includes the "intertrial interval" or "baseline" periods between stimulus presentations. In this setting, blocked and event-related designs are viewed simply as different ways of arranging periods of "rest" (or no stimulus) with respect to other sorts of conditions. (For a more complete exploration of these concepts, see Friston.[23])

The prototypical fMRI experiment is a blocked approach in which two conditions alternate over the course of a scan. For most hypotheses of interest, these periods of time will not be utterly homogeneous but will consist of several trials of some kind presented together. For example, a given block might present a series of faces to be passively perceived, or a sequence of words to be remembered, or a series of pictures to which the subject must make a living/nonliving judgment and press a button to indicate the response. Blocked designs have superior statistical power compared to all other experimental designs. This is because the fundamental frequency of the boxcar can be positioned at an optimal location with respect to the filtering properties of the hemodynamic response function and the low-frequency noise.

Event-related designs model signal changes associated with individual trials as opposed to blocks of trials. This makes it possible to ascribe changes in signal to particular events, allowing one to randomize stimuli, assess relationships between behavior and neural responses, and engage in retrospective assignment of trials. Conceptually, the simplest type of event-related design to consider is one which uses only a single stimulus type and uses sufficient temporal spacing of trials to permit the complete rise and fall of the hemodynamic response to each trial; a briefly presented picture of a face once every 16 s, for example. Importantly, while this prototypical experiment has only one stimulus, it has *two* experimental conditions (the stimulus and the intertrial interval). If one is willing to abandon the fixed ordering and spacing of these conditions, more complex designs become possible. For example, randomly ordered picture presentations and rest periods could be presented as rapidly as once a second. The ability to present rapid alternations between conditions initially seems counterintuitive, given the temporal smoothing effects of the hemodynamic response function. While BOLD fMRI is insensitive to the particular high-frequency alternation between one trial and the next, it is still sensitive to the low-frequency "envelope" of the design. In effect, with closely spaced, randomly ordered trials, one is detecting the low-frequency consequences of the random assortment of trial types.

The discussion thus far regarding event-related designs has assumed an ability to randomize perfectly the order of presentation of different event types. There are certain types of behavioral paradigms, however, that do not permit a random ordering of the events. For example, the delay period of a working memory experiment always follows the presentation of a stimulus to be remembered. In this case, the different events of the trial cannot be placed arbitrarily close together without risking the possibility of false-positive results that accrue from the hemodynamic response to one trial event (e.g., the stimulus presentation) being interpreted as resulting from neural activity in response to another event (e.g., the delay period). It turns out that, given the shape typically observed for hemodynamic responses, events within a trial as close together as 4 s can be reliably discriminated.[18] Thus, event-related designs can be used to examine directly, for example, the hypothesis that certain cortical areas increase their activity during the delay period of a working memory paradigm without requiring the problematic assumptions traditionally employed in blocked, subtractive designs.

As a final example of event-related design, consider an experiment that aims to identify a neural onset asynchrony. As noted above, the hemodynamic response observed for a subject during a scanning session is highly reliable in its shape and is relatively smooth (i.e., is not composed of high-frequency components). As a result, it might be possible to use fMRI to detect small neural onset asynchronies. Such a design might present one of two different behavioral trials (in a random order) every 16 s. Because of the reliability of the hemodynamic transformation, differences in the mean time to peak of the responses to the two different types of stimuli could be identified and ascribed to an asynchrony in onset of neural activity.[24] Such a design might allow one, for example, to test the hypothesis that a cortical area that responds to pictures of faces responds with a slightly longer latency (on the order of 100 ms) to pictures of inverted faces.

CONCLUSION

There is an enormous variety of experimental designs that may be used to ask cognitive neuropsychology questions with neuroimaging methods. I have provided here frameworks for organizing these approaches into inferential categories, methods of manipulating evoked cognitive processes, and ways of arranging different experimental conditions in time. Hopefully, the general principles enumerated here will be of use not only for BOLD fMRI, the preeminent neuroimaging method of today, but also for whatever leap in neuroimaging methodology awaits us tomorrow.

REFERENCES

1. Leniger-Follert E, Hossmann K-A: Simultaneous measurements of microflow and evoked potentials in the somatomotor cortex of the cat brain during specific sensory activation. *Pflugers Arch* 380:85–89, 1979.
2. Malonek D, Grinvald A: Interactions between electrical activity and cortical microcirculation revealed by imaging spectroscopy: implications for functional brain mapping. *Science* 272:551–554, 1996.
3. Jezzard P, Song A: Technical foundations and pitfalls of clinical fMRI. *Neuroimage* 4:S63–S75, 1996.
4. Moonen CTW, Bandettini PA (eds): *Functional MRI.* Berlin: Springer-Verlag, 1999.
5. Detre JA, Alsop DC: Perfusion fMRI with arterial spin labeling. In: Bandettini PA, Moonen C (eds): *Functional MRI.* Berlin: Springer-Verlag, 1999, pp 47–62.
6. Aguirre GK, Detre JA, Alsop DC: Experimental design and the relative sensitivity of BOLD and perfusion fMRI. *Neuroimage* 15:488–500, 2002.
7. Sternberg S: The discovery of processing stages: extensions of Donder's method. *Acta Psychol* 30:276–315, 1969.
8. Rees G, Frith CD, Lavie N: Modulating irrelevant motion perception by varying attentional load in an unrelated task. *Science* 278:1616–1619, 1997.
9. Tong F, Nakayama K, Vaughan JT, Kanwisher N: Binocular rivalry and visual awareness in human extrastriate cortex. *Neuron* 21:753–759, 1998.
10. Buchel C, Friston K: Assessing interactions among neural systems using functional neuroimaging. *Neural Networks* 13:871–882, 2000.
11. Jarrard LE: On the role of the hippocampus in learning and memory in the rat. *Behav Neural Biol* 60:9–26, 1993.
12. Feeney DM, Baron J-C: Diaschisis. *Stroke* 17:817–830, 1986.
13. Binder JR, Swanson SJ, Hammeke TA: Determination of language dominance using functional MRI: a comparison with the Wada test. *Neurology* 46:978–984, 1996.
14. Jayakar P, Bernal B, Medina LS, Altman N: False lateralization of language cortex on functional MRI after a cluster of focal seizures. *Neurology* 58:490–492, 2002.
15. Donders FC: On the speed of mental processes. *Acta Psychologia* 30:412–431, 1969.
16. Posner MI, Petersen SE, Fox PT, Raichle ME: Localization of cognitive operations in the human brain. *Science* 24:1627–1631, 1988.
17. Boynton G, Engel S, Glover G, Heeger D: Linear systems analysis of functional magnetic resonance imaging in human V1. *J Neurosci* 16:4207–4221, 1996.
18. Zarahn E, Aguirre GK, D'Esposito M: A trial-based experimental design for fMRI. *Neuroimage* 6:122–138, 1997.
19. Friston KJ, Price CJ, Fletcher P, et al: The trouble with cognitive subtraction. *Neuroimage* 4:97–104, 1996.
20. Price CJ, Friston KJ: Cognitive conjunctions: a new experimental design for fMRI. *Neuroimage* 5:261–270, 1997.
21. Aguirre GK, Zarahn E, D'Esposito M: The variability of human BOLD hemodynamic responses. *Neuroimage* 8:360–369, 1998.
22. Worsley KJ, Friston KJ: The analysis of fMRI time-series revisited—again. *Neuroimage* 2:173–182, 1995.
23. Friston KJ, Zarahn E, Josephs O, et al: Stochastic designs in event-related fMRI. *Neuroimage* 10:607–619, 1999.
24. Menon RS, Luknowsky DC, Gati JC: Mental chronometry using latency-resolved functional MRI. *Proc Natl Acad Sci USA* 95:10902–10907, 1998.
25. Engel S, Zhang X, Wandell B: Colour tuning in human visual cortex measured with functional magnetic resonance imaging. *Nature* 388:68–71, 1997.
26. Ogawa S, Menon RS, Tank DW, et al: Functional brain mapping by blood oxygenation level–dependent contrast magnetic resonance imaging. A comparison of signal characteristics with a biophysical model. *Biophys J* 64:803–812, 1993.

Chapter 8

FUNCTIONAL NEUROIMAGING STUDIES OF NEUROPSYCHOLOGICAL PATIENTS

Cathy J. Price
Karl J. Friston

In this chapter, we consider the types of questions that can be addressed with functional neuroimaging investigations of neuropsychologically impaired patients. In particular, we consider the contributions that can be made to normal and abnormal cognitive and anatomic models of behavior. To this end, Sec. I starts with a brief overview of the advantages of functional imaging relative to behavioral measures. Section II highlights the constraints functional imaging places on cognitive models of normal and abnormal processing. Sections III and IV describe how functional imaging studies of neurologically impaired patients can contribute to models of normal functional anatomy and recovery; and Sec. V concludes by emphasizing some of the critical limitations related to patient studies.

SECTION I: ADVANTAGES OF FUNCTIONAL IMAGING STUDIES OF PATIENTS

Relative to behavioral measurements—which usually rely on the accuracy or speed of vocal responses and finger movements—PET and fMRI have several advantages. The first advantage is that neurophysiologic changes at the neural level always precede the motor output/muscular activity required for vocal responses and finger movements. Thus, PET and fMRI can detect significant responses even when there are no behavioral manifestations. The obvious benefit with neuropsychologically impaired patients is that neural activity can be measured in patients who are unable to make vocal or manual responses. For example, a patient could be scanned with PET or fMRI while listening to stories, a task that does not involve behavioral responses. If semantic areas activate normally, some residual semantic processing might be implied. Another advantage of PET and fMRI is that the hemodynamic response is multidimensional, measured in thousands of voxels across the brain, irrespective of whether the brain regions are involved in task performance or not. By simultaneously recording thousands of data sequences across the whole brain, abnormal effects can be categorized in terms of which neural area or cognitive stage they arise in. For instance, a patient listening to stories may show normal responses in auditory processing areas but no activation in semantic areas.

Multidimensional recordings also have the advantage of tapping into processing that is superfluous to task requirements times. For instance, face naming may elicit emotional responses that do not affect naming times but do change the distribution and composition of hemodynamic responses. Functional imaging can therefore detect activation related solely to changes in facial expression.[1] In this context, we argue that the effect of facial expression is not involved in the task but induced by the stimulus change. It is therefore incidental to the task requirements. Detecting incidental processing of this sort can be particularly useful in the study of patients with limited behavioral responses. For example, Morris et al.[2] have recently reported a functional imaging study of a patient with blind sight. Although the patient was not aware that fearful faces were being presented, discriminatory amygdala responses were detected with functional imaging.

In summary, PET and fMRI provide a measure of cognitive function that is independent of behavioral responses because condition effects are measured by hemodynamic changes (blood flow or deoxyhemoglobin content) rather than the speed and accuracy of overt motor responses. Whereas behavioral measurements are primarily determined by factors that affect task performance (response time and accuracy), functional imaging can reveal significant effects in the absence of any task or when the task/stimulus change has no effect on reaction times and accuracy.

SECTION II: THE CONSTRAINTS THAT FUNCTIONAL NEUROIMAGING PLACES ON COGNITIVE MODELS

The contribution that PET and fMRI provide for understanding the functional anatomy of cognitive processes is undisputed. What is often less clear is how an understanding of normal and abnormal functional anatomy contributes to the corresponding cognitive models. The answer is that functional imaging provides physiologic constraints on cognitive models. In particular it distinguishes between functions associated with specific neural areas from those that emerge from changes in the way a set of areas interact with one another. Without neuroanatomic constraints, an infinite number of cognitive modules can be hypothesized. Although computational approaches have emphasized the explanatory power and biological efficiency associated with implementing functions via changes in connection strengths, connectionist models seldom conform to biological constraints. A classic illustration of the importance of this issue is provided by cognitive models of reading. In the 1980s, the most influential cognitive models of reading (e.g., Patterson and Shewell[3]) emphasized multiple cognitive modules including (1) orthographic analysis, (2) an orthographic input lexicon, (3) a phonologic output lexicon, (4) an orthographic output lexicon, (5) semantic processing, and (6) a subword orthographic to phonologic conversion route. In the 1990s, connectionist models emphasized that the same set of functions could be implemented by only three modules (orthography, semantics, and phonology) and changes in the interactions between these modules (see Seidenberg and McClelland[4]). Functional neuroimaging can evaluate the validity of these models by identifying which neural areas are activated for reading and what the functions of these regions correspond to. For instance, is reading implemented by interactions between neural systems specialized for orthography, semantics, and phonology or are there also neural areas that can be associated with the input and output lexicons?

Studies of neuropsychologically impaired patients can also establish the physiologic validity of cognitive models of normal and abnormal function. Returning to cognitive models of reading, a key factor in their formulation was the observation that brain damage can have remarkably selective effects on reading ability. The well-documented double dissociation[5] is between patients (e.g., surface dyslexics) who have less difficulty reading words and pseudowords with regular/consistent spelling to sound relationships (e.g., *pond* and *yeeping*) than words with irregular spellings (e.g., *yacht*). These patient sometimes attempt to read on the basis of sublexical spelling to sound relationships (e.g., pronouncing *yacht* as *yatched*). In contrast, other patients (e.g., phonologic dyslexics) have more difficulty reading pseudowords (e.g., *yeeping*) that rely on sublexical spelling to sound relationships but are relatively better at reading familiar words with strong semantic associations even when the spelling is irregular (e.g., *yacht* and *choir*). To account for this double dissociation in function, all cognitive models of reading include two or more possible reading routes: one that incorporates sublexical spelling to sound relationships and one that can retrieve the sounds linked to familiar words irrespective of their spelling.

The potential that functional imaging studies of dyslexia offer can be appreciated in light of a limitation with functional imaging studies with normal subjects. The limitation is that irrespective of whether normal subjects are engaged in reading pseudowords or words with regular and irregular spellings, the same set of reading areas are activated with very little effect of word type.[6–12] The most likely explanation is that, irrespective of word type, normal subjects engage all potential reading systems to ensure robust and veridical lexical processing. Scanning patients, with brain damage to one or another reading route, provides a means to segregate these different pathways. An example of such a study is provided by Small and Flores,[13] who report that the left angular gyrus was activated in a patient who presented with "phonologic dyslexia"; after therapy, however, when the patient had learned to read words on the basis of sublexical spelling to sound relationships, there was increased activation in the left lingual gyrus. Further studies of this sort may help to segregate the different reading strategies and explain how they are compromised and then recover following brain damage.

Another way that functional imaging can contribute to abnormal models of cognitive function is through a clear understanding of the role that the damaged area normally plays. Neuropsychological assessments of patients usually focus on deficits that interfere with a normal lifestyle or deficits that the investigator has particular interest in. Understanding normal functional anatomy can motivate and guide other behavioral assessments. Thus, if a patient has a lesion in an area that is known to participate in a particular function, then assessment of that function would be indicated. For example, functional imaging has shown that the right cerebellum is engaged by verbal fluency tasks, although patients with right cerebellar damage do not present with behavioral deficits on standardized language tasks. Motivated by this discrepancy, Feiz et al.[14] investigated the verbal fluency performance of a patient with a right cerebellar infarct and revealed that the patient had subtle deficits learning and completing the task. However, as described in the next section, damage to an area activated in normal subjects does not always impair the patient's performance on the activating task.

SECTION III: NORMAL FUNCTIONAL ANATOMY

In the previous sections, we described how the multidimensional measurements afforded by functional imaging make it sensitive to processes that are "incidental" to task requirements. Incidental processing reflects processes that are elicited in parallel with the task. This may arise because there are multiple routes for performing the same task (e.g., semantic and sublexical word processing) or because the stimuli trigger processing that is not involved in the task (e.g., the effects of facial expression during face naming). Incidental processing has advantages when the aim of the experiment is to detect cognitive responses in patients who have limited motor output (see Sec. I) but disadvantages when the aim is to segregate processes that are either necessary or not necessary for intact task performance (see Sec. II). The problem disentangling "necessary" and "incidental" activation can be partially resolved by investigating the effect of damage to areas that activate in normal subjects. In the example given above, Feiz et al.[14] demonstrated that damage to the right cerebellum (activated by verbal fluency tasks) did impair verbal fluency performance. However, if the right cerebellar activation in normal subjects was incidental to task requirements, then no effect of damage would have been detected. Thus, the combination of (1) functional imaging studies of normal subjects and (2) neuropsychological studies of patients with damage to the activated areas should help to refine our models of normal functional anatomy by distinguishing "necessary" from "incidental" activations.

The combination of functional imaging and neuropsychological studies can also help to distinguish different types of incidental processing. Incidental processing can be of two types: (1) involved in the task but "not necessary" because there are other systems/areas that can subserve the same function and (2) not involved in the task but triggered by the same stimuli. Although impaired performance may not be detectable following selective damage to areas involved in either type of incidental processing, damage to an area that is involved in the task would change the necessity of the remaining intact areas. For example, if there are two possible neural mechanisms for the same function, damage to one mechanism should not impair performance but would result in increased reliance on the surviving mechanism. In other words, the surviving mechanism would become necessary for the function. A second lesion affecting the surviving system (or a large lesion incorporating both) would then be expected to impair performance. Incidental processing that is involved in the task can therefore be identified by the differential effects of selective and multiple lesions.[15]

The segregation of different types of activation involved in a task is facilitated in two important ways by functional imaging studies of patients.[16] First, functional imaging studies of patients can identify neural systems that are not activated by normal subjects. For instance, it may be the case that a patient may retain task performance despite damage to all the areas activated by normal subjects. This situation could arise if the patient engaged neural systems that are not normally involved because they are either "inhibited" or "untrained." Functional imaging studies of patients with damage to areas that activate in normal subjects are therefore important for revealing alternative neural systems for the same task. Once a neural system becomes involved in a function, it may also become "necessary" even if it was not necessary in the normal system. This has been demonstrated using the Wada test following lesions to the right hemisphere in the context of a previous lesion to the left hemisphere. For example, injection of sodium amytal in the right hemisphere does not normally disrupt language, but Kinsbourne[19] reported impaired language capabilities in patients who had recovered from aphasia following a left hemisphere lesion.

Functional imaging studies of patients are also required to moderate conclusions that an area is not necessary to complete the task. This is because functional imaging allows pathologic damage to be characterized in a way that cannot be deduced from structural scans (e.g., CT and conventional use of MRI). Residual responsiveness within or around the site of brain damage (i.e., perilesional activation; see Heiss et al.,[17] Warburton et al.[18]) can therefore be detected and indicates that the damaged area may retain some functionality. It would therefore be wrong to conclude that the damaged area was not required for performing the task.

In summary, behavioral studies of patients cannot detect when patients are using atypical neural mechanisms when there are alternative systems for performing the same task. By contrast, functional imaging studies of normal subjects can not distinguish whether activation is (1) necessary to complete the task; (2) involved in the task but "not necessary" because there are other systems/areas that can subsume the same function; or (3) not involved in the task but triggered by the same stimuli. Functional imaging studies of patients with selective and multiple lesions to each component of the normal system can help to overcome these limitations by revealing alternative neural systems for the same task and discriminating among the different types of activation observed in normal subjects.

Another contribution that functional imaging studies of patients can provide for normal models of functional anatomy concerns our understanding of "functional integration" or "functional connectivity" among brain regions. This is because, unlike structural imaging (CT and conventional MRI), functional imaging can detect abnormal neuronal responses distant to the site of brain damage. These distant effects can either be expressed as an under- or an overactivation relative to normal. In either case, we assume that the cause of the abnormality relates to the damaged area perturbing responses elsewhere in the system. The distant effect of lesions has been referred to as "diaschisis." Classical diaschisis, demonstrated by early anatomic studies and more recently by neuroimaging studies of resting brain activity, refers to regionally specific reductions in metabolic activity at sites that are remote from damaged regions but connected to them. The clearest example is "crossed cerebellar diaschisis," in which abnormalities of cerebellar metabolism are characteristically seen following cerebral lesions involving the motor cortex.[20] Crossed cerebellar diaschisis highlights the strong connections between the (e.g., right) cerebellum and the (e.g., left) motor cortex.

We have introduced the term *dynamic diaschisis*[21] to refer to the context-sensitive and task-specific effects that a lesion can have on the *evoked* responses of distant cortical regions. The basic idea is that an undamaged area can have abnormal responses when it relies on interactions with the damaged area but normal responses when neural dynamics depend only upon integration with undamaged regions. This effect can arise because normal responses in any given region depend upon driving and modulatory inputs from many other regions and reciprocal interactions with them. The regions involved will depend on the cognitive and sensorimotor operation engaged at any particular time. For example, we report a patient with left frontal damage who activated the left posterior temporal cortex normally during a semantic task but abnormally during a reading task.[21] These results suggest that left posterior temporal activation depended on interaction with the damaged area during the reading task but not during the semantic task. Thus, dynamic diaschisis can contribute to our understanding of normal functional anatomy, connectivity, and functional integration among brain regions. Critically, abnormal activation distant to the site of brain damage can only be fully characterized with whole-brain functional neuroimaging studies of patients.

SECTION IV: COGNITIVE AND ANATOMIC MODELS OF RECOVERY

The clinical literature[22,23] offers several popular theories of recovery (see Chaps. 5 and 13) that can be tested with functional neuroimaging studies of patients. These theories have been referred to as (1) redundancy, (2) unmasking, (3) vicarious redundancy, (4) perilesional activation, (5) reversal of diaschisis, and (6) compensatory cognitive strategies. Each of these is considered in turn.

Redundancy

The term *redundancy* has been used to refer to the availability of more than one neural mechanism for performing the same function/task. More recently, however, Edelman and colleagues have emphasized the distinction between redundancy and degeneracy.[24,25] The term *degeneracy* has been defined as "the ability of elements that are structurally different to perform the same function or yield the same output." In contrast, *redundancy* refers to the same structures performing the same function. Since neuropsychological and neuroimaging studies are concerned with cortical and subcortical structures that have a spatial scale of millimeters or centimeters, there will be no redundancy because no two areas have the same structure. Nevertheless, irrespective of terminology, if there are several neural systems for the same task with each being able to substitute for another, functional competence will be protected from selective damage to any one system. Functional imaging studies of patients who recover solely by virtue of the availability of redundant or alternative systems should reveal activation in only a subset of the normally activated regions. There may also be enhanced activation in undamaged areas of the normal system because, if one neuronal system engaged by a task is damaged, intact task performance may become increasingly dependent on the surviving systems.

Unmasking

The term *unmasking* has been used in the clinical literature to refer to neural systems that are "inhibited" in normal subjects but "disinhibited" following damage to the inhibiting system or its adaptation. Functional imaging studies of patients who recover by virtue of "unmasking" or "disinhibition" should reveal activation in regions that are not normally observed. The most likely systems to be disinhibited are those in regions of the contralateral hemisphere that are homologous to the damaged areas. This is because the functional role played by any brain component (cortical area, subarea, neuronal population, or neuron) is defined by the connections and interactions it has with other cortical areas. Therefore, functional similarities between neuronal systems depend on the similarity in their connection profiles. These similarities are likely to be greatest within a cytoarchitectonic region or in the homologous area of the contralateral hemisphere (by virtue of transcollosal interhemispheric connections). Although there is empiric evidence for inhibition in the motor system,[26,27] the role it plays in other neuronal systems is less clear. Some functional imaging studies have revealed right hemisphere activation during language tasks following recovery from left hemisphere damage,[28–31] but the role of disinhibition in these studies is not clear because right hemisphere activation may also be seen following compensatory cognitive strategies (below). Nevertheless, it might be expected that disinhibition would occur earlier in the reorganization process than learning-related compensatory strategies and be less dependent on rehabilitation therapy.

Vicarious Redundancy

Vicarious redundancy has been used to imply that patients might recover by engaging neural systems that were previously unrelated to the task (i.e., "equipotential" systems). This would necessitate the growth of new neuronal processes (neurogenesis). Recently it has been demonstrated that even in the adult brain, there are mitotically competent cells that can divide and create new cells.[32,33] However, despite these recent observations, it is still generally accepted that long-range extrinsic axonal connections do not form de novo in the mature brain. This means that it is unlikely that patients recover by engaging neural systems that were previously unrelated to the task. Demonstrating vicarious redundancy with functional imaging studies of patients would involve demonstrating that abnormal neural systems were engaged by the patient and that normal subjects did not activate these neural systems under any other conditions. In other words, an infinite number of experiments with normal subjects would be required.

Perilesional Activation

Perilesional activation has already been discussed in Sec. III above. It refers to residual functional responsiveness at the site of damage and indicates that the damaged area may retain some functionality. This residual function may emerge during the acute stages of recovery when edema is controlled and circulation is reestablished in areas subject to partial ischemia. Functional neuroimaging of the patient would demonstrate normal activation everywhere except at the site of lesion where it is "patchy."[17,18]

Reversal of Diaschisis

Reversal of diaschisis results when basal activity in an undamaged area is reestablished following a temporary lesion-dependent reduction (see Sec. III for a definition of diaschisis). If evoked responses return to normal, activation in the patient should be normal after recovery and, indeed, monitored with longitudinal studies.

Compensatory Cognitive Strategies

A compensatory cognitive strategy may involve either learning a new strategy or using a preestablished strategy. Learning a new strategy is mediated by changes in the function or number of synapses (i.e., synaptic plasticity) that follow attempts to perform the task. With respect to functional neuroimaging, compensatory cognitive strategies could change activation patterns in contralateral, ipsilateral, or subcortical brain systems. An example of how activation can change with relearning is provided by Small and Flores[13] and described in Sec. II above. They demonstrate how the activation pattern for reading changed after the patient was taught a sublexical phonologic reading strategy. Critically, to demonstrate the involvement of a compensatory cognitive strategy, functional imaging of the patient is required before and after retraining.

In summary, there are several different theories of functional recovery that can be tested with functional imaging studies of neurologically impaired patients. These theories emphasize differential effects from (1) reestablishing the normal neuronal system (periinfarct activation and the reversal of diaschisis), (2) neuronal reorganization (e.g., following disinhibition, or neuroplasticity), and (3) cognitive reorganization (following learning-related synaptic changes). However, it should be emphasized that distinguishing among cognitive or neuronal reorganization is not always easy. This is because to infer neuronal reorganization, one has to demonstrate that the cognitive processes are the same; to infer that a patient is using a different cognitive strategy, one has to demonstrate that the neuronal processing for this cognitive strategy is normal. These inferences rest on (1) a detailed cognitive analysis of the task, (2) a detailed assessment of the patient's and normal subjects' strategies during the task, and (3) neuroimaging experiments to identify the neuronal systems engaged. For instance, abnormal cognitive processing might be assumed if (1) extensive behavioral testing suggested abnormal cognitive processes, (2) normal subjects could be enticed to use the same cognitive processes as the patient, and (3) the normal subjects activated the same set of brain regions as the patient when using this abnormal cognitive strategy. On the other hand, neuronal reorganization in the absence of abnormal cognitive processing might be assumed if the criteria outlined above were not evident—i.e., that there was no evidence that the patient was performing the task differently from normals and no evidence that normal subjects could ever use the alternative neuronal system to perform the task.

SECTION V: LIMITATIONS

In the previous sections, we focused on the advantages of functional imaging studies of neurologically impaired patients. There are, however, two critically important limitations of such studies that have led to many misguided applications. The first limitation is that the interpretation of abnormal activations relies upon our understanding of normal activation patterns. Thus, patient studies will inevitably lag behind and will depend upon developments made in the normal domain. In particular, we need a good understanding of normal variability before inferring patient activation profiles are abnormal. The second limitation is that to make inferences about abnormal neuronal responses, the patient must enact the same set of cognitive, sensory, and motor processes as normal subjects do. Obviously, this is not possible if the processes engaged by the task are impaired. For example, if a patient cannot make speech production responses, the corresponding neuronal correlates will not be expressed. It may be tempting to infer that reduced activation relative to normals is the physiologic cause of the deficit (e.g., with speech production), but fully functional areas may simply not activate when the task is not being performed.

Debate in the current functional imaging literature about developmental dyslexia highlights the issues discussed above. For example, most functional imaging studies of developmental dyslexia have reported abnormal activation in a posterior region of the left temporoparietal junction, in the vicinity of the left angular gyrus.[34–36] Consequently, it has been argued that developmental dyslexics have a dysfunctional or "disconnected" left angular gyrus.[37,38] However, in all of these studies, the developmental dyslexics had reduced accuracy and slower response times than the normal subjects. In contrast, when response accuracy for the dyslexics and controls is matched, no abnormality in the left angular gyrus has been detected.[9,39] Furthermore, functional imaging studies of normal subjects suggest that the left posterior temporoparietal junction is involved in semantic processing (see Price[40] for a review). An alternative interpretation of the abnormal temporoparietal responses in developmental dyslexia could therefore be that there was less semantic activation consequent on less accurate reading.

In summary, when performance is impaired, the neuronal and cognitive abnormalities are confounded and we cannot determine whether abnormal neuronal responses are (1) the physiologic cause or (2) the consequence of impaired performance. Functional imaging studies of patients therefore require that the patients perform the task with the same level of performance as the normal controls. This is counterintuitive from the perspective of neuropsychological studies, where the focus is usually on testing selective deficits in cognitive function. Some functional imaging studies of patients have attempted to match performance by using different experimental parameters for the patients and the normals. For example, stimulus presentation can be made slower for the patient than the normal controls. However, this only substitutes one problem for another, because even subtle changes in stimulus parameters can have highly significant effects on the pattern of activation.[41,42]

In conclusion, although functional imaging studies of neurologically impaired patients are limited to paradigms that the patient can perform, they offer several advantages relative to behavioral tests and functional imaging studies of normals. This chapter has focused on the contributions that imaging studies of patients offer normal and abnormal cognitive and anatomic models, particularly the insights afforded to the mechanisms that sustain functional recovery.

REFERENCES

1. Morris JS, Ohman A, Dolan RJ: Concious and unconscious emotional learning in the human amygdala. *Nature* 93:467–470, 1998.
2. Morris JS, DeGelder B, Weiskrantz L, Dolan RJ: Differential extrageniculostriate and amygdala responses to blind field presentation of emotional faces. *Brain* 124:1241–1252, 2001.
3. Patterson K, Shewell C: Speak and spell: Dissociations and word class effects, in Coltheart M, Sartori G, Job R (eds): *The Cognitive Neuropsychology of Language.* London: Erlbaum, 1987, pp 273–294.
4. Seidenberg MS, McClelland JL: Distributed developmental model of word recognition and naming. *Psychol Rev* 96:523–568, 1989.
5. Marshall JC, Newcombe F: Patterns of paralexia: A psycholinguistic approach. *J Psycholinguist Res* 2:175–199, 1973.
6. Price CJ, Wise RJS, Frackowiak RSJ: Demonstrating the implicit processing of visually presented words and pseudowords. *Cerebr Cortex* 6:62–70, 1996.
7. Herbster AN, Mintun MA, Nebes RD, Becker JT: Regional cerebral blood flow during word and nonword reading. *Hum Brain Map* 5:84–92, 1997.
8. Rumsey JM, Horwitz B, Donohue C, et al: Phonologic and orthographic components of word recognition: A PET-rCBF study. *Brain* 120:739–759, 1997.
9. Brunswick N, McCrory E, Price CJ, et al: Explicit and implicit processing of words and pseudowords by adult developmental dyslexics: A search for Wernicke's Wortschatz. *Brain* 122:1901–1917, 1998.
10. Fiez JA, Balota DA, Raichle ME, Petersen SE: Effects of lexicality, frequency, and spelling-to-sound consistency

on the functional anatomy of reading. *Neuron* 24:205–218, 1999.

11. Hagoort P, Indefrey P, Brown C, et al: The neural circuitry involved in the reading of German words and pseudowords: A PET study. *J Cogn Neurosci* 11(4):383–398, 1999.
12. Tagamets MA, Novick JM, Chalmers ML, Friedman RB: A parametric approach to orthographic processing in the brain: An fMRI study. *J Cogn Neurosci* 12:281–297, 2000.
13. Small SL, Flores DK: Different neural circuits subserve reading before and after therapy for acquired dyslexia. *Brain Lang* 62:298–308, 1998.
14. Fiez JA, Petersen SE, Cheney, MK, Raichle ME: Impaired nonmotor learning and error detection associated with cerebellar damage. *Brain* 115:155–178, 1992.
15. Price CJ, Friston KJ: Functional imaging studies of neuropsychological patients: Applications and limitations. *Neurocase*. In press.
16. Price CJ, Mummery CJ, Moore CJ, et al: Delineating necessary and sufficient neural systems with functional imaging studies of neuropsychological patients. *J Cogn Neurosci* 11(4):371–382, 1999.
17. Heiss WD, Karber H, Weber-Luxenburger G, et al: Speech-induced cerebral metabolic activation reflects recovery from aphasia. *J Neurol Sci* 145(2):213–217, 1997.
18. Warburton EA, Price CJ, Swinburn K, Wise RJS: Mechanisms of recovery from aphasia: evidence from positron emission tomography studies. *J Neurol Neurosurg Psychiatry* 66:155–161, 1999.
19. Kinsbourne M: The minor cerebral hemisphere as a source of aphasic speech. *Arch Neurol* 15:530–535, 1971.
20. Feeney DM, Baron JC: Diaschisis. *Stroke* 17:317–377, 1986.
21. Price CJ, Warburton EA, Moore CJ, et al: Dynamic diaschisis: Context sensitive human brain lesions. *J Cogn Neurosci* 13:419–429, 2001.
22. Kertesz A: Recovery and treatment, in Heilman KM, Valenstein E (eds): *Clinical Neuropsychology,* 3d ed. New York: Oxford University Press, 1993.
23. Hallett M: Plasticity, in Frackowiak RSJ, Mazziotta JC, Toga A (eds): *Mapping: The Disorders*. San Diego, CA: Academic Press, 2000, pp 569–585.
24. Edelman GM, Gally JA: Degeneracy and complexity in biological systems. *Proc Natl Acad Sci U S A* 98:13763–13768, 2001.
25. Tononi G, Sporns O, Edelman GM: Measures of degeneracy and redundancy in biological networks. *Proc Natl Acad Sci U S A* 96:3257–3262, 1999.
26. Geffen GM, Jones DL, Geffen LB: Inter-hemispheric control of manual motor activity. *Behav Brain Res* 64:131–140, 1994.
27. Meyer BU, Roricht S, Woiciechowsky C: Topography of fibres in the human corpus callosum mediating interhemispheric inhibition between the motor cortices. *Ann Neurol* 43:360–369, 1998.
28. Weiller C, Isenee C, Rijntjes M, et al: Recovery from Wernicke's aphasia: A positron emission tomography study. *Ann Neurol* 37:723–732, 1995.
29. Gold BT, Kertesz A: Right hemisphere semantic processing of visual words in an aphasic patient: An fMRI study. *Brain Lang* 73:456–465, 2000.
30. Miura K, Nakamura Y: Functional magnetic resonance imaging to word generation task in a patient with Broca's aphasia. *J Neurol* 246:939–942, 1999.
31. Calvert GA, Brammer MJ: Using fMRI to study recovery from acquired dysphasia. *Brain Lang* 71:391–399, 2000.
32. Barinagh M: No-new-neurons dogma loses ground. *Science* 279:2041–2042, 1998.
33. Gross CG: Neurogenesis in the adult brain: Death of a dogma. *Nat Neurosc Rev* 1:67–73, 2000.
34. Rumsey JM, Nace K, Donohue BC, et al: A positron emission tomographic study of impaired word recognition and phonological processing in dyslexic men. *Arch Neurol* 54:562–573, 1997.
35. Shaywitz SE, Shaywitz BA, Pugh KR, et al: Functional disruption in the organization of the brain for reading in dyslexia. *Proc Natl Acad Sci U S A* 95:2636–2641, 1998.
36. Temple E, Poldrack RA, Protopapas A, et al: Disruption of the neural response to rapid acoustic stimuli in dyslexia: Evidence from functional MRI. *Proc Natl Acad Sci U S A* 97:13907–13912, 2000.
37. Horwitz B, Rumsey JM, Donohue BC: Functional connectivity of the angular gyrus in normal reading and dyslexia. *Proc Natl Acad Sci U S A* 95:8939–8944, 1998.
38. Rumsey JM, Horwitz B, Donohue BC, et al: A functional lesion in developmental dyslexia: Left angular blood flow predicts severity. *Brain Lang* 70:187–204, 1999.
39. Paulesu E, Demonet JF, Fazio F, et al: Dyslexia: Cultural diversity and biological unity. *Science* 291:2165–2167, 2001.
40. Price CJ: The anatomy of language: Contributions from functional neuroimaging. *J Anat* 197:335–359, 2000.
41. Price CJ, Moore CJ, Frackowiak RSJ: The effect of varying stimulus rate and duration on brain activity during reading. *Neuroimage* 3:40–52, 1996.
42. Price CJ, Friston KJ: The temporal dynamics of reading: A PET study. *Proc R Soc Lond Ser B* 264:1785–1791, 1997.

Chapter 9

ELECTROPHYSIOLOGIC METHODS AND TRANSCRANIAL MAGNETIC STIMULATION IN BEHAVIORAL NEUROLOGY AND NEUROPSYCHOLOGY*

Leon Y. Deouell
Richard B. Ivry
Robert T. Knight

Electrophysiologic recording techniques are widely employed to study cognitive processing in normal and clinical populations.[1–3] Frequency analysis of the ongoing electroencephalogram (EEG) and extraction of event-related potentials (ERPs) embedded in the ongoing EEG provide information on tonic and phasic changes in brain activity during cognitive processing. Analysis of EEG frequencies is particularly valuable for the study of alterations in regional neural activity in a time domain extending from one to several seconds, approximating the time scale of blood-flow–based physiologic techniques described in Chap. 7, such as positron emission tomography (PET) or functional magnetic resonance imaging (fMRI). Metabolic techniques such as PET and fMRI currently provide better spatial resolution of cognitive activity, but their temporal resolution is limited to the second (fMRI) or minute (PET) range.

ERP methods can extract stimulus, response, or cognition-related neural activity from the ongoing EEG in the millisecond-to-second range, providing a method for real-time assessment of changes in neural activity during cognitive processing. Recent efforts to record EEG and fMRI simultaneously represent a promising approach to linking neuronal and regional blood-flow changes during mental activity.[4–8] Converging data from ERP, PET, and fMRI will likely provide the strongest insights into the neural regions and mechanisms involved in mental activity. This review focuses predominantly on the use of event-related potentials in behavioral neurology (for discussions of frequency-based methods, see, for example, Refs. 9 to 15).

While metabolic and electrophysiologic measurements allow researchers to "eavesdrop" on neural activity, it has long been recognized that an alternative physiologic approach to understanding the function of specific brain regions would be to manipulate neural activity directly. By applying an electrical current, neural discharge can be induced, and the effects of this stimulation can be observed in the resulting behavior. The classic example of this approach is Penfield's work in the 1950s, in which the somatotopic organization of sensorimotor cortex was revealed through direct cortical stimulation applied during the course of neurosurgery.[16] The direct stimulation of human neural tissue is naturally limited to relatively rare situations, however—surgical situations in which the individuals suffer from neurologic conditions such as epilepsy, Parkinson's disease, or tumors.

Transcranial magnetic stimulation (TMS) allows either activation or disruption of activity in neural tissue through the intact skull, providing a more widely applicable method. Rapid improvements in the methodology and safety of these methods provide an exciting way for testing the integrity of neural pathways[17] and for testing hypotheses regarding the role of cortical areas in sensory, motor, and higher cognitive functions.[18] By

* **ACKNOWLEDGMENTS:** Special thanks to Clay C. Clayworth for skillful technical assistance. Supported by NINDS Grants NS21135, NS30256, and NS33504.

producing brief deactivation of cortical areas, TMS results in highly selective "virtual lesions" within healthy brains. It thus has the potential to pinpoint the critical areas responsible for specific functional deficits found in patients with naturally occurring (and permanent) lesions.

EVENT-RELATED POTENTIALS

Neural activity in axonal pathways and inhibitory (IPSPs) and excitatory (EPSPs) postsynaptic potentials on the soma and dendrites of active neurons contribute to scalp-recorded field potentials, with the brunt of scalp EEG activity due to summed IPSPs and EPSPs. A major limitation of scalp electrical and (to a lesser degree) magnetic recording is uncertainty about the precise brain locations of the signal sources. However, intracranial source localization is improved by using mathematical dipole modeling constrained by information obtained from intracranial recordings in surgical patients, event-related fMRI studies, the study of brain-damaged patients, and animal models (see Refs. 19 to 21 for reviews).

ERPs are classified as either exogenous (sensory) or endogenous (cognitive). The latency and amplitude of exogenous responses are determined predominantly by stimulus parameters such as intensity and rate. Examples of exogenous responses include the brainstem auditory evoked response (BAEP), the pattern shift P100 visual evoked potential (VEP), and primary somatosensory evoked potentials (SEP). Since these responses are largely resistant to cognitive influences, they are widely employed in a variety of neurologic conditions to measure neural activity in sensory pathways.

In contrast, endogenous potentials are sensitive to the cognitive parameters of the task. The degree of attention [P300 (P for positive, 300 for latency in milliseconds)], effort [contingent negative variation (CNV)], movement preparation [movement-related potentials (MRPs)], and linguistic analysis [N400 (N for negative, 400 for latency in milliseconds)] are examples of cognitive factors determining the amplitude, latency, and scalp distribution of different types of endogenous brain potentials (see Refs. 22 to 24 for reviews). Since endogenous potentials reflect mental processes not immediately evoked by an external stimulus, the term *evoked potentials* has been replaced by the term *event-related potentials* in describing these signals. However, the borderline between a truly exogenous (presumably sensory, data-driven, hard-wired, and automatic) response and one involving higher cognitive functions is frequently blurred, as several "exogenous" components are modulated by top-down processes (see below). Moreover, some potentials may be regarded as being "exogenous" in some respects and "endogenous" in others [e.g., the mismatch negativity (MMN); visual N170]. Therefore the term *event-related potential* (ERP) may be used for all time-locked scalp potentials, as is done in this chapter.

General Technical Considerations

The local intracranial geometry of intracranial neural sources places an important constraint on scalp or extracranial EEG or magnetoencephalography (MEG) recording. Neural sources must have an open-field configuration to generate dipole sources recordable at a distance.[19,25] Simply put, an open-field geometry occurs when neurons assume a local organized cellular structure wherein neurons are oriented in the same direction. Examples of open-field geometry would include the laminar structure of the cortex or the hippocampus where electromagnetic fields of synchronously active pyramidal neurons are aligned and sum to produce a dipole field recordable at the scalp. A closed-field geometry occurs when a neuronal structure lacks a clear local cellular anatomic substructure (e.g., the intralaminar thalamic nuclei). In this situation, neurons may fire synchronously but the local extracellular fields are not well aligned, and the dipoles will cancel out locally and not generate a summed dipole field recordable at a distance.

This constraint of open-versus closed-field geometry is shown schematically in Fig. 9-1. On the left are two neurons that are aligned in the same direction in an open-field configuration. If these neurons fire synchronously, their extracellular fields will sum and this activity can be propagated by volume conduction and recorded at a distant site such as the scalp. On the right are the same two neurons firing synchronously but aligned 180 degrees out of phase in a closed-field configuration. In this situation their extracellular fields

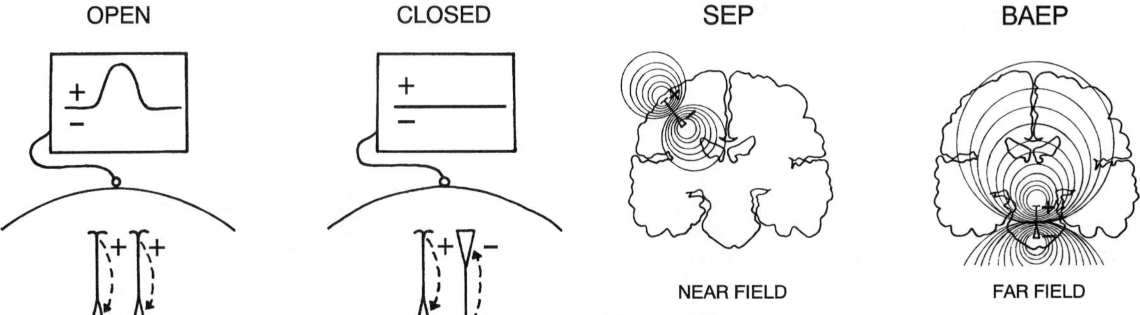

Figure 9-1
Schematic of an idealized open- and closed-field neuronal configuration. In the open-field situation, extracellular fields sum and can be recorded at a distance. In the closed-field condition, the extracellular fields of the two synchronously active neurons cancel and no evoked field is recorded at a distance.

Figure 9-2
On the left is the near field of the primary SEP. The evoked field changes rapidly over small distances on the scalp. On the right is an example of the far-field response of the BAEP. Note that the field is broadly distributed over the scalp, since the neural source is deep in the brainstem. See text for details. (Modified from Knight,[53] with permission.)

would cancel and no electrical field would be recorded at a distance. A single-unit recording electrode would record equivalent activity in both the open- and closed-field condition, and metabolic techniques would also record comparable activity in each situation.

The distance of an active neuronal source from the recording site has a major influence on the strength of the signal recorded at the scalp. This is due to the fact that electric and magnetic fields drop in amplitude as an inverse power function of the distance of the active neuronal elements from a recording site. Intracranial neuronal generators can be classified as near- or far-field sources. An example of a near-field source would be the primary SEP generated in the depths and crown of the postcentral gyrus. Since this neuronal source is on the surface of the hemisphere, the scalp field will be strong and focally distributed in parietal scalp electrodes situated over the postcentral gyrus (Fig. 9-2). A classic far-field source would be the BAEP. The BAEP is generated by sequential activity of auditory structures located in the brainstem extending from the eighth nerve to the inferior colliculus. The dipole field of these generators is broadly distributed over the scalp and small in amplitude due to its distance from the scalp (Fig. 9-2). Because of this biophysical constraint, the brunt of electrical activity recorded at scalp sites arises in near-field generators in neocortical regions. This selectivity for near-field sources may be sharpened using scalp current-density (SCD) derivations of scalp potentials.[26] The SCD is calculated by taking the second spatial derivative (the Laplacian) of the potential distribution over the scalp. Therefore it reflects the rate of change of potential between nearby electrodes. Since far-field sources will not result in large differences between adjacent electrodes (Fig. 9-2), their contribution will be effectively filtered out, providing a finer resolution of more superficial (cortical) sources. Figure 9-3 provides a demonstration of potential maps and SCD maps from the same data set.[103] Whereas the potential maps reveal a broad frontocentral negativity and posterior positivity which is quite similar across conditions, the SCD maps reveal more localized foci of activity, highlighting differences between the conditions (see legend for Fig. 9-3).

Event-related potentials range in amplitude from 0.5 μV for the exogenous BAEP to 10 to 20 μV for longer-latency endogenous potentials such as the P300, N400, and CNV. These signals are buried in the ongoing EEG, which typically varies from 10 to 200 μV, depending in large part on the arousal state of the subject. In order to extract these signals from the ongoing EEG, the event-related response to a discrete sensory stimulus or cognitive manipulation must be averaged over multiple trials. Since the background EEG can be approximated as random noise, the average of repetitive EEG epochs will approximate zero.

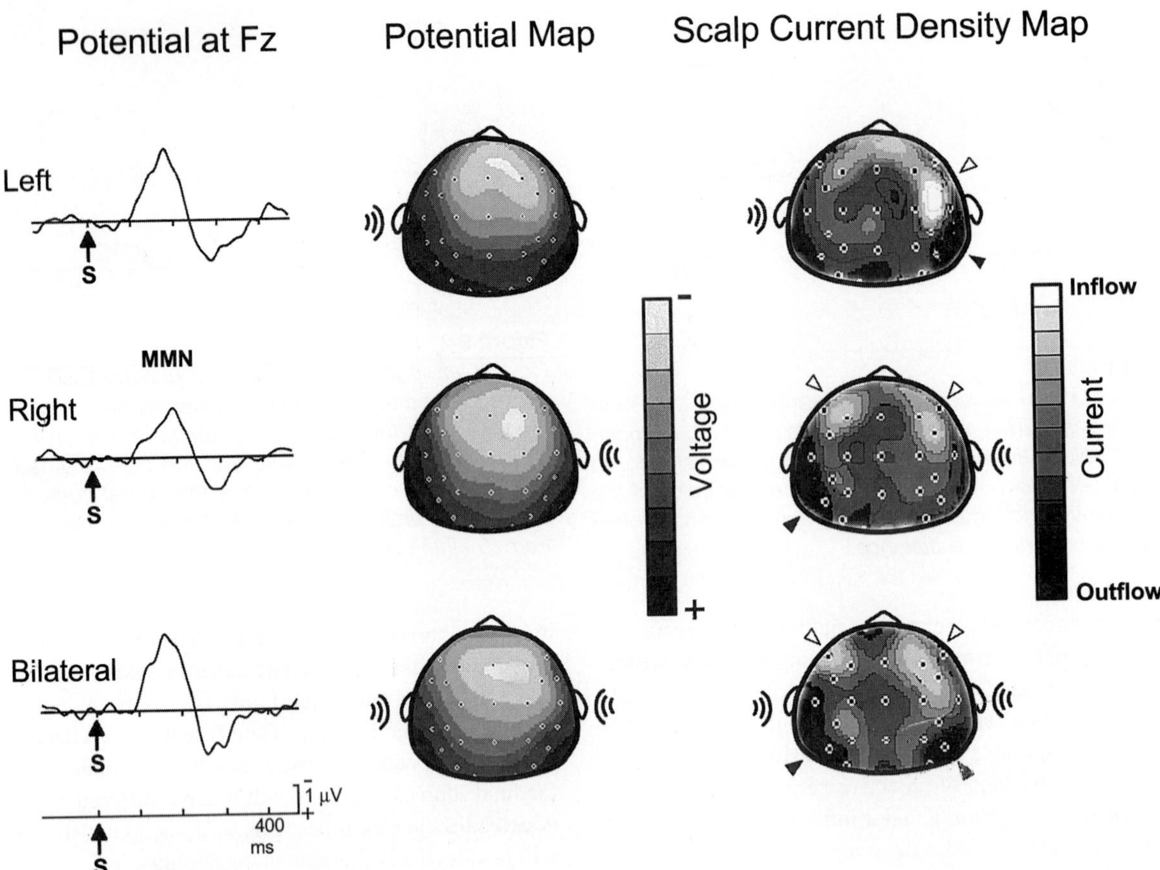

Figure 9-3

Waveforms, potential maps, and scalp current density (SCD) maps for the same data. Fifteen subjects heard sequences of two different tones presented simultaneously, one to each ear. The waveforms show the difference, at the Fz site, between the event-related potential (ERP) elicited by a standard pair and the ERP elicited by a change in the pitch of the left, right, or both tones. The deviants elicited the typical mismatch negativity. The potential maps around the peak of the MMN for each condition show a broad frontocentral negativity, skewed rightward, regardless of the side of deviation, and a bilateral temporal positivity. The SCD maps, which are the laplacian derivations of the same data, show more circumscribed foci of activity with different patterns dependent on side of deviation. The temporal foci (black arrowheads) were significantly stronger contralateral to the side of deviation (symmetrical for the bilateral condition). The frontal scalp foci (open arrowheads) were significantly right lateralized in the left-deviant condition but were symmetrical when the deviant was on the right or bilateral (see Deouell et al.[103] for details).

Conversely, the event-related response, time-locked to a specific stimulus or response, is assumed to repeat itself across trials and therefore emerges by averaging from the background EEG. The signal-to-noise ratio, which can be viewed as a measure of the ability to confidently identify the evoked signal in the background EEG "noise," is proportional to the square root of the number of epochs averaged. Consequently, smaller signals require many more trials before a reliable potential is seen. The effects of signal averaging for the small, far-field, exogenous BAEP is shown in Fig. 9-4. Note that no signal is apparent in the evoked potential

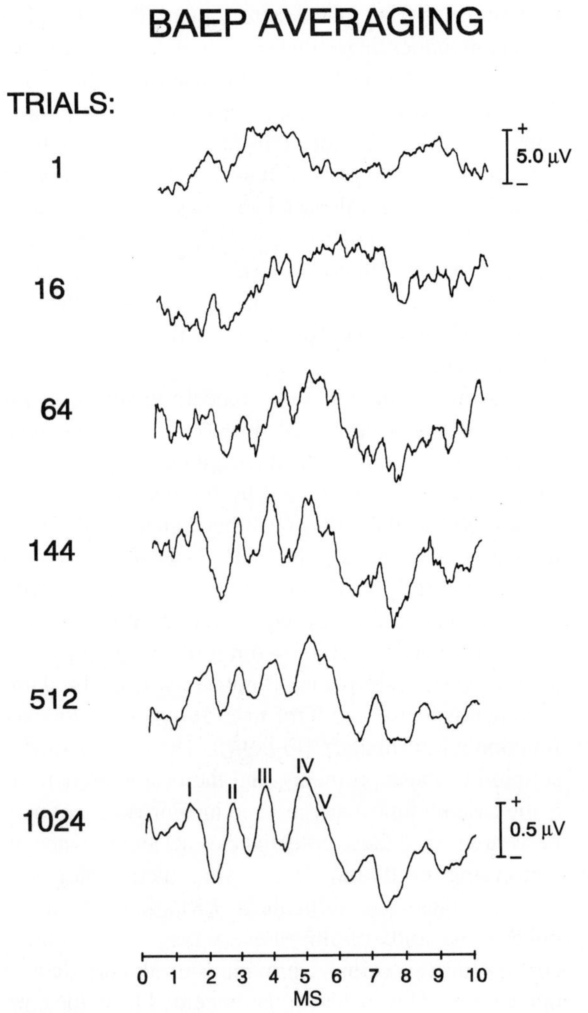

Figure 9-4
The signal averaging of the BAEP. Note that a clear signal is not observable for at least 144 trials, since the BAEP is small (~0.5 μV) and buried in the background EEG activity.

average of the first 16 trials. A clear but noisy signal is seen after 144 trials. By 1024 trials, a clean signal is obtained, revealing the principal five components of the BAEP as well as two additional potentials that reflect thalamocortical activity projecting from the inferior colliculus to primary auditory cortex. A different pattern is seen in Fig. 9-5, which shows the averaging of a P300 response to unexpected novel sounds over 1 to 36 trials in two subjects. Since the P300 to these

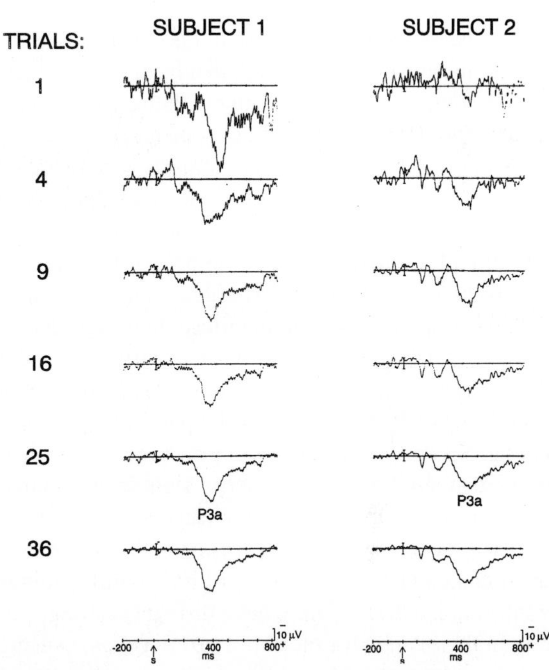

Figure 9-5
The signal averaging of novelty P3a responses in two subjects. Since the P3a amplitude is large (~10 μV), the signal is well seen in only a few trials.

unexpected sounds is in the range of 10 to 30 μV for a single stimulus, it can be readily distinguished from the background EEG noise after just a few trials. Indeed, it can be seen after a single trial in subject 1 and after four trials in subject 2. Note that the superimposed EEG noise continues to flatten out with repetitive trials, especially apparent in the prestimulus epoch. Several techniques have been developed to extract single trials from the ongoing EEG during cognitive tasks that generate large responses (see Refs. 19 and 27 for reviews of signal processing techniques).

Special Considerations in Studying Brain-Damaged Patients with ERPs

Chapter 8 reviews some of the advantages and special challenges of functional neuroimaging with brain-damaged patients. Many of these special considerations arise with the use of ERPs with neurological populations, along with others unique to electrophysiologic methods.

The recording of ERPs requires considerable cooperation from the subject, both in minimizing artifacts and, in some cases, in complying with the task requirements. These limitations may be especially pronounced for brain-damaged patients, particularly when studied in relative proximity to the onset of their illness. The difficulties result from several factors. First, it is often difficult to make sure that the patient fully understands the procedure, aim, and significance of the test, especially when he or she manifests language disturbances (aphasia), disorientation, or confusion. Under these circumstances, the environment and equipment used in an ERP study may also be particularly intimidating. Second, with or without psychoactive medications, patients frequently undergo significant fluctuations in their arousal. This may cause both problems in performance and interference from slow waves (in the alpha band or slower) in the EEG. Third, patients with motor weakness may have difficulty sitting quietly in their chairs for the entire test duration, causing excessive artifacts of muscular activity. Fourth, patients may suffer from general attention deficits, making it difficult for them to stay alert, focused, and compliant throughout a prolonged testing session. The last problem is especially evident in patients with right hemisphere damage (RHD).

The above difficulties require the adjustment of experimental paradigms to shorten the testing sessions as much as possible and to minimize the patient's discomfort and apprehension. Alternatively, patients can be tested in a more chronic phase, when many of the above concerns are alleviated. However, if the goal is to correlate ERPs with behavioral deficits that may subside with time (e.g., unilateral neglect or aphasia), one must attempt to deal with the problems inherent in studying acute patients. Unfortunately, even if these precautions are taken, patients are occasionally excluded a priori from ERP studies because of failure to cooperate fully, and considerable amounts of data may often have to be discarded because of excessive noise (cf. Ref. 28). Of course, this procedure increases the risk of a selection bias toward less severely affected patients.

An additional problem (not unique to ERPs) is that the comparison of patients with normal controls is confounded by many factors other than the phenomenon under investigation. Such factors are, for example, the hospitalization, the use of medications, concomitant affective components such as depression, and the level of alertness. In fact, even the comparison between patients is complicated by inescapable variability in lesion sites and volumes, general medical condition, and uncontrolled premorbid differences. A possible partial remedy is to prefer designs in which each patient serves as his or her own control ("within subject" designs; see, for example, the studies of neglect patients below).

A major methodologic concern involves the interpretation of scalp-recorded ERPs in brain-damaged patients. The amplitude and spatial distribution of the ERP signals may be altered by the lesion in at least three ways: (1) there may be direct damage to the electrical source generating the ERP, (2) the damaged area may modulate the activity of an electrical source distant from the lesion, and (3) altered electrical conduction in the damaged tissue may diminish or augment the amplitude of scalp-recorded potentials over the damaged hemisphere even if the underlying generators are functioning normally[29] (Fig. 9-6). There is no simple solution to these problems, and the best approach (as is the case in almost any method in neuroscience) may be awareness of these potential caveats and reliance on converging information from several methodologies.

Despite these difficulties, ERPs have been applied to the study of almost every functional problem covered in this volume, providing invaluable data in many cases. This endeavor has benefited from the convergence of better understanding of the cognitive correlates and anatomic substrate of different ERP components (e.g., Refs. 20, 22, and 30), improved localization of lesions with the advent of MRI and computerized reconstructions (e.g., Refs. 31 to 33), and increasingly refined neuropsychological methods. This combination of ERPs, lesion analysis, and cognitive neuropsychology is informative in at least two complementary ways. First, by examining the effect of discrete lesions on specific components of ERPs, it is possible to discern the neural elements of large-scale networks controlling, for example, attention and memory in the healthy brain.[34] Second, by using electrophysiologic components whose correlation with specific cognitive operations is reasonably clear, it is possible to shed light on the cognitive, anatomic, and physiologic mechanisms

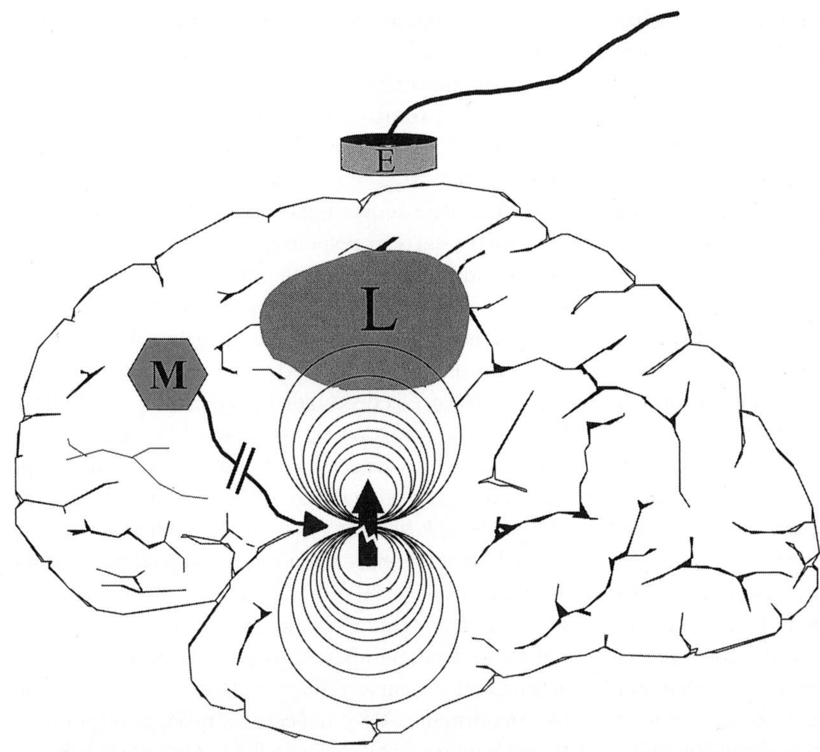

Figure 9-6
Schematic model depicting three possible ways in which a lesion can change the pattern of a scalp recorded potential: (1) The lesion destroys the neural generator (broken arrow); (2) the conductivity of the damaged parenchyma (L) is altered, distorting the amplitude recorded at the scalp electrode (E); (3) The lesion is remote from the neural generator of the recorded potential, but it disrupts modulatory input (M) to the generator by ablating the source of the modulatory input or by disconnection.

of specific functional deficits, information that cannot be obtained by traditional behavioral methods.[35,36]

In the following, we attempt to demonstrate some of these insights through examination of three cardinal neurobehavioral domains—prefrontal damage, unilateral neglect following right hemisphere damage, and aphasia following left hemisphere damage.

Prefrontal Damage and Executive Control

As discussed in Chaps. 32 and 33, prefrontal cortex is crucial for executive control and efficient goal-directed activity. Through its attentional, inhibitory and/or working memory functions, prefrontal cortex enables us to suppress irrelevant information and facilitate the processing of relevant information. These functions may be bound under the headings of sustained and selective attention. For attention to be flexible, we must also be able to respond to potentially important events (e.g., a threat) outside the focus of attention and to detect and further process targets within the focus of attention (phasic attention). Lateral prefrontal cortex is crucial for the control of sustained and phasic attention to environmental events, as well as to novelty and target detection.[37,38] Attention and orienting ability have been studied using ERP techniques in neurologic patients with damage centered in Brodmann's areas 9 and 46 and in patients with posterior cortical and mesial temporal damage. Both the electrophysiologic and behavioral data from these patients have indicated that problems with inhibitory control of sensory inputs, reduced facilitation of processing of relevant information (sustained attention), and abnormalities in the detection of novel events are central concomitants of prefrontal disease.[39] At the same time, these data reveal the dynamic interaction between bottom-up and top-down processes that is necessary for normal function.

Inhibitory Modulation and Sensory Gating

The attention deficits of patients with prefrontal lesions and the behavioral phenomena of perseveration in advanced prefrontal disease have been linked to problems with inhibitory control of posterior sensory and perceptual mechanisms.[40,146] Inability to inhibit internal representations of previous responses that are now incorrect, coupled with random inappropriate shifts of attention, contributes to the poor performance of patients with prefrontal damage on the Wisconsin Card Sorting Task and on the Stroop task.[41,77] Problems with tasks involving "working memory" (operationally defined as the holding of information needed for the execution of action over short delays) may be due to intrusion of irrelevant information coupled with failures to sustain neural activity in distributed task-dependent neural circuits.[43] Physiologic data indicates that this lack of inhibitory control may extend to early sensory processing in primary cortical regions.

Neural inhibition by prefrontal regions has been reported in a variety of mammalian preparations. A net inhibitory output to both subcortical[44] and cortical regions has been documented.[45] Cryogenic blockade of a prefrontal-thalamic gating system in cats results in enhancement of amplitudes of primary sensory cortex evoked responses.[46,47] This system is modulated by an excitatory lateral prefrontal projection to the nucleus reticularis thalami, although the precise course of anatomic projections between these structures is not well understood. The nucleus reticularis thalami, in turn, sends inhibitory GABAergic projections to sensory relay nuclei, providing a neural substrate for selective sensory suppression.[48]

This prefrontal-thalamic inhibitory system provides a potential mechanism for modality-specific suppression of irrelevant inputs at an early stage of sensory processing. Support for a similar mechanism in humans has been obtained from the observation of patients with prefrontal damage due to stroke.[49,50] Task-irrelevant auditory and somatosensory stimuli were delivered to patients with damage to lateral prefrontal cortex (PFC) and to others with comparably sized lesions in the temporoparietal junction or the lateral parietal cortex. Evoked responses from primary auditory and somatosensory cortices were recorded in these patients and in age-matched controls (Fig. 9-7). The stimuli consisted of either monaural clicks or brief electric shocks to the median nerve, eliciting a small opponens pollicis twitch.

Lesions of the posterior association cortex invading either the primary auditory or somatosensory cortex reduced early latency (20 to 40 ms) evoked responses generated in these regions. Lesions in posterior association cortex, sparing primary sensory regions, had no effects on the amplitudes or latencies of the primary cortical evoked responses; such patients served as a brain-lesioned control group. Lateral prefrontal damage resulted in enhanced amplitude of both the primary auditory and somatosensory evoked responses generated from 20 to 40 ms poststimulation.[43,49–51] Spinal cord and brainstem potentials were unaffected by prefrontal damage, indicating that amplitude enhancement of primary cortical responses was due to abnormalities in either prefrontal-thalamic or direct prefrontal-sensory cortical mechanisms. Chronic disinhibition of sensory inputs may contribute to many of the behavioral sequelae of prefrontal damage. For instance, decision confidence is decremented by a noisy internal milieu, and the orienting response would be expected to habituate.[52,53] A direct correlation between disinhibition and decreased performance in a delayed matching to sample task has been now demonstrated in a group of prefrontal patients, required to compare two sounds separated by a 5-s delay.[43,54] Patients' performance was significantly degraded when the delay period was filled with tone pips, and these tone pips, in turn, elicited an augmented primary auditory potentials (Na, Pa) relative to normals. The enhancement of Pa in response to the distracting tones also correlated with the number of delay errors. Similarly, in patients with right prefrontal damage, sounds presented to an unattended ear in a dichotic paradigm reduce the attentional enhancement (see next section) of subsequent to-be-attended sounds. The unattended sounds have no such effect in healthy controls.[55]

Attentional Facilitation In addition to suppressing irrelevant information, normal function involves facilitation of processing of relevant information. A "biased competition" model suggests that excitatory signals to neurons result in inhibition of nearby task-irrelevant neurons, resulting in a sharpening of the attentional focus.[56] Selective attention to a sensory channel such as an ear, a portion of the visual field, or a finger increases the amplitude of evoked potentials generated to all stimuli delivered to that region[57–60] and induces a slow negative potential spanning several hundreds of milliseconds following the presentation of the stimulus [known, in different contexts, as negative difference (Nd), selection negativity (SN), or processing negativity (PN)].[22] There is evidence that attention reliably modulates neural activity at early sensory

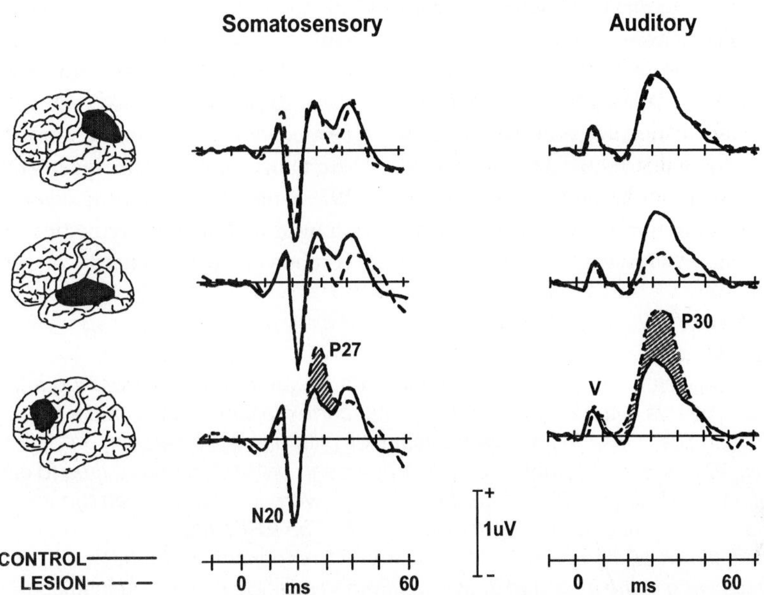

Figure 9-7
Primary cortical auditory and somatosensory event-related potentials are shown for controls (solid line) and patients (dashed line) with focal damage in the lateral parietal cortex (top, n = 8), temporoparietal junction (middle, n = 13), or dorsolateral prefrontal cortex (bottom, n = 13). Reconstructions of the center of damage in each patient group are shown on the left. Somatosensory event-related responses were recorded from area 3b (N20) and areas 1 and 2 on the crown of the postcentral gyrus (P26). Stimuli were square-wave pulses of 0.15 ms duration delivered to the median nerve at the wrist. Stimulus intensity was set at 10 percent above opponens twitch threshold, and stimuli were delivered at a rate of 3/s. Damage in posterior cortical regions sparing primary somatosensory cortex had no effect on the N20 or earlier spinal cord potentials. Prefrontal damage resulted in a selective increase in the amplitude of the P26 response (hatched area). Auditory stimuli were clicks delivered at a rate of 13/s at intensity levels of 50 dB HL. Unilateral damage in the temporoparietal junction extending into primary auditory cortex reduces P30 responses. Lateral parietal damage sparing primary auditory cortex has no effect on P30 responses. Dorsolateral prefrontal damage results in normal inferior collicular potentials (wave V) but an enhanced P30 primary cortical response (hatched area). The shaded area in each modality indicates the area of event-related potential amplitude enhancement.

cortices, including secondary and perhaps primary sensory cortex.[61–65] Visual attention involves modulation in the excitability of extrastriate neurons through descending projections from hierarchically ordered brain structures.[66] Single-cell recordings in monkeys,[67,68] lesion studies in humans[34,39,42] and monkeys,[69] and blood-flow data[70–76] have linked PFC to control of extrastriate cortex during visual attention.

ERP studies in patients with lateral PFC damage suggests that human lateral PFC regulates extrastriate neural activity through three distinct mechanisms: (1) by enhancement of extrastriate cortex response to attended information; (2) through a tonic excitatory influence on ipsilateral posterior areas for all sensory information, including attended and nonattended sensory inputs; and (3) by a phasic excitatory influence of ipsilateral posterior areas to correctly perceived task relevant stimuli. In a series of ERP studies, patients with unilateral PFC lesions (centered in Brodmann's areas 9 and 46) were required to detect inverted triangles (targets) among a series of upright triangles (distractors). In one experiment, patients and age-matched controls were asked to press a button whenever a target appeared at fixation.[34] In another, the target appeared in either visual field[42] while both visual fields were similarly attended. In a third experiment, subjects were instructed to attend to only one visual field.[79]

An interesting pattern of results emerged from these experiments (Figs. 9-8 and 9-9). First, the experiments revealed that lateral PFC provides a tonic excitatory influence to ipsilateral extrastriate cortex. When the stimuli appear centrally the PFC patients showed a significant reduction of the extrastriate N1 component (with a latency of 170 ms).[34,78] When the

Figure 9-8

Visual event–related potentials in patients with lateral frontal lobe damage and healthy controls. Patients with dorsolateral prefrontal cortex lesions and controls had to detect upright triangles in a series of inverted triangles (standards, 70 percent), upright triangles (targets, 20 percent), and novel stimuli (10 percent) presented one at time to either side of fixation. Patients (n = 8) and controls (n = 11) were instructed to attend and respond to targets on the left or on the right of fixation. **A:** *The ERPs elicited by the contralesional standard stimuli elicited significantly reduced P1 responses in the patients whether the standards were in the attended or the unattended side.* **B:** *The attention effect (extracted by subtracting the response to unattended standards from the response to the attended ones) reveals a significantly smaller effect for contralesional standards in patients relative to controls, starting around 200 ms postonset. POi = The ipsilesional of P7 and P8. POc = The contralesional of the two. For controls POi/POc = P7/P8, respectively. (Modified from Yago and Knight.[79])*

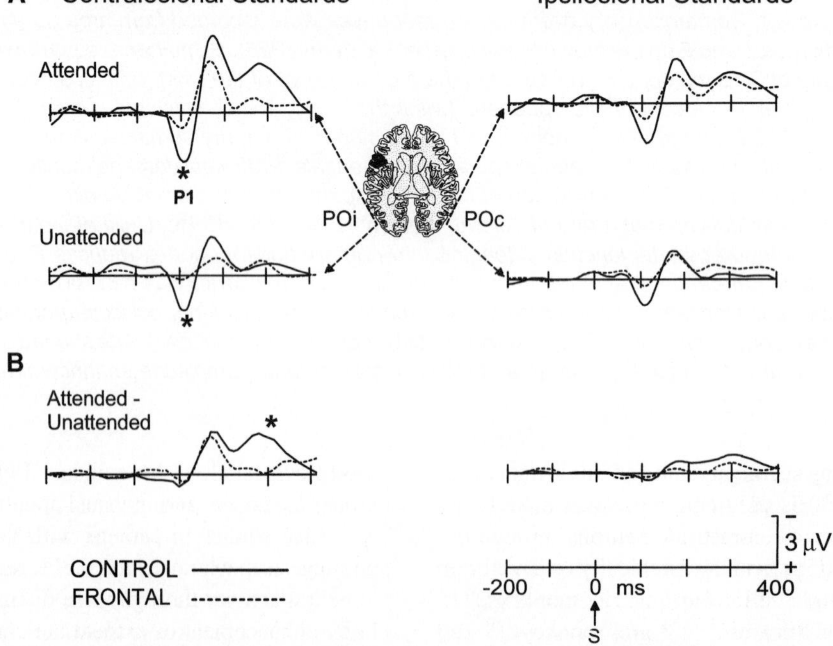

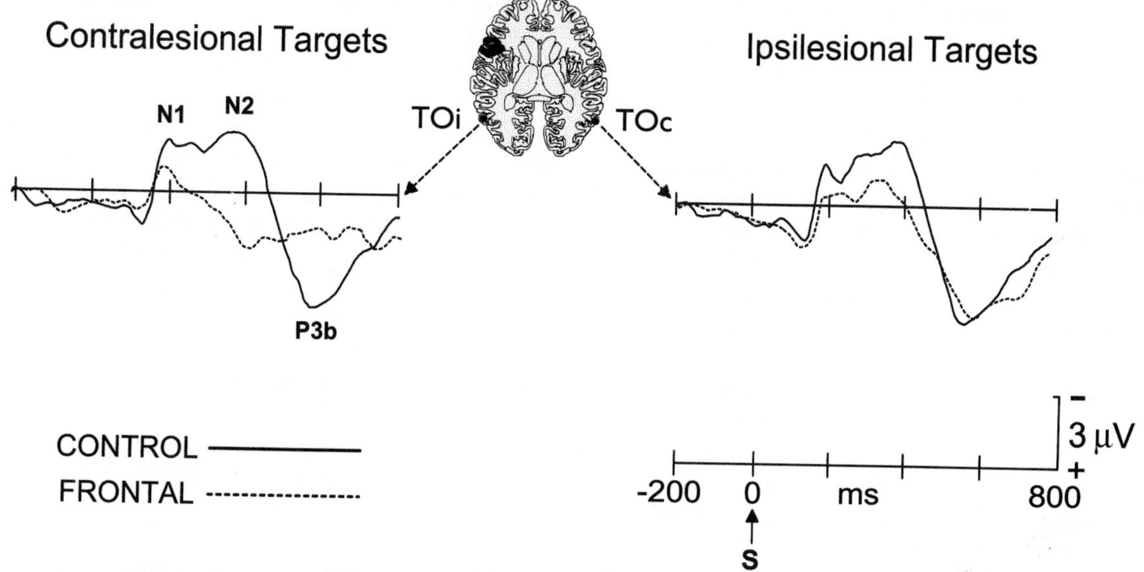

Figure 9-9

Same paradigm as Fig. 9–8, only that the patients (n = 10) and controls (n = 10) were attending to both right and left sides in this case. The N1, N2, and P3b peaks, seen in the controls' waveform, were significantly reduced in the patients in response to contralesional targets but not for ipsilesional targets (see Ref. 42 for more details). TOi = T5 or T6, the one ipsilateral to the lesion in patients; T5 in controls. TOc = T5 or T6, the one contralateral to the lesion in patients, T6 in controls.

stimuli were lateralized, the P1 component of the visual ERP was markedly reduced in amplitude for all stimuli presented to the contralesional field.[42,79] Importantly, this tonic influence was attention-independent, since a reduced P1 potential in extrastriate cortex was found ipsilateral to PFC damage for all visual stimuli (attended and nonattended targets and nontargets) presented to the contralesional field (Fig. 9-8a.).[79] This tonic component may be viewed as a modulatory influence on extrastriate activity. In the auditory modality, the patients elicited a reduced N1 component peaking 100 ms after the onset of the stimulus.[43] The auditory N1 has several sources in the superior temporal plane[20] providing additional evidence or prefrontal modulation of early sensory processing. Second, when the attention was directed to only one visual field, attention effects on extrastriate cortex were normal in the first 200 ms for the PFC patients and severely disrupted after 200 ms (Fig 9-8b).[79] This finding suggests that other cortical areas, possibly the posterior parietal cortex, are responsible for attention-dependent regulation of extrastriate cortex in the first 200 ms. The PFC facilitation appears to begin after 200 ms. It is conceivable that inferior parietal cortex is responsible for the early reflexive component of attention, whereas PFC is responsible for more controlled and sustained aspects of visual attention beginning after the parietal signal to extrastriate cortices.

Third, in addition to the observation of channel-specific enhancement, another distinct electrophysiologic event (including the N2-P3b complex) was observed when a relevant target event was detected in an attended channel (Fig. 9-9).[79] The latency of this top-down signal was about 200 ms after a correct detection, and it extended throughout the ensuing 500 ms, superimposed on the channel-specific ERP attention enhancement.[80] Damage to lateral PFC results in marked decrements in the top-down signal, accompanied by behavioral evidence of impaired detection ability.[42] The N2, a component which is generated in the inferior temporal lobe in response to targets and which is therefore assumed to reflect postselection processing, was abolished over the lesioned hemisphere for targets in both visual fields. Behaviorally, the patients reacted more slowly to targets in the contralesional visual field and missed more targets than the controls did. The frontal patients also showed reduced P3b over the temporooccipital electrodes, but not at parietal sites.[42]

The P3b has been proposed to underlie a range of cognitive processes. One proposal is that the P3b is generated during closure of a perceptual task.[81] According to this theory, the P3b represents inhibition of a discrete epoch of stimulus processing. More precisely, this theory posits that the P3b is generated by inhibition of regional negativity in activated neocortex or mesial temporal sites associated with the termination of voluntary processing of an expected stimulus.[82,83] Alternatively, the P3b may index the updating of information in working memory.[84] Other proposals, such as those linking P3b and template matching, may be subsumed under the concept of context updating in working memory.[85] Most likely, the P3b includes contributions from multiple intracranial sources and processes (for reviews see Refs. 30, 86, and 87), which may include also modality-specific components.[88] This is highlighted by the fact that, in the PFC patients, the parietal P3b was intact, but at the same latency positivity was reduced over ipsilateral occipitotemporal sites.

Auditory selective attention capacity has also been examined in patients with lateral PFC lesions. In dichotic selective attention tasks, normal subjects generate an enhanced ("selection") negativity to all stimuli in an attended channel with onset from 25 to 50 ms after delivery of an attended auditory stimulus. Prefrontal patients generated reduced attention effects depending on the side of the lesion. Patients with left hemisphere lesions showed a reduced attention effect regardless of which ear was attended. In contrast, patients with right prefrontal damage showed reduced enhancement effect mainly when the contralateral ear was to be attended, consistent with the symptoms of unilateral neglect (see below).[89] Posterior association cortex lesions in the temporoparietal junction have comparable attention deficits for left- and right-sided lesions.[90] This suggests that some aspects of hemineglect subsequent to temporoparietal damage may be due to remote effects of disconnection from asymmetrically organized prefrontal regions.

The CNV is a negative-polarity brain potential maximal over frontal-central scalp sites generated during a delay period initiated by a warning stimulus. The CNV is terminated by a behavioral response that is contingent on information delivered in the warning stimulus.[91] The behavioral structure of tasks that generate a CNV shares attributes with paradigms associated with working memory in monkeys and humans.[92,93] The CNV potentials are focally reduced by discrete prefrontal damage, supporting a generator of the CNV in prefrontal cortex[94–96] (Fig. 9-10). These data provide a further link between prefrontal regions and sustained attention and working memory capacity.

Novelty Detection The earliest brain potential directly reflecting the detection of deviance is the mismatch negativity (MMN). The MMN[97] is elicited in response to small deviations from regularities in the acoustic environment (e.g., a pitch change in a series of tones). The MMN can be observed for events outside the focus of attention and peaks 100 to 250 ms following the deviant event. It reflects an "error signal" generated automatically by a neural mechanism comparing a perceived stimulus to a sensory "memory trace" formed by the standard stimuli[98] or the updating of the existing model of the environment.[99] The mismatch response is presumed to trigger an involuntary reorientation of attention.[98,100] The MMN is generated mainly in the secondary auditory cortex (see Ref. 101 for review) but may have a second frontal generator, presumably related to the triggering of an attention switch.[102,103] The distribution of this frontal generator is reminiscent of the distribution of the visual attention mechanism, whereby the left frontal generator is active in response to contralateral deviancies while the right frontal generator responds to events on either side (Fig. 9-3).[103,104]

The MMN in response to pitch and pattern changes[51,105] is reduced in patients with prefrontal lesions, indicating an early deficit in automatic detection of deviance outside the focus of attention. Whereas temporoparietal lesions caused an MMN reduction

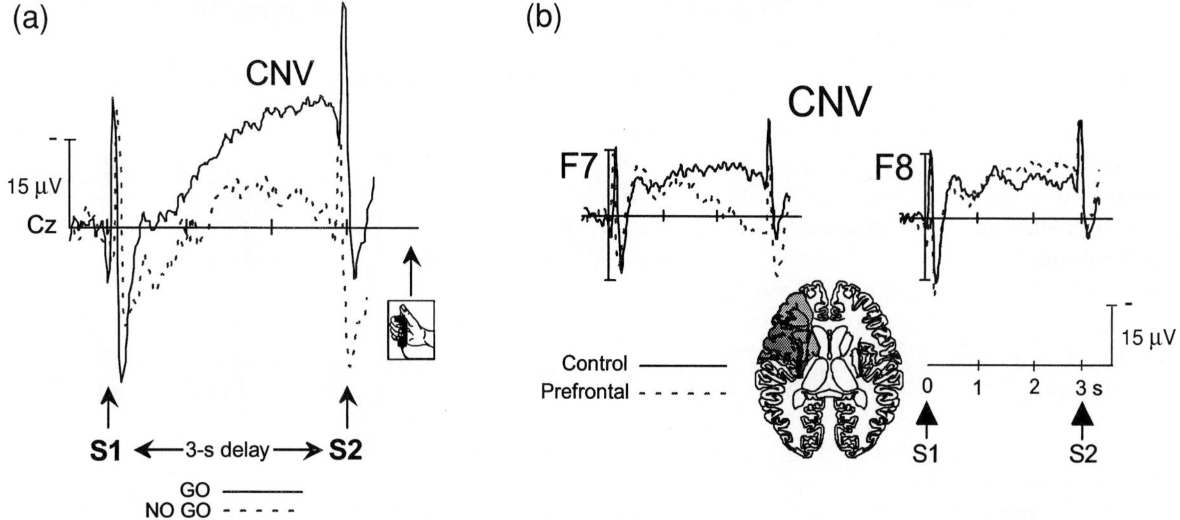

Figure 9-10

This figure shows the results of a classic auditory contingent negative variation (CNV) experiment in patients with focal prefrontal (PFCx) damage. On the left (a) are the results of a CNV task in normals. A warning stimulus (S1) triggers either a GO or NO/GO trial, which is terminated by the imperative S2 stimulus. GO trials generate a large DC shift maximal over frontocentral scalp sites, referred to as the CNV. Damage to the PFCx results in severe attenuation in the CNV over lesioned cortex (b), reductions observed throughout the lesioned hemisphere (see Rosahl and Knight[95] for details). On the bottom right are the group-averaged lesion reconstructions in 10 patients with prefrontal damage. Posterior lesions focally reduce the CNV over lesioned cortex but do not result in widespread hemispheric declines. These data provide evidence of PFCx involvement in sustaining distributed neural activity during delay periods.

mainly to contralesional stimuli, dorsolateral prefrontal lesions elicited comparable deficits regardless of stimulus side in one study[105] and more to ipsilesional sounds in another.[51] In addition, there was a tendency for right prefrontal lesions to be associated with larger MMN reductions than left frontal lesions, while no such asymmetry was found for the temporoparietal lesions.[105] These results suggest different contributions of the temporoparietal region and the prefrontal region to the MMN. It is yet to be determined whether reduced MMN following prefrontal damage reflects a weakened memory trace of the previous regularity due to disinhibition of irrelevant information, reduced frontal facilitation of a comparator mechanism in the secondary auditory cortex, a failure to initiate an attention switch following the detection of the change, or a damage to the postulated frontal generator of MMN.

Delivery of an unexpected and novel stimulus generates a P300 response (P3a) that is observed over widespread anterior and posterior scalp sites. The P3a potential has an earlier latency and a more frontocentral scalp distribution than the P3b in all sensory modalities and has been proposed to be a central marker of the orienting response.[52,53,106,107] Intracranial recordings in the visual, auditory, and somatosensory modalities have shown that multiple neocortical and limbic regions are activated during tasks that generate scalp novelty-dependent P3a potentials.[108–111] Intracranial P3a activity has been recorded in widespread areas of frontal and posterior association cortex in addition to cingulate and mesial temporal regions.[112] These intracranial novelty-related P3a potentials have been proposed to reflect neural activity in a distributed multimodal corticolimbic orienting

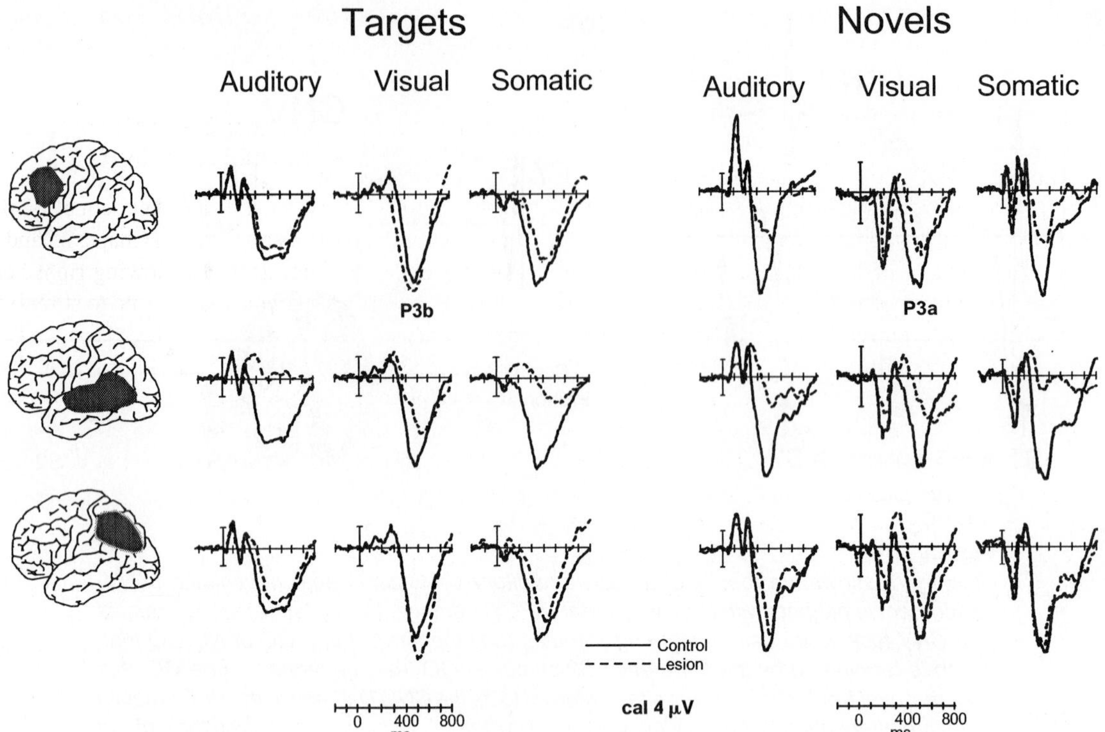

Figure 9-11
Summary of the target P3b and novelty P3a effects in controls and three patient groups with focal cortical damage. The center of the damage in each group is shown on the left. The waveforms from selected electrodes with maximal response amplitude (Pz for targets, Fz for novels) are shown for both target and novel stimuli in the auditory, visual, and somatosensory modalities in patients and controls. Prefrontal and lateral parietal lesions had no significant effect on the latency or amplitude of the target P3b generated in this simple detection task in the auditory, somatosensory, or visual modalities, implying that substantial regions of dorsolateral, prefrontal, and parietal association cortex are not critical for the parietal maximal P3b. Conversely, focal infarction in the temporoparietal junction resulted in marked P3b reductions in the auditory and somatosensory modalities and partial reductions in the visual modality. On the right are the results of the novelty experiments. Lateral parietal damage again had no significant effect on the P3 to novel stimuli and served as a brain lesioned control. Both prefrontal and temporoparietal damage resulted in multimodal reductions of the novelty P3a.

system. Similar theories have been suggested for the scalp P3a response.[53,106,113] fMRI studies using both blocked and event-related designs indicate distributed regions of activation during novelty and target detection, including the inferior frontal gyri, inferior parietal regions, the insula, the lateral temporal lobe,[114,115] and, in certain paradigms, also in the hippocampus.[116]

Novelty P3a responses generated over prefrontal scalp sites to unexpected novel stimuli are reduced by prefrontal lesions, with reductions observed throughout the lesioned hemisphere.[34] Comparable P3a decrements have been observed in the auditory,[53,117] visual,[34] and somatosensory modalities in humans with prefrontal damage[118] (Fig. 9-11). Reductions appear to be more severe after right prefrontal damage.[119]

Galvanic skin response (GSR), a peripheral marker of the orienting response, is also reduced by damage to the prefrontal and posterior association cortex.[120] These findings support a prefrontal source for the frontal scalp component of the novelty P300 and converge with both clinical observations and animal experimentation supporting a critical role of prefrontal structures in the detection of novel stimuli.[121,122] The combination of data from patients with lesions in anterior and posterior lesions suggest distributed interaction between prefrontal and posterior regions during both voluntary and involuntary attention and working memory,[123,124] with a special role for the right prefrontal region.[2]

Unilateral damage centered in the posterior hippocampal region has no effect on parietal P3b activity generated to auditory, visual, and somatosensory stimuli but reduces frontocentral P3 activity to both target and novel stimuli in all modalities. Reductions are most prominent over frontal regions and for novel stimuli[87,126] (Figs. 9-12 and 9-13). These reductions are comparable in amplitude to those observed after focal prefrontal damage. However, unilateral hippocampal damage reduces P300 potentials over both prefrontal cortices, whereas prefrontal damage results in predominantly unilateral reductions over the lesioned hemisphere. Studies with PET have also documented frontal hypometabolism in patients with medial temporal amnesia.[127] These observations support involvement of a prefrontal-hippocampal system in the detection of deviancies in the ongoing sensory stream and indicate that the hippocampal formation has bilateral facilitatory input to prefrontal cortex. Reciprocal pathways coursing through the caudomedial lobule of the mesial temporal lobe provide a potential anatomic substrate for prefrontal-hippocampal interactions during sensory and mnemonic processing.[128]

These results, in conjunction with the data from intracranial and functional imaging studies, provide further evidence that the P300 phenomenon is not a unitary phenomenon but represents distributed neural activity in corticolimbic regions engaged during both voluntary and involuntary response to discrete environmental events. Although this view is more complicated than initial proposals of a unitary nature of P300 activity, it strengthens the potential utility of scalp ERP recording, since it provides a means for the measurement of neural activity in distributed brain regions in the time domain of cognitive processing.

Unilateral Neglect and Extinction after Right Hemisphere Damage

Unilateral neglect (UN) is a frequent sequel of right hemisphere damage. As reviewed in Chaps. 25 and 26, patients suffering from neglect following right hemisphere damage fail to orient and respond to stimuli and events occurring on the left side of their personal or extrapersonal space.[129] In extinction, a related disorder, the failure to notice a contralesional stimulus occurs only when a competing stimulus is simultaneously presented more toward the side of the lesion.[130–132] Unilateral neglect (UN) may manifest itself in the visual, auditory, or tactile modalities.[133–135] Examination of UN patients has been widely used to explore mechanisms of attention and awareness. Yet, despite the ubiquity of such patients and the grave implications for their recovery after stroke, the cognitive and anatomic underpinnings of UN are not clear (see Chaps. 25 and 26). Since UN and extinction may occur in the absence of primary sensory deficits, theoretical accounts of UN have emphasized higher-order processes associated with the allocation of attention, representation of space, or motor preparation. These theories are based almost exclusively on clinical observations and studies employing behavioral methods. Recently, functional neuroimaging methods including ERP and fMRI have begun to provide new insights that might necessitate modification of current theories.

A major question in neglect research is still whether early perceptual processes are really unaltered, as suggested by theories that emphasize higher-order deficits in neglect. Normal SEPs (including N9, N13, P15, N20, and P25) were observed in three UN patients with lesions in the right frontotemporo-parietal regions and in one patient with damage in the right occipital periventricular region, even though the patients were not aware of the electrical shocks applied to the left median nerve.[136,137] Moreover, in two of the patients whose primary visual cortex was largely spared, the visual evoked potentials (VEPs) including N75, P100, and N145 were within normal range.[136] In contrast, SEPs and VEPs were absent or reduced in patients suffering from hemianesthesia or hemianopsia,

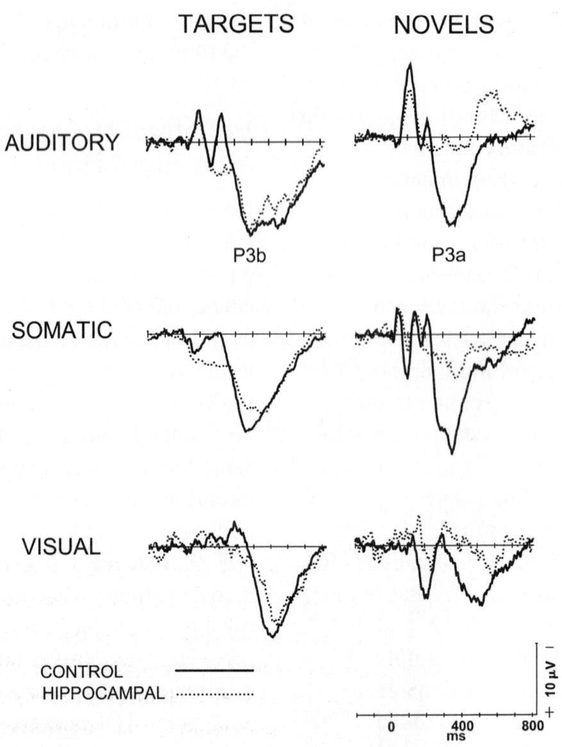

Figure 9-12
Group-averaged event-related potential (ERP) data from controls and patients with hippocampal lesions (n =7) for auditory, visual, and somatosensory target and novel stimuli. Subjects were seated in a sound-attenuated booth and instructed to press a button upon detection of a designated target stimulus during each experiment. Auditory stimuli consisted of blocks of repetitive standard 1000-Hz monaural tone bursts (60 dB HL; 50 ms duration, 1 s ISI). Tone bursts of 1500 Hz occurred randomly on 10 percent of the trials and served as targets. Unexpected novel tones consisting of complex computer-generated sounds, and environmental noises such as bells or barks were randomly delivered on 10 percent of the trials. A similar paradigm was employed in the visual modality. Visual stimuli consisted of repetitive presentation of triangles. On 10 percent of the trials, inverted triangles served as target stimuli. On an additional 10 percent of trials, random line drawings or pictures of irrelevant stimuli served as novel events. Somatosensory stimuli consisted of repetitive taps to the index finger, with targets being random taps to the ring finger that occurred on 10 percent of the trials. Novel stimuli consisted of brief random shocks to the median nerve on 6 percent of the trials. The ERPs shown are from the electrode where maximal responses were recorded (Pz for targets; Fz for novels). The novelty P3a is markedly reduced at prefrontal sites in all three modalities, and the target P3b is spared.

respectively—syndromes that resulted from damage to the left primary somatosensory and visual cortices, respectively. Analogous results were reported by Viggiano and colleagues, who recorded steady-state VEPs in 10 neglect patients, 10 brain-damaged patients without neglect, and 6 healthy subjects.[138] No differences in right-left amplitude were observed in the neglect patients. These data support the view that the impairment in neglect stems from "defective access of the output of *preserved* primary sensory analyses to successive processes involved in conscious perception and in overt verbal response" (Vallar et al.,[137] p. 1921, our italics). However, more recent findings suggest that early sensory analysis may not be completely intact.

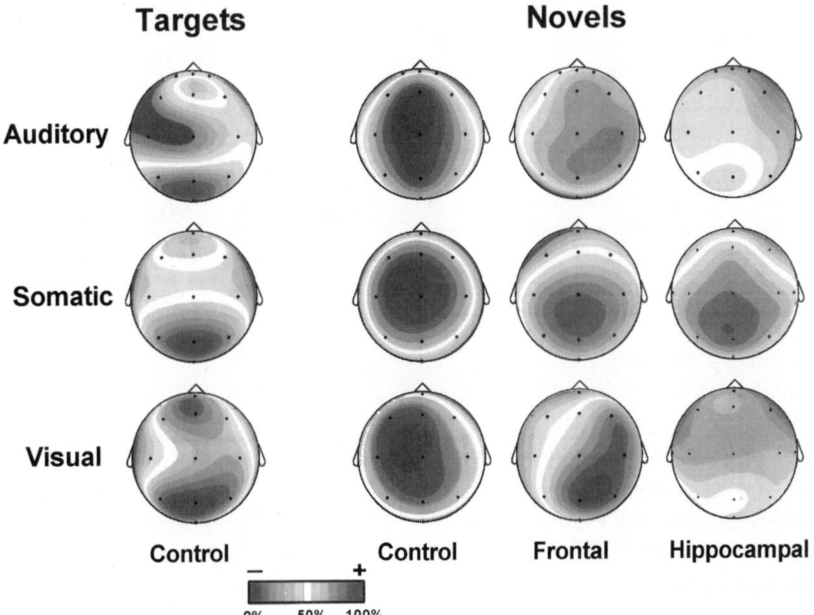

Figure 9-13
This figure shows the scalp voltage topographies for target and novel stimuli in controls. Note the marked increase in prefrontal activity to the novel stimuli in all sensory modalities. The effects of prefrontal or hippocampal lesions on the brain novelty response are shown on the right. Unilateral prefrontal damage results in multimodal decreases in the novelty response. Unilateral hippocampal damage results in severe bilateral reductions in the novelty response, maximal at prefrontal sites. These findings implicate a prefrontal-hippocampal network in the detection of perturbations in the environment (see text for details).

Abnormal sensory function in neglect was found in studies reporting that the visual and auditory N1 components are smaller over the damaged relative to the intact hemisphere of neglect patients regardless of the side of stimulation.[35,139] In contrast, the N1 in normal subjects is larger over the hemisphere contralateral to the stimulus side.[140] The enhanced left hemisphere (relative to right hemisphere) auditory N1, irrespective of the side of the stimuli, may contribute to the tendency of patients with left-side auditory neglect to err localizing auditory stimuli as coming more to the right of their true source.[141]

Drawing from the putative association between the N1 and the orienting response,[142] it has been suggested that the N1 reduction over the damaged hemisphere reflects the patients' difficulty in orienting toward the contralesional side of space.[139] This is consistent with two single-case studies in which the visual N1 and P1 components were reduced in trials in which the left-sided stimulus was extinguished, but not when it was recognized[143,144] (see also Ref. 145). Recent fMRI studies comparing detected versus extinguished stimuli revealed reduced activation in right occipital cortex (as well as in bilateral fusiform and left parietal sites) when stimuli were extinguished in patients with right hemisphere damage.[144,145] The fact that in these fMRI studies extinguished faces seemed to activate the so-called fusiform face area suggests that the lack of awareness may not result from a breakdown of the object recognition pathway of the visual system but from a failure of its interaction with parietal and frontal mechanisms.[35,144,146,147]

Steady-state VEPs revealed an intriguing pattern in neglect patients. Latencies are increased for steady-state VEPs elicited by stimulation in the neglected side compared with those elicited by similar stimulation in the intact side.[28,148–150] This delay was absent in brain-damaged patients who did not show signs of neglect. Even more revealing is the fact that the latency increase was found with relatively high frequency luminance-contrast gratings but not with chromatically modulated contrasts,[151] suggesting a specific deficit related to the magnocellular system (luminance sensitive but color blind) and sparing the parvocellular part of the visual system.[152] The possibility of a feature specific deficit in preattentive processing has also been investigated in the auditory modality using the MMN.

As noted previously, the MMN is an electrical brain manifestation elicited by infrequently occurring oddball stimuli interspersed among repetitive stimuli. Several characteristics of the MMN make it an especially interesting measure in the study of UN and extinction. First, the MMN is assumed to reflect an automatically elicited preattentive process.[153–155] Second, the process underlying the MMN has a potential role in triggering an involuntary attention switch,[98,156–158] and such a process is likely disrupted in UN. Third, the MMN paradigm allows one to examine separately the feature-specific processing of auditory stimuli[159–162] (see Ref. 163 for a discussion of the feature-specificity). Fourth, elicitation of the MMN does not require the subject to perform a task or impose any attentional requirements. Therefore it is an ideal probe for comparing preattentive processing of left- and right-sided stimuli and for evaluating the processing of different dimensions of the auditory stimulus.

In a study of 10 patients with auditory and visual UN, deviations on either side of space were examined, with the stimulus differences defined in terms of spatial location, duration, or the pitch of sounds presented from loudspeakers.[35] The most robust finding was that the MMN elicited by deviation in sound-source location was considerably reduced when the stimuli were on the left (neglected) compared to the right side. Pitch deviance also tended to exhibit right-side advantage, but this effect was not as robust as for location. In contrast, no right-left difference was found for the MMN elicited by duration deviance (Fig. 9-14). Since the magnocellular visual pathway is the main contributor to the dorsal stream of the visual system, which is involved with the processing of spatial information, the results from the studies in vision[151] and audition[35] suggest a specific, preattentive deficit in encoding spatial attributes of sensory events. A possible reason for the lack of awareness in UN despite implicit processing of the neglected stimuli is that perceived events cannot be placed in a spatial framework, which is necessary for conscious awareness and for adequately shifting attention towards the stimuli.[35]

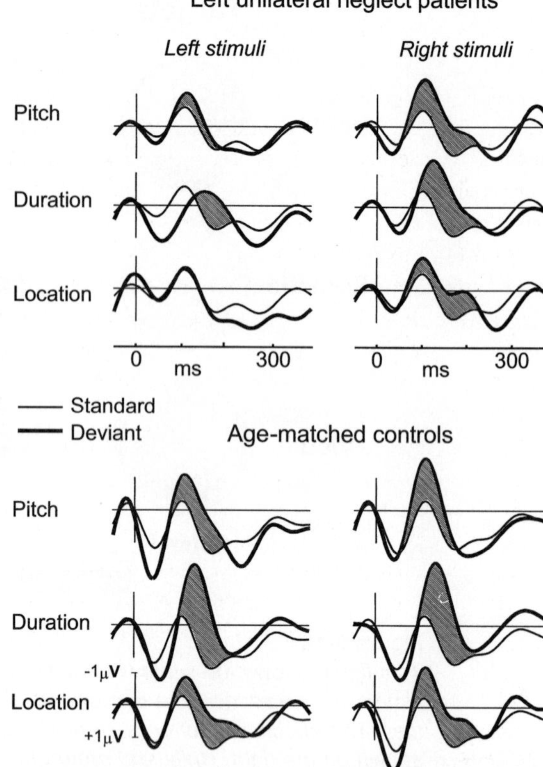

Figure 9-14

Mismatch negativity (hatched area) to deviation in pitch, duration, and location of stimuli in 10 patients with damage to the right hemisphere and with unilateral left visual and auditory neglect and 10 age-matched controls. Stimuli were presented in different blocks 60 degrees to the right or to the left of the subjects through loudspeakers. Standard stimuli were 75-ms-long harmonic tones (600-Hz fundamental). The probability of the pitch deviants (60 Hz lower), duration deviants (50 ms shorter), and location deviants (30 degrees more medial) was 0.1 each. Data presented are for Fz electrode referenced to averaged mastoids. There was a significant decrement in MMN to left location deviants (comparing within patient to the response to right side stimuli). The decrement approached significance for pitch and was not significant for duration (see Ref. 35 for details).

The "Posner paradigm"[164] was used to explore the effect of neglect on the allocation of attention as reflected by the P3 and Nd.[139] It has been previously shown that in right temporoparietal patients, a misleading (invalid) cue on the ipsilesional side dramatically slows down the reaction time to contralesional targets more than the normal effect of such a cue and more than the effect of a contralesional invalid cue on the reaction time to an ipsilesional target,[164,165] suggesting that patients with these lesions fail to "disengage" from stimuli (e.g., the invalid cue) on the ipsilesional side. This conjecture was corroborated by the finding that in right parietal patients the Nd, an ERP manifestation of selective attention, was significantly smaller following right-sided (invalid) cues than any other cue-target combination.[139] This effect was evident as early as 200 ms after target onset, suggesting that even if the underlying deficit may originate in the higher-order attention mechanism, it affects "the very processing of perceptual input" (Verleger et al.,[139] p. 455).

A more complex pattern of results was obtained regarding the patients' P3 component in the Posner paradigm.[139] The late positive potential (LAP or P3f, denoting a P3 recorded at Fz[166]) was largest for the critical combination of right cue and left target. This pattern resembles the enhanced P3 observed in monkeys with frontoparietal damage and signs of UN.[167] Post hoc, the P3f enhancement was interpreted as reflecting the patients' attempt to reorient attention toward the left-side target following late detection. Direct tests of this hypothesis are needed. In contrast to the P3f, the P3b (recorded at a central parietal site) was reduced in patients irrespective of the cue and target location, corroborating earlier observations.[125] This general reduction was ascribed to damage to P3 generators, especially those centered in the temporoparietal junction.

The use of electrophysiological and hemodynamic functional imaging sheds new light on intact and impaired processes in UN. The extant studies show that the lesion may induce specific impairments in an early stage of processing to which behavioral methods may be blind.

Linguistic Processing in Aphasic Patients

Whereas language deficits following brain damage are traditionally classified into crude clinical syndromes such as Broca's or Wernicke's aphasia, advances in neurolinguistics suggest that a finer-grain analysis, based on individual symptoms, may be more fruitful (see Chap. 12). Distinct ERP components have been linked to stages of language comprehension including (1) early left anterior negativity (ELAN), a marker of syntactic violations[168,169]; (2) The N400, related to lexical/semantic integration (N400)[170]; and (3) the "late positivity" or P600, which has been attributed to reprocessing of linguistic information (P600).[171] The N400 was first described by Kutas and Hillyard as being elicited by violations of semantic expectancies at the end of sentences ("She takes her coffee with cream and *dog*" rather than ". . . cream and *sugar*").[170] The N400 amplitude is modulated by the extent to which a word is related to its prior context ("N400 effect"), being more negative the more unexpected the word is.[172] The effect is not limited to sentences but can be seen both when comparing words primed or not primed by a previous semantically related or associated word[173] or when a word in a sentence is incompatible with the general context of a discourse.[174] In fact, even nonverbal stimuli such as faces,[175] pictures,[176–178] and environmental noises[85] (but not endings of melodies[179,180]) have been reported to elicit N400-type components, suggesting a link to lexical access[181] or postlexical integration of a stimulus into the semantic context.[182] It is conceivable that multiple intracranial regions contribute to the scalp N400 with different subcomponents related to various aspects of cognitive processing, as has been suggested for P300 phenomena.[183] The N400 amplitude was reduced in patients with lesions of the left temporoparietal cortex exhibiting symptoms of Wernicke's aphasia. Conversely, N400 amplitudes were reported to be less affected in patients with frontal lesions exhibiting symptoms of Broca's aphasia.[184] Intracranial recordings in the anterior medial temporal lobe (MTL) have revealed potentials resembling the scalp N400 in verbal recognition memory, lexical decision, semantic priming, and picture-naming tasks.[183,185,186] MTL-N460 amplitudes have been reported to be largest in the left MTL following new words, while an MTL-P620 potential was largest to repeated words and was reduced in a passive condition. Puce and colleagues[187] found similar MTL potentials to both verbal stimuli and abstract "nonverbalizable" patterns during recognition memory. These data suggest that a posterior cortical-mesial-temporal network is engaged during N400 generation.

Elderly controls and patients with Broca's aphasia demonstrated semantic and associative priming effects, manifest by a decreased N400 to related targets versus unrelated targets, while patients with Wernicke's aphasia failed to show this priming effect.[184] However, the N400 effect was found to correlate significantly with the degree of comprehension in a group of aphasic patients irrespective of their diagnosis as Broca's or Wernicke's aphasia.[36,184] Whereas the hallmark of Broca's aphasia is an expressive problem, it is now believed that these patients also have some problems with comprehension. For example, agrammatic nonfluent aphasics have difficulty in understanding sentences involving atypical syntactic constructions.[188] An interesting double dissociation was found between a "Broca" patient with a frontal lesion including the frontal operculum and the insula, and a "Wernicke" patient with posterior-temporal/inferior-parietal lesion.[189] The patient with the frontal lesion failed to elicit the "early left anterior negativity" (ELAN) effect following a phrase structure (grammatical) violation but showed a normal N400 effect for a semantic violation of the sort outlined in the previous paragraph. The patient with the posterior lesion showed the opposite result. This supports the existence of distinct mechanisms for grammatical parsing and lexical-semantic integration, with the former dependent on the inferior frontal and insular cortex and the latter dependent on posterior parietotemporal cortex. Patients with anterior lesions fail to exhibit a differential ERP response to closed-class (e.g., pronouns) and open-class (e.g., nouns) words, possibly reflecting a deficit in the rapid categorization of words into their syntactic roles.[190] However, the semantic processing in patients with anterior lesions may not be completely intact. When an ambiguous word (e.g., *bank*) is placed as the last word in a sentence, the sentence may disambiguate the word in one direction (e.g., "the man called the bank"). In normal controls, a target word (e.g., *river*) following the disambiguated word elicits a smaller N400 if it is associated with the selected meaning than if it is unrelated or is related to the alternative meaning (the N400 effect). The same result was obtained in a group of patients with frontal lesions and Broca's aphasia as long as the time between the disambiguated word and the target word was long (1250 ms).[190] When this gap was short (100 ms), the alternative meaning primed the target word significantly (although to a smaller degree than the selected meaning). Age-matched controls showed the normal pattern for both gaps. This has been interpreted as a slowing of lexical integration in the aphasic patients, with both meanings of the ambiguous word remaining "active" for a longer time and thus hampering comprehension. In addition to higher-order linguistic deficits, ERP studies using the MMN component revealed a lower level deficit of phonetic discrimination in patients with comprehension deficits following left posterior temporal lesions, including Wernicke's area, but not in patients with anterior lesions and signs of Broca's aphasia.[159,191–193] Thus, some of the deficit in comprehension may reflect difficulty in deciphering the phonetic stream, resulting in degraded input to higher-order linguistic processes.

Although the results of these pioneering studies of language impairment may be open to different interpretations based on competing theories of language processing, they nevertheless demonstrate the potential benefits of using ERPs to investigate normal and impaired language processes. Initial attempts have also been made to use ERPs as a diagnostic aid in examining the comprehension of patients with global aphasia, which cannot be examined behaviorally.[194,195]

TRANSCRANIAL MAGNETIC STIMULATION

Merton and Morton provided the first demonstration of transcranial electrical stimulation (TES) in 1980.[196] By applying a brief, high-voltage electric shock to the scalp over motor cortex, they were able to elicit focal muscle activity, or what has come to be called the motor evoked response (MER). This technique had obvious utility for clinicians, offering a tool for measuring the integrity of efferent pathways in a manner analogous to that provided by the somatosensory evoked potential. However, TES had one serious drawback: the shocks were very painful because the stimulus also activated pain receptors in the scalp. Transcranial magnetic stimulation (TMS) was developed as a painless alternative to TES[197] (for recent reviews, see Refs. 198 and 199).

Technical Considerations

The TMS device consists of a tightly wrapped wire coil that is encased in an insulated sheath and connected to a power source of electrical capacitors. When triggered, the capacitors send a large electric current through the coil, resulting in the generation of a large yet compact magnetic field (up to 3 tesla) with lines of flux perpendicular to the plane of the coil. The magnetic field peaks within about 150 μs and decays within 1 ms. This rapid change induces electric eddy currents in conductive tissue. The skull presents low impedance to magnetic fields of this frequency; thus there is minimal current induction in extracerebral tissue, including pain receptors. However, eddy currents are produced within the brain, thus stimulating neural tissue. The exact mechanism is unknown. It may be that the current leads to the generation of action potentials in the soma; alternatively, the current may directly stimulate axons or involve a mixture of cell body and axonal stimulation.

The current generated is strongest under the edges of the coil; it become weak near the center. Thus, with circular coils, the area of activation is dispersed and not homogenous across the region spanned by the coil. To obtain more focal stimulation, figure-eight coils are commonly employed, with the current strongest at the point where the two circles intersect (Fig. 9-15). With such coils, the primary activation can be restricted to an area of about 1 to 1.5 cm. The extent and intensity of the induced neural activity varies with the intensity of the generated current and falls off fairly rapidly as the distance from the coil increases. As such, TMS is primarily targeted at cortical areas that lie along the gyri, although deeper structures such as the supplementary motor area have been successfully stimulated.[200] In addition, the resistance of white matter is greater than that of gray matter, further reducing the likelihood that TMS can be targeted to deep structures of the cortex or subcortical nuclei.

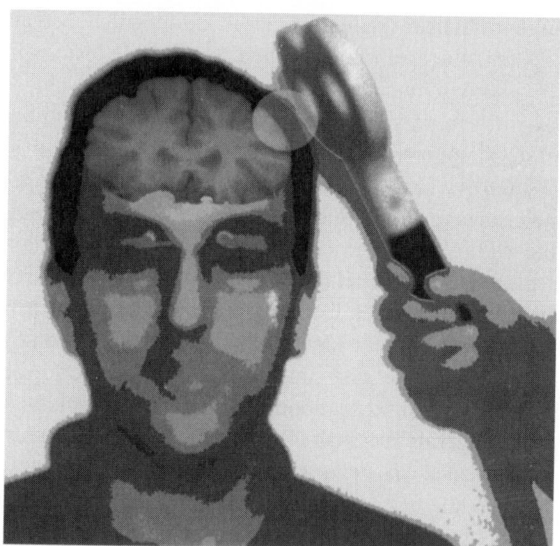

Figure 9-15
Transcranial magnetic stimulation (TMS). The figure shows a figure-eight-shaped TMS stimulator applied to the head; the region of stimulated cortex is indicated schematically.

Applications of TMS

TMS has become a relatively standard clinical tool for evaluating the speed of conduction in motor pathways. For example, activation of the abductor digiti minimi muscle (fifth finger) can be elicited by placing the stimulator over the ulnar nerve at the wrist, at the C7 level of the spinal cord, or over the contralateral motor cortex.[17] In this manner, it is possible to determine if abnormal latencies arise from central or peripheral pathology in a disease such as multiple sclerosis or when monitoring corticospinal function during spinal cord surgery. While clinical uses of this kind are primarily diagnostic, TMS has also been studied as a possible therapeutic device. Preliminary studies have indicated that repetitive TMS (rTMS; with rates varying from 0.5 Hz for 10 s to 10 Hz for 5 s) applied over prefrontal cortex may prove effective for treating major depression.[201,202] The mechanism of such treatment is unclear, but it may offer a more focal and less debilitating treatment than electroshock therapy for patients with resistant mood disorders.

TMS offers a new experimental approach for cognitive neuroscience. With this method, an experimenter can disrupt neural function in a selected region of the cortex and, as with lesion studies, the resulting changes in behavior can shed light on the normal function of the targeted tissue. What makes this method appealing is that, appropriately applied, the technique is safe and noninvasive. Moreover, since the principal use is with neurologically healthy individuals, TMS allows for the creation of "virtual" reversible lesions in an otherwise intact brain.[18]

Virtual lesions have been created over a number of disparate cortical areas. A functional scotoma can be created by a single TMS pulse applied over the occipital pole, presumably reflecting the disruption of processing within primary visual cortex.[203,204] An important feature of TMS is that the effect shows a high degree of temporal specificity. Corthout et al.[205] found that performance on a letter-identification task was essentially abolished for one subject when the TMS pulse followed the stimulus onset by about 100 ms. For stimulus-to-TMS intervals less than 60 ms or greater than 140 ms, performance was near perfect.

While it is tempting to conclude that the critical activity within primary visual cortex for letter identification occurs about 100 ms after stimulus presentation, it is also possible that there is a delay between the onset of the TMS-induced activity and the actual neural disruption in task performance. For example, it is quite possible that a silent period follows the TMS volley, and it may be that this silent period is what leads to the scotoma. Nonetheless, TMS can be useful for examining the relative timing of processing within different visual areas. For example, Beckers and Zeki[206] reported that stimulation over either V1 or V5 (MT) impaired performance on a motion discrimination task. Interestingly, the disruptive effects in V1 occurred with much longer stimulus-to-TMS intervals than found for V5, a result that would seem at odds with conventional notions that processing proceeds in a serial manner from V1 to higher visual areas. The TMS results would suggest that back projections from V5 to V1 might be an important part of the discrimination process (see also Ref. 207).

A second example of the use of TMS for exploring functional connectivity comes from a study in which subjects were trained to perform sequential finger movements.[200] When the coil was centered over the hand area of motor cortex, the next response in the sequence was frequently disturbed, either because the movement was halted in midstream or because the wrong key was pressed. The subjects perceived the problem as a temporary loss of coordination, commenting that the finger suddenly seemed to jerk in the wrong direction. In contrast, when the coil was targeted to affect the supplementary motor area (SMA), the effects were delayed, occurring about three key presses after the TMS pulse. Here, the subjects reported that they lost track of their place in the sequence or that they temporarily forgot the order of responses. Thus, TMS demonstrated the differential role of supplementary motor area and primary motor cortex in motor planning and execution, respectively. It is important to note that TMS pulses in this study were applied in a rapid series (3 Hz). It is unclear whether measurable effects on higher-level aspects of cognition such as motor programming can be obtained with single-pulse TMS. Unfortunately, there have been a few reported cases of induced seizure activity with rapid TMS (>1 Hz), thus limiting the use of this method.[216]

There have recently been a number of impressive reports in which TMS and functional neuroimaging have been used in combination. A long-standing debate in cognitive neuroscience has centered on the question of whether visual imagery requires the engagement of neural regions involved in visual perception. Evidence in favor of a shared medium for imagery and perception comes from imaging studies; as measured by PET, activation in visual areas including primary visual cortex have been reported when subjects were asked to image visual patterns and then make judgments about properties such as length and orientation.[208]

However, as with all imaging studies, the evidence is correlational, making it difficult to draw conclusions about causation. Connections from higher-order visual areas (or even nonvisual areas) to primary visual cortex due to long-term perceptual experience may have led to the activation of primary visual cortex even though this activity was not essential for task performance. To test this possibility, Kosslyn and colleagues used a novel TMS method. Prior to performing a second session on the imagery task, 1-Hz TMS was applied over the occipital pole for 10 min.[208] Previous studies had shown that the efficacy of neural activity is depressed for an extended period after such repetitive TMS, allowing performance to be assessed under conditions in which the nonspecific effects such as the noise from the stimulator or muscle twitches are not present.[209] Indeed, performance on the imagery task was impaired following this stimulation in comparison to a sham TMS control condition in which the coil was oriented perpendicular to the skull. Thus it appears that disruption of normal activity in primary visual cortex can impair imagery, providing experimental evidence that converges with the correlational results obtained in the PET phase of the study. In a similar way, TMS over visual cortex has been shown to disrupt tactile perception of shape in both sighted[210] and blind individuals,[211] indicating that the activation observed in these areas during neuroimaging studies[212,213] is not an epiphenomenon.

TMS has recently been used to reproduce phenomena naturally observed after brain damage. The line bisection task is a common test for unilateral neglect (see above and Chap. 25). In a variant of this task known as the landmark task, subjects are asked to judge whether a line is correctly bisected into two equal segments. Single-pulse TMS applied within 200 ms following the stimulus over posterior parietal area of healthy volunteers slowed down reaction times when the bisecting landmark was to the right of the midline[214] and biased perception toward underestimating the left segments.[215] Left-sided pulses or sham pulses did not alter performance. Notably, patients with right parietal lesions bisect lines to the right of the midline. Thus, the posterior parietal region stimulated (corresponding to Brodman's area 7 and the intraparietal sulcus) may indeed have a critical role in this task. In addition, this procedure suggests the possibility of a human model for studying some visuospatial deficits found in unilateral neglect.

CONCLUSIONS

The use of event-related potentials to study patients with localized brain damage and with specific behavioral dysfunctions continues to provide invaluable information on the underlying mechanisms of normal and pathologic cognition and its neural mechanism. TMS provides a new and promising method of inducing virtual lesions in healthy subjects, thus providing a method to test functional hypotheses regarding the contribution of targeted neural areas to particular tasks. The combination of these methods with traditional neuropsychological and hemodynamic imaging methods is likely to transform our understanding of brain function. Hopefully, this will yield better diagnostic as well as restorative procedures for neurologic patients.

REFERENCES

1. Hillyard SA, Picton TW: Electrophysiology of cognition, in Plum F (ed): *Handbook of Physiology: The Nervous System.* Baltimore: American Physiological Society, 1987, pp 519–584.
2. Knight RT: Attention regulation and human prefrontal cortex, in Thierry AM, Glowinski J, Goldman-Rakic P, Christen Y (eds): *Motor and Cognitive Functions of the Prefrontal Cortex: Research and Perspectives in Neurosciences.* Berlin and Heidelberg: Springer-Verlag, 1994, pp 160–173.
3. Egan MF, Duncan CC, Suddath RL, et al: Event-related potential abnormalities correlate with structural brain alterations and clinical features in patients with chronic schizophrenia. *Schizophr Res* 11:259–271, 1994.
4. Bonmassar G, Schwartz DP, Liu AK, et al: Spatiotemporal brain imaging of visual-evoked activity using interleaved EEG and fMRI recordings. *Neuroimage* 13:1035–1043, 2001.
5. Goldman RI, Stern JM, Engel J, et al: Acquiring simultaneous EEG and functional MRI. *Clin Neurophysiol* 111:1974–1980, 2000.
6. Allen PJ, Josephs O, Turner R: A method for removing imaging artifact from continuous EEG recorded during functional MRI. *Neuroimage* 12:230–239, 2000.
7. Kruggel F, Herrmann CS, Wiggins CJ, et al: Hemodynamic and electroencephalographic responses to illusory figures: Recording of the evoked potentials during functional MRI. *Neuroimage* 14:1327–1336, 2001.
8. Lazeyras F, Zimine I, Blanke O, et al: Functional MRI with simultaneous EEG recording: Feasibility and application to motor and visual activation. *J Magn Reson Imaging* 13:943–948, 2001.
9. König P, Engel AK: Correlated firing in sensory-motor systems. *Curr Opin Neurobiol* 5:511–519, 1995.
10. Basar-Eroglu C, Strüber D, Schürmann M, et al: Gamma-band responses in the brain: a short review of psychophysiological correlates and functional significance. *Int J Psychophysiol* 24:101–112, 1996.
11. Llinas R, Ribary U, Contreras D, et al: The neuronal basis for consciousness. *Philos Trans R Soc Lond B Biol Sci* 353:1841–1849, 1998.
12. Pfurtscheller G, Lopes da Silva FH: Event-related EEG/MEG synchronization and desynchronization: Basic principles. *Clin Neurophysiol* 110:1842–1857, 1999.
13. Sannita WG: Stimulus-specific oscillatory responses of the brain: A time/frequency-related coding process. *Clin Neurophysiol* 111:565–583, 2000.

14. Tallon-Baudry C, Bertrand, O, Peronnet F, et al: Induced gamma-band activity during the delay of a visual short-term memory task in humans. *J Neurosci* 18:4244–4254, 1998.
15. Herrmann CS, Knight R: Mechanisms of human attention: event-related potentials and oscillations. *Neurosci Biobehav Rev* 25:465–476, 2001.
16. Penfield W. Jasper H: *Epilepsy and the Functional Anatomy of the Human Brain*. Boston: Little, Brown, 1954.
17. Brunholzl C, Claus D: Central motor conduction time to upper and lower limbs in cervical cord lesions. *Arch Neurol* 51:245–249, 1994.
18. Pascual-Leone A, Bartres-Faz D, Keenan JP: Transcranial magnetic stimulation: Studying the brain-behaviour relationship by induction of "virtual lesions." *Philos Trans R Soc Lond B Biol Sci* 354:1229–1238, 1999.
19. Picton TW, Lins OG, Scherg M: The recording and analysis of event-related potentials, in Boller F, Graffman J (eds): *Handbook of Neuropsychology*. New York: Elsevier, 1995, pp 3–73.
20. Picton TW, Alain C, Woods DL, et al: Intracerebral sources of human auditory-evoked potentials. *Audiol Neurootol* 4:64–79, 1999.
21. Swick D, Kutas M, Neville HJ: Localizing the neural generators of event-related brain potentials, in Kertesz A (ed): *Localization in Neuroimaging in Neuropsychology.* New York: Academic Press, 1994, pp 73–121.
22. Näätänen R: *Attention and Brain Function*. Hillsdale, NJ: Erlbaum, 1992.
23. Knight RT: Electrophysiology in behavioral neurology, in Mesulam M-M (ed): *Principles of Behavioral Neurology*. Philadelphia: Davis, 1985, pp 327–346.
24. Picton TW: Human event-related potentials, in *Handbook of Electroencephalography and Clinical Neurophysiology*. Philadelphia: Elsevier, 1987, vol 3.
25. Klee M, Rall W: Computed potentials of cortically arranged populations of neurons. *J Neurophysiol* 40:647–666, 1977.
26. Pernier J, Perrin F, Bertrand O: Scalp current density fields: Concept and properties. *Electroencephalogr Clin Neurophysiol* 69:385–589, 1998.
27. Gevins A, Smith ME, McEvoy LK, et al: Electroencephalographic imaging of higher brain function. *Philos Trans R Soc Lond B Biol Sci* 354:1125–1133, 1999.
28. Angelelli P, De Luca M, Spinelli D: Early visual processing in neglect patients: A study with steady-state VEPs. *Neuropsychologia* 34:1151–1157, 1996.
29. Aboud S, Bar L, Rosenfeld M, et al: Left-right asymmetry of visual evoked potentials in brain-damaged patients: a mathematical model and experimental results. *Ann Biomed Eng* 24:75–86, 1996.
30. Knight RT, Scabini D: Anatomic bases of event-related potentials and their relationship to novelty detection in humans. *J Clin Neurophysiol* 15:3–13, 1998.
31. Damasio H, Damasio AR: *Lesion Analysis in Neuropsychology*. New York: Oxford University Press, 1989.
32. Fiez JA, Damasio H, Grabowski TJ: Lesion segmentation and manual warping to a reference brain: Intra- and interobserver reliability. *Hum Brain Mapp* 9:192–211, 2000.
33. Brett M, Leff AP, Rorden C, et al: Spatial normalization of brain images with focal lesions using cost function masking. *Neuroimage* 14:486–500, 2001.
34. Knight RT: Distributed cortical network for visual attention. *J Cogn Neurosci* 9:75–91, 1997.
35. Deouell LY, Bentin S, Soroker N: Electrophysiological evidence for an early (pre-attentive) information processing deficit in patients with right hemisphere damage and unilateral neglect. *Brain* 123:353–365, 2000.
36. Swaab T, Brown C, Hagoort T: Spoken sentence comprehension in aphasia: Event-related potential evidence for a lexical integration deficit. *J Cogn Neurosci* 9:39–66, 1997.
37. Knight RT, Stuss DT: Prefrontal cortex: the present and the future, in Stuss DT, Knight RT (eds): *Principles of Frontal Lobe Function*. New York: Oxford University Press, 2002, pp 573–597.
38. Knight RT, D'Esposito M: The lateral prefrontal syndrome: A deficit in executive control, in D'Esposito M (ed): *Neurological Foundations of Cognitive Neuroscience.* Cambridge, MA: MIT Press. In press.
39. Knight, RT, Staines WR, Swick D, et al: Prefrontal cortex regulates inhibition and excitation in distributed neural networks. *Acta Psychol* 101:159–178, 1999.
40. Lhermitte F: Human autonomy and the frontal lobes: Part II. Patient behavior in complex and social situations: The "environmental dependency syndrome." *Ann Neurol* 19:335–343, 1986.
41. Shimamura AP: Memory and the frontal lobe, in Gazzaniga M (ed): *The Cognitive Neurosciences.* Cambridge, MA: MIT Press, 1994, pp 803–813.
42. Barcelo F, Suwazono S, Knight RT: Prefrontal modulation of visual processing in humans. *Nat Neurosci* 3:399–403, 2000.
43. Chao LL, Knight, RT: Contribution of human prefrontal cortex to delay performance. *J Cogn Neurosci* 10:167–77, 1998.

44. Edinger HM, Siegel A, Troiano R: Effect of stimulation of prefrontal cortex and amygdala on diencephalic neurons. *Brain Res* 97:17–31, 1975.
45. Alexander GE, Newman JD, Symmes D: Convergence of prefrontal and acoustic inputs upon neurons in the superior temporal gyrus of the awake squirrel monkey. *Brain Res* 116:334–338, 1976.
46. Skinner JE, Yingling CD: Central gating mechanisms that regulate event-related potentials and behavior, in Desmedt JE (ed): *Progress in Clinical Neurophysiology.* Basel: Karger, 1977, vol 1, pp 30–69.
47. Yingling CD, Skinner JE: Gating of thalamic input to cerebral cortex by nucleus reticularis thalami, in Desmedt JE (ed): *Progress in Clinical Neurophysiology.* Basel: Karger, 1977, vol I, pp 70–96.
48. Guillery RW, Feig SL, Lozsadi DA: Paying attention to the thalamic reticular nucleus. *Trends Neurosci* 21:28–32, 1998.
49. Knight RT, Scabini D, Woods DL: Prefrontal cortex gating of auditory transmission in humans. *Brain Res* 504:338–342, 1989.
50. Yamaguchi S, Knight RT: Gating of somatosensory inputs by human prefrontal cortex. *Brain Res* 521:281–288, 1990.
51. Alho K, Woods DL, Algazi A, et al: Lesions of frontal cortex diminish the auditory mismatch negativity. *Electroencephalogr Clin Neurophysiol* 91:353–362, 1994.
52. Sokolov EN: Higher nervous functions: The orienting reflex. *Annu Rev Physiol* 25:545–580, 1963.
53. Knight RT: Decreased response to novel stimuli after prefrontal lesions in man. *Electroencephalogr Clin Neurophysiol* 59:9–20, 1984.
54. Chao L, Knight RT: Human prefrontal lesions increase distractibility to irrelevant sensory inputs. *Neuroreport* 6:1605–1610, 1995.
55. Woods DL, Knight RT: Electrophysiological evidence of increased distractibility after dorsolateral prefrontal lesions. *Neurology* 36:212–216, 1986.
56. Desimone R: Visual attention mediated by biased competition in extrastriate visual cortex. *Philos Trans R Soc Lond B Biol Sci* 353:1245–1255, 1998.
57. Hillyard SA, Hink RF, Schwent UL, et al: Electrical signs of selective attention in the human brain. *Science* 182:177–180, 1973.
58. Heinze HJ, Mangun GR, Burchert W, et al: Combined spatial and temporal imaging of brain activity during visual selective attention in humans. *Nature* 372:543–546, 1994.
59. Mangun GR: Neural mechanisms of visual selective attention. *Psychophysiology* 32:4–18, 1995.
60. Martínez A, Anllo-Vento L, Sereno MI, et al: Involvement of striate and extrastriate visual cortical areas in spatial attention. *Nat Neurosci* 2:364–369, 1999.
61. Woldorff MG, Gallen CC, Hampson SA, et al: Modulation of early sensory processing in human auditory cortex during auditory selective attention. *Proc Natl Acad Sci U S A* 90:8722–8726, 1993.
62. Grady CL, Van Meter JW, Maisog JM, et al: Attention-related modulation of activity in primary and secondary auditory cortex. *Neuroreport* 8:2511–2516, 1997.
63. Somers DC, Dale AM, Seiffert AE, et al: Functional MRI reveals spatially specific attentional modulation in human primary visual cortex. *Proc Natl Acad Sci U S A* 96:1663–1668, 1999.
64. Steinmetz PN, Roy A, Fitzgerald PJ, et al: Attention modulates synchronized neuronal firing in primate somatosensory cortex. *Nature* 404:187–190, 2000.
65. Roelfsema PR, Lamme VAF, Spekreijse H: Object-based attention in the primary visual cortex of the macaque monkey. *Nature* 395:376–381, 1998.
66. Hillyard SA, Anllo-Vento L: Event-related brain potentials in the study of visual selective attention. *Proc Natl Acad Sci U S A* 95:781–787, 1998.
67. Fuster JM, Bodner M, Kroger JK: Cross-modal and cross-temporal association in neurons of frontal cortex. *Nature* 405:347–351, 2000.
68. Funahashi S, Bruce CJ, Goldman-Rakic PS: Dorsolateral prefrontal lesions and oculomotor delayed-response performance: Evidence for mnemonic "scotomas." *J Neurosci* 13:1479–1497, 1993.
69. Rossi AF, Rotter PS, Desimone R, et al: Prefrontal lesions produce impairments in feature-cued attention. *Soc Neurosci Abstr* 29:2, 1999.
70. McIntosh AR, Grady CL, Ungerleider LG, et al: Network analysis of cortical visual pathways mapped with PET. *J Neurosci* 14:655–666, 1994.
71. Büchel C, Friston KJ: Modulation of connectivity in visual pathways by attention: Cortical interactions evaluated with structural equation modeling and fMRI. *Cereb Cortex* 7:768–778, 1997.
72. Chawla D, Rees G, Friston KJ: The physiological basis of attentional modulation in extrastriate visual areas. *Nat Neurosci* 2:671–676, 1999.
73. Rees G, Frackowiak R, Frith C: Two modulatory effects of attention that mediate object categorization in human cortex. *Science* 275:835–838, 1997.
74. Kastner S, Pinsk MA, de Weerd P, et al: Increased activity in human visual cortex during directed attention in the absence of visual stimulation. *Neuron* 22:751–761, 1999.

75. Corbetta M: Frontoparietal cortical networks for directing attention and the eye to visual locations: Identical, independent, or overlapping neural systems? *Proc Natl Acad Sci U S A* 95:831–838, 1998.
76. Hopfinger JP, Buonocore MH, Mangun GR: The neural mechanisms of top-down attentional control. *Nat Neurosci* 3:284–291, 2000.
77. Barcelo F, Knight RT: Both random and perseverative errors underlie WCST deficits in prefrontal patients. *Neuropsychologia* 40:349–356, 2001.
78. Swick D: Effects of prefrontal lesions on lexical processing and repetition priming: An ERP study. *Brain Res Cogn Brain Res* 7:143–157, 1998.
79. Yago E, Knight RT: Tonic and phasic prefrontal modulation of extrastriate processing during visual attention. *Soc Neurosci Abstr* 30:8397, 2000.
80. Suwazono S, Machado L, Knight RT: Predictive value of novel stimuli modifies visual event-related potentials and behavior. *Clin Neurophysiol* 111:29–39, 2000.
81. Verleger R: Event-related potentials and cognition: A critique of the context updating hypothesis and an alternative interpretation of P3. *Behav Brain Sci* 11:343–356, 1988.
82. Heit G, Smith ME, Halgren E: Neuronal activity in the human medial temporal lobe during recognition memory. *Brain* 113:1093–1112, 1990.
83. Schupp HT, Lutzenberger W, Rau H, Birbaumer N: Positive shifts of event-related potentials: A state of cortical disfacilitation as reflected by the startle reflex probe. *Electroencephalogr Clin Neurophysiol* 90:135–144, 1994.
84. Donchin E, Coles MGH: Is the P300 component a manifestation of context updating? *Behav Brain Sci* 11:357–427, 1988.
85. Chao L, Nielsen-Bohlman L, Knight RT: Auditory event-related potentials dissociate early and late memory processes. *Electroencephalogr Clin Neurophysiol* 96:157–168, 1995.
86. Soltani M, Knight RT. The neural origins of P3. *Crit Rev Neurobiol.* In press.
87. Knight RT, Nakada, T: Cortico-limbic circuits and novelty: A review of EEG and blood flow data. *Rev Neurosci* 9:57–70, 1998.
88. Verleger R, Heide W, Butt C, Kompf D: Reduction of P3b potentials in patients with temporo-parietal lesions. *Cogn Brain Res* 2:103–116, 1994.
89. Knight RT, Hillyard SA, Woods DL, et al: The effects of frontal cortex lesions on event-related potentials during auditory selective attention. *Electroencephalogr Clin Neurophysiol* 52:571–582, 1981.
90. Woods DL, Knight RT, Scabini D: Anatomical substrates of auditory selective attention: behavioral and electrophysiological effects of temporal and parietal lesions. *Cogn Brain Res* 1:227–240, 1993.
91. Walter WG, Cooper R, Aldridge V, et al: Contingent negative variation: An electrical sign of sensorimotor association and expectancy in the human brain. *Nature* 203:380–384, 1964.
92. Levy R, Goldman-Rakic PS: Segregation of working memory functions within the dorsolateral prefrontal cortex. *Exp Brain Res* 133:23–32, 2000.
93. McCarthy G, Puce A, Constable RT, et al: Activation of human prefrontal cortex during spatial and nonspatial working memory tasks measured by functional MRI. *Cereb Cortex* 6:600–611, 1996.
94. Chao LL, Knight RT: Age related prefrontal changes during auditory memory. *Soc Neurosci Abstr* 20:1003, 1994.
95. Rosahl S, Knight RT: Prefrontal cortex contribution to the contingent negative variation. *Cereb Cortex* 5:123–134, 1995.
96. Zappoli R, Versari A, Zappoli F, et al: The effects on auditory neurocognitive evoked responses and contingent negative variation activity of frontal cortex lesions or ablations in man: three new case studies. *Int J Psychophysiol* 38:109–144, 2000.
97. Näätänen R, Gaillard AW, Mäntysalo S: Early selective-attention effect on evoked potential reinterpreted. *Acta Psychol* 42:313–29, 1978.
98. Näätänen R: The role of attention in auditory information processing as revealed by event-related potentials and other brain measures of cognitive function. *Behav Brain Sci* 13:201–288, 1990.
99. Winkler I, Karmos G, Näätänen R: Adaptive modeling of the unattended acoustic environment reflected in the mismatch negativity event-related potential. *Brain Res* 742:239–252, 1996.
100. Schröger E: A neural mechanism for involuntary attention shifts to changes in auditory stimulation. *J Cogn Neurosci* 8:527–539, 1996.
101. Alho K: Cerebral generators of mismatch negativity (MMN) and its magnetic counterpart (MMNm) elicited by sound changes. *Ear Hearing* 16:38–51, 1995.
102. Giard M-H, Perrin F, Pernier J, et al: Brain generators implicated in the processing of auditory stimulus deviance: A topographic event related potential study. *Psychophysiology* 27:627–640, 1990.
103. Deouell LY, Bentin S, Giard M-H: Mismatch negativity in dichotic listening: Evidence for interhemispheric differences and multiple generators. *Psychophysiology* 35:355–365, 1998.
104. Kaiser J, Lutzenberger W, Birbaumer N: Simultaneous bilateral mismatch response to right- but not leftward sound lateralization. *Neuroreport* 11:2889–2892, 2000.

105. Alain C, Woods DL, Knight RT: Distributed cortical network for sensory memory in humans. *Brain Res* 812:23–37, 1998.
106. Courchesne E, Hillyard SA, Galambos R: Stimulus novelty, task relevance, and the visual evoked potential in man. *Electroencephalogr Clin Neurophysiol* 39:131–143, 1975.
107. Yamaguchi S, Knight RT: P300 generation by novel somatosensory stimuli. *Electroencephalogr Clin Neurophysiol* 78:50–55, 1991.
108. Paller KA, McCarthy G, Wood CC: Event-related potentials elicited by deviant endings to melodies. *Psychophysiology* 29:202–206, 1992.
109. Halgren E, Baudena P, Clarke JM, et al: Intracerebral potentials to rare target and distractor auditory and visual stimuli: I. Superior temporal plane and parietal lobe. *Electroencephalogr Clin Neurophysiol* 94:191–220, 1995.
110. Smith ME, Halgren E, Sokolik ME, et al: The intracranial topography of the P3 event-related potential elicited during auditory oddball. *Electroencephalogr Clin Neurophysiol* 76:235–248, 1990.
111. Scabini D, McCarthy G: Hippocampal responses to novel somatosensory stimuli. *Soc Neurosci Abstr* 19: 564, 1993.
112. Halgren E, Marinkovic K, Chauvel P: Generators of the late cognitive potentials in auditory and visual oddball tasks. *Electroencephalogr Clin Neurophysiol* 106:156–164, 1998.
113. Squires N, Squires K, Hillyard SA: Two varieties of long-latency positive waves evoked by unpredictable auditory stimuli in man. *Electroencephalogr Clin Neurophysiol* 38:387–401, 1975.
114. Opitz B, Mecklinger A, Friederici AD, et al: The functional neuroanatomy of novelty processing: integrating ERP and fMRI results. *Cereb Cortex* 9:379–391, 1999.
115. Kiehl KA, Laurens KR, Duty TL, et al: Neural sources involved in auditory target detection and novelty processing: An event-related fMRI study. *Psychophysiology* 38:133–142, 2000.
116. Zeineh MM, Engel SA, Bookheimer SY: Application of cortical unfolding techniques to functional MRI of the human hippocampal region. *Neuroimage* 11:668–683, 2000.
117. Scabini D, Knight RT: Frontal lobe contributions to the human P3a. *Soc Neurosci Abstr* 15:477, 1989.
118. Yamaguchi S, Knight RT: Anterior and posterior association cortex contributions to the somatosensory P300. *J Neurosci* 11:2039–2054, 1991.
119. Scabini D: Contribution of anterior and posterior association cortices to the human P300 cognitive event related potential. PhD dissertation. University of California, Davis: University Microfilms International, 1992.
120. Tranel D, Damasio H: Neuroanatomical correlates of electrodermal skin conductance responses. *Psychophysiology* 31:427–438, 1994.
121. Kimble DP, Bagshaw MH, Pribram KH: The GSR of monkeys during orienting and habituation after selective partial ablations of the cingulate and frontal cortex. *Neuropsychology* 3:121–128, 1965.
122. Knight RT, Grabowecky M: Escape from linear time: Prefrontal cortex and conscious experience, in Gazzaniga M (ed): *The Cognitive Neurosciences.* Cambridge, MA: MIT Press, 1995, pp 1357–1371.
123. Mesulam MM: A cortical network for directed attention and unilateral neglect. *Ann Neurol* 10:309–325, 1981.
124. Friedman HR, Goldman-Rakic PS: Coactivation of prefrontal and inferior parietal cortex in working memory tasks revealed by 2DG functional mapping in the rhesus monkey. *Neuroscience* 14:2775–2788, 1994.
125. Lhermitte F, Turell E, LeBrigand D, et al: Unilateral neglect and wave P300. A study of nine cases with unilateral lesions of the parietal lobes. *Arch Neurol* 42:567–573, 1985.
126. Knight, RT: Contribution of human hippocampal region to novelty detection. *Nature* 383:256–259, 1996.
127. Perani D, Bressi S, Cappa SF, et al: Evidence of multiple memory systems in the human brain: A 18F FDG PET metabolic study. *Brain* 116:903–919, 1993.
128. Goldman-Rakic PS, Selemon LD, Schwartz ML: Dual pathways connecting the dorsolateral prefrontal cortex with the hippocampal formation and parahippocampal cortex in the rhesus monkey. *Neuroscience* 12:719–743, 1984.
129. Heilman KM, Watson RT, Valenstein E: Neglect and related disorders, in Heilman KM, Valenstein E (eds): *Clinical Neuropsychology,* 3d ed. New York: Oxford University Press, 1993, pp 279–336.
130. Rapcsak SZ, Watson R, Heilman KM: Hemispace-visual field interactions in visual extinction. *J Neurol Neurosurg Psychiatry* 50:1117–1124, 1987.
131. De Renzi E, Gentilini M, Pattacini F: Auditory extinction following hemispheric damage. *Neuropsychologia* 22:733–744, 1984.
132. Heilman KM, Pandya DN, Geschwind N: Trimodal inattention following parietal lobe ablations. *Trans Am Neurol Assoc* 95:259–261, 1970.
133. De Renzi E, Gentilini M, Barbieri C: Auditory neglect. *J Neurol Neurosurg Psychiatry* 52:613–617, 1989.
134. Soroker N, Calamaro N, Glickson J, et al: Auditory inattention in right-hemisphere-damaged patients with and without visual neglect. *Neuropsychologia* 35:249–256, 1997.

135. Gainotti G, De Bonis C, Daniele A, et al: Contralateral and ipsilateral tactile extinction in patients with right and left focal brain lesions. *Int J Neurosci* 45:81–89, 1989.
136. Vallar G, Sandroni P, Rusconi ML, et al: Hemianopia, hemianesthesia, and spatial neglect: a study with evoked potentials. *Neurology* 41:1918–22, 1991.
137. Vallar G, Bottini MD, Sterzi R, et al: Hemianesthesia, sensory neglect, and defective access to conscious experience. *Neurology* 41:650–652, 1991.
138. Viggiano MP, Spinelli D, Mecacci L: Pattern reversal visual evoked potentials in patients with hemineglect syndrome. *Brain Cogn* 27:17–35, 1995.
139. Verleger R, Heide W, Butt C, et al: On-line correlates of right parietal patients' attention deficits. *Electroencephalogr Clin Neurophysiol* 99:444–457, 1996.
140. Näätänen R, Picton TW: The N1 wave of the human electric and magnetic response to sound: A review and an analysis of the component structure. *Psychophysiology* 24: 375–425, 1987.
141. Bisiach E, Cornacchia L, Sterzi R, et al: Disorders of perceived auditory lateralization after lesions of the right hemispheres. *Brain* 107:37–52, 1984.
142. Luck SJ, Heinze HJ, Mangun GR, et al: Visual event related potentials index focused attention within bilateral stimulus arrays: II. Functional dissociation of P1 and N1 components. *Electroencephalogr Clin Neurophysiol* 75:528–542, 1990.
143. Marzi CA, Girelli M, Miniussi C, et al: Electrophysiological correlates of conscious vision: Evidence from unilateral extinction. *J Cog Neurosci*, 12:869–877, 2000.
144. Vuilleumier P, Sagiv N, Hazeltine E, et al: Neural fate of seen and unseen faces in visuospatial neglect: A combined event-related fMRI and ERP study. *Proc Natl Acad Sci U S A* 98:3495–3500, 2001.
145. Driver J, Vuilleumier P, Eimer M, et al: Functional magnetic resonance imaging and evoked potential correlates of conscious and unconscious vision in parietal extinction patients. *Neuroimage* 14:S68–S75, 2001.
146. Lhermitte F, Pillon B, Serdaru M: Human anatomy and the frontal lobes: Part I. Imitation and utilization behavior: A neuropsychological study of 75 patients. *Ann Neurol* 19:326–334, 1986.
147. Driver J, Vuilleumier P: Perceptual awareness and its loss in unilateral neglect and extinction. *Cognition* 79:39–88, 2001.
148. Pitzalis S, Spinelli D, Zoccolotti P: Vertical neglect: Behavioral and electrophysiological data. *Cortex* 33:679–88, 1997.
149. Spinelli D, Burr DC, Morrone MC: Spatial neglect is associated with increased latencies of visual evoked potentials. *Vis Neurosci* 11:909–18, 1994.
150. Spinelli D, Di Russo F: Visual evoked potentials are affected by trunk rotation in neglect patients. *Neuroreport* 7:553–556, 1996.
151. Spinelli D, Angelelli P, De Luca M, et al: VEP in neglect patients have longer latencies for luminance but not for chromatic patterns. *Neuroreport* 7:815–859, 1996.
152. Doricchi F, Angelelli P, De Luca M, et al: Neglect for low luminance contrast stimuli but not for high colour contrast stimuli: A behavioural and electrophysiological case study. *Neuroreport* 31:1360–1364, 1996.
153. Alho K, Sams M, Paavilainen P, et al: Event related potentials reflecting processing of relevant and irrelevant stimuli during selective listening. *Psychophysiology* 26:514–528, 1989.
154. Alho K, Woods DL, Algazi A, et al: Intermodal selective attention: II. Effects of attentional load on processing of auditory and visual stimuli in central space. *Electroencephalogr Clin Neurophysiol* 82:356–368, 1992.
155. Näätänen R: Mismatch negativity outside strong attentional focus: A commentary on Woldorff et al (1991). *Psychophysiology* 28:478–484, 1991.
156. Alho K, Escera C, Diaz R, et al: Effects of involuntary auditory attention on visual task performance and brain activity. *Neuroreport* 8:3233–3237, 1997.
157. Novak G, Ritter W, Vaughan HG Jr: The chronometry of attention-modulated processing and automatic mismatch detection. *Psychophysiology* 29:412–430, 1992.
158. Schröger E: A neural mechanism for involuntary attention shifts to changes in auditory stimulation. *J Cogn Neurosci* 8:527–539, 1996.
159. Aaltonen O, Tuomainen J, Laine M, et al: Cortical differences in tonal versus vowel processing as revealed by an ERP component called mismatch negativity (MMN). *Brain Lang* 44:628–640, 1993.
160. Deacon D, Nousak JM, Pilotti M, et al: Automatic change detection: does the auditory system use representations of individual stimulus features or gestalts? *Psychophysiology* 35:413–419, 1998.
161. Deouell LY, Bentin S: Variable cerebral responses to equally distinct deviance in four auditory dimensions: A mismatch negativity study. *Psychophysiology* 35:745–754, 1998.
162. Schröger E: Processing of auditory deviants with changes in one versus two stimulus dimensions. *Psychophysiology* 32:55–65, 1995.
163. Ritter W, Deacon D, Gomes H, et al: The mismatch negativity of event-related potentials as a probe of transient auditory memory: A review. *Ear Hear* 16:52–57, 1995.

164. Posner MI, Walker JA, Friedrich FJ, et al: Effects of parietal lobe injury on covert orienting of visual attention. *J Neurosci* 4:1863–1874, 1984.
165. Friedrich FJ, Egly R, Rafal RD, et al: Spatial attention deficits in humans: A comparison of superior parietal and temporal-parietal junction lesions. *Neuropsychology* 12:193–207, 1998.
166. Donchin E, Ritter W, McCallum WC: Cognitive psychophysiology: The endogenous components of the ERP, in Callaway E, Tueting P, Koslow SH (eds): *Event-Related Potentials in Man.* New York: Academic Press, 1978, pp 349–442.
167. Watson RT, Miller BD, Heilman KM: Evoked potential in neglect. *Arch Neurol* 34, 224–227, 1977.
168. Neville H, Nicole JL, Barss A, et al: Syntactically based sentence processing classes: Evidence form event related brain potentials, *J Cogn Neurosci* 3:155–170, 1991.
169. Friederici AD, Pfeifer E, Hahne A: Event-related brain potentials during natural speech processing: Effects of semantic, morphological and syntactic violations. *Brain Res Cogn Brain Res* 1:183–192, 1993.
170. Kutas M, Hillyard SA: Reading senseless sentences: Brain potentials reflect semantic incongruity. *Science* 207:203–205, 1980.
171. Osterhout L, Holcomb PJ: Event-related brain potentials elicited by syntactic anomaly. *J Mem Lang* 31:785–806, 1992.
172. Van Petten C, Kutas M: Influences of semantic and syntactic context on open- and closed-class words. *Mem Cognit* 19:95–112, 1991.
173. Bentin S, McCarthy G, Wood CC: Event-related potentials, lexical decision and semantic priming. *Electroencephalogr Clin Neurophysiol* 60:343–355, 1985.
174. van Berkum JJ, Hagoort P, Brown CM: Semantic integration in sentences and discourse: Evidence from the N400. *J Cogn Neurosci* 11:657–671, 1999.
175. Barrett SE, Rugg MD, Perrett DI: Event-related potentials and the matching of familiar and unfamiliar faces. *Neuropsychology* 26:105–117, 1988.
176. Nielsen-Bohlman LC, Knight RT: Rapid memory mechanisms in man. *Neuroreport* 5:1517–1521, 1994.
177. Friedman D: Cognitive event-related potential components during continuous recognition memory for pictures. *Psychophysiology* 27:136–148, 1990.
178. Nigam A, Hoffman JE, Simons RF: N400 to semantically anomalous pictures and words. *J Cogn Neurosci* 4:15–22, 1992.
179. Paller KA, McCarthy G, Roessler E, et al: Potentials evoked in human and monkey medial temporal lobe during auditory and visual oddball paradigms. *Electroencephalogr Clin Neurophysiol* 84:269–279, 1992.
180. Besson M, Macar F: An event-related potential analysis of incongruity in music and other nonlinguistic contexts. *Psychophysiology* 24:14–25, 1987.
181. Deacon D, Hewitt S, Yang C, et al: Event-related potential indices of semantic priming using masked and unmasked words: evidence that the N400 does not reflect a post-lexical process. *Brain Res Cog Brain Res* 9:137–146, 2000.
182. Brown C, Hagoort P: The processing nature of the N400: Evidence from masked priming. *J Cogn Neurosci* 5:34–44, 1993.
183. Nobre AC, McCarthy G: Language-related ERPs: Scalp distributions and modulation by word type and semantic priming. *J Cogn Neurosci* 6:233–255, 1994.
184. Hagoort P, Brown CM, Swaab T: Lexical-semantic event-related potential effects in left hemisphere patients with aphasia and right hemisphere patients without aphasia. *Brain* 119:627–649, 1996.
185. Smith ME, Stapleton JM, Halgren E: Human medial temporal lobe potentials evoked in memory and language tasks. *Electroencephalogr Clin Neurophysiol* 63:145–159, 1986.
186. McCarthy G, Nobre AC, Bentin S, et al: Language-related field potentials in the anterior-medial temporal lobe: I. Intracranial distribution and neural generators. *J Neurosci* 15:1080–1089, 1995.
187. Puce A, Andrewes DG, Berkovic SF, et al: Visual recognition memory: neurophysiological evidence for the role of temporal white matter in man. *Brain* 114:1647–1666, 1991.
188. Berndt RS, Mitchum CC, Haendiges AN: Comprehension of reversible sentences in "agrammatism": A meta-analysis. *Cognition* 58:289–308, 1996.
189. Friederici AD, Hahne A, von Cramon DY: First-pass versus second-pass parsing processes in a Wernicke's and a Broca's aphasic: Electrophysiological evidence for a double dissociation. *Brain Lang* 62:311–341, 1998.
190. ter Keurs M, Brown CM, Hagoort P, et al: Electrophysiological manifestations of open- and closed-class words in patients with Broca's aphasia with agrammatic comprehension. An event-related brain potential study. *Brain* 122:839–854, 1999.
191. Swaab TY, Brown C, Hagoort P: Understanding ambiguous words in sentence contexts: Electrophysiological evidence for delayed contextual selection in Broca's aphasia. *Neuropsychologia* 36:737–761, 1998.
192. Auther LL, Wertz RT, Miller, et al: Relationships among the mismatch negativity (MMN) response, auditory

comprehension and site of lesion in aphasic adults. *Aphasiology* 14:461–470, 2000.
193. Wertz RT, Auther LL, Burch-Sims GP, et al: A comparison of the mismatch negativity (MMN) event-related potential to tone and speech stimuli in normal and aphasic adults. *Aphasiology* 12:499–507, 1998.
194. Connolly JF, D'Arcy RC, Lynn Newman R, et al: The application of cognitive event-related brain potentials (ERPs) in language-impaired individuals: review and case studies. *Int J Psychophysiol* 38:55–70, 2000.
195. Revonsuo A, Laine M: Semantic processing without conscious understanding in a global aphasic: Evidence from auditory event-related brain potentials. *Cortex* 32:29–48, 1996.
196. Merton PA, Morton HB: Stimulation of the cerebral cortex in the intact human subject. *Nature* 285:227, 1980.
197. Barker AT, Jalinous R, Freeston IL: Noninvasive magnetic stimulation of human motor cortex. *Lancet* 1:1106–1107, 1985.
198. Hallett M: Transcranial magnetic stimulation and the human brain. *Nature* 406:147–150, 2000.
199. Walsh V, Cowey A: Transcranial magnetic stimulation and cognitive neuroscience. *Nat Rev Neurosci* 1:73–79, 2000.
200. Gerloff C, Corwell B, Chen R, et al: Stimulation over the human supplementary motor area interferes with the organization of future elements in complex motor sequences. *Brain* 120:1587–1602, 1997.
201. Loo C, Mitchell P, Sachdev P, et al: Double-blind controlled investigation of transcranial magnetic stimulation for the treatment of resistant major depression. *Am J Psychiatry* 156:946–948, 1999.
202. Menkes DL, Bodnar P, Ballesteros RA, et al: Right frontal lobe slow frequency repetitive transcranial magnetic stimulation (SF r-TMS) is an effective treatment for depression: a case-control pilot study of safety and efficacy. *J Neurol Neurosurg Psychiatry* 67:113–115, 1999.
203. Amassian VE, Cracco RQ, Maccabee PJ, et al: Suppression of visual perception by magnetic coil stimulation of human occipital cortex. *Electroencephalogr Clin Neurophysiol* 74:458–462, 1989.
204. Kastner S, Demmer I, Ziemann U: Transient visual field defects induced by transcranial magnetic stimulation over human occipital pole. *Exp Brain Res* 118:19–26, 1998.
205. Corthout E, Uttl B, Ziemann U, et al: Two periods of processing in the (circum)striate visual cortex as revealed by transcranial magnetic stimulation. *Neuropsychologia* 37:137–145, 1999.
206. Beckers G, Zeki S: The consequences of inactivating areas V1 and V5 on visual motion perception. *Brain* 118:49–60, 1995.
207. Pascual-Leone A, Walsh V: Fast backprojections from the motion to the primary visual area necessary for visual awareness. *Science* 292:510–512, 2001.
208. Kosslyn SM, Pascual-Leone A, Felician O, et al: The role of area 17 in visual imagery: Convergent evidence from PET and rTMS. *Science* 284:167–170, 1999.
209. Pascual-Leone A, Tormos JM, Keenan J, et al: Study and modulation of human cortical excitability with transcranial magnetic stimulation. *J Clin Neurophysiol* 15:333–343, 1998.
210. Zangaladze A, Epstein CM, Grafton ST, et al: Involvement of visual cortex in tactile discrimination of orientation. *Nature* 401:587–590, 1999.
211. Cohen LG, Celnik P, Pascual-Leone A, et al: Functional relevance of cross-modal plasticity in blind humans. *Nature* 389:180–183, 1997.
212. Deibert E, Kraut M, Kremen S, et al: Neural pathways in tactile object recognition. *Neurology* 52:1413–1417, 1999.
213. Sathian K, Zangaladze A, Hoffman JM, et al: Feeling with the mind's eye. *Neuroreport* 8:3877–3881, 1997.
214. Pourtois G, Vandermeeren Y, Olivier E, et al: Event-related TMS over the right posterior parietal cortex induces ipsilateral visuo-spatial interference. *Neuroreport* 12:2369–2374, 2001.
215. Fierro B, Brighina F, Piazza A, et al: Timing of right parietal and frontal cortex activity in visuo-spatial perception: a TMS study in normal individuals. *Neuroreport* 12:2605–2607, 2001.
216. Wasserman EM: Risk and safety of repetitive transcranial magnetic stimulation: Report and suggested guidelines from the International Workshop on the Safety of Repetitive Transcranial Magnetic Stimulation, June 5–7, 1996. *Electroencephalogr Clin Neurophysiol* 108:1–16, 1998.

Chapter 10

COMPUTATIONAL MODELING IN BEHAVIORAL NEUROLOGY AND NEUROPSYCHOLOGY

Martha J. Farah

COGNITION AS COMPUTATION

If the insights of cognitive psychology had to be boiled down to a single statement, a good candidate would be "cognition is computation." Starting with the work of Allen Newell and Herbert Simon (1972) in the sixties and seventies, psychologists have been able to explain a wide range of human behavior in terms of information encoded from the environment, information stored in memory, and mechanisms for combining these two sources of information to select appropriate actions.

Viewing cognition as computation freed the field of psychology from the constraints of Skinnerian behaviorism, in which all psychological explanation was confined to directly observable entities such as stimulus and response. According to behaviorism, to hypothesize about the internal mental states intervening between stimulus and response was unscientific, nonexplanatory, and downright mystical. The information processing of computers provided a concrete demonstration that the states intervening between stimulus and response could also be within the domain of objective science. Hypothesizing about the knowledge that caused a person to act one way rather than another is no more mystical than hypothesizing about the stored data in a computer that caused it to give one output rather than another. The computational view of the mind made it possible to have a *psychological* level of explanation—dealing with entities such as memory, knowledge, inference and decision—that could be understood as a function of perfectly nonmystical *physical* mechanisms.

There are many different ways in which physical mechanisms can process information. The best-known, and in many ways the most powerful, is the way computers work. Symbolically coded information is retrieved from a particular physical memory location, operated upon in a physically distinct central processing unit according to stored instructions, and then reentered into memory. Most of the early theories of cognitive psychology assumed this type of computational architecture. More recently, a very different computational architecture has been explored by computer scientists, psychologists, and neuroscientists, which has more in common with brains than with office computers. This is the parallel distributed processing (PDP) architecture. Because PDP is similar in many ways to neural information processing, PDP models have increasingly come to be used in neuropsychology.

Computation has played two roles in cognitive psychology and neuropsychology. In some cases theories are simply expressed in terms of the concepts of computation: the informational content and format of representations, the parallel or serial nature of searches, and the like. In other cases, researchers implement their theories as running computer simulations. With the advent of the PDP architecture, computer simulation is increasingly used. One reason for this is that the behavior of PDP systems is not always obvious or predictable by intuition alone.

PARALLEL DISTRIBUTED PROCESSING

PDP systems consist of a large number of highly interconnected neuron-like units. These units are connected to one another by weighted connections that determine how much activation from one unit flows to another. There is no central controller governing the behavior of the network. Rather, each part of the network functions locally and in parallel with the other parts, hence the first P in PDP. Representations consist of the pattern of activation distributed over a population of units, and long-term memory knowledge is encoded in the pattern of connection strengths distributed among a population of units, hence the D. Alternative terms for PDP include connectionism (not to be confused with the center-and-pathway approach of Wernicke and his followers, which has also been called connectionism), brain-style computation, and artificial neural networks. For more than the brief overview offered here, the reader is directed to O'Reilly and Munakata's (2000) recent textbook on computational modeling in cognitive neuroscience.

There are many types of PDP networks with different computational properties. Among the features that determine network type are the activation rule, connectivity, and learning rule. The activation rule governs how the activation values of units are updated given a certain input activation. Units' activations can be discrete or continuous, and activations may be increased in direct proportion to the sum of the inputs (a *linear activation function*) or as a nonlinear function of the inputs (generally a sigmoid shaped function). The activation rule has a variety of consequences for network behavior, some of which are not immediately obvious. For example, as noted below, purely linear networks will not be able to learn certain kinds of associations.

A major distinguishing feature is connectivity, which can be unidirectional, in which case the network is called *feedforward,* or bidirectional, in which case it is called *interactive.* Feedforward networks may consist simply of a set of input units and a set of output units. A pattern associator can be made from such a network if the weights between the first and second layer units are set so that each of a set of patterns of activation over the units in the first layer evokes an associated pattern over the units in the second layer. Some feedforward networks have an additional set of so-called *hidden units* interposed between the input and output units. With nonlinear systems, the additional set of units is useful in transforming the input patterns of activation to the desired output patterns; indeed certain types of problems (such as associating input patterns 00 and 11 with one output and 01 and 10 with another, the "XOR" problem) can be solved only with hidden units. In *recurrent networks,* later layers loop back to earlier layers. In interactive networks, some or all connections are bidirectional. In recurrent and interactive networks, "downstream" units can influence "upstream" units; more than one processing step is therefore needed to arrive at their final activation state. These networks are said to "settle into" a stable state after the addition of an input pattern of activation.

Learning in neural networks consists of adjusting the weights between units so that, given a set of input activation patterns, in each case the network ends up in the desired activation state. For example, for a network to learn that a certain name goes with a certain face, the weights among units in the network are adjusted so that presentation of any one of the face patterns in the units representing faces or any one of the name patterns in the units representing names causes the corresponding other patterns to become activated.

There is a wide variety of learning algorithms; the choice depends in part on the type of network and the task to be learned. A learning rule proposed many decades ago by the neuroscientist Donald Hebb (1949) forms the basis for many current learning algorithms. The gist of the *Hebb Rule* is: Neurons that fire together wire together. In other words, when there is a positive correlation in the activity of two units, their connection should be strengthened, so that future activation of one will be even more likely to activate the other. This form of the rule enables *unsupervised learning,* that is, learning without an external source of feedback about right and wrong performance. Networks that use unsupervised learning are called *self-organizing,* as they develop their own representations of regularities in their input, for example, developing edge representations from center-surround–like inputs (Ritter, 1990), or semantic representations from patterns of word co-occurrence. (See Kohonen, 1995 for additional information on self-organizing systems.)

The Hebb rule can also be used to learn to associate patterns, but only if the input patterns are orthogonal, a rather stringent requirement. When the object is to learn to associate or complete patterns, then *supervised* learning is normally used. The *Delta Rule* is an example of a supervised learning rule that can be viewed as a variant of the Hebb rule. Both learning rules change weights proportionate with a comparison between activation values; in the case of supervised learning, the comparison is between desired activation value and actual activation value, an error measure. Networks with hidden units demand yet a further modification of the learning rule, as the weights to be changed do not directly link the input with the output units from which the error measure is derived. The *Generalized Delta Rule,* or *Backpropagation,* is often used in this case. With this rule the error in the output units is propagated back to alter the weights of the (nonadjacent) input units.

Further discussion of learning rules is beyond the scope of this chapter, except to note that learning in PDP models is often not intended to simulate real learning. Rather, it is frequently used as a tool for setting the weights in a network so that the network can simulate some aspect of cognition in its mature end-state. Backpropagation is sometimes criticized for being physiologically implausible. This may or may not be a valid criticism, depending on the goal of the simulation. For example, if one were interested in studying the effects of damage to the face recognition system, one would need a model of face recognition that embodied a set of associations between facial appearance and other knowledge about people, on which one could inflict damage. As it is virtually impossible to "hand wire" networks of more than a few units, learning rules would be used to build in these associations. However, they would not be simulating the way in which people learn face recognition. For this reason it might be less confusing to refer to learning algorithms for neural networks as weight-setting algorithms, unless the learning process is explicitly being modeled.

How Realistic are PDP Models?

Of course, there are cases when real human learning is the subject of the model, and then we are right to inquire whether or in what sense the model's learning is similar to human learning. More generally, it is important to consider whether PDP is a reasonable model for human brain function.

PDP models differ from real neural networks, including the human brain, in numerous ways: even the biggest PDP networks are tiny compared to the brain, PDP models have just one kind of unit compared to a variety of types of neurons, and just one kind of activation (which can act excitatorily or inhibitorily) rather than a multitude of different neurotransmitters, and so on. Yet these differences are not necessarily a cause to reject the PDP approach. No model is identical in all respects to the system being modeled; models possess theory-relevant and theory-irrelevant attributes. Furthermore, science must often simplify nature in order to understand it. PDP models should be viewed as simplifications of the brain, possessing enough theory-relevant attributes of the brain to be informative on many questions but clearly leaving out or even contradicting many known aspects of brain function.

Among the theory-relevant aspects of PDP models are the use of distributed representations, the large number of inputs to and outputs from each unit, the modifiable connections between units, the existence of both inhibitory and excitatory connections, summation rules, bounded activations, and thresholds. PDP models allow us to find out what aspects of behavior, normal and pathologic, can be explained by this set of theory-relevant attributes. Of course, some behavior may be explainable only with the incorporation of other features of neuroanatomy and neurophysiology not currently used in PDP models. This seems quite likely, and the discovery of such instances will be extremely informative with respect to the functional significance of these features of our biology. However, note that this problem does not apply to cases in which the current models perform well. In such cases, the only danger associated with nonrealism is that the model's success might depend on a theory-irrelevant simplification. For example, scale is generally treated as theory-irrelevant, but it is possible that certain mechanisms will work only for small networks or small amounts of knowledge. We must be on the lookout for such cases, but also recognize that it is unlikely that the success of most models will happen to depend critically on their unrealistic features.

Spatial Analogies for Understanding the Behavior of PDP Networks

Spatial analogies are useful for visualizing certain aspects of network dynamics, including the way in which the network's patterns of activation change under the influence of an input and the way in which the ensemble of weights changes during learning. The activation state of the network at any point in time can be represented as a point in a high-dimensional space called *activation space.* The dimensions of this space represent the level of activation of each unit in the network, assuming a fixed set of weights. In addition to the dimensions representing the activation levels of the units, there is one additional dimension, representing the overall "fit" between the current activation pattern and the weights.

When units that are both active have a large positive weight between them, so that they reinforce each other's activation, this is an example of a good fit. If both units are active and the weight between them is negative (i.e., inhibitory), the fit would be poor. This measure of fit is called *energy,* with low energy representing a better fit. The energy value associated with each pattern of activation defines a surface in activation space.

When an input pattern is presented to the network, the corresponding initial position in activation space is defined by the activation levels on the input units, along with resting level values for the dimensions representing the other units in the network. The weights in the rest of the network will not fit well with uniform resting level activation values over their portion of the network. Thus, the initial point in activation space will be in a region of high energy. As activation propagates through the network, the pattern of activation changes and the point representing this pattern moves along the energy surface in activation space. The movement will be generally downward, as the network lowers its energy, much as a ball rolls down a hill to lower its potential energy. To see why this would happen in terms of network dynamics, rather than by analogy with rolling balls, consider the examples given earlier of high- and low-energy activation states. For example, active units connected by negative weights (a poor fit, high energy pattern) will tend to change their activations until one is active and the other not (a good fit, low energy pattern).

The energy minima toward which the network tends are termed *attractors.* Attractors are useful in network computation not only for associating patterns and completing partial patterns but also for their ability to "clean up" a noisy input, by transforming a pattern similar to a known pattern into that known pattern (i.e., a pattern just uphill from an attractor will roll down into the attractor). So long as the input is sufficiently similar to (in the spatial analogy, close to) the attractor that it falls within the attractor's "basin," it will be pulled into the attractor.

The shape of the energy landscape is determined by the network's weights. In an untrained network, the landscape will be generally flat, with random hills and valleys. When the network has learned a certain association, its weights will create an energy landscape in activation space in which the point corresponding to the input pattern and the attractor point corresponding to the complete associated pattern are connected by a smoothly and steeply sloping path that causes the one state to "roll" down into the other.

The weights that determine the attractor structure of activation space can themselves be used to define a space, and this space is useful for visualizing the process of learning. In *weight space,* each of the weights in a network corresponds to one dimension of a space, so that we can represent the sum total of the network's knowledge as a point in this high-dimensional space. If one additional dimension is now added to the space, representing the performance of the network at associating names and faces (an error measure of some sort), then there will be a surface defined by each combination of weights and their associated error measure. Learning consists of moving along this surface in weight space and changing weight values until a sufficiently low point has been reached.

APPLICATIONS OF COMPUTATIONAL MODELING TO BEHAVIORAL NEUROLOGY AND NEUROPSYCHOLOGY

For most of the history of behavioral neurology and neuropsychology, the lesion method has been our primary source of insights into human brain organization. Yet the interpretation of lesion effects is not always as transparent as one would like. As early as the nineteenth century, authors such as John Hughlings-Jackson (1873) cautioned that the brain is a distributed and highly interactive system, such that local damage to one part can unleash new modes of functioning in the remaining parts of the system. As a result, one cannot assume that a patient's behavior following brain damage is the direct result of a simple subtraction of one or more components of the mind, with those that remain functioning normally. More likely, it results from a combination of the subtraction of some components, and changes in the functioning of other components that had previously been influenced by the missing components.

PDP provides a conceptual framework and concrete tools for reasoning about the effects of local lesions in distributed, interactive systems. It has already proven helpful in understanding a number of different neuropsychological disorders. Each of the examples reviewed here constitutes a reinterpretation of a well-known disorder, with qualitatively different implications for the normal organization of the brain and the functional locus of damage within that organization.

Neglect Dyslexia: A Pre- or Postlexical Impairment?

Patients with left visual neglect omit or misidentify letters on the left side of letter strings. When the letter string is a word, this pattern of performance is termed *neglect dyslexia* (see Chap. 14). Surprisingly, neglect dyslexics are more likely to report the initial letters of a word than of a nonword letter string, even when the initial letters of the word cannot simply be guessed on the basis of the end of the word (Sieroff et al., 1988). This seems to imply that the breakdown in the processing of neglected stimuli comes at a late stage, after word recognition, for how else could lexical status (word versus nonword) affect performance? Yet there are other good reasons to believe that neglect affects the early stages of visual perception, prior to recognition (see Chaps. 25 and 26).

It is possible to reconcile these two apparently conflicting observations, that neglect is sensitive to lexical status and that neglect affects prerecognition visual processing, within the context of a network model. Mozer and Behrmann (1990) simulated neglect dyslexia with a model in which spatial attention operates at an early stage, prior to visual recognition. Specifically, in this model, attention gates the flow of information out of early visual feature maps into higher-order letter and letter string representations. Neglect consists of an asymmetrical distribution of attention over letter strings; in the case of left neglect, a reduction of the attention normally allocated to the initial letter positions within the string. Neglect therefore results in full information from the right side of a letter string, but only partial information from the left, being transmitted to word representations.

According to this model, the errors that occur with nonword letter strings result from partial visual information about the letter features on the left side of the string, which is not sufficient to identify precisely which letters are present. In contrast, the same partial information about the initial letters of a word, with good-quality information about the remaining letters of a word, will result in an activation pattern that is similar to the activation pattern for that word. A key aspect of the model, which explains the relative preservation of word reading in neglect, is that known words are attractor states for the network. Therefore, given enough information about the letters in word, even if not complete information, the network will settle into the pattern of the word, including the initial letters. In this way, it is possible to explain why neglect dyslexics read words better than nonwords without giving up the hypothesis that neglect is a disorder of visual perception, affecting stimulus processing prior to the recognition stage.

Computational models make predictions that can be tested empirically. According to this model of neglect dyslexia, if the asymmetry of attention is too extreme, no information about the initial letters will get through to word representations and the resulting activation state will not fall within the basin of attraction for the word. Behrmann and colleagues tested this prediction with a patient who had severe neglect (Behrmann et al., 1990). As predicted, he did not show better perception of the initial letters of words than nonwords. Furthermore, when his attention was drawn to the left, and the attentional asymmetry thereby made less extreme, he then showed the usual difference between word and nonword letter strings. Conversely, a patient who normally showed this difference between words and nonwords was stopped from doing so by attentional manipulations that increased his attentional asymmetry.

In general, this model demonstrates how the interaction between lower- and higher-level representations is influenced by attractors and the implications such interactions have for our interpretation of neuropsychological data. This general approach has been used to interpret other neuropsychological findings. For example, Mozer (2000) has extended his model to account for findings of object-centered neglect (i.e., neglect in which attention appears to be directed to objects rather than spatial locations; see Chap. 26) in terms of a purely spatial attentional process. The attractors representing objects bias the top-down activation to early visual representations in a way that respects the grouping or object information present at the higher levels. Other examples of the explanatory power of top-down effects of attractors can be found in models of reading and reading disorders, in which phenomena such as regularization by surface dyslexics (see Chap. 14) are explained in terms of a weakened attractor structure in the widest and deepest attractors are the most robust to damage (see Plaut et al., 1996, for a review).

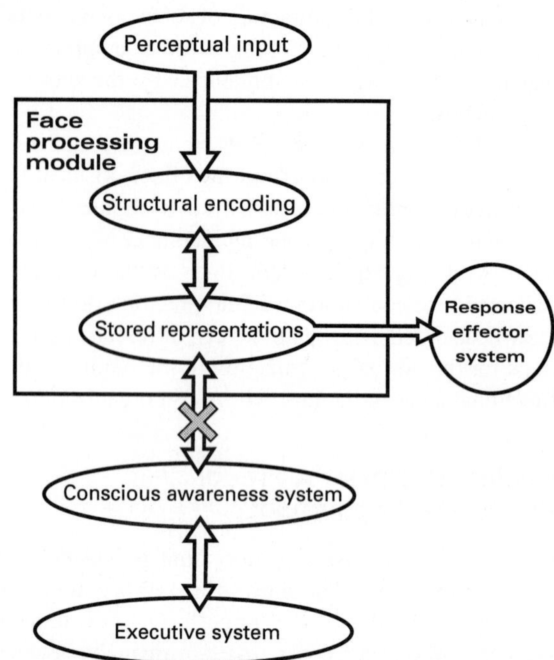

Figure 10-1
A model proposed by De Haan et al. (1992) to account for covert face recognition in prosopagnosia. There is a separate mechanism hypothesized for conscious awareness, distinct from the mechanisms of face recognition, and covert recognition is explained by a lesion at location 1, disconnecting the two parts of the model.

Covert Face Recognition: Evidence for a "Consciousness Module"?

Prosopagnosia is an impairment of face recognition that can occur relatively independently of impairments in object recognition (see Chap. 19). A number of recent findings seem to suggest that the underlying impairment, in at least some patients, is not in face recognition per se but in conscious awareness of recognition. This would seem to imply that recognition and consciousness depend on dissociable and distinct brain systems, as shown in Fig. 10-1. My colleagues and I built a computer simulation that is able to account for covert recognition across a number of very different tasks (Farah et al., 1993; O'Reilly and Farah, 1999). The network is shown in Fig. 10-2 and consists of face recognition units, semantic knowledge units, and name units (embodying knowledge of people's facial appearance, general information about them, and their names, respectively). Hidden units were interposed between these layers to assist the network in learning to associate faces and names by way of semantic information. There is no part of the network that is dedicated to awareness.

The first finding to be simulated was that some prosopagnosics can learn to associate facial photographs with names faster when the pairings are true (e.g., Harrison Ford's face with Harrison Ford's name) than when they are false (e.g., Harrison Ford's face with Michael Douglas's name) (De Haan et al., 1987). This result was initially taken to imply that these patients were recognizing the faces normally, and that the breakdown in processing lay downstream from vision, as shown in Fig. 10-1. However, when some of the face units were eliminated from our model, thus simulating a lesion in the visual system, the network also relearned old face–name pairings faster than new ones. Why should this be? Recall that learning can be viewed as a process of moving through weight space. After damage, the network is in a high-error region of weight space for both old face–name pairings and new ones, and for this reason the network cannot overtly associate any faces with any names. However, that region of weight space is closer to a low-error region for the old pairings than for the new ones, because the residual weights (connecting intact units) have the correct

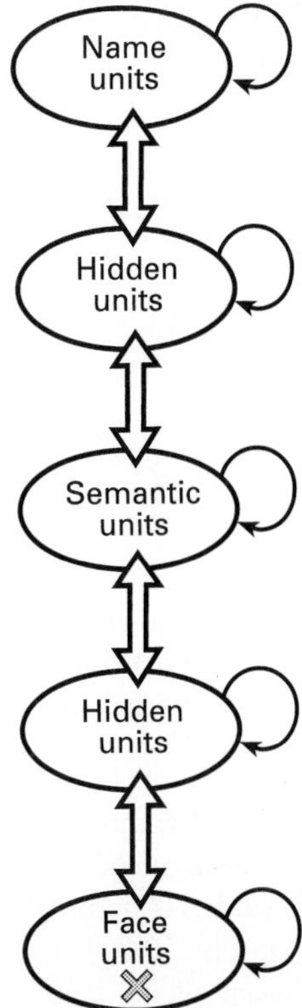

Figure 10-2
A model proposed by Farah et al. (1993) to account for covert face recognition in prosopagnosia. The dissociation between overt and covert face recognition emerges when the face recognition system is damaged.

values for the old pairings, and the learning process is therefore shorter.

A second finding, that previously familiar faces are perceived more quickly in the context of a same/different matching task, has also been interpreted as evidence for intact visual face processing (De Haan et al., 1987). However, after lesions to the face units in our model, the remaining face units settled into a stable state faster for previously familiar face patterns. This can be understood in terms of the distortion of the network's attractor structure after damage. The original structure was designed to take familiar face patterns as input and settle quickly to a stable state. After damage, these patterns will still find themselves on downward sloping parts of the energy landscape more often than novel patterns, even if the energy minima into which they roll have changed.

In yet another task, which requires classifying a printed name as belonging to an actor or a politician, a face from the opposite occupation category shown in the background has been found to slow the responses of both normal subjects and a prosopagnosic (De Haan et al., 1987). This seems to imply that the face is recognized despite prosopagnosia. In simulating this finding, face units were removed until the network's overt performance at classifying faces according to occupation was as poor as the patient's. At this level of damage, wrong-category faces slowed performance in the name classification task. This can be understood in terms of the distributed nature of representation in neural networks, which allows for partial representation of information when some but not all units representing a face have been eliminated. The partial information generally raises the activation of the appropriate downstream occupation units, thus biasing their responses to the printed names, but is not generally able to raise their activations above threshold to allow an explicit response to faces.

The basic principle at work in this model of covert recognition is that neural network representations are graded in quality, not all-or-none, and that the representations remaining in a damaged network may be sufficient to support performance in some tasks but not others. This principle has also been used to explain dissociations within the realm of visual word recognition (Mayall and Humphreys, 1996), and wide range of other behavioral dissociations in developmental psychology as well as neuropsychology (Munakata, 2001).

Optic Aphasia: How Many Semantic Modules are There?

Optic aphasia is a puzzling disorder in which patients cannot name visually presented objects despite demonstrating good visual recognition nonverbally (e.g., by pantomiming the use of a seen object or sorting semantically related objects together) and good naming (e.g., by naming palpated objects or objects they hear described verbally). If they can get from vision to semantics (intact visual recognition) and from semantics

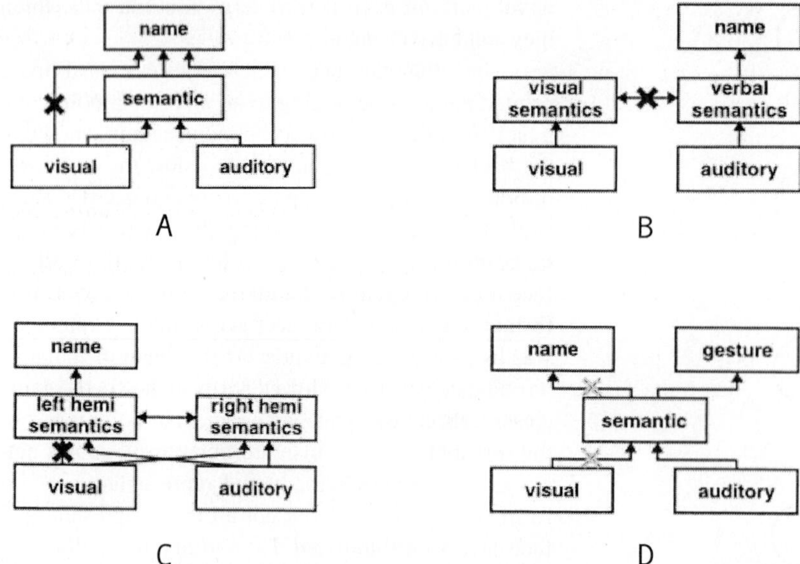

Figure 10-3
Four different models intended to account for optic aphasia. See text for explanation.

to naming (intact object naming of nonvisual inputs), why can they not name visually presented objects?

In response to this counterintuitive dissociation among tasks, traditional accounts of optic aphasia in cognitive neuropsychology have invoked additional processing components for visual naming, beyond vision, semantics, and name retrieval. For example, Ratcliff and Newcombe (1982) hypothesized a system for accessing names from vision directly, shown in Fig. 10-3*A*, which they proposed might be needed to supplement the semantically mediated processing. Beauvois (1982) hypothesized two separate semantic systems, as shown in Fig.10-3*B*, one used for visual input and the other used for verbal input and output. Coslett and Saffran (1989) proposed separate right and left hemisphere semantic systems, with only the latter accessing verbal output, as shown in Fig. 10-3*C*. On the face of things, it seems that optic aphasia requires additions of one sort or another to the simplest model of visual naming, whereby visual inputs activate a unified semantic system, which in turn activates verbal output.

An alternative account of optic aphasia preserves this simple model, by adding a hypothesized second lesion instead of adding components to the brain's functional architecture. Sitton and coworkers (2000) showed that multiple lesions can have synergistic effects, resulting in impaired performance only when more than one lesioned component is required for a task. Specifically, we simulated visual naming and the other tasks used in studies of optic aphasia with the simple model shown in Fig. 10-3*D*. When a small lesion is introduced into one of the pathways, the system's attractors are able to "clean up" the resulting noisy representations; the representations are still within the system's basins of attraction. However, two lesions' worth of damage to the representations exceed the system's clean-up abilities and performance suffers. Given that visual naming is the only task requiring both the vision-to-semantics pathway and the semantics to naming pathway, small lesions in these two parts of the system will result in a selective impairment in visual naming.

Many dissociations in neuropsychology have been interpreted as evidence for highly specific modules, yet the possibility of multiple synergistic lesion effects suggests that simpler interpretations may be possible. For example, Young et al. (1990) report a case of neglect confined to faces. The most straightforward interpretation of this case involves a specialized spatial attention module that is dedicated to face processing. However, a pair of small but synergistic lesions in a general spatial attention module and in face processing will also produce this effect (Mozer and Farah, 2001). In principle this same approach could be taken to the explanation of highly specific neurolinguistic dissociations, such as the case of impaired verb production in the face of preserved verb comprehension and preserved production of other parts of speech (Caramazza and Hillis, 1991).

REFERENCES

Beauvois MF: Optic aphasia: A process of interaction between vision and language. Philos Trans R Soc Lond Ser B 298:35–47, 1982.

Behrmann M, Moscovitch M, Black S, Mozer M: Perceptual and conceptual mechanisms in neglect dyslexia: Two contrasting case studies. *Brain*113:1163–1183, 1990.

Caramazza A, Hillis A: Lexical organization of nouns and verbs in the brain. *Nature* 349:788–790, 1991.

Coslett HB, Saffran EM: Preserved object recognition and reading comprehension in optic aphasia. *Brain* 112:1091–1110, 1989.

De Haan EHF, Bauer RM, Greve KW: Behavioral and physiological evidence for covert recognition in a prosopagnosic patient. *Cortex* 28:77–95, 1992.

De Haan EHF, Young AW, Newcombe F: Face recognition without awareness. *Cogn Neuropsychol* 4:385–415, 1987.

Farah MJ, O'Reilly RC, Vecera SP: Dissociated overt and covert recognition as on emergent property of lesioned attractor networks. *Pychol Rev* 100:751–788, 1993.

Hebb DO: *Organization of Behavior.* New York: Wiley, 1949.

Hinton GE, Shallice T: Lesioning an attractor network: Investigations of acquired dyslexia. *Psychol Rev* 98:96–121, 1991.

Jackson JH: On the anatomical and physiological localization of movements in the brain. *Lancet* 1:84–85, 162–164, 232–234, 1873.

Kohonen T: *Self-Organizing Maps.* New York: Springer-Verlag, 1995.

Linsker R: From basic network principles to neural architecture: Emergence of orientation-selective cells. *Proc Natl Acad Sci U S A* 83:8390–8394, 1986.

Mozer MC, Behrmann M: On the interaction of selective attention and lexical knowledge: A connectionist account of neglect dyslexia. *J Cogn Neurosci* 2:96–123, 1990.

Mozer M, Farah MJ: Content-specific neglect syndromes and the modularity of attention. *J Cogn Neurosci* 2001 Suppl.

Munakata Y: Graded representations in behavioral dissociations. *Trends Cogn Sci* 5:309–314, 2001.

Newell A, Simon HA: *Human Problem Solving.* Englewood Cliffs, NJ: Prentice-Hall, 1972.

O'Reilly RC, Farah MJ: Simulation and explanation in neuropsychology and beyond. *Cogn Neuropsychol* 16:1–48, 1999.

O'Reilly RC, Munakata Y: *Computational Explorations in Cognitive Neuroscience.* Cambridge, MA: MIT Press, 2000.

Plaut DC: Understanding normal and impaired word reading: Computational principles in quasi-regular domains. *Psychol Rev* 103:56–115, 1996.

Plaut DC, Shallice T: Deep dyslexia: A case study of connectionist neuropsychology. *Cogn Neuropsychol* 10:377–500, 1993.

Ritter H: Self-organizing maps for internal representations. *Psychol Res* 52:128–136, 1990.

Sieroff E, Pollatsek A, Posner MI: Recognition of visual letter strings following injury to the posterior visual spatial attention system. *Cogn Neuropsychol* 5:427–449, 1988.

Sitton M, Mozer MC, Farah MJ: Superadditive effects of multiple lesions in a connectionist architecture: implications for the neuropsychology of optic aphasia. *Psychol Rev* 107:709–734, 2000.

Young AW, De Haan EH, Newcombe F, Hay DC: Facial neglect. *Neuropsychologia* 28:391–415, 1990.

Part 2

APHASIA AND OTHER DOMINANT HEMISPHERE SYNDROMES

Chapter 11

APHASIA: CLINICAL AND ANATOMIC ISSUES

Michael P. Alexander

The clinical study of aphasia began in 1861 with the observations of Paul Broca.[1] Within 40 or 50 years, all of the basic clinical phenomena reviewed here had been described and many of the major flash points of clinical and theoretical disagreement had been identified. In the past 20 years, fresh interest has come to clinical aphasia research from two directions: modern neuroimaging and cognitive neurosciences. Together, they have additionally provided tools to carry out aphasia-related language experiments in normals. Furthermore, old questions such as cerebral laterality, the influence of handedness, the effects of gender and bilingualism on aphasia, and the mechanisms of recovery have been re-explored. Much of this chapter–which reviews the basic clinical features of aphasia–could have been written 20, 50, or even 100 years ago. In 2002, it is possible to consider this material with greater appreciation of the variability found in the basic syndromes, of their anatomic complexities, of the natural history of recovery, and (although here only briefly) of the cognitive and linguistic deficits that fundamentally underlie the classic syndromes. The chapters on neuroimaging (Chaps. 7–9) and on cognitive analysis of aphasia (Chap. 12) should be read along with this chapter.

CLINICAL SYNDROMES

The description of syndromes of aphasia arose out of much the same motivation as the identification of other clinical neurologic syndromes: the need to identify clinically useful associations between specific clusters of signs and the likely anatomy of the lesion producing them. The most clinically transparent signs of aphasia have generally been taken to be independent signs of brain damage. Thus, syndromes have been constructed out of reduced language output as well as impaired comprehension, repetition, and naming. Disorders of written language have been divided into additional syndromes only as reading and writing have been impaired beyond spoken language impairments. The use of three independent signs generates eight syndromes, assuming naming to be impaired in all aphasic patients.

Although these syndromes have reasonable clinical validity, there are numerous limitations to this type of syndrome construction. First, the syndromes depend on a sign being normal or not, much as a hemiparesis is present or absent; but the complexity of impairments in comprehension and language production are less amenable to simple dichotomous judgments. Thus, distinctions come to depend on the statistical properties and structural assumptions of the test. Second, there is no certainty that signs all have the same pathophysiologic mechanism in all patients. For comprehension at the sentence level, in particular, there may be several independent pathways to impairment.[2] Third, the syndromes are not stable even when the anatomy is. A patient with a temporoparietal stroke may have an initial Wernicke's aphasia, but, over weeks, language improves to reach the clinical diagnosis of conduction aphasia.[3] Does one conclude that the behavioral-anatomic correlations are with Wernicke's or conduction aphasia? Can one be certain that there are two distinct syndromes if they blur into each other? Should one conclude that only the early-phase correlations hold, that all correlations have built in corollaries about recovery, or that both are true? Fourth, most syndromes are polytypic–that is, they are defined by several criteria.[4] What do we conclude if only some of the criteria are met? Would this be a less severe syndrome? A subsyndrome? A different syndrome altogether?

Despite these limitations, the classic syndromes do have utility. They serve as a type of shorthand for clinical communications. If told that a patient has a particular aphasic syndrome 2 weeks after a stroke, one would know approximately what to expect of language examinations, what the range of possible brain lesions would be, what the prognosis should be, and what some reasonable treatments might be. And although the clinical-anatomic correlations are imperfect, certainly nothing as robust as the brainstem syndromes, they are a good first fit.[5] Any alleged scientific account of aphasia must be compatible with the syndrome-lesion correlations. If so inclined, one could suggest directly from the classic syndrome which interesting cognitive neuroscience issues the patient might illuminate.

Broca's Aphasia

In Broca's aphasia, language output is nonfluent–that is, it is reduced in phrase length and grammatical complexity. This reduction can range from no recognizable output or repeated meaningless utterances to short, truncated phrases using only the most meaning-laden words (substantives). When truncated, the sentence structure is poor; articles, modifiers, complex verb forms, etc., are missing, and the overall structure of sentences is simplified. This is referred to as *agrammatism* when it is dominated by simplifications, elisions, and omissions. *Paragrammatism* is incorrect grammar, such as incorrect pronoun use, wrong verb tense, number disagreement, etc. Few patients with severe Broca's aphasia produce enough language to be paragrammatic. Numerous theories have been proposed to account for agrammatism; none is universally accepted. It is also possible that agrammatism/paragrammatism in these patients represents the loss of schematic procedural knowledge for the implementation of grammar and syntax. Kolk has demonstrated substantial similarities in the grammatical capacities of patients with chronic agrammatic aphasia and normal young children who have the lexical capacity to produce complex sentences but not the practiced ("proceduralized") subroutines of producing complexity.[6]

There is also usually considerable hesitation and delay in production. Speech quality is impaired. Articulation is poor (dysarthria). Melodic line is disrupted (dysprosody), partly due to dysarthria but often more than just secondary to it. Volume is usually reduced at first (hypophonia). With time, speech takes on hyperkinetic (dystonic and spastic) qualities. Language comprehension is adequate although rarely normal. Response to word-recognition tasks, simple commands, and routine conversation is generally good. Response to multistep commands and complex syntactic requests is generally poor. Repetition is poor, although often better than speech. Relational words (functors–articles, conjunctions, modifiers, etc.) may be produced in repetition, but they are exceedingly uncommon in spontaneous speech. Written language parallels spoken, although some patients, while never regaining useful speech, develop writing that is telegraphic. Oral reading is usually agrammatic; so-called deep dyslexia (see Chap. 14) may emerge with this.[7] Naming is usually poor, but it may be surprisingly good in chronic patients. All types of errors can occur, although semantic errors are most typical for substantive words.[8] Objects are frequently named better than are actions.[9]

Broca's aphasia is commonly accompanied by right hemiparesis, buccofacial apraxia, and ideomotor apraxia of the left arm (or both arms in the nonparetic case). Right-sided sensory loss and right visual field impairments (extinction and/or lower-quadrant deficit) are less frequent. Depression, frequently major, develops in approximately 40 percent of patients with Broca's aphasia.[10]

Many patients have fractional syndromes of Broca's aphasia. Because all of these fractional disorders are still taxonomically closer to Broca's aphasia than to any of the other seven classic diagnoses, many aphasia systems will classify them all as Broca's aphasia.[11] In analyzing reports of Broca's aphasia, it is crucial to understand the taxonomic rules of the report's assessment tool. If all fractional cases are considered Broca's aphasia, the clinicoanatomic correlations will seem imprecise. This is an example of the difficulty inherent in building syndromes with polytypic qualities. Analysis of the clinicoanatomic relationships within these fractional cases may be much more informative than lumping them all together on the basis of some overlap with the full syndrome.

Chronic Broca's Aphasia This syndrome, as described above, often emerges out of global aphasia.[12] Damage can vary in extent; there does not seem to be a necessary and sufficient lesion profile. The most common pattern is extensive dorsolateral frontal, opercular, rolandic, and anterolateral parietal cortical damage plus lateral striatal and extensive paraventricular white matter damage (Fig. 11-1).[13] Particularly critical to

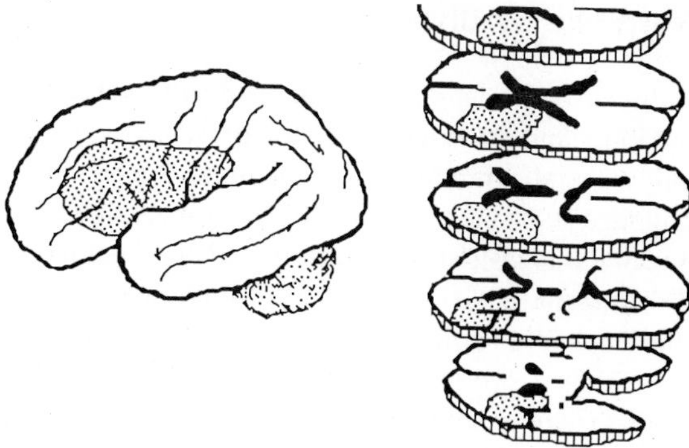

Figure 11-1
Typical lesion associated with severe chronic Broca's aphasia.

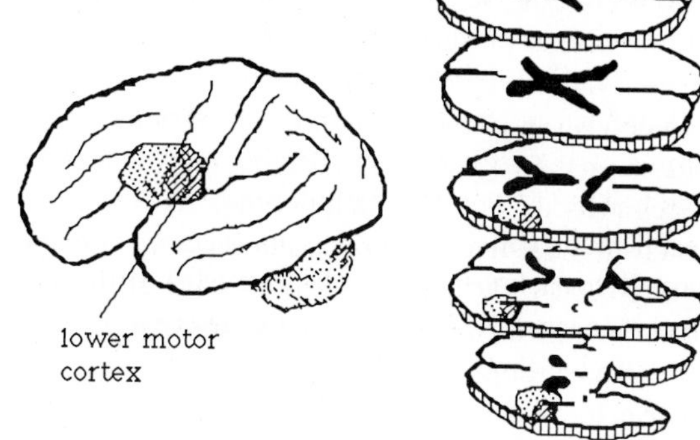

Figure 11-2
Lesion distributions of incomplete forms of Broca's aphasia. The entire lesion would produce "acute" Broca's aphasia. The anterior component involved alone (stippled area) *would typically evolve toward transcortical motor aphasia. The posterior component involved alone would typically evolve toward aphemia. In either case, the residual aphasia would be mild.*

chronic Broca's aphasia is the subcortical extension of the lesion.[14] Long-lasting mutism can be seen after anterior deep lesions, undercutting supplementary motor area and cingulate-caudate projections.[15] Deep anterior periventricular white matter lesions disrupt dorsolateral frontal-caudate systems involved in ready access to complex output procedures.[16] They may also disrupt ascending anterior thalamic-frontal projections. Anterior supraventricular deep white matter lesions disrupt callosal frontal projections. Large periventricular and subcortical white matter lesions can disrupt all of the long, bidirectional parietotemporal-to-frontal projection pathways. All the distant corticocortical systems will be disrupted. A combination of these systems' disruptions seems to be the structural basis of persistent Broca's aphasia even with subcortical lesions only.

Acute Broca's Aphasia Infarctions or trauma that produce acute Broca's aphasia often involve the frontal operculum, lower motor cortex, lateral striatum, and subcortical white matter (Fig. 11–2).[17] These patients recover over weeks to months, with variable mixtures of initiation delay, syntactic simplification, paraphasias, speech impairment, and usually with impaired repetition.

"Broca's Area" Lesion Damage to the frontal operculum (areas 44 and 46) produces an acute aphasic disorder roughly compatible with Broca's aphasia (Fig. 11–2), but there is quite rapid improvement, usually to transcortical motor aphasia or even just mild anomic aphasia.[11,17] Damage to the dorsolateral frontal cortex (areas 44, 46, 6, and 9) produces classic transcortical motor aphasia[15] (discussed in detail below). Damage to the subcortical frontal white matter or perhaps even to the dorsolateral caudate nuclei may produce the same deficit.[16,18] These observations suggest the existence of a "frontal-caudate" regional network required for construction of complex output procedures of language–syntax and narrative discourse at a minimum. Damage to this system is part of classic Broca's aphasia.

Lower Motor Cortex Lesion Damage to the lower 50 percent of the prerolandic gyrus can acutely produce a deficit pattern roughly compatible with mild Broca's aphasia, but there is rapid recovery to a much more limited disorder of speech–predominantly of articulation and prosody–sometimes called aphemia (Fig. 11–2).[19] Damage to the subcortical outflow of lower motor cortex can produce the same speech deficit, suggesting the existence of a local (rolandic) network for articulation and some aspects of prosody that project to the brainstem. Some investigators consider this to be "apraxia of speech," a disruption in motor planning for speech movements.[20] This, too, is part of classic Broca's aphasia.

A rare variant of this restricted damage to motor systems of speech production is the foreign-accent syndrome.[21] A small number of cases have been described, usually emerging out of mild Broca's aphasia. In these patients, the predominant deficit is in speech prosody, but the quality of the prosodic deficit sounds to the listener like a foreign accent, not pathologic prosody. The reported lesions have all been in some component of the motor system for speech, either lower motor cortex[19] or putamen or deep connections between lower motor cortex and basal ganglia.[22,23] The precise speech impairment has not been consistent, and the foreign-accent syndrome probably represents a heterogeneous group with partial damage to the motor speech apparatus.

For all of these variants and fractional syndromes of Broca's aphasia, some improvement can be expected. The severe cases that often emerge from global aphasia typically have better recovery of comprehension than of speech; this recovery that may continue over a very long time.[3,24] Minimal recovery of spoken or written output from essentially none to classic telegraphic output is usually accompanied by lesion extent throughout the deep frontal white matter from the middle periventricular region to the region anterior and superior to the frontal horn.[14] The outcome of the milder cases is partly determined by lesion size,[11] but for these smaller lesions, precise lesion site seems to best account for evolution into the various fractional systems.[12,17,19] In both severe and milder cases, some patients may recover by reorganizing cerebral functions to allow some right-brain control of speech. Most current evidence comes from functional activation studies. Additional evidence comes from patients with serial frontal lesions[25] and from temporary inactivation of the right brain (Wada test) after left-brain stroke has produced severe nonfluent aphasia.[26] Recovery through increased compensatory regions in the right hemisphere is not uniformly present or definitively valuable. Some language tasks (semantic decision) may involve more distributed neural networks, and increased right opercular activity may compensate for left-sided damage.[27] Other functions (e.g., phonology) may be neurally restricted to a limited left hemisphere region, and right sided compensation cannot recreate the normal level of function. Only adjacent regions in the left hemisphere can compensate.

Wernicke's Aphasia

In this disorder, language output is fluent–that is, normal in mean phrase length, generally sentence-length, and using all grammatical elements available in the language. Content may be extremely paraphasic[8] or empty. Paraphasic speech conforms to the general rules of the language but contains substitutions at the phonemic level (phonemic paraphasias such as *smoon* for *spoon*), the word level (semantic paraphasias such as *cup* for *spoon*), or entirely novel but phonologically legal words (neologisms such as *snopel*). Empty speech may consist of either vague circumlocutions or single words (*thing, one, unit, it, going,* etc.). Lengthy, complex, phonologically rich output with varied neologisms is jargonaphasia. Although statements may be of sentence length, grammar may become quite imprecise, usually because of semantic ambiguity; this is paragrammatism.[2] Speech is normal. Language comprehension is poor at the levels of word recognition, simple commands, and simple conversation. Repetition is very poor. Written language is comparable to spoken. Naming is very poor. Errors are paraphasias, circumlocutions, and nonresponses.

Apraxia to command is common, but when the patient is given a model to imitate, performance can be extremely variable, from persistently severe apraxia to normal performance.[28] Deficits in the right visual field are common. In the acute phase, patients may be anosognosic; but with awareness of deficits, agitation and suspiciousness may emerge.

Fractional syndromes of Wernicke's aphasia are less common but can occur. Some patients have relatively better auditory comprehension (and usually repetition); others have relatively better reading comprehension. Severe limb apraxia (both ideomotor, even with imitation of gestures, and ideational) is sometimes seen.

The minimal lesion producing Wernicke's aphasia is damage to the superior temporal gyrus back to the end of the sylvian fissure (Fig. 11–3).[13] If damage includes additional adjacent structures, either the deep temporal white matter or the supramarginal gyrus or both, problems will be more persistent.[29–31] If damage includes middle and interior temporal gyri, initial deficits will be more severe, anomia will be more persistent, and reading comprehension will be poor even

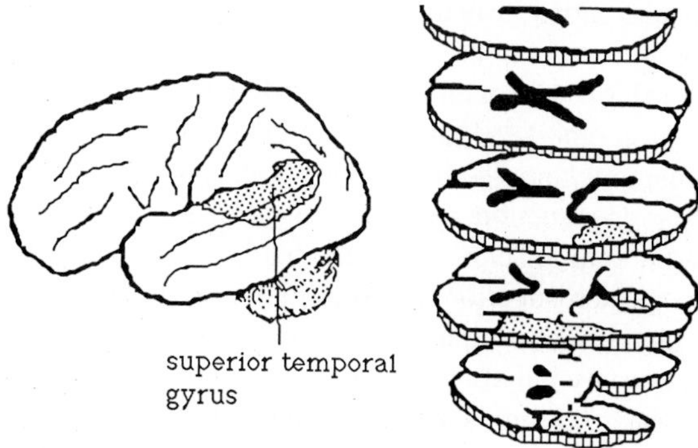

Figure 11-3
Typical lesion producing Wernicke's aphasia. Persistence and severity would depend on lesion extent (see text).

if auditory comprehension improves. Patients with lesions restricted to the superior temporal gyrus may have predominantly auditory comprehension difficulties with relatively little anomia and much less reading impairment. The differential effects of lesion placement in the posterior temporal lobe certainly reflect variable damage to converging regional networks for several language processing systems. The auditory language system may be more specifically temporal, thus the relatively greater impairment of auditory comprehension. Visual language processing surely emerges out of the more posterior temporooccipitoparietal association cortex.[32] Cross-modal lexical and semantic knowledge emerges out of a broad range of regions in the posterior association cortex, but available evidence highlights the inferior temporal and middle temporal/angular gyrus transition as the particularly key regions for word retrieval.[33]

Severe and persistent Wernicke's aphasia seems to require damage to all of these regions or to their deep functional connections. The mechanisms of recovery are not completely known. As noted above, the brain regions involved in lexical-semantic function are broadly distributed in posterior association cortex. Size of lesion in these regions, extent of involvement of the superior temporal gyrus,[30,31] and extent of coincident damage to supramarginal and angular gyri[29] have all been implicated as factors in recovery of comprehension. Studies with positron emission tomography (PET) have demonstrated a variety of effects related to recovery. Heiss and colleagues, studying subacute recovery in a mixed group of aphasic syndromes, demonstrated that recovery of comprehension was proportional to recovery of resting blood flow in the surviving left hemisphere, particularly the temporoparietal junction.[34] Weiller and coworkers demonstrated that recovery in Wernicke's aphasia is closely related to a shift in PET activation to semantic tasks from left temporal in normals to right temporal in patients with Wernicke's aphasia who recover.[35] Using a different paradigm with functional magnetic resonance imaging (fMRI), Cao et al. also demonstrated increased right-sided activation during lexical-semantic tasks in a mixed group of patients with aphasia, but the best recovery of comprehension was associated with the greatest activation of left-sided cortex adjacent to the lesion.[36] Heise et al. have reported identical results for comprehension, also in a mixed group of aphasic patients.[37] The precise meaning of these related studies is not known, but they all converge on the importance of posterior association cortex, either left or, if it is too damaged, right for recovery of comprehension.

Pure word deafness is sometimes considered a separate syndrome reflecting exclusive impairment to the auditory language processing system.[38] Most patients are only relatively "pure," emerging out of Wernicke's aphasia with relatively better recovery of reading comprehension for anatomically specific reasons proposed above. Some patients have had only small left temporal lesions[38]; others have had bilateral temporal lesions.[39] Depending upon the relative size and location of the bilateral lesions, these patients may be effectively deaf (cortical deafness: bilateral Heschl gyrus lesions) or have agnosia for the meaning of all sounds (machinery, animals, musical instruments, etc.), even though they hear them (auditory environmental agnosia: large right lesion, whatever the left lesion).[40] Also, depending on specific lesion sites, language output can be variably abnormal, although to be "pure," it should be normal. In this case, the implication is that underlying knowledge of word phonology is preserved because spontaneous production is normal. Depending on lesion site, patients with "relatively pure" Wernicke's aphasia may have considerable phonemic paraphasia or anomia.

The mechanism of pure word deafness is presumably damage to a system that converts the acoustic signal into a phonologically meaningful stimulus.[39] This is necessary but not sufficient for comprehension; for example, normals can repeat sentences in languages phonologically similar to their native one without understanding anything. There must still be a merger of the processed acoustic signal with a semantic system. In some patients with Wernicke's aphasia, the phonologic process seems very impaired; in others, the mapping to semantics; and in yet others, both are impaired.

Conduction Aphasia

In conduction aphasia, language output is fluent. Content is paraphasic, usually predominantly phonemic.[8] There may be frequent hesitations and attempts to correct ongoing phonemic errors (so-called *conduit d'approche*). Speech is normal. Language comprehension is good except for auditory span. Repetition is poor, not always worse than spontaneous output but dominated by phonemic paraphasias on substantive words, particularly phonologically complex target words (*happy hippopotamus*) or words embedded in phonologically complex sentences ("Dogs chase but rarely catch clever cats"). Written language is extremely variable in this syndrome. Writing is rarely better than speech, but it can be much more impaired. Oral reading is usually comparable to speech but can be better or worse. Reading comprehension is usually comparable to auditory but can be worse. Patients with the agraphia-with-alexia syndrome usually have conduction aphasia. Naming is also extremely variable, from extremely poor to nearly normal. Errors are paraphasias (phonemic especially).

Limb ideomotor apraxia is common initially but clears in most patients.[28] Right-sided sensory loss and visual field impairment (extinction and/or lower-quadrant deficit) are common.

Most patients with conduction aphasia have prominently reduced auditory verbal short-term memory (STM), tested as digit-span, word-span, or sentence-length effect in repetition. There is, however, little specificity of the STM problem, as many patients with perisylvian aphasias have a similar problem. The STM deficit also has little relevance to the language production problem, as similar output occurs in spontaneous output, oral reading and naming, and repetition. There is converging evidence that the inferior parietal lobule, particularly the supramarginal gyrus, is critical for all aspects of phonologic processing. Thus, lesions there have been blamed for pure STM deficits,[41] phonologic agraphia,[42,43] and phonologic alexia, all of which commonly emerge from conduction aphasia.

Conduction aphasia is usually due to a lesion in the inferior parietal lobule, but lesions restricted to the posterosuperior temporal gyrus may also present with conduction aphasia.[44] As might be gathered from the discussion above of Wernicke's aphasia, involvement of the infrasylvian structures produces conduction aphasia with greater comprehension deficit than a purely suprasylvian one. Within the inferior parietal lobule, the classic lesion is in the supramarginal gyrus[45] (Fig. 11–4), involving the arcuate fasciculus, putatively connecting the temporal lobe to the frontal lobe.[46] Lesions in subcortical parietal white matter disrupt this fasciculus and may represent the classic correlation.[47] Lesions in white matter deep to sensory cortex or in the subinsular extreme capsule, as well as supramarginal cortex lesions, may also produce conduction aphasia.[48] These observations suggest that temporoparietal short association pathways (i.e., a regional network) may support the phonologic output structure of speech. This network is required for phonologic accuracy in spontaneous output, repetition, oral reading, and naming. If disturbed phonologic structure of output is the hallmark of conduction aphasia, this would be the criterion structural basis.

Figure 11-4
Typical lesion producing conduction aphasia. Smaller lesions within this region may also produce similar aphasia (see text).

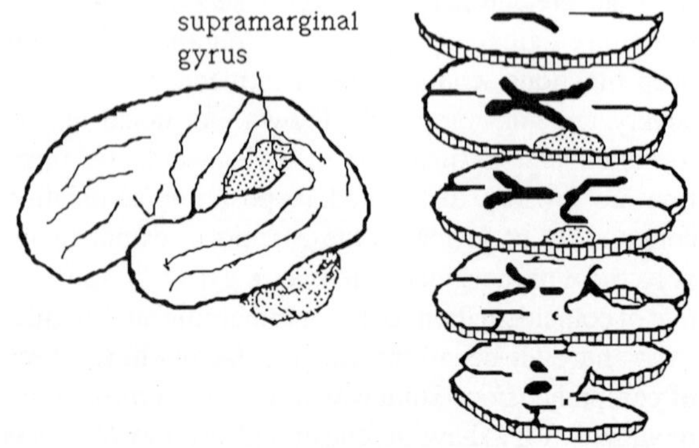

Some patients have very extensive parietal lesions with more severe anomia, agraphia, and limb ideomotor apraxia. Partial involvement of the superior temporal gyrus can produce initial Wernicke's aphasia that evolves into conduction aphasia with very paraphasic output and severe anomia. Again, the overlap of syndromes should be evident. Patients whose perisylvian arterial architecture just happens to catch the superior temporal lobe in a predominantly parietal stroke will have elements of pure word deafness (decreased auditory comprehension) with conduction aphasia (phonemic paraphasias, anomia, and agraphia). That combination would be indistinguishable from Wernicke's aphasia; in fact, it probably is Wernicke's aphasia except that recovery of comprehension would be "surprisingly" good.

Most patients with acute conduction aphasia have good recovery over a few weeks, although residual writing impairments, mild anomia, and occasional phonemic errors can be observed. For the more severe cases with marked anomia and very paraphasic output, recovery is less complete. The combination of significant phonologic and semantic deficits despite good comprehension can be very long lasting. Over time, patients become less neologistic and more empty and circumlocutory, even if the basic deficits do not improve.[49]

Global Aphasia

In many ways global aphasia is the easiest syndrome to define. By definition, patients have significant impairments in all aspects of language. Language output is severely limited—there is no more than "yes," "no," and a recurring stereotypic utterance ("da, da," "no way, no way," etc.). In some patients with global aphasia (and Broca's aphasia) the recurring utterance may be repeated rapidly in a richly inflected manner that suggests fluent output if only it could be comprehended.[50] This is not jargonaphasia; it has none of the phonologic richness or preservation of grammatical infrastructure of jargonaphasia. The mechanism of this richly inflected stereotype is unknown, and it has no known prognostic significance.

Comprehension is very impaired. The Boston Diagnostic Aphasia Examination (BDAE) definition allows comprehension up to the 30th percentile for an aphasic population.[51] This is compatible with considerable single-word comprehension. The language comprehension tasks most likely to be preserved in global aphasia are pointing to a named location on a map,[52] pointing to personally highly familiar names from multiple choice or acknowledging them when they are presented auditorily, and a small subset of commands ("take off your glasses," "close your eyes," "stand up").[28] Some patients with global aphasia can do those tasks but little else. There is no repetition, naming, or writing.

Buccofacial and limb apraxia, to command and imitation, are nearly universal.[28] Right hemiplegia, hemisensory loss, and visual field impairments are all common but not invariable.

The most typical lesion involves or substantially undercuts the entire perisylvian region.[11,53] At least, this would require a combination of the Broca's and Wernicke's aphasia lesions, but much clinical variability is seen. Some patients with Broca's aphasia lesions present as having global aphasia without evident temporal lesions.[54] The mechanism of severe comprehension loss without a temporal lesion in a substantial fraction of patients with global aphasia is not known. The coincident frontal lesion may produce additional cognitive problems—such as inattention, underactivation, unconcern, poor problem solving (particularly relevant when the Token Test is the defining tool of comprehension), or perseveration—that interact with more modest phonologic/semantic deficits to produce more profound functional comprehension deficits.

A sufficiently great lesion of the deep temporal white matter might undercut connections to the temporal lobe.[55] Naeser and colleagues found these deep temporal lesions to be associated with poor comprehension in patient's with Wernicke's aphasia.[30] There was good recovery of comprehension in patients with deep temporal lesions but intact temporal cortex. As noted above, Heisse and coworkers have demonstrated a very high correlation between reduced temporoparietal blood flow in resting PET and poor comprehension, whatever the anatomic limits of the infarction.[34] Vignolo and associates[54] and DeRenzi and colleagues,[53] who have provided the most meticulous description of global aphasia without temporal lesions, have not found that temporal white matter lesions easily account for the deficits in comprehension. Conversely, some patients with very extensive posterior lesions that extend into subrolandic white matter present with global aphasia without any definite frontal or even anterior periventricular lesion.[11] The mechanism is not known.

Some patients with global aphasia have no hemiparesis. As a group, they are likely to have only a large frontal lesion or separate frontal and temporal lesions.[56] The purely frontal lesions are again presumably causing a "quasi"-comprehension deficit due to inattention, activation, perseveration, and so on. Many evolve into transcortical motor aphasia (see below).[57] These patients are also likely to have a better prognosis, but absence of hemiparesis is not a guarantee of a good outcome, as the absence of hemiparesis means only that a small portion of paraventricular white matter has been spared.[58]

When caused by infarction, global aphasia has a poor prognosis. Patients with smaller lesions (some without hemiparesis) will improve quickly. After infarction, patients still meeting taxonomic criteria for global aphasia at 1 month postonset have a very low probability of improving substantially.[3] Large hemorrhages may be associated with more late recovery, but by 2 months without improvement, the prognosis remains grim. Many patients show gradually improving comprehension over weeks and months and eventually reach taxonomic criteria for severe Broca's aphasia. Even with severe deficits in language comprehension, patients with global aphasia may have considerable retained capacity to understand the emotional intonation of speech.[59] Recognition of the gist or of the key words in an utterance, such as proper names, combined with accurate discrimination of emotional intent may be sufficient to power substantial social interaction. Many experienced clinicians have the impression that numerous patients with chronic global aphasia are even sensitive to the inflections of sarcasm.

Transcortical Motor Aphasia

In this syndrome, language output is commonly viewed as nonfluent because there is substantial initiation block, reduction in average phrase length, and simplification of grammatical form.[15] Many patients with transcortical motor aphasia (TCMA) are initially mute and may remain mute or nearly so for days or weeks. Note that if they are mute, repetition is obviously absent and, by strict taxonomic criteria, such patients would initially be seen to have Broca's aphasia. Frank agrammatism is uncommon; responses are simply terse and delayed. Echolalia in various forms is frequently observed. Completely uninhibited echolalia is unusual, but fragmentary echoing, particularly of commands, may be observed. Incorporation echolalia is more common. The patient incorporates a portion of a question into the initial portion of his response. Speech quality is normal in the classic case. Repetition is, by definition, normal or at least vastly superior to spontaneous output. Recitation of even very complex overlearned material (e.g., the Lord's Prayer) may be flawless. Language comprehension is supposed to be normal, but, as observed above, the large frontal lesions most often associated with TCMA may produce substantial impairment of comprehension. Writing is usually similar to spoken output, but patients rarely write to dictation as well as they repeat. Reading comprehension parallels auditory. Oral reading may be quite normal if initial prompts are provided. Naming is quite variable. It may be quite normal. If not, errors are nonresponses, semantic paraphasias, or perseverations.

Transcortical motor aphasia may have any range of associated motor deficits, depending upon lesion site. The classic case has no motor deficit. Hemiparesis accompanies many cases of subcortical TCMA.[16] Inverted hemiparesis (leg worse than arm) and a contralateral grasp reflex accompany medial frontal TCMA.[15] Sensory loss and visual field deficits are not usually seen except in subcortical cases. Buccofacial apraxia may be seen, but limb ideomotor apraxia is less common.[28]

The classic patient has a large dorsolateral frontal lesion, typically extending into the deep frontal white matter (Fig. 11–5).[15] Identical cases have been reported with just a white matter lesion abutting the frontal horn of the lateral ventricle.[55] Very similar cases involve the capsulostriatal region, particularly the dorsolateral caudate and adjacent paraventricular white matter (Fig. 11–6).[16] The similarity of the aphasia associated with these disparate lesions is paralleled by the nearly identical reduction in blood flow seen on resting PET or single proton emission computed tomography (SPECT) in dorsolateral frontal cortex, whatever the lesion site.[60,61] The more posterior the lesion extends along the paraventricular white matter, the likelier the presence of dysarthria (see discussion of transcortical

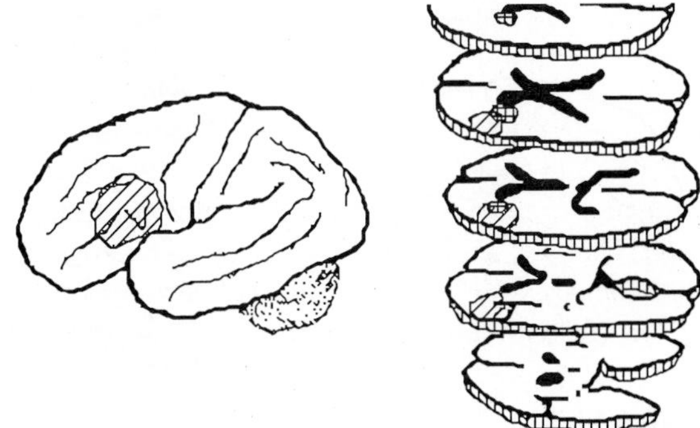

Figure 11-5
Typical lesions producing transcortical motor aphasia. Note overlap with lesions in Broca's area (Fig. 11–2).

motor aphasia, above) and hemiparesis. Damage to the medial frontal lobe, particularly the supplementary motor area, produces TCMA-like disturbance.[62,63] Mutism may be more prolonged. When patients begin to speak, they rarely show any frankly aphasic qualities. They simply do not speak much.

Analysis of cortical and subcortical cases with TCMA suggests that one fundamental deficit is in generative language tasks.[16,64,65] The patients seem to have very limited capacity to generate complex syntax. They may reuse the syntax in a question they are asked (incorporation echolalia). They may produce short responses,

Figure 11-6
Large lenticulostriate lesion, which is often associated with transcortical motor aphasia, frequently accompanied by speech disturbance and hemiparesis. Smaller lesion (cross-hatched area) *may produce mild transcortical motor aphasia without motor deficits.*

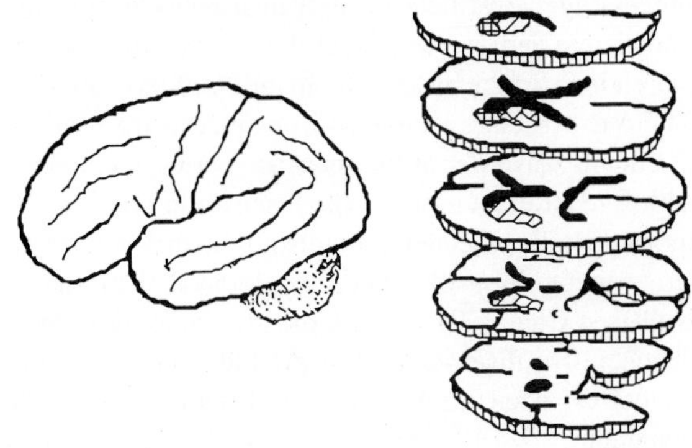

even short sentences, quite well. When asked an open-ended question, however, they do not have timely access to the range of syntax needed to answer. Patients with this profile—essentially normal responsive language but deeply limited open-ended language—have been said to have "dynamic aphasia." Several analyses of patients with this disorder point to disruption in the recruitment or deployment of schemas for complex language constructions, particularly when the utterance is not constrained in any way. That is, the speaker must generate an action plan for how the utterance will unfold, and this must happen over seconds.[66,67] Bedside generative tasks—word-list generation, storytelling, or producing sentences using provided main verbs—will be impaired out of proportion to other language tasks. Patients with large dorsolateral frontal lesions may have little or no aphasia on standard tests but will still be unable to tell a story or recite a narrative in normal fashion. This level of language is called discourse.[68] In parallel with claims for utilization of learned schemas (procedures) for grammar and syntax, it has been claimed that discourse requires recruitment and utilization of a schema for unfolding a very complex utterance. All of these systems for utilizing language are embedded in related frontal structures.[69] Neither the functional nor anatomic boundaries are sharp between sentence structure and story structure. There is a series of interactive effector systems from conception and organization to rules of narrative to complex language to common grammar to speech. Their organization runs from prefrontal to lower motor cortex.

A second fundamental deficit in TCMA is reduction in activation to speak (or to write). Analysis of lesion site effects, particularly the profound mutism that occurs with medial frontal damage, suggests that reduced activation is due to loss of ascending dopaminergic pathways. The medial frontal regions are primary targets of the nonnigral dopaminergic system.[70] Bilateral damage to this system anywhere from the upper midbrain to the frontal cortex results in akinetic mutism,[71] evolving into less flagrant forms often called abulia.[72] Transcortical motor aphasia may represent a subsyndrome of akinetic mutism with more rapid clearing of mutism and less global akinesia because the lesion is only unilateral. The improvement in fluency and speech rate after administration of direct dopamine agonists supports this proposition.[73,74] Improvement with bromocriptine is almost uniquely seen in TCMA or in other nonfluent aphasias that also include significant speech and language initiation block [75,76]

Transcortical Sensory Aphasia

In transcortical sensory aphasia (TCSA), language output is fluent. Content is very empty, with semantic paraphasia predominating. All patients make abundant use of one-word circumlocutions and nonspecific filler words, such as *one, things, does,* etc. Phonemic paraphasias and neologistic jargon are less common, so that output is more accurately described as extended English jargon. Content is also often perseverative. Speech quality is normal. Repetition is, by definition, normal. Language comprehension is impaired. In particular, single-word comprehension may be quite poor. When accompanied by accurate repetition of the test words and even their incorporation in sentences ("A watch? I should know that. Is one of these a watch?"), the behavior has been called alienation of word meaning.[77] There may be category-specific comprehension impairments with particularly good performance at following commanded actions and very poor performance at pointing to named targets. Many patients will accept incorrect names or quibble over accuracy. ("You could call it a watch, but I don't think it is one.") Naming is poor, and again some category specificity may be observed. Some patients are worse at naming animals, insects, and other animate objects than tools and other inanimate objects.[78] There is no important discrepancy between naming performance to different sensory modalities. Many patients respond quickly to phonemic cues but will then reject or be uncertain about the correct response. This behavior has been called a two-way naming impairment.[79] Written output may be similar to spoken, but patients usually do not write extensively and are very perseverative. Reading aloud and reading comprehension are both abnormal. In many patients, reading comprehension is even worse than auditory comprehension.

Transcortical sensory aphasia has been described after lesions in middle and inferior temporal gyri (Fig. 11–7).[77] The temporal lesion may produce a right visual field defect if white matter extent reaches the geniculocalcarine pathways. Many cases of TCSA have unexpected lesion sites involving the entire perisylvian cortex, a lesion much likelier to produce global aphasia.[80] The mechanism for this is unknown, although some variant on bilateral language representation is usually recruited. Some cases with temporal lesions may also involve the inferior temporo-occipital region—for instance, after posterior cerebral artery infarction. These patients will certainly have very impaired reading.[32] Many have associative agnosia.[81] As reviewed in Chap. 18, not only can they not name an object or point to a named object but they cannot indicate its use or sort it into a correct functional category (i.e., put a pencil with chalk rather than with a knife). Thus, the deficit is not restricted to *lexical* semantic knowledge but involves actual semantic knowledge. This may be modality-specific, with visually presented tasks more impaired,[81] or it may affect all modalities equally.[81]

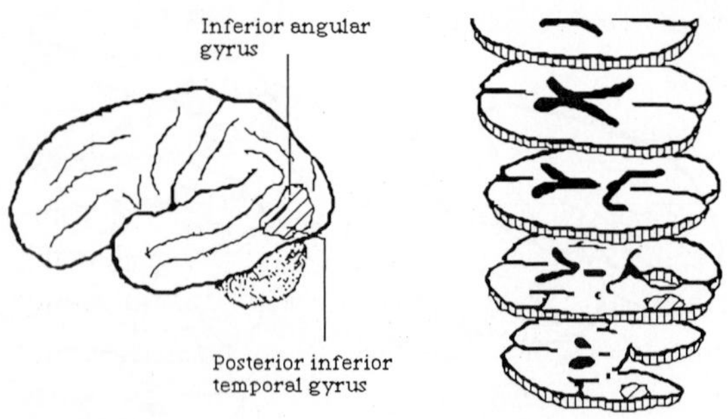

Figure 11-7
Typical lesion producing transcortical sensory aphasia. Lesions more medial and inferior, usually posterior cerebral artery infarctions, may produce similar aphasia (see text).

Transcortical sensory aphasia is almost monotypic in that it is fundamentally a disorder of semantic processing. Nevertheless, different aspects of semantic knowledge and access to such knowledge may be impaired in different cases. The inability of patients with TCSA to associate a name with an object is the result of a semantic disorder at the interface between language and semantic memory. When semantic memory is more globally affected, patients are unable to demonstrate recognition of objects by nonverbal means as well (see Chap. 39). This is most commonly seen in degenerative diseases with a predilection for temporal cortex, such as Alzheimer's disease or semantic dementia.[33,78,82–84]

Anomic Aphasia

Anomic aphasia is a much less homogeneous grouping than any of the other classic syndromes. By definition, language is fluent, comprehension good, and repetition good. The only deficit in spoken language is in word retrieval. Paraphasias are infrequent. Word-finding problems usually produce filler words[8] or circumlocutions. Other impairments vary with lesion site.

Anomic aphasia is the residual state of many aphasic disorders after time for improvement.[3] As a primary diagnosis, anomic aphasia usually accompanies lesions in the same regions as TCMA or TCSA or the anterior thalamus.

As noted, most patients with TCMA are or at least become basically fluent but with terse, unelaborated utterances. When it is accompanied by word-finding deficits, this condition would qualify as anomic aphasia. Anomic aphasia is also the mildest form of TCSA, representing a deficit only in lexical retrieval from semantic stores. Thus, when anomic aphasia is caused by a dorsolateral frontal lesion, there are no accompanying neurologic signs. When it is caused by a deep frontostriatal lesion, there may be dysarthria, hemiparesis, and buccofacial apraxia, depending upon lesion extent. When it is caused by a posterior association cortex lesion, there may be a visual field deficit and alexia, depending upon lesion extent. When anomic aphasia is the residual of partly recovered conduction or Broca's aphasia, the accompanying signs are as expected for those disorders.

Mixed Transcortical Aphasia

In mixed transcortical aphasia (MTA), language output is nonfluent. Comprehension is impaired. Naming is poor. Repetition is preserved. Echolalia and fragmentary sentence starters ("I don't . . . ," "Not with the . . .") are common. Speech quality is normal. Writing and reading are similarly reduced.

In the patient whose case report defined this syndrome, MTA was due to bilateral hypoxic neuronal loss in the arterial border zones,[85] but ischemic damage in the left border zones could presumably cause the same disorder. The implication is that MTA requires a combination of the lesions of TCMA and TCSA, with perisylvian structures allowing repetition preserved. Most cases are actually due to large frontal lesions in the region of TCMA lesions. The comprehension defect is probably due to a mixture of frontal impairments, exactly as described for restricted frontal lesions and global aphasia. Comprehension improves, and patients evolve toward TCMA. Associated lesions are as described for TCMA.

Large anterior thalamic lesions also produce MTA.[86–88] Most cases have involved the anterior, ventrolateral, and dorsomedian nuclei at a minimum. Damage to those three nuclei effectively deprives the frontal lobe of thalamic input and modulation. Patients are often mute initially. When they speak, the reduction in narrative and terseness of structure are similar to those of TCMA. The impairment in comprehension may be due to the speculative "frontal" mechanisms. The associated signs depend upon lesion extent out of the thalamus. Recovery of language is usually good.

CROSSED APHASIA AND APHASIA IN LEFT-HANDERS

The foregoing review is valid for most right-handers with lesions of the left hemisphere. For the 10 percent of the population that is left-handed and for the approximately 2 to 5 percent of the right-handed population that becomes aphasic after a right-brain lesion (crossed aphasia), some modifications of the clinical rules are required. For left-handers, the phenomenology of aphasia is complicated by the very issue of left-handedness. More than right-handers, all left-handers are not created equal; they vary greatly in degree and nature of hemispheric specialization for language. For both populations, the phenomenology is further complicated by irregularities in lateral dominance for other typically lateralized functions, such as praxis and some aspects of visuospatial function. Only a brief summary of these issues is possible here.

Crossed Aphasia

The incidence of crossed aphasia has been reported as anywhere from 1 to 13 percent.[89–91] The stroke population is least contaminated by possible bilateral lesions, but in all populations methodologic limitations (defining handedness and aphasia testing strategies) leave the actual incidence uncertain. A reasonable estimate is 2 to 5 percent.

Patients with crossed aphasia fall into two broad categories. About 70 percent have a standard aphasia syndrome associated with, at least approximately, the lesion site expected in the left hemisphere.[92] All types of aphasia profiles can occur with the expected lesions (albeit in the right hemisphere). The other 30 percent have striking anomalies in the aphasia-lesion relationship.[92] In this group, unexpectedly mild aphasia syndromes occur despite large lesions that would typically cause a more severe aphasia. Conduction aphasia or phonologic agraphia have been seen despite large perisylvian lesions.[92,93] In other patients with large perisylvian lesions, transcortical sensory aphasia or anomic aphasia has been described.[80,94] Alexander and Annett have suggested that these anomalous cases point to possible discrepant lateralizations of phonologic and semantic functions.[95] Patients with crossed aphasia, particularly if anomalous, may have a better capacity for recovery.

Lateralization of praxis and visuospatial functions in crossed aphasia has not been as definitely addressed as the language functions. Castro-Caldos and coworkers claim that these functions show anomalous lateralization less frequently than language, asserting that praxis remains in the left hemisphere contralateral to the preferred right hand and that visuospatial functions remain in the right hemisphere.[91] Others have disputed this, arguing from case reports that all functions show a high rate of anomalous lateralization.[94,96] Alexander and coworkers have reviewed the case reports of anomalous visuospatial lateralization to the left hemisphere in right-handers.[97] They have proposed that there is a subset of right-handers who have chance lateralization of all functions. These authors, among others, have even proposed that a genetic basis for the inheritance of handedness and laterality of cognitive functions, such as the right shift theory of Annett,[89,95] can account for the rates of all anomalies. The biological basis of crossed aphasia, however, remains unknown.

Aphasia in Left-Handers

Left-handers make up 10 percent of the population, but they are a much more heterogeneous group than right-handers. If a strict criterion for left-handedness is used, most of the left-handed population becomes relabeled as being mixed-handed.[89] Thus, some authorities simply refer to non-right-handers. The rate of cerebral lateralization of left-handers depends to some extent on the criteria used to define the group. Large studies of left-handed aphasics have been reasonably consistent, however, in finding that about 70 percent have left-brain lesions and 30 percent have right-brain lesions.[98] Hécaen computed that approximately 15 percent probably would be aphasic after a lesion of either hemisphere; that is, they have bilateral language representation. Whether aphasic after left or right brain lesions, the proportion of cases with anomalous aphasia-lesion relationships is higher than in right-handers.[99] It has been claimed that left-handers have better recovery than right-handers,[98] but, as with crossed aphasia, this question is muddied by the higher proportion of mild aphasics.[99] It is also unclear if better recovery means bilateral language capacity, so that all functions have higher potential for recovery, or divergent lateralization of functions, so that some are left uninvolved by any lateralized lesion.[90,95,100] Both factors are probably operative, but in different patients.

Lateralization of praxis and visuospatial function shows anomalies at a rate similar to those of crossed aphasia. Every possible arrangement of impaired and preserved functions has been reported after left or right lesions.[94] Since the biological basis of neither handedness nor the lateralization of cognitive functions has been established, it remains an open question how these anomalies occur in left-handers as well as right-handers.

EFFECT OF ETIOLOGY

Infarctions

Almost all of the foregoing is based on the literature accumulated from strokes. Infarcts have numerous advantages for clinicoanatomic correlations. They are sudden in onset, and there is therefore no accommodation and compensation prior to clinical presentation. Boundaries between damaged and nondamaged brain are fairly precise, so correlations are clearer. Nevertheless, the vascular system cannot provide every topographic variation of brain injury; therefore much of what has come to us as classic syndromes could easily be partially artifactual correlations produced by the limited independence of lesions sites from infarctions.

There are some aphasic syndromes that are commonly believed to be caused by emboli because the distribution of infarction seems most plausibly to be in the territory of a branch of the middle cerebral artery. The fractional Broca's aphasias, conduction aphasia, and Wernicke's aphasia all seem likely to have an embolic basis when due to infarction. Global aphasia and Broca's aphasia require more extensive damage in the territory of the middle cerebral artery. There is, however, no basis for presuming an infarction mechanism simply on the basis of these aphasia types.

Hemorrhages

All of the rules established for infarctions apply for hemorrhages if the hemorrhage happens to be in the same brain topography as an infarction pattern. Patients with hemorrhages may be much more impaired initially because of physiologic deficits not primarily related to aphasia–mass effects, intraventricular blood, and so on. Hemorrhages are not constrained by vascular patterns, so entirely novel arrangements of lesions can be seen. This may be exemplified most clearly with lesions of the lenticulostriate region. Infarctions tend to be partially or completely limited to the middle cerebral artery perforators, but hemorrhages can dissect out of that limited region. Much of the variability reported after lenticulostriate lesions[101] may be due to idiosyncratic extensions of hemorrhages.[102]

Trauma

Focal contusions can occur anywhere, depending upon the direction of the blow, skull fragments, and so forth. When the contusion is in a perisylvian region, the resulting aphasia will usually follow the rules established by infarctions. Conduction and Wernicke's aphasias may result from relatively superficial cortical lesions; thus traumatic contusions, which are also predominantly cortical, may produce typical profiles. Cortical contusions rarely cause injury deep enough to damage all of the required deep structures (see above) to produce lasting nonfluent aphasia. There is a strong tendency for traumatic contusions to arise from basal structures due to inertial effects. Focal contusions of the inferior temporal lobe will cause anomic aphasia. If the lesions are large and extend into lateral temporal lobe or hemorrhage dissects up into the deep temporal white matter, patients may present with Wernicke's aphasia or TCSA. Trauma can also cause large epidural or subdural hematomas that do not directly affect language zones. They cause cerebral herniation with entrapment of the posterior cerebral artery, causing occipitotemporal infarctions with alexia and anomia. This herniation-caused infarction can be superimposed on direct temporal contusion, resulting in a very severe fluent aphasia.

Tumors

The lesson for aphasia due to tumors is no different than that for any cognitive function. In general, large tumors produce relatively much less cognitive impairment than an infarction of the same size would produce, but tumors produce symptoms qualitatively appropriate for the region involved. Primary brain tumors tend to infiltrate and gradually disrupt function, allowing substantial compensation as the disorder progresses. The conformity with patterns established by infarctions will be correlated largely with the malignancy and speed of growth of the tumor.

Herpes Simplex Encephalitis

Although rare, herpes simplex encephalitis (HSE) has a predilection for the medial temporal lobes, basal-medial frontal lobes, and insular cortices. Survivors of HSE frequently have severe amnesia. Patients with extensive left-sided HSE lesions, including the inferotemporal lobe, commonly show category-specific semantic deficits.[78,103]

Dementia

The most common dementing illnesses—dementia of the Alzheimer's type (DAT) and multi-infarct dementia (MID)–both cause language impairments. As reviewed in Chaps. 44 and 45, DAT typically presents with memory and language disturbances.[83] The language problem begins as anomia and is often misidentified by families as memory impairment. With time, the language disorder evolves toward TCSA, and the patient's semantic memory erodes.[104] The structure of this erosion is fairly predictable. Highly typical semantic associations survive longer than the semantic associations and attributes of low typicality.[104] For instance, the patients may still recognize the words and concepts behind *cat* but not the words and then even the concepts of *leopard, fang*, or *litter*. It has been proposed that this slow erosion of semantic knowledge—first words and then concepts—is the fundamental cognitive deficit of DAT.[105] Its presumed pathologic basis is the loss of neurons in posterior association cortex.

If one of the infarcts is in the language zone, MID may cause aphasia directly. The more typical pathology of MID is, however, numerous small infarcts in subcortical regions. These lesions may produce a variety of motor speech impairments such as articulatory problems, hypophonia, dysprosody, and rate disturbances. A recognizable aphasic syndrome does not occur, but patients may show cognitive deficits similar to those seen with frontal lobe lesions, including disturbances in all aspects of generative language: reduced word-list generation, terse or unelaborate utterances, and poor narrative ability. It has been suggested that a single small infarct in the genu of the left internal capsule is sufficient to disconnect frontothalamic circuitry and produce these deficits.[106]

A less common but hardly rare form of degenerative dementia, frontotemporal dementia, often presents with primary progressive aphasia. By definition, this disorder is characterized by a gradual decline that is essentially limited to language deficits.[107] The most common form is progressive loss of semantics and has therefore also been called semantic dementia (see Chap. 39). The presentation is usually similar to the language impairments of DAT–anomia initially progressing to TCSA and finally to loss of semantic concepts and knowledge. Unlike DAT, other cognitive functions remain are initially and often remain intact in these cases. Pathology is restricted to the anterior inferior temporal lobes. Two different "nonfluent" forms of primary progressive aphasia have also been described.[108–110] In one, the deficit is identical to dynamic aphasia described above, and imaging shows focal atrophy in the left prefrontal regions. In the other, the deficit is a progressive speech disorder, a mixture of articulation problems, stuttering, rate abnormalities, phonemic paraphasias, and facial apraxia. All forms are commonly associated with extrapyramidal disorders, either corticobasal degeneration or progressive supranuclear palsy.[111,112] In all forms of this disorder, the histopathology has been similar, although the distribution of the pathology has reflected the focal language profiles. Many patients would be labeled as having Pick's disease or a near variant.[113,114] A sizable minority is inherited, usually due to an abnormality on chromosome 17 in the gene for the tau protein, a critical element of axonal function.[111,115] For the neuroscientist, it should be fascinating to contemplate a single gene critical for language functions. What should be most interesting for students of aphasia is how closely the focal and multifocal degenerative disorders recapitulate the localization matrix created through the study of stroke.

REFERENCES

1. Broca P: Perte de la parole. Ramollissement chronique et destruction partielle du lobe anterieur gauche du cerveau. *Bull Soc Anthropol* 2:235, 1861.
2. Goodglass H: *Understanding Aphasia*. San Diego, CA: Academic Press, 1993.
3. Kertesz A, McCabe P: Recovery patterns and prognosis in aphasia. *Brain* 100:1–18, 1977.
4. Caramazza A: The logic of neuropsychological research and the problem of patient classification in aphasia. *Brain Lang* 21:9–20, 1984.
5. Kreisler A, Godefroy O, Delmaire C, et al: The anatomy of aphasia revisited. *Neurology* 54:1117–1123, 2000.
6. Kolk H: Does agrammatic speech constitute a regression to child language? A three-way comparison between agrammatic, child and normal ellipsis. *Brain Lang* 77:340–350, 2001.
7. Marshall JC, Newcombe F: Patterns of paralexia. *J Psycholinguist Res* 2:175–199, 1973.
8. Ardila A, Rosselli M: Language deviations in aphasia: A frequency analysis. *Brain Lang* 44:165–180, 1993.
9. Kohn SE: Verb finding in aphasia. *Cortex* 25:57–69, 1989.
10. Robinson RG, Kubos KL, Starr LB, et al: Mood disorders in stroke patients: Importance of location of lesion. *Brain* 107:81–93, 1984.

11. Mazzocchi F, Vignolo LA: Localisation of lesions in aphasia: Clinical–CT scan correlations in stroke patients. *Cortex* 15:627–654, 1979.
12. Mohr JP, Pessin MS, Finkelstein S, et al: Broca's aphasia: Pathologic and clinical. *Neurology* 28:311–324, 1978.
13. Naeser MA, Hayward RW: Lesion location in aphasia with cranial computed tomography and the Boston Diagnostic Aphasia Exam. *Neurology* 28:545–551, 1978.
14. Naeser MA, Palumbo CL, Helm-Estabrooks N, et al: Severe nonfluency in aphasia: Role of the medial subcallosal fasciculus and other white matter pathways in recovery of spontaneous speech. *Brain* 112:1–38, 1989.
15. Freedman M, Alexander MP, Naeser MA: Anatomic basis of transcortical motor aphasia. *Neurology* 34: 409–417, 1984.
16. Mega MS, Alexander MP: Subcortical aphasia: The core profile of capsulostriatal infarction. *Neurology* 44:1824–1829, 1994.
17. Alexander MP, Naeser MA, Palumbo C: Broca's area aphasia. *Neurology* 40:353–362, 1990.
18. Nadeau S, Crosson B: Subcortical aphasia. *Brain Lang* 58:355–402, 1995.
19. Schiff HB, Alexander MP, Naeser MA, Galaburda AM: Aphemia: Clinical-anatomic correlation. *Arch Neurol* 40:720–772, 1983.
20. Fox RJ, Kasner SE, Chatterjee AC, Chalela JA: Aphemia: An isolated disorder of articulation. *Clin Neurol Neurosurg* 103:123–126, 2001.
21. Monrad-Krohn GH: Dysprosody or altered "melody of language." *Brain* 70:405–415, 1947.
22. Blumstein SE, Alexander MP, Ryalls JH: The nature of the foreign accent syndrome: A case study. *Brain Lang* 31:215–244, 1987.
23. Graff-Radford NR, Cooper WE, Colsher PL, Damasio AR: An unlearned foreign "accent" in a patient with aphasia. *Brain Lang* 28:86–94, 1986.
24. Prin RS, Snow E, Wagenaar E: Recovery from aphasia: Spontaneous speech versus language comprehension. *Brain Lang* 6:192–211, 1978.
25. Basso A, Gardelli M, Grassi MP, et al: The role of the right hemisphere in recovery from aphasia: Two case studies. *Cortex* 25:555–566, 1989.
26. Kinsbourne M: The minor hemisphere as a source of aphasic speech. *Trans Am Neurol Assoc* 96:141–145, 1971.
27. Calvert GA, Brammer MJ, Morris RG, et al: Using fMRI to study recovery from acquired dysphasia. *Brain Lang* 71:391–399, 2000.
28. Alexander MP, Baker E, Naeser MA, Kaplan E: Neuropsychological and neuroanatomical dimensions of ideomotor apraxia. *Brain* 118:87–107, 1992.
29. Kertesz A, Lau WK, Polk M: The structural determinants of recovery in Wernicke's aphasia. *Brain Lang* 44:153–164, 1993.
30. Naeser MA, Helm-Estabrooks N, Haas G, et al: Relationship between lesion extent in Wernicke's area on computed tomographic scan and predicting recovery of comprehension in Wernicke's aphasia. *Arch Neurol* 44:73–82, 1987.
31. Selnes OA, Knopman DS, Niccum N, et al: Computed tomographic scan correlates of auditory comprehension deficits in aphasia: A prospective recovery study. *Ann Neurol* 13:558–566, 1983.
32. Henderson VW, Friedman RB, Teng EL, Weiner JM: Left hemisphere pathways in reading: Inference from pure alexia without hemianopia. *Neurology* 35:962–968, 1985.
33. Damasio AR: Synchronous activation in multiple cortical regions: A mechanism for recall. *Semin Neurosci* 2:287–296, 1990.
34. Heiss W, Kessler J, Karbe H, et al: Cerebral glucose metabolism as a predictor of recovery from aphasia in ischemic stroke. *Arch Neurol* 50:958–964, 1993.
35. Weiller C, Isensee C, Rijintjes M, et al: Recovery from Wernicke's aphasia: A positron emission tomography study. *Ann Neurol* 37:723–732, 1995.
36. Cao Y, Vikingstad EM, George KP, et al: Cortical language activation in stroke patients recovering from aphasia with functional MRI. *Stroke* 30:2331–2340, 1999.
37. Heise WD, Karbe H, Weber-Luxenburger G, et al: Speech-induced cerebral metabolic activation reflects recovery from aphasia. *J Neurol Sci* 145:213–217, 1997.
38. Takahashi N, Kawamura M, Shinotou H, et al: Pure word deafness due to left hemisphere damage. *Cortex* 28:295–303, 1992.
39. Auerbach SH, Allard T, Naeser MA, et al: Pure word deafness: Analysis of a case with bilateral lesions and a defect at the prephonemic level. *Brain* 105:271–300, 1982.
40. Fujii T, Fukatsu, Watabe S, et al: Auditory sound agnosia without aphasia following a right temporal lobe lesion. *Cortex* 26:263–268, 1990.
41. Paulesu E, Frith CD, Frackowiack RSJ: The neural correlates of the verbal component of working memory. *Nature* 362:342–345, 1993.
42. Alexander MP, Friedman RB, Loverso F, Fischer RF: Lesion localization in phonological agraphia. *Brain Lang* 43:83–95, 1992.

43. Roeltgen DP, Sevush S, Heilman KM: Phonological agraphia: Writing by the lexical semantic route. *Neurology* 33:755–765, 1983.
44. Axer H, von Keyserlingk AG, Berks G, von Keyserlingk DG: Supra- and infrasylvian conduction aphasia. *Brain Lang* 76:317–331, 2001.
45. Palumbo CL, Alexander MP, Naeser MA: CT scan lesion sites associated with conduction aphasia, in Kohn S (ed): *Conduction Aphasia*. Hillsdale NJ: Erlbaum, 1992, pp 51–75.
46. Benson DF, Sheremata WA, Bouchard R, et al: Conduction aphasia: A clinicopathological study. *Arch Neurol* 28:339–346, 1973.
47. Mendez MF, Benson DF. Atypical conduction aphasia: A disconnection syndrome. *Arch Neurol* 42:886–891, 1985.
48. Damasio H, Damasio AR: The anatomical basis of conduction aphasia. *Brain* 103:337–350, 1980.
49. Kertesz A, Benson DF: Neologistic jargon: A clinicopathological study. *Cortex* 6:362–386, 1970.
50. Poeck K, de Bleser R, von Keyserlingk DG: Neurolinguistic status and localization of lesions in aphasic patients with exclusively consonant vowel recurring utterances. *Brain* 107:199–217, 1984.
51. Goodglass H, Kaplan E: *The Assessment of Aphasia and Related Disorders*. Philadelphia: Lea & Febiger, 1983.
52. Wapner W, Gardner H. A note on patterns of comprehension and recovery in global aphasia. *J Speech Hear Res* 29:765–771, 1979.
53. DeRenzi E, Colombo A, Scarpa M: The aphasic isolate. *Brain* 114:1719–1730,1991.
54. Vignolo LA, Boccardi E, Caverni L: Unexpected CT-scan finding in global aphasia. *Cortex* 22:55–69, 1986.
55. Alexander MP, Naeser MA, Palumbo CL: Correlations of subcortical CT lesion sites and aphasia profiles. *Brain* 110:961–991, 1987.
56. Tranel D, Biller J, Damasio H, Damasio AR: Global aphasia without hemiparesis. *Arch Neurol* 44:304–308, 1987.
57. Hanlon RE, Lux WE, Dromerick AW: Global aphasia without hemiparesis: Language profiles and lesion distribution. *J Neurol Neurosurg Psychiatry* 66:365–369, 1999.
58. Legatt AD, Rubin AJ, Kaplan LR, et al: Global aphasia without hemiparesis. *Neurology* 37:201–205, 1987.
59. Barrett AM, Crucian GP, Raymer AM, Heilman KM: Spared comprehension of emotional prosody in a patient with global aphasia. *Neuropsychiatry Neuropsychol Behav Neurosci* 12:117–120, 1999.
60. Alexander MP: Speech and language deficits after subcortical lesions of the left hemisphere: A clinical, CT, and PET study, in Vallar G CS, Wallesch C-W (eds): *Neuropsychological Disorders Associated with Subcortical Lesions*. Oxford: Oxford Science Publications, 1991, pp 454–477.
61. Démonet JF, Puel M: "Subcortical" aphasia: Some proposed pathophysiological mechanisms and their rCBF correlates revealed by SPECT. *J Neuroling* 6:319–344, 1991.
62. Alexander MP: Disturbances in language initiation: Mutism and its lesser forms, in Joseph AB, Young RR (eds): *Movement Disorders in Neurology and Psychiatry*. Boston: Blackwell, 1992, pp 389–396.
63. Rubens AB: Transcortical motor aphasia. *Stud Neuroling* 1:293–306, 1976.
64. Costello AL, Warrington EK: Dynamic aphasia. The selective impairment of verbal planning. *Cortex* 25:103–114, 1989.
65. Luria AR, Tsvetkova LS: Towards the mechanism of "dynamic aphasia." *Acta Neurol Psychiatr Belg* 67:1045–1067, 1967.
66. Robinson G, Blair J, Cipolotti L: Dynamic aphasia: An inability to select between competing verbal responses? *Brain* 121:77–89, 1998.
67. Thompson-Schill SL, Swick D, Farah MJ, et al: Verb generation in patients with focal frontal lesions: A neuropsychological test of neuroimaging findings. *Proc Natl Acad Sci U S A* 95:15855–15860, 1998.
68. Chapman SB, Culhane KA, Levin HS, et al: Narrative discourse after closed head injury in children and adolescents. *Brain Lang* 43:42–65, 1992.
69. Sirigu A, Cohen L, Zalla T, et al: Distinct frontal regions for processing sentence syntax and story grammar. *Cortex* 34:771–778, 1998.
70. Lindvall O, Bjorklund A, Moore RY, Stenevi U: Mesencephalic dopamine neurons projecting to neocortex. *Brain Res* 81:325–331, 1974.
71. Alexander MP: Chronic akinetic mutism after mesencephalic-diencephalic infarction: Remediated with dopaminergic medications. *Neurorehabil Neural Repair.* 15:151–156, 2001.
72. Fisher CM: Abulia minor vs agitated behavior. *Clin Neurosurg* 1985;31:9–31, 1985.
73. Albert ML, Bachman DL, Morgan A, Helm-Estabrooks N: Pharmacotherapy for aphasia. *Neurology* 38:877–879, 1988.
74. Saba L, Leiguarda R, Starkstein SE: An open-label trial of bromocriptine in nonfluent aphasia. *Neurology* 42:1637–1638, 1992.

75. Bragoni M, Altieri M, DiPiero V, Padovani A, et al: Bromocriptine and speech therapy in non-fluent chronic aphasia after stroke. *Neurol Sci* 21:19–22, 2000.
76. Gold M, VanDam D, Silliman ER: An open-label trial of bromocriptine in non-fluent aphasia: A qualitative analysis of word storage and retrieval. *Brain Lang* 74:141–156, 2000.
77. Alexander MP, Hiltbrunner B, Fischer RF: The distributed anatomy of transcortical sensory aphasia. *Arch Neurol* 46:885–892, 1989.
78. Warrington EK, Shallice T: Category-specific semantic impairment. *Brain* 107:829–854, 1984.
79. Benson DF: Neurologic correlates of anomia, in Whitaker HWH (ed): *Studies in Neurolinguistics*. New York: Academic Press, 1979, pp 293–328.
80. Berthier ML, Starkstein SE, Leiguarda R, et al: Transcortical aphasia. *Brain* 114:1409–1427, 1991.
81. Feinberg TE, Dyckes-Berke D, Miner CR, Roane DM: Knowledge, implicit knowledge and metaknowledge in visual agnosia and pure alexia. *Brain* 118:789–800, 1995.
82. Graff-Radford NR, Damasio AR, Hyman BT, et al: Progressive aphasia in a patient with Pick's disease. *Neurology* 40:620–626, 1990.
83. Price BH, Gurvit H, Weintraub S, et al: Neuropsychological patterns and language deficits in 20 consecutive cases of autopsy-confirmed Alzheimer's disease. *Arch Neurol* 50:931–937, 1993.
84. Riddoch MJ, Humphreys GW, Coltheart M, Funnell E: Semantic systems or system? Neuropsychological evidence re-examined. *Cogn Neuropsychol* 5:3–25, 1988.
85. Geschwind N, Quadfasel FA, Segarra JM: Isolation of the speech area. *Neuropsychologia* 6:327–340, 1968.
86. Cappa SF, Vignolo LA: "Transcortical" features of aphasia following left thalamic hemorrhage. *Cortex* 19:227–241, 1979.
87. Graff-Radford NR, Damasio H, Yamada T, et al: Nonhemorrhagic thalamic infarction. *Brain* 108:485–516, 1985.
88. McFarling D, Rothi LJ, Heilman KM: Transcortical aphasia from ischemic infarcts of the thalamus. *J Neurol Neurosurg Psychiatry* 45:107–112, 1982.
89. Annett M: *Left, Right, Hand and Brain: The Right Shift Theory.* Hillsdale, NJ: Erlbaum, 1985.
90. Bryden MP, Hécaen H, DeAgostini M: Patterns of cerebral organization. *Brain Lang* 20:249–262, 1983.
91. Castro-Caldas A, Confraria A, Poppe P: Nonverbal disturbances in crossed aphasia. *Aphasiology* 1:403–413, 1987.
92. Alexander MP, Fischette MR, Fischer RS: Crossed aphasia can be mirror image or anomalous. *Brain* 112:953–973, 1989.
93. Basso A, Capitani E, Laiacona M, Zanobio ME: Crossed aphasia: One or more syndromes? *Cortex* 25:25–45, 1985.
94. Alexander MP, Annett M: Crossed aphasia and related anomalies of cerebral organization: case reports and a genetic hypothesis. *Brain Lang* 55:213–239, 1996.
95. Annett M, Alexander MP: Atypical cerebral dominance: Predictions and tests of the RS theory. *Neuropsychologia* 34:1215–1227, 1996.
96. Trojano L, Balbi P, Russo G, Elefante R: Patterns of recovery in verbal and nonverbal function in a case of crossed aphasia. *Brain Lang* 46:637–661, 1994.
97. Fischer RS, Alexander MP, Gabriel C, Milione J: Reversed lateralization of cognitive functions in right handers. *Brain* 114:245–261, 1991.
98. Hécaen H, DeAgostini M, Monzon-Montes A: Cerebral organization in lefthander. *Brain Lang* 12:261–284, 1981.
99. Basso A, Farabola M, Grassi MP, et al: Aphasia in lefthanders. *Brain Lang* 38:233–252, 1990.
100. Naeser MA, Borod JC: Aphasia in lefthanders. *Neurology* 36:471–488, 1986.
101. Puel M, Démonet JF, Cardebat I, et al: Aphasies souscorticales: Étude neurolinguistigue avec scanner x de 25 cas. *Rev Neurol* 140:695–710, 1984.
102. D'Esposito M, Alexander MP: Subcortical aphasia: Distinct profiles following left putaminal hemorrhages. *Neurology* 45:33–37, 1995.
103. DeRenzi E, Lucchelli F: Are semantic systems separately represented in the brain? The case of living category impairment. *Cortex* 30:3–25, 1994.
104. Smith S, Faust M, Beeman M, et al: A property level analysis of lexical semantic representation in Alzheimer's disease. *Brain Lang* 49:263–279, 1995.
105. Hodges JR, Salmon DP, Butters N: Semantic memory impairment in Alzheimer's disease: Failure of access or degraded knowledge? *Neuropsychologia* 30:301–314, 1992.
106. Tatemichi TK, Desmond DW, Prohovnik I, et al: Confusion and memory loss from capsular genu infarction: A thalamocortical disconnection syndrome? *Neurology* 42:1966–1979, 1992.
107. Hodges JR, Patterson K, Oxbury S, Funnell E: Semantic dementia. *Brain* 115:1783–1806, 1992.
108. Mesulam M-M: Slowly progressive aphasia without generalized dementia. *Ann Neurol* 1982;11:592–598, 1982.

109. Mesulam M-M: Primary progressive aphasia. *Ann Neurol* 49:425–432, 2001.
110. Weintraub S, Rubin NP, Mesulam M-M: Primary progressive aphasia: Longitudinal course, neuropsychological profile and language features. *Arch Neurol* 47:1329–1335, 1990.
111. Foster NL, Wilhelmsen KC, Sima AAF, et al: Frontotemporal dementia and Parkinsonism linked to chromosome 17: A consensus conference. *Ann Neurol* 41:706–715, 1997.
112. Kertesz A, Martinez-Lage P, Davidson W, Munoz DG: The corticobasal degeneration syndrome overlaps progressive aphasia and frontotemporal dementia. *Neurology* 55(9):1368–1375, 2000.
113. Kertesz A, Davidson W, Munoz DG: Clinical and pathological overlap between frontotemporal dementia, primary progressive aphasia and corticobasal degeneration: The Pick complex. *Dement Geriatr Cogn Disord* 10 (Suppl 1):46–49, 1999.
114. Kertesz A, Hudson L, MacKenzie IRA, Munoz DG: The pathology and nosology of primary progressive aphasia. *Neurology* 44:2065–2072, 1994.
115. van Slegtenhorst M, Lewis J, Hutton M: The molecular genetics of the tauopathies. *Exp Gerontol* 35(4): 461–471, 2000.

Chapter 12

APHASIA: COGNITIVE NEUROPSYCHOLOGICAL ISSUES*

Eleanor M. Saffran

As is evident from the preceding chapter, much was known about aphasia prior to the emergence of cognitive neuropsychology in the 1970s. Symptoms had been described, diagnostic and treatment protocols developed, anatomic correlates established, and models proposed that interpreted aphasic phenomena within an anatomic theory based on aphasic data (see Ref. 1 for review). The cognitive neuropsychological approach represents a shift from clinical and anatomic concerns to an emphasis on functional architecture. One assumption that underlies this approach is that language breakdown patterns reflect the natural divisions of the language system and hence that the disorders reveal its componential structure. This school of neuropsychological research is closely tied to developments in cognitive psychology and psycholinguistics. Normative models guide the investigation of pathologic phenomena, which, in turn, provide fertile ground for testing and extending theories of language function.

The concern with functional architecture has implications not only for the types of questions that are addressed by aphasia research but also for methodology. Earlier investigators had relied extensively on the classic aphasia syndrome categories (e.g., Broca's aphasia, Wernicke's aphasia) as the basis for identifying and grouping subjects. While useful as behavioral descriptors and pointers to lesion site, the syndrome designations allow a considerable amount of variability.[2,3] Moreover, these fairly gross breakdown patterns did not map very neatly onto the models of normal language processing that psycholinguists were developing. The investigative focus therefore moved from what might be regarded as "typical" aphasic manifestations[†]—for example, the combination of receptive and expressive symptoms that define Wernicke's aphasia—to deficits that were (1) of a more circumscribed nature and (2) had some clear relationship to models of language processing.[‡] An early statement of the assumptions underlying the approach was provided by Marin and colleagues[4]:

> . . . *the behavior of the patient with organic brain disease largely reflects capacities which existed in the premorbid state. We should therefore be able to make some inferences about the organization of normal language function from* patterns of functional preservation and impairment: *if process X is intact where process Y is severely compromised or absent, and especially if the converse is found in other patients, there is reason to believe that X and Y reflect different underlying mechanisms in the normal state. At the very least, the resulting matrix of intact and impaired functions should yield a taxonomy of functional subsystems. It may not tell us* how *these subsystems interact—but it should identify and describe what distinct capacities are available (e.g., it might, to take a hypothetical instance, describe a semantic process that is distinct from a syntactic process). The method is, of course, limited by the functional topology of the brain. Because functions may overlap in their anatomical*

* **ACKNOWLEDGMENT:** Preparation of this chapter was supported by grant DC00191 from the National Institutes of Health.

[†] Although any experienced clinician would agree that many patients are not easily assigned to classic syndrome categories.

[‡] This is not to imply that the cognitive neuropsychology approach is without clinical relevance. The assumption is that analyses of disorders in terms of loci of disruption within processing models should provide the basis for developing treatment programs tailored to the underlying disturbance (e.g., Chap. 12 in Ref. 105).

> *substrates, we cannot state with assurance that every functional system which* could *be observed* will *be observed. But* positive *evidence that functions are organized independently should be significant for a theory of the language process [pp. 869–870].*

It follows from this emphasis on dissociations that, for investigative purposes, greater value is placed on the purity of the impairment than on its frequency of occurrence in the aphasic population. Since circumscribed deficits are relatively rare, studies of single patients are not only admissible but, in the view of some investigators (e.g., Ref. 5), constitute the only valid source of neuropsychological data for the purpose of testing models of cognitive function (see Chap. 10 in Ref. 6 for discussion). Many cognitive neuropsychologists do not subscribe to this position, and group studies that involve sets of patients identified as having a particular cognitive impairment (e.g., "asyntactic" comprehension; see below) are not uncommon. Moreover, although the case study approach clearly departs from the random sampling from a population that is standard for behavioral research, the data are nevertheless cumulative. Delineation of an impairment in a single case report often leads to the identification of other patients with similar impairments and ultimately to compilations of data from a number of cases whose deficits appear quite similar.[7,8]

The cognitive neuropsychological approach is clearly well suited to the investigation of cognitive systems with modular architectures, that is, systems with components that are discrete and isolable, both functionally and anatomically.[9] In a system so constituted, the effects of damage to a single component should be quite local; other components should continue to function much as they did before the damage was incurred.[6] According to this view, the behavioral deficit should directly reflect the nature of the underlying impairment; Caramazza[2] refers to this as the "transparency" assumption. We will return to this point again at the end of the chapter, after reviewing the major contributions of cognitive neuropsychology to the study of aphasia.*

*Although the approach was first applied in the study of acquired dyslexia,[7] reading disorders are the subject of another chapter in this volume (Chap. 14) and are not discussed here.

COMPONENTS OF LANGUAGE PROCESSING

Most psycholinguists would agree that a model of language processing should include the components identified in Fig. 12-1. The model distinguishes among three types of information—semantic, syntactic, and phonologic; it does not, however, specify the extent to which these forms of information are processed independently, a matter that is still much debated.[10–12] The model includes procedures for recognizing and producing spoken words and for recovering and generating syntactic structures; the extent to which components are shared by the comprehension and production streams is another open question.[13,14] Language breakdown patterns are germane to both of these issues.

Assuming that the model is correct and that the processes and components identified in Fig. 12-1 can be disrupted independently, it should be possible to find patients with deficits that reflect breakdown at particular loci in the model. We will examine evidence for such disorders in the sections that follow.

DISORDERS OF LANGUAGE PROCESSING

Processing of Single Words: Comprehension

Impairments in the comprehension of spoken words are common in aphasia, and it is evident from Fig. 12-1 that there are a number of ways in which comprehension might fail: faulty phonologic processing prior to lexical access; loss of or impaired access to the phonologic forms of words; and/or loss of or impaired access to word meanings. Disorders of the first type can be ruled out by tests of phoneme perception and the second by lexical decision tasks in which the patient is asked to determine whether a string of phonemes is or is not a word. If a semantic deficit is present, it should be manifest not only on tests of auditory word comprehension but on written word comprehension and

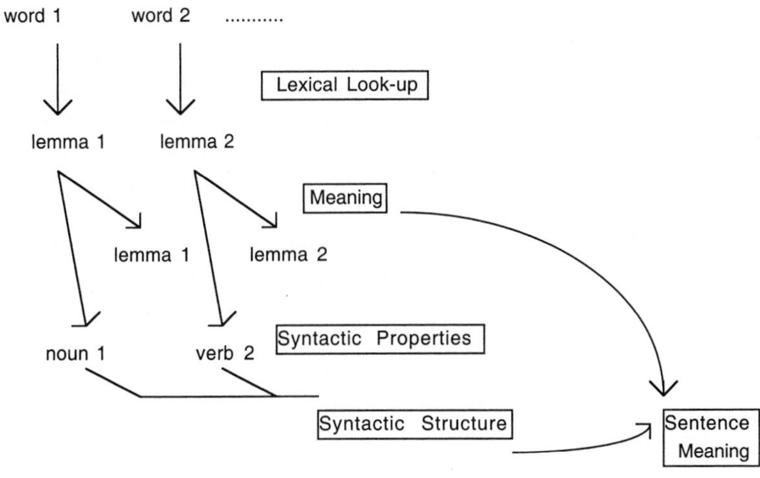

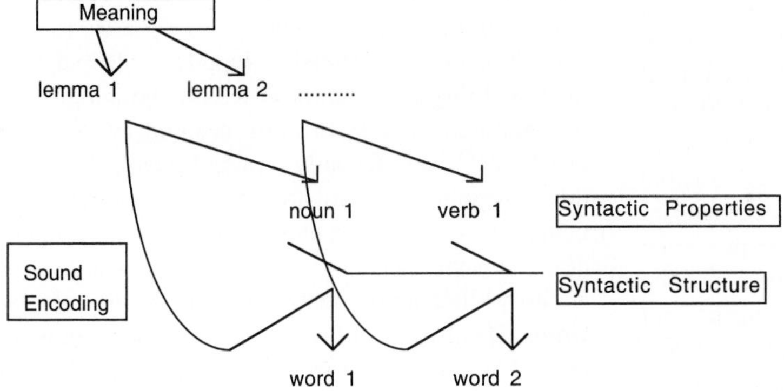

Figure 12-1
Stages in language processing. A. Processing of single words. The lemma refers to a processing level at which the word is specified with respect to meaning and grammatical class but not encoded phonologically. B. Processing of sentences.

production tasks as well. This follows from the widely held assumption that comprehension and production in both oral and written modalities rely on a common conceptual base.[14]

Phonologic Processing

The task for the perceiver of spoken language is to recover meaningful units (words) from the complex and variable sound patterns produced by the human vocal tract. Phonemes, such as *d*, *ow*, and *t*, which are the basic building blocks of words, consist of several distinct frequency bands (formants) that may differ in their relative onset times as well as undergo transient shifts in frequency. These acoustic properties can vary depending on the context in which the phoneme occurs; compare the *d* sound in the word *ride* with the *d* sound in *rider*. A further complication is that the boundaries between words are not systematically marked by gaps in the acoustic stimulus, as they are in written text. Thus the processing of speech input is a complicated matter, which, it has been argued, requires specialized mechanisms that are distinct from those used to process other types of acoustic stimuli.[15]

The fact that the processing of speech sounds can be selectively disrupted by brain damage supports this view. Disorders that meet this description are labeled *pure word deafness*. They are the product of small lesions, usually embolic in nature, that affect the superior temporal lobe on the left or, in other cases, that occur bilaterally. In its pure form, the disorder is relatively rare. In most cases the lesion is more extensive, resulting in the set of symptoms associated with Wernicke's aphasia, which may include features of word deafness.[16]

The hallmark of pure word deafness is that the patient has great difficulty comprehending and repeating what he or she hears but can read and speak virtually normally. The audiometric exam is essentially normal, and nonspeech sounds are interpreted without difficulty. Some patients have shown suppression of right-ear input under dichotic listening conditions, suggesting that auditory input is being processed in the right hemisphere[17,18] (but see Ref. 19). Auditory comprehension improves significantly when lip reading is allowed,[19] speech is slowed down,[17] and/or contextual constraints are provided. For example, Saffran and coworkers[18] described a patient whose ability to repeat words was better with semantically constrained than random word lists. These observations suggest that the auditory information available for word identification is in some way inadequate or degraded. Studies in which speech perception has been carefully examined have demonstrated deficits in the discrimination and identification of phonemes.[18–20] Vowels, made up of steady-state formants, tend to be better preserved than consonants, in which there are transient frequency shifts.[20] The processing of nonspeech sounds has not been examined as systematically. Although word-deaf patients are generally able to identify environmental stimuli such as the sounds of animals and musical instruments, they have seldom been called upon to make fine-grained judgments outside the speech domain, involving, for example, the temporal and waveform parameters that are manipulated in speech perception tasks. In the few studies that have included such investigations, deficits in the resolution of repetitive click stimuli have been identified.[17,19,21] This finding points to an impairment in auditory processes that are essential to phoneme perception but are not necessarily specific to speech. Auerbach and coworkers[19] have suggested that there may, in fact, be two forms of word deafness, one reflecting impairment of prephonetic auditory processing and the other specific to phonetic operations. This proposal requires further investigation.

Lexical Processing

Lexical access entails matching of the acoustic input to an entry in lexical memory that represents the word's phonologic form. Loss or degradation of lexical phonology is a possible cause of comprehension failure. Deciding whether a speech sound is a word or not (auditory lexical decision) should be impaired under these conditions, but it should still be possible to repeat words, treating them as one would normally treat nonwords. Lexical decision and comprehension of written words should be preserved. Deficits in word comprehension, with relatively preserved repetition, have been described under the label *word-meaning deafness.*[22–24] These patients are reported to have no comparable difficulty with written words and may resort to writing down spoken words in order to understand them. However, data on lexical decision have not been provided, and evidence for the critical phenomenon—failure to comprehend spoken words that can be understood in written form—are limited to a small number of examples.

The model outlined in Fig. 12-1 also suggests the possibility of preserved access to phonologic form with failure of access to word meaning. Franklin and associates[25] have recently reported a case that meets this description, at least for abstract words. This patient performed well on phonologic processing and auditory lexical decision tasks but was impaired in the auditory—but not written—comprehension of abstract words. He also had difficulty repeating abstract words as well as nonwords. Word meaning was clearly a significant factor in his repetition performance, as further indicated by a tendency to produce semantic errors in repeating single words. This pattern of repetition performance is termed *deep dysphasia* (for case reports, see Refs. 26 to 28). As shown below, this is but one of several disorders in which particular types of words are disproportionately affected.

Semantic Processing

Deficits that involve the loss of word meaning are frequently reported, although often in the context of other impairments (e.g., as in Wernicke's aphasia). Relatively pure cases have been described under the label *transcortical sensory aphasia,* a disorder in which repetition is spared relative to comprehension and spontaneous production.[29,30] Semantic disturbances are also found in cases of herpes encephalitis[31,32] and, in progressive form (*semantic dementia*), in association with degenerative brain disease[33,34]; these disorders involve damage to middle and inferior temporal lobe structures that lie outside the perisylvian zone usually associated with language function (see Chap. 39).

In some cases, the deficit is remarkably selective, affecting some categories of words more than others. The pattern that has been most frequently reported is a disproportionate loss of knowledge of biological kinds, such as animals, fruits, and vegetables; knowledge of artifacts, such as tools and furniture, is at least relatively preserved (see Ref. 35 for review). The semantic deficit is manifest on naming tasks as well as on a variety of measures of word comprehension. This "category-specific" disorder has most often been described in cases of herpes encephalitis but has also been found in one case of semantic dementia.[36] There have been attempts to account for this pattern in terms of confounding factors such as the greater visual complexity and lesser familiarity of animals relative to objects such as tools,[37,38] but the category differences have been shown to persist even when these factors are well controlled.[39] Moreover, the opposite pattern—better performance on living things—has been demonstrated in patients with frontoparietal lesions (see Ref. 35 for review). One possible account of this double dissociation is that biological kinds and artifacts depend in different degrees on different types of semantic information.[31,40] For example, animals are distinguished largely on the basis of perceptual characteristics such as shape and color (compare *lion* and *tiger,* for example), while artifacts are defined primarily by their function (namely, the diverse objects that qualify as radios).

These considerations are compatible with the view that semantic memory is distributed across subsystems specialized for different types of knowledge (but see Ref. 41). Figure 12-2, from Allport,[42] illustrates such a model: the shape of a telephone is stored in one subsystem, its sound in another, its function (not shown) in still another. Although represented in different subsystems, the properties of an object are linked in memory by virtue of the fact that they consistently occur together. When some features of an object (e.g., its shape) are accessed, properties that reside in other

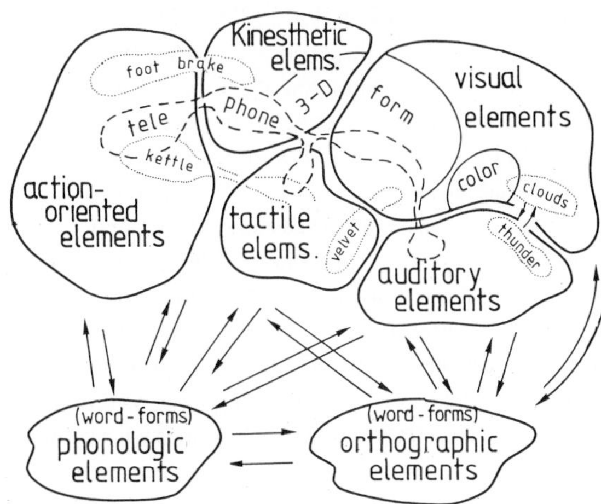

Figure 12-2
Schematic of a distributed model of conceptual representation. (From Allport,[42] with permission.)

subsystems (e.g., function) are automatically activated, instantiating the distributed activation pattern that corresponds to full knowledge of the object.

Semantic breakdown also occurs along the abstractness/concreteness dimension. Normal subjects show an advantage for concrete words,[43] and it would not be surprising if brain damage magnified this effect. This is, in fact, the result that is most frequently reported. For example, repetition of abstract words is disproportionately impaired in deep dysphasia,[26–28] a pattern that also holds for oral reading in deep dyslexia.[7] It is unlikely, however, that this effect simply reflects the greater difficulty of abstract words, as there are patients who show the reverse pattern, performing better on abstract than concrete words.[36,44,45] There is some evidence that abstract word superiority is associated with differential impairment within the class of concrete words, specifically, worse performance on words denoting living things than those denoting artifacts.[32,36] This would suggest that both patterns reflect disproportionate loss of perceptual components of meaning, which are irrelevant to abstract words and more salient for some categories of concrete words than others.

Processing of Single Words: Production

Psycholinguists conceive of production as a multistage process that begins with a concept and ends with movement of the articulators.[11,46,47] Here we concern ourselves only with the processes exemplified in Fig. 12-1, which involve selection of a lexical entry (lemma) that corresponds to the concept to be communicated, followed by access to the phonologic form of the word. The evidence that supports the two-stage retrieval process is not reviewed here (see Refs. 11, 46, and 47), but consideration of the tip-of-the-tongue phenomenon—knowing that one knows a word without being able to encode it phonologically—suggests that there is a stage of lexicalization that precedes access to phonology. The second stage, phonologic encoding, is a complex process involving retrieval of a set of phonemes, arranging them in the correct serial order, and specifying their stress pattern.[11]

Although there is general agreement that word retrieval is a two-step process, the nature of the relationship between the two stages is controversial. Some theorists maintain that lemma selection precedes and is entirely uninfluenced by phonologic encoding.[11] Others view lexical retrieval as an interactive process, involving feedback from phonology as well as activation in the forward direction, with the result that phonology can affect lemma selection.[10,48] Observations that favor the latter account include the fact that mixed errors that bear both a semantic and a phonologic relationship to the target word (e.g., *carrot*, *cabbage*) are more frequent than would be expected by chance.[49,50] This finding suggests that phonologic feedback interacts with feed-forward activation from semantics to promote the selection of alternatives that bear both a semantic and a phonologic relationship to the target.

Models of word production are based to a large extent on normal speech error patterns.[46,47] It should be possible to account for aphasic speech errors within the same theoretical framework. The errors produced by normal speakers include word substitutions that are semantically (e.g., *fork; spoon*) or phonologically related to the target (e.g., *index; insect*) as well as the mixed errors referred to above. Semantic errors are common in aphasics, and although the literature suggests that phonologically related word substitutions are rare (cf. Ref. 51), there are some patients who do produce high rates of these "formal paraphasias"[52,53] Perhaps the major difference between aphasic and normal speech errors (aside from the increase in overall rate of error production) is the frequency with which aphasic patients generate errors that are not words; these are referred to as phonemic paraphasias, or neologisms. Some of these errors bear a clear phonologic relationship to the target (e.g., *scout; scut*); others, sometimes referred to as abstruse neologisms,[54] do not.

Although patients generally produce both semantic and phonologic errors, there are cases in which one type of error dominates. For example, Caramazza and Hillis[55] describe a patient who produced only semantic errors, while Caplan and coworkers[56] report a case in which errors were exclusively phonologic. In general, the error patterns of aphasics are consistent with the two-stage model, with indications that semantic and phonologic processes can, on occasion, be disrupted independently.

Recently, there have been efforts to bring aphasic data to bear on the question of independent stage versus interactive models of lexical retrieval. As noted earlier, the interactive model predicts that mixed (semantic + phonologic) errors should exceed levels expected by chance; this prediction should hold for aphasic individuals as well as for normals. Martin and coworkers[57] examined a corpus of errors elicited from aphasic patients in a picture-naming task and found that it does. Martin and colleagues[53] were also able to simulate error patterns of a patient who produced a high rate of form-based word substitutions by altering parameter settings on an implemented version of an interactive computational model.[10]

Grammatical class is another important variable in lexical retrieval. It is not unusual to find patients who show significant differences in their ability to retrieve nouns versus verbs.[58,59] Case studies include those of McCarthy and Warrington,[60] of a patient with a selective disturbance in verb production and comprehension, and Zingeser and Berndt,[61] whose patient showed preservation of action naming relative to object naming. Different lesion sites have been implicated in these selective impairments—specifically, a frontal locus for verbs and a temporal locus for nouns.[62] But the functional basis for these grammatical class effects is not entirely clear. As grammatical class reflects a conceptual distinction, one might expect this factor to be operative early in word retrieval; indeed, the lemma is assumed to specify grammatical class.[11] However, Caramazza and Hillis[63] have argued that phonologic output from the lexicon is also organized with respect to grammatical class. This proposal follows from their study of two patients who showed selective deficits for verbs in a single modality—oral production in one case and written production in the other. They interpret these patterns to reflect selective impairment for verbs at the level of orthographic or phonologic encoding.

Sentence-Level Processing: Comprehension

As inspection of the sentences below indicates, the meaning of a sentence is not solely a function of its lexical content. Failure to comprehend such sentences—interpreting sentence 1 to indicate that the cat was the chaser or that the dog was black—is not uncommon in aphasic individuals, even when they understand all of the individual words. In an influential study, Caramazza and Zurif[64] demonstrated such an impairment in patients with Broca's aphasia. Although their subjects had no difficulty understanding sentences like sentence 2, they performed at chance on sentences like sentence 1.

1. The cat that the dog chased was black.
2. The apple that the boy ate was red.

The difference between the two sentences, which have the same syntactic structure, is that the second one is semantically constrained (apples cannot eat boys), while the first is not. In order to interpret sentence 1 correctly, it is necessary to recover the syntax of the sentence and to use this information to assign the nouns to the thematic roles specified by the verb (i.e., *dog* to the role of agent, or chaser, and *cat* to the role of theme, or the entity being chased). Caramazza and Zurif's experiment showed that the aphasic subjects had difficulty utilizing syntactic information for this purpose, although they were clearly able to make use of semantic constraints. These authors showed, further, that performance was a function of syntactic complexity: although the patients did relatively well on simple active declarative sentences, their performance broke down on more complex structures, such as passives and object relatives (sentence 1, for example). Caramazza and Zurif interpreted this result to indicate that the patients were using heuristics such as "assign the preverbal noun the agent role and the postverbal noun the role of theme." Reliance on heuristics, together with semantic constraints, would account for the fact that sentence comprehension appears relatively preserved in those with Broca's aphasia.

Difficulty in sentence production—the pattern known as "agrammatism"—is also part of the symptom complex in Broca's aphasia. The fact that syntactic impairments in comprehension and production occurred in the same patients gave rise to the hypothesis that the co-occurring deficits were due to a central syntactic deficit, characterized as a loss of grammatical knowledge.[65] Another influential view was that both disturbances reflect impairment to the closed class vocabulary, consisting of elements such as prepositions and tense markers, which convey syntactic information.[66] Both hypotheses were subsequently challenged by two sources of evidence: reports of cases in which production was agrammatic but comprehension was intact[67] and the demonstration that patients with agrammatic Broca's aphasia with the "asyntactic" comprehension pattern described by Caramazza and Zurif[64] were able to detect grammatical violations such as those in sentences 3a and 3b.[68,69]

3a. How many did you see birds in the park?

3b. John was finally kissed Louise.

These results, subsequently replicated in other laboratories,[70,71] present difficulty for both accounts of the agrammatic impairment. The ability to detect such violations requires knowledge of the grammar as well as sensitivity to the absence or presence and identity of the grammatical morphemes on which most of them depend.

What, then, is the basis for the "asyntactic" comprehension pattern? Linebarger and coworkers[68] suggested two possible accounts. The first of these is the limited capacity hypothesis. The patients have limited processing resources that will not suffice for parsing and interpretive operations; if they parse, they cannot interpret, and vice versa. Schwartz and coworkers[72] tested this hypothesis in a study in which patients judged the plausibility of sentences such as sentences 4a and 4b. The "padding" in sentence 4b should increase the difficulty of parsing relative to sentence 4a; on the limited capacity hypotheses, one might therefore expect worse performance on the padded sentences.

4a. The chicken killed the farmer.

4b. In the early part of the day, the chicken drank some water and then killed and ate the farmer.

4c. The farmer was killed by the chicken.

The results showed, however, that the effect of padding was negligible for the "asyntactic" comprehenders (though not for other aphasic patients); in contrast, the effect of the syntactic manipulation in sentence 4c, which involves movement of the nouns from their canonical (preverbal agent, postverbal theme) positions, was seriously detrimental. The second account is the mapping hypothesis. The patients are able to parse sentences but cannot carry out additional operations on the structures computed by the parser, such as mapping from a syntactic representation to thematic roles.

Interpretation of the "asyntactic" comprehension pattern remains controversial. The mapping and limited capacity hypotheses are still debated, as are other interpretations motivated by recent developments in linguistic theory (see Ref. 69 for discussion). The mapping hypothesis has led to the development of treatment programs directed at the mapping operation (see Refs. 73 and 74 and Chap. 13, this volume), which have produced gains in some patients with chronic aphasia. The capacity limitation hypothesis has received support from studies conducted with normal subjects; it turns out that a variety of manipulations that might be expected to tax processing capacity (e.g., rapid serial visual presentation of the words in a sentence; divided attention; elimination of grammatical morphemes) result in comprehension patterns that mirror those of the aphasic individuals.[75–77] However, this evidence in itself is not compelling. Assuming that it is the recovery of syntactic information and/or the mapping from syntactic to semantic structures that are most vulnerable under these conditions, one would expect other factors that contribute to sentence interpretation to be more influential; these include a tendency to assign the preverbal noun the role of agent, which it often is in English sentences.[78] Other proposals have come from linguists, who have attempted to interpret the asyntactic comprehension pattern in terms of constructs in linguistic theory (see Ref. 69 and other papers in that volume). To a large extent, these accounts emphasize the difficulty that these aphasic patients have in comprehending sentences with moved arguments; these structures are marked with "traces" (indicated by *t*) linked to the argument that has been moved, as in sentence 5:

5. The farmer was killed *t* by the chicken.

It is assumed that the necessity to link the moved argument (the farmer, in sentence 5) to the trace complicates sentence processing for those with aphasia. Often ignored by proponents of these views, however, is the fact that "asyntactic" patients frequently have difficulty with sentences that (at least according to most theories) lack traces, such as the simple active declarative[79,80] and locative[79,81] sentences exemplified by sentences 6a and 6b.

6a. The boy follows the girl.

6b. The paper is on the book.

Thus, while the basic phenomena are well established, there is as yet no generally accepted interpretation of the "asyntactic" comprehension pattern.

Short-Term Memory and Sentence Processing

Other studies of aphasia have focused on the role of short-term memory (STM) in sentence processing. Although most aphasic patients show some degree of short-term verbal memory impairment (see Ref. 82 for review), there are cases in which STM capacity, as measured by digit and word span, is markedly deficient in the context of relatively preserved language abilities.[83,84] The STM deficit appears to reflect impairment of a phonologic component of STM.[8] Most STM patients have difficulty with sentence comprehension, demonstrating the performance pattern characteristic of agrammatical aphasia that was described above.[85] It has proved difficult, however, to specify the relationship between these two impairments. One complicating factor is that the two are not perfectly correlated; there are instances in which reduced memory span is not accompanied by impairment in comprehension.[86,87] Studies of normal sentence processing indicate, moreover, that syntactic and semantic encoding occur on line,[88] so that there would seem to be no need to maintain the input in phonologic form. But while phonologic memory may not be necessary for first-pass encoding operations, it may serve as a backup store that allows the listener to revise interpretations in light of information that comes later in the sentence (for discussion, see Refs. 89 and 90).

Sentence-Level Processing: Production

A schema for sentence production is outlined in Fig. 12-1. Although not explicitly represented in the diagram, most psycholinguists assume that sentence production involves retrieval of a syntactic frame that stipulates word order (e.g., determiner-noun-auxiliary-verb. . .) and serves as a template into which phonologically specified words are later inserted (e.g., Refs. 47 and 48). While there are other aphasic patients who are impaired in some aspects of sentence production,[91] it is the deficits of agrammatical Broca's aphasia that have drawn most attention. The production of such patients is characterized by the limited use of syntactic structures and the omission of grammatical morphemes, such as tense markers (e.g., *-ed*), determiners (e.g., *the*), and prepositions (e.g., *to*). It seems likely that frame retrieval is seriously impaired in such patients, reflecting a reduction in the inventory of syntactic structures, their inaccessibility, or both.[92] The fact that patients occasionally produce utterances that are more complex than those constituting the bulk of their corpora suggests that inaccessibility of these structures is at least part of the problem.[93] In light of evidence from normals that use promotes further use,[94,95] it seems likely that a tendency to rely on a limited set of structures will render other structures progressively less accessible. There is some evidence that frame retrieval can be disrupted independently of access to grammatical morphology[67,96] and that bound (i.e., inflectional) and free-standing grammatical morphemes can be selectively affected.[97,98]

NEW DIRECTIONS

Cognitive neuropsychology adopted the box-and-arrow information processing models that were favored by cognitive psychologists in the 1970s. The boxes stood for modules whose internal operations were largely unknown; the arrows symbolized the flow of information between them. More recently, cognitive theorists have turned to computer-implemented (neural network or "connectionist") models that specify more precisely how information is represented and processed (see Chap. 10). These models are networks of units that represent information; the informational significance of the units is either specified by the modeler (in "localist" models; e.g., Ref. 48) or acquired during learning trials [in parallel distributed processing (PDP) models; e.g., Refs. 40 and 99]. In the latter, inner layers of units are initially connected randomly to input and output layers in which units are specified for content. Thus, for example, models that learn to read aloud have input units that stand for individual letters or groups of letters and output units that stand for specific phonemes or groups of phonemes. Explorations of effects of "lesioning" these models (for example, by randomly eliminating units or altering the strength of connections between units) have revealed some interesting properties that have implications for fundamental assumptions in cognitive neuropsychology.

One major result of the simulation studies is that symptoms are not necessarily a direct reflection of the type of representation that is lesioned. For example, Shallice and colleagues[99,100] have developed a connectionist model of reading in which learning procedures are used to train graphemic units to activate units of meaning ("sememes" such as "brown," "has legs," etc.) that ultimately activate phoneme units. In other words, the model learns to pronounce written words by looking up their meanings. Lesioning of this model can result in semantic errors (e.g., reading *night* as *sleep*) of the sort that are produced by patients with deep dyslexia (see Chap. 14, this volume). These errors were generally thought to reflect impairment at the semantic level.[101] The simulations on this model demonstrate, however, that semantic errors can be generated by lesions elsewhere in the network. A related point is made by data from a study by Farah and McClelland,[40] who lesioned a semantic network to simulate the disorders involving living and nonliving things. The model included two semantic subsystems, one representing functional properties and the other visual properties, which predominated for living things. As a result of the connectivity patterns within the network, damage to the visual subsystem rendered the functional properties of living things inaccessible. The "symptoms" therefore reflected perturbations that extended well beyond the subsystem targeted by the lesion. The implication of these findings is that the relationship between symptom and deficit may not be as direct as it is often taken to be (cf. Ref. 102).

Other simulation studies demonstrate that performance patterns that appear selective can be generated by lesions that are widespread. Employing a localist model of word retrieval,[10] which allows activation to feed back from phonemes to lemma to semantic units as well as to proceed in the forward direction, our group has shown that shifts in the dominant error types can be produced by altering different parameters of the model.[53,103] The two parameters are connection strength, which affects the ease with which activation flows (in both directions) from one level to another, and decay rate, which affects the persistence of activation within representational levels. Different error patterns result from connection weight and decay rate lesions, both applied uniformly throughout the lexical system. A decrease in connection strength reduces the flow of activation to target-related units, resulting in an increase in nonword errors. Decay rate lesions have a different effect on the distribution of activation, shifting error production in the direction of semantic and formal substitutions. Lest it be thought that this is merely a formal exercise, manipulation of these two parameters closely simulated the individual error patterns of almost all (20 of 23) of the patients with fluent aphasia tested by us.

How seriously should we take these demonstrations of nonlocal effects of lesions, and do they in any way invalidate the 20-year research program in cognitive neuropsychology? Computational modeling in the language domain is relatively new, and it is too soon to determine how useful this approach will prove to be. However, recent psycholinguistic studies indicate that normal language processing is characterized by a good deal of interaction among processing components.[10,95,104] Interactive processing architectures complicate the task of inferring the locus of the deficit from a patient's performance. As Farah[102] has observed, the relationship between symptom and impaired process is no longer transparent; semantic errors, for example, need not necessarily reflect perturbation of a semantic process. But while it will be necessary to interpret new data more cautiously and, perhaps, to reexamine earlier conclusions, the effort to tie phenomena of language breakdown to models of normal language function remains useful and valid. Neuropsychological data extend the database and testing ground for normative models, and the models, in turn, provide a coherent framework for the investigation and interpretation of clinical phenomena.

REFERENCES

1. Goodglass H, Geschwind N: Language disorders (aphasia), in Carterette EC, Friedman MP (eds): *Handbook of Perception.* New York: Academic Press, 1976.
2. Caramazza A: The logic of neuropsychological research and the problem of patient classification in aphasia. *Brain Lang* 21:9–20, 1984.
3. Schwartz MF: What the classical aphasia categories can't do for us and why. *Cognit Neuropsychol* 21:3–8, 1984.
4. Marin OSM, Saffran EM, Schwartz MF: Dissociations of language in aphasia: Implications for normal function. *Ann NY Acad Sci* 280:868–884, 1976.
5. Caramazza A: On drawing inferences about the structure of normal cognitive systems from the analysis of patterns of impaired performance: the case for single-patient studies. *Brain Cogn* 5:41–66, 1986.
6. Shallice T: *From Neuropsychology to Mental Structure.* Cambridge, England: Cambridge University Press, 1988.
7. Coltheart M, Patterson KE, Marshall JC (eds): *Deep Dyslexia.* London: Routledge, 1980.
8. Vallar G, Shallice T (eds): *Neuropsychological Deficits in Short-Term Memory.* Cambridge, England: Cambridge University Press, 1990.
9. Fodor JA: *The Modularity of Mind.* Cambridge, MA: MIT Press, 1983.
10. Dell GS, O'Seaghdha PG: Mediated and convergent lexical priming in language production: A comment on Levelt et al. *Psychol Rev* 98:604–614, 1991.
11. Levelt WJM: Accessing words in speech production: Stages, processes and representations. *Cognition* 42: 1–21, 1992.
12. Mitchell DC: Sentence parsing, in Gernsbacher MA (ed): *Handbook of Psycholinguistics.* San Diego, CA: Academic Press, 1994.
13. Allport DA: Speech production and comprehension: One lexicon or two? in Prinz W, Sanders AF (eds):

Cognition and Motor Processes. Berlin: Springer-Verlag, 1984.

14. Monsell S: On the relation between lexical input and output pathways for speech, in Allport A, MacKay D, Prinz W, Sheerer E (eds): *Language Perception and Production.* London: Academic Press, 1987.
15. Liberman AM, Studdert-Kennedy M: Phonetic perception, in Held R, Lebowitz H, Teuber H-L (eds): *The Handbook of Sensory Physiology: Perception.* Heidelberg: Springer-Verlag, 1978, vol 8, pp. 143–178.
16. Caramazza A, Berndt RS, Basili AG: The selective impairment of phonological processing: A case study. *Brain Lang* 18:128–174, 1983.
17. Albert ML, Bear D: Time to understand: A case study of word deafness with reference to the role of time in auditory comprehension. *Brain* 97:373–384, 1974.
18. Saffran EM, Marin OSM, Yeni-Komshian G: An analysis of speech perception in word deafness. *Brain Lang* 3:209–228, 1976.
19. Auerbach SH, Allard T, Naeser M, et al: Pure word deafness: Analysis of a case with bilateral lesions and defect at the prephonemic level. *Brain* 105:271–300, 1982.
20. Denes G, Semenza C: Auditory modality-specific anomie: Evidence from a case of pure word deafness. *Cortex* 14:41–49, 1975.
21. Tanaka Y, Yamadori A, Mori E: Pure word deafness following bilateral lesions. *Brain* 110:381–403, 1987.
22. Bramwell B: Illustrative cases of aphasia (case 11). *Lancet* 1:1256–1259, 1897. [Reprinted with an introduction by AW Ellis. *Cognit Neuropsychol* 1:245–258, 1984.]
23. Kohn SE, Friedman RB: Word-meaning deafness: A phonological semantic dissociation. *Cognit Neuropsychol* 3:291–308, 1986.
24. Schacter DL, McGlynn SM, Milberg WP, Church BA: Spared priming despite impaired comprehension: Implicit memory in a case of word-meaning deafness. *Neuropsychology* 7:107–118, 1993.
25. Franklin S, Howard D, Patterson K: Abstract word meaning deafness. *Cogn Neuropsychol* 11:1–34, 1994.
26. Howard D, Franklin S: *Missing the Meaning? A Cognitive Neuropsychological Study of Processing of Words by an Aphasic Patient.* Cambridge, MA: MIT Press, 1988.
27. Katz R, Goodglass H: Deep dysphasia: an analysis of a rare form of repetition disorder. *Brain Lang* 39:153–185, 1990.
28. Martin N, Saffran EM: A computational account of deep dysphasia: Evidence from a single case study. *Brain Lang* 43:240–274, 1992.
29. Berndt RS, Basili A, Caramazza A: Dissociation of functions in a case of transcortical sensory aphasia. *Cognit Neuropsychol* 4:79–101, 1987.
30. Martin N, Saffran EM: Factors underlying repetition and short-term memory in transcortical sensory aphasia. *Brain Lang* 37:440–479, 1990.
31. Warrington EK, Shallice T: Category-specific semantic impairments. *Brain* 107:829–854, 1984.
32. Sirigu A, Duhamel J-R, Poncet M: The role of sensorimotor experience in object recognition. *Brain* 114:2555–2573, 1991.
33. Snowden JS, Goulding PJ, Neary D: Semantic dementia: a form of circumscribed cerebral atrophy. *Behav Neurol* 2:167–182, 1989.
34. Hodges JR, Patterson K, Oxbury S, Funnell E: Semantic dementia: progressive fluent aphasia, with temporal lobe atrophy. *Brain* 115:1783–1806, 1992.
35. Saffran EM, Schwartz MF: Of cabbages and things: semantic memory from a neuropsychological perspective—a tutorial review, in Umilta C, Moscovitch M (eds): *Attention and Performance: XV. Conscious and Nonconscious Processes.* Cambridge, MA: MIT Press, 1994.
36. Breedin SD, Saffran EM, Coslett HB: Reversal of the concreteness effect in a patient with semantic dementia. *Cognit Neuropsychol* 11:617–660, 1994.
37. Funnell E, Sheridan J: Categories of knowledge? Unfamiliar aspects of living and non-living things. *Cognit Neuropsychol* 9:135–154, 1992.
38. Stewart F, Parkin AJ, Hunkin NM: Naming impairments following recovery from herpes simplex encephalitis: category specific? *Q J Exp Psychol* 44A:261–284, 1992.
39. Farah MJ, McMullen PA, Meyer MM: Can recognition of living things be selectively impaired? *Neuropsychologia* 29:185–193, 1991.
40. Farah MJ, McClelland JL: A computational model of semantic memory impairment: Modality specificity and emergent category. *J Exp Psychol (Gen)* 120:339–357, 1991.
41. Caramazza A, Hillis AE, Rapp B, Romani C: The multiple semantics hypothesis: Multiple confusion? *Cognit Neuropsychol* 7:161–189, 1990.
42. Allport DA: Distributed memory, modular subsystems and dysphasia, in Newman SK, Epstein R (eds): *Current Perspectives in Dysphasia.* Edinburgh: Churchill Livingstone, 1985, pp 32–60.
43. Paivio A: Dual coding theory: Retrospect and current status. *Can J Psychol* 45:255–258, 1991.
44. Warrington EK: The selective impairment of semantic memory. *Q J Exp Psychol* 27:635–657, 1975.

45. Cipolotti L, Warrington EK: Semantic memory and reading abilities: A case report. *J Int Neuropsychol Soc* 1:104–110, 1995.
46. Fromkin VA: The non-anomalous nature of anomalous utterances. *Language* 47:27–52, 1971.
47. Garrett MF: Levels of processing in sentence production, in Butterworth B (ed): *Language Production.* New York: Academic Press, 1980, vol 1.
48. Dell GS: A spreading activation theory of retrieval in language production. *Psychol Rev* 93:283–321, 1986.
49. Dell GS, Reich PA: Stages in sentence production: An analysis of speech error data. *J Verb Learn Verb Behav* 20:611–629, 1981.
50. Martin N, Weisberg R, Saffran EM: Variables influencing the occurrence of naming errors: Implications for models of lexical retrieval. *J Mem Lang* 28:462–485, 1989.
51. Ellis AW: The production of spoken words, in Ellis AW (ed): *Progress in the Psychology of Language.* London: Erlbaum, 1985, vol 2.
52. Blanken G: Formal paraphasias: A single case study. *Brain Lang* 38:534–554, 1990.
53. Martin N, Dell GS, Saffran EM, Schwartz MF: Origins of paraphasias in deep dysphasia: Testing the consequences of a decay impairment to an interactive spreading activation model of lexical retrieval. *Brain Lang* 47:609–660, 1994.
54. Schwartz MF, Saffran EM, Bloch DE, Dell GS: Disordered speech production in aphasic and normal speakers. *Brain Lang* 47:52–88, 1994.
55. Caramazza A, Hillis AE: Where do semantic errors come from? *Cortex* 26:95–122, 1990.
56. Caplan D, Vanier M, Baker C: A case study of reproduction conduction aphasia: I. Word production. *Cognit Neuropsychol* 3:99–128, 1986.
57. Martin N, Gagnon DA, Schwartz MF, et al: Phonological facilitation of semantic errors in normal and aphasic speakers. *Lang Cogn Process* 11:257–282, 1996.
58. Miceh G, Silveri MC, Romani C, Caramazza A: On the basis for the agrammatic's difficulty in producing main verbs. *Cortex* 20:207–220, 1984.
59. Kohn SE, Lorch MP, Pearson DM: Verb finding in aphasia. *Cortex* 25:57–69, 1989.
60. McCarthy R, Warrington EK: Category specificity in an agrammatic patient: The relative impairment of verb retrieval and comprehension. *Neuropsychologia* 23:709–727, 1985.
61. Zingeser LB, Berndt RS: Retrieval of nouns and verbs in agrammatism and anomia. *Brain Lang* 39:14–32, 1990.
62. Daniele A, Giustolisi L, Silveri MC, et al: Evidence for a possible neuroanatomical basis for lexical processing of nouns and verbs. *Neuropsychologia* 32:1325–1341, 1994.
63. Caramazza A, Hillis AE: Lexical organization of nouns and verbs in the brain. *Nature* 349:788–790, 1991.
64. Caramazza A, Zurif EB: Dissociations of algorithmic and heuristic processes in language comprehension: Evidence from aphasia. *Brain Lang* 3:572–582, 1976.
65. Caramazza A, Berndt RS: Semantic and syntactic processes in aphasia: A review of the literature. *Psychol Bull* 85:898–918, 1978.
66. Bradley DC, Garrett MF, Zurif EB: Syntactic deficits in Broca's aphasia, in Caplan D (ed): *Biological Studies of Mental Processes.* Cambridge, MA: MIT Press, 1980.
67. Miceli G, Mazzuchi A, Menn L, Goodglass H: Contrasting cases of Italian agrammatic aphasia without comprehension disorder. *Brain Lang* 19:65–97, 1983.
68. Linebarger MC, Schwartz MF, Saffran EM: Sensitivity to grammatical structure in so-called agrammatic aphasics. *Cognition* 13:641–662, 1983.
69. Linebarger MC: Agrammatism as evidence about grammar. *Brain Lang* 50:52–91, 1995.
70. Berndt RS, Salasoo A, Mitchum CC, Blumstein S: The role of intonation cues in aphasic patients' performance of the grammaticality judgment task. *Brain Lang* 34:65–97, 1988.
71. Shankweiler D, Crain S, Gorrell P, Tuller B: Reception of language in Broca's aphasia. *Lang Cogn Process* 4: 1–33, 1989.
72. Schwartz MF, Linebarger M, Saffran EM, Pate DS: Syntactic transparency and sentence interpretation in aphasia. *Lang Cogn Process* 2:85–113, 1987.
73. Byng S: Sentence comprehension deficit: theoretical analysis and remediation. *Cognit Neuropsychol* 5:629–676, 1988.
74. Schwartz MF, Saffran EM, Fink RB, et al: Mapping therapy: A treatment program for agrammatism. *Aphasiology* 8:19–54, 1994.
75. Miyake A, Carpenter PA, Just MA: A capacity approach to syntactic comprehension disorders: Making normal adults perform like aphasics. *Cognit Neuropsychol* 11:671–717, 1994.
76. Blackwell A, Bates E: Inducing agrammatic profiles in normals: evidence for the selective vulnerability of morphology under cognitive resource limitation. *J Cogn Neurosci* 7:228–257, 1995.
77. Pulvermüller F: Agrammatism: Behavioral description and neurobiological explanation. *J Cogn Neurosci* 7:165–181, 1995.
78. Bever TG: The cognitive basis for linguistic structures, in Hayes JR (ed): *Cognition and the Development of Language.* New York: Wiley, 1970.

79. Schwartz MF, Saffran EM, Marin OSM: The word order problem in agrammatism: 1. Comprehension. *Brain Lang* 10:263–288, 1980.
80. Berndt RS, Mitchum CC, Haendiges AN: Comprehension of reversible sentences in "agrammatism." *Cognition*. In press.
81. Kolk H, Van Grunsven MJE: Agrammatism as a variable phenomenon. *Cogn Neuropsychol* 2:347–384, 1985.
82. Saffran EM: Short-term memory impairment and language processing, in Caramazza A (ed): *Advances in Cognitive Neuropsychology and Neurolinguistics.* Hillsdale, NJ: Erlbaum, 1990.
83. Saffran EM, Marin OSM: Immediate memory for word lists and sentences in a patient with deficient auditory short-term memory. *Brain Lang* 2:420–433, 1975.
84. Vallar G, Baddeley AD: Phonological short-term store, phonological processing and sentence comprehension: A neuropsychological case study. *Cognit Neuropsychol* 1:121–142, 1984.
85. Saffran EM, Martin N: Short-term memory impairment and sentence processing, in Vallar G, Shallice T (eds): *Neuropsychological Impairments of Short Term Memory.* Cambridge, England: Cambridge University Press, 1990.
86. Butterworth B, Campbell R, Howard D: The uses of short-term memory: A case study. *Q J Exp Psychol* 38:705–737, 1986.
87. Martin RC: Articulatory and phonological deficits in short-term memory and their relation to syntactic processing. *Brain Lang* 32:159–192, 1987.
88. Marslen-Wilson W, Tyler LK: The temporal structure of spoken language understanding. *Cognition* 8:1–71, 1980.
89. Caplan D: *Language: Structure, Processing and Disorders.* Cambridge, MA: MIT Press, 1992.
90. Gathercole SE, Baddeley AD: *Working Memory and Language*. Hillsdale, NJ: Erlbaum, 1993.
91. Butterworth B, Howard D: Paragrammatisms. *Cognition* 26:1–38, 1987.
92. LaPointe S, Dell GS: A synthesis of some recent work on sentence production, in Tanenhaus MK, Carlson G (eds): *Linguistic Structure in Language Processing.* Dordrecht: Kluwer, 1988.
93. Menn L, Obler LK (eds): *Agrammatic Aphasia: A Cross-Language Narrative Sourcebook.* Philadelphia: John Benjamins, 1990.
94. Bock JK: Syntactic persistence in language production. *Cognit Psychol* 18:355–387, 1986.
95. Bock JK: Structure in language: Creating form in talk. *Am Psychol* 45:1221–1236, 1990.
96. Saffran EM, Schwartz MF, Marin OSM: Evidence from aphasia: Isolating the components of a production model, in Butterworth B (ed): *Language Production.* London: Academic Press, 1980, pp 221–240.
97. Nespoulous J-L, Dordain M, Perron C, et al: Agrammatism in sentence production without comprehension deficits: reduced variability of syntactic structures and/or of grammatical morphemes? A case study. *Brain Lang* 33:273–295, 1988.
98. Saffran EM, Berndt RS, Schwartz MF: A scheme for the quantitative analysis of agrammatic production. *Brain Lang* 37:440–479, 1989.
99. Plaut D, Shallice T: Deep dyslexia: A case study of connectionist neuropsychology. *Cognit Neuropsychol* 10:377–500, 1993.
100. Hinton GE, Shallice T: Lesioning an attractor network: Investigations of acquired dyslexia. *Psychol Rev* 98:74–95, 1991.
101. Shallice T, Warrington EK: Single and multiple component central dyslexic syndromes, in Coltheart M, Patterson KE, Marshall JC (eds): *Deep Dyslexia.* London: Routledge, 1980, pp 119–145.
102. Farah MJ: Neuropsychological inference with an interactive brain: a critique of the "locality assumption." *Behav Brain Sci* 17:43–104, 1994.
103. Dell GS, Schwartz MF, Martin N, et al: Lesioning a connectionist model of lexical retrieval to simulate naming errors in aphasia. Presented at conference on Neural Modeling of Cognitive and Brain Disorders; June 9, 1995; College Park, MD.
104. MacDonald MC, Pearlmutter NJ, Seidenberg MS: Lexical nature of syntactic ambiguity resolution. *Psychol Rev* 101:676–703, 1994.
105. Howard D, Hatfield FM: *Aphasia Therapy: Historical and Contemporary Issues.* Hillsdale, NJ: Erlbaum, 1987.
106. Heilman KM, Scholes RJ: The nature of comprehension errors in Broca's conduction, and Wernicke's aphasics. *Cortex* 12:258–265, 1976.
107. Grodzinsky Y: The syntactic characterization of agrammatism. *Cognition* 16:99–120, 1984.
108. Kay J, Lesser R, Coltheart M: *Psycholinguistic Assessment of Language Processing in Aphasia (PALPA).* London: Erlbaum, 1992.

Chapter 13

REHABILITATION OF APHASIA*

Myrna F. Schwartz
Ruth B. Fink

It is widely accepted that the goal of aphasia rehabilitation is to maximize functional communication skills. There is less agreement on the optimal route to that goal. Speech-language pathologists are exposed to a broad range of approaches and are expected to make informed decisions about the best treatment for an individual patient based on a number of factors (e.g., etiology, severity, and type of aphasia). They are trained to view aphasia as a complex cognitive/linguistic/communication disorder requiring intervention that addresses the social, as well as the linguistic, needs of the client,[1,2] and they work with patients in a variety of settings (acute care hospitals, rehabilitation units, home care, and outpatient facilities) throughout the phases of recovery.

Differences aside, speech-language pathologists typically perform three basic functions: assessment, treatment, and outcome evaluation. The initial assessment is critical for establishing the diagnosis of aphasia and differentiating it from other neuropathologies such as dementia and dysarthria, communicating with other professionals and the patient's family, and setting goals and developing a treatment plan. Following a program of treatment, an outcome evaluation is performed to determine how well the goals have been met. Each of these three functions (assessment, treatment, and outcome evaluation) is carried out at several levels of analysis.

LEVELS OF ANALYSIS: IMPAIRMENT, ACTIVITY LIMITATION, PARTICIPATION RESTRICTION

The World Health Organization (WHO)[3] has proposed a useful framework which distinguishes three levels at which functioning and disability may be described and explained: *impairment, activity limitation,* and *participation restriction*. These levels replace those used in the 1980 *WHO International Classification of Impairment, Disability and Handicap* (ICIDH)[4] and reflect a revision in the classification system. The new (ICIDH-2)[3] terminology extends the meanings to include descriptions of positive as well as negative experiences, as shown below.

ICIDH	*ICIDH-2*
Impairment	Body structure and function (impairment)
Disability	Activity (activity limitation)
Handicap	Participation (participation restriction)

Impairment refers to "problems in body function or structure such as significant deviation or loss" (Ref. 3, p. 13). The classic taxonomy of aphasia (Broca's aphasia, Wernicke's aphasia, conduction aphasia, anomic aphasia) rests on a mix of anatomic-psychological impairment symptoms [e.g., disruption of auditory-phonologic images caused by lesions in the left posterior temporal gyrus (Wernicke's area)]. The contemporary cognitive neuropsychological approach, which we focus on in later sections, derives its impairment categories from cognitive and psycholinguistic theories of the normal language system.

Activity limitation (formerly *disability*) refers to an individual's competence in executing a skill or activity. While the characterization of impairments is theory dependent, *activity limitation* refers to categories of behavior that have strong face validity, such as producing and understanding speech, reading, or writing. When speech pathologists characterize an aphasic disturbance, they generally do so in terms of its impact on skills like these. On the other hand, such

* **ACKNOWLEDGMENTS:** Preparation of this manuscript was supported by NIH grants 1R01 DC01825 and DC00191. Jessica Myers and Jennifer Bender provided invaluable assistance.

characterizations often also make reference to the units affected (e.g., word, phrase, sentence), in which case it becomes difficult to distinguish this level of description from the impairment level. In general, however, activity limitations are observable at the level of the person while the presence of an impairment is inferred from diagnostic tests that reflect on the functioning of a body organ or system.

Participation restriction (formerly *handicap*) refers to involvement in life situations or capacity to function in society. When communication is compromised by a speech/language disability (e.g., nonfluent speech) such that the individual can no longer function effectively in his or her role as parent, spouse, lawyer, etc., a participation restriction is present. The degree of restriction depends upon factors both within and external to the individual. These include the severity of the disability; the intactness of other avenues of communication, such as writing or gesturing; the readiness of others to shoulder the burden of communication; and the ability to use, and to afford, alternate communication systems like computers or communication boards. Participation restrictions are thus affected by social factors or barriers (structural or attitudinal) which limit fulfillment of roles or deny access to services and opportunities. They are observed at the interface of the individual and environment.

THE TRADITIONAL LANGUAGE-ORIENTED SCHOOL OF APHASIA THERAPY

In aphasia rehabilitation, any one of these three levels may be targeted for assessment, treatment, and outcome evaluation. The impairment-activity-participation matrix shown in Fig. 13-1 represents the various possibilities[5] and the shaded cells locate the endeavor we term the *traditional language-oriented school*. The majority of clinicians in the United States would probably identify themselves with this school, which is eclectic in its approach to assessment and treatment. Assessment draws upon standardized instruments that measure loss at both the activity and impairment level (e.g., Boston Diagnostic Aphasia Examination,[6] Western Aphasia Battery,[7] Minnesota Test for Differential Diagnosis of Aphasia[8]). The assessment serves as a guide to treatment, which might target several impairments concurrently or bypass the impairment level altogether in favor of direct retraining or stimulation of the compromised language skill. Both the target of treatment and the treatment techniques are tailored to the needs of the individual patient. The clinician may chose from several approaches. For example, the "stimulation" approach advocated by Schuell and colleagues[9] uses intensive auditory or multimodality input to elicit language production through a variety of means (e.g., repetition, phonemic cueing, reading) and in a variety of contexts (linguistic and situational). Helm-Estabrooks developed a variant of this technique to facilitate sentence production. Helm's Elicited Language Program for Syntax Stimulation (HELPSS)[10] uses a combined delayed repetition/story elicitation procedure to stimulate production of specific syntactic structures (e.g., yes-no questions; passive voice constructions) in aphasics with grammatical disturbances. The rationale behind the stimulation approach is that aphasia represents reduced access or efficiency. An alternative view is that specific aspects of the language system are lost or disrupted. This view is represented in Shewan and Bandur's "language-oriented therapy,"[11] a comprehensive, psycholinguistically based treatment program that aims to strengthen the impaired function(s) using training methods derived from behavioral learning theory. The common thread among these different approaches is the focus on restoration of language skills as the route to improved functional communication.

The same language-oriented assessments used to evaluate the patient's initial status are generally used as well to measure the gains made in treatment. But this alone does not constitute outcome evaluation. Also required is an assessment of the extent to which the *functional goals* projected for the patient at the outset have been met.

Medicare guidelines[12] specifically require that a plan of treatment state functional goals and estimated rehabilitation potential: "Functional goals must be written by the speech and language pathologist to reflect the level of communicative independence the patient is expected to achieve, outside of the therapeutic environment. The long-term functional goals must

Figure 13-1
The impairment-activity-participation (ICIDH-2) matrix. Assessment, treatment, and outcome evaluation can be directed at any of the three levels. The traditional, language-oriented school of aphasia rehabilitation focuses primarily on the impairment and activity levels.

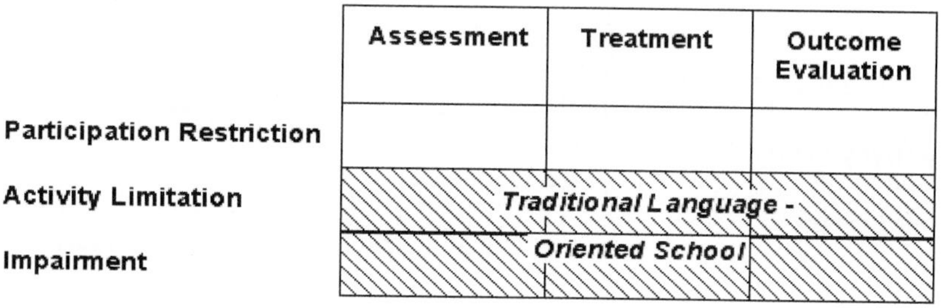

	Assessment	Treatment	Outcome Evaluation
Participation Restriction			
Activity Limitation	*Traditional Language -*		
Impairment	*Oriented School*		

reflect the final level the patient is expected to achieve, be realistic, and have a positive effect on the quality of the patient's everyday functions."

To assess whether functional goals have been met, clinicians often rely on anecdotal reports from patients and family members. While formal assessments of functional communication are available (e.g., Functional Communication Profile,[13] Communicative Abilities in Daily Living,[14] Communicative Effectiveness Index,[15] ASHA's Functional Communication Scales for Adults[16]), many clinicians find that these instruments lack the requisite sensitivity or are too cumbersome to administer.[17] A new generation of functional assessments is being developed to better meet the needs of the clinic in documenting change associated with communication training. For example, conversational analysis[18,19] and discourse assessments (Assessment Profile of Pragmatic Language Skills,[20] Discourse Abilities Profile[21]) offer structured ways of assessing change in narrative and conversational discourse. Rating scales[15,22] and questionnaires[23] measure quality of life, ability to perform various communication tasks, and participation in social activities and social functioning.

That language-oriented therapy succeeds in enhancing the language skills of treated patients is demonstrated in a number of large-scale group studies,[24–28] as well as smaller, more focused studies.[29–33] There is less evidence that these gains translate into expanded participation and enhanced quality of life. Indeed, the general view is that language gains evident in the clinic do not generalize well to less constrained tasks or settings.[34] This is one problem with the traditional, language-oriented school of aphasia therapy. A second is its weak theoretical base. Two newer schools have arisen in response to these perceived weaknesses: the functional/pragmatic/social school and the cognitive neuropsychological school.

THE FUNCTIONAL/PRAGMATIC/SOCIAL SCHOOL OF APHASIA THERAPY

If linguistic gains made in the clinic do not automatically translate into improved functional communication, then perhaps functional carryover should be programmed in as an integral part of the rehabilitation process. For adherents of the functional/pragmatic/social school, this means gearing therapy toward the enhancement of *communication*, nonverbal as well as verbal, in functional settings and/or with functional materials. Functional/pragmatic approaches typically capitalize on the patients' strengths and seek to train patients to use compensatory strategies when communicating. They may also involve use of behavioral methodology to achieve changes in pragmatic skills, as Doyle et al.[35] demonstrated in a study aimed at teaching patients with Broca's aphasia to make requests. The point of functional/pragmatic treatments is to develop communication skills that can be used in everyday life. The most widely known program of this type is Promoting Aphasics Communicative Effectiveness (PACE),[36] which fosters the communication of new information (the patient conveys a message unknown to the therapist, who must then figure it out) using whatever combination of strategies (verbal, written, gestural, graphic) achieves success. Another functional/pragmatic program, conversational coaching,[37]

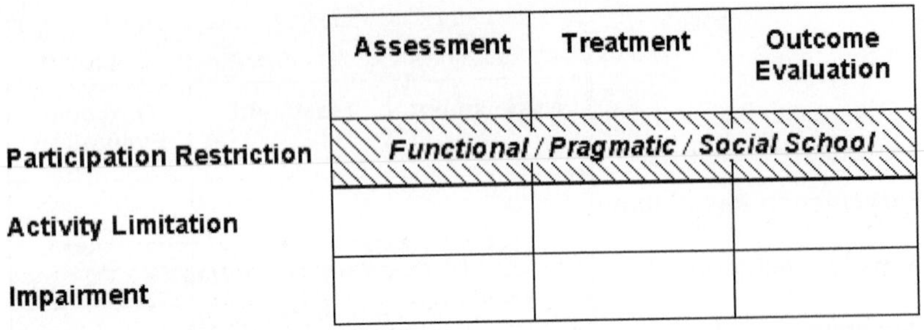

	Assessment	Treatment	Outcome Evaluation
Participation Restriction	*Functional / Pragmatic / Social School*		
Activity Limitation			
Impairment			

Figure 13-2
The functional/pragmatic/social school of aphasia rehabilitation focuses primarily on the level of participation restriction.

develops compensatory strategies in treatment sessions that simulate conversations that might take place outside the clinic. These include conversations with unfamiliar listeners to further extend generalization. Ultimately, the patient and his or her relatives are trained to use these strategies to communicate with maximum effectiveness.

Training aphasic patients to get their message across using compensatory strategies and multiple modalities is now a staple of most treatment programs. In recent years, however, there has been a growing movement toward "social" or "life participation" approaches to aphasia. These approaches have developed in response to the unmet needs and rights of those affected by aphasia and are in keeping with the disability movement and the revised WHO ICIDH-2 classification. The social approach, as we will call it, is a natural outgrowth of the functional/pragmatic school. It addresses activity and participation issues directly, by emphasizing the context in which communication occurs and involving family members and/or peers within the community. Treatment is not intended to make the person "talk" better. It is designed to improve the quality of interactions between individuals with aphasia and their communication partners. To this end, programs such as Communication Partners,[38] Supported Conversation for Adults with Aphasia (SCA),[39] family member training,[40,41] and Family Intervention in Chronic Aphasia (FICA)[42,43] train family members and other partners to take greater responsibility for facilitating and supporting the communicative exchanges. For example, in the FICA program, partners learn to identify facilitative and nonfacilitative behaviors, first in videotaped conversations, and then in actual conversations. (Nonfacilitative behavior includes such things as asking questions whose answers are already known; interrupting and correcting the aphasic partner during a successful communication effort.) Subsequently, partners engage in "negative practice," wherein they deliberately employ nonfacilitative behaviors and explore the degree to which these behaviors impede the success of the interaction.

Preliminary research on the FICA program indicates that (1) education (e.g., disseminating and discussing information) alone is not sufficient for altering interaction patterns; (2) an increase in facilitative behaviors and decrease in nonfacilitatory behaviors occurs within 3 to 5 weeks of direct behavior training; and (3) changes in the quality of communicative interactions are recognized by uninvolved observers.[42,43]

In its pure form (depicted in Fig. 13-2), the functional/pragmatic/social school replaces the traditional emphasis on language impairment and disability with an emphasis on minimizing handicap through enhanced communication, activity, and participation. In actuality, however, even its strongest proponents advocate that pragmatic techniques be used in combination with language-based approaches.[37,44,45]

THE COGNITIVE NEUROPSYCHOLOGY (CN) SCHOOL

Cognitive neuropsychologists apply information-processing models of normal cognition to the analysis of disorders of higher cortical function, including language. Until recently, CN's major contribution to rehabilitation was the development of model-driven assessments for describing impairments. With increasing frequency, though, cognitive neuropsychologists are involving themselves in treatment. Speech-language pathologists have also begun to apply cognitive models

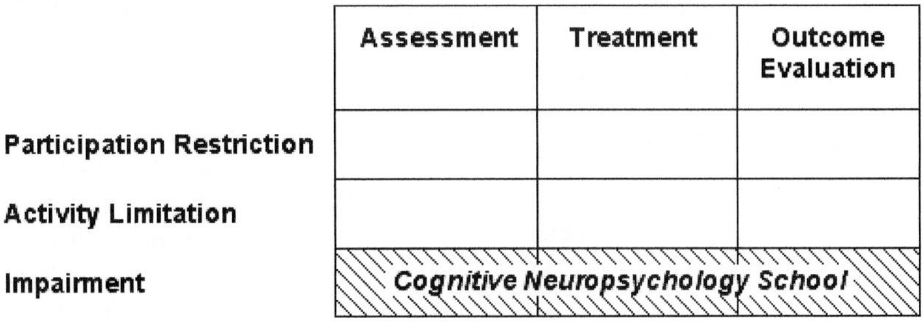

	Assessment	Treatment	Outcome Evaluation
Participation Restriction			
Activity Limitation			
Impairment	*Cognitive Neuropsychology School*		

Figure 13-3
The cognitive neuropsychology school of aphasia rehabilitation focuses primarily on the impairment level.

in the clinic. The basic idea is to pursue a more "rational" approach to treatment, in which the goals of the treatment program are informed by theory-based assessment of the patient's language capabilities.[46–48*]

CN assessments identify and measure impairments. It is not surprising, therefore, that impairments are also the focus of CN treatments and outcome evaluations. This restricted focus is in no way a necessary consequence of using cognitive theory to guide treatment, however. As noted by Caramazza,[49] the outcome of a cognitive assessment does not constrain the choice of therapeutic strategy; having characterized the patient's deficit at the level of impairment, one is perfectly free to target the level of activity or participation as the focus of treatment and/or outcome. Nevertheless, the bias in CN treatment research, if not in clinical practice, has been to target the impairment level as the focus for assessment, treatment, and outcome evaluation (Fig. 13-3).

Cognitive Neuropsychological Analysis Applied to Disorders of Word Retrieval (Anomia)

CN assessment begins where traditional assessment ends. For example, having identified a primary disorder of word retrieval, the CN-oriented clinician attempts to locate the deficit within the "functional architecture" of the language production system. The basic assumption is that one must probe for the explanation of a surface symptom like anomia; two patients with the same surface symptom may have very different underlying deficits. Probing for underlying deficits proceeds with reference to an information processing model, using tests and procedures specifically developed with the model in mind.

Figure 13-4 presents a schematic version of a model that has been very influential in the analysis of word retrieval deficits and, in particular, deficits in picture naming.[50–52] The model subdivides word retrieval into two temporally distinct stages, each of which accomplishes a transcoding, or "mapping," from one type of representation to another. The first stage takes place within the "semantic lexicon"; here, the semantic code that defines the word's meaning is mapped into a phonologic address that provides key information about the word's pronunciation, for example, the initial sound in the word, the number of syllables it contains, and its stress pattern. The second stage takes place

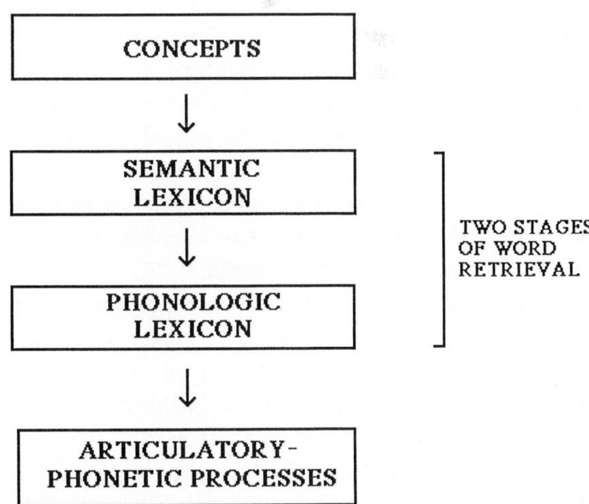

Figure 13-4
Schematic version of the two-stage model of word retrieval.

* The journal *Neuropsychological Rehabilitation* has devoted two special issues to the topic of cognitive neuropsychology and language rehabilitation: volume 5, issue 1/2 (March 1995) and volume 10, issue 3 (June 2000).

within the "phonologic lexicon." Here, the phonologic address for each known word is mapped onto an ordered string of phonemes specifying the full pronunciation, albeit still in a form more abstract than what the articulatory-motor system can take as input. The transcoding from a phonemic to articulatory-motor representation occurs at a subsequent step of word production. Disruption of this last step results in verbal "apraxia" of the sort we see in nonfluent (Broca's) aphasia. The types of word retrieval disorders that are of concern to us here are those that arise earlier in the process, at the first or second word-retrieval stage.

Various diagnostic tests are used to locate a picture naming deficit at one or the other of these stages (or both). Briefly, when we find that a patient's comprehension of pictures is unimpaired but he or she nevertheless makes semantic errors in naming (e.g., *horse* for *cow*), we immediately think of a problem in the semantic lexicon. If the patient makes semantic errors in comprehension as well as production, it is likely that the meaning representations in the semantic lexicon are degraded.[53] A patient studied by Howard and Orchard-Lisle[54] could not generate any names unless cued with the first phoneme of the target; when this patient was cued with the first phoneme of a semantically related word (e.g., shown a lion and cued with *t*), she showed a reliable tendency to produce the semantic substitution (*tiger*) and to accept that as the correct response. The implication of this "miscueing" effect is that degradation of semantic lexical entries resulted in the subthreshold activation of multiple entries in the semantic lexicon, and hence multiple phonologic addresses. Phonemic cues raised the activation value of corresponding addresses to threshold level; when the cue corresponded to the target, the correct name was produced; when it corresponded to a semantic coordinate, a semantic error was produced.

Many anomic patients can be cued phonemically to the correct target but do not show miscueing. Such patients are frequently able to provide partial information about the names they are unable to retrieve (e.g., that it is a long word or short word), and their errors, when they make them, bear a phonologic, rather than semantic, relation to the target.[55] These are indications that the problem arises in the retrieval of the full phonologic form, at the level of the phonologic lexicon.

Implications for Treatment of Word-Retrieval Deficits

The previous section illustrates the type of evidence that is used to locate a naming deficit within a functional model of the intact system. Reasoning about the treatment implications of such an analysis might proceed as follows: Patients whose deficits are centered in the semantic lexicon, i.e., in the semantic specification of words or the phonologic addressing mechanism, should benefit from interventions that encourage semantic processing of pictures in conjunction with phonologic processing of their names. A standard way of accomplishing this is to have the patient match pictures to written words, at least some of which bear a semantic relationship to the target name. The semantic component of such tasks should be less important for patients whose deficits are centered in the phonologic lexicon. These patients should benefit as much from purely phonologic techniques, such as oral reading, repeating the target name, or making a rhyme judgment.

A few studies have tested this model-driven prediction directly.[56–58] The conclusion at this point seems to be that patients with pure phonologic deficits do, as predicted, benefit from purely phonologic treatments. However, at least some patients with semantic involvement also benefit from phonologic techniques, which, if not pure, require only minimal semantic processing (e.g., responding to sentence-completion cues). It may be the key ingredient in phonologic techniques for patients with semantic or multilevel impairments is having some opportunity to strengthen the connections between corresponding entries in the semantic and phonologic lexicons.

Most CN treatment studies have not tested the model-based predictions directly. A number have assessed the short- and long-term effects of semantic and phonologic techniques in groups of subjects with undifferentiated naming deficits.[59,60] The results of these studies have generally favored semantic over phonologic techniques. Other studies have used the model-driven analysis to suggest the type of intervention called for (semantic or phonologic) in single cases or small homogeneous groups, but without examining whether the alternative approach would have been less successful. (Examples of these model-driven studies can be found in Refs. 56 to 58 and 61 to 71.)

Cumulatively, these CN-based studies provide conclusive evidence that anomia is amenable to treatment by a variety of semantic and phonologic techniques and that these benefits are maintained long after treatment ceases—as much as 1 year in the follow-up study reported by Pring and colleagues.[68] They also show that contrary to the findings of earlier single-exposure ("facilitation") studies[59,72] phonologic treatments have the potential to produce long-lasting effects and some degree of generalization. Further research is still needed to better understand who benefits from what treatment and what constitutes the "active ingredient" in each treatment.

Cognitive Neuropsychological Analysis Applied to Agrammatism

The term *agrammatism* refers to the simplification and fractionation of morphosyntactic structure in the speech of patients with nonfluent Broca's aphasia (see Table 13-1). The traditional, language-oriented approach to treating agrammatism uses combinations of

Table 13-1

Examples of G.R.'s picture description performance at three points in time[a]

TARGET	**THE BOY IS SLEEPING IN THE BED.**
PRE M	Sleep . . . boy . . . bed . . .
POST M	The man is sleeping.
POST V	The boy is sleeping.
TARGET	**THE GIRL IS GIVING FLOWERS TO THE TEACHER.**
PRE M	Girl and woman . . . flowers . . .
POST M	The . . . girls is washing . . . daisies.
POST V	The girl is . . . giving the papsies [poppies] to the teacher.
TARGET	**THE ROCK IS FALLING ON THE BOY.**
PRE M	Rock . . .
POST M	The . . . the rock is small big . . . big . . .
POST V	The rock is . . . putting on the man.
TARGET	**THE BOY IS GIVING A VALENTINE TO THE GIRL.**
PRE M	Boy is . . . valentine . . . and . . . girl . . .
POST M	The man . . . valentine's day . . .
POST V	1. The boy is giving the girl to the no . . . 2. The boy is holding the card to the girl . . . valentine. 3. The boy is holding the valentine of the girl.
TARGET	**THE TRUCK IS TOWING THE CAR.**
PRE M	One grutch [truck] and one car . . .
POST M	The truck is . . . the car . . .
POST V	The truck is towing the car.
TARGET	**THE BOY IS WATCHING TELEVISION.**
PRE M	Television and man . . .
POST M	The man is TV opening the TV.
POST V	The boy is . . . putting on the TV.
TARGET	**THE BALL IS HITTING THE BOY IN THE HEAD.**
PRE M	Baseball hit . . .
POST M	The baseball is . . . ah no . . .
POST V	The . . . ball is striking the . . . boy.

Source: From Fink et al,[94] with permission.

[a]Pre-mapping therapy (Pre M), 1/20/90; post-mapping therapy (Post M), 5/11/90; post-verb studies (Post V), 12/7/90.

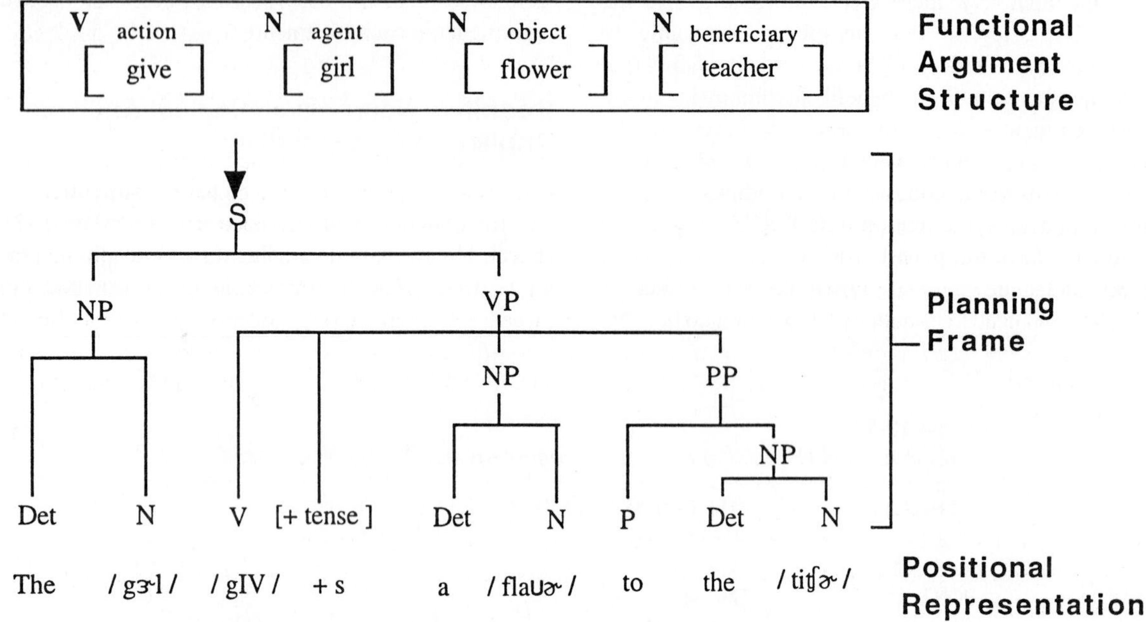

Figure 13-5
Schematic interpretation of Garrett's model of sentence production, applied to the sentence "The girl gives a flower to the teacher." The functional level contains content words only, and these are represented in the abstract format of the semantic lexicon. At the positional level, content words are represented in a phonologic format, while grammatical morphemes are represented more abstractly. S, sentence; NP, noun phrase; VP, verb phrase; PP, prepositional phrase; Det, determiner; N, noun; V, verb; P, preposition.

stimulation, repetition, and shaping techniques to facilitate production of affected structures. The CN approach aims deeper, at the underlying causes of the impaired production.

Psycholinguist Merrill Garrett[51,73] produced an account of sentence planning in normal speakers that has been very influential in the CN analyses of agrammatism. The model is illustrated in Fig. 13-5. The first stage involves formulation of the "functional argument structure" (alternatively, predicate- or verb-argument structure), which encodes the "who-is-doing-what-to whom" information in the sentence. The "positional representation" encodes the surface form of the sentence, including the left-to-right order of the content words and the form as well as placement of the grammatical morphemes. Mapping from the functional to positional level is accomplished by means of "planning frames."

The diverse symptoms of agrammatism are associated with one or another stage of sentence planning. Problems in selecting or pronouncing grammatical morphemes are thought to arise at or after the creation of the positional level. Problems in retrieving verbs and their associated argument structures arise earlier, at the functional level, or in the mapping from the functional to the positional level. Schwartz and colleagues[74,75] have also identified faulty mapping between functional and positional representations as the basis for the syntactic comprehension disorder that often accompanies agrammatic speech.

The notion that a deficit in functional-positional level mapping is responsible for production and comprehension impairments in agrammatic aphasics motivated a number of treatment studies aimed at remediating the mapping deficit.[76–84] These "mapping treatments" represent a radical departure from traditional treatments for agrammatism. We illustrate the mapping-based approach with a 1986 case study by speech pathologist E. Jones.[80]

Jones's patient (B.B.) was a severely nonfluent agrammatic aphasic patient, who remained essentially at a single-word level 6 years after a left cerebrovascular accident despite many years of speech therapy. B.B.'s attempts at connected speech contained almost no verbs, but he was able to produce verbs on an action-naming test. Asked to describe pictures of simple transitive events, he had difficulty communicating the correct verb-argument structure. Even when supplied with the verb, he continued to have difficulty, for example, leaving out the subject (agent) or reversing the order of agent and object. Referring to the Garrett model, Jones interpreted these findings as evidence of a problem in the early stages of sentence planning, i.e., prior to the positional level.

In comprehension testing, B.B. was found to make errors in comprehending reversible sentences, ordering printed noun and verb constituents to convey the meaning of a picture, and rearranging printed phrases into sentences. Together with the production data, the findings are indicative of a deficit in mapping between sentence form (positional level) and sentence meaning (functional level).

To address this mapping deficit, Jones developed a highly structured treatment program using written sentences. B.B. was first trained to identify the verb in simple sentences, then to identify the arguments of the verb in response to probe questions: "Who (or what) is doing the action? To whom? Where?" After 3 months of this purely receptive treatment, B.B. demonstrated improved sentence comprehension for both written and spoken sentences. Moreover, his production improved as well, as indexed by increased use of correctly inflected verb phrases and increased use of prepositions, particles, and determiners. This improvement in production was noted in the home setting as well as on formal testing.

Jones's report was one of the first in a series of mapping therapy studies (see Refs. 76 to 79 and 81 to 84; for review, see Refs. 85 and 86). Most of these studies involved subjects with chronic aphasia who underwent detailed, model-driven assessments that yielded evidence consistent with a mapping deficit (e.g., impaired access to verbs and failure to comprehend semantically reversible sentences). In each case a program was designed to remediate the mapping deficit. The specifics of the programs differed, but the strategy employed by most was to focus the patient's attention on the verb (or preposition, as in the case of locative sentences like "The pencil is *in* the sink.") and the roles it assigns to other constituents in the sentence (for an alternative approach, see Refs. 79 and 82). In most of the studies, production was not trained directly. Nevertheless, there were posttreatment gains in production, particularly those measures of production that reflect functional-level processes (i.e., production of verb, number of arguments produced, reduction in word-order errors).

That a treatment program involving no production training can nonetheless improve production is a striking finding. One possible explanation is that mapping therapy reeducates patients in mapping rules,[76] which can then be applied across tasks. However, since mapping rules are at least partly verb-specific, one would expect only limited generalization to untrained verbs, which is contrary to the findings of Jones's and other mapping therapy studies (e.g., Ref. 76, case 1; Ref. 84). A more plausible explanation is that the knowledge needed to map correctly is present prior to training, but not fully utilized. By drawing the patient's attention to the verb and the meaning it confers on sentence constituents, mapping therapy may shift or facilitate the allocation of processing resources to these aspects of sentence processing. Future studies should help resolve these issues. In any case, it is worth underscoring that the extent of the generalization to untrained materials and tasks that has been reported in some mapping therapy studies is substantially greater than what has been found with more traditional approaches that seek to train production directly.

The effect of mapping therapy on sentence comprehension is less impressive. While a number of subjects showed gains in syntactic comprehension of active reversible sentences, the gains and generalization patterns were variable within and across studies. Furthermore, half of the subjects studied did not show notable gains in syntactic comprehension in spite of their gains in production. This finding has both theoretical and practical implications regarding the underlying nature of the mapping disorder and how best to treat it (see Refs. 82, 84, and 87 for discussion).

Although the results of mapping therapy studies have been generally promising, a number of points are worth mentioning. First, the sentence query approach is not suitable for those with more complicated impairments, and it has yet to be shown that a standardized mapping protocol can benefit the wide range of agrammatic presentations that come through the clinic. Indeed, since agrammatism is a multifaceted condition, no single approach is likely to benefit all that carry this diagnosis. For example, depending on the nature of the verb retrieval problem, different approaches may be called for. Consequently, a complete program for agrammatism will likely require not one, but a series of targeted interventions. (We return to this point below, in the section on modular treatments.)

COGNITIVE NEUROPSYCHOLOGY AND APHASIA REHABILITATION: AN EVALUATION

While the CN approach has much to offer the rehabilitation enterprise, it is not a panacea. Cognitive models are of great value in specifying the locus of impairment in a particular patient, as well as the residual areas of strength, but it still falls to the clinician to use her or his judgment and experience to arrive at the optimal program of treatment, that is, whether to attempt to remediate the impaired process(es) and, if so, how. Rehabilitationists are being challenged to develop theories of how the damaged brain relearns and reorganizes itself,[88,89] and it is not clear whether and how cognitive models can contribute to this process (but see Ref. 90 for an encouraging step in this direction).

The length of CN assessments and the need to tailor such assessments to individual patients is poorly suited to the exigencies of the clinic. The development of model-driven language assessments that are standardized and normed [e.g., Psycholinguistic Assessment of Language Processing in Aphasia (PALPA)][91] has been of great help in this regard. Even so, the CN approach is probably not appropriate for all individuals with aphasia. Pinpointing the functional locus of a deficit rests on a fair degree of selectivity: the more global the deficit, the more problematic the endeavor.

CN interventions may be of greatest value when used as part of a more comprehensive treatment program that aims to achieve maximal carryover to real-world settings.[92] Toward this end, we advocate an approach that uses CN-motivated treatments as the building blocks or "modules" of a comprehensive treatment program.[93]

THE MODULAR-TREATMENTS APPROACH

In preceding sections we have enumerated a set of impairment symptoms that derive from contemporary models of spoken language production. At the level of the lexicon there are symptoms bearing on the representation and retrieval of meaning, and of phonology. At the sentence level there are symptoms having to do with the verb and its argument structure, the mapping between this and surface syntax, and the retrieval and/or phonologic realization of grammatical morphemes. In other domains, too—spoken language comprehension, written language production and comprehension—CN studies have elucidated a relatively small set of impairment symptoms that accounts for much of the variability in how disabilities in these domains are expressed.

Most aphasic patients display multiple impairments in more than one domain. The particular combination of impairment symptoms determines the patient's clinical classification. But most impairment symptoms are not restricted to a single clinical classification. For example, the lexical-semantic impairment that compromises word retrieval is found in patients with Broca's, Wernicke's, and anomic aphasia.

The goal of a CN assessment is to determine which impairment symptoms are present in the patient and which are amenable to treatment. For many patients, treatment will then aim to strengthen the impaired processes, one at a time or concurrently. To assist the therapist in this enterprise, we advocate the development of semistandardized treatment "modules," each of which targets a different impairment symptom. Such treatments should be designed to serve as broad a segment of the aphasia population as evinces the target symptom. This can be accomplished by graduating the demands of the treatment task and using multimodality treatment materials whenever possible. In Schwartz et al.,[93] we illustrated the requirements of treatment modules with experimental and clinical protocols already in use.

The basic idea behind this modular approach is that model-driven treatments that target specific impairments may produce narrow gains; however, the cumulative impact of multiple treatments can be substantial. Consider the case of G.R., a severely agrammatical patient who was 7 years postonset when he joined our mapping therapy study.[84] Comparison of his sentence production before and after mapping therapy revealed nontrivial gains on a 20-item picture description test: the percentage of words in sentences increased from 52 to 88; and the percentage of syntactically well-formed sentences increased from 30 to 44. He continued to experience difficulty retrieving verbs, however: the number of verbs produced was 10 before training and 11 after training (maximum 18). We therefore followed mapping therapy with a verb-treatment program designed to facilitate verb retrieval in the context of sentence production.[94] In this study, we compared the effects of two facilitation techniques: a repetition priming technique and a direct production technique that employs cueing and modeling in the context of mapping-type probe questions. The second technique proved more effective in facilitating acquisition of a small set of training verbs and carryover to untrained verbs.

At the end of the verb-treatment study, the number of verbs in G.R.'s picture description attempts increased from 11 to 18, and the number of appropriate verbs increased from 9 to 14. Examples of his picture description attempts at each stage of the treatment program are shown in Table 13-1. Although this was not designed as a test of the modular treatment approach, the results demonstrate the cumulative effects of treatments targeted at specific impairment symptoms.

CONCLUSION

The ICIDH-2 matrix serves as a reminder that the components of aphasia rehabilitation—assessment, treatment, and outcome evaluation—take place at multiple levels of analysis. The different schools of aphasia rehabilitation assign particular emphasis to one or another level, but, in reality, they are not as distinct from one another as Figs. 13-1 to 13-3 suggest. CN is really a branch of the language-oriented school that advocates using cognitive and psycholinguistic theory to direct rehabilitation activities. And as language-oriented therapists turn their attentions to the upper right-hand cell of the ICIDH-2 matrix, which insurance providers are increasingly requiring them to do, they are likely to draw on the theoretical and practical tools of the functional/pragmatic/social school.

What should be clear even from this brief discussion is that the future of aphasia rehabilitation will be shaped by interactions among clinicians and researchers with diverse perspectives and expertise. And there is much that we have not touched upon: research in neural plasticity is changing the way we think about the brain's capacity for recovery and reorganization after damage (e.g., Refs. 95 and 96); neural models that learn, and that relearn after "lesioning," provide a testing ground for theories of cognitive rehabilitation[90]; and advances in psychopharmacology[97–100] and computer technology[101–106] offer new avenues for treatment. Translating these promising trends into improved care for the individual with aphasia requires opportunities for clinicians, cognitive scientists, and neuroscientists to interact with one another and funding mechanisms to support and sustain such interdisciplinary collaborations.

REFERENCES

1. Chapey R: An introduction to language intervention strategies in adult aphasia, in Chapey R (ed): *Language Intervention Strategies in Adult Aphasia,* 2d ed. Baltimore: Williams & Wilkins, 1986, pp 2–11.
2. Wepman J: Aphasia therapy: Some "relative" comments and some purely personal prejudices, in Sarno M (ed): *Aphasia: Selected Readings*. New York: Appleton-Century-Crofts, 1972.
3. World Health Organization: *International Classification of Functioning, Disability and Health* (prefinal draft). Geneva: 2000.
4. World Health Organization: *International Classification of Impairments, Disabilities, and Handicaps: A Manual of Classification Relating to the Consequences of Diseases*. Geneva: World Health Organization, 1980.
5. Schwartz MF, Whyte J: *Methodological Issues in Aphasia Treatment Research: The Big Picture*. NIDCD Monograph, vol 2. Publication No. 93-3424:17–23. Bethesda, MD: National Institutes of Health, 1992.

6. Goodglass H, Kaplan E: *Assessment of Aphasia and Related Disorders*. Philadelphia: Lea & Febiger, 1983.
7. Kertesz A: *Western Aphasia Test Battery*. New York: The Psychological Corporation, 1982.
8. Schuell H: *Minnesota Test for Differential Diagnosis of Aphasia*. Minneapolis: University of Minnesota Press, 1965.
9. Schuell H, Jenkins JJ, Jimenez-Pabon E: *Aphasia in Adults: Diagnosis, Prognosis, and Treatment*. New York: Harper and Row, 1964.
10. Helm-Estabrooks NA: *Helm Elicited Language Program for Syntax Stimulation (HELPSS)*. Austin, TX: Exceptional Resources, 1981.
11. Shewan C, Bandur D: *Treatment of Aphasia: A Language-Oriented Approach*. Boston: College-Hill Press, 1986.
12. *Medicare Intermediary Manual, Billing Procedures for Part B Outpatient Speech and Language Services, 3905.3*. Washington, DC: US Government Printing Office.
13. Sarno MT: *Functional Communication Profile*. New York: Institute of Rehabilitation Medicine, 1969.
14. Holland AL, Frattali C, Fromm, D: *Communicative Abilities in Daily Living: Manual*. Austin, TX: Pro-Ed, 1999.
15. Lomas J, Pickard L, Bester S, et al: The communicative effectiveness index: Development and psychometric evaluation of a functional communication measure for adult aphasia. *J Speech Hear Disord* 54:113–124, 1989.
16. Frattali C, Thompson C, Holland A, et al: The FACS of Life. ASHA FACS: A functional outcome measure for adults. *ASHA* 37:40–46, 1995.
17. Frattali C, Thompson CK, Wohl CB: Trends in functional assessment. *Am Speech Lang Hear Assoc Newsl* 4:4–9, 1994.
18. Boles L, Bombard T: Conversational discourse analysis: Appropriate and useful sample sizes. *Aphasiology* 12:547–670, 1998.
19. Damico JS, Oelschlager M, Simmons-Mackie N: Qualitative methods in aphasia research: Conversational analysis. *Aphasiology* 13:667–679, 1999.
20. Gerber SK, Gerland GB: Applied pragmatics in the assessment of aphasia. *Semin Speech Lang* 10:14–25, 1989.
21. Terrell BY, Ripich DN: Discourse competence as a variable in intervention. *Semin Speech Lang* 10:282–297, 1989.
22. Sarno JE, Sarno MT, Levita E: The functional life scale. *Arch Phys Med Rehabil* 54:214–220, 1973.
23. Willer B, Rosenthal M, Kreutzer JS, et al: Assessment of community integration following rehabilitation for traumatic brain injury. *J Head Trauma Rehabil* 8:75–87, 1993.
24. Basso A, Capitani E, Vignolo LA: Influence of rehabilitation on language skills in aphasic patients: A controlled study. *Arch Neurol* 36:190–196, 1979.
25. Poeck K, Huber W, Williams K: Outcome of intensive language treatment in aphasia. *J Speech Hear Disord* 54:471–479, 1989.
26. Shewan CM, Kertesz A: Effects of speech and language treatment on recovery of aphasia. *Brain Lang* 23:272–299, 1984.
27. Wertz RT, Collins MJ, Weiss D, Kurtze JF, et al: Veterans administration cooperative study on aphasia: A comparison of individual and group treatment. *J Speech Hear Res* 24:580–594, 1981.
28. Wertz RT, Weiss DG, Aten JL, et al: Comparison of clinic, home, and deferred language treatment for aphasia. *Arch Neurol* 43:653–658, 1986.
29. Doyle PJ, Bourgeois MJ: The effect of syntax training on adequacy of communication in Broca's aphasia: A social validation study, in Brookshire RH (ed): *Clinical Aphasiology*. Minneapolis: BRK Publishers, 1986, vol 16, pp 123–132.
30. Doyle PJ, Goldstein H, Bourgeois M: Experimental analysis of syntax training in Broca's aphasia: A generalization and social validation study. *J Speech Hear Disord* 52:143–156, 1987.
31. Fink RB, Schwartz MF, Rochon E, et al: Syntax stimulation revisited: An analysis of generalization of treatment effects. *Am J Speech Lang Pathol* 4:99–104, 1995.
32. Helm-Estabrooks NA, Ramsberger G: Treatment of agrammatism in long-term Broca's aphasia. *Br J Disord Commun* 21:39–45, 1986.
33. Thompson CK, McReynolds LV: Wh-interrogative production in agrammatic aphasia: An experimental analysis of auditory-visual stimulation and direct-production treatment. *J Speech Hear Res* 29:193–206, 1986.
34. Thompson CK: Generalization research in aphasia: A review of the literature, in Prescott T (ed): *Clinical Aphasiology*. Boston: College-Hill Publications, 1989, vol 18, pp 195–222.
35. Doyle P, Goldstein H, Bourgeois M, Nakles K: Facilitating generalized requesting behavior in Broca's aphasia: a generalization and social validation study. *J Speech Hear Disord* 22:157–170, 1989.
36. Davis GA, Wilcox MJ: *Adult Aphasia Rehabilitation: Applied Pragmatics*. San Diego, CA: College Hill, 1985.

37. Holland AL: Pragmatic aspects of intervention in aphasia. *J Neuroling* 6:197–211, 1991.
38. Lyon JG, Cariski D, Keisler L, et al: Communication partners: enhancing participation in life and communication for adults with aphasia in natural settings. *Aphasiology* 11:693–708, 1997.
39. Kagen A: Supported conversation for adults with aphasia: Methods and resources for training conversation partners. *Aphasiology* 12:816–831, 1998.
40. Hinckley JJ, Packard MEW: Family education seminars and social functioning of adults with chronic aphasia. *J Commun Disord* 34:241–254, 2001.
41. Simmons N, Kearns K, Potechin G: Treatment of aphasia through family member training, in Prescott T (ed): *Clinicial Aphasiology*. Austin, TX: Pro-Ed, 1987, vol 17, pp 106–116.
42. Rogers MA, Alarcon NB, Olswang LB: Aphasia management considered in the context of the World Health Organization model of disablements. *Phys Med Rehabil Clin North Am* 13:907–923, 1999.
43. Hickey E, Rogers MA, Alaron NB, et al: Social validity measures for family-based intervention for chronic aphasia (FICA): presentation. Clinical Aphasiology Conference. Asheville, NC, 1998.
44. Davis A: Pragmatics and treatment, in Chapey R (ed): *Language Intervention Strategies in Adult Aphasia,* 2d ed. Baltimore: Williams & Wilkins, 1986, pp 251–265.
45. Springer L, Glindemann R, Huber W, Williams K: How efficacious is PACE therapy when "language systematic training" is incorporated? *Aphasiology* 5:391–399, 1991.
46. Coltheart M: Editorial. *Cogn Neuropsychol* 1:1–8, 1984.
47. Mitchum CC, Berndt RS: Aphasia rehabilitation: An approach to diagnosis and treatment of disorders of language production, in Eisenbert MG (ed): *Advances in Clinical Rehabilitation*. New York: Springer-Verlag. 1989.
48. Seron X, Deloche G: Introduction, in Seron X, Deloche G (eds): *Cognitive Approaches in Neuropsychological Rehabilitation*. Hillsdale, NJ: Erlbaum, 1989, pp 1–16.
49. Caramazza A: Cognitive neuropsychology and rehabilitation: An unfulfilled promise? in Seron X, Deloche G (eds): *Cognitive Approaches in Neuropsychological Rehabilitation*. Hillsdale, NJ: Erlbaum, 1989, pp 383–398.
50. Butterworth B: Lexical access in speech production, in Marslen-Wilson W (ed): *Lexical Representation and Process*. Cambridge, MA: MIT Press, 1989, pp 108–135.
51. Garrett MF: Production of speech: observations from normal and pathological language use, in Ellis A (ed): *Normality and Pathology in Cognitive Functions*. London: Academic Press, 1982.
52. Levelt WJM: *Speaking: From Intention to Articulation*. Cambridge, MA: MIT Press, 1989.
53. Hillis A, Rapp B, Romani C, Carramazza A: *Selective Impairments of Semantics in Lexical Processing: Reports of the Cognitive Neuropsychology Laboratory*. Baltimore: Johns Hopkins University, 1989.
54. Howard D, Orchard-Lisle V: On the origin of semantic errors in naming: evidence from the case of a global aphasic. *Cogn Neuropsychol* 1:163–190, 1984.
55. Kay J, Ellis A: A cognitive neuropsychological case study of anomia. *Brain* 110:613–629, 1987.
56. Greenwald ML, Raymer AM, Richardson ME, Rothi LJG: Contrasting treatments for severe impairments of picture naming. *Neuropsychol Rehabil* 5:17–49, 1995.
57. Hillis AE, Caramazza A: Theories of lexical processing and rehabilitation of lexical deficits, in Riddoch MJ, Humphreys GW (eds): *Cognitive Neuropsychology and Cognitive Rehabilitation*. Hove, Sussex: Erlbaum: 1994, pp 449–484.
58. LeDorze G, Pitts C: A case study evaluation of the effects of different techniques for the treatment of anomia. *Neuropsychol Rehabil* 5:51–65, 1995.
59. Howard D, Patterson K, Franklin S, et al: The facilitation of picture naming in aphasia. *Cogn Neuropsychol* 2:48–80, 1985.
60. Howard D, Patterson K, Franklin S, et al: Treatment of word retrieval deficits in aphasia: A comparison of two therapy methods. *Brain* 108:817–829, 1985.
61. Fink RB, Brecher A, Schwartz MF: A computer implemented protocol for treatment of naming disorders: Evaluation of clinician-guided and partially self-guided instruction. *Aphasiology*. In press.
62. Hillis AE: Efficacy and generalization of treatment for aphasic naming errors. *Arch Phys Med Rehabil* 70:632–636, 1989.
63. Hillis AE: Effects of separate treatments for distinct impairments within the naming process, in Prescott T (ed): *Clinicial Aphasiology*. Austin, TX: Pro-Ed, 1991, vol 19, pp 255–265.
64. Marshall J, Pound C, White-Thomson M, Pring T: The use of picture/word matching tasks to assist word retrieval in aphasic patients. *Aphasiology* 4:167–184, 1990.
65. Miceli G, Amitrano A, Capasso R, Caramazza A: The remediation of anomia resulting from output lexical damage: analysis of two cases. *Brain Lang* 52:150–174, 1996.

66. Nettleton J, Lesser R: Therapy for naming difficulties in aphasia: Application of a cognitive neuropsychological model. *J Neuroling* 6:139–154, 1991.
67. Nickels L, Best W: Therapy for naming disorders: Part 2. Specifics, surprises and suggestions. *Aphasiology* 10:109–136, 1996.
68. Pring T, White-Thomson M, Pound C, et al: Short report: picture/word matching tasks and word retrieval. Some follow-up data and second thoughts. *Aphasiology* 4:479–483, 1990.
69. Raymer AM, Thompson CK, Jacobs B, LeGrand HR: Phonological treatment of naming deficits in aphasia: model-based generalization analysis. *Aphasiology* 7:27–53, 1993.
70. Robson J, Marshall J, Pring T, Chiat S: Phonological naming therapy in jargon aphasia: positive but paradoxical effects. *J Int Neuropsychol Soc* 4:675–686, 1998.
71. Wambaugh J, Doyle P, Linebaugh C: Effects of deficit oriented treatments on lexical retrieval in a patient with semantic and phonological deficits. *Brain Lang* 69:446–450, 1999.
72. Patterson KE, Purell C, Morton J: Facilitation of word retrieval in aphasia, in Code C, Muller DJ (eds): *Aphasia Therapy.* London: Arnold, 1983, pp 76–87.
73. Garrett MF: Levels of processing in sentence production, in Butterworth B (ed): *Language Production*. New York: Academic Press, 1980, vol 1, pp 177–220.
74. Linebarger MC, Schwartz MF, Saffran EM: Sensitivity to grammatical structure in so-called agrammatic aphasics. *Cognition* 13:361–392, 1983.
75. Schwartz MF, Linebarger MC, Saffran EM: The status of the syntactic deficit theory of aggrammatism, in Kean MC (ed): *Agrammatism.* New York: Academic Press, 1985, pp 83–124.
76. Byng S: Sentence processing deficits: theory and therapy. *Cogn Neuropsychol* 1988; 5:629–676.
77. Byng S, Nickels L, Black M: Replicating therapy for mapping deficits in agrammatism: remapping the deficit. *Aphasiology* 8:315–341, 1994.
78. Fink RB, Schwartz MF, Myers, JL: Investigations of the sentence-query approach to mapping therapy. *Brain Lang* 65:203–207, 1998.
79. Haendiges AN, Berndt RS, Mitchum CC: Assessing the elements contributing to a "mapping deficit": A targeted treatment study. *Brain Lang* 52:276–302, 1996.
80. Jones EV: Building the foundations for sentence production in a non-fluent aphasic. *Br J Disord Commun* 21:63–82, 1986.
81. LeDorze G, Jacob A, Coderre L: Aphasia rehabilitation with a case of agrammatism: A partial replication. *Aphasiology* 5:63–85, 1991.
82. Mitchum, CC, Haendiges AN, Berndt RS: Treatment of thematic mapping in sentence comprehension: Implications for normal processing. *Cogn Neuropsychol* 12:503–547, 1995.
83. Nickels L, Byng S, Black M: Sentence processing deficits: A replication of therapy. *Br J Disord Commun* 26:175–199, 1991.
84. Schwartz MF, Saffran EM, Fink RB, et al: Mapping therapy: A treatment program for agrammatism. *Aphasiology* 8:19–54, 1994.
85. Fink RB: Mapping treatment: an approach to treating sentence level impairments in agrammatism. *Am Speech Lang Hear Assoc Newsl* 11:14–23, 2001.
86. Marshall J: The mapping hypothesis and aphasia therapy. *Aphasiology* 9:517–539, 1995.
87. Mitchum CC, Greenwald ML, Berndt RS: Cognitive treatments of sentence processing disorders: What have we learned? *Neuropsychol Rehabil* 10(3):311–336, 2000.
88. Byng S: A theory of the deficit: A prerequisite for a theory of therapy? *Clin Aphasiol* 22:265–273, 1994.
89. Holland AL: Cognitive neuropsychological theory and treatment for aphasia: Exploring the strengths and limitations. *Clin Aphasiol* 22:275–282, 1994.
90. Plaut DC: Relearning after damage in connectionist networks: Toward a theory of rehabilitation. *Brain Lang* 52:25–82, 1996.
91. Kay J, Lesser R, Coltheart M: *Psycholinguistic Assessment of Language Processing in Aphasia*. East Sussex, England: Erlbaum, 1992.
92. Lesser R, Algar L: Towards combining the cognitive neuropsychological and the pragmatic in aphasia therapy. *Neuropsychol Rehabil* 5:67–92, 1995.
93. Schwartz MF, Fink RB, Saffran EM: The modular treatment of agrammatism. *Neuropsychol Rehabil* 5:93–127, 1995.
94. Fink RB, Martin N, Schwartz MF, et al: Facilitation of verb retrieval skills in aphasia: A comparison of two approaches. *Clin Aphasiol* 21:263–275, 1992.
95. Thomas C, Altenmuller E, Marckmann G, et al: Language processing in aphasia: Changes in lateralization patterns during recovery reflect cerebral plasticity in adults. *Electroencephalogr Clin Neurophysiol* 102:86–97, 1997.
96. Thulborn KR, Carpenter PA, Just MA: Plasticity of language-related brain function during recovery from stroke. *Stroke* 30:749–754, 1999.
97. Bragoni M, Altieri M, DiPiero V, et al: Bromocriptine and speech therapy in non-fluent chronic aphasia after stroke. *Neuroscience* 21:10–22, 2000.

98. Gold M, VanDam D, Silliman ER: An open label trial of Bromocriptine in non-fluent aphasia: A qualitative analysis of word storage and retrieval. *Brain Lang* 74:141–156, 2000.
99. Kessler J, Thiel A, Karbe H, Heis WD: Piracetam improves activated blood flow and facilitates rehabilitation of post stroke aphasic patients. *Stroke* 31:2112–2116, 2000.
100. Walker-Batson D, Curtis S, Natarajan R, et al: A double blind placebo-controlled study of the use of amphetamine in the treatment of aphasia. *Stroke* 32:2093–2098, 2001.
101. Aftonomos LB, Steele R, Wertz R: Promoting recovery in chronic aphasia with an interactive technology. *Arch Phys Med Rehabil* 78:841–846, 1997.
102. Crerar M, Ellis A, Dean E: Remediation of sentence processing deficits in aphasia using a computer-based microworld. *Brain Lang* 52:229–275, 1996.
103. Katz RC, Wertz T: The efficacy of computer-provided reading treatment for chronic aphasic adults. *J Speech Lang Hear Res* 40:493–507, 1997.
104. Linebarger MC, Schwartz MF, Kohn SE: Computer-based training of language production: An exploratory study. *Neuropsychol Rehabil* 11(1):57–96, 2001.
105. Linebarger MC, Schwartz MF, Romania JR, et al: Grammatical encoding in aphasia: Evidence from a "processing prosthesis." *Brain Lang* 75:416–427, 2000.
106. Weinrich M, McCall D, Weber C, et al: Training on an iconic communication system for severe aphasia can improve natural language production. *Aphasiology* 9(4):343–364, 1995.

Chapter 14

ACQUIRED DISORDERS OF READING

H. Branch Coslett

The study of acquired dyslexia or disorders of reading dates at least to the contributions of Déjerine, who, in 1891 and 1892, described two patients with quite different patterns of reading impairment. Déjerine's first patient[1] developed an impairment in reading and writing subsequent to an infarction involving the left parietal lobe. Déjerine termed this disorder "alexia with agraphia" and attributed the disturbance to a disruption of the "optical image for words," which he thought to be supported by the left angular gyrus. In an account that in some respects presages contemporary psychological accounts, Déjerine concluded that reading and writing required the activation of these "optical images" and that the loss of the images resulted in an inability to recognize or write familiar words.

Déjerine's second patient[2] was quite different. This patient was unable to read aloud or for comprehension but could write, a disorder that Déjerine designated "alexia without agraphia" (also known as agnosic alexia and pure alexia). The patient had a right homonymous hemianopia from a left occipital lesion, which included the fibers carrying visual information from the right to the left hemisphere. Déjerine explained alexia without agraphia in terms of a "disconnection" between visual information confined to the right hemisphere and the left angular gyrus, which he assumed to be critical for the recognition of words.

After the seminal contributions of Déjerine, the study of acquired dyslexia languished for decades, during which the relatively few investigations that were reported focused primarily on the anatomic underpinnings of the disorders. The study of acquired dyslexia was revitalized, however, by the elegant and detailed investigation by Marshall and Newcombe,[3] demonstrating that by virtue of a careful investigation of the pattern of reading deficits exhibited by dyslexic subjects, distinctly different and reproducible types of reading deficits could be elucidated. These investigators described a patient (GR) who read approximately 50 percent of concrete nouns but was severely impaired in the reading of abstract nouns and all other parts of speech. The most striking aspect of GR's performance, however, was his tendency to produce errors that appeared to be semantically related to the target word (e.g., *speak* read as "talk"). Marshall and Newcombe[3] designated this disorder "deep dyslexia." These investigators also described two patients whose primary deficit appeared to be an inability to derive the pronunciation of irregularly spelled words, such as "yacht." This disorder was designated "surface dyslexia."

On the basis of these data, Marshall and Newcombe[3] concluded that the meaning of written words could be accessed by two separate and distinct procedures. The first was a lexical (whole-word) procedure whereby familiar words activated the appropriate stored representation (or visual word form), which, in turn, activated meaning; reading in deep dyslexia was assumed to involve this procedure, labeled A in Fig. 14-1.

The second procedure was assumed to be a phonologically based process in which "grapheme-to-phoneme" (hereafter termed "print-to-sound") correspondences were employed to derive the appropriate phonology (that is, "sound out" the word); the reading of surface dyslexics was assumed to be mediated by this nonlexical procedure, labeled B in Fig. 14-1. Although a number of Marshall and Newcombe's specific hypotheses have been criticized, their argument that reading may be mediated by two distinct procedures has received considerable empirical support. Indeed, although it has occasionally been questioned,[4,5] the dual-route model of reading has provided the conceptual framework that has motivated most subsequent studies of acquired dyslexias and animates the present discussion.

In this chapter we briefly summarize the clinical features and conceptual basis of the major types of acquired dyslexia. Additionally, the possible role of

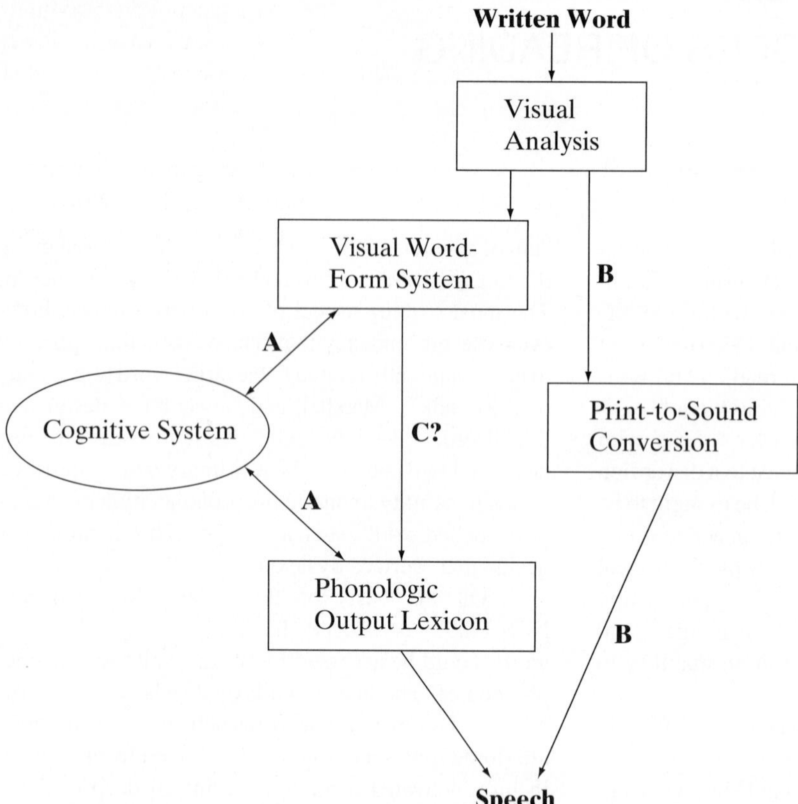

Figure 14-1
A diagram of an information-processing model of reading incorporating three procedures for oral reading.

the right hemisphere in reading is briefly discussed. Finally, recent efforts to develop computational models of normal reading and acquired dyslexia are briefly described.

PERIPHERAL DYSLEXIAS

A useful starting point in the discussion of the dyslexias is the distinction offered by Shallice and Warrington[6] between "peripheral" and "central" dyslexias. The former are conditions characterized by a deficit in the processing of visual aspects of the stimulus that interferes with matching the familiar word to its stored orthographic representation or "visual word form."[6] Central dyslexias, in contrast, are attributable to an impairment of "deeper" or "higher" reading mechanisms by means of which visual word forms gain access to meaning or speech production mechanisms. The major types of peripheral dyslexia are briefly described below.

Alexia without Agraphia (Pure Alexia)

The classic syndrome of alexia without agraphia or pure alexia is perhaps the prototypical peripheral dyslexia. As noted above, the traditional account[2,7] of this disorder attributes the syndrome to a "disconnection" of visual information, which is restricted to the right hemisphere, from the left-hemispheric word-recognition system.

Though these patients do not appear to be able to read in the sense of fast, automatic word recognition, many are able to use a compensatory strategy that involves naming the letters of the word in serial fashion; they read, in effect, letter by letter. Using the slow and inefficient letter-by-letter procedure, pure alexics typically exhibit significant effects of word length, requiring more time to read long as compared to short words. In contrast to the central dyslexias, performance is typically not influenced by linguistic factors such as parts of speech (e.g., noun versus functor), the extent to which the referent of the word is concrete (e.g., *table*) or abstract (e.g., *destiny*), or whether the word is orthographically regular (that is, can be "sounded out").

A number of alternative accounts of the processing deficit in pure alexia have been proposed. Thus, some investigators have proposed that the impairment is attributable to a limitation in the transmission of letter identity information to the visual word system,[8] an inability to directly encode visual letters as abstract orthographic types,[9,10] or an inability to encode multiple visual shapes of any sort in rapid succession.[11,12] Other investigators have argued that the disorder is attributable to a disruption of the visual word-form system itself.[13,14]

Although most reports of pure alexia have emphasized the profound nature of the reading deficit, often stating that patients were utterly incapable of reading without recourse to a letter-by-letter strategy,[7,8] a number of investigators have reported data demonstrating that at least some pure alexic patients are able to comprehend words that they are unable to explicitly identify.[15–17] This capacity has been attributed by some investigators (e.g., Ref. 17) to the operation of a reading procedure based in the right hemisphere.

The anatomic basis of pure alexia has been extensively investigated. Although on rare occasions associated with lesions that "undercut" or disconnect the posterior perisylvian cortex on the left,[18] the disorder is typically associated with a lesion in the posterior portion of the dominant hemisphere, which compromises visual pathways in the dominant hemisphere and disrupts white matter tracts (such as the splenium of the corpus callosum or forceps major) critical for the interhemispheric transmission of visual information.[19,20]

Neglect Dyslexia

Neglect dyslexia, which is most commonly encountered in patients with left-sided neglect, is characterized by a failure to explicitly identify the initial portion of a letter string. Interestingly, the performance of patients with neglect dyslexia is often influenced by the nature of the letter string; thus, patients with this disorder may fail to report the initial letters in nonwords (e.g., the "ti-" in a nonword such as "tiggle") but read real words (e.g., "giggle") correctly (Ref. 21; see also Refs. 22 and 23). The fact that performance is affected by the lexical status of the stimulus has been taken to suggest that neglect dyslexia is not attributable to a failure to register letter information but reflects an attentional impairment at a higher level of representation (see also Chap. 10).

Although neglect dyslexia is generally seen in the context of the neglect syndrome (see Chaps. 25 and 26), it has occasionally been observed in isolation or even in the context of neglect of the opposite side of space.[24]

Attentional Dyslexia

Perhaps the least studied of the acquired dyslexias, attentional dyslexia is characterized by the relative preservation of single-word reading in the context of a gross disruption of reading when words are presented in text or in the presence of other words or letters.[25–28] Patients with this disorder may also exhibit difficulties identifying letters within words, even though the words themselves are read correctly,[25] and be impaired in identifying words flanked by extraneous letters (e.g., "lboat"). We[28] have recently investigated a patient with attentional dyslexia secondary to autopsy-proven Alzheimer disease who produced frequent "blend" errors in which letters from one word of a two-word display intruded into the other word (e.g., "take lime" read as "tame"). Although several accounts for this disorder have been proposed, the disorder has been attributed by several investigators to an impairment in visual attention or a loss of location information. As visual attention may be critical to mapping the location of visually presented objects, these accounts are not clearly distinguishable.

CENTRAL DYSLEXIAS

In this section we briefly describe the clinical features and conceptual basis of the major types of central dyslexia including "deep," "phonologic," and "surface" dyslexia. Additionally, the phenomenon of "reading without meaning" is discussed.

Deep Dyslexia

Deep dyslexia, the most extensively investigated central dyslexia (see, for example, Coltheart and colleagues[29]) is in many respects the most compelling. The allure of deep dyslexia is due in large part to the intrinsically interesting hallmark of the syndrome, *semantic errors*. When shown the word *castle*, a deep dyslexic may respond "knight"; similarly, these interesting patients may read *bird* as "canary." At least for some deep dyslexics, it is clear that these errors are not circumlocutions and that the patients are not even aware that they have erred.

While semantic errors are typically regarded as essential for the diagnosis of deep dyslexia, the frequency with which deep dyslexics produce them is quite variable; for some patients, semantic errors may represent the most frequent error type, whereas for others they constitute a small proportion of reading errors. These patients also produce a variety of other types of reading errors, including "visual" errors in which the response bears a clear visual similarity to the target (e.g., *skate* read as "scale") and "morphologic" errors, in which a prefix or suffix is added, deleted, or substituted (e.g., *scolded* read as "scolds"; *governor* read as "government").

Additional hallmarks of the syndrome include a greater success in reading words of high as compared to low imageability. Thus, words such as *table, chair, ceiling,* and *buttercup,* the referents of which are concrete or imageable, are read more successfully by deep dyslexics than words such as *fate, destiny, wish,* and *universal,* the referents of which are abstract.

Also characteristic of the syndrome is part-of-speech effect, such that nouns are read more reliably than modifiers (adjectives and adverbs), which are, in turn, read more accurately than verbs. Deep dyslexics manifest particular difficulty in the reading of functors (a class of words that includes pronouns, prepositions, conjunctions, and interrogatives such as *that, which, they, because, under,* etc.). The striking nature of the part-of-speech effect is illustrated by the patient reported by Saffran and Marin[30] who correctly read the word *chrysanthemum* but was unable to read the *the*! Many errors to functors involve the substitution of a different functor (*that* read as *which*) rather than the production of words of a different class, such as nouns or verbs.

As functors are, in general, less imageable than nouns, verbs, or abjectives, some investigators have claimed that the apparent effect of part of speech is in reality a manifestation of the pervasive imageability effect described above.[31] We have reported a patient,[32] however, whose performance suggests that the part-of-speech effect is not simply a reflection of a more general deficit in the processing of low-imageability words, as the difference remained after functors and content words were matched for imageability.

Finally, all deep dyslexics exhibit a substantial impairment in the reading of nonwords; when confronted with letter strings such as *flig* or *churt,* deep dyslexics are typically unable to employ print-to-sound correspondences to derive phonology; nonwords frequently elicit "lexicalization" errors (e.g., *flig* read as "flag"), perhaps reflecting a reliance on lexical reading in the absence of access to reliable print-to-sound correspondences.

How can deep dyslexia be accommodated by the model of reading depicted in Fig. 14-1? Several alternative explanations have been proposed. Most investigators agree that multiple processing deficits must be hypothesized to account for the full range of symptoms found in deep dyslexia. First, the strikingly impaired performance in reading nonwords and other tasks assessing phonologic function suggests that the print-to-sound conversion procedure is disrupted. Second, the presence of semantic errors and the effects of imageability (a variable usually thought to influence processing at the level of semantics) have been interpreted by many investigators as evidence that these patients also suffer from a semantic impairment; it should be noted in this context, however, that some deep dyslexic patients perform well on tests of comprehension with words they are unable to read aloud. Semantic errors in these patients have been attributed to a deficit in or access to representations in the output phonologic lexicon (Ref. 33; see also Ref. 6). Last, the production of visual errors has been interpreted by some to suggest that these patients suffer from an impairment in the visual word-form system. Other investigators (e.g., Coltheart,[34] Saffran and coworkers[35]) have argued that deep dyslexics' reading is mediated by a system not normally used in reading—that is, the right hemisphere. We will return to the issue of reading with the right hemisphere below.

Although deep dyslexia has occasionally been associated with posterior lesions, this disorder is typically encountered in association with large perisylvian lesions extending into the frontal lobe. As might be expected given the lesion data, deep dyslexia is usually associated with global or Broca's aphasia but may rarely be encountered in patients with fluent aphasia.

Phonological Dyslexia: Reading without Print-to-Sound Conversion

First described in 1979 by Derouesne and Beauvois,[36] phonological dyslexia is, perhaps, the "purest" of the central dyslexias in that the syndrome appears to be attributable to a selective deficit at some stage in the procedure mediating the translation from print to sound. Thus, although in many respects less arresting than deep dyslexia, phonological dyslexia is of considerable theoretical import. It is of interest to note that the existence of this syndrome was *predicted* by dual-route accounts of reading similar to that proposed by Marshall and Newcombe[3] and subsequently identified when dyslexic patients were assessed with theoretically motivated tasks. It has since become the subject of intensive study by cognitive neuropsychologists interested in the organization of reading in the brain.[37]

Phonological dyslexia is a relatively mild disorder in which reading of real words may be only slightly impaired. Many patients with this disorder, for example, correctly read 85 to 95 percent of real words (e.g., Refs. 32, 36, 38). Some patients with this disorder read all different types of words with equal facility,[38–40] whereas other patients are relatively impaired in the reading of functors.[41,42] Unlike patients with surface dyslexia, described below, the regularity of print-to-sound correspondences is not relevant to the performance of phonological dyslexics; thus, these patients typically pronounce orthographically irregular words such as *colonel* and words with standard print-to-sound correspondences such as *administer* with equal facility. Most errors in response to real words appear to have a visual basis, often involving the substitution of visually similar real words (e.g., *topple* read as "table").

The striking and theoretically relevant aspect of the performance of phonological dyslexics is a substantial impairment in the oral reading of nonword letter strings. A number of investigators have described patients with this disorder, for example, who read more than 90 percent of real words of all types yet correctly pronounce only about 10 percent of nonwords.[32,36] Most errors in nonword reading involve the substitution of a visually similar real word (e.g., *phope* read as "phone") or the incorrect application of print-to-sound correspondences (e.g., *stime* read as "stim," rhyming with "him").

Within the context of the reading model depicted in Fig. 14-1, the account for this disorder is relatively straightforward. The patients' good performance with real words suggests that the processes involved in normal "lexical" reading—that is, visual analysis, the visual word-form system, semantics, and the phonological output lexicon—are at least relatively preserved. The impairment in nonword reading suggests that the print-to-sound translation procedure is disrupted.

A final point of interest is that a number of phonological dyslexics exhibit substantial deficits in processing morphologically complex words—that is, words with prefixes and suffixes.[38,42] The explanation for this association is not clear.

Phonological dyslexia has been observed in association with lesions in a number of sites in the dominant perisylvian cortex and, on occasion, with lesions of the right hemisphere (e.g., Ref. 42). Damage to the superior temporal lobe and angular and supramarginal gyri in particular is found in most but not all patients with this disorder. Although quantitative data are lacking, the lesions associated with phonological dyslexia appear to be smaller on average than those associated with deep dyslexia.

Just as there is variability with respect to the lesion site associated with phonological dyslexia, there is variability with respect to the type and severity of aphasia observed in these patients. A phonological dyslexic reported by Derouesne and Beauvois,[36] for example, did not exhibit a significant aphasia, whereas Funnell's patient W.B.[38] appears to have had a severe nonfluent aphasia.

Surface Dyslexia

Surface dyslexia is a disorder characterized by the inability to read words with "irregular" or exceptional print-to-sound correspondences. Patients with surface dyslexia are thus unable to read aloud words such as *colonel, yacht, island, have,* and *borough,* the pronunciation of which cannot be derived by phonological or "sounding out" strategies. In contrast, these patients read words containing regular correspondences (e.g., *state, hand, mint, abdominal*) as well as nonwords (e.g., *blape*) quite well.

As noted above, normal subjects may read familiar words by matching the letter string to a stored representation of the word and retrieving the pronunciation by means of a mechanism linked to semantics (or, as discussed below, by means of a nonsemantic "direct" route). As this procedure involves the activation of stored representations, the pronunciation of the word is not computed by rules but is retrieved; consequently, the regularity of print-to-sound correspondences would not be expected to play a major role in performance.

In the context of a dual-route model of reading, the sensitivity to the regularity of the print-to-sound correspondences provides prima facie evidence that the impairment in surface dyslexia is in the mechanism(s) mediating lexical reading. Similarly, the preserved ability to read regular words and nonwords provides compelling support for the claim that the procedures by which pronunciations are computed by the application of print-to-sound correspondences are at least relatively preserved.

Noting that there is substantial variability in the performance of surface dyslexics with respect to leading latencies as well as accuracy, Shallice and McCarthy[43] suggested that the syndrome of surface dyslexia be fractionated. Type 1 surface dyslexia, they suggested, is characterized by effortless and accurate reading of nonwords and regular words with poor performance with irregular words only. Type 2 surface dyslexia, in contrast, is characterized by slow, effortful reading; although these patients read irregular words less well than regular words and nonwords, they make errors with all types of stimuli. More recently, Shallice[44] suggested that at least for patients with type 2 surface dyslexia, the syndrome may reflect an attempt to compensate for damage to early stages of the reading process.

Other investigators have suggested that the syndrome may be fractionated even more. Thus, for example, surface dyslexia may be associated with disruption of the visual word-form system,[3] with a disruption of semantics (in conjunction with deficit in the "direct" route),[45,46] or with a lesion involving the phonological output lexicon.[47] Indeed, Coltheart and Funnell[48] proposed that within the context of a multiroute model of reading, surface dyslexia might be associated with as many as seven distinct types of impairment.

Finally, if as suggested above, patients with surface dyslexia are unable to access semantics by means of a direct lexical procedure, one might ask how these patients derive word meaning. At least for some surface dyslexics, access to a word's meaning appears to occur only after the phonological form of the word has been derived. Thus, when presented the word *listen,* a patient described by Marshall and Newcombe[3] responded "Liston" and added "that's the boxer."

The anatomic correlate of surface dyslexia has not been well established. Indeed, in recent years the syndrome has been reported most frequently in the context of dementia.[46,49–54] Accordingly, surface dyslexia in demented patients is sometimes termed "semantic dyslexia." Many of these patients have exhibited brain atrophy most prominent in the temporal lobes (e.g., Refs. 50 and 53).

Reading without Meaning

In 1979, Schwartz and coworkers[45] reported a patient (WLP) who exhibited a profound loss of semantics in the context of dementia. Her performance was of particular interest because, unlike patients with surface dyslexia, she correctly read aloud both regular and irregular words that she was unable to comprehend. Thus, for example, when asked to sort written words into their appropriate semantic categories, she correctly classified only 7 of 20 animal names; critically, WLP correctly read aloud 18 of these animal names, including such orthographically ambiguous or irregular words as *hyena* and *leopard*. The same basic phenomenon—that is, the ability to read aloud regular and irregular words that the patient does not understand—has subsequently been reported by a number of investigators (see Refs. 55 and 56).

The pattern of performance exhibited by WLP and similar patients is of considerable theoretical interest. Recall that to this point, two procedures have been described by which written words may be pronounced. The first (labeled A in Fig. 14-1) involves the activation of an entry in the visual word-form system, access to semantic information, and ultimately activation of an entry in the phonological output lexicon. The second (B in Fig. 14-1) involves the nonlexical print-to-sound translation process. Reading without semantics is of interest precisely because it cannot readily be accommodated by such an account. The fact that these patients do not comprehend the words they correctly pronounce indicates that their oral reading is not mediated by the semantically based reading procedure. Additionally, the fact that these patients can read irregular words suggests that they are not relying on a sublexical print-to-sound conversion procedure.

How, then, do these patients read aloud? Several explanations have been proposed. One response was to suggest that oral reading may be mediated by a third mechanism or route (e.g., Ref. 57). This mechanism was assumed to be lexically based, involving the activation of an entry in the visual word-form system and the "direct" activation of an entry in the phonological output lexicon (C in Fig. 14-1); note that this procedure differs from the lexical procedure described above in that there is no intervening activation of semantic information. Based on the analysis of a phonological dyslexic's performance across a variety of reading, writing, and repetition tasks, we[32] have reported data providing additional support for the existence of a lexical but nonsemantic reading procedure. An alternative hypothesis was proposed by Shallice and colleagues (Refs. 44 and 46; see also Ref. 58). These investigators attempted to explain reading without semantics within the context of a dual-route model by proposing that the phonological reading procedure employs not only grapheme-to-phoneme correspondences but also correspondences based on larger units including syllables and even morphemes. Thus, on this account, WLP and similar patients are assumed to compute the pronunciation of irregular words they cannot understand by relying on the multiple levels of print-to-sound correspondences available in the phonological system. Finally, Hillis and Caramazza[59] have suggested that the apparent ability to read without meaning is attributable to the fact that, while the patient is impaired, the semantic and phonological reading procedures provide partial information that constrains the subject's responses. Thus, on this account, neither the semantic nor phonological procedure is assumed to be capable of generating the correct response, but the combination of partial phonological and incomplete semantic information is often sufficient to identify the stimulus.

READING AND THE RIGHT HEMISPHERE

One important and controversial issue regarding reading concerns the putative reading capacity of the right hemisphere. For many years investigators argued that the right hemisphere was "word blind."[2,6,7] In recent years, however, several lines of evidence have suggested that the right hemisphere may possess the capacity to read. One seemingly incontrovertible line of evidence comes from the performance of a patient who underwent a left hemispherectomy at age 15 for treatment of seizures caused by Rasmussen's encephalitis;[60] after the hemispherectomy, the patient was able to read approximately 30 percent of single words and exhibited an effect of part of speech; she was also utterly unable to use a print-to-sound conversion process. Thus, in many respects this patient's performance was similar to that of a person with deep dyslexia, a pattern of reading impairment that has been hypothesized to reflect the performance of the right hemisphere.[34,35]

The performance of some split-brain patients is also consistent with the claim that the right hemisphere is literate. These patients may, for example, be able to match printed words presented to the right hemisphere with an appropriate object.[61,62] Interestingly, the patients are apparently unable to derive sound from the words presented to the right hemisphere; thus, they are unable to determine if a word presented to the right hemisphere rhymes with an auditorially presented word.

Another line of evidence supporting the claim that the right hemisphere is literate comes from evaluation of the reading of patients with pure alexia and optic aphasia.[17,63] We reported data, for example, from four patients with pure alexia who performed well above chance on a number of lexical decision and semantic categorization tasks with briefly presented words that they could not explicitly identify. Three of the patients who regained the ability to identify rapidly presented words explicitly exhibited a pattern of performance consistent with the right-hemisphere reading hypothesis. These patients read nouns better than functors and words of high (e.g., *chair*) better than words of low (e.g., *destiny*) imageability. Additionally, both patients for whom data were available demonstrated a deficit in the reading of suffixed (e.g., *flowed*) as opposed to pseudo-suffixed (e.g., *flower*) words. These data are consistent with a version of the right-hemisphere reading hypothesis postulating that the right-hemisphere lexical-semantic system primarily represents high imageability nouns. On this account, functors, affixed words, and low imageability words are not adequately represented in the right hemisphere.

Finally, we reported data from an investigation with a patient with pure alexia in which transcranial magnetic stimulation (TMS) was employed to directly test the hypothesis that the right hemisphere mediates the reading of at least some patients with acquired dyslexia.[64] We reasoned that if the right hemisphere provides the neural substrate for reading, the transient, localized disruption of cortical processing caused by TMS of the right hemisphere would interfere with reading. An extensively investigated patient with pure alexia who exhibited the reading pattern described above was asked to read aloud briefly presented words, half of which were presented in association with TMS. Consistent with the hypothesis that his reading was mediated by the right hemisphere, stimulation of the right hemisphere interfered with oral reading, whereas left-hemisphere stimulation had no significant effect.

Although a consensus has not yet been achieved, there is mounting evidence that, at least for some people, the right hemisphere is not word-blind but may support the reading of some types of words. The full extent of this reading capacity and whether it is relevant to normal reading, however, remain unclear.

COMPUTATIONAL MODELS OF THE DYSLEXIAS

To this point, the discussion of acquired reading disorders has been motivated by a widely though not universally (see Refs. 4 and 5) accepted multiroute information processing model of reading. In recent years, however, computer-implemented parallel distributed processing (PDP) models of cognitive processing have made important contributions in many domains of cognitive science, including reading (see Chap. 10). These models, which differ from traditional information processing models in that they offer (and in fact require) greater specification of the manner in which information is represented and processed, have called into question the necessity of hypothesizing two routes to account for the syndromes reviewed here. Although a detailed discussion of these models is beyond the scope of this chapter, several PDP accounts of reading are briefly summarized below.

Seidenberg and McClelland[65] have reported a PDP model of single-word reading in which the procedure for computing pronunciation directly from orthography (that is, without semantic mediation) is assumed to be mediated by a single network in which orthographic patterns are linked to phonological representations by means of an intermediate "hidden layer."[65] In contrast to the information processing accounts described above, this model does not postulate a discrete "lexical" or word-representation procedure or distinct lexical and sublexical procedures for the computation of phonology. Of particular relevance in the present context is the fact that investigators have attempted to simulate the performance of dyslexic patients by modifying or "lesioning" this PDP model. Patterson and colleagues,[66] for example, have attempted to model the performance of surface dyslexics by eliminating a proportion of the connections or units at different "lesion" sites. Although the simulations do not appear to capture all of the characteristic features of the performance of surface dyslexics, the lesioned models generate data that are in many interesting and important respects similar to those of patients. More recently, Plaut and Shallice[67] have reported a series of simulations of different PDP architectures in an attempt to model the performance of patients with deep dyslexia.

Finally, Seidenberg and Joanisse have recently extended their computational approach to reading to an issue of considerable theoretical importance: the reading of prefixed and suffixed (that is, "multimorphemic") words.[68] On the basis of empiric studies with normals as well as data from a computational model, Gonnerman et al.[69,70] argue that morphologic structure is an "emergent, interlevel representation that mediates computations between form and meaning" rather than an explicit level of representation.

An alternative computational account of reading has been developed by several investigators. Reggia and coworkers[71] developed a model that incorporates both lexical and nonlexical procedures for the computation of phonology. This model, which employs a competitive distribution of activation to govern interaction between competing concepts, simulates many aspects of normal reading performance. In a series of elegant investigations, Coltheart and colleagues[72,73] have described a computationally instantiated version of dual-route theory similar to that presented in Fig. 14-1, the "dual-route cascaded" model. This account incorporates a "lexical" route (similar to C in Fig. 14.1) as well as a "nonlexical" route by which the pronunciation of graphemes is computed on the basis of position-specific correspondence rules. Like the PDP models described above, the dual-route cascaded model accommodates a wide range of findings from the literature on normal reading. And as with the PDP models, "lesioning" the dual-route cascaded model produces disorders that are, at least in many respects, similar to acquired dyslexias described earlier in this chapter.[74]

A full discussion of the relative merits of these models as well as other approaches to the understanding of reading and acquired dyslexia (e.g., Ref. 75) is beyond the scope of this chapter. It would appear likely, however, that investigations of acquired dyslexia will help to adjudicate between competing accounts of reading and that these models will continue to offer critical insights into the interpretation of data from brain-injured subjects.

REFERENCES

1. Déjerine J: Sur un cas de cécité verbale avec agraphie, suivi d'autopsie. *C R Séances Soc Biol* 3:197–201, 1891.
2. Déjerine J: Contribution à l'étude anatomo-pathologique et clinique des différentes variétés de cécité verbale. *C R Séances Soc Biol* 4:61–90, 1892.
3. Marshall JC, Newcombe F: Patterns of paralexia: A psycholinguistic approach. *J Psycholinguist Res* 2:175–199, 1973.
4. Marcel AJ: Surface dyslexia and beginning reading: A revised hypothesis of the pronunciation of print and its impairments, in Coltheart M, Patterson KE, Marshall JC (eds): *Deep Dyslexia*. London: Routledge, 1980.
5. Van Orden GC, Pennington BF, Stone GO: Word identification in reading and the promise of subsymbolic psycholinguistics. *Psychol Rev* 97:488–522, 1990.
6. Shallice T, Warrington EK: Single and multiple component central dyslexic syndromes, in Coltheart M, Patterson K, Marshall JC (eds): *Deep Dyslexia*. London: Routledge, 1980.
7. Geschwind N: Disconnection syndromes in animals and man. *Brain* 88:237–294, 585–644, 1965.
8. Patterson K, Kay J: Letter-by-letter reading: Psychological descriptions of a neurological syndrome. *Q J Exp Psychol* 34A:411–441, 1982.
9. Arguin M, Bub DN: Pure alexia: Attempted rehabilitation and its implications for interpretation of the deficit. *Brain Lang* 47:233–268, 1994.
10. Arguin M, Bub DN: Single-character processing in a case of pure alexia. *Neuropsychologia* 31:435–458, 1993.
11. Kinsbourne M, Warrington EK: A disorder of simultaneous form perception. *Brain* 85:461–486, 1962.
12. Farah MJ, Wallace MA: Pure alexia as a visual impairment: A reconsideration. *Cognit Neuropsychol* 8:313–334, 1991.
13. Warrington EK, Shallice T: Word-form dyslexia. *Brain* 103:99–112, 1980.
14. Warrington EK, Langdon D: Spelling dyslexia: A deficit of the visual word-form. *J Neurol Neurosurg Psychiatry* 57:211–216, 1994.
15. Landis T, Regard M, Serrat A: Iconic reading in a case of alexia without agraphia caused by a brain tumor: A tachistoscopic study. *Brain Lang* 11:45–53, 1980.
16. Shallice T, Saffran EM: Lexical processing in the absence of explicit word identification: Evidence from a letter-by-letter reader. *Cognit Neuropsychol* 3:429–458, 1986.
17. Coslett HB, Saffran EM: Evidence for preserved reading in pure alexia. *Brain* 112:327–329, 1989.
18. Greenblatt SH: Subangular alexia without agraphia or hemianopia. *Brain Lang* 3:229–245, 1976.
19. Binder JR, Mohr JP: The topography of callosal reading pathways: A case-control analysis. *Brain* 115:1807–1826, 1992.
20. Damasio AR, Damasio H: The anatomic basis of pure alexia. *Neurology* 33:1573–1583, 1983.
21. Sieroff E, Pollatsek A, Posner MI: Recognition of visual letter strings following injury to the posterior visual spatial attention system. *Cognit Neuropsychol* 5:427–449, 1988.
22. Behrman M, Moscovitch M, Black SE, Mozer M: Perceptual and conceptual mechanisms in neglect dyslexia. *Brain* 113:1163–1183, 1990.

23. Berti A, Frassinetti F, Umilta C: Nonconscious reading? Evidence from neglect dyslexia. *Cortex* 30:181–197, 1994.
24. Costello AD, Warrington EK: The dissociation of visual neglect and neglect dyslexia. *J Neurol Neurosurg Psychiatry* 50:110–116, 1987.
25. Shallice T, Warrington EK: The possible role of selective attention in acquired dyslexia, *Neuropsychologia* 15:31–41, 1977.
26. Price CJ, Humphreys GW: Attentional dyslexia: The effects of co-occurring deficits. *Cognit Neuropsychol* 6:569-592, 1993.
27. Warrington EK, Cipolotti L, McNeil J: Attentional dyslexia: A single case study. *Neuropsychologia* 31:871–886, 1993.
28. Saffran EM, Coslett HB: "Attentional dyslexia" in Alzheimer's disease: A case study. *Cognit Neuropsychol.* In press.
29. Coltheart M, Patterson K, Marshall JC (eds): *Deep Dyslexia*. London: Routledge, 1980.
30. Saffran EM, Marin OSM: Reading without phonology: Evidence from aphasia. *Q J Exp Psychol* 29:515–525, 1977.
31. Allport DA, Funnell E: Components of the mental lexicon. *Phil Trans R Soc Lond B* 295:397–410, 1981.
32. Coslett HB: Read but not write "idea": Evidence for a third reading mechanism. *Brain Lang* 40:425–443, 1991.
33. Caramazza A, Hillis AE: Where do semantic errors come from? *Cortex* 26:95–122, 1990.
34. Coltheart M: Deep dyslexia: A right hemisphere hypothesis, in Coltheart M, Patterson K, Marshall JC (eds): *Deep Dyslexia*. London: Routledge, 1980.
35. Saffran EM, Bogyo LC, Schwartz MF, Marin OSM: Does deep dyslexia reflect right-hemisphere reading? in Coltheart M, Patterson K, Marshall JC (eds): *Deep Dyslexia*. London: Routledge, 1980.
36. Derouesne J, Beauvois M-F: Phonological processing in reading: Data from alexia. *J Neurol Neurosurg Psychiatry* 42:1125–1132, 1979.
37. Coltheart M (ed): *Special Issue on Phonological Dyslexia, Cognit Neuropsychol,* 13, 1996.
38. Funnell E: Phonological processes in reading: New evidence from acquired dyslexia. *Br J Psychol* 74:159–180, 1983.
39. Bub D, Black SE, Howell J, Kertesz A: Speech output processes and reading, in Coltheart M, Sartori G, Job R (eds): *Cognitive Neuropsychology of Language*. Hillsdale, NJ: Erlbaum, 1987.
40. Friedman RB, Kohn SE: Impaired activation of the phonological lexicon: Effects upon oral reading. *Brain Lang* 38:278–297, 1990.
41. Glosser G, Friedman RB: The continuum of deep/ phonological dyslexia. *Cortex* 26:343–359, 1990.
42. Patterson KE: The relation between reading and psychological coding: Further neuropsychological observations, in AW Ellis (ed): *Normality and Pathology in Cognitive Functions*. London: Academic Press, 1982.
43. Shallice T, McCarthy R: Phonological reading: From patterns of impairment to possible procedures, in Patterson KE, Coltheart M, Marshall JC (eds): *Surface Dyslexia*. London: Erlbaum, 1985.
44. Shallice T: *From Neuropsychology to Mental Structure*. Cambridge, England: Cambridge University Press, 1987.
45. Schwartz MF, Saffran EM, Marin OSM: Dissociation of language function in dementia: A case study. *Brain Lang* 7:277–306, 1979.
46. Shallice T, Warrington EK, McCarthy R: Reading without semantics. *Q J Exp Psychol* 35A:111–138, 1983.
47. Howard D, Franklin S: Three ways for understanding written words, and their use in two contrasting cases of surface dyslexia (together with an odd routine for making "orthographic" errors in oral word production), in Allport A, Mackay D, Prinz W, Scheerer E (eds): *Language Perception and Production*. New York: Academic Press, 1987.
48. Coltheart M, Funnell E: Reading writing: One lexicon or two? in Allport DA, MacKay DG, Printz W, Scheerer E (eds): *Language Perception and Production: Shared Mechanisms in Listening, Speaking, Reading and Writing*. London: Academic Press, 1987.
49. Warrington EK: The selective impairment of semantic memory. *Q J Exp Psychol* 27:635–657, 1975.
50. Hodges JR, Patterson K, Oxbury S, Funnell E: Semantic dementia: Progressive fluent aphasia with temporal lobe atrophy. *Brain* 115:1783–1806, 1992.
51. Patterson K, Hodges J: Deterioration of word meaning: Implications for reading. *Neuropsychologia* 30:1025–1040, 1992.
52. Graham KS, Hodges JR, Patterson K: The relationship between comprehension and oral reading in progressive fluent aphasia. *Neuropsychologia* 32:299–316, 1994.
53. Breedin SD, Saffran EM, Coslett HB: Reversal of the concreteness effect in a patient with semantic dementia. *Cognit Neuropsychol* 11:617–660, 1994.
54. Cipolotti L, Warrington EK: Semantic memory and reading abilities: A case report. *J Int Neuropsychol Soc* 1:104–110, 1994.
55. Friedman RB, Ferguson S, Robinson S, Sunderland T: Dissociation of mechanisms of reading in Alzheimer's disease. *Brain Lang* 43:400-413, 1992.

56. Raymer AM, Berndt RS: Models of word reading: Evidence from Alzheimer's disease. *Brain Lang* 47:479–482, 1994.
57. Morton J, Patterson KE: A new attempt at an interpretation, or an attempt at a new interpretation, in Coltheart M, Patterson K, Marshall JC (eds): *Deep Dyslexia*. London: Routledge, 1980.
58. McCarthy RA, Warrington EK: Phonological reading: Phenomena and paradoxes. *Cortex* 22:359–380, 1986.
59. Hillis AE, Caramazza A: Mechanisms for accessing lexical representations for output: Evidence from a category-specific semantic deficit. *Brain Lang* 40:106–144, 1991.
60. Patterson K, Vargha-Khadem F, Polkey CF: Reading with one hemisphere. *Brain* 112:39–63, 1989.
61. Zaidel E: Lexical organization in the right hemisphere, in Buser P, Rougeul-Buser A(eds): *Cerebral Correlates of Conscious Experience*. Amsterdam: Elsevier, 1978.
62. Zaidel E, Peters AM: Phonological encoding and ideographic reading by the disconnected right hemisphere: Two case studies. *Brain Lang* 14:205–234, 1981.
63. Coslett HB, Saffran EM: Preserved object recognition and reading comprehension in optic aphasia. *Brain* 12:1091–1110, 1989.
64. Coslett HB, Monsul N: Reading and the right hemisphere: Evidence from transcranial magnetic stimulation. *Brain Lang* 46:198–211, 1994.
65. Seidenberg MS, McClelland JL: A distributed, developmental model of word recognition and naming. *Psychol Rev* 96:522–568, 1989.
66. Patterson KE, Seidenberg MS, McClelland JL: Connections and disconnections: Acquired dyslexia in a computational model of reading processes, in Morris RGM (ed): *Parallel Distributed Processing: Implications for Psychology and Neurobiology*. Oxford, England: Oxford University Press, 1989.
67. Plaut D, Shallice T: Deep dyslexia: A case study of connectionist neuropsychology. *Cognit Neuropsychol* 10:377–500, 1993.
68. Joanisse MF, Seidenberg MS: Impairments in verb morphology after brain injury: A connectionist model. *Proc Natl Acad Sci U S A* 96:7592–7597, 1999.
69. Plaut DC, Gonnerman LM: Are non-semantic morphological effects incompatible with a distributed connectionist approach to lexical processing? *Lang Cogn Proc* 15:445–485, 2000.
70. Gonnerman M, Devlin JT, Andersen ES, Seidenberg MS: Derivational morphology as an emergent interlevel representation (personal communication, 2002).
71. Reggia J, Marsland P, Berndt R: Competitive dynamics in a dual-route connectionist model of print-to-sound transformation. *Complex Systems* 2:509–547, 1988.
72. Rastle K, Coltheart, M: Serial and strategic effects in reading aloud. *J Exp Psychol Hum Percept Perform* 25:482–503, 1999.
73. Coltheart M, Rastle, K, Perry C, et al: DRC: A dual route cascaded model of visual word recognition and reading aloud. *Psychol Rev* 108:204–256, 2001.
74. Coltheart M, Langdon R, Haller M: Simulations of acquired dyslexias by the DRC model, a computational model of visual word recognition and reading aloud, in Proceedings of the 1995 Workshop on Neural Modeling of Cognitive and Brain Disorders, College Park, MD: University of Maryland, June 8–10, 1995.
75. Van Orden GC, Jansen op de Haar MA, Bosman AM: Complex dynamic systems also predict dissociations but they do not reduce to autonomous components. *Cognit Neuropsychol* 14:131–165, 1997.

Chapter 15

ACALCULIA AND NUMBER PROCESSING DISORDERS

Stanislas Dehaene

The foundation for the amazing successes of our species in science and technology lies in our ability to do mathematics. Although little is known about the cerebral substrates of mathematics in general, one of its subareas, elementary arithmetic, has received considerable attention from cognitive neuroscientists. The present chapter reviews the organization of the number system from the point of view of cognitive neuropsychology. Brain lesions can selectively affect several components of the number processing system, revealing a highly organized brain architecture for arithmetic that is now being confirmed and refined by brain imaging methods. Current results indicate that (1) the number system is segregated from other symbolic processing systems at multiple levels; (2) parietal lobe lesions can interfere with the semantic component of number processing; (3) dissociations between operations are frequently observed, suggesting that multiple parietal circuits contribute to arithmetic; and (4) developmental disorders of calculation, possibly of genetic origin, can be traced to pre- or perinatal pathology often affecting the parietal lobe.

THE ISOLATION OF THE NUMBER PROCESSING SYSTEM

The specialization of the number processing system can be inferred from the observation that, at virtually all levels of processing, dissociations have been observed between numbers and the rest of language. For instance, high-level calculation abilities may be spared in patients with severe global aphasia (Rossor et al., 1995) or impaired short-term memory (Butterworth et al., 1996). At the visual identification level, pure alexic patients who fail to read words often show a largely preserved ability to read and process digits (Cohen and Dehaene, 1995; Déjerine, 1891; Déjerine, 1892). Conversely, a case of impaired number reading with preserved word reading is on record (Cipolotti et al., 1995). In the writing domain, severe agraphia and alexia may be accompanied by a fully preserved ability to write and read arabic numbers (Anderson et al., 1990). Even within the speech production system, patients who suffer from random phoneme substitutions, thus resulting in the production of an incomprehensible jargon, may produce jargon-free number words (Cohen et al., 1997).

Most importantly, numbers may doubly dissociate from other categories of words at the semantic level, suggesting the existence of a category-specific semantic system for numerical quantities. Spared calculation and number comprehension abilities have been described in patients with grossly deteriorated semantic processing (Thioux et al., 1998) or semantic dementia (Butterworth et al., 2001; Cappelletti et al., 2001). The converse dissociation is also on record. Cipolotti and coworkers (1991) first reported a striking case of a patient with a small left parietal lesion and an almost complete deficit in all spheres of number processing, sparing only the numbers 1 through 4, in the context of otherwise largely preserved language and semantic functions. Although such a severe degradation of the number system has never been replicated, other cases, discussed further below, confirm that the understanding of numbers and their relations can be specifically impaired in the context of preserved language and semantics (e.g., Dehaene and Cohen, 1997; Delazer and Benke, 1997).

THE CENTRAL ROLE OF THE PARIETAL LOBE AND ACALCULIA

The parietal lobe appears to play a central role in number processing. It has been known since the beginning of this century that parietal lesions, usually in the dominant hemisphere, can cause calculation deficits. Gerstmann (1940) reported the frequent co-occurence of agraphia, acalculia, finger agnosia, and left-right confusion in parietal cases, a tetrad of deficits referred to as Gerstmann's syndrome (although the elements of the syndrome are now known to be dissociable; see Benton, 1992). The lesions that cause acalculia of the Gerstmann's type are typically centered on the portion of the left intraparietal sulcus that sits immediately behind the angular gyrus (Brodman's area 39) (Mayer et al., 1999; Takayama et al., 1994). In many cases, the deficit can be extremely incapacitating. Patients may fail to compute operations as simple as $2 + 2$, $3 - 1$, or 3×9. Several characteristics indicate that the deficit arises at a rather abstract level of processing. First, patients may remain fully able to comprehend and to produce numbers in all formats. Second, they show the same calculation difficulties whether the problem is presented to them visually or auditorily and whether they have to respond verbally or in writing, or even merely have to decide whether a proposed operation is true or false. Thus, the calculation deficit is not due to an inability to identify the numbers or to produce the operation result. Rather, patients with inferior parietal lesions and acalculia of the Gerstmann type suffer from a category-specific impairment of the semantic representation and manipulation of numerical quantities (Dehaene and Cohen, 1995, 1997).

One patient, Mr. Mar (Dehaene and Cohen, 1997), experienced severe difficulties in calculation, especially with single-digit subtraction (75 percent errors). He failed on problems as simple as $3 - 1$, with the comment that he no longer knew what the operation meant. His failure was not tied to a specific modality of input or output, because the problems were simultaneously presented visually and read out loud and because he failed in both overt production and covert multiple-choice tests. Moreover, he also erred on tasks outside of calculation per se, such as deciding which of two numbers is the larger (16 percent errors) or what number falls in the middle of two others (bisection task: 77 percent errors). He easily performed analogous comparison and bisection tasks in nonnumerical domains such as days of the week, months, or the alphabet (What is between Tuesday and Thursday? February and April? B and D?), indicating that he suffered from a category-specific deficit for numbers. This and similar patients (Delazer and Benke, 1997; Takayama et al., 1994) suggest that parietal lesions can cause a selective disturbance to the central representation of numerical quantity.

BRAIN-IMAGING STUDIES OF NUMBER PROCESSING

The involvement of parietal cortex in number processing is confirmed by brain imaging studies in normal subjects. Roland and Friberg (1985) were the first to monitor blood-flow changes during calculation as opposed to rest. When subjects repeatedly subtracted 3 from a given number, activation increased bilaterally in inferior parietal and prefrontal cortex. These localizations were later confirmed using functional magnetic resonance imaging (fMRI) (Burbaud et al., 1995; Rueckert et al., 1996). A positron emission tomography (PET) study of multiplication and comparison of digit pairs revealed bilateral parietal activation confined to the intraparietal region (Dehaene et al., 1996), in agreement with lesion data. Several recent brain-imaging studies all confirm the involvement of bilateral parietal cortices in calculation (Burbaud et al., 1999; Chochon et al., 1999; Dehaene et al., 1999; Pesenti et al., 2000; Rueckert et al., 1996; Zago et al., 2001).

Several features of the inferior parietal contribution to number processing have been clarified by imaging methods. First, the parietal region is active whenever an arithmetic operation or the mere comprehension of the size of a number is called for (Chochon et al., 1999; Dehaene et al., 1999). Second, its activation is proportional to the number of calculations performed per unit of time (Menon et al., 2000). Third, its activation is independent of the particular input or output modalities used to convey the numbers, such as arabic or spelled-out numerals, suggesting that parietal cortex may be coding the abstract meaning of numbers rather than the numerical symbols themselves (Dehaene, 1996; Kiefer and Dehaene, 1997; Pinel et al., 2001). Fourth, the amount of activation correlates directly with the complexity of an arithmetic operation. Thus, event-related potentials (ERPs) and fMRI recordings in a number comparison task reveal that intraparietal activity is modulated by the numerical distance separating the numbers to be compared

(Dehaene et al., 1996; Pinel et al., 2001). Moreover, inferior parietal activity is larger and lasts longer during operations with large numbers than with small numbers (Kiefer and Dehaene, 1997; Stanescu-Cosson et al., 2000). Fifth, parietal activation during number processing can be found even when the subject is not aware of having been presented with a subliminal number (Dehaene et al., 1998; Naccache and Dehaene, 2001). I suggest that parietal cortices provide us with a "numerical intuition," a permanent and often implicit reference to the meaningful size of a numerical quantity in relation to others on the "mental number line" (Dehaene, 1992; Dehaene, 1997). Patients in whom this unconscious reference is impaired suffer a drastic loss of stable reference in the numerical domain.

DISSOCIATIONS BETWEEN OPERATIONS

Although the inferior parietal region seems to play a crucial role in number sense, it is important to note that it is not the only brain region involved in number processing in adults. The phrenologic notion that a single area can hold all the knowledge about an entire domain such as arithmetic has to give way to a more parallel view of number processing in the brain. Multiple brain areas are involved, whether for identifying arabic numerals, writing them down, understanding spoken number words, retrieving multiplication facts from memory, or organizing a sequence of multidigit calculations (Caramazza and McCloskey, 1987; Dehaene and Cohen, 1995; McCloskey and Caramazza, 1987; McCloskey et al., 1992). Correspondingly, a great variety of brain-lesioned patients with number processing deficits, too broad to be reviewed here, have been described.

One of the most striking dissociations occurs among different arithmetic operations. It is not rare for a patient to be much more severely impaired in multiplication than in subtraction (Cohen and Dehaene, 2000; Dagenbach and McCloskey, 1992; Dehaene and Cohen, 1997; Lampl et al., 1994; Pesenti et al., 1994), while other patients are much more impaired in subtraction than in multiplication (Dehaene and Cohen, 1997; Delazer and Benke, 1997). It may not be necessary, however, to postulate as many brain circuits as there are arithmetical operations (although see van Harskamp and Cipolotti, 2001). Rather, such dissociations may reflect a basic distinction between overlearned arithmetic facts such as the multiplication table, which are stored in rote verbal memory, and the genuine understanding of number meaning that underlies non-table operations such as subtraction (Dehaene and Cohen, 1997; Delazer and Benke, 1997; Hittmair-Delazer et al., 1995). Indeed, patients with impaired multiplication often have associated aphasia and lesions within the left perisylvian areas (Cohen et al., 2000) or left basal ganglia (Dehaene and Cohen, 1997), while patients with impaired subtraction tend to have lesions in the left intraparietal region outside of language cortex per se.

Brain imaging has confirmed that different operations rely on partially dissociable parietal circuits, with bilateral intraparietal activation during subtraction and more posterior and left-lateralized subangular activation during multiplication (Chochon et al., 1999; Lee, 2000). Brain imaging also indicates that those parietal circuits are differentially called upon during exact calculation and approximation (Dehaene et al., 1999): exact calculation of addition problems is dependent on language and causes relatively greater activation of the left anterior inferior frontal region and the angular gyrus, while approximation of quantities is independent of language and causes greater activation of the bilateral intraparietal sulci. This finding may explain why some patients with severe deficits of exact calculation may remain able to compute approximations of the desired result (Dehaene and Cohen, 1991; Warrington, 1982).

HEMISPHERIC SPECIALIZATION

There is an as yet unresolved discrepancy between brain imaging and neuropsychological findings. On the one hand, the parietal activations during number processing tend to be bilateral, though often with increasingly greater left lateralization as the task requires exact calculation and arithmetic tables (e.g., Chochon et al., 1999). On the other hand, the lesion site for acalculia and Gerstmann's syndrome appears strictly lateralized to the dominant left parietal lobe. Although this is not fully understood yet, the issue may be partially clarified by studies of split-field presentations in callosal patients (Cohen and Dehaene, 1996; Gazzaniga and Hillyard, 1971; Gazzaniga and Smylie, 1984; Seymour et al., 1994). Those studies confirm that both hemispheres can process digits and quantities at the semantic level. When two digits are presented simultaneously *within* the same hemifield, split-brain patients experience no difficulty deciding whether they are the same or different (while their disconnection renders them completely unable to compare two digits *across* the two hemifields). Hence, both hemispheres can analyze digit shapes. Furthermore, both hemispheres can also point to the larger digit (or to the smaller), and both can classify digits or even two-digit numbers as larger or smaller than some reference. Hence, both hemispheres seem to possess a quantity representation of numbers.

There are, however, at least two striking differences between the numerical abilities of the left and the right hemispheres. First, digits presented to the left hemisphere can be named normally by the patients, but digits presented to the right hemisphere cannot. This is in keeping with the well-known lateralization of speech production abilities to the left hemisphere. Second, split-brain patients can calculate only with digits presented to their left hemisphere. When digits are presented to their right hemisphere, the patients fail with operations as simple as adding 2, multiplying by 3, subtracting from 10, or dividing by 2. This is the case even when they merely have to point to the correct result among several possible results or to indicate nonverbally whether a proposed result is correct or not. The only calculation ability that seems to be available to an isolated right hemisphere, at least occasionally, is approximation. A patient might not be able to decide whether $2 + 2$ makes 4 or 5, but might still easily notice that $2 + 2$ cannot make 9 (Cohen and Dehaene, 1996; Dehaene and Cohen, 1991). It has been suggested that the right hemisphere may have a special role in the "abstraction of numerical relations" (Langdon and Warrington, 1997).

DEVELOPMENTAL DYSCALCULIA

Deficits of number processing can be observed in adults with acquired brain lesions, but also in young children. Developmental dyscalculia, coarsely defined as a failure on standardized tests of arithmetic independently of IQ or social factors, is not rare. Kosc (1974) reported an incidence of 6.4 percent in a sample of 375 children between the age of 10 and 12. Badian (1983) studied 1476 children between 7 and 14 years of age and observed that 2.7 percent had both reading and mathematical deficits, another 3.6 percent only had difficulties in mathematics, and yet another 2.5 percent only in reading. In another study in Great Britain, those figures were 2.3, 1.3, and 3.9 percent (Lewis et al., 1994). Other family members are frequently affected, suggesting that genetic factors may contribute to the disorder (Shalev et al., 2001).

A variety of systems of classification of developmental dyscalculia have been proposed. Badian (1983) used a terminology initially proposed for adult acalculia cases (Hécaen et al., 1961) to distinguish dyscalculia due to a reading or writing deficit, spatial dyscalculia due to an inability to organize the figures on a page, dyscalculia due to attentional disorders, and anarithmia proper. Kosc (1974) adopted a similar though more complex classification. Simpler categories were achieved by Temple (1991, 1994) on the basis of Caramazza and McCloskey's model of number processing (Caramazza and McCloskey, 1987; McCloskey and Caramazza, 1987; McCloskey et al., 1992). She distinguished dyscalculia due to a failure to process the number notations (e.g., difficulties in reading or in writing arabic numerals); arithmetic fact dyscalculia, or a failure to store and retrieve arithmetic tables; and procedural dyscalculia, or an inability to execute a multidigit calculation in the correct sequence. A particularly striking double dissociation between arithmetic fact and procedural dyscalculia was reported, strengthening the hypothesis that cases of developmental dyscalculia can be as selective as adult neuropsychological cases (Temple, 1991). A similar approach has been adopted to analyze a single case of number-notation dyscalculia (Sullivan et al., 1996) and two series of cases with various subtypes of developmental dyscalculia (Ashcraft et al., 1992; Sokol et al., 1994).

In a series of publications, Geary and colleagues have focused on developmental calculation deficits and have attempted to characterize their origins (Geary, 1990, 1993, 1994; Geary et al., 1992; Geary and Brown, 1991; Geary et al., 1991; Geary et al., 1986; Geary et al., 1987). In comparison to normal children, they report that dyscalculic children use immature calculation strategies, largely based on counting; make an improper choice of strategy; and show a slower evolution in their strategies with time. Dyscalculic children also have a poorer short-term memory span for digits (Geary et al., 1991; Hitch and McAuley, 1991). Most interestingly, some dyscalculic children may suffer from a lack of understanding of the counting principles proposed by Gelman and Gallistel (1978), suggesting that some of them at least may have a fundamental deficit in understanding the conceptual bases of arithmetic (Geary et al., 1992).

The notion that at least some children with developmental dyscalculia may suffer from a core conceptual deficit is supported by the existence of a "developmental Gerstmann syndrome" in children (Benson and Geschwind, 1970; Kinsbourne and Warrington, 1963; Spellacy and Peter, 1978; Temple, 1989; Temple, 1991). Like in adults, the calculation deficit is accompanied by most or all of the following symptoms: dysgraphia, left-right disorientation, and finger agnosia, which suggest a neurologic involvement of the parietal lobe. Interestingly, even in a sample of 200 normal children, a test of finger knowledge appears to be a better predictor of later arithmetic abilities than is a test of general intelligence (Fayol et al., 1998), again supporting a tight correlation between number knowledge and finger knowledge in the parietal lobe.

Very few imaging studies to date have been dedicated to developmental dyscalculia. Levy et al. (1999) report the case of an adult with lifelong isolated dyscalculia together with superior intelligence and reading ability, in whom the standard anatomic MRI appeared normal, yet MR spectroscopy techniques revealed a metabolic abnormality in the left inferior parietal area, exactly where a lesion would be expected in an adult Gerstmann syndrome case. Similarly, Isaacs and coworkers used voxel-based morphometry to compare gray matter density in adolescents born at equally severe grades of prematurity, half of whom suffered from dyscalculia (Isaacs et al., 2001). They found a single region of reduced gray matter in the left intraparietal sulcus, coinciding precisely with the site of fMRI activations during calculation in normal subjects. Those studies strengthen the hypothesis that early parietal dysfunction may underlie isolated developmental dyscalculia.

TURNER'S SYNDROME: DYSCALCULIA OF GENETIC ORIGIN?

If the parietal lobe involvement for arithmetic results at least in part from a genetic predisposition, then one would expect to find genetic diseases targeting the parietal region and causing dyscalculia. Although the search for such dyscalculias of genetic origin has only very recently begun, the possibility that Turner syndrome may conform to this typology has recently attracted attention. Turner syndrome is a genetic disorder characterized by partial or complete absence of one X chromosome in a female individual. The disorder occurs in approximately 1 girl in 2000 and is associated with well-documented physical disorders and abnormal estrogen production and pubertal development. The cognitive profile includes deficits in visual memory, visuospatial and attentional tasks, and social relations, in the context of a normal verbal IQ (Rovet, 1993). Most interestingly in the present context is the documentation of a mild to severe deficit in mathematics, particularly clear in arithmetic (Mazzocco, 1998; Rovet et al., 1994; Temple and Marriott, 1998). Anatomically, the data suggest possible bilateral parietooccipital dysfunction. A positron emission tomography study of five adult women demonstrated a glucose hypometabolism in bilateral parietal and occipital regions (Clark et al., 1990). Two anatomic MRI studies, one with 18 and the other with 30 affected women, demonstrated bilateral reductions in parietooccipital brain volume, together with other subcortical regions (Murphy et al., 1993; see also Reiss et al., 1993, 1995). Interestingly, the phenotype of Turner syndrome can differ depending on whether the remaining X chromosome is of paternal or maternal origin (Xm or Xp subtypes) (Bishop et al., 2000; Skuse, 2000; Skuse et al., 1997). Such a genomic imprinting effect was first demonstrated on tests of social competence (Skuse et al., 1997). It will be interesting to see if a similar effect exists in the arithmetic domain.

CONCLUSION

In this review, we have focused on the large empirical database of patients with number processing deficits. Detailed theoretical models of those deficits have been published (see, e.g., Caramazza and McCloskey, 1987; Dehaene and Cohen, 1995; McCloskey and Caramazza, 1987; McCloskey et al., 1992) and have been related to cognitive psychological, developmental, and animal research (Dehaene, 1997). As our knowledge of the normal and pathological organization of the number processing system increases, it may eventually become possible to design cognitive rehabilitation programs based on a more accurate anatomic and functional characterization of the impairment (for early attempts, see Girelli et al., 1996; Sullivan et al., 1996).

REFERENCES

Anderson SW, Damasio AR, Damasio H: Troubled letters but not numbers. Domain specific cognitive impairments following focal damage in frontal cortex. *Brain* 113, 749–766, 1990.

Ashcraft MH, Yamashita TS, Aram DM: Mathematics performance in left and right brain-lesioned children and adolescents. *Brain Cogn* 19:208–252, 1992.

Badian NA: Dyscalculia and nonverbal disorders of learning, in Myklebust HR (ed): *Progress in Learning Disabilities* New York: Stratton, 1983, vol 5, pp 235–264.

Benson DF, Geschwind N: Developmental Gerstmann syndrome. *Neurology* 20:293–298, 1970.

Benton AL: Gerstmann's syndrome. *Arch Neurol* 49:445–447, 1992.

Bishop DV, Canning E, Elgar K, et al: Distinctive patterns of memory function in subgroups of females with Turner syndrome: Evidence for imprinted loci on the X-chromosome affecting neurodevelopment. *Neuropsychologia* 38(5):712–721, 2000.

Burbaud P, Camus O, Guehl D, et al: A functional magnetic resonance imaging study of mental subtraction in human subjects. *Neurosci Lett* 273(3):195–199, 1999.

Burbaud P, Degreze P, Lafon P, et al: Lateralization of prefrontal activation during internal mental calculation: A functional magnetic resonance imaging study. *J Neurophysiol* 74:2194–2200, 1995.

Butterworth B, Cappelletti M, Kopelman M: Category specificity in reading and writing: The case of number words. *Nat Neurosci* 4(8):784–786, 2001.

Butterworth B, Cipolotti L, Warrington EK: Short-term memory impairment and arithmetical ability. *Q J Exp Psychol* 49A:251–262, 1996.

Cappelletti M, Butterworth B, Kopelman M: Spared numerical abilities in a case of semantic dementia. *Neuropsychologia* 39(11):1224–1239, 2001.

Caramazza A, McCloskey M: Dissociations of calculation processes, in Deloche G, Seron X (eds): *Mathematical Disabilities: A Cognitive Neuropsychological Perspective.* Hillsdale, NJ: Erlbaum, 1987, 221–234.

Chochon F, Cohen L, van de Moortele PF, Dehaene S: Differential contributions of the left and right inferior parietal lobules to number processing. *J Cogn Neurosci* 11:617–630, 1999.

Cipolotti L, Butterworth B, Denes G: A specific deficit for numbers in a case of dense acalculia. *Brain* 114:2619–2637, 1991.

Cipolotti L, Warrington EK, Butterworth B: Selective impairment in manipulating arabic numerals. *Cortex* 31:73–86, 1995.

Clark C, Klonoff H, Hadyen M: Regional cerebral glucose metabolism in Turner syndrome. *Can J Neurol Sci* 17:140–144, 1990.

Cohen L, Dehaene S: Number processing in pure alexia: The effect of hemispheric asymmetries and task demands. *Neurocase* 1:121–137, 1995.

Cohen L, Dehaene S: Cerebral networks for number processing: Evidence from a case of posterior callosal lesion. *Neurocase* 2:155–174, 1996.

Cohen L, Dehaene S: Calculating without reading: Unsuspected residual abilities in pure alexia. *Cogn Neuropsychol* 17(6):563–583, 2000.

Cohen L, Dehaene S, Chochon F, et al: Language and calculation within the parietal lobe: A combined cognitive, anatomical and fMRI study. *Neuropsychologia* 38:1426–1440, 2000.

Cohen L, Verstichel P, Dehaene S: Neologistic jargon sparing numbers: A category specific phonological impairment. *Cogn Neuropsychol* 14:1029–1061, 1997.

Dagenbach D, McCloskey M: The organization of arithmetic facts in memory: Evidence from a brain-damaged patient. *Brain Cogn* 20:345–366, 1992.

Dehaene S: Varieties of numerical abilities. *Cognition* 44:1–42, 1992.

Dehaene S: The organization of brain activations in number comparison: Event-related potentials and the additive-factors methods. *J Cogn Neurosci* 8:47–68, 1996.

Dehaene S: *The Number Sense.* New York: Oxford University Press, 1997.

Dehaene S, Cohen L: Two mental calculation systems: A case study of severe acalculia with preserved approximation. *Neuropsychologia* 29:1045–1074, 1991.

Dehaene S, Cohen L: Towards an anatomical and functional model of number processing. *Math Cogn* 1:83–120, 1995.

Dehaene S, Cohen L: Cerebral pathways for calculation: Double dissociation between rote verbal and quantitative knowledge of arithmetic. *Cortex* 33:219–250, 1997.

Dehaene S, Naccache L, Le Clec'H G, et al: Imaging unconscious semantic priming. *Nature* 395:597–600, 1998.

Dehaene S, Spelke E, Stanescu R, et al: Sources of mathematical thinking: Behavioral and brain-imaging evidence. *Science* 284:970–974, 1999.

Dehaene S, Tzourio N, Frak V, et al: Cerebral activations during number multiplication and comparison: A PET study. *Neuropsychologia* 34:1097–1106, 1996.

Déjerine J: Sur un cas de cécité verbale avec agraphie suivi d'autopsie. *Mem Soc Biol* 3:197–201, 1891.

Déjerine J: Contribution à l'étude anatomo-pathologique et clinique des différentes variétés de cécité verbale. *Mem Soc Biol* 4:61–90, 1892.

Delazer M, Benke T: Arithmetic facts without meaning. *Cortex* 33(4):697–710, 1997.

Fayol M, Barrouillet P, Marinthe X: Predicting arithmetical achievement from neuropsychological performance: A longitudinal study. *Cognition* 68:B63–B70, 1998.

Gazzaniga MS, Hillyard SA: Language and speech capacity of the right hemisphere. *Neuropsychologia* 9:273–280, 1971.

Gazzaniga MS, Smylie CE: Dissociation of language and cognition: A psychological profile of two disconnected right hemispheres. *Brain* 107:145–153, 1984.

Geary DC: A componential analysis of an early learning deficit in mathematics. *J Exp Child Psychol* 49:363–383, 1990.

Geary DC: Mathematical disabilities: Cognitive, neuropsychological and genetic components. *Psychol Bull* 114:345–362, 1993.

Geary DC: *Children's Mathematical Development.* Washington DC: American Psychological Association, 1994.

Geary DC, Bow-Thomas CC, Yao Y: Counting knowledge and skill in cognitive addition: A comparison of normal and mathematically disabled children. *J Exp Child Psychol* 54:372–391, 1992.

Geary DC, Brown SC: Cognitive addition: strategy choice and speed-of-processing differences in gifted, normal, and mathematically disabled children. *Dev Psychol* 27:398–406, 1991.

Geary DC, Brown SC, Samaranayake VA: Cognitive addition: A short longitudinal study of strategy choice and speed-of-processing differences in normal and mathematically disabled children. *Dev Psychol* 27:787–797, 1991.

Geary DC, Widaman KF, Little TD: Cognitive addition and multiplication: Evidence for a single memory network. *Mem Cogn* 14:478–487, 1986.

Geary DC, Widaman KF, Little TD, Cormier P: Cognitive addition: Comparison of learning disabled and academically normal elementary school children. *Cogn Dev* 2:249–269, 1987.

Gelman R, Gallistel CR: *The Child's Understanding of Number.* Cambridge, MA: Harvard University Press, 1978.

Gerstmann J: Syndrome of finger agnosia, disorientation for right and left, agraphia, and acalculia. *Arch Neurol Psychiatry* 44:398–408, 1940.

Girelli L Delazer M, Semenza C, Denes G: The representation of arithmetical facts: Evidence from two rehabilitation studies. *Cortex* 32(1):49–66, 1996.

Hécaen H, Angelergues R, Houillier S: Les variétés cliniques des acalculies au cours des lésions rétro-rolandiques: approche statistique du problème. *Rev Neurol* 105:85–103, 1961.

Hitch GJ, McAuley E: Working memory in children with specific arithmetical difficulties. *Br J Psychol* 82:375–386, 1991.

Hittmair-Delazer M, Sailer U, Benke T: Impaired arithmetic facts but intact conceptual knowledge—a single case study of dyscalculia. *Cortex* 31:139–147, 1995.

Isaacs EB, Edmonds CJ, Lucas A, Gadian DG: Calculation difficulties in children of very low birthweight: A neural correlate. *Brain* 124(Pt 9):1701–1707, 2001.

Kiefer M, Dehaene S: The time course of parietal activation in single-digit multiplication: Evidence from event-related potentials. *Math Cogn* 3:1–30, 1997.

Kinsbourne M, Warrington EK: The developmental Gerstmann syndrome. *Arch Neurol* 8: 490, 1963.

Kosc L: Developmental dyscalculia. *J Learn Disabil* 7:165–177, 1974.

Lampl Y, Eshel Y, Gilad R, Sarova-Pinhas I: Selective acalculia with sparing of the subtraction process in a patient with left parietotemporal hemorrhage. *Neurology* 44:1759–1761, 1994.

Langdon DW, Warrington EK: The abstraction of numerical relations: A role for the right hemisphere in arithmetic? *J Int Neuropsychol Soc* 3:260–268, 1997.

Lee KM: Cortical areas differentially involved in multiplication and subtraction: A functional magnetic resonance imaging study and correlation with a case of selective acalculia. *Ann Neurol* 48:657–661, 2000.

Levy LM, Reis IL, Grafman J: Metabolic abnormalities detected by H-MRS in dyscalculia and dysgraphia. *Neurology* 53:639–641, 1999.

Lewis C, Hitch GJ, Walker P: The prevalence of specific arithmetic difficulties and specific reading difficulties in 9- and 10-year-old boys and girls. *J Child Psychol Psychiatry* 35:283–292, 1994.

Mayer E, Martory MD, Pegna AJ, et al: A pure case of Gerstmann syndrome with a subangular lesion. *Brain* 122 (Pt 6):1107–1120, 1999.

Mazzocco MM: A process approach to describing mathematics difficulties in girls with Turner syndrome. *Pediatrics* 102(2 Pt 3):492–496, 1998.

McCloskey M, Caramazza A: Cognitive mechanisms in normal and impaired number processing, in Deloche G, Seron X (eds): *Mathematical Disabilities: A Cognitive Neuropsychological Perspective.* Hillsdale, NJ: Erlbaum, 1987, pp 201–219.

McCloskey M, Macaruso P, Whetstone T: The functional architecture of numerical processing mechanisms: Defending the modular model, in Campbell JID (ed): *The Nature and Origins of Mathematical Skills.* Amsterdam: Elsevier, 1992, pp 493–537.

Menon V, Rivera SM, White CD, et al: Dissociating prefrontal and parietal cortex activation during arithmetic processing. *Neuroimage* 12(4):357–365, 2000.

Murphy DG, DeCarli C, Daly E, et al: X-chromosome effects on female brain: A magnetic resonance imaging study of Turner's syndrome [see comments]. *Lancet* 342(8881):1197–1200, 1993.

Naccache L, Dehaene S: The priming method: imaging unconscious repetition priming reveals an abstract representation of number in the parietal lobes. *Cereb Cortex* 11(10):966–974, 2001.

Pesenti M, Seron X, van der Linden M: Selective impairment as evidence for mental organisation of arithmetical facts: BB, a case of preserved subtraction? *Cortex* 30(4):661–671, 1994.

Pesenti M, Thioux M, Seron X, De Volder A: Neuroanatomical substrates of arabic number processing, numerical comparison, and simple addition: a PET study. *J Cogn Neurosci* 12(3): 461–479, 2000.

Pinel P, Rivière D, Le Bihan D, Dehaene S: Modulation of parietal activation by semantic distance in a number comparison task. *Neuroimage* 14(5):1013–1026, 2001.

Reiss AL, Freund L, Plotnick L, et al: The effects of X monosomy on brain development: monozygotic twins discordant for Turner's syndrome. *Ann Neurol* 34(1):95–107, 1993.

Reiss AL, Mazzocco MM, Greenlaw R, et al: Neurodevelopmental effects of X monosomy: A volumetric imaging study. *Ann Neurol* 38(5):731–738, 1995.

Roland PE, Friberg L: Localization of cortical areas activated by thinking. *J Neurophysiol* 53:1219–1243, 1985.

Rossor MN, Warrington EK, Cipolotti L: The isolation of calculation skills. *J Neurol* 242(2):78–81, 1995.

Rovet J, Szekely C, Hockenberry MN: Specific arithmetic calculation deficits in children with Turner syndrome. *J Clin Exp Neuropsychol* 16(6):820–839, 1994.

Rovet JF: The psychoeducational characteristics of children with Turner syndrome. *J Learn Disabil* 26(5):333–341, 1993.

Rueckert L, Lange N, Partiot A, et al: Visualizing cortical activation during mental calculation with functional MRI. *Neuroimage* 3:97–103, 1996.

Seymour SE, Reuter-Lorenz PA, Gazzaniga MS: The disconnection syndrome: Basic findings reaffirmed. *Brain* 117:105–115, 1994.

Shalev RS, Manor O, Kerem B, et al: Developmental dyscalculia is a familial learning disability. *J Learn Disabil* 34:59–65, 2001.

Skuse DH: Imprinting, the X-chromosome, and the male brain: Explaining sex differences in the liability to autism. *Pediatr Res* 47(1):9–16, 2000.

Skuse DH, James RS, Bishop DV, et al: Evidence from Turner's syndrome of an imprinted X-linked locus affecting cognitive function [see comments]. *Nature* 387(6634):705–708, 1997.

Sokol SM, Macaruso P, Gollan TH: Developmental dyscalculia and cognitive neuropsychology. *Dev Neuropsychol* 10:413–441, 1994.

Spellacy F, Peter B: Dyscalculia and elements of the developmental Gerstmann syndrome in school children. *Cortex* 14:197–206, 1978.

Stanescu-Cosso, R, Pinel P, van de Moortele PF, et al: Cerebral bases of calculation processes: Impact of number size on the cerebral circuits for exact and approximate calculation. *Brain* 123:2240–2255, 2000.

Sullivan K S, Macaruso P, Sokol SM: Remediation of arabic number processing in a case of developmental dyscalculia. *Neuropsychol Rehabil* 6:27–53, 1996.

Takayama Y, Sugishita M, Akiguch I, Kimura J, et al: Isolated acalculia due to left parietal lesion. *Arch. Neurol* 51:286–291, 1994.

Temple CM: Digit dyslexia: A category-specific disorder in development dyscalculia. *Cogn Neuropsychol* 6:93–116, 1989.

Temple CM: Procedural dyscalculia and number fact dyscalculia: double dissociation in developmental dyscalculia. *Cogn Neuropsychol* 8:155–176, 1991.

Temple CM: The cognitive neuropsychology of the developmental dyscalculias. *Cah Psychol Cogn /Curr Psychol Cogn* 13:351–370, 1994.

Temple CM, Marriott AJ: Arithmetic ability and disability in Turner's syndrome: A cognitive neuropsychological analysis. *Dev Neuropsychol* 14:47–67, 1998.

Thioux M, Pillon A, Samson D, et al: The isolation of numerals at the semantic level. *Neurocase* 4:371–389, 1998.

van Harskamp NJ, Cipolotti L: Selective impairments for addition, subtraction and multiplication. Implications for the organisation of arithmetical facts. *Cortex* 37(3):363–388, 2001.

Warrington EK: The fractionation of arithmetical skills: A single case study. *Q J Exp Psychol* 34A:31–51, 1982.

Zago L, Pesenti M, Mellet E, et al: Neural correlates of simple and complex mental calculation. *Neuroimage* 13(2): 314–327, 2001.

Chapter 16

DISORDERS OF SKILLED MOVEMENTS: LIMB APRAXIA

Kenneth M. Heilman
Robert T. Watson
Leslie J. Gonzalez Rothi

Apraxia is an inability to correctly perform learned skilled movements. In part, it is defined by what it is not.[1] Patients with impaired motor performance induced by weakness, sensory loss, tremors, dystonia, chorea, ballismus, athetosis, myoclonus, ataxia, and seizures are not considered apraxic. Patients with severe cognitive, memory, motivational, and attentional disorders may have difficulty performing skilled motor acts because they cannot comprehend, cooperate, remember, or attend, but these deficits are also not considered apraxic.

Limb apraxia may be the most frequently unrecognized behavioral disorder associated with cerebral disease. It is most often associated with strokes and degenerative dementia of the Alzheimer type but also occurs with a variety of other diseases. For example, apraxia may be the presenting symptom and sign in corticobasal ganglionic degeneration.

Apraxia may go unrecognized for several reasons. The apraxia associated with strokes is often accompanied by weakness of the preferred arm. In attempting to perform skilled acts with the nonpreferred arm, apraxic patients may recognize that they are not performing well, but they may attribute their difficulty in performing skilled acts to the inexperience of this nondominant arm or to premorbid clumsiness of the nonpreferred arm. However, even when using their dominant limb, apraxic patients may be anosognosic for their apraxia[2] and therefore will not complain of a problem in performing skilled movements. Finally, many physicians and other health professionals do not test for limb apraxia and are not aware of the nature of the errors associated with it or that it may be a disabling disorder.

The types of limb apraxia are defined by the nature of errors made by the patient and the means by which these errors are elicited. Liepmann[3] subdivided limb apraxic disorders into three types: melokinetic (or limb kinetic), ideomotor, and ideational. In addition to discussing these forms of apraxia, three additional forms of apraxia are discussed below, which we have called *disassociation apraxia, conduction apraxia,* and *conceptual apraxia*.

APRAXIA TESTING

The physician must perform a thorough neurologic examination to be certain that abnormal performance is not induced by the nonapraxic motor, sensory, or cognitive disorders mentioned above. The presence of elemental motor defects does not prohibit apraxia testing; however, the examiner must interpret the results with the knowledge gained from the neurologic examination.

Both the right and left forelimbs should be tested independently. Patients should be requested to pantomime to verbal command (e.g., "Show me how you would use a pair of scissors"). All patients should also be asked to imitate the examiner's gestures. The examiner may want to perform both meaningful and meaningless gestures for the patient to imitate. Independent of the results of the pantomime and imitation tests, the patient should be given actual objects and tools and asked to demonstrate how to use the tool or object. One should test transitive movements (i.e., using a tool or instrument) and intransitive movements (i.e., communicative gestures not using tools, such as waving good-bye). When having a patient pantomime, in addition to giving verbal commands, the examiner may also want to show the patient a tool or a picture of the tool or object that the patient is required to pantomime. It may be valuable to see if the patient can recognize transitive and intransitive pantomimes performed by the examiner and discriminate between those that are well and poorly performed. To assess deftness (dexterity) the examiner measures speed, precision, and independent finger movement (e.g., rapid finger tapping; pegboard coin rotation between the thumb, index, and middle finger). The patient should be given a task that requires several motor acts in sequence. Finally, one may want to learn if the patient knows what tools operate on what objects (e.g., hammer and nail), what action is associated with each tool or object, and how to fabricate tools to solve mechanical problems.

LIMB KINETIC APRAXIA

In limb kinetic apraxia, there is a loss of the ability to make finely graded, precise, individual finger movements—a loss of deftness. Limb kinetic apraxia occurs primarily in the limb contralateral to a hemispheric lesion. Right-handed people who have left hemispheric dysfunction may also develop limb kinetic apraxia of their left ipsilesional forelimb.[4,5] Lawrence and Kuypers[6] demonstrated that monkeys with lesions confined to the corticospinal system show similar errors. We have noted that patients with convexity premotor lesions also have limb kinetic apraxia.

IDEOMOTOR APRAXIA

Clinical Findings

Patients with ideomotor apraxia (IMA) make the most errors when asked to pantomime transitive acts. They typically improve with imitation and may perform the best when using actual tools with actual objects.

We classify apraxic errors as errors of content or of production.[7] In order to be considered as having IMA, a patient should make primarily production errors. Content errors occur when a patient substitutes an incorrect but recognizable pantomime for the target pantomime. For example, when asked to pantomime using scissors, a patient may demonstrate hammering movements. Occasionally, a patient's performance is so profoundly impaired that the examiner cannot recognize the intent of the movements. When patients with IMA pantomime, their pantomimes may be incorrectly produced, but the goal or intent of the act can usually be recognized as correct.

Patients with IMA make two major types of production errors: spatial and temporal. Spatial errors can be divided into several subtypes, including postural (or internal configuration), spatial movement, and spatial orientation. Regarding postural errors, Goodglass and Kaplan[8] noted that when patients with IMA are asked to pantomime, they often use a body part as the tool. For example, when these patients are asked to pantomime using a pair of scissors, they may use their fingers as if they were the blades. Many normal subjects make a similar error; therefore, it is imperative that the patient be instructed not to use a body part as a tool. Patients with IMA may continue to make errors using body parts as tools in spite of these instructions. Patients with IMA will often fail to position their hands as if they were holding the tool or object they were requested to pantomime.

When normal subjects are asked to use a tool, they will orient that tool to the target of that tool's action (whether real or imaginary). Patients with IMA often fail to orient their forelimbs to a real or imaginary target. For example, when asked to pantomime cutting a piece of paper in half with a scissors, rather than keeping the scissors oriented in the sagittal plane, the patient may orient the scissors laterally.[7]

When making spatial movement errors, patients with IMA will often make the correct core movement (e.g., twisting, pounding, cutting) but will not move their limb correctly through space.[7,9] These spatial movement errors are associated with incorrect joint movements such that the apraxic patients will stabilize a joint that should be moving and move joints that should be stabilized. For example, in pantomiming the use of a screwdriver, the patient with IMA may rotate his arm at the shoulder joint and fix his elbow. Shoulder rotation moves the hand in circles rather than rotating the hand on a fixed axis. When multiple joint movements must be coordinated, the patient may be unable to coordinate the movement to get the desired spatial trajectory. For example, when pantomiming sawing wood, the shoulder and elbow joints must be alternatively flexed and extended. When the joint movements are not well coordinated, the patient may make primarily chopping or stabbing movements.

Poizner and colleagues[9] have noted that patients with IMA may make timing errors, including a long delay before initiating a movement and brief multiple stops (stuttering movements). Patients with IMA often do not demonstrate a smooth sinusoidal hand speed when they perform cyclic movements, such as slicing bread with a knife.

Pathophysiology

Whereas in right-handed individuals, IMA is almost always associated with left hemisphere lesions, in left-handers IMA is usually associated with right hemisphere lesions. Ideomotor apraxia can be induced by lesions in a variety of structures, including the corpus callosum, inferior parietal lobe, and supplementary motor area (SMA). IMA has also been reported with subcortical lesions that involve basal ganglia and white matter. Below, each of these anatomic areas is discussed and an attempt is made to develop a model of how the brain mediates learned skilled motor activity of the limbs.

Corpus Callosum In 1907 Liepmann and Maas[10] described a patient with a right hemiparesis from a lesion of the pons and a lesion of the corpus callosum. This patient was unable to pantomime correctly to command with his left arm. Because this patient had a right hemiparesis, his right hand could not be tested. Since the work of Broca and Wernicke, neurologists have known that right-handers' left hemisphere is dominant for language. Liepmann and Maas could have attributed their patient's inability to pantomime to a disconnection between language and motor areas, such that the left hemisphere, which mediates comprehension of the verbal command, could not influence the right hemisphere, which is responsible for controlling the left hand. However, this patient could also not imitate gestures or use actual objects correctly, and language-motor disconnection could not account for these findings. Liepmann and Maas therefore posited that the left hemisphere of right-handers contains movement formulas (or spatiotemporal representations of movements) and that the callosal lesion disconnects these movement formulas from the motor areas of the right hemisphere.

Geschwind and Kaplan[11] as well as Gazzaniga and coworkers[12] found that their patients with callosal disconnection, unlike the callosal patient of Liepmann and Maas, could not correctly pantomime to command with the left hand but could imitate and correctly use actual objects with this hand, suggesting that the apraxia of callosal disconnection in these patients was induced by a language-motor disconnection. Watson and Heilman,[13] however, described a patient with an infarction of the body of the corpus callosum. This patient, however, had no weakness in her right hand and performed all tasks flawlessly with that hand; but with her left hand, she could not correctly pantomime to command, imitate, or use actual objects. Although early in her course she made content errors, she subsequently made the spatial and temporal errors associated with IMA. Her performance indicated that not only language but also movement representations were stored in the left hemisphere and her callosal lesion disconnected these movement representations from the right hemisphere.

Inferior Parietal Lobe Whereas Geschwind[9] proposed that the ideomotor apraxia associated with left-sided parietal lesions induced a language motor disconnection, Heilman and colleagues[14] and Rothi and coworkers[15] proposed that the movement representations or movement formulas were stored in the left parietal lobe of right-handers and that destruction of the left parietal lobe should induce not only a production deficit (apraxia) but also a gesture comprehension/discrimination disorder. Apraxia induced by premotor lesions, lesions of the pathways that connect premotor areas to motor areas, or the pathways that lead to the premotor areas from the parietal lobe may also cause a production deficit. In contrast to parietal lesions, however, these lesions should not induce gesture comprehension/discrimination disorders. Heilman and colleagues[14] and Rothi and associates[15] tested patients with anterior and posterior lesions and found that while both groups were apraxic, the patients with a damaged parietal lobe had comprehension-discrimination disturbances and those with more anterior lesions did not.

Liepmann proposed that handedness was related to the hemispheric laterality of the movement representations. It is not unusual, however, to see right-handed patients with left hemisphere lesions who are not apraxic. Although it is possible that these patients' lesions did not destroy a critical left hemisphere area, it is also possible that not all right-handers have movement representations stored entirely in their left hemisphere. Some people may have either bilateral movement representations or even right hemisphere representations. Apraxia from a right hemisphere lesion in a right-hander is rare but has been reported, suggesting that hand preference is not entirely determined by the laterality of the movement representations and may be multifactorial. Whereas the laterality of the movement formula may be the most important factor, there are other factors, including more elemental motor factors such as strength, speed, precision, attentional factors, and even environmental factors.

Supplementary Motor Area Muscles move joints, and motor nerves from the spinal cord activate these muscles. The motor nerves are activated by corticospinal neurons. The corticospinal tract neurons are, in turn, activated by neurons in the premotor areas.

For each specific skilled movement there is a set of spatial loci that must be traversed in a specific temporal pattern. We proposed that movement formulas that are represented in the inferior parietal lobe are stored in a three-dimensional supramodal code. Although Geschwind[11] thought that the convexity premotor cortex was important for praxis, its function in the control of praxis remains uncertain. The convexity premotor cortex may be important in motor learning or in adapting the program to environmental pertubations.

The medial premotor cortex or supplementary motor area (SMA), however, appears to play an important role in mediating skilled movements. Whereas electrical stimulation of the primary motor cortex induces simple movements, SMA stimulation induces complex movements of the fingers, arms, and hands. The SMA receives projections from parietal neurons and projects to motor neurons in the primary motor cortex. The SMA neurons appear to discharge before neurons in the primary motor cortex. Studies of cerebral blood flow, an indicator of synaptic activity, have revealed that a single repetitive movement increases activation of the contralateral motor cortex, but complex movements increase flow in the contralateral motor cortex and in SMA. When subjects remained still and thought about making complex movements, blood flow to the SMA increased but the blood flow to the motor

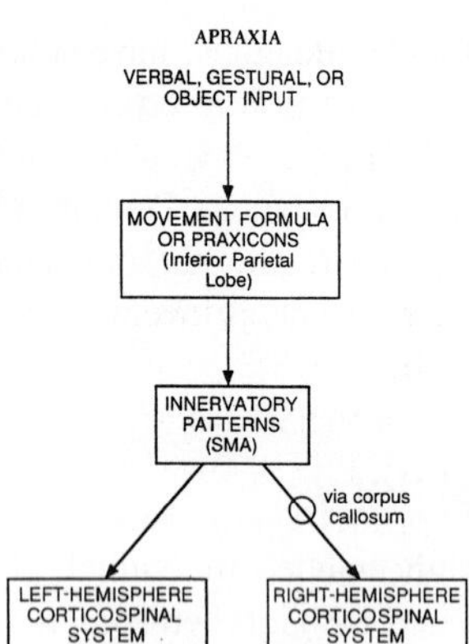

Figure 16-1
Diagrammatic model of ideomotor apraxia. SMA, supplementary motor area. (From Heilman and Rothi,[27] with permission.)

cortex remained unchanged. Watson and coworkers[16] reported several patients with left-sided mediofrontal lesions that included the SMA who demonstrated an ideomotor apraxia when tested with either arm. Unlike patients with parietal lesions, these patients could both comprehend and discriminate pantomimes.

The model we have discussed so far is illustrated in Fig. 16-1. The praxicon is a theoretical store of the temporospatial representations of learned skill movements. When a skilled act is being performed, these representations are transcoded into innervatory patterns by the SMA. When the right hand acts, the SMA programs the motor cortex (Brodmann's area 4) of the left hemisphere, and when the left hand acts, these innervatory patterns activate the motor regions of the right hemisphere via the corpus callosum.

Basal Ganglia and Thalamus Portions of the basal ganglia such as the putamen receive projections from premotor cortex including the SMA. Several investigators have reported that injury to the basal ganglia can induce IMA.[17,18] Pramstaller and Marsden,[19] however, thought that the evidence supporting the basal ganglia apraxia postulate was weak and that the apraxia reported to be associated with basal ganglia lesions was probably related to damage to other areas of the brain. More recently, Hanna-Pladdy not only reported additional patients with IMA from basal ganglia lesions but also demonstrated that these patients made primarily postural errors.

DeRenzi et al.[18] also reported that patients with thalamic lesions might demonstrate IMA. In regard to the intrathalamic localization, Shuren et al.[20] as well as Nadeau et al.[21] reported that these lesions might involve the pulvinar. The pulvinar thalamic nucleus projects primarily to the parietal lobe, where movement representation are stored, and these pulvinar lesions might interfere with the activation of these movement representations.

DISASSOCIATION APRAXIAS

Clinical Findings

Heilman[22] described several patients who, when asked to pantomime to command, looked at their open hands or would slowly pronate and supinate their arms but would not perform any recognizable action. Unlike the patients with ideomotor apraxia described above, these patients' imitations and use of objects were flawless. DeRenzi and colleagues[23] reported patients similar to those reported by Heilman[22] and also other patients who had a similar defect in other modalities. For example, when asked to pantomime in response to visual or tactile stimuli, they may have been unable to do so, but they could pantomime to verbal command.

Pathophysiology

While callosal lesions may be associated with an ideomotor apraxia, callosal disconnection may also cause disassociation apraxia. The subjects of Gazzaniga and associates[12] and the patients described by Geschwind and Kaplan[11] had disassociation apraxia. We posit that language in these patients was mediated by the left hemisphere and movement representations were bilaterally represented. A callosal lesion induced a dissociation between the portions of the left hemisphere, which are important in language comprehension, and the motor cortex of the right hemisphere, which controls the left hand. Thus, the patient with callosal disassociation apraxia will not be able to correctly carry out skilled learned movements of the left arm to command, but he or she will be able to imitate and use actual objects with the left hand because these tasks do not require language and these patient's right hemisphere contains the movement formula as well as the other apparatus needed to transcode the time-space movement representations to motor acts.

Right-handed patients who have both language and movement formula represented in their left hemisphere may show a combination of disassociation and ideomotor apraxia with callosal lesions.[13] When asked to pantomime with their left hands, they may look at them and perform no recognizable movement (disassociation apraxia); but when imitating or using actual objects, they may demonstrate the spatial and temporal errors seen with ideomotor apraxia.

Left-handers may demonstrate an ideomotor apraxia without aphasia from a right hemisphere lesion. These left-handers are apraxic because their movement representations were stored in their right hemispheres and their lesions destroyed these representations.[24,25] These left-handers were not aphasic because language was mediated by their left hemispheres (as is the case in the majority of left-handers). If these left-handers had a callosal lesion, they may have demonstrated a disassociation apraxia of the left arm and an ideomotor apraxia of the right arm.

The disassociation apraxia described by Heilman[22] from left hemisphere lesions was unfortunately incorrectly termed "ideational apraxia." The patients reported by Heilman[22] and those of DeRenzi and associates[23] probably have an intrahemispheric language-movement formula, a visual-movement formula, or a somesthetic-movement formula disassociation. The locations of the lesions that cause these intrahemispheric disassociation apraxias are not known.

CONDUCTION APRAXIA

Clinical Findings

Ochipa and coworkers[26] reported a patient who was unlike patients with ideomotor apraxia because, rather than improving with imitation, this patient was more impaired when imitating than when pantomiming to command.

Pathophysiology

Because this patient with conduction apraxia could comprehend the examiner's pantomime and gestures, we believe that the patient's visual system could access the movement representations, or what we have termed *praxicons,*[27] and that the activated movement representations, or praxicons, could activate semantics. It is possible that decoding a gesture requires the accessing of different movement representations or praxicons than does programming an action. Therefore, Ochipa and colleagues[26] and Rothi and coworkers[28] suggested that there may be two different stores of movement representations, an input praxicon and output praxicon. In the verbal domain, a disconnection of the hypothetical input and output lexicons induces conduction aphasia; in the praxis domain, a disconnection between the input and output praxicons could induce conduction apraxia.

Whereas the lesions that induce conduction aphasia are usually in the supramarginal gyrus or Wernicke's area, the location of lesions that induce conduction apraxia are unknown.

IDEATIONAL APRAXIA

Unfortunately, there has been much confusion about the meaning of the term *ideational apraxia.* The inability to carry out a series of acts, an ideational plan, has been called ideational apraxia.[29,30] In performing a task that requires a series of acts, these patients have difficulty sequencing the acts in the proper order (for example, instead of cleaning the pipe, putting tobacco in the bowl, lighting the tobacco, and smoking, the patient might attempt to light the empty bowl, put the tobacco in the bowl, and then clean it). Pick[30] noted that most of the patients with this type of ideational apraxia have a dementing disease.

Whereas most patients with apraxia improve when they are using objects. DeRenzi and colleagues[31] reported patients who made errors with the use of actual objects. Although the inability to use actual objects may be associated with a conceptual disorder, a severe production disorder may also impair object use.[32] However, as discussed in the next section, production and conceptual disorders may be associated with different types of errors.

CONCEPTUAL APRAXIA

Clinical Findings

To perform a skilled act, two types of knowledge are needed: conceptual knowledge and production knowledge. Dysfunction of the praxis production system induces ideomotor apraxia. Defects in the knowledge needed to successfully select and use the tools or objects we term *conceptual apraxia.* Whereas patients with ideomotor apraxia make production errors (e.g., spatial and temporal errors), patients with conceptual apraxia make content and tool-selection errors. The patients with conceptual apraxia may not recall the types of actions associated with specific tools, utensils, or objects (tool–object action knowledge) and therefore make content errors.[33,34] For example, when asked to demonstrate the use of a screwdriver, either pantomining or using the tool, the patient may pantomime a hammering movement or use the screwdriver as if it were a hammer.

The patient with ideomotor apraxia may make production errors by moving the hand in circles rather than twisting the hand on its own axis. Although such patients make production errors by moving the hand in circles, they are demonstrating knowledge of the turning action of screwdrivers. Content errors (i.e., using a tool as if it were another tool) can also be induced by an object agnosia. However, Ochipa and associates[35] reported a patient who could name tools (and therefore was not agnosic) but often used them inappropriately.

Patients with conceptual apraxia may be unable to recall which specific tool is associated with a specific object (tool–object association knowledge). For example, when shown a partially driven nail, they may select a screwdriver rather than a hammer from an array of tools. This conceptual defect may also be in the verbal domain, such that when an actual tool is shown to a patient with conceptual apraxia, the patient may be able to name it (e.g., hammer); but when the patient is asked to name or point to a tool when its function is discussed, he or she cannot. The patient may also be unable to describe the functions of tools.

Patients with conceptual apraxia may also have impaired mechanical knowledge. For example, if they are attempting to drive a nail into a piece of wood and there is no hammer available, they may select a screwdriver rather than a wrench or pliers (which are hard, heavy, and good for pounding).[35] Mechanical knowledge is also important for tool development, and patients with conceptual apraxia may be unable to develop tools correctly.[35]

Pathophysiology

Liepmann[3] thought that conceptual knowledge was located in the caudal parietal lobe, and DeRenzi and Luccelli[33] placed it in the temporoparietal junction. The patient reported by Ochipa and coworkers[34] was left-handed and rendered conceptually apraxic by a lesion in the right hemisphere, suggesting that both production and conceptual knowledge have lateralized representations and that such representations are contralateral to the preferred hand. Further evidence that these conceptual representations are stored in the hemisphere contralateral to the preferred hand comes from a study of right-handed patients who had unilateral strokes of either their right or left hemisphere. This study revealed that left hemisphere but not right hemisphere injury is associated with conceptual apraxia.[36] We also studied a patient who had a callosal disconnection and demonstrated conceptual apraxia and ideomotor apraxia of her nonpreferred (left) hand.[13] Conceptual apraxia, however, is most commonly seen in degenerative dementia of the Alzheimer type.[35] Ochipa and colleagues noted that the severity of conceptual and ideomotor apraxia did not always correlate. The observation that patients with ideomotor apraxia may not demonstrate conceptual apraxia and patients with conceptual apraxia may not demonstrate ideomotor apraxia provides support for the postulate that the praxis production and praxis conceptual systems are independent. For normal function, however, these two systems must interact.

CONCLUSIONS

Lesions of the motor cortex and perhaps convexity premotor cortex induces a loss of hand deftness called limb-kinetic apraxia. In right handed people left hemisphere injury can cause ipsilateral deficits.

Movement representations (praxicons) are stored in the left inferior parietal lobe of right-handers. These representations code the spatial and temporal patterns of learned skilled movements. Injury to the left parietal lobe induces a production deficit in both hands termed ideomotor apraxia. Patients with ideomotor apraxia make spatial and temporal errors. Patients with injury to these representations are not only impaired at pantomiming, imitating, and using actual objects but also cannot discriminate between well- and poorly performed gestures. These patients may also not be able to comprehend gestures. Patients with injury to premotor cortex and the basal ganglia also have IMA but these patients can discriminate and comprehend gestures.

There are patients who are more impaired at imitation of gestures than they are when gesturing to command (conduction apraxia), suggesting that movement representations (praxicons) may be divided into input and output subdivisions. In conduction apraxia, there is a dissociation between these input and output praxicons.

In order to perform learned skilled acts, abstract movement representations have to be transcoded into motor programs. This transcoding appears to be performed by a premotor (supplementary motor area)—basal ganglia (putamen-globus pallidus-thalamus) system. Injuries to the brain that interrupt the connections between the movement representations stored in the parietal lobe and the portions of the brain that develop the innervatory patterns or the parts of the brain that allow the innervatory patterns to gain access to the motor system may also produce a praxis production deficit (ideomotor apraxia).

A patient may have intact representations of learned skilled movements but have modality-specific deficits in accessing these representations. For example, a patient with dissociation apraxia may be unable to pantomime to command but be able to pantomime correctly when seeing the tool.

Finally, some patients, when pantomiming or using actual tools, may make content errors. Whereas spatial and temporal errors are related to deficits in the praxic production system, content errors are related to deficits in a hypothetical praxis conceptual system or action semantics. Dysfunction of this system, termed *conceptual apraxia,* may produce deficits of associative knowledge, such as tool-action or tool-object knowledge (i.e., knowing that a hammer is used to pound and that a hammer is associated with a nail). Defects in action semantics may also be associated with deficits in mechanical knowledge (i.e., knowing how to use alternative tools and how to fabricate tools).

REFERENCES

1. Geschwind N: Disconnection syndromes in animals and man. *Brain* 88:237–294, 585–644, 1965.
2. Rothi LJG, Mack L, Heilman KM: Unawareness of apraxic errors. *Neurology* 40(suppl 1):202, 1990.
3. Liepmann H: Apraxia. *Erbgn Ges Med* 1:516–543, 1920.
4. Heilman KM, Meador KJ, Loring DW: Hemispheric asymmetries of limb-kinetic apraxia: A loss of deftness. *Neurology* 55:523–526, 2000.
5. Hanna-Pladdy B, Daniels SK, Fieselman MA, et al: Praxis lateralization: Errors in right and left hemisphere stroke. *Cortex* 37:219–230, 2001.
6. Lawrence DG, Kuypers HGJM: The functional organization of the motor system in the monkey. *Brain* 91:1–36, 1968.
7. Rothi LJG, Mack L, Verfaellie M, et al: Ideomotor apraxia: Error pattern analysis. *Aphasiology* 2:381–387, 1988.
8. Goodglass H, Kaplan E: Disturbance of gesture and pantomime in aphasia. *Brain* 86:703–720, 1963.
9. Poizner H, Mack L, Verfaellie M, et al: Three dimensional computer graphic analysis of apraxia. *Brain* 113:85–101, 1990.
10. Liepmann H, Mass O: Fall von Linksseitiger Agraphie und Apraxie bei Rechsseitiger Lahmung. *Z Psychol Neurol* 10:214–227, 1907.
11. Geschwind N, Kaplan E: A human cerebral disconnection syndrome. *Neurology* 12:675–685, 1962.
12. Gazzaniga M, Bogen J, Sperry R: Dyspraxia following diversion of the cerebral commisures. *Arch Neurol* 16:606–612, 1967.
13. Watson RT, Heilman KM: Callosal apraxia. *Brain* 106:391–403, 1983.
14. Heilman KM, Rothi LJ, Valenstein E: Two forms of ideomotor apraxia. *Neurology* 32:342–346, 1982.
15. Rothi LJG, Heilman KM, Watson RT: Pantomime comprehension and ideomotor apraxia. *J Neurol Neurosurg Psychiatry* 48:207–210, 1985.
16. Watson RT, Fleet WS, Rothi LJG, Heilman KM: Apraxia and the supplementary motor area. *Arch Neurol* 43:787–792, 1986.
17. Agostoni E, Coletti A, Orlando G, Tredici G: Apraxia in deep cerebral lesions. *J Neurol Neurosurg* Psychiatry 46(9):804–808, 1983.
18. DeRenzi E, Faglioni P, Scarpa M, Crisi G: Limb apraxia in patients with damage confined to the left basal ganglia and thalamus. *J Neurol Neurosurg Psychiatry* 49(9):1030–1038, 1986.
19. Pramstaller PP, Marsden CD: The basal ganglia and apraxia. *Brain* 119(pt 1):319–340, 1996.
20. Shuren JE, Maher LM, Heilman KM: Role of the pulvinar in ideomotor praxis. *J Neurol Neurosurg Psychiatry* 57(10):1282–1283, 1994.
21. Nadeau SE, Roeltgen DP, Sevush S, et al: Apraxia due to a pathologically documented thalamic infarction. *Neurology* 44(11):2133–2137, 1994.
22. Heilman KM: Ideational apraxia–A re-definition. *Brain* 96:861–864, 1973.
23. DeRenzi E, Faglioni P, Sorgato P: Modality-specific and supramodal mechanisms of apraxia. *Brain* 105:301–312, 1982.
24. Heilman KM, Coyle JM, Gonyea EF, Geschwind N: Apraxia and agraphia in a left-hander. *Brain* 96:21–28, 1973.
25. Valenstein E, Heilman KM: Apraxic agraphia with neglect induced paragraphia. *Arch Neurol* 36:506–508, 1979.
26. Ochipa C, Rothi LJG, Heilman KM: Conduction apraxia. *J Clin Exp Neuropsychol* 12:89, 1990.
27. Heilman KM, Rothi LJG: Apraxia, in Heilman KM, Valenstein E (eds): *Clinical Neuropsychology*, 3d ed. New York: Oxford University Press, 1993.
28. Rothi LJG, Ochipa C, Heilman KM: A cognitive neuropsychological model of limb praxis. *Cogn Neuropsychol* 8:443–458, 1991.
29. Marcuse H: Apraktiscke Symotome bein linem Fall von seniler Demenz. *Zentralbl Mervheik Psychiatr* 27:737–751, 1904.
30. Pick A: *Studien über Motorische Apraxia und ihre Mahestenhende Erscheinungen*. Leipzig: Deuticke, 1905.
31. DeRenzi E, Pieczuro A, Vignolo L: Ideational apraxia: A quantitative study. *Neuropsychologia* 6:41–52, 1968.
32. Zangwell OL: L'apraxie ideatorie. *Nerve Neurol* 106:595–603, 1960.
33. DeRenzi E, Lucchelli F: Ideational apraxia. *Brain* 113:1173–1188, 1988.
34. Ochipa C, Rothi LJG, Heilman KM: Ideational apraxia: A deficit in tool selection and use. *Ann Neurol* 25:190–193, 1989.
35. Ochipa C, Rothi LJG. Heilman KM: Conceptual apraxia in Alzheimer's disease. *Brain* 115:1061–1071, 1992.
36. Heilman KM, Maher LM, Greenwald ML, Rothi LJG: Conceptual apraxia from lateralized lesions. *Neurology* 49:457–464, 1997.

Part 3

AGNOSIA AND DISORDERS OF PERCEPTION

Chapter 17

VISUAL PERCEPTION AND VISUAL IMAGERY

Martha J. Farah

Primates are visual creatures, and humans are no exception to this generalization. If one surveys our cortex and asks which areas are either partially or exclusively devoted to processing information from our eyes, one finds that about half of the cortex is involved in vision. Vision is the main function of occipital cortex and occupies much of parietal and temporal cortex as well. Even the most anterior parts of the brain include areas dedicated to eye-movement programming and visual working memory. One consequence of having this far-flung visual network is that lesions to many different parts of the brain can affect vision. The nature of the visual disturbance depends on the particular contribution that the damaged area would normally have made to vision.

Several chapters in this book are devoted to specific visual disorders that result from damage to high-level visual areas—that is, visual areas that are several synapses past primary visual cortex. These disorders include visual object agnosia (Chap. 18); prosopagnosia (Chap. 19); certain disorders of reading (Chap. 14), color processing (Chap. 20), and neglect (Chaps. 25 and 26); Balint's syndrome (Chap. 27), and visual spatial disorders (Chap. 24). The goal of this chapter is to review cortical visual processing at stages prior to these high-level functions. The chapter also considers cognitive disorders of mental imagery, or the activation of these visual representations endogenously as a medium of thought. In each case, the disorders arising from damage to these stages of vision is reviewed with respect to their main behavioral features, associated lesion sites, and implications for our understanding of normal vision.

VISUAL PERCEPTION

Damage to Primary Visual Cortex and Its Afferents

Although considerable information processing is carried out in the retina and thalamus, the visual disorders relevant to behavioral neurology generally involve brain damage at the level of primary visual cortex and beyond. Because the vast majority of visual information is processed through primary visual cortex on its way to higher-level perceptual areas, destruction of primary visual cortex causes cortical blindness. Partial destruction causes partial blindness, and the location of the lesion within primary visual cortex corresponds to the location of the blind spot, or visual field defect, in a highly systematic way that reflects the retinotopy of primary visual cortex. With vascular lesions, it is common for some or all of the primary cortex in one hemisphere to be damaged while the opposite hemisphere is unaffected. This results in blindness restricted to one-half of the visual field, or *hemianopia*. It is sometimes called *homonymous hemianopia* to indicate that the blind regions are the same regardless of which eye is used to see.

As shown in Fig. 17-1, visual field defects can be used to deduce the location of the lesion and were regularly used in this way before the days of computed tomography (CT). Homonymous visual field defects imply that the lesion is posterior, because input from the two eyes merges anteriorly. Because the left optic radiation projecting to left visual cortex represent only the right visual field, and vice versa, visual field

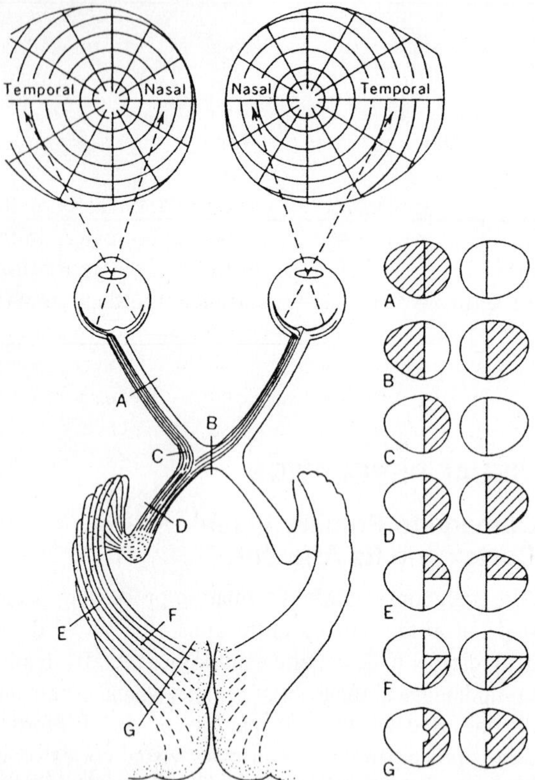

Figure 17-1
Correspondences between location of lesion within the visual system and pattern of visual field defects. (From Homans J: A Textbook of Surgery. *Springfield, IL: Charles C Thomas, 1945, with permission.)*

defects also reveal the side of the lesion. The altitude of the visual field defect is also informative, with lower-quadrant blindness, or *quadrantanopia,* suggesting a parietal or superior occipital lesion, because of the dorsal course of the pathways from thalamus to cortex, and upper quadrantanopia suggesting a temporal or inferior occipital lesion, because of the ventral course.

Prosopagnosia (see Chap. 19) was first localized on the basis of the visual field defects reported in a large set of cases (Meadows, 1974). Most cases reported a upper-left quadrantanopia, some with defects in the upper right as well. From this, Meadows was able to infer that the critical substrates for face recognition are in the right temporal cortex or bilateral temporal cortices in most people—a conclusion that has withstood the tremendous increase in localizing capability as structural and functional brain imaging became available.

Although hemianopia and quadrantanopia are, by definition, blindness in the regions of the visual field represented by damaged visual cortex or its afferents, there are patients who retain some visual functions in these regions. *Blindsight* is the appropriately oxymoronic term applied to this puzzling phenomenon. The preserved perceptual abilities may be limited to localization of light and movement, but in some cases the limitations go well beyond this.

In one very thoroughly studied case of blindsight, Weiskrantz and colleagues (1986) found relatively preserved ability to point to the locations of visual stimuli, to detect movement, to discriminate the orientations of lines and gratings, and to discriminate large shapes such as X and O despite the patient's denial that he could see anything. The mechanism of blindsight has been a controversial topic. One possibility is that it simply reflects incomplete damage to visual cortex (see, e.g., Fendrich and coworkers, 2001), although this seems unlikely given that hemidecorticate patients have shown blindsight. Other explanations involve pathways to visual association cortex that bypass primary visual cortex. One such possibility is that blindsight is mediated by the subcortical visual system, which consists of projections from the retina to the superior colliculus and pulvinar and its projections to secondary cortical visual areas (e.g., Rafal et al., 1990). Alternatively, there may be sparse projections within the cortical visual system, from the lateral geniculate nucleus directly to visual association cortex (Stoerig and Cowey, 1997).

Damage to Surrounding Association Cortex

Surrounding primary visual cortex is additional modality-specific visual cortex that receives its input principally from primary visual cortex. From single-cell recording and other invasive measures used in animals, it is known that this region is functionally a mosaic of areas, each of which represents the visual field with some degree of retinotopy and has largely reciprocal projections to particular sets of other visual areas (see Zigmond et al., 1999). It is assumed that this multiplicity of areas is there for some purpose and that each area probably analyzes different aspects of the input, although this assumption has been fully validated in only a couple of cases—areas that subserve color vision and motion vision.

Primate neurophysiology has shown that neurons in area V4 of the monkey brain are highly selective for color and indeed respond to color per se rather than wavelength (Zeki, 1983). (The difference can be appreciated by considering that the green color of a plant, for instance, remains at least roughly constant across ambient lighting conditions containing widely differing wavelengths, which result in different wavelengths reflecting off the plant's surface and stimulating the retina.) That a homologous area exists in humans and is vulnerable to damage is suggested by the disorder *cerebral achromatopsia,* color blindness due to brain damage (see Chap. 20). Achromatopsic patients report that the world seems drained of color, like a black-and-white movie. In other respects, their vision may be at least roughly normal. For example, they may have good acuity, motion and depth perception, and object recognition. It should be added that problems with face, object and printed word recognition do sometimes accompany achromatopsia, but they are often transient and are likely to be caused by impairment to areas neighboring the color area. Cases in which the color vision impairment is truly selective imply that there is a brain region dedicated to color perception—that is, necessary for color perception and not for other aspects of vision.

In some cases, a unilateral lesion will result in color loss in just one hemifield, consistent with retinotopic mapping of the area responsible for color vision. A particularly selective and well-studied case of this was described by Damasio et al. (1980). Although acuity, depth perception, motion perception, and object recognition was normal in both hemifields, they differed strikingly for color perception:

> *He was unable to name any color in any portion of the left field of either eye, including bright reds, blues, greens and yellows. As soon as any portion of a colored object crossed the vertical meridian, he was able instantly to recognize and accurately name its color. When an object such as a red flashlight was held so that it bisected the vertical meridian, he reported that the hue of the right half appeared normal while the left half was gray.*

He was also unable to match colors in the left visual field.

The lesions in achromatopsia are usually on the inferior surface of the temporooccipital region, in the lingual and fusiform gyri. In full achromatopsia they are bilateral, and in hemiachromatopsia they are confined to the hemisphere contralateral to the color vision defect. This localization accords well with functional neuroimaging studies in which the substrates of color perception have been isolated by comparing cerebral activation patterns while subjects view colored displays to patterns resulting when gray-scale versions of the same displays are viewed (e.g., Zeki et al., 1991). Chapter 20 reviews achromatopsia in further detail, as well as distinguishing it from a number of other disorders of color cognition.

Single-cell recording has also been used to elucidate the neural systems of motion perception in the monkey. Area MT (for middle temporal) contains neurons whose response properties suggest a primary role in motion perception. Consistent with this, humans with damage in the homologous region have developed *cerebral akinotopsia* (see Zeki, 1993, for a review). By far the best-studied case is that of Zihl et al. (1983). This was case L.M., a 43-year-old woman who, following bilateral strokes in the posterior parietotemporal and occipital regions, was left with but one major impairment, namely the complete inability to perceive visual motion. Zihl et al. (1983) tested L.M.'s visual perception in a variety of simple experimental tasks and compared her performance with that of normal subjects. In her color and depth perception, object and word recognition, and a variety of other visual abilities tested by these authors, L.M. did not differ significantly from normal subjects. In addition, her ability to judge the motion of a tactile stimulus (wooden stick moved up or down her arm) and an auditory stimulus (tone-emitting loudspeaker moved through space) was also normal. In contrast, her perception of direction and speed of visual motion in horizontal and vertical directions within the picture plane and in depth was grossly impaired.

In her everyday life she was profoundly affected by her visual impairment. When she was pouring tea or coffee, the fluid appeared to be frozen, like a glacier. Without being able to perceive movement, she could not stop pouring at the right time and frequently filled the cup to overflowing. She found it difficult to follow conversations without being able to see the facial and mouth movements of each speaker, and gatherings of more than two other people left her feeling unwell and insecure. She complained that "People were suddenly here or there but I have not seen them moving." The patient could not cross the street because of her inability to judge the speed of a car. "When I see the car at first, it seems far away. But then, when I want to cross the road, suddenly the car is very near." She gradually learned to estimate the distance of moving vehicles by means of the sound as it became louder.

As with achromatopsia, the existence of akinotopsia implies a high degree of cerebral specialization, with one cortical area being necessary for motion perception and not necessary for other aspects of perception. Although L.M.'s lesions were fairly large and encompassed both parietal and temporal cortex, the critical lesion site has been inferred to be the posterior middle temporal gyrus. Functional neuroimaging studies of motion perception, comparing brain activation patterns to moving and static displays, show their maximum in this same region (Zeki et al., 1991).

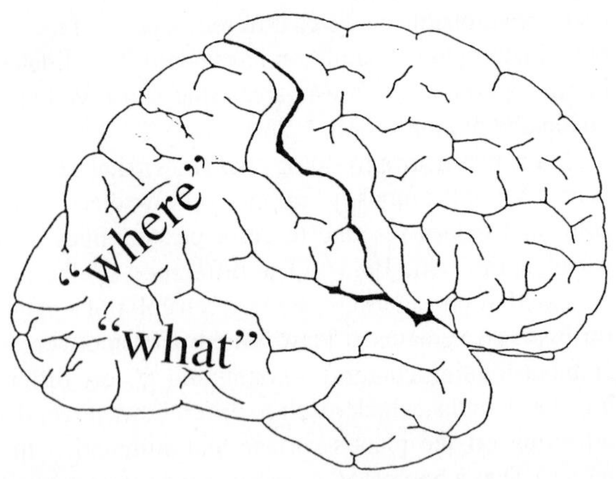

Figure 17-2
The two cortical visual systems: Dorsal visual areas are particularly important for spatial or "where" processing, and ventral visual areas are particularly important for appearance or "what" processing.

An Organizing Framework for Higher-Level Visual Disorders

Vision has two main goals, the identification of stimuli and their localization. Although a bit of an oversimplification, this dichotomy has provided a useful organizing framework for the neuropsychology of high-level vision. The two goals, sometimes abbreviated as *what* and *where,* are achieved by relatively independent and anatomically separate systems, located in ventral and dorsal visual cortices, respectively, as shown in Fig. 17-2. These have been termed *the two cortical visual systems* (Ungerleider and Mishkin, 1972).

Note that the color and motion disorders discussed in the previous section fit naturally into this framework: color is an aspect of appearance that is useful for object recognition but plays little role in spatial function. The critical lesion site for achromatopsia lies on the ventral surface of the brain. Motion is, by its very nature, a spatial property—change of location over time—and is one of the most powerful cues for summoning spatial attention. The critical lesion site for akinotopsia is dorsolateral to this, in the posterior temporal lobe.

Damage further along the dorsal and ventral visual streams is responsible for a variety of neurobehavioral syndromes. The disorders of spatial perception and attention discussed in Chaps. 24 to 27 result from damage to posterior parietal cortex, part of the dorsal *where* route, whereas the disorders of object and face recognition discussed in Chaps. 18 and 19 result from damage to inferior temporal cortex, part of the ventral *what* route.

VISUAL MENTAL IMAGERY

The most obvious function of the cortical visual system is the analysis of retinal inputs. Yet under some circumstances it is also used in thinking, as when we generate a visual image from memory. Brain damage can affect the process of generating a visual mental image in two ways: by impairing the visual representations themselves or by impairing the process of activating those representations in the absence of a stimulus.

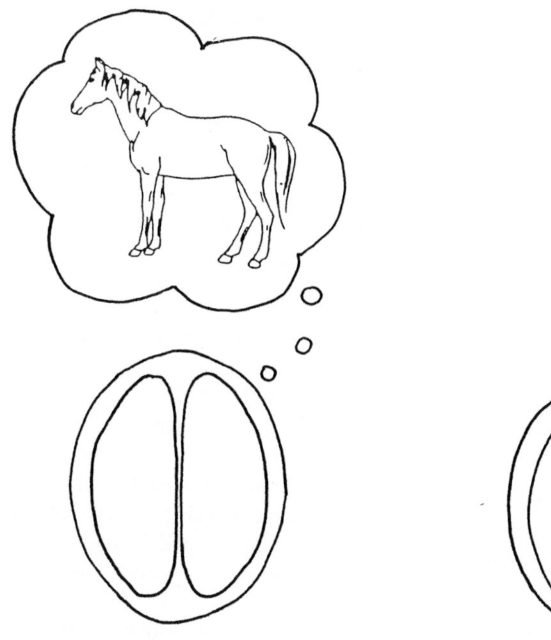
"I can get to within 15 feet of the horse in my imagination before it starts to overflow"

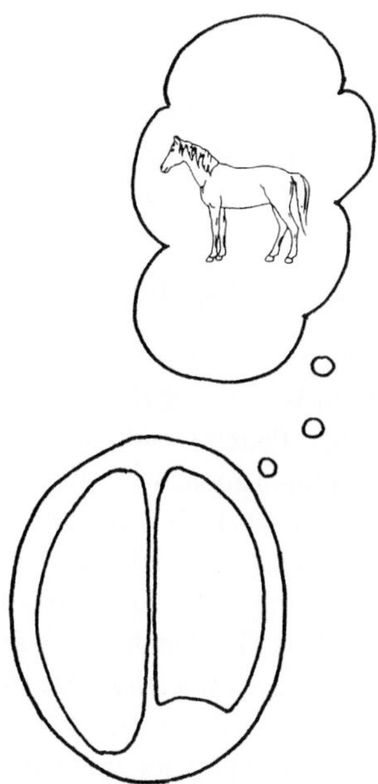

Figure 17-3

Depiction of the effects of unilateral occipital lobectomy on the visual angle of the mind's eye. (From Farah MJ, in Gazzaniga MS (ed): The Cognitive Neurosciences. *Cambridge, MA: MIT Press, 1996, with permission.)*

Disorders of Image Representation

If imagery and perception are both impaired after brain damage, this suggests that the functional locus of damage is the representations of visual appearance used by both. There are many reports of parallel impairments of imagery and perception, and these have attracted interest for what they can tell us about mental image representation. Specifically, they imply that mental imagery shares representations with the cortical visual system.

A clear-cut example of parallel imagery-perception impairment comes from a study comparing visual and "imaginal" fields. We were able to test an epileptic woman before and after a right occipital lobectomy. If mental imagery consists of activating representations in the occipital lobe, then it should be impossible to form images in regions of the visual field that are blind due to occipital lobe destruction. This predicts that after surgery, she should have both a narrower visual field and a narrower imaginal field. By asking her to report the distance of imagined objects such as a horse, breadbox, or ruler when they are visualized as close as possible without "overflowing" her imaginal field, we could compute the visual angle of that field. We found that the size of her biggest possible image was reduced after surgery, as represented in Fig. 17-3. Furthermore, by measuring maximal image size in the vertical and horizontal dimensions separately, we found that only the horizontal dimension of her imaginal field was significantly reduced. These results provide strong evidence for the use of occipital visual representations during imagery.

Other parallels have been noted as well—for example, between disorders of color perception and disorders of color imagery, between left visual neglect and inattention to the left sides of mental images, and between the ability to recognize objects from their visual appearance and the ability to imagine their appearance. A fuller discussion of these findings, as well as cases of visual impairment in which imagery ability is not affected, may be found in Farah (2000).

Disorders of Image Generation

In the absence of visual perceptual disorder, visual imagery may be impaired because of damage affecting image generation ability. Patients with an image generation deficit are disproportionately impaired at answering questions such as "Which is bigger, a grapefruit or a cantaloupe?" or "Does a kangaroo have a short or a long tail?" compared to questions that do not evoke imagery such as "Do kangaroos wash their food before eating it?" Other indications are that their drawing from memory is sketchy despite good copying ability, and their ability to report the color of objects from memory depends upon the availability of verbal associations (e.g., the colors of the sky, lemons, and fire engines can be retrieved without imagery, but the color of a coke can, a mailbox, or a peanut cannot). Some typical cases include those of Farah and coworkers (1988), Goldenberg (1992), Grossi and colleagues (1986), and Riddoch (1990). The critical lesion site in these cases appears to be left temporooccipital cortex (see Farah, 1995, for a review of lesion and neuroimaging data).

REFERENCES

Damasio AR, Yamada T, Damasio H, et al: Central achromatopsia: behavioral, anatomic, and physiologic aspects. *Neurology* 30:1064–1071, 1980.

Farah MJ: Current issues in the neuropsychology of mental image generation. *Neuropsychologia* 33:1445–1471, 1995.

Farah MJ: *The Cognitive Neuroscience of Vision*. Oxford, UK: Blackwell, 2000.

Farah MJ, Hammond KL, Levine DN, Calvanio R: Visual and spatial mental imagery: Dissociable systems of representation. *Cogn Psychol* 20:439–462, 1988.

Fendrich R, Wessinger CM, Gazzaniga MS: Speculations on the neural basis of islands of blindsight. *Prog Brain Res* 134:353–366, 2001.

Goldenberg G: Loss of visual imagery and loss of visual knowledge—a case study. *Neuropsychologia* 30:1081–1099, 1992.

Grossi D, Orsini A, Modafferi A: Visuoimaginal constructional apraxia: On a case of selective deficit of imagery. *Brain Cogn* 5:255–267, 1986.

Meadows JC: The anatomical basis of prosopagnosia. *J Neurol Neurosurgery Psychiatry* 37:489–501, 1974.

Rafal R, Smith J, Krantz J, et al: Extrageniculate vision in hemianopic humans: saccade inhibition by signals in the blind field. *Science* 250:118–121, 1990.

Riddoch JM: Loss of visual imagery: A generation deficit. *Cogn Neuropsychol* 7:249–273, 1990.

Stoerig P, Cowey A: Blindsight in man and monkey, *Brain* 120:535–559, 1997.

Ungerleider LG, Mishkin M: Two cortical visual systems, in Ingle DJ, Goodale MA, Mansfield RJW (eds): *Analysis of Visual Behavior*. Cambridge, MA: MIT Press, 1982.

Weiskrantz L: *Blindsight: A Case Study and Implications*. Oxford, UK: Oxford University Press, 1986.

Zeki S: Colour coding in the cerebral cortex: The reaction of cells in monkey visual cortex to wavelengths and colours. *Neuroscience* 9:741–756, 1983.

Zeki S: *A Vision of the Brain*. Oxford, UK: Blackwell, 1993.

Zeki S, Watson JDG, Lueck CJ, et al: A direct demonstration of functional specialization in human visual cortex. *J Neurosci* 11:641–649, 1991.

Zigmond M, Floom FE, Landis SC (eds): *Fundamental Neuroscience*. New York: Academic Press, 1998.

Zihl J, von Cramon D, Mai N: Selective disturbance of movement vision after bilateral brain damage. *Brain* 106:313–340, 1983.

Chapter 18

VISUAL OBJECT AGNOSIA

Martha J. Farah
Todd E. Feinberg

The term *visual object agnosia* refers to the impairment of object recognition in the presence of relatively intact elementary visual perception, memory, and general intellectual function. This chapter reviews the different subtypes of agnosia, their major clinical features and associated neuropathology, and their implications for cognitive neuroscience theories of visual object recognition.

The study of agnosia has a long history of controversy, with some authors doubting that the condition even exists. For example, Bay[1] suggested that the appearance of disproportionate difficulty with visual object recognition could invariably be explained by synergistic interactions between mild perceptual impairments on the one hand and mild general intellectual impairments on the other. The rarity of visual object agnosia has contributed to the slowness with which this issue has been resolved, but several decades of careful case studies have now shown, to most people's satisfaction, that agnosic patients may be no more impaired in their elementary visual capabilities and their general intellectual functioning than many patients who are not agnosic. Therefore, most current research on agnosia focuses on a new set of questions. Are there different types of visual object agnosia, corresponding to different underlying impairments? At what level of visual and/or mnestic processing do these impairments occur? What can agnosia tell us about normal object recognition? What brain regions are critically involved in visual object recognition?

APPERCEPTIVE AGNOSIA

Lissauer[2] reasoned that visual object recognition could be disrupted in two different ways: by impairing visual perception, in which case patients would be unable to recognize objects because they could not see them properly, and by impairing the process of associating a percept with its meaning, in which case patients would be unable to recognize objects because they could not use the percept to access their knowledge of the object. He termed the first kind of agnosia *apperceptive agnosia* and the second kind *associative agnosia*. This terminology is still used today to distinguish agnosic patients who have frank perceptual impairments from those who do not, although the implicit assumption that the latter have an impairment in "association" is now questioned.

Behavior and Anatomy

One might wonder whether apperceptive agnosics should be considered agnosics at all, given that the definition of agnosia cited at the beginning of this article excludes patients whose problems are caused by elementary visual impairments. The difference between apperceptive agnosics and patients who fall outside of the exclusionary criteria for agnosia is that the former have relatively good acuity, brightness discrimination, color vision, and other so-called elementary visual capabilities. Despite these capabilities, their perception of shape is markedly abnormal. For example, in the classic case of Benson and Greenberg,[3] pictures, letters, and even simple geometric shapes could not be recognized. Figure 18-1 shows the attempts of their patient to copy a column of simple shapes. Recognition of real objects may be somewhat better than recognition of geometric shapes, although this appears to be due to the availability of additional cues such as size and surface properties such as color, texture, and specularity rather than object shape. Facilitation of shape perception by motion of the stimulus has been noted in several cases of apperceptive agnosia. In most cases of apperceptive

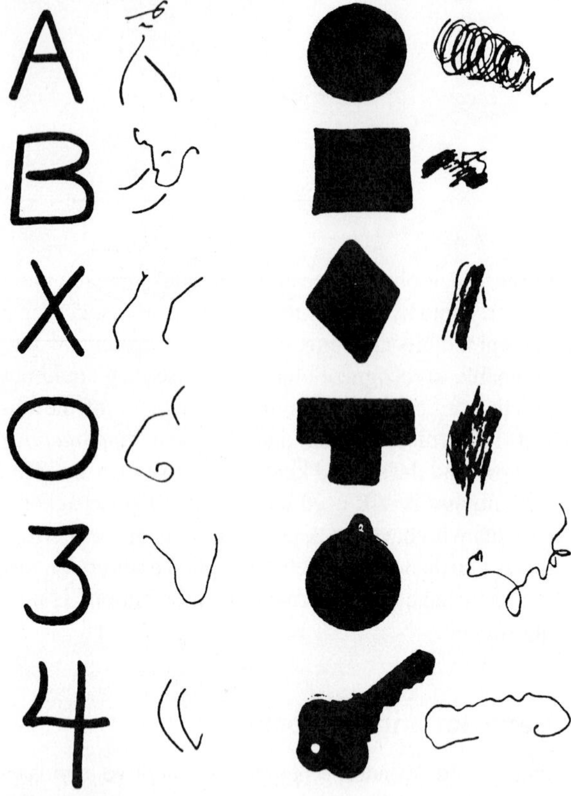

Figure 18-1
The attempts of an apperceptive agnosic patient to copy simple shapes. (From Benson and Greenberg,[3] with permission.)

agnosia, the brain damage is diffuse, often caused by carbon monoxide poisoning. For a review of other cases of apperceptive visual agnosia, see Ref. 4.

Interpretation of Apperceptive Agnosia

One way of interpreting apperceptive agnosia is in terms of a disorder of grouping processes that normally operate over the array of local features representing contour, color, depth, and so on.[4] Outside of their field defects, apperceptive agnosics have surprisingly good perception of local visual properties. They fail when they must extract more global structure from the image. Motion is helpful because it provides another cue to global structure in the form of correlated local motions. The perception of form from motion may also have different neural substrates from the perception of form from static contour,[5] and may therefore be spared in apperceptive agnosia.

Relation to Other Disorders

Some authors have used the term *apperceptive agnosia* for other, quite different types of visual disorders, including two forms of simultanagnosia and an impairment in recognizing objects from unusual views or under unusual lighting conditions. *Simultanagnosia* is a term used to describe an impairment in perception of multielement or multipart visual displays. When shown a complex picture with multiple objects or people, simulanagnostics typically describe them in a piecemeal manner, sometimes omitting much of the material entirely and therefore failing to interpret the overall nature of the scene being depicted.

Dorsal simultanagnosia is a component of Balint's syndrome (see Chap. 27), in which an attentional limitation prevents perception of more than one object at a time.[4,6–8] Occasionally attention may be captured by just one part of an object, leading to misidentification of the object and the appearance of perception confined to relatively local image features. The similarity of dorsal simultanagnosia to apperceptive agnosia is limited, however. Once they can attend to an object, dorsal simultanagnosics recognize it quickly and accurately, and even their "local" errors encompass much more global shape information than is available to apperceptive agnosics. Their lesions are typically in the posterior parietal cortex bilaterally.

Despite some surface similarity to apperceptive agnosia and dorsal simultanagnosia, *ventral simultanagnosia* represents yet another disorder.[4,9] Ventral simultanagnosics can recognize whole objects, but are limited in how many objects can be recognized in a given period of time. Their descriptions of complex scenes are slow and piecemeal, but unlike apperceptive agnosics their recognition of single shapes is not obviously impaired. The impairment of ventral simultanagnosics is most apparent when reading, because the individual letters of words are recognized in an abnormally slow and generally serial manner (letter-by-letter reading, see Chap. 14). Unlike the case with dorsal simultanagnosics, their detection of multiple stimuli appears normal; the bottleneck is in recognition per se.

Unlike apperceptive agnosics, they perceive individual shapes reasonably well. Their lesions are typically in the left inferior temporooccipital cortex.

Some patients have roughly normal perception and recognition of objects except when viewed from unusual perspectives or under unusual lighting. Their impairment has also been grouped with apperceptive agnosia by some, but for clarity's sake can also be called *perceptual categorization deficit* because they cannot categorize together the full range of images cast by an object under different viewing conditions. This disorder does not have great localizing value, although the lesions are generally in the right hemisphere and frequently include the inferior parietal lobe.[4,10]

ASSOCIATIVE AGNOSIA

Behavior and Anatomy

In associative agnosia, visual perception is much better than in apperceptive agnosia. Compare, for example, the copies made by the associative agnosics shown in Figs. 18-2 and 18-3 with the copies shown in Fig. 18-1. Nevertheless, object recognition is impaired. Associative agnosic patients may be able to recognize an object by its feel in their hand or from a spoken definition, demonstrating that they have intact general knowledge of the object in addition to being able to see it well enough to copy it, but they cannot recognize the same

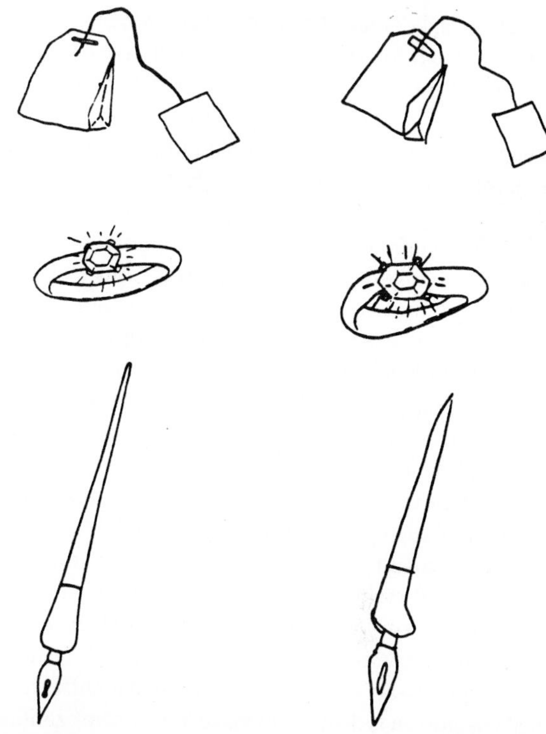

Figure 18-2
The copies of an associative agnosic patient with prosopagnosia and object agnosia. The patient did not recognize any of the original drawings. (From Farah et al.,[31] with permission.)

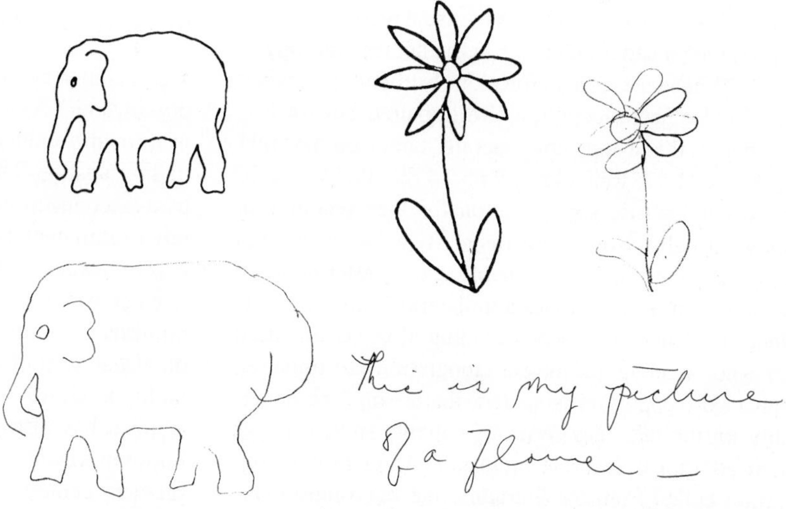

Figure 18-3
The copies of associative visual agnosic patients with alexia and object agnosia. The patients did not recognize the original drawings. Also shown is a sample of a patient's writing to dictation. After a delay, her own handwriting could not be read. (From Feinberg et al.,[16] with permission.)

object by sight alone. The impairment is not simply a naming deficit for visual stimuli; associative agnosics cannot indicate their recognition of objects by nonverbal means, as by pantomiming the use of an object or by grouping together dissimilar-looking objects from the same semantic category[11–16] (see Ref. 4 for a review of representative cases).

The scope of the recognition impairment varies from case to case of associative agnosia. Some patients encounter difficulty mainly with face recognition (see Chap. 19), while others demonstrate better face recognition than object recognition. Printed-word recognition is similarly impaired in some cases but not others. The selectivity of these impairments suggests that there is more than one system involved in visual recognition. According to one analysis,[17] there are two underlying forms of visual representation, one of which is required for face recognition, used for object recognition but not for word recognition, and the other of which is required for word recognition, used for object recognition and not required for face recognition. Indeed, if one regards associative agnosia as a single undifferentiated category, it is difficult to make any generalizations about the brain regions responsible for visual object recognition. Although the intrahemispheric location of damage is generally occipitotemporal, involving both gray and white matter, cases of associative agnosia have been reported following unilateral right-hemispheric lesions,[18] unilateral left-hemispheric lesions,[15,16,19,20] and bilateral lesions.[21–23] However, if one considers impairments in face and word recognition as markers for different underlying forms of visual recognition disorder, then a pattern emerges in the neuropathology.

When face recognition alone is impaired or when face and object recognition are impaired but reading is spared, the lesions are generally either on the right or bilateral. De Renzi has proposed that the degree of right-hemispheric specialization for face recognition may normally cover a wide range, such that most cases of prosopagnosia become manifest only after bilateral lesions, but in some cases a unilateral lesion will suffice (see Chap. 19). When reading alone is impaired or when reading and object recognition are impaired but face recognition is spared, the lesions are generally on the left. In a series of patients studied by us and additional cases of agnosia sparing face recognition culled from the literature, the maximum overlap in lesion locus was in the left inferior medial region involving parahippocampal, fusiform, and lingual gyri.[16] When recognition of faces, objects, and words is impaired, the lesions are generally bilateral.

The hypothesis of two underlying systems explains the pairwise dissociations among three different stimulus categories—words, objects, and faces—in a parsimonious way, with only two systems. In addition, it reveals a systematicity in lesion sites not previously apparent. Nevertheless, the hypothesis has been questioned following more recent reports of patients with patterns of spared and impaired recognition abilities that are inconsistent with an impairment in one of just two underlying systems. One patient with impaired face and word recognition but relatively less impaired object recognition has been reported.[24] The presence of a degree of object agnosia precludes strong inferences, however. Another patient with an isolated object recognition impairment has also been reported.[25] In this case, however, the object recognition impairment was evident to a degree on purely verbal tasks, limiting its relevance to visual agnosia.

Functional neuroimaging of normal subjects has largely supported the idea of a bilateral- or right-lateralized system for face recognition and a left-lateralized system for word recognition, with object recognition using both,[26] but has also raised the possibility of additional specialization within those systems, for example, specialization for orthography per se.[27]

Interpreting Associative Agnosia

Is associative agnosia a problem with perception, memory, or both? Associative agnosia has been explained in three different ways that suggest different answers to this question. The simplest way to explain agnosia is by a disconnection between visual representations and other brain centers responsible for language or memory. For example, Geschwind[28] proposed that associative agnosia is a visual–verbal disconnection. This hypothesis accounts well for agnosics' impaired naming of visual stimuli, but it cannot account for their inability to convey recognition nonverbally. Associative agnosia has also been explained as a disconnection between visual representations and medial temporal memory centers.[23] However, this would account for a modality-specific impairment in new learning, not the inability to access old knowledge through vision.

The inadequacies of the disconnection accounts lead us to consider theories of associative agnosia in which some component of perception and/or memory has been damaged. Perhaps the most widely accepted account of associative agnosia is that stored visual memory representations have been damaged. According to this type of account, stimuli can be processed perceptually up to some end-state visual representation, which would then be matched against stored visual representations. In associative agnosia, the stored representations are no longer available and recognition therefore fails. Note that an assumption of this account is that two identical tokens of the object representation normally exist, one derived from the stimulus and one stored in memory, and that these are compared in the same way as a database might be searched in a present-day computer. This account is not directly disconfirmed by any of the available evidence. However, there are some reasons to question it and to suspect that subtle impairments in perception may underlie associative agnosia.

Although the good copies and successful matching performance of associative agnosics might seem to exonerate perception, a closer look at the manner in which these tasks are accomplished suggests that perception is not normal in associative agnosia and suggests yet a third explanation of associative agnosia. Typically, these patients are described as copying drawings "slavishly"[29] and "line by line."[30] In matching tasks, they rely on slow, sequential feature-by-feature checking. It therefore may be premature to rule out faulty perception as the cause of associative agnosia.

Recent studies of the visual capabilities of associative agnosic patients confirm that there are subtle visual perceptual impairments present in all cases studied.[4] If the possibility of impaired recognition with intact perception is consistent with the use of a computational architecture in which separate perceptual and memory representations are compared, then the absence of such a case suggests that a different type of computational architecture may underlie object recognition. Parallel distributed processing (PDP) systems exemplify an alternative architecture in which the perceptual and memory representations cannot be dissociated (see Chap. 10; see also Refs. 4 and 5 for discussions of computational approaches to agnosia). In a PDP system, the memory of the stimulus would consist of a pattern of connection strengths among a number of neuronlike units. The "perceptual" representation resulting from the presentation of a stimulus will depend upon the pattern of connection strengths among the units directly or indirectly activated by the stimulus. Thus, if memory is altered by damaging the network, perception will be altered as well. On this account, associative agnosia is not a result of an impairment to perception *or* to memory; rather, the two are in principle inseparable, and the impairment is better described as a loss of high-level visual perceptual representations that are shaped by, and embody the memory of, visual experience. It will thus be of great interest to see whether future studies of associative agnosics will ever document a case of impaired recognition with intact perception.

Relation to Other Disorders

As with apperceptive agnosia, a number of distinct disorders have been labeled associative agnosia by different authors. Visual modality–specific naming disorders exist and are usually termed *optic aphasia* (see Chap. 10), but they may on occasion be called *associative visual agnosia. Impairments of semantic memory* (see Chap. 39) will affect object-recognition ability (as well as entirely nonvisual abilities such as verbally defining spoken words) and perhaps for this reason have also sometimes been called *associative visual agnosia.*

REFERENCES

1. Bay E: Disturbances of visual perception and their examination. *Brain* 76:515–530, 1952.
2. Lissauer H: Ein Fall von Seelenblindheit nebst einem Beitrage zur Theori derselben. *Arch Psychiatr Nervenkrankh* 21:222–270, 1890.
3. Benson R, Greenberg JP: Visual form agnosia. *Arch Neurol* 20:82–89, 1969.
4. Farah MJ: *Visual Agnosia: Disorders of Object Recognition and What They Tell Us about Normal Vision*, 2d ed. Cambridge, MA: MIT Press, 2003.
5. Farah MJ: *The Cognitive Neuroscience of Vision.* Oxford: Blackwells, 2000.
6. Williams M: *Brain Damage and the Mind.* Baltimore: Penguin Books, 1970.

7. Girotti F, Milanese C, Casazza M, et al: Oculomotor disturbances in Balint's syndrome: Anatomoclinical findings and electrooculographic analysis in a case. *Cortex* 18:603–614, 1982.
8. Tyler HR: Abnormalities of perception with defective eye movements (Balint's syndrome). *Cortex* 3:154–171, 1968.
9. Kinsbourne M, Warrington EK: A disorder of simultaneous form perception. *Brain* 85:461–486, 1962.
10. Warrington EK: Agnosia: The impairment of object recognition, in Vinken PJ, Bruyn GW, Klawans HL (eds): *Handbook of Clinical Neurology*. Amsterdam: Elsevier, 1985.
11. Rubens AB, Benson DF: Associative visual agnosia. *Arch Neurol* 24:305–316, 1971.
12. Bauer RM, Rubens AB: Agnosia, in Heilman KM, Valenstein E (eds): *Clinical Neuropsychology,* 2d ed. New York: Oxford University Press, 1985.
13. Albert ML, Reches A, Silverberg R: Associative visual agnosia without alexia. *Neurology* 25:322–326, 1975.
14. Hécaen H, de Ajuriaguerra J: Agnosie visuelle pour les objets inanimes par lesion unilateral gauche. *Rev Neurol* 94:222–233, 1956.
15. McCarthy RA, Warrington EK: Visual associative agnosia: A clinico-anatomical study of a single case. *Neurol Neurosurg Psychiatry* 48:1233–1240, 1986.
16. Feinberg TE, Schindler RJ, Ochoa E, et al: Associative visual agnosia and alexia without prosopagnosia. *Cortex* 30:395–412, 1994.
17. Farah MJ: Patterns of co-occurrence among the associative agnosias: Implications for visual object representation. *Cognit Neuropsychol* 8:1–19, 1991.
18. Levine DN: Prosopagnosia and visual object agnosia: A behavioral study. *Neuropsychologia* 5:341–365, 1978.
19. Pilon B, Signoret JL, Lhermitte F: Agnosie visuelle associative rôle de l'hemisphere gauche dans la perception visuelle. *Rev Neurol* 137:831–842, 1981.
20. Feinberg TE, Heilman KM, Gonzalez-Rothi L: Multimodal agnosia after unilateral left hemisphere lesion. *Neurology* 36:864–867, 1986.
21. Alexander MP, Albert ML: The anatomical basis of visual agnosia, in Kertesz A (ed): *Localization in Neuropsychology*. New York: Academic Press, 1983.
22. Benson DF, Segarra J, Albert ML: Visual agnosia-prosopagnosia: A clinicopathologic correlation. *Arch Neurol* 30:307–310, 1973.
23. Albert ML, Soffer D, Silverberg R, Reches A: The anatomic basis of visual agnosia. *Neurology* 29:876–879, 1979.
24. Buxbaum LJ, Glosser G, Coslett HB: Relative sparing of object recognition in alexia-prosopagnosia. *Brain Cognit.*
25. Humphreys GW, Rumiati RI: Agnosia without prosopagnosia or alexia. *Cognit Neuropsychol* 15:243–277, 1998.
26. Farah MJ, Aguirre GK: Imaging visual recognition. *Trends Cognit Sci* 3:179–186, 1999.
27. Polk TA, Stallcup M, Aguirre G et al: Neural specialization for letter recognition. *J Cognit Neurosci* 14:145–159, 2001.
28. Geschwind N: Disconnexion syndromes in animals and man: Part II. *Brain* 88:585–645, 1965.
29. Brown JW: *Aphasia, Apraxia and Agnosia: Clinical and Theoretical Aspects*. Springfield, IL: Charles C Thomas, 1972.
30. Ratcliff G, Newcombe F: Object recognition: Some deductions from the clinical evidence, in Ellis AW (ed): *Normality and Pathology in Cognitive Functions*. New York: Academic Press, 1982.
31. Farah MJ, Hammond K, Levine DN, et al: Visual and spatial mental imagery. *Cognit Neuropsychol* 20:439–462, 1988.

Chapter 19

PROSOPAGNOSIA

Martha J. Farah

Visual object agnosia, discussed in the previous chapter, does not always affect the recognition of all types of stimuli equally. Quite often, the recognition of faces seems disproportionately or even exclusively impaired, a condition known as *prosopagnosia*. Prosopagnosia can be so severe that the patient cannot recognize close friends, family members, or even his or her own face in a photograph. Yet nonfacial knowledge of people is preserved, and prosopagnosics typically resort to recognizing individuals by their voices or even by nonfacial visual cues such as clothing. Of course, such strategies have only very limited effectiveness. Prosopagnosia is therefore a serious problem for patients and is usually discovered because of the patient's complaint rather than by testing or examination.

The most straightforward explanation of prosopagnosia is that a specialized brain system for recognizing faces has been damaged. In recent years, much of the research on prosopagnosia has been aimed at testing this explanation against various alternative explanations. The reason that so much attention has been paid to this issue is that it bears directly on a larger controversy in cognitive science concerning the unity versus modularity of cognitive processes (e.g., Fodor, 1982). Does the brain support intelligent behavior with a relatively small set of general-purpose information processing mechanisms, or has it evolved to carry out its many functions by the use of dedicated, special-purpose mechanisms?

THE FUNCTIONAL DEFICIT IN PROSOPAGNOSIA: FACE-SPECIFIC?

The most straightforward interpretation of prosopagnosia is consistent with anatomically separate recognition systems for faces and objects. More precisely, prosopagnosia suggests that there is some system that is necessary for face recognition and either unnecessary or less important for object recognition. An alternative interpretation is that faces and all other types of objects are recognized using a single recognition system and that faces are simply the most difficult type of object for the recognition system. Prosopagnosia can then be explained as a mild form of agnosia, in which the impairment is detectable only on the most taxing form of recognition task.

The first researchers to address this issue directly were McNeil and Warrington (1993). They studied case W.J., a middle-aged professional man who became prosopagnosic following a series of strokes. After becoming prosopagnosic, W.J. made a career change and went into sheep farming. He eventually came to recognize many of his sheep, although he remained unable to recognize most humans. The authors noted the potential implications of such a dissociation for the question of whether human face recognition is "special" and designed an ingenious experiment exploiting W.J.'s new-found career. They assembled three groups of photographs—human faces, sheep faces of the same breed kept by W.J., and sheep faces of a different breed—and attempted to teach subjects names for each face. Normal subjects performed at intermediate levels between ceiling and floor in all conditions. They performed better with the human faces than with sheep faces, even those who, like W.J., worked with sheep. In contrast, W.J. performed poorly with the human faces and performed normally with the sheep faces.

The issue of whether prosopagnosia is selective for faces relative to common objects was addressed by my colleagues and myself with patient L.H., a well-educated professional man who has been prosopagnosic since an automobile accident in college (Farah et al., 1995). We employed a recognition memory paradigm in which L.H. and control subjects first studied a set of photographs of faces and nonface objects, such as forks, chairs, and eyeglasses. Subjects were then given a larger set of photographs, and asked to make "old"/"new" judgments on them. Whereas normal subjects performed equally well with the faces and nonface objects, L.H. showed a significant performance disparity, performing worse with faces than with objects. In a second experiment, we used a similar method to contrast L.H. and normal subjects' recognition performance with 40 faces and 40 eyeglass frames and again found that L.H. was disproportionately impaired at face recognition. This, as well as the results of testing W.J. with human and sheep faces, implies that prosopagnosia is not a problem with recognizing specific exemplars from any visually homogeneous category but is specific to faces.

Another source of evidence for the independence of face and object recognition comes from patients who show the opposite dissociation—namely, more difficulty with object recognition than with face recognition (Feinberg et al., 1994; Moscovitch et al., 1997). The existence of such cases also supports the interpretation that prosopagnosia is not simply a mild general visual agnosia, because such an interpretation is inconsistent with the possibility of relatively preserved face recognition with object agnosia.

A different kind of alternative interpretation of prosopagnosia does not deny that visual recognition involves some specialized subsystems that are necessary for face recognition. However, according to this alternative, the nature of the specialization is subtly different from that discussed so far. Gauthier and collaborators have proposed that we have a recognition system that is specialized for objects that require expertise to discriminate from one another and which share an overall configuration. Faces fall into this category, but other objects can as well. These include birds or dogs for expert bird watchers and dog show judges (Tanaka and Taylor, 1991) and a set of artificial creatures devised by Gauthier and Tarr (1997) called "greebles." Greeble recognition has been shown to have many similarities to face recognition, and recent efforts to teach a prosopagnosic to recognize Greebles were unsuccessful, adding further support to Gauthier's hypothesis. Of course, it is possible to view such demonstrations as evidence that people occasionally recruit their specialized face recognition system for use with other stimuli.

ANATOMIC BASES OF FACE RECOGNITION

If we are interested in knowing precisely where, in the human brain, face recognition is carried out, individual cases are rarely very informative. L.H. sustained head injuries followed by surgery and W.J. suffered at least three strokes, resulting in widely distributed damage in both cases. Surveys of the lesions in larger groups of prosopagnosics are more helpful for localization, as the regions of overlap among different patients can be identified. Damasio et al. (1982) conducted a survey of the literature for autopsied cases of prosopagnosia, and studied three of their own patients, concluding that the critical lesion site is in ventral occipitotemporal cortex bilaterally. De Renzi and colleagues (1994) reviewed much of the same case material, along with more recent cases and data from living patients whose brain damage was mapped using both structural magnetic resonance imaging (MRI) and positron emission tomography (PET). Their findings supported the ventral localization of face recognition but called for a revision of the idea that bilateral lesions are necessary. Some patients became prosopagnosic after unilateral right hemisphere damage. The possibility of hidden left hemisphere dysfunction in these cases was reduced by the finding of normal metabolic activity in the left hemisphere by PET scan. De Renzi et al. conclude that there is a spectrum of hemispheric specialization for face recognition in normal right-handed adults. Although the right hemisphere may be relatively better at face recognition than the left, most people have a degree of face recognition ability in both hemispheres. Nevertheless, in a minority of cases, face recognition is so focally represented in the right hemisphere that a unilateral lesion will lead to prosopagnosia. The lesion sites associated with prosopagnosia are, as a group, clearly different from the lesions associated with object agnosia in the absence of prosopagnosia. The latter syndrome is almost invariably the result of a unilateral left hemisphere lesion, although confined to roughly the same intrahemispheric region (Feinberg et al., 1994).

Converging evidence about the localization of face recognition in the human brain comes from functional neuroimaging of normal individuals. The most relevant experimental design for comparison with prosopagnosics' lesions is one in which brain activity while viewing faces is contrasted with brain activity while viewing nonface objects. Kanwisher and coworkers (1996) used functional MRI to compare regional brain activity while subjects viewed photographs of faces and of objects. An objects-minus-faces subtraction revealed areas more responsive to objects than faces and the reverse subtraction revealed an area more responsive to faces than objects. Both types of stimuli activated inferior temporooccipital regions, with face-specific activation confined to part of the right fusiform gyrus. A follow-up study identified the same fusiform face area and systematically verified its specificity for faces by comparing its response to faces and to scrambled faces, houses, and hands (Kanwisher et al., 1997). Similar conclusions were reached by McCarthy and coworkers (1997), who found right fusiform activation unique to passive viewing of faces relative to objects or scrambled objects, and left fusiform activation unique to flowers relative to scrambled objects.

REFERENCES

Damasio AR, Damasio H, Van Hoesen GW: Prosopagnosia: anatomic basis and behavioral mechanisms. *Neurology* 32:331–341, 1982.

De Renzi E, Perani D, Carlesimo GA, et al: Prosopagnosia can be associated with damage confined to the right hemisphere—an MRI and PET study and a review of the literature. *Neuropsychologia* 32:893–902, 1994.

Farah MJ, Levinson KL, Klein KL: Face perception and within-category discrimination in prosopagnosia. *Neuropsychologia* 33:661–674, 1995.

Feinberg TE, Schindler RJ, Ochoa E, et al: Associative visual agnosia and alexia without prosopagnosia. *Cortex* 30:395–411, 1994.

Fodor JA: *The Modularity of Mind*. Cambridge, MA: MIT Press, 1983.

Gauthier I, Tarr MJ: Becoming a "greeble" expert: Exploring mechanisms for face recognition. *Vis Res* 37:1673–1682, 1997.

Kanwisher N, Chun MM, McDermott J, Ledden PJ: Functional imaging of human visual recognition. *Cogn Brain Res* 5:55–67, 1996.

Kanwisher N, McDermott J, Chun MM: The fusiform face area: A module in human extrastriate cortex specialized for face perception. *J Neurosci* 17:4302–4311, 1997.

McCarthy G, Puce A, Gore JC, Allison T: Face-specific processing in human fusiform gyrus. *J Cogn Neurosci* 9:605–610, 1997.

McNeil JE, Warrington EK: Prosopagnosia: a face-specific disorder. *Q J Exp Psychol Hum Exp Psychol* 46A:1–10, 1993.

Tanaka JW, Taylor M: Object categories and expertise: Is the basic level in the eye of the beholder? *Cogn Psychol* 23:457–482, 1991.

Chapter 20

DISORDERS OF COLOR PROCESSING*

Daniel Tranel

The "higher" or "central" processing of color information in the human brain takes place at the level of primary visual cortex, visual association cortices, and beyond. The principal neural regions important for color processing include primary visual cortex and early visual association cortices in the lingual and fusiform gyri (Fig. 20-1). The primary visual cortex corresponds to Brodmann area 17, while the association cortices correspond to areas 18/19, respectively; these areas are also known as V1, V2/V3, and V4 (cf. Felleman and Van Essen, 1991). Acquired damage to these neural structures or to the higher-order visually related cortices in the transition zone between the ventral occipital and posterior temporal region can produce disturbances in various aspects of color processing, including color perception, color imagery, color recognition, and color naming. Impairments in these four aspects of color processing are reviewed in this chapter, with a focus on both the neuropsychological and neuroanatomic features of each condition. It should be noted that what is covered here are disorders of *central* processing of color that occur as a consequence of acquired brain injury and not impairments of color vision that are peripheral, developmental, or congenital in nature. This is an important distinction, because a large number of persons, especially males, have some degree of inherited color "blindness." In fact, it has been estimated that nearly 1 percent of males are red-blind and nearly 2 percent are green-blind (Gouras, 1991). The reader is referred to Roorda and Williams (1999) for an intriguing summary of the peripheral processing of color.

Terminology

Although the distinctions are somewhat arbitrary, it is possible to specify four more or less separate aspects of central color processing: color perception, color imagery, color recognition, and color naming. *Color perception* is the capacity to perceive color; hence this is a basic visual perceptual capacity, akin to perceiving form or texture. *Color imagery* is the capacity to imagine colors or to imagine entities in color—i.e., bringing images of colors or colorful entities into the mind's eye. *Color recognition* refers to the assignment of psychological meaning to color information—i.e., capacities such as knowing the difference between various colors, knowing the colors in which various entities normally appear, and knowing that colors can vary as functions of properties such as brightness, saturation, and hue. From a psychological perspective, color knowledge is remarkably robust: for example, individuals show a lot of consensus about typical colors for entities (Joseph and Proffitt, 1996; Saunders and van Brakel, 1997) and make very reliable judgments about which colors are characteristic of particular entities (Siple and Springer, 1983). *Color naming* is the capacity to apply a lexical term to a color—e.g., naming the color of corn as yellow.

Measurement

A critical prerequisite to diagnosing and quantifying disorders of color processing is the availability of reliable and valid measurement instruments. The reader is referred to Rizzo et al. (1993) for a nice summary of state-of-the-art testing procedures for quantifying various color-related processing capacities. Here, the procedures for measuring color perception, color recognition, and color naming are summarized. Measurement of color imagery essentially depends on the self-report of the patient: there is no quantitative, objective means by which it can be quantified.

Color Perception Color perception can be tested with color-plate tests (e.g., the Ishihara Color Plate

* **ACKNOWLEDGMENT:** Supported by Program Project Grant NINDS NS19632.

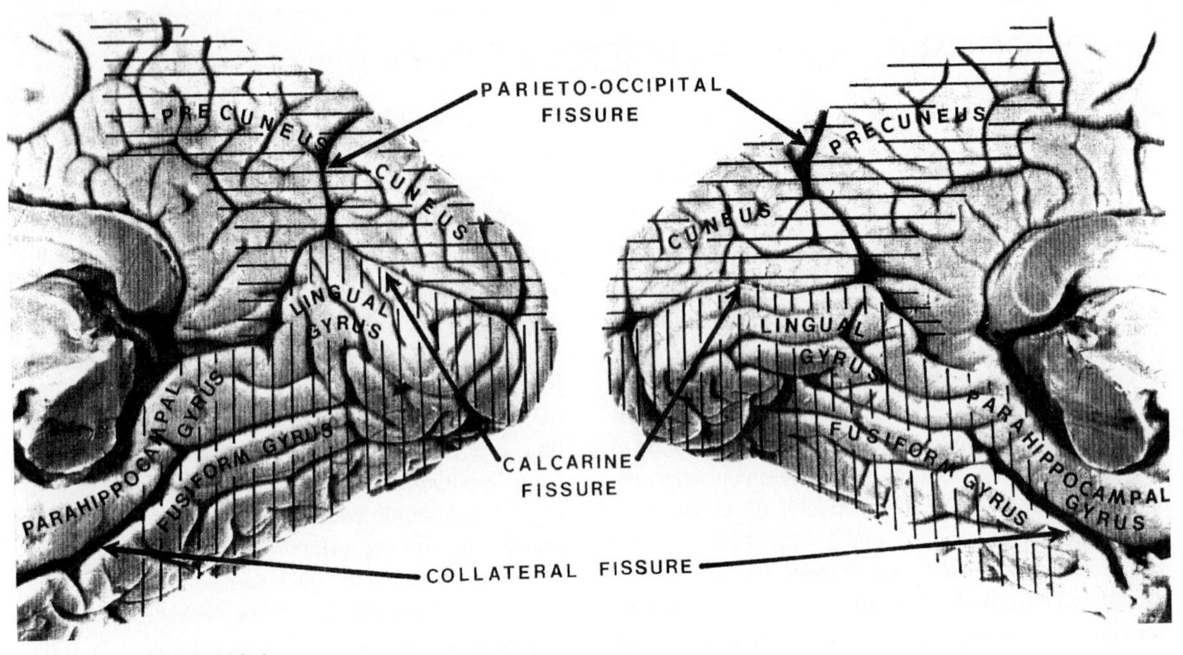

Figure 20-1
A mesial view of the posterior right (left side of figure) *and left* (right side of figure) *hemispheres of the human brain, showing major sulci and gyri. Regions important for various aspects of color processing include the lingual gyrus and the posterior part of the fusiform gyrus, located below the calcarine fissure in the medial and ventral aspects of the hemispheres.*

Test) and color arrangement tests (e.g., the Farnsworth-Munsell 100-Hue Test). For patients with naming impairments (especially aphasic patients), color arrangement tests are particularly useful, since the tests do not depend on the production of a verbal response. Color perception should be measured separately in all four quadrants of vision, since the most common disorders of color perception affect either a quadrant or hemifield. Also, both peripheral and central vision should be tested. For example, the examiner can slowly pass a highly saturated colored object (e.g., the color chips from the Token Test of the Multilingual Aphasia Examination) back and forth between a patient's quadrants of vision and inquire as to whether the color of the object appears to change when the horizontal and vertical midlines are crossed. When the object moves from peripheral to central vision or crosses one of the midlines, patients with color perception defects will typically indicate that the color of the object has "dimmed," "changed," or even "disappeared."

Color Recognition Color recognition should be tested with both verbal and nonverbal procedures. In verbal tasks, patients are questioned about color knowledge. Questions in which a color name constitutes the answer (e.g., "What color is a radish?") as well as questions in which a color name is in the question (e.g., "What are some things that are blue?") should be used. In nonverbal tasks, patients are presented with black-and-white line drawings of characteristically colored entities (e.g., an apple or a tire), and asked to select from an array of foils (patches of color) the correct color for the entity. It is important to include at least some items whose color names are uncommon verbal associates (e.g., eggplant), to provide a rigorous test of color knowledge, because for many common entities, the verbal association between the color name and object name can be fairly prepotent (e.g., *white,* snow; *orange,* pumpkin), and may be sufficient for the patient to answer the question accurately even if basic color knowledge is impaired.

Color Naming Two types of tasks can be used to assess color naming, one in which the patient is asked to produce color names to colored stimuli [e.g., "What color is this (a *green* grape)?"], and one in which the patient is asked to point to colored stimuli given a color name (e.g., "Point to all the *brown* objects in this picture."). It is worthwhile to request both oral and written responses in the first task, particularly with aphasic patients, because patients can demonstrate remarkable dissociations between the ability to produce color names orally versus in writing (e.g., one output modality is relatively normal while the other is severely impaired). Testing should cover the basic set of 6 to 10 colors that are widely known by normal individuals (cf. Berlin and Kay, 1969; Bornstein, 1985). Unless warranted by the particulars of a given case, more extensive investigation is usually not productive because the effects of expertise become the predominant influence on performance (e.g., testing a visual artist).

DISORDERS OF COLOR PERCEPTION (CENTRAL ACHROMATOPSIA)

Definition

Impaired color perception related to brain damage, known as *central achromatopsia,* is an impairment of color perception caused by an acquired cerebral lesion (see also Chap. 17). Several putative mechanisms for central achromatopsia have been proposed, such as reduced hue discrimination (e.g., Heywood et al., 1987; Victor et al., 1989) and defective color constancy (Zeki, 1990), but so far, this issue remains unresolved (Hurlbert et al., 1998; Ruttiger et al., 1999). In this vein, Wray and Edelman (1996) proposed an interesting neurobiological model of central color processing. In any event, the defining feature of central achromatopsia is an inability to perceive colors normally, despite relatively intact processing of other aspects of the visual world, such as form, motion, and depth (e.g., Heywood et al., 1998).

Clinical Presentation

In the most common presentation, central achromatopsia affects a quadrant or hemifield of vision; it is very rare for the entire visual field to be affected (Damasio et al., 1980; Kolmel, 1988; Meadows, 1974; Paulson et al., 1994; Rizzo et al., 1993). Within the affected part of the field, it is common for the periphery to be more affected than central vision. In fact, the portion of the visual field near the fovea may be entirely spared. Patients usually present with complaints that colors look "washed out," "dim," or "dirty," and in more severe cases may note that their entire visual world has turned to shades of black and white. It is intriguing to note that patients often complain about the ambient lighting being poor; however, the complaint is usually unrelated to the actual quality of the lighting. Patients with achromatopsia tend to be very sensitive to dim lighting, and such conditions invariably exacerbate the severity of their color perception problems. Increasing the level of ambient lighting can, in fact, be very helpful to achromatopsic patients, even if the effect is mostly psychological—i.e., the patients have the sense that they are "seeing" more accurately with brighter lighting.

Neuro-ophthalmologic Features

Detailed neuro-ophthalmological assessment is mandatory in the evaluation of patients presenting with complaints of altered color perception. This testing will help determine what is and is not wrong with the patient's vision in different parts of the visual fields. Most patients with central achromatopsia have blindness (anopsia) in at least part of their visual field, typically a hemifield or quadrant, because the lesions that cause central achromatopsia generally take out some nearby regions that are necessary for basic form vision. A common pattern is that the patient has blindness in one quadrant of a hemifield, and achromatopsia in the other quadrant of the same hemifield. In the colorless but sighted portion of the field, other aspects of vision, such as spatial contrast sensitivity, flicker and motion perception, and depth perception, are typically preserved (Cavanagh et al., 1998; Rizzo et al., 1993).

Neuropsychological Features

With some circumscribed lesions, achromatopsia may occur as a fairly isolated manifestation of acquired cerebral disease. More commonly, the patient will have other neuropsychological deficits, and the most frequent symptoms occur in the domains of object recognition and reading. Object recognition impairments are classified under the term *visual agnosia* (see Chaps. 18 and 19), which refers to impaired recognition of entities that are perceived more or less normally. Visual agnosia frequently affects certain categories of entities more than others. Impaired recognition of familiar faces—known as *prosopagnosia*—is the most common manifestation of visual agnosia. *Visual object agnosia* refers to impaired recognition of stimuli from other categories, such as animals, fruits/vegetables, or tools. A considerable body of evidence has accumulated, indicating that visual recognition impairments can have a remarkable degree of category relatedness—that is, patients show striking defects in recognition of animals but not tools, or vice versa (Damasio et al., 1990; Farah et al., 1996; Hillis and Caramazza, 1991; Sartori et al., 1993; Tranel et al., 1997a, 1997c; Warrington and McCarthy, 1994; Warrington and Shallice, 1984).

The fact that achromatopsia and visual agnosia tend to occur together should not be taken as evidence of a cause-and-effect relationship. In fact, patients with severely impaired color perception often have normal visual recognition of concrete entities. Furthermore, most entities are recognized nearly as well when they are presented in black-and-white as when they are presented in color (although color can have an influence on recognition, especially latency; see Joseph and Proffitt, 1996; Siple and Springer, 1983). The reason why achromatopsia and visual agnosia tend to co-occur is based on neuroanatomy—the neural structures important for color perception are very close to those important for visual recognition of concrete entities; hence, a single lesion can easily damage both sets of structures and impair both types of functions. Figure 20-2, Plate 8, provides neuroanatomic details for a patient who developed achromatopsia and prosopagnosia following bilateral occipitotemporal lesions.

Another neuropsychological sign that occurs frequently in patients with central achromatopsia is impaired reading, which is generally known as *acquired alexia* (see Chap. 19). The type of reading deficit most commonly manifested by achromatopsic patients is "pure alexia" or what is also known as "alexia without agraphia." Pure alexia involves the inability to read while retaining the capacity to write. Pure alexia is caused by left-sided inferior occipital/occipitotemporal lesions. As in the case of visual agnosia, the co-occurrence of pure alexia and achromatopsia has a neuroanatomic explanation: the close proximity of neural structures important for reading and for color perception means that these two functions can easily be disrupted by a single, focal lesion (Damasio and Damasio, 1983). It is worth noting that the reading deficits that develop following acquired brain injury can be fairly subtle, especially in the chronic phase of recovery (i.e., months or years after the onset of brain injury), making it important to use sensitive tests to measure reading. An example of one such test is the Iowa-Chapman Reading Test, which we recently developed and standardized (Manzel and Tranel, 1999). This test has a stringent time demand, which contributes to its capacity to detect fairly mild reading defects that are typically missed by simpler assessment techniques (including those that typify the standard aphasia batteries, such as the Boston Diagnostic Aphasia Examination and the Multilingual Aphasia Examination).

A neuropsychological impairment that sometimes occurs together with achromatopsia is *topographical disorientation*. This condition involves the inability to navigate familiar routes or to learn new ones (Barrash, 1998; see also Chap. 24). As in the cases of visual agnosia and alexia, the co-occurrence of this disorder with achromatopsia is attributable to the closeness of neural structures required for topographical knowledge and color perception. For example, we found in a large-scale lesion study that topographic learning is highly dependent on structures in right and left mesial occipitotemporal regions (Barrash et al., 2000). Functional imaging studies have demonstrated consistent activation, usually bilateral, of the mesial occipital/occipitotemporal cortices during learning and recall of topographical knowledge (e.g., Aguirre and D'Esposito, 1997; Aguirre et al., 1996; Maguire et al., 1998). While the ability to perceive color is probably not critical for normal topographic orientation, the extent to which topographical learning and recall may depend to some extent on color knowledge remains an unanswered question.

Neuroanatomic Correlates

Lesion Studies Full-field achromatopsia can be produced by bilateral lesions in the inferior occipital

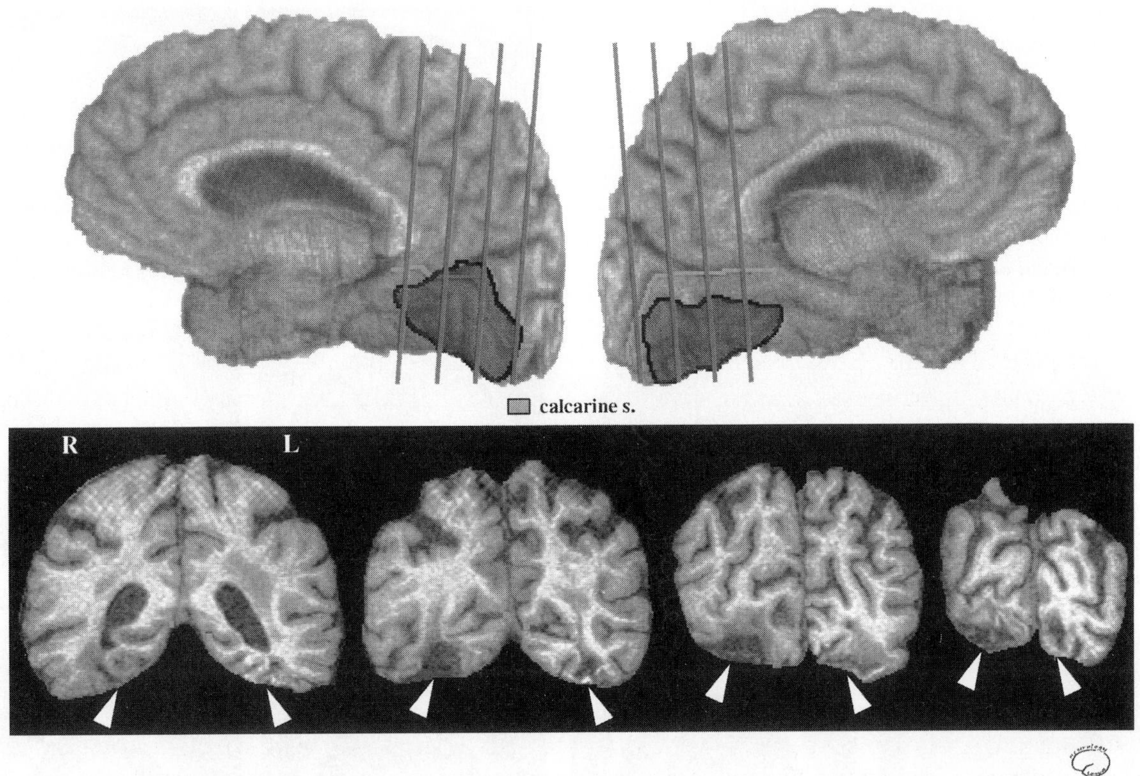

Figure 20-2 (Plate 8)
Top: Mesial views of a three-dimensional MRI reconstruction of a patient who sustained bilateral infarcts in the infracalcarine visual association cortices (the right hemisphere is on the left, and vice versa*).* Bottom*: The lesions are shown in coronal MRI sections* (arrows), *which correspond to the four planes marked with red lines in the mesial hemispheric views. The patient had a superior altitudinal hemianopia. In the lower fields, form vision was normal, but color perception was impaired—i.e., the patient was achromatopsic. The patient also had prosopagnosia in connection with these lesions.*

region and in the occipitotemporal junction, in and near the lingual and fusiform gyri (Damasio et al., 1980). Unilateral inferior occipital or occipitotemporal lesions produce hemiachromatopsia in the contralateral field. However, the most frequent presentation of central achromatopsia is a combination of quadrantanopia and quadrantachromatopsia. In the hemifield contralateral to the lesion, the patient is blind in the upper quadrant and has a loss of color perception in the lower quadrant. On either the left or right side, occipital/occipitotemporal lesions commonly cause some degree of visual agnosia and topographic disorientation; in addition, left-sided lesions typically produce alexia. In general, lesion studies suggest that damage to the middle third of the lingual gyrus is the most consistent neuroanatomic correlate of central achromatopsia (Rizzo et al., 1993). Damage to white matter immediately behind the posterior tip of the lateral ventricle is another common neural correlate of central achromatopsia. Figure 20-3, Plate 9, presents the neuroanatomic findings in a patient who developed right-field hemiachromatopsia, "pure" alexia, and category-related visual object agnosia following a left occipitotemporal lesion.

The relationship between color perception and motion perception has been investigated in detail in

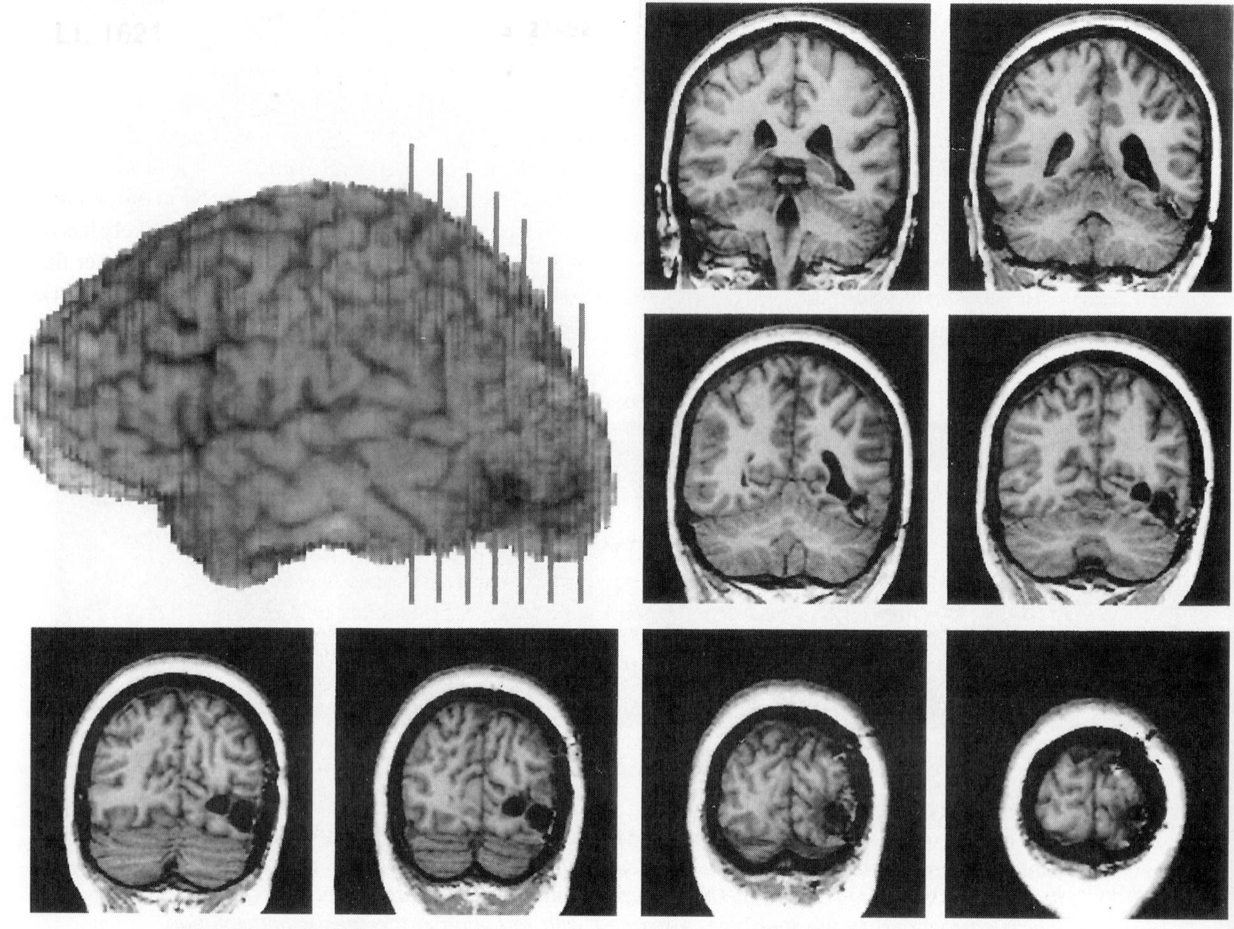

Figure 20-3 (Plate 9)
Three-dimensional reconstruction of a T1-weighted MRI in a patient with hemiachromatopsia, pure alexia, and category-specific visual object agnosia. The lesion, centered in the left occipitotemporal region, involves parts of the lingual and fusiform gyri.

several lesion studies (Cavanagh et al., 1998; Heywood et al., 1998). The findings indicate a clear anatomic separation for color perception and motion perception, consistent with a large body of experimental neurophysiologic work in nonhuman primates (e.g., Hubel and Livingstone, 1987; Livingstone and Hubel, 1984, 1987; see also Chap. 17). Also, Merigan et al. (1997) reported a patient who suffered a circumscribed lesion in the right fusiform gyrus, and developed impairments of color and form perception in the left superior quadrant while maintaining normal motion perception in this quadrant. In fact, there has been a considerable amount of recent work on the neural correlates of motion perception and of other related aspects of the processing of movement and action knowledge (e.g., H. Damasio et al., 2001; Kourtzi and Kanwisher, 2000; Senior et al., 2000; Tranel et al., 2001).

Functional Imaging Studies Findings from the lesion work summarized above have been replicated and extended in recent functional imaging approaches to the investigation of the neural basis of color processing [positron emission tomography (PET), magnetic resonance imaging (fMRI)]. For example, when subjects are viewing colored stimuli, there is selective activation (relative to a non-color-viewing baseline) of areas in the region of the lingual and fusiform gyri, or the putative human area V4 (Chao and Martin, 1999; Clark et al., 1997; Corbetta et al., 1990, 1991; Lueck et al., 1989; Sakai et al., 1995; Zeki et al., 1991). Moreover, Clark et al. (1997) emphasized the finding that face- and color-processing tasks both tended to activate ventral occipitotemporal cortices, suggesting that the neural structures used for processing faces and colors have considerable overlap. This finding is very reminiscent of the lesion work, which has consistently demonstrated a strong association between achromatopsia and prosopagnosia. These findings have also been corroborated with paradigms using electrophysiologic measures (Allison et al., 1993; Plendl et al., 1993; Rosler et al,. 1995).

It is important to note that while the bulk of the lesion work has pointed to the lingual gyrus as being especially important for color perception, the functional imaging work has tended to emphasize the importance of the fusiform gyrus. The discrepancy may have to do with the nature of the task demands in the functional imaging studies, or, relatedly, to the types of "control" tasks employed. On the other hand, there is a certain degree of imprecision in the lesion work, inasmuch as studies tend to rely on patients with relatively large lesions, where it is difficult to separate the relative contributions of the lingual and fusiform gyri (the right hemisphere lesion in the patient displayed in Fig. 20-2 is a good example of this problem). In any event, the discrepancies remain unresolved, and they are worth exploring in more detail.

DISORDERS OF COLOR IMAGERY

It was noted earlier that the assessment of color imagery depends on the self-report of the patient. Typically, patients complain that they can no longer imagine colors, imagine entities with characteristic colors, or remember the colors that objects should have. Such complaints can be probed by asking the patient what the world looks like in the patient's "mind's eye." Responses absent of color information are suggestive of a color imagery defect. Another useful approach is to ask the patient to describe, from imagery, entities that do not have characteristic colors—e.g., "What color is your car? Your winter coat? Your living-room sofa?" It is also informative to ask about items whose color is determined by social convention rather than as an inherent property—e.g., "What color is a school crossing sign? A mile-marker sign? The diamonds suit in a deck of cards?" In these tasks, since the coloration of the entities is idiosyncratic or arbitrary, the patient likely has to imagine the entities—in color—in order to answer the questions accurately (De Vreese, 1991; Farah, 1984). Hence, patients who struggle to answer such questions can be suspected as having color imagery defects. The examiner should also inquire about dreaming—does the patient dream in color? The examiner should also ask the patient whether he or she has experienced any *change* in the presence of color in dreams since the onset of the brain injury (since there are wide individual differences in the extent to which persons dream in color). A major decrease of color in dreams following brain damage is suggestive of color imagery deficits.

There is an intimate—perhaps inseparable—association between color imagery and color perception. In fact, a contentious and unresolved issue in this field is the question of whether the same neural structures are used for both color perception and color imagery. In earlier work based on lesion studies, several investigators suggested that achromatopsia is virtually always accompanied by impaired color imagery (Beauvois and Saillant, 1985; De Renzi and Spinnler, 1967). If correct, this would support the claim that the perception of color is dependent upon the same neural regions that subserve color imagery (Farah, 1988). This position has also received some support from functional imaging studies, which have demonstrated that when subjects imagine and name the colors associated with various entities, similar neural regions are activated—specifically, sectors in the left and right fusiform gyri. On the other hand, there are a number of lesion and functional imaging studies that are at variance with this position and that suggest, instead, that color perception and color imagery can be dissociated. De Vreese (1991) reported a patient who had preserved color perception but impaired color imagery. Patients with the opposite dissociation—impaired color perception but intact color imagery—have also been reported (Bartolomeo et al., 1997; Shuren et al., 1996), completing a double dissociation in this regard. Chao and Martin (1999), using a PET approach, found that the retrieval of color knowledge (presumably related to some extent to color imagery) activated different neural regions from those activated by color perception. These results are consistent with the idea that color imagery and color perception do not depend on exactly the same neural structures.

At this point, it is probably safe to conclude that the processes of color perception and color imagery must rely on neural structures that are very close if not identical. These structures very likely include part of the fusiform gyrus and perhaps part of the lingual gyrus. This issue is unresolved, though, and deserving of further study. Functional imaging approaches may shed further light on this question, given their powerful spatial resolution. Event-related fMRI, in particular, has the kind of spatial and temporal resolution that could very well help resolve this debate. And it should be added that a comparable debate has been waged in regard to other aspects of visual perception— for instance, the extent to which the perception of objects and the imagery of objects depend on the same neural structures (e.g., D'Esposito et al., 1997; see Kosslyn, 1994, for a fuller discussion of this issue).

DISORDERS OF COLOR RECOGNITION (COLOR AGNOSIA)

Definition

Earlier, color recognition was defined as the assignment of psychological meaning to color information—i.e., knowing what colors are. Disorders of color recognition, properly known as *color agnosia,* are rare. Moreover, the study of this condition has been hampered by the confusing and sometimes contradictory ways in which the condition has been defined. For example, some investigators have designated patients who cannot name colors correctly as having color agnosia, which is incorrect and a direct confusion of color naming with color recognition. In other cases, patients who were designated as having color agnosia clearly had significant defects in color perception, making rather questionable the application of the term *agnosia.* However, several well studied cases of color agnosia have been reported (Farah et al., 1988; Kinsbourne and Warrington, 1964; Luzzatti and Davidoff, 1994; Schnider et al., 1992), although the neuropsychological specification of these cases is far and away superior to the neuroanatomic description.

Here, a strict definition of agnosia is adopted, namely, *a normal percept stripped of its meaning* (cf. Teuber, 1968; Tranel and Damasio, 1996). Accordingly, *color agnosia* is defined as the loss of the ability to retrieve color knowledge pertinent to a given stimulus—a loss that cannot be attributed to impaired perception or to a naming defect. Patients with color agnosia manifest impairments on tasks in which the retrieval of color knowledge is crucial—e.g., remembering the characteristic colors of various entities, recalling entities that appear in certain colors, choosing the correct color for an entity, and retrieving basic knowledge about color (e.g., knowing that mixing red and yellow will make orange).

Neuropsychological Correlates

Impairments in the ability to recognize objects presented through the visual modality—i.e., visual object agnosia—is the most common neuropsychological correlate of color agnosia. As mentioned earlier, visual object agnosia frequently affects some categories of entities more than others. The most common pattern is a defect in the recognition of living entities (e.g., animals), with relative or complete sparing of recognition of artifactual entities (e.g., tools and utensils). These findings converge well with recent studies of the neuroanatomic correlates of object recognition, which have suggested a crucial role for mesial occipital and occipitotemporal structures in the retrieval of conceptual (semantic) knowledge for animals (Tranel et al., 1997a). By contrast, the retrieval of conceptual knowledge for tools has been associated with structures in the left occipito-temporo-parietal junction (Tranel et al., 1997a). Another, less frequent correlate of color agnosia is a defect in object naming to visual confrontation—i.e., anomia (or what has sometimes been called *optic aphasia*). Anomia, like visual agnosia, often affects some conceptual categories more than others—for example, patients may evince a marked impairment in tool naming and yet be able to name animals normally (Tranel et al., 1997b; H. Damasio et al., in press).

Neuroanatomic Correlates

The neuroanatomic correlates of color agnosia are obscure. They would appear to include the occipitotemporal region, either unilaterally on the left or bilaterally, but if this is true, it is not clear how this pattern would differ from what has been described in connection with central achromatopsia (e.g., Benton and Tranel, 1993; see "Disorders of Color Perception," above). Presumably, color agnosia and achromatopsia have at least partially separable neuroanatomic substrates, but the studies available to date do not permit an unequivocal separation. Luzzatti and Davidoff (1994) reported two patients with color agnosia, one of whom had a "left temporal" lesion and the other a "left temporo-parieto-occipital" lesion; no further anatomic details were provided. Schnider et al. (1992) reported a patient whose color agnosia was noted to be caused by a "left inferotemporo-occipital" lesion; again, further details about the lesion were not provided. The best guess at this point is that color agnosia is probably associated with lesions that are somewhat anterior to those responsible for central achromatopsia; however, until further studies provide better clarification of this issue, it must be concluded that the neuroanatomic correlates of color agnosia remain elusive.

Studies using functional imaging techniques have begun to provide some pertinent information on this topic. Martin and colleagues, using PET, have reported activations in the left inferotemporal region, bilateral fusiform gyrus, and right lingual gyrus during a condition in which subjects were asked to retrieve previously acquired color knowledge (Chao and Martin, 1999; Martin et al., 1995). The investigators emphasized that these regions are probably somewhat anterior and lateral to color perception substrates and do not overlap, at least entirely, with those that have been identified as being activated by color perception per se. In general, the functional imaging work reported so far tends to support the same conclusion hinted at by lesion studies—namely, that the neural substrates for color perception and color knowledge are at least partially separable.

A Case Study

We studied a patient who, premorbidly, was an expert in painting with oils. Following bilateral occipitotemporal lesions, the patient found that he was unable to mix different colors of paints to obtain the desired colors. A detailed evaluation indicated that the patient did not have achromatopsia or color anomia; he performed normally on all standard tests of color perception and could name colors accurately. In fact, he even remained capable of articulating verbally the recipe he should follow to obtain certain colors (e.g., "I need to mix this dark red with this light blue and a hint of black to get the color I want for the shaded portion of this mountain scene..."); however, he could not perform this process "intuitively," i.e., by mixing just the right amounts together to achieve desired colors. We have reasoned that this patient has a genuine loss of color knowledge—i.e., color agnosia—albeit in the setting of a certain level of special expertise insofar as color knowledge is concerned. This patient had bilateral occipitotemporal lesions that were just anterior to those that have been associated most frequently with achromatopsia. Thus, this case provides some additional support for the notion that this lesion locus may be a reasonable correlate of color agnosia and that color recognition and color perception can be dissociated.

DISORDERS OF COLOR NAMING (COLOR ANOMIA)

Definition

Color anomia is an impairment in the ability to name colors, which cannot be attributed to faulty color perception or to aphasia. Typically, the defect is bidirectional—that is, the patient cannot name colors when presented colored stimuli, and cannot point to colors, given their names. The former direction (naming the colors of colored stimuli), though, is often more severely impaired. General cognitive disturbance (e.g., dementia), or severe impairments in visual attention and perception, preclude the diagnosis of color anomia; also, severe aphasia, which will often disrupt the naming of all manner of categories, is another exclusion criterion.

Neuropsychological Correlates

A right homonymous hemianopia, with intact color and form perception in the left hemifield, is the most typical presentation in patients with color anomia. Pure alexia (as defined earlier) is another very frequent neuropsychological correlate of color anomia (Damasio and Damasio, 1983). In fact, it has been argued that color anomia rarely occurs without some degree of acquired reading impairment (Davidoff and De Bleser, 1994; Mohr et al., 1971). By definition, the naming of colors can be impaired selectively in relationship to other aspects of color processing, that is, patients with color anomia can present with no accompanying defects in the perception, imagery, and recognition of colors (Damasio et al., 1979; Geschwind and Fusillo, 1966; Rizzo and Damasio, 1989; Rizzo et al., 1993).

It was noted earlier that naming defects are frequently category-related—that is, patients manifest a more severe impairment in naming some categories than others. In this context, it is intriguing to note that the ability to name colors is frequently *spared* in patients who otherwise have pronounced defects in naming for many other categories of stimuli. In an early large-scale study of this issue, Goodglass et al. (1986) found that in aphasic patients, color naming was often unimpaired, even when patients had severe naming defects for other stimuli. This finding is consistent with an older case study (Yamadori and Albert, 1973). We have made similar observations in several studies of naming disorders; specifically, the vast majority of patients with naming defects—even patients with very severely impaired naming—do not have impaired naming of colors (Damasio et al., 1990; Damasio and Damasio, 1992; Tranel et al., 1997b, 1998).

Neuroanatomic Correlates

Color anomia has been linked to lesions in the left mesial occipitotemporal region, in a subsplenial position (Damasio et al., 2000; Davidoff and De Bleser, 1994). This lesion locus typically affects visual cortex and/or optic radiations, so that the patient develops a right hemianopia; thus, the processing of visual information is confined to the right visual cortex. In addition, the lesion is situated in such a way that primary language regions in the left hemisphere are prevented from receiving information related to color, yielding the color naming impairment. An interesting implication of this pattern is that the right hemisphere cannot support, by itself, the naming of colors. To the extent that color naming is a relatively basic ability, is restricted to a fairly narrow range of items, and is frequently spared in aphasia, this conclusion is somewhat counterintuitive. However, it is fair to say that this issue has barely been studied, and further investigation may provide new insights into the manner in which higher-order processing of color knowledge, and its link to color naming, is subserved by various neural sectors.

Other Considerations

In fact, it is intriguing to note that the condition of color anomia has received very little attention in the scientific literature in recent years, insofar as lesion studies are concerned. Since the widely cited paper by Damasio et al. (1979), which is now more than two decades old, very few studies have been published. One can speculate about some of the potential explanations for this scarcity. Color anomia is very rare—in many patients, as noted earlier, the ability to name colors is often preserved in the face of severe naming deficits for many other categories of stimuli. One factor that probably contributes to the relative invulnerability of color naming is the fact that color names comprise a very small, and essentially closed, set of items. Most individuals can name reliably less than a dozen or so colors, and beyond this, hybrid terms such as "blueish-green" or "light red" are usually applied. And by and large, new terms (and new stimuli) are not being added to the prevailing cultural repertoire (cf. Saunders and van Brakel, 1997), that is, the class is "closed." It is interesting in this context to draw comparisons with other categories. Take prepositions, for example: this is also a "closed" class, and it is generally considered to be relatively small—however, it contains upwards of a 100 different items (Landau and Jackendoff, 1993), or nearly an order of magnitude more than vernacular color terms. And in the better-studied categories of nouns or even verbs, there are literally thousands of members, and more items are added on a regular basis (i.e., the classes are "open"). It figures that color naming may be highly resistant to impairment by virtue of its simplicity and circumscribed nature.

Also, it is very difficult to separate experimentally the processes of word retrieval and conceptual knowledge retrieval, particularly in functional imaging studies. It is well established, in lesion studies, that the processes of knowing and naming can be clearly dissociated. That is, there is a basic distinction between *recognition,* on the one hand, and *naming,* on the other. The former refers to knowing and retrieving the meaning of a concept—its functions, features, characteristics, relationships to other concepts; the latter refers to knowing and retrieving the name of that concept—what it is called. It is true that the recognition of an entity, under normal circumstances, is frequently indicated by naming, but this need not be the case. In functional imaging studies with normal subjects, though, the typical method of assessing knowledge retrieval is to ask the subjects to name various stimuli (at least covertly), but this directly confounds the processes of naming and recognition. Even in the best studies available to date, this problem cannot be dismissed (cf. Chao and Martin, 1999; Martin et al., 1995). For example, in the Chao and Martin study, which is one of the best studies of this type available so far, the investigators found that naming the color of colored objects, relative to naming the colored objects, activated the left lingual gyrus and the inferior temporal cortex bilaterally. The authors pointed out, correctly, that these areas are virtually identical to those that are activated by tasks requiring color perception (lingual gyrus) or retrieving color knowledge (inferior temporal cortex). The experimental design, however, does not allow an unequivocal separation of color naming from other aspects of color processing, because the subjects could not be prevented from engaging different aspects of color processing—including naming and knowing—while performing the experimental tasks. Functional imaging paradigms have yet to yield unequivocal insights regarding the neural underpinnings of color naming, distinct from the processes of color perception and retrieving other knowledge about color.

SUMMARY

The scientific investigation of several different disorders of color processing, including achromatopsia, color agnosia, and color anomia, has generated a number of important insights into neuropsychological and neuroanatomical correlates of visual processing. Lesion studies furnished many intriguing and testable hypotheses regarding color processing, and functional imaging approaches have begun to corroborate many of the clues derived from lesion work. Many details have yet to be worked out, but the evidence available so far points consistently to a role for mesial and ventral occipital and occipitotemporal regions in color processing. Moreover, for several aspects of color processing, a predominant role for left-hemisphere occipital and occipitotemporal structures has been consistently supported. And perhaps the most important finding thus far, and one for which there is considerable convergent evidence from several different experimental approaches (e.g., lesion studies, functional imaging studies, neurophysiology), is that color processing depends on neural structures which are separable, at least in part, from those that support other aspects of vision, including processing of form, depth, and motion.

REFERENCES

Aguirre GK, D'Esposito M: Environmental knowledge is subserved by separable dorsal/ventral neural areas. *Neurosci* 17:2512–2518, 1997.

Aguirre GK, Detre JA, Alsop DC, D'Esposito M: The parahippocampus subserves topographical learning in man. *Cereb Cortex* 6:823–829, 1996.

Allison T, Begleiter A, McCarthy G, et al: Electrophysiological studies of color processing in human visual cortex. *Electroencephalogr Clin Neurophysiol* 88:343–355, 1993.

Barrash J: A historical review of topographical disorientation and its neuroanatomical correlates. *J Clin Exp Neuropsychol* 20:807–827, 1998.

Barrash J, Damasio H, Adolphs R, Tranel D: The neuroanatomical correlates of route learning impairment. *Neuropsychologia* 38:820–836, 2000.

Bartolomeo P, Bachoud-Levi A-C, Denes G: Preserved imagery for colours in a patient with cerebral achromatopsia. *Cortex* 33:369–378, 1997.

Beauvois MF, Saillant B: Optic aphasia for colours and colour agnosia: A distinction between visual and visuo-verbal impairments in the processing of colours. *Cogn Neuropsychol* 2:1–48, 1985.

Benton AL, Tranel D: Visuoperceptual, visuospatial, and visuoconstructive disorders, in Heilman KM, Valenstein E (eds): *Clinical Neuropsychology,* 3d ed. New York: Oxford University Press. 1993, pp. 165–213.

Berlin B, Kay P: *Basic Color Terms.* Berkeley, CA: University of California Press, 1969.

Bornstein MH: On the development of color naming in young children: Data and theory. *Brain Lang* 26:72–93, 1985.

Cavanagh P, Henaff M-A, Michel F, et al: Complete sparing of high-contrast color input to motion perception in cortical color blindness. *Nat Neurosci* 1:242–247, 1998.

Chao LL, Martin A: Cortical regions associated with perceiving, naming, and knowing about colors. *J Cogn Neurosci* 11:25–35, 1999.

Clark VP, Parasuraman R, Keil K, et al: Selective attention to face identity and color studied with fMRI. *Hum Brain Map* 5:293–297, 1997.

Corbetta M, Miezin FM, Dobmeyer S, et al: Attentional modulation of neural processing of shape, color, and velocity in humans. *Science* 248:1556–1559, 1990.

Corbetta M, Miezin FM, Dobmeyer S, et al: Selective and divided attention during visual discriminations of shape, color, and speed: Functional anatomy by positron emission tomography. *J Neurosci* 11:2383–2402, 1991.

Damasio AR, Damasio H: The anatomic basis of pure alexia. *Neurology* 33:1573–1583, 1983.

Damasio AR, Damasio H: Brain and language. *Sci Am* 267:88–95, 1992.

Damasio AR, Damasio H, Tranel D, Brandt JP: The neural regionalization of knowledge access: Preliminary evidence. *Quant Biol* 55:1039–1047, 1990.

Damasio AR, McKee J, Damasio H: Determinants of performance in color anomia. *Brain and Lang* 7:74–85, 1979.

Damasio AR, Tranel D, Rizzo M: Disorders of complex visual processing, in Mesulam M-M (ed): *Principles of Behavioral and Cognitive Neurology*. Philadelphia: Davis, 2000, pp. 332–372.

Damasio AR, Yamada T, Damasio H: Central achromatopsia: Behavioral, anatomic and physiologic aspects. *Neurology* 30:1064–1071, 1980.

Damasio H, Grabowski TJ, Tranel D, et al: Neural correlates of naming actions and of naming spatial relations. *Neuroimage* 13:1053–1064, 2001.

Damasio H, Tranel D, Grabowski TJ, et al: Uncovering neural systems behind word and concept retrieval. *Cognition* In Press.

Davidoff J, De Bleser R: Impaired picture recognition with preserved object naming and reading. *Brain Cogn* 24:1–23, 1994.

De Renzi E, Spinnler H: Impaired performance on color tasks in patients with hemispheric lesions. *Cortex* 3:194–217, 1967.

D'Esposito M, Detre JA, Aguirre GK, et al: A functional MRI study of mental image generation. *Neuropsychologia* 35:725–730, 1997.

De Vreese LP: Two systems for colour-naming deficits: Verbal disconnection vs colour imagery disorder. *Neuropsychologia* 29:1–18, 1991.

Farah MJ: The neurological basis of mental imagery: A componential analysis. *Cognition* 18:245–272, 1984.

Farah MJ: Is visual imagery really visual? Overlooked evidence from neuropsychology. *Psychol Rev* 95:307–317, 1988.

Farah MJ, Levine DN, Calvanio R: A case study of mental imagery deficit. *Brain and Cogn* 8:147–164, 1988.

Farah MJ, Meyer MM, McMullen PA: The living/nonliving dissociation is not an artifact: Giving an a priori implausible hypothesis a strong test. *Cogn Neuropsychol* 13:137–154, 1996.

Felleman DJ, Van Essen DC: Distributed hierarchical processing in the primate cerebral cortex. *Cereb Cortex* 1: 1–47, 1991.

Geschwind N, Fusillo M: Color naming defects in association with alexia. *Arch Neurol* 15:137–146, 1966.

Goodglass H, Wingfield A, Hyde MR, Theurkauf JC: Category specific dissociations in naming and recognition by aphasic patients. *Cortex* 22:87–102, 1986.

Gouras P: The perception of color, in Gouras P (ed): *Vision and Visual Dysfunction* London: Macmillan, 1991, vol VI.

Heywood CA, Kentridge RW, Cowey A: Form and motion from colour in cerebral achromatopsia. *Exp Brain Res* 123:145–153, 1998.

Heywood CA, Wilson B, Cowey A: A case study of cortical colour "blindness" with relatively intact chromatic discrimination. *J Neurol Neurosurg Psychiatry* 50:22–29, 1987.

Hillis AE, Caramazza A: Category-specific naming and comprehension impairment: A double dissociation. *Brain* 114:2081–2094, 1991.

Hubel DH, Livingstone MS: Segregation of form, color, and stereopsis in primate area 18. *J Neurosci* 7:3378–3415, 1987.

Hurlbert AC, Bramwell DI, Heywood C, Cowey A: Discrimination of cone contrast changes as evidence for colour constancy in cerebral achromatopsia. *Exp Brain Res* 123:136–144, 1998.

Joseph JE, Proffitt DR: Semantic versus perceptual influences of color in object recognition. *J Exp Psychol Learn Mem Cogn* 22:407–429, 1996.

Kinsbourne M, Warrington EK: Observations on colour agnosia. *J Neurol Neurosurg Psychiatry* 27:296–299, 1964.

Kolmel HW: Pure homonymous hemiachromatopsia: Findings with neuro-ophthalmologic examination and imaging procedures. *Eur Arch Psychiatry Neurol Sci* 237:237–243, 1988.

Kosslyn SM: *Image and Brain: The Resolution of the Imagery Debate.* Cambridge, MA: MIT Press, 1994.

Kourtzi Z, Kanwisher N: Activation in human MT/MST by static images with implied motion. *J Cogn Neurosci* 12:48–55, 2000.

Landau B, Jackendoff R: "What" and "where" in spatial language and spatial cognition. *Behav Brain Sci* 16:217–265, 1993.

Livingstone MS, Hubel DH: Anatomy and physiology of a color system in the primate visual cortex. *J Neurosci* 4:309–356, 1984.

Livingstone, MS, Hubel DH: Psychophysical evidence for separate channels for the perception of form, color, movement, and depth. *J Neuroscience* 7:3416–3468, 1987.

Lueck CJ, Zeki S, Friston KJ, et al: The color centre in the cerebral cortex of man. *Nature* 340:386–389, 1989.

Luzzatti C, Davidoff J: Impaired retrieval of object-colour knowledge with preserved colour naming. *Neuropsychologia* 32:933–950, 1994.

Maguire EA, Burgess N, Donnett JG, et al: Knowing where and getting there: A human navigation network. *Science* 280:921–924, 1998.

Manzel K, Tranel D: Development and standardization of a reading test for brain-damaged patients. *Dev Neuropsychol* 15:407–420, 1999.

Martin A, Haxby JV, Lalonde FM, et al: Discrete cortical regions associated with knowledge of color and knowledge of action. *Science* 270:102–105, 1995.

Meadows JC: Disturbed perception of colors assocaited with localized cerebral lesions. *Brain* 97:615–632, 1974.

Merigan W, Freeman A, Meyers SP: Parallel processing streams in human visual cortex. *Neuroreport* 8:3985–3991, 1997.

Mohr JP, Leicester J, Stoddard LT, Sidman M: Right hemianopia with memory and color deficits in circumscribed left posterior cerebral artery territory infarction. *Neurology* 21:1104–1113, 1971.

Paulson HL, Galetta SL, Grossman M, Alavi A: Hemiachromatopsia of unilateral occipitotemporal infarcts. *Am J Ophthalmol* 118:518–523, 1994.

Plendl H, Paulus W, Roberts IG, et al: The time course and location of cerebral evoked activity associated with the processing of colour stimuli in man. *Neurosci Lett* 150:9–12, 1993.

Rizzo M, Damasio AR: Acquired central achromatopsia, in Kulikowski J J, Dickinson C M, Murray I J (eds.): *Seeing Contour and Color.* Oxford, England: Pergamon Press, 1989, pp 758–763.

Rizzo M, Smith V, Pokorny J, Damasio AR: Color perception profiles in central achromatopsia. *Neurology* 43:995–1001, 1993.

Roorda A, Williams DR: The arrangement of the three cone classes in the living human eye. *Nature* 397:520–522, 1999.

Rosler F, Heil M, Henninghausen E: Distinct cortical activation patterns during long-term memory retrieval of verbal, spatial, and color information. *J Cogn Neurosci* 7:51–65, 1995.

Ruttiger L, Braun DI, Gegenfurtner KR, et al: Selective color constancy deficits after circumscribed unilateral brain lesions. *J Neurosci* 19:3094–3106, 1999.

Sakai K, Watanabe E, Onodera Y, et al: Functional mapping of the human colour centre with echo-planar magnetic resonance imaging. *Proc R Soc Lond B,* 261:89–98, 1995.

Sartori G, Job R, Miozzo M, et al: Category-specific form-knowledge deficit in a patient with herpes simplex virus encephalitis. *J Clin Exp Neuropsych* 15:280–299, 1993.

Saunders BAC, van Brakel J: Are there nontrivial constraints on colour categorization? *Behav Brain Sci* 20:167–228, 1997.

Schnider A, Landis T, Regard M, Benson D F: Dissociation of color from object in amnesia. *Arch Neurol* 49:982–985, 1992.

Senior C, Barnes J, Giampietro V, et al: The functional neuroanatomy of implicit-motion perception or "representational momentum." *Curr Biol* 10:16–22, 2000.

Shuren JE, Brott TG, Schefft BK, Houston W: Preserved color imagery in an achromatopsic. *Neuropsychologia* 34:485–489, 1996.

Siple P, Springer RM: Memory and preference for the colors of objects. *Percept Psychophys* 34:363–370, 1983.

Teuber HL: Alteration of perception and memory in man, in Weiskrantz L (ed): *Analysis of Behavioral Change.* New York: Harper & Row, 1968, pp 268–375.

Tranel D, Adolphs R, Damasio H, Damasio AR: A neural basis for the retrieval of words for actions. *Cogn Neuropsychol* 18:655–670, 2001.

Tranel D, Damasio AR: The agnosias and apraxias, in Bradley WG, Daroff RB, Fenichel GM, Marsden CD (eds.): *Neurology in Clinical Practice,* 2d ed. Stoneham, MA: Butterworth, 1996, pp 119–129.

Tranel D, Damasio H, Damasio AR: A neural basis for the retrieval of conceptual knowledge. *Neuropsychologia* 35:1319–1327, 1997a.

Tranel D, Damasio H, Damasio AR: On the neurology of naming, in Goodglass H, Wingfield A (eds): *Anomia: Neuroanatomical and Cognitive Correlates.* New York: Academic Press, 1997b, pp 65–90.

Tranel D, Damasio H, Damasio AR: The neural basis of lexical retrieval, in Parks, Levine R W, D S, Long D L (eds): *Fundamentals of Neural Network Modeling: Neuropsychology and Cognitive Neuroscience.* Cambridge, MA: MIT Press. 1998, pp 271–296.

Tranel D, Logan CG, Frank RJ, Damasio AR: Explaining category-related effects in the retrieval of conceptual and lexical knowledge for concrete entities: Operationalization and analysis of factors. *Neuropsychologia* 35:1329–1339, 1997c.

Victor JD, Maiese K, Shapley R et al: Acquired central dyschromatopsia: analysis of a case with preservation of color discrimination. *Clin Vis Sci* 4:183–196, 1989.

Warrington EK, McCarthy RA: Multiple meaning systems in the brain: A case for visual semantics. *Neuropsychologia* 32:1465–1473, 1994.

Warrington, EK, Shallice T: Category specific semantic impairments. *Brain* 107:829–853, 1984.

Wray J, Edelman GM: A model of color vision based on cortical reentry. *Cereb Cortex* 6:701–716, 1996.

Yamadori A, Albert ML: Word category aphasia. *Cortex* 9:83–89, 1973.

Zeki S: A century of cerebral achromatopsia. *Brain* 113: 1727–1777, 1990.

Zeki SM, Watson JDG, Lueck CJ, et al: A direct demonstration of functional specialization in human visual cortex. *J Neurosci* 11:641–649, 1991.

Chapter 21

AUDITORY AGNOSIA AND AMUSIA

Russell M. Bauer
Carrie R. McDonald

Auditory agnosia refers to an impaired capacity to recognize sounds in the presence of otherwise adequate hearing as measured by standard audiometry. Historically, the term has been used broadly to refer to impaired capacity to recognize sounds in general and in a narrow sense to refer to a selective deficit in recognizing nonverbal sounds only. Terminological confusion abounds, with such terms as *cortical auditory disorder,*[1,2] *auditory agnosia,*[3,4] and *auditory agnosia and word deafness*[5] all being used to describe similar phenomena. In most cases, impairment in the recognition of both speech and nonspeech sounds is present to some degree. The relative severity of these impairments depends on lesion localization, on premorbid lateralization of linguistic and nonlinguistic skills in the individual patient, and on which hemisphere is first or more seriously damaged[6] (but see Ref. 7). Complicating the picture even further is the fact that many patients evolve from one disorder to another as recovery takes place.[8]

In regard to generalized auditory agnosia, we prefer the theoretically neutral term *cortical auditory disorder,* and we first discuss this entity together with *cortical deafness.* We then discuss more "selective" deficits, including *pure word deafness* (a selective impairment in speech-sound recognition), *auditory sound agnosia* (selective impairment in recognizing nonspeech sounds), and *paralinguistic agnosias* (in which recognition of prosodic features of spoken language is impaired). We then describe patients with *receptive (sensory) amusia,* loss of the ability to appreciate various characteristics of heard music. Table 21-1 lists the major clinical features of each syndrome. In the final section of the chapter, we consider recent functional neuroimaging studies that have begun to shed important new light on the functional neuroanatomy of auditory abilities and disorders.

CORTICAL DEAFNESS AND CORTICAL AUDITORY DISORDER

Patients with cortical deafness show profound impairments in processing auditory stimuli of any kind and often have electrophysiologic signs of primary impairment in auditory-perceptual acuity. The behavior of patients with cortical auditory disorders is similar, though auditory evoked responses are more often normal in this population. Both groups show a range of impairments in auditory perception, discrimination, and recognition that affect verbal and nonverbal material.[9,10] Aphasic signs, if present, are mild and do not prevent the patient from identifying visual or somesthetic stimuli. Difficulties in elementary auditory function, including temporal auditory analysis and localization of sounds in space, are common.

In our view, cortical auditory disorders and cortical deafness are related in much the same way as visual agnosia is related to cortical blindness. If so, then cortical auditory disorders can take apperceptive or associative[11] forms, though some degree of perceptual deficit is apparent in nearly all cases where the evaluation of auditory abilities has been sufficiently comprehensive. This statement is true even in cases where pure tone audiometry is relatively normal. Jerger and coworkers[12,13] reported impairments in auditory perception (ear suppression in dichotic listening, abnormal click fusion thresholds, and impaired discrimination of basic sound attributes) in patients with cortical auditory disorders. It is important to note that cortical auditory disorders sometimes evolve from a state of cortical deafness, and it is difficult to distinguish between the two entities. Michel and colleagues[14] argued that the cortically deaf patient looks and feels deaf, whereas the patient with cortical auditory disorders insists that he or she is not deaf. This turns out

Table 21-1
Clinical features of various forms of auditory agnosia

	Cortical deafness	Cortical auditory disorder	Pure word deafness	Auditory sound agnosia	Sensory/ receptive amusia
Audiometric sensitivity	−	+/−	+	+	+
Speech comprehension	−	−	−	+	+
Speech repetition	−	−	−	+	+
Spontaneous speech	+	+*	+*	+	+
Reading comprehension	+	+	+	+	+
Written language	+	+	+	+	+
Recognition of familiar sounds	−	−	+	-	?
Musical perception	−	−	−†	−	+/−
Recognition of vocal prosody	−	−	+	?	−

Key: + = spared ability; − = impaired ability; ? = insufficient information in literature to generalize.

*May be some paraphasia.

†When tested (rarely), musical perception has been shown to be impaired in these patients.

Sources: Adapted from Buchman et al.[7] and Oppenheimer and Newcombe,[3] with permission.

to be a poor criterion, because the subjective experience of deafness in the former condition is typically so transient, and patients in both groups are "deaf" when subjected to appropriate tests. Although it was once believed that bilateral cortical lesions involving primary auditory cortex resulted in total hearing loss, evidence from animal experiments,[15,16] cortical mapping of the auditory area,[17] and clinicopathologic studies in humans[18,19] indicate that complete destruction of primary auditory cortex does not lead to permanent loss of audiometric sensitivity. Thus, clinical, pathologic, and electrophysiologic data question the distinctive nature of cortical deafness[1,9,10] and suggest that it is one of a spectrum of auditory impairments that runs from generalized disturbances in detecting and discriminating basic sound attributes to more complex and selective impairments in auditory recognition.

Recent behavioral studies of cortical deafness focused on deficits in attention and behavioral response, rather than entirely on perceptual deficits, as underlying the disorder. Engelien and colleagues[20] studied "deaf behavior" in a patient diagnosed with cortical deafness and found that under conditions of selective attention to audition, their patient achieved normal awareness of sounds, despite persistent impairment in sound localization and identification. In addition, the patient showed no orienting or startle response to unexpected, sudden sounds unless attention was focused exclusively on audition. This patient, however, had damage to the frontal operculum, in addition to bilateral lesions of the superior temporal gyri, which may have contributed to his auditory attentional deficits. Garde and Cowey[21] described a cortically deaf patient following pontine and bitemporal cortical lesions whose detection *and* localization of auditory stimuli both improved when attention was directed on audition. Their patient, unlike the patient of Engelien et al.,[20] responded reflexively to sounds that she denied hearing.

Cortical deafness is most often seen in bilateral cerebrovascular disease. A recent case of cortical deafness resulting from moyamoya disease (a vascular disorder in which the main cerebral arteries at the base of the brain are replaced by a fine network of vessels) has been reported in the Japanese literature.[22] The course is usually biphasic, with an initial deficit (often aphasia and hemiparesis) related to unilateral damage, followed by a second (contralateral) deficit associated with sudden transient total deafness.[12,13,20,21] A biphasic course is also typical of cortical auditory disorders. In cortical deafness, bilateral destruction of the auditory radiations or the primary auditory cortex (Heschl's gyrus) has been a constant finding.[20] Bilateral temporal lobe damage is generally reported, which in most cases involves the primary auditory cortex, although this area may be partially or completely spared. When the cortex is spared, underlying white matter pathology is a consistent finding.[25] Several researchers[26,27] have claimed that true "cortical" deafness does not result from isolated lesions of the cortex, but more often results from bilateral disconnection of the pathway to the auditory cortices. To date, the importance of cortical versus subcortical involvement in the etiology of cortical deafness is unclear, although this controversy will likely be resolved by studies using detailed MRI and comparison with probabilistic atlases.[28] The anatomic basis of cortical auditory disorder is more variable. Lesions can be quite extensive,[3] though the superior temporal gyrus and efferent connections of Heschl's gyrus are aften involved. Several case reports[29–31] suggest that cortical auditory disorder can result from bilateral lesions sparing the cortex entirely. Thus, the lesions in cortical auditory disorder seem to involve either intrinsic or disconnecting lesions involving the auditory association cortex, with relative sparing of Heschl's gyrus. A recent report[32] suggests that a generalized auditory agnosia may even result from circumscribed bilateral damage to the inferior colliculi.

PURE WORD DEAFNESS (AUDITORY AGNOSIA FOR SPEECH, AUDITORY VERBAL AGNOSIA)

The patient with pure word deafness is unable to comprehend spoken language although he or she can read, write, and speak in a *relatively* normal manner.[7] As such, it can be discussed as a form of aphasia (as in Chap. 11) as well as an impairment of high-level auditory function. Writing to dictation is typically impaired, though copying of written material is not. By definition, comprehension of nonverbal sounds is *relatively* spared, but nonverbal auditory recognition is impaired in the majority of cases in which it has been evaluated.[7] Thus, the syndrome is "pure" in that (1) the patient is *relatively* free of signs of posterior aphasia (see Chap. 11) and (2) the impairment in speech sound recognition is disproportionately severe. The disorder was first described by Kussmaul.[33] Lichteim[34] later defined it as an isolated deficit and postulated a bilateral subcortical interruption of fibers from ascending auditory projections to the left "auditory word center." With few exceptions, pure word deafness has been associated with bilateral, symmetric cortical-subcortical lesions of the anterior part of the superior temporal gyri with some sparing of Heschl's gyrus, particularly on the left. Some patients have subcortical lesions of the dominant temporal lobe only, presumably destroying the ipsilateral auditory radiation as well as callosal fibers from the contralateral auditory region.[35–37] It is generally agreed that the lesion profile results in a bilateral disconnection of Wernicke's area from auditory input.[38] The fact that it involves an unusually placed, circumscribed lesion explains the low incidence of pure word deafness. In the review performed by Buchman and colleagues,[7] the lesions in 30 of 37 reviewed cases were of cerebrovascular origin. Other etiologies include encephalitis[39] and neoplasm.[40] Childhood forms of pure word deafness have also been associated with Landau-Kleffner syndrome,[41,42] although the course and prognosis in patients with Landau-Kleffner syndrome are highly variable. Kaga[41] reports that patients with Landau-Kleffner syndrome often show a sequential and hierarchical language disorder that commonly begins with sensory aphasia, followed by generalized auditory agnosia, and finally pure word deafness. Language disturbances in Landau-Kleffner syndrome may improve with anticonvulsant medication[43] or may be long lasting.[44]

When first seen, the patient is often recovering from a Wernicke's aphasia, though occasionally pure word deafness may actually give way to a Wernicke's aphasia.[45–48] As the paraphasias and writing and reading disturbances disappear, the patient still does not comprehend spoken language but can communicate by writing. Deafness can be ruled out by normal audiometric pure-tone thresholds. In some cases, however, mild bilateral neurosensory hearing loss is detected in patients with pure word deafness.[49,50] At this point, the patient may experience auditory hallucinations[51] or may exhibit transient euphoric[52] or paranoid[53,54] ideation. The inability to repeat poorly comprehended speech stimuli distinguishes pure word deafness from transcortical sensory aphasia; the absence of florid paraphasia and of reading and writing disturbance distinguishes it from Wernicke's aphasia. This having been said, it should be recognized that "aphasic" and "agnosic" symptoms may both be present, though different in degree, in the individual case.[7]

Many patients are responsive to speech input but complain of dramatic, sometimes aversive changes in their subjective experience of speech sounds.[8] The pure word deafness patient may complain that speech is muffled or sounds like a foreign language. Hemphill and Stengel's[55] patient stated that "voices come but no words." Klein and Harper's[46] patient described speech as "an undifferentiated continuous humming noise without any rhythm" and "like foreigners speaking in the distance." Albert and Bear's[30] patient said "words come too quickly" and, "they sound like a foreign language." The patient of Wee and colleagues[56] described voices as "distorted and cartoonlike." The speech of these patients is often slightly louder than normal and can be dysprosodic. Performance on speech perception tests is inconsistent and highly dependent upon context[57] and linguistic complexity.[58]

Many studies of pure word deafness have emphasized the role of auditory-perceptual processing in the genesis of the disorder.[1,8,12,45,58] Problems with temporal resolution[45] and phonemic discrimination[59–61] have also received attention. Auerbach and coworkers[58] suggest that the disorder may take two forms: (1) a prephonemic temporal auditory acuity disturbance associated with bilateral temporal lesions or (2) a disorder of phonemic discrimination attributable to left temporal lesions and closely linked to Wernicke's aphasia. Wang and colleagues[62] have challenged this division and suggested that prephonemic processing may also be affected following left unilateral lesions with subcortical involvement in patients with pure word deafness. Albert and Bear[45] suggested that the problem in pure word deafness is one of temporal resolution of auditory stimuli rather than specific phonetic impairment. Their patient demonstrated abnormally long click-fusion thresholds, and improved in auditory comprehension when speech was presented at slower rates. Wang et al.[62] provided additional support for impaired temporal processing in the genesis of pure word deafness. They described a patient with a lesion involving the cortical and subcortical white matter of the left temporal lobe who was unable to process sound elements or dynamic acoustic changes that occurred in a short period of time (less than 300 ms). They concluded that the inability to detect even moderately rapid acoustic changes make it unlikely that these patients can process syllables in speech (which last only several hundred milliseconds) in any meaningful way.

Other researchers have also emphasized the role of poor temporal resolution in pure word deafness associated with Landau-Kleffner's syndrome[42] and progressive neuropathology.[49,63] Klein and others[42] studied electrophysiological abnormalities in six young adults who exhibited "verbal auditory agnosia" associated with Landau-Kleffner syndrome. They found that, compared to a control group, the cortical evoked potentials (CEPs) of their patient group were characterized by a delay in the N1 component to both tones and to speech sounds. This delay in N1 was consistently found over the lateral temporal cortex, despite a normal latency of the N1 component recorded over the frontocentral region of the scalp. These results suggest slowed processing of auditory stimuli within the secondary auditory cortex of the lateral temporal lobes for both speech and tones. The authors concluded that the perceptual impairment associated with verbal auditory agnosia is not speech-specific, rather speech is disproportionately affected since perception of speech sounds involves the analysis of brief acoustic transients that rapidly change in their spectral content. Otsuki et al.[49] described a patient with pure word deafness associated with generalized, progressive cortical atrophy, particularly in the left superior temporal region. Similar to the patient of Albert and Bear, this patient exhibited abnormally long click-fusion thresholds suggestive of an impairment in the temporal processing of auditory information.

Saffran, Marin, and Yeni-Komshian,[61] on the other hand, showed that informing their patient of the nature of the topic under discussion significantly facilitated comprehension. Thus, the disorder appeared to arise at different levels in these two patients. Other researchers have suggested that aside from deficits in temporal resolution and phonemic discrimination, a deficit in the processing of syllable sequences may contribute to pure word deafness.[64] This variability supports Buchman et al.'s[7] contention that pure word deafness describes a spectrum rather than an individual disorder.

On tests of phonemic discrimination, patients with bilateral lesions tend to show distinctive deficits for the feature of place of articulation.[58,59,65] Those with unilateral left hemispheric disease (LHD) show either impaired discrimination of voicing[41] or no distinctive pattern.[60] In dichotic listening, some patients show extreme suppression of right-ear perception,[45,61] suggesting the inaccessibility of the left hemispheric phonetic decoding areas (Wernicke's area) to auditory material that had already been acoustically processed by the right hemisphere. Several studies have reported brainstem and cortical auditory evoked responses in pure word deafness patients.[14] Brainstem auditory evoked potentials (BAEPs) are almost always normal, suggesting intact processing up to the level of the auditory radiations.[42,45,56,58,62,64,66] One study of progressive pure word deafness, however, reported normal amplitudes, but prolonged brainstem auditory evoked response latencies after wave.[63] Results from studies of cortical auditory evoked potentials (AEPs) are more variable, consistent with variable pathology.[58] For example, the patient of Jerger and colleagues[12] had no appreciable AEP, yet heard sounds. The patient of Auerbach and associates[58] showed normal P1, N1, and P2 responses to right-ear stimulation but had minimal response over either hemisphere to left-ear stimulation. A recent study measuring auditory evoked magnetic fields[67] revealed no N100 m detected in the left temporal lobe with the right ear stimulation in two patients with putaminal hemorrhages: one bilateral, the other only on the left. However, normal N100 m was obtained in the right hemisphere with the left ear stimulation in both cases. The location of the equivalent current dipole (ECD) of the intact N100 m in the right hemisphere was superimposed on the Heschl gyrus in brain MRI. These results are consistent with other studies[40] that support the disconnection view of pure word deafness.

Although patients with pure word deafness are supposed to perform relatively well with environmental sounds, many show subnormal performances when such abilities are formally tested.[7] Similarly, the appreciation of music is often disturbed.[7,56] Some patients may recognize foreign languages by their distinctive prosodic characteristics, and others can recognize *who* is speaking, suggesting preserved ability to comprehend paralinguistic aspects of speech. Coslett and associates[68] described a word-deaf patient who showed a remarkable dissociation between the comprehension of neutral and affectively intoned sentences. He was asked to point to pictures of males and females depicting various emotional expressions. When instructions were given in a neutral voice, he performed poorly, but when instructions were given with affective intonations appropriate to the target face, he performed normally (at a level commensurate to his performance with written instructions). This patient had bilateral destruction of primary auditory cortex with some sparing of auditory association cortex, suggesting at least some direct contribution of the auditory radiations directly to association cortex without initial decoding in Heschl's gyrus.[68] It has been found that patients with pure word deafness generally comprehend better when they can lip-read, although isolated cases have been reported in which lipreading did not improve performance.[62] Coslett and others[68] speculate that one reason why patients with pure word deafness improve their auditory comprehension with lipreading is that face-to-face contact allows them to take advantage of visual cues (gesture and facial expression that are processed by different brain systems). Another explanation is that lipreading provides visual information about place of articulation, a linguistic feature that is markedly impaired at least in the bilateral cases.[58] In either case, the preserved comprehension of paralinguistic aspects of speech in pure word deafness patients further reinforces the widely held belief that comprehension of speech and nonspeech sounds are dissociable abilities.

Although distinctions have been made between basic defects in auditory perception vs. defects in linguistic processing, few studies of pure word deafness have analyzed the defect in terms of the apperceptive-associative distinction so prominent in discussing visual agnosia (see Chap. 18).[69] It has been suggested that word deafness may represent the apperceptive counterpart of a very rare and ill-defined disorder called "pure word meaning deafness," in which the patient can hear and repeat words, but do not know their meaning.[70,71] Franklin and others[71] suggest that in "classic" cases of word meaning deafness, patients present with preserved repetition, phoneme discrimination, and lexical decision, but with impaired comprehension of spoken words alone. This "associative" form of the disorder results in errors that are generally semantic in nature and patients show poorer comprehension of abstract compared to concrete words. While an abstract/concrete dissociation suggests a "language-specific" explanation of word meaning deafness, Tyler and Moss[72] proposed an account of how a more general impairment in auditory processing would affect abstract words more than concrete words. Therefore, apperceptive and associative forms of verbal auditory agnosia have yet to be clearly delineated.

AUDITORY SOUND AGNOSIA (AUDITORY AGNOSIA FOR NONSPEECH SOUNDS)

Patients with auditory sound agnosia have selective difficulty recognizing and identifying nonverbal sounds. The disorder is rare, less common by far than pure word deafness, but its existence has raised interest because it suggests the same type of "domain-specificity" in the auditory system that has received much recent attention in the study of visual recognition disorders.[45–47,74,75] The lower incidence of auditory sound agnosia may be due in part to the fact that such patients are less likely seek medical advice than are those with a disorder of speech comprehension and also because on specific auditory complaints may be discounted when pure tone audiometric and speech discrimination thresholds are normal. This is unfortunate, since normal audiometry does not rule but the possibility of primary auditory perceptual defects.[76,77]

Vignolo[9] argued that there may be two forms of auditory sound agnosia: (1) a perceptual-discriminative type associated mainly with right hemisphere damage and (2) an associative-semantic type associated with left hemisphere damage and linked with posterior aphasia. The former group makes predominantly acoustic (e.g., "man whistling" for birdsong) errors on picture-sound matching tasks, while the latter makes predominantly semantic (e.g., "train" for automobile engine) errors. This division follows the original classification of Kliest,[78] who distinguished between the ability to detect/perceive isolated sounds or noises and the inability to understand the meaning of sounds. In the verbal sphere, the analogous distinction (at least on the input side) is between pure word deafness (perceptual-discriminative) and transcortical sensory aphasia (semantic-associative). Relatively few cases of "pure" auditory sound agnosia have been reported.[79–84] Sometimes a patient's condition evolves into auditory sound agnosia from a more generalized agnosia for both verbal and nonverbal sounds,[85–87] and occasionclly this evolves from an auditory sound agnosia into an auditory recognition defect that encompasses speech sounds and other auditory stimuli.[41]

The patient of Spreen and colleagues[83] is a paradigm case. He was a 65-year-old right-handed male who complained of "nerves" and headache when seen 3 years after a left hemiparetic episode. Audiometric testing revealed moderate bilateral high-frequency loss and speech reception thresholds of 12 dB for both ears. The outstanding abnormality was the inability to recognize common sounds. There was neither aphasia nor any other agnosic deficit. Sound localization was normal, but scores on the pitch subtest of the Seashore Tests of Musical Talent were at chance level. The patient performed well on a matching-to-sample test, suggesting that his sound recognition disturbance could not be attributed to serious acoustic disturbance. He claimed no musical experience or talent and refused to cooperate with further testing of musical ability. Postmortem examination revealed a sharply demarcated old infarct of the right hemisphere centering around the parietal lobe and involving the superior temporal and angular gyri as well as a large portion of the inferior parietal, inferior, and middle frontal gyri and the insula. Other cases with unilateral pathology were reported by Clark and associates[80] (four patients with variable left temporal lobe lesions), Fuji and coworkers[81] (small posterior right temporal hemorrhagic lesion of the middle and superior temporal gyri), Neilsen and Sult[82] (right thalamus and parietal lobe), and Wortis and Pfeffer[84] (large lesion of the right temporoparietooccipital junction).

These data suggest that an inability to recognize environmental sounds can occur after unilateral right hemisphere damage. Such a defect is less commonly seen in the context of bilateral disease,[79] but these cases are less "pure" at least in the acute stage. The association of auditory sound agnosia with right hemisphere damage implies that acoustic processors within the right hemisphere are preferentially involved in dealing with nonlinguistic sounds. The left hemisphere is likely involved in providing linguistic labels for identified sounds, and in performing semantic-associative functions supporting sound recognition and identification.

Other cases of auditory sound agnosia have been reported following bilateral subcortical lesions[30,87] and bilateral ventricular enlargement[86] in the absence of cortical pathology. The patient of Motomura et al.[30] presented following a thalamic hemorrhage with a generalized auditory agnosia that evolved to an auditory sound agnosia. Their patient showed a temporal discrimination impairment on click fusion tests that is often described in patients following bilateral temporal lobe lesions. Tanawaki and colleagues[87] describe a patient who presented initially with generalized cortical deafness, which then evolved to a generalized auditory agnosia, and finally to an auditory sound agnosia. Neuroradiological examination of their patient revealed bilateral subcortical lesions involving the acoustic radiations following a bilateral putaminal hemorrhage. This patient made errors on tests of sound recognition that were discriminative rather than associative in nature. An unusual case of auditory sound agnosia following head injury was reported by Lambert and others.[86] In their patient, CT and MRI did not provide evidence of cortical or subcortical pathology, but CT showed an intraventricular hemorrhage without parenchymal lesion, resulting in ventricular enlargement. The patient showed deficits on a loudness discrimination test with no deficit observed in temporal auditory acuity.

Clarke and associates[80] described four patients with unilateral, left hemisphere damage who had deficits in auditory recognition, sound localization, or both. Based on lesion analysis, they propose that two anatomically distinct pathways exist for auditory sound recognition and auditory sound localization. The authors suggest that auditory recognition is mediated by the lateral auditory cortex and temporal convexity, whereas auditory localization is mediated by posterior auditory areas, the insula, and the parietal convexity. These anatomically distinct pathways parallel the distinctions made of distinct "what" and "where" pathways described in the human visual system. Additional support for anatomically distinct auditory systems comes from a functional MRI study with healthy individuals which showed greater activation in the auditory cortex and inferior frontal gyrus during sound identification tasks (pitch processing) and greater activation in bilateral posterior temporal, and inferior and superior parietal regions during sound localization tasks.[88] These studies and others provide convincing evidence that auditory pattern and object recognition are processed along the temporal lobes—specifically, the anterior superior temporal gyrus and sulcus and parts of the middle temporal gyrus.[89]

In summary, case studies of auditory sound agnosia have suggested significant variability in both the localization and lateralization of neuropathology. As with pure word deafness, perceptual and associative forms of the disorder have been proposed, although these subtypes are not well defined. Evidence for distinct "what" and "where" pathways in the auditory modality is increasing with the use of functional imaging techniques.[88] In addition, recent neuroimaging studies have revealed that both the primary auditory cortex and the auditory association cortex may be needed to integrate environmental sounds, with a strong rightward asymmetry,[89] whereas the left temporal and frontal cortical regions are necessary for the analysis of speech information.[90] A review of recent neuroimaging studies of human audition will be presented at the end of this chapter.

"PARALINGUISTIC AGNOSIAS": AUDITORY AFFECTIVE AGNOSIA AND PHONAGNOSIA

The auditory speech signal conveys not only linguistic meaning but also—through variations in volume, timbre, pitch, and rhythm—information about the emotional state of the speaker (see Chap. 59). Recent clinical evidence suggests that comprehension of affective tone can be selectively impaired. Heilman and coworkers[91] showed that patients with hemispatial neglect from right temporoparietal lesions were impaired in the comprehension of affectively intoned speech (a deficit they called "auditory affective agnosia") but showed normal comprehension of linguistic speech content. Patients with left temporoparietal lesions and fluent aphasia showed normal comprehension of both linguistic and affective (paralinguistic) aspects of speech. Whether this defect is "agnosic" in nature remains to be seen, since auditory sensory/perceptual skills were not assessed. It is possible that auditory affective agnosia is a subtype of auditory sound agnosia (i.e., that it represents a category-specific auditory agnosia), but further studies are necessary before this can be asserted with any certainty.

Studies by Van Lancker and associates[92–94] have revealed another type of paralinguistic deficit after right hemisphere damage. In these studies, patients with unilateral right hemisphere damage showed deficits in discriminating and recognizing familiar voices, while patients with left hemisphere damage were impaired only on a task that required a discrimination between two famous voices. Although the exact nature of this distinction is elusive, it seems to parallel that between episodic (personally experienced) versus semantic (generally known) memory in amnesia research. Evidence from computed tomography (CT) suggested that right parietal damage resulted in voice-recognition impairment, while temporal lobe damage in either hemisphere led to deficits in voice discrimination. The authors refer to this deficit as "phonagnosia," but, like auditory affective agnosia, it remains to be seen whether it is truly agnosic in nature.

SENSORY (RECEPTIVE) AMUSIA

The subject of amusia has been reviewed in detail by Wertheim,[95] Critchley and Henson,[96] and Gates and Bradshaw.[97] *Sensory amusia* refers to an inability to appreciate various characteristics of heard music. Impairment of music perception occurs to some extent in all cases of auditory sound agnosia and in the majority of cases of aphasia[97] and pure word deafness, though its exact prevalence in such populations is unknown. Loss of musical perceptual ability is probably underreported because a specific musical disorder rarely interferes with everyday life.

Wertheim[95] believed that receptive amusia occurs more frequently with left hemisphere damage, while expressive musical disabilities are more apt to be associated with right hemisphere damage. More recent evidence suggests that music perception is a multicomponent process to which both hemispheres contribute in complex ways. Dichotic listening studies show that the right hemisphere plays a more important role than the left in the processing of musical and nonlinguistic sound patterns.[98,99] However, the left hemisphere appears to be important in the processing of sequential (temporally organized) material of any kind, including musical series. The dominant hemisphere may process heard music more analytically or with more attention to specific features of the music, such as temporal order or rhythm.[97,100] According to Gordon,[99] melody recognition becomes more dependent on sequential processing as time and rhythm factors become more important for distinguishing tone patterns (see Ref. 101).

Many clinical studies distinguish between "instant" perceptual processes governing judgments of pitch, harmony, timbre, and intensity (loudness) and more "sequential," time-dependent processes governing melody recognition and judgments of rhythm and duration. Tentative clinical support for this kind of distinction exists in a double dissociation between the perceptual processing of pitch and the processing of temporal sequences,[102] dissociations that also hold true for reading music and for singing. There is further evidence that aspects of musical denotation (the "real-world" events referred to by lyrics) and musical connotation (the formal expressive patterns indicated by pitch, timbre, and intensity) are selectively vulnerable to focal brain lesions.[103,104] Gordon and Bogen[105] reported that during the right hemispheric anesthesia by the Wada procedure, singing was impaired with disrupted pitch production but preserved rhythmic expression. Hallucinations of voices and musical sounds have been reported with electrical stimulation of the lateral and superior surfaces of the first temporal convolutions in either hemisphere with more frequent occurrence on the nondominant side.[106] These complexities make it difficult to define receptive amusia and to localize the deficit to a particular brain region. Further complicating the picture is the fact that pitch, harmony, timbre, intensity, and rhythm may be affected to different degrees and in various combinations in the individual patient.

Peretz and colleagues[103] applied comprehensive nonverbal auditory testing to two patients with bilateral lesions of auditory cortex. In their patients, the perception of speech and environmental sounds was spared, but the perception of tunes, prosody, and voice was impaired. Based on these behavioral dissociations, they argue that music processing is distinct from the processing of speech or environmental sounds. Their data led them to argue for a task- and process-specific approach to the analysis of cases of auditory agnosia. They suggest that nominally "auditory" tasks should be broken down into their functional subcomponents and that more extensive component-based analysis of auditory processing deficits is warranted. For example, they distinguish between processes involved in the recognition of specific voices or musical instruments (which is timbre-dependent), and processes involved in recognition of tunes (which is pitch-dependent). The notion that nominally distinct classes of auditory material (e.g., melodies, prosody, and voice) share common processes may be critically important in developing a functional taxonomy of auditory recognition disorders in general and of amusia in particular.

This suggestion points out certain significant deficiencies in the evaluation of amusic patients. Although theories linking brain function to music perception have long been available,[95,107,108] such theories do not often contain sufficient process specificity to guide the clinical evaluation of amusic patients. Thus, for example, relatively little is known regarding which musical features will be most informative in constructing a neuropsychological model of music perception. Another obstacle to systematic study of acquired amusia is the variability of preillness musical abilities, interests, and experience (see Wertheim[95] for a system of classifying musical ability level). The cerebral organization of musical perception has been suggested to be dependent upon the degree of these preillness characteristics.[107]

NEUROIMAGING THE FUNCTIONAL ANATOMY OF AUDITORY PROCESSING

Recent advances in neuroimaging have contributed significantly to our understanding of auditory processing in both healthy and neurologically impaired individuals. While a thorough review of neuroimaging studies is beyond the scope of this chapter, an overview of the methods can be found in Chaps. 7 to 9, and an excellent review of recent positron emission tomography (PET), functional magnetic resonance imaging (fMRI), and magnetoencephalogram (MEG) studies of human auditory perception has been provided by Engelien and colleagues.[89] In addition, studies of human audition using EEG techniques have been reviewed in detail by Nuwer.[109] Here, we briefly describe some of the recent neuroimaging studies of auditory processing as they relate to our understanding of the cortical auditory disorders presented in this chapter. These studies provide evidence for specific neural networks that underlie the clinical dissociations observed in patients with selective impairments in speech versus nonspeech sounds as well as those with impairments in attention to auditory information. In addition, we discuss neuroanatomical changes that may underlie recovery from auditory agnosia.

Tzourio and associates[110] used PET to investigate the functional anatomy of auditory selective attention in healthy males. Evoked response potentials were simultaneously recorded with PET, with regional cerebral blood flow (rCBF) measurements obtained during tasks of both passive listening and auditory selective attention to tones. Analysis of the results revealed that two different networks were recruited during passive listening and auditory selective attention. When passively listening to tones, bilateral activations were observed in Heschl's gyrus and the planum temporale, with a strong rightward asymmetry, and in the posterior part of the superior temporal gyrus. In addition, right precentral and right anterior cingulate rCBF increases were observed in the frontal lobe. A second "attentional" network was activated during selective attention to tones, which was composed of the anterior cingulum, the right precentral gyrus, and the right prefrontal cortex. These findings are consistent with studies of auditory sound agnosia which emphasize bilateral involvement, with a disproportionate contribution of the right temporal cortex in the processing of nonspeech sounds.[81] In addition, right frontal activations appear to comprise an auditory "attentional network" which may be additionally impaired in patients with cortical deafness whose performance is aided when attention is directed to auditory stimuli.[89]

Other researchers have used PET to identify the distributed neuronal systems activated by words, syllables, and environmental sounds in healthy individuals. Using this method, Giraud and Price[111] found that central regions in the superior temporal sulcus were equally responsive to speech (words and syllables) and environmental sounds, whereas the posterior and anterior regions of the left superior temporal gyrus were more active for speech. This study is consistent with other neuroimaging studies that have implicated the left temporal and frontal cortical regions in the analysis of speech information, and with clinical studies of patients with pure word deafness who generally have bilateral cortical-subcortical lesions involving the superior temporal gyrus and/or sulcus or unilateral damage to superior temporal regions on the left.

While many functional imaging studies have focused on identifying hemispheric and site-specific processing of verbal and nonverbal information, few studies have focused on the basis of this specialization. Zatorre and Belin[112] used PET to examine the response of human auditory cortex to spectral and temporal variations. They found that distinct subareas of auditory cortex respond to spectral and temporal features, with a leftward and rightward bias, respectively. Temporal changes recruited Heschl's gyrus in both hemispheres, with a greater activation on the left. Spectral changes recruited anterior superior temporal gyrus regions bilaterally, with greater activations on the right. The authors conclude that the left hemisphere's predominant role in complex linguistic function may be related to its ability to process the rapidly changing acoustic features involved in decoding speech sounds. As discussed above, impaired temporal processing of auditory information is one of the prevailing theories of pure word deafness.

Alternatively, Zatorre and Belin suggested that the role of the right hemisphere in spectral processing may underlie its importance in many aspects of musical perception and decoding affectively intoned speech which could explain some accounts of amusia, sound agnosia, and affective agnosia. These findings support a unified theory of complex sound processing disorders proposed by Griffiths and colleagues.[25] These authors suggested that the marked overlap observed among the various auditory agnosias may not be related to impairments in sound perception at the level of words, environmental sounds, or music. Rather, they propose that the auditory agnosias may best be described as "spectrotemporal disorders" in which there is a disruption in the interaction among temporal, spectral, and spatial properties of auditory stimuli. Additional neuroimaging and lesion studies designed to isolate spectral and temporal processing in healthy individuals and in patients are needed to clarify this issue.

Finally, studies examining the functional anatomy associated with recovery from auditory disorders are beginning to advance our understanding of cortical reorganization that may correspond to symptom resolution in many patients. Engelien and others[113] used PET to study the recovery from generalized auditory agnosia in a patient with bilateral perisylvian lesions who partially recovered the ability to recognize environmental sounds. During passive listening to sounds, activations were observed in the spared auditory cortex and in the right inferior parietal lobe and regions adjacent to the perisylvian lesion in the left hemisphere. During sound categorization (the "recovered function"), activations were observed in a bilateral distributed neural network comprising prefrontal, middle temporal, and inferior parietal cortices. In normal controls, sound categorization was associated with activation of a left network alone. This study suggests that bilateral activation and the recruitment of perilesional regions may constitute a functional recovery, or an attempt to compensate for, auditory processing deficits in patients recovering from auditory agnosia and auditory spectrum disorders.

SUMMARY

In this chapter, we have briefly reviewed major types of auditory recognition disorders. Although certain identifiable syndromes exist, our review suggests a bewildering array of clinical symptoms and assessment methods. A fundamental problem concerns the lack of a comprehensive theory of auditory cognition. Compared to vision, for example, we know relatively little about the cognitive architecture underlying auditory identification of voices or environmental sounds. This theoretical anarchy has led to terminologic confusion and has slowed development of a cognitive taxonomy of auditory disorders because it has been unsafe to assume that different authors are using such terms in the same way. Another problem is that relatively little agreement exists regarding necessary and sufficient methods of testing in patients with auditory recognition disturbances. Thus, for example, it is not uncommon for claims of a specific defect in one area of auditory processing to be made when, in fact, such specificity is a spurious result of incomplete testing. This problem has been noted by others,[9] and it is obvious that further theoretical development in the area of auditory recognition disturbances will depend on the ability of researchers to devise more comprehensive and theoretically driven assessments of auditory function.[103]

Despite these problems, some progress has been made in identifying potentially important dissociations within auditory recognition disturbances that may eventually reveal the underlying structure of higher auditory processes. Dissociations between verbal (pure word deafness) and nonverbal (auditory sound agnosia) deficits and between perceptual-discriminative and semantic-associative forms of recognition disturbance have been described. Recent findings of impairments in recognizing affective prosody, tunes, and voice are exciting because they raise the further possibility of "category-specificity"[75,114,115] (or process-specificity) in auditory recognition, as has been described for vision (see Chaps. 19 and 20).

It seems clear at this point that further divisions within the concept of auditory agnosia are necessary and that a more comprehensive, process-based approach to evaluating auditory function is required. If this approach is developed further, the important building blocks in the structure of auditory cognition will eventually become apparent through behavioral dissociations. In our view, the clinical approach to a patient suspected of auditory agnosia should consist, at a minimum, of the following steps. First, extensive testing of nonauditory language functions and of general neuropsychological status should be conducted in order to rule out the contribution of aphasia or dementia to the auditory recognition deficit. Second, detailed testing of auditory-perceptual abilities should be conducted, including but not necessarily limited to pure tone audiometry, speech-detection thresholds, temporal auditory acuity (e.g., click fusion thresholds), auditory discrimination,[116] and sound-localization tasks. When possible, brainstem and cortical auditory evoked responses should be evaluated in order to ascertain the "level" at which the patient's deficit occurs. Third, a broad evaluation of auditory capacities should be conducted, including evaluation of the patient's ability to recognize speech, environmental sounds, and music. Performance in other areas not typically assessed in these patients (e.g., voice recognition, singing and related expressive behavior, and evaluation of the patient's ability to recognize linguistic and nonlinguistic prosody) should be assessed. In order to sharpen the hazy distinctions between auditory agnosia (identification and recognition disturbances) and auditory comprehension deficits associated with aphasia, it might also be fruitful to routinely subject aphasic groups to the same kind of comprehensive auditory testing instead of assuming that their impairment in speech comprehension is a straightforward consequence of linguistic impairment.

REFERENCES

1. Kanshepolsky J, Kelley J, Waggener J: A cortical auditory disorder. *Neurology* 23:699–705, 1973.
2. Miceli G: The processing of speech sounds in a patient with cortical auditory disorder. *Neuropsychologia* 20: 5–20, 1982.
3. Oppenheimer DR, Newcombe F: Clinical and anatomic findings in a case of auditory agnosia. *Arch Neurol* 35:712–719, 1978.
4. Rosati G, DeBastiani P, Paolino E, et al: Clinical and audiological findings in a case of auditory agnosia. *J Neurol* 227:21–27, 1982.
5. Goldstein MN, Brown M, Holander J: Auditory agnosia and word deafness: Analysis of a case with three-year follow up. *Brain Lang* 2:324–332, 1975.
6. Ulrich G: Interhemispheric functional relationships in auditory agnosia: An analysis of the preconditions and a conceptual model. *Brain Lang* 5:286–300, 1978.
7. Buchman AS, Garron DC, Trost-Cardamone JE, et al: Word deafness: One hundred years later. *J Neurol Neurosurg Psychiatry* 49:489–499, 1986.
8. Mendez MF, Geehan GR: Cortical auditory disorders: Clinical and psychoacoustic features. *J Neurol Neurosurg Psychiat* 51:1–9, 1988.
9. Vignolo LA: Auditory agnosia: A review and report of recent evidence. In Benton AL (ed): *Contributions to Clinical Neuropsychology*. Chicago: Aldine, 1969.
10. Lhermitte F, Chain F, Escourolle R, et al: Etudo des troubles per-ceptifs auditifs dans les lesion temporales bilaterales. *Rev Neurol* 128:329–351, 1971.
11. Teuber H-L: Alteration of perception and memory in man, in Weiskrantz L (ed): *Analysis of Behavior Change*. New York: Harper & Row, 1968.
12. Jerger J, Weikers N, Sharbrough F, Jerger S: Bilaeral lesions of the temporal lobe: A case study. *Acoto-Laryngologica,* 258(suppl):1–51, 1969.
13. Jerger J, Lovering L, Wertz M: Auditory disorder following bilateral temporal lobe insult: Report of a case. *J Speech Hearing Dis* 37:523–535, 1972.
14. Michel J, Peronnet F, Schott B: A case of cortical deafness: Clinical and electrophysiological data. *Brain Lang* 10:367–377, 1980.
15. Massopoust LC, Wolin LR: Changes in auditory frequency discimination thresholds after temporal cortex ablation. *Exp Neurol* 19:245–251, 1967.

16. Dewson JH, Pribram KH, Lynch JC: Effects of ablation of temporal cortex upon speech sound discrimination in the monkey. *Exp Neurol* 24:279–291, 1969.
17. Celesia GG: Organization of auditory cortical areas in man. *Brain* 99:403–414, 1976.
18. Mahoudeau D, Lemoyne J, Dubrisay J, Caraes J: Sur un cas dagnosie auditive. *Rev Neurol* 95:57, 1956.
19. Wohlfart G, Lindgren A, Jernelius B: Clinical picture and morbid anatomy in a case of "pure word deafness." *J Nerv Ment Dis* 116:818–827, 1952.
20. Engelein A, Huber W, Silbersweig D, et al: The neural correlates of 'deaf-hearing' in man: Conscious sensory awareness enabled by attentional modulation. *Brain* 123:532–545, 2000.
21. Garde MM, Cowey A: "Deaf hearing": Unacknowledged detection of auditory stimuli in a patient with cerebral deafness. *Cortex* 36:71–80, 2000.
22. Wakabayashi Y, Nakano T, Isono M, Hori S: Cortical deafness due to bilateral temporal subcortical hemorrhages associated with moyamoya disease: Report of a case. *No Shinkei Geka* 27:915–919, 1999.
23. Leicester J: Central deafness and subcortical motor aphasia. *Brain Lang* 10:224–242, 1980.
24. Earnest MP, Monroe PA, Yarnell PA: Cortical deafness: Demonstration of the pathologic anatomy by CT scan. *Neurology* 27:1172–1175, 1977.
25. Griffiths TD, Rees A, Green GGR: Disorders of human complex sound processing. *Neurocase* 5:365–378, 1999.
26. Mendez MF, Geehan GR: Cortical auditory disorders: Clinical and psychoacoustic features. *J Neurol Neurosurg Psychiatry* 51:1–9, 1988.
27. Tanaka Y, Kamo T, Yoshida M, Yamadori A: "So-called" cortical deafness. Clinical, neurophysiological, and radiological observations. *Brain* 114:2385–2401, 1991.
28. Penhune VB, Zatorre RJ, MacDonald JD, Evans AC: Interhemispheric anatomical differences in human primary auditory cortex: Probabilistic mapping and volume measurement from magnetic resonance scans. *Cereb Cortex* 6:661–672, 1966.
29. Kazui S, Naritomi H, Sawada T, Inque N: Subcortical auditory agnosia. *Brain Lang* 38:476–487, 1990.
30. Motomura N, Yamadori A, Mori E, Tamaru F: Auditory agnosia: Analysis of a case with bilateral subcortical lesions. *Brain* 109:379–391, 1986.
31. Hasegawa M, Bando M, Iwata M, et al: A case of auditory agnosia with the lesion of bilateral auditory radiation. *Rinsho Shinkeigaku* 29:180–185, 1989.
32. Johkura K, Matsumoto S, Hasegawa O, Kuroiwa Y: Defective auditory recognition after small hemorrhage in the inferior colliculi. *J Neurol Sci* 161:91–96, 1988.
33. Kussmaul A: Disturbances of speech, in von Ziemssien H (ed): *Cyclopedia of the Practice of Medicine*. New York: William Wood, 1877.
34. Lichteim L: On aphasia. *Brain* 7:433–484, 1885.
35. Kanter SL, Day AL, Heilman KM, Gonzalez-Rothi LJ: Pure word deafness: A possible explanation of transient-deterioration after extracranial-intracranial bypass grafting. *Neurosurgery* 18:186–189, 1986.
36. Liepmann H, Storch E: Der mikroskopische Gehirnbefund bei dem Fall Gorstelle. *Monatsschr Psychiatr Neurol* 11:115–120, 1902.
37. Schuster P, Taterka H: Beitrag zur Anatomie und Klinik der reinen Worttaubbeit. *Z Neurol Psychiatr* 105:494, 1926.
38. Geschwind N: Disconnexion syndromes in animals and man. *Brain* 88:237–294, 585–644, 1965.
39. Arias M, Requena I, Ventura M, et al: A case of deafmutism as an expression of pure word deafness: Neuroimaging and electrophysiological data. *Eur J Neurol* 2:583–585, 1995.
40. Karibe H, Yonemori T, Matsuno F, et al: A case of tentorial meningioma presented with pure word deafness. *No To Shinkei* 52:997–1001, 2000.
41. Kaga M: Language disorders in Landau-Kleffner syndrome. *J Child Neurol* 14:118–122, 1999.
42. Klein SK, Kurtzberg D, Brattson A, et al: Electrophysiologic manifestations of impaired temporal lobe auditory processing in verbal auditory agnosia. *Brain Lang* 51:383–405, 1995.
43. Pearce PS, Darwish H: Correlation between EEG and auditory perceptual measures in auditory agnosia. *Brain Lang* 22:41–48, 1984.
44. Baynes K, Kegl JA, Brentari D, et al: Chronic auditory agnosia following Landau-Kleffner syndrome: A 23 year outcome study. *Brain Lang* 63:381–425, 1988.
45. Albert ML, Bear D: Time to understand: A case study of word deafness with reference to the role of time in auditory comprehension. *Brain* 97:373–384, 1974.
46. Klein R, Harper J: The problem of agnosia in the light of a case of pure word deafness. *J Mental Sci* 102:112–120, 1956.
47. Gazzaniga M, Glass AV, Sarno MT: Pure word deafness and hemispheric dynamics: A case history. *Cortex* 9:136–143, 1973.
48. Ziegler DK: Word deafness and Wernicke's aphasia: Report of cases and discussion of the syndrome. *Arch Neurol Psychiatry* 67:323–331, 1942.
49. Otsuki M, Soma Y, Sato M, et al: Slowly progressive pure word deafness. *Eur Neurol* 39:135–140, 1988.

50. Yaqub BA, Gascon GG, Al-Nosha M, Whitaker H: Pure word deafness (acquired verbal auditory agnosia) in an Arabic speaking patient. *Brain* 111:457–466, 1988.
51. Anegawa T, Hara K, Yamamoto K, Matsuda M: Unilateral auditory hallucinations due to left temporal lobe ischemia: A case report. *Rinsho Shinkeigaku* 35:1137–1141, 1995.
52. Shoumaker RD, Ajax ET, Schenkenberg T: Pure word deafness (auditory verbal agnosia). *Dis Nerv Sys* 38: 293–299, 1977.
53. Mendez MF, Rosenberg S: Word deafness mistaken for Alzheimer's disease: Differential characteristics. *J Amer Geriat Soc* 39:209–211, 1991.
54. Reinhold M: A case of auditory agnosia. *Brain* 73:203–223, 1950.
55. Hemphill RC, Stengel E: A study of pure word deafness. *J Neurol Psychiatry* 3:251–262, 1940.
56. Wee J, Menard MR: "Pure word deafness": Implications for assessment and management in communication disorder—a report of two cases. *Arch Phys Med Rehabil* 80:1106–1109, 1999.
57. Caplan LR: Variability of perceptual function: The sensory cortex as a categorizer and deducer. *Brain Lang* 6:1–13, 1978.
58. Auerbach SH, Allard T, Naeser M, et al: Pure word deafness: Analysis of a case with bilateral lesions and a defect at the prephonemic level. *Brain* 105:271–300, 1982.
59. Chocholle R, Chedru F, Bolte MC, et al: Etude psychoacoustique d'un cas de surdite corticale. *Neuropsychologia* 13:163–172, 1975.
60. Denes G, Semenza C: Auditory modality-specific anomia: Evidence from a case of pure word deafness. *Cortex* 11:401–411, 1975.
61. Saffran EB, Marin OSM, Yeni-Komshian GH: An analysis of speech perception in word deafness. *Brain Lang* 3:255–256, 1976.
62. Wang E, Peach RK, Xu Y, et al: Reception of dynamic acoustic patterns by an individual with unilateral verbal auditory agnosia. *Brain Lang* 73:442–455, 2000.
63. Croisile B, Laurent B, Michel D, et al: Different clinical types of degenerative aphasia. *Rev Neurol* 147:192–199, 1991.
64. Nakakoshi S, Kashino M, Mizobuchi A, et al: Disorder in sequential speech perception: A case study on pure word deafness. *Brain Lang* 76:119–129, 2001.
65. Naeser M: The relationship between phoneme discrimination, phoneme/picture perception, and language comprehension in aphasia. Presented at the Twelfth Annual Meeting of the Academy of Aphasia, Warrenton, Virginia, October 1974.
66. Stockard JJ, Rossiter VS: Clinical and pathologic correlates of brainstem auditory response abnormalities. *Neurology* 27:316–325, 1977.
67. Makino M, Takanashi Y, Iwamoto K, et al: Auditory evoked magnetic fields in patients of pure word deafness. *No To Shinkei* 50:51–55, 1998.
68. Coslett HB, Brashear HR, Heilman KM: Pure word deafness after bilateral primary auditory cortex infarcts. *Neurology* 34:347–352, 1984.
69. Polster MR, Rose SB: Disorders of auditory processing: Evidence for modularity in audition. *Cortex* 34:47–65, 1998.
70. Corballis MC: Neuropsychology of perceptual functions, in Zaidel E (ed), *Neuropsychology*. New York: Academic Press, 1994, pp 83–104.
71. Franklin S, Turner J, Ralph M, Morris J, Bailey PL: A distinctive case of word-meaning deafness. *Cognit Neuropsychol* 13:1139–1162, 1996.
72. Tyler LK, Moss HE: Imageability and category specificity. *Cognit Neuropsychol* 14:293–318, 1977.
73. Bauer RM: Agnosia, in Heilman KM, Valenstein E (eds): *Clinical Neuropsychology,* 3d ed. New York: Oxford University Press, 1993, pp 215–278.
74. Farah MJ: *Visual Agnosia: Disorders of Object Vision and What They Tell Us about Normal Vision,* 2d ed. Cambridge, MA: MIT Press/Bradford, 2003.
75. Farah MJ, Meyer M, McMullen PA: The living/nonliving dissociation is not an artifact. *Cognit Neuropsychol* 13:137–154, 1996.
76. Buchtel HA, Stewart JD: Auditory agnosia: Apperceptive or associative disorder? *Brain Lang* 37:12–25, 1989.
77. Goldstein MN: Auditory agnosia for speech ("pure word deafness"): A historical review with current implications. *Brain Lang* 1:195–204, 1974.
78. Kliest K: Gehirnpathologische und Lokalisatorische Ergebnisse uber Horstorungen, Geruschtaubheiten und Amusien. *Monatsschr Psychiatr Neurol* 68:853–860, 1928.
79. Albert ML, Sparks R, von Stockert T, Sax D: A case study of auditory agnosia: Linguistic and nonlinguistic processing. *Cortex* 8:427–433, 1972.
80. Clarke S, Bellmann A, Meuli RA, Assal, et al: Auditory agnosia and auditory spatial deficits following left hemispheric lesions: Evidence for distinct processing pathways. *Neuropsychologia* 38:797–807, 2000.
81. Fujii T, Fukatsu R, Watabe S, et al: Auditory sound agnosia without aphasia following a right temporal lobe lesion. *Cortex* 26:263–268, 1990.
82. Nielsen JM, Sult CW Jr: Agnosia and the body scheme. *Bull LA Neurol Soc* 4:69–81, 1939.

83. Spreen O, Benton AL, Fincham R: Auditory agnosia without aphasia. *Arch Neurol* 13:84–92, 1965.
84. Wortis SB, Pfeffer AZ: Unilateral auditory-spatial agnosia. *J Nerv Ment Dis* 108:181–186, 1948.
85. Habib M, Daquin G, Milandre L, et al: Mutism and auditory agnosia due to bilateral insular damage—role of the insula in human communication. *Neuropsychologia* 33:327–339, 1995.
86. Lambert J, Eustache F, Lechevalier B, et al: Auditory agnosia with relative sparing of speech perception. *Cortex* 25:71–82, 1989.
87. Taniwaki T, Tagawa K, Sato F, Iino K: Auditory agnosia restricted to environmental sounds following cortical deafness and generalized auditory agnosia. *Clin Neurol Neurosurg* 102:156–162, 2000.
88. Alain C, Arnott, SR, Hevenor S, et al: "What" and "where" in the human auditory system. *Proc Natl Acad Sci U S A* 98:12301–12306, 2001.
89. Engelien A, Stern E, Silbersweig DA: Functional neuroimaging of human central auditory processing in normal subjects and patients with neurological and neuropsychiatric disorders. *J Clin Exp Neuropsychol* 23:94–120, 2001.
90. Binder JR: Neuroanatomy of language processing studied with functional MRI. *Clin Neurosci* 4:87–94, 1997.
91. Heilman KM, Scholes R, Watson RT: Auditory affective agnosia. Disturbed comprehension of affective speech. *J Neurol Neurosurg Psychiatry* 38:69–72, 1975.
92. Van Lancker DR, Kreiman J: Unfamiliar voice discrimination and familiar voice recognition are independent and unordered abilities. *Neuropsychologia* 25:829–834, 1988.
93. Van Lancker DR, Kreiman J, Cummings J: Voice perception deficits: Neuroanatomical correlates of phonagnosia. *J Clin Exp Neuropsychol* 11:665–674, 1989.
94. Van Lancker DR, Cummings JL, Kreiman J, Dobkin BH: Phonagnosia: A dissociation between familiar and unfamiliar voices. *Cortex* 24:195–209, 1988.
95. Wertheim N: The amusias, in Vinken PJ, Bruyn GW (eds): *Handbook of Clinical Neurology*. Amsterdam: North-Holland, 1969, vol 4.
96. Critchley MM, Henson RA: *Music and the Brain: Studies in the Neurology of Music*. Springfield, IL: Charles C Thomas, 1977.
97. Gates A, Bradshaw JL: The role of the cerebral hemispheres in music. *Brain Lang* 4:403–431, 1977.
98. Blumstein S, Cooper W: Hemispheric processing of intonation contours. *Cortex* 10:146–158, 1974.
99. Gordon HW: Auditory specialization of the right and left hemispheres, in Kinsbourne M, Smith WL (eds): *Hemispheric Disconnection and Cerebral Function*. Springfield, IL: Charles C Thomas, 1974.
100. Krashen SD: Mental abilities underlying linguistic and nonlinguistic functions. *Linguistics* 115:39–55, 1973.
101. Mavlov L: Amusia due to rhythm agnosia in a musician with left hemisphere damage: A nonauditory supramodal defect. *Cortex* 16:331–338, 1980.
102. Peretz I: Processing of local and global musical information by unilateral brain-damaged patients. *Brain* 113:1185–1205, 1990.
103. Peretz I, Kolinsky R, Tramo M, et al: Functional dissociations following bilateral lesions of auditory cortex. *Brain* 117:1283–1301, 1994.
104. Gardner H, Silverman H, Denes G, et al: Sensitivity to musical denotation and connotation in organic patients. *Cortex* 13:242–256, 1977.
105. Gordon HW, Bogen JE: Hemispheric lateralization of singing after intracarotid sodium amylobarbitone. *J Neurol Neuorsurg Psychiatry* 37:727–738, 1974.
106. Penfield W, Perot P: The brain's record of auditory and visual experience. *Brain* 86:595–696, 1963.
107. Bever TG, Chiarello RJ: Cerebral dominance in musicians and nonmusicians. *Science* 185:137–139, 1974.
108. Hecaen H: Clinical symptomotology in right and left hemispheric lesions, in Mountcastle VB (ed): *Interhemispheric Relations and Cerebral Dominance*. Baltimore: Johns Hopkins University Press, 1962.
109. Nuwer MR: Fundamentals of evoked potentials and common clinical applications today. *EEG Clin Neurophysiol* 106:142–148, 1998.
110. Tzourio N, Massioui FE, Crivello F, et al: Functional anatomy of human auditory attention studied with PET. *Neuroimage* 5:63–77, 1997.
111. Giraud AL, Price CJ: The constraints functional neuroimaging places on classical models of auditory word processing. *J Cogn Neurosci* 13:754–765, 2001.
112. Zattore RJ, Belin P: Spectral and temporal processing in human auditory cortex. *Cereb Cortex* 11:946–953, 2001.
113. Engelien A, Silbersweig D, Stern E, et al: The functional anatomy of recovery from auditory agnosia. A PET study of sound categorization in a neurological patient and normal controls. *Brain* 118:1395–1409, 1995.
114. Warrington EK, Shallice T: Category-specific semantic impairments. *Brain* 107:829–854, 1984.
115. Damasio AR: Category-related recognition defects as a clue to the neural substrates of knowledge. *Trends Neurosci* 13:95–98, 1990.
116. Chedru F, Bastard V, Efron R: Auditory micropattern discrimination in brain damaged subjects. *Neuropsychologia* 16:141–149, 1978.

Chapter 22

TACTILE AGNOSIA AND DISORDERS OF TACTILE PERCEPTION

Richard J. Caselli

As with the recognition of objects through sight or sound (see Chaps. 18 and 21), tactile object recognition requires the integrity of transducers, primary sensory processes, and higher-order perceptual processes in association cortex. Damage at any of these levels will impair object recognition in different ways. For tactile object recognition, transduction most commonly occurs on the glabrous skin of the digits and palms, which has been called the "fovea" of the human somatosensory system.[1] This skin contains four major types of low-threshold mechanoreceptors, each with its own submodal specificity that contributes in some measure to somesthetic perception. For most types of object recognition, spatial acuity, or form perception, would seem to be of special importance. The slowly adapting type I (SAI) receptor-afferent unit is the critical peripheral limb of the spatial system concerned with somesthetic processing of form.[1–5] SAI responses are isomorphic at the peripheral afferent fiber level[3–5] and produce isomorphic responses in the cortical neurons of area 3b.[6] The sensations evoked by stimulation of such single receptor units alone, however, are not "natural" sensations, and even the most basic somesthetic sensations (like touch) probably result from highly specific combinations of various receptor inputs.[7] Active exploration confers no advantage over passive touch in spatial resolution of SAI units,[8] despite known tactual exploration strategies.[9,10] In short, the spatial properties of tactual stimuli are transduced by the SAI system, which is necessary and may be sufficient (for at least some natural objects) for the high-fidelity reproduction of form in area 3b, primary somatosensory cortex. Additional processing in primary and somatosensory association cortices will be required, however, for the somesthetic percept to be incorporated into our ongoing behavior.

SOMATOSENSORY CORTICES

Primary Somatosensory Cortex

All motor and koniocortical sensory systems are composed of multiple cortical areas, each defined by its own somatotopic representations, cytoarchitecture, and thalamocortical/corticocortical connectivity patterns. Within the somatosensory system, the "first somatosensory area" or SI, located on the postcentral gyrus, is considered the primary sensory area. SI receives a dense thalamocortical projection from the ventrobasal complex, which contains the somatosensory relay nuclei. Reciprocal corticocortical connections of SI include primary motor cortex (Brodmann area 4) and somatosensory association cortices (see below). Broadly defined, SI has included Brodmann areas 3a, 3b, 1, and 2. SI was originally defined as a somatotopically unitary area in laboratory animals[11,12] and subsequently in humans.[13] More recent studies, however, have shown that there are approximate mirror-image somatotopic representations in Brodmann areas 3b and 1, as well as additional somatotopies in Brodmann areas 2 and 3a.[14–16] Though more relative than absolute, there are functional differences between these areas: areas 3b and 1 respond to cutaneous stimuli and areas 3a and 2 respond to muscle, visceral, and joint afferent stimulation.[16] Area 3b contains the greatest number of neurons with isomorphic responses to peripheral tactual stimulation of SAI afferents and hence the greatest spatial fidelity.[6] Area 3b also contains some neurons that respond in a nonisomorphic fashion, but these occur in increasing numbers in area 1 (and beyond), suggesting progressively increasing degrees of abstraction as the stimulus moves away from area 3b.[6] With these differences in mind, comparative neuroanatomic studies have led to the more modern interpretation that area 3b is the one and only SI which is homologous in humans, monkeys, and lower mammals.[16]

Somatosensory Association Cortices

SI is bounded ventrolaterally by SII (parietal operculum), which has been mapped in many animal species[12,16,17] and in humans.[13,18–20] In cats[21–23] and monkeys,[24,25] two other somatosensory areas contiguous to SII have been described and labeled SIII (inferior parietal cortex, Brodmann area 7 in monkeys) and SIV (posterior insula and retroinsular cortex). In humans, area 7 is the posterior portion of the superior parietal lobule. Studies of learned movement in humans have shown that cortices bounding the intraparietal sulcus, including a portion of area 7, work in conjunction with lateral premotor regions as part of a sensorimotor network that is functionally rather than somatotopically mapped.[26] A recent study of the insula in patients with temporal lobe epilepsy demonstrated contralateral somesthetic symptoms caused by an insular epileptic focus.[27] Each region appears to contain its own representation of the body, and the somatotopic schema differ between regions.

SI is bounded dorsomedially by another SAC originally defined by Penfield during intraoperative stimulation studies in humans; he called it the supplementary sensory area (SSA).[13] Anatomic studies in monkeys suggest that it encompasses mesial Brodmann area 5 and possibly the anterior portion of mesial area 7.[28–30] Supplementary motor area (SMA) stimulation[13,31–33] and ablation[34] experiments during brain surgery in humans have sometimes elicited somesthetic sensations, suggesting that this motor association cortex may also be a dorsomedial SAC.

Ventrolateral and dorsomedial SACs are topographically disparate (Fig. 22-1) but share a prokoniocortical cytoarchitecture, bridge a limbic or paralimbic cortex with a koniocortical sensory cortex, and derive phylogenetically from the parinsular/paralimbic growth ring.[35] Ventrolateral SAC, however, derives phylogenetically from olfactocentric paleocortex, while dorsomedial SAC derives from hippocampocentric archicortex.[35] Anatomically, ventrolateral SAC appears more closely related than SSA to SI in terms of corticocortical reciprocity and thalamocortical connectivity,[36] whereas SSA is more closely related than ventrolateral SAC to the supplementary motor area (SMA)[29] and posterior parietal cortices.[37] Physiologic studies have also suggested a strong functional distinction between ventrolateral and dorsomedial SAC. Ablation studies have shown that SII activity can depend entirely upon SI and not thalamic input, providing evidence for serial cortical processing between SI and SII.[38] Receptive field properties of neurons in SII are similar in size and sensitivity to

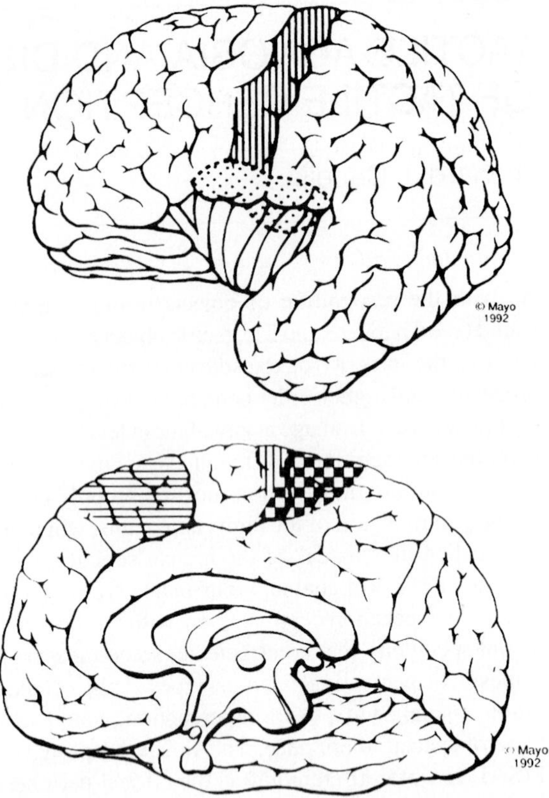

Figure 22-1
Ventrolateral and dorsomedial somatosensory association cortices depicted in a human brain. (Reproduced with permission from Caselli.[65]) Homologies between humans and monkeys are inferred (see text). Top figure: small dots demarcate SII and posterior insula. Bottom figure: checkerboard demarcates SSA, and horizontal lines demarcate SMA. Vertical lines in both figures demarcate SI.

neurons in SI.[12] Neurons in SSA, however, have much larger receptive fields, and some SSA neurons are sensitive to pain.[29] Therefore, ventrolateral and dorsomedial SACs have different phylogenetic derivations, anatomic connections, and physiologic properties (Table 22-1).

NORMAL SOMATOSENSORY FUNCTION

The definition of normal somatosensory function, and conversely abnormal, depends as much upon the individual's neurologic status as on the task used to probe the status of a particular function. Psychophysics has

Table 22-1
Ventrolateral and dorsomedial somatosensory association cortices

	Ventrolateral somatosensory association cortex	*Dorsomedial somatosensory association cortex*	
	SII	*SSA*	*SMA*
Phylogenetic derivation	Insulolimbic paleocortical	Mediolimbic archicortical	Mediolimbic archicortical
Cytoarchitecture	Prokoniocortex (good lamina iv)	Prokoniocortex (poor lamina iv)	Prokoniocortex
Thalamic projections	VPL, VPM, LP	VL, LP, DM, intralaminar, pulvinar	VL, LP, DM, intralaminar, VA
Corticocortical/reciprocal			
Motor connections		Premotor and SMA (area 6), area 4	Area 4, premotor, prefrontal (area 9), area 44
Sensory connections	SI, contralateral SII, area 7b (monkey SIII), retroinsular (monkey SIV)	Area 5	
Corticocortical/afferent			
Motor connections		Areas 1 and 2	Area 1
Sensory connections			SII, insula, superior temporal gyrus
Corticocortical/efferent			
Motor connections	Area 4		
Sensory connections			
Somatotopic interface with SI	Face	Hindlimb	None (hindlimb with MI)
Sensory receptive fields	Same size as SI; touch, tap	Larger than SI and SII; touch, pain	
Human stimulation studies	Contralateral and bilateral tingling	Contra- and bilateral tingling, total body aura	Mainly movement-related; some "sensory phenomena"
Human lesion studies	Transient numbness acutely; tactile agnosia	Transient relief of thalamic pain; SSA and SMA combined ablation produces dorsomedial syndrome (see text)	Acute akinesis; bilateral grasp reflex; slowed rapid alternating movement

Abbreviations: DM = dorsal medial nucleus; LP = lateral posterior nucleus; MI = first motor area; SI = first somatosensory area; SII = second somatosensory area; SIII = third somatosensory area; SIV = fourth somatosensory area; SMA = supplementary motor area; VA = ventral anterior nucleus; VL = ventral lateral nucleus; VPL = ventral posterior lateral nucleus; VPM = ventral posterior medial nucleus.

probed the limits of somesthetic perception in neurologically healthy subjects and has demonstrated how slight a stimulus or change in stimulus is required for touch,[39,40] two-point discrimination (gap detection),[41] vibratory detection,[42–44] shape recognition,[8,41,43] texture discrimination (which includes both roughness and hardness),[5,45–48] and how one property (such as size) influences the perception of another property (such as shape).[49,50] Behavioral syndromes discussed here, such as tactile agnosia, have not been defined or studied using psychophysical techniques, although such would represent a logical extension of somesthetic research. Rather, clinical somatosensory disorders have been defined, by and large, with cruder "bedside" techniques that vary somewhat between examiners and are rarely highly standardized.[51–53] Nonetheless these techniques have been used over many years with great practical success.[51]

From a clinical standpoint, somatosensory testing can be classified as outlined below.

Basic Somesthetic Functions

As noted above, microneurographic stimulations of single afferent units result in pure sensations that are not identical to naturally experienced sensations such as light touch.[7] With that caveat in mind, those "basic" somesthetic functions that are tested clinically include light touch (with, for instance, a wisp of cotton or von Frey hairs), vibratory sensation (generally over a bony prominence such as a joint), proprioception (the examiner simply moves the patient's joint a small distance and asks him or her to guess the direction of movement), superficial pain (pinprick), temperature (a cold or warm object applied to the skin), and two-point discrimination (generally with a lower limit of 3 mm, which is approximately three times greater than the psychophysical threshold for gap detection).

Intermediate Somesthetic Functions

These include weight discrimination (e.g., differentially weighted objects of identical size, shape, and exterior substance), texture discrimination (e.g., relative grades of sandpaper from very fine to very coarse), dimension perception (e.g., length, width, and height of four rectangular wooden blocks), generic shape recognition (e.g., square, circle, triangle, rectangle, sphere), substance recognition (e.g., plastic, metal, wood, glass, styrofoam, rubber, paper, wax), and double-simultaneous stimulation (right and left sides of the patient).

Complex Somesthetic Functions

Tactile object recognition is tested with familiar objects.[53,54] Familiar objects handled unimanually by a blindfolded patient are normally recognized quickly (within 5 s in over 90 percent[54]), accurately (87 to 99 percent[53,54]), and symmetrically between the two hands.[54] Braille and other types of letter/digit recognition techniques (e.g., Optacon[55]) serve as aids to the visually impaired and can sometimes be used to assess somesthetic perception. Graphesthesia,[51] the ability to recognize familiar patterns such as letters or digits when traced on the skin, can also be used, but is less reliable than object recognition.

Clinical Laboratory Assessment Nerve conduction studies and needle electromyography (EMG) are used to evaluate peripheral nerve function, and somatosensory evoked potentials serve to evaluate central somatosensory conduction pathways in patients with somatosensory abnormalities. Computer assisted sensory examinations (CASE) are used occasionally to determine vibratory and temperature thresholds.[56]

CLINICAL SOMATOSENSORY DISORDERS RESULTING FROM CORTICAL LESIONS

Parietal lobe damage is capable of producing a wealth of possible somesthetic problems. Critchley[57] summarized these based on his own considerable experience and an extensive literature, including the seminal contributions of Head and Holmes[58]: (1) focal sensory epilepsy, (2) tactile perseveration and hallucinations of touch (e.g., feeling two points when only one is applied; e.g, feeling a nonexistent object in an anesthetic hand), (3) cortical sensory loss: impaired recognition of objects, texture, two-point discrimination, stimulus localization, barognosis, vibratory sensation, position sense, graphesthesia, (4) hemianesthesia, (5) tactile inattention (to double simultaneous stimulation), (6) altered sensory adaptation time (the time it takes for a continued monotonous somesthetic stimulus, such as clothing, to cease engaging the perceiver's attention), (7) "anestho-agnosia" (bilateral sensory alterations following a unilateral lesion), (8) asymboly for pain (failure to be bothered by an otherwise correctly perceived painful stimulus), and (9) "pseudothalamic syndrome" (hemianesthesia with spontaneous pain and painful perception of normally nonpainful stimuli in the anesthetic areas, akin to the Roussy-Dejerine thalamic pain syndrome, but occurring on a parietal basis).

Following parietal lobe infarction in patients with minimal hemiparesis, a typical, routine neurologic examination is more likely to reveal a more modest number of somesthetic syndromes: (1) faciobrachiocrural elementary sensory loss (or pseudothalamic sensory syndrome) which essentially means impairment of all modalities tested in the face and upper limb contralateral to the side of the stroke; (2) isolated discriminative sensory loss (or cortical sensory syndrome) which means impaired stereognosis, graphesthesia, and position sense in some combination of face-hand; and (3) complete sensory loss with partial distribution (or atypical sensory syndrome) which is the same as the first type but topographically incomplete.[59]

The following classification of cortical somatosensory disorders is based upon modern anatomic concepts, and attempts at once to be both simplified and comprehensive.

The SI Syndrome: Astereognosis

An early description of stereognosis as a complex sensory function that perceived images rather than the simple sensory functions of pain, touch, and temperature was that of Verger in 1897.[60] According to an early classification (Delay), astereognosis is a complex somatosensory disorder that has three subsidiary parts: amorphognosia, the inability to recognize size and shape; ahylognosia, the inability to decipher density, weight, thermal conductivity, and roughness; and tactile asymbolia, which is the same as tactile agnosia, the inability to to identify an object in the absense of amorphognosis and ahylognosis.[61] Because the existence of tactile agnosia was disputed and in 1965 disavowed,[62] until recently there was little reason to specify the precise boundaries of astereognosis. However, with the reemergence of tactile agnosia as a plausible behavioral entity,[53,63–65] the term *astereognosis* needs to be distinguished from tactile agnosia. Astereognosis should be restricted to mean impaired tactual spatial perception due to severe basic somatosensory perceptual impairment. In contrast, tactile agnosia is a selective disturbance of tactile object recognition (TOR) in the absence of more basic somatosensory perceptual impairment.[53]

In this light, astereognosis reflects cortical deafferentation arising from damage to any level of the somatosensory system including the peripheral nerves (particularly severe large-fiber peripheral neuropathies such as Guillain-Barré syndrome), spinal cord (especially posterior column pathways), brainstem (interruption of the medial lemniscus), and thalamus (VPL nucleus), or SI destruction.[53,62,66,67] Patients with astereognosis typically have severe impairment of most of the basic and intermediate sensory modalities listed above; if it results from a right hemispheric lesion, they may also have extinction on the left to double simultaneous stimulation due to concurrent hemineglect (see below). TOR impairment is generally more severe when caused by a cortical lesion than by a peripheral nerve, spinal cord, or thalamic lesion.

Though not considered sensory disorders, there is increasing evidence that focal dystonias may result from physiologic alterations in SI neurons. Chronic repetitive hand movements in monkeys lead to enlarged receptive fields of SI neurons,[68] and there is some evidence in patients as well of abnormal finger representations.[69] Functional imaging studies of patients with writer's cramp show activation of SI cortex,[70] and psychophysical studies of such patients have demonstrated reduced gap detection and single-touch localization.[71]

The Ventrolateral Somatosensory Association Cortex Syndrome: Tactile Agnosia

Behavioral Considerations

Definition The selective impairment of TOR in the absence of more basic somesthetic impairment is called tactile agnosia. The inability to recognize a previously known object must be distinguished from the inability to simply name the object,[72] including the modality-specific naming disorder tactile aphasia (analogous to optic aphasia, see Chaps. 10 and 39), and from "tactile inexperience," in which the target object might not be familiar to the subject.[57] Psychophysical analyses are few in tactile agnosia research to date, and the statement that impaired TOR occurs in the *absence* of more basic somesthetic impairment should be modified currently to state that impaired TOR occurs in the absence of *clinically demonstrable* or *clinically significant* basic somesthetic impairment.

Properties Tactile agnosia is a unilateral disorder (it affects only the left or only the right hand) that results from a unilateral lesion.[53,63–65] It is not a source of great disability for the affected patients. (One such patient complained that she had to take an object out of her pocket and look at it to be certain it was her key.) Several types of misidentifications commonly occur in tactile agnosia which are analogous to the error types, found in visual agnosia (see Chap. 18). First, an object may be described in spatially approximate terms: "pencil-like with a string" for an artist's paintbrush. Second, an object may be confused with a spatially similar object: "safety pin" for a paper clip. In this example, the patient correctly identifed the supraordinate spatial category (small wiry pin-like items) but misjudged the specific subordinate member. Third, an object may be identified in a more generic way: "a tool" for a wrench. In this example, the supraordinate spatial/functional category was correctly identified, but the patient failed to access taxonomically deeper subordinate members of that category. Tactile agnosics can draw the object they are feeling (Fig. 22-2), providing further demonstration of their preserved ability to decipher the salient somesthetic characteristics of the object they fail to recognize.[73] In tactile agnosia, unlike prosopagnosia, the ability to associate tactually defined objects and their parts with episodic memory is preserved. This is based upon the finding that in tactile agnosia, personal items are recognized with greater success than impersonal items.[63]

Tactual exploration strategies are normal in tactile agnosics[63] and in fact seem unimportant for TOR. Hemiparetic patients without damage to somatosensory-related structures have normal TOR despite an impaired (and in hemiplegic cases, nonexistent) search strategy.[53,65,74]

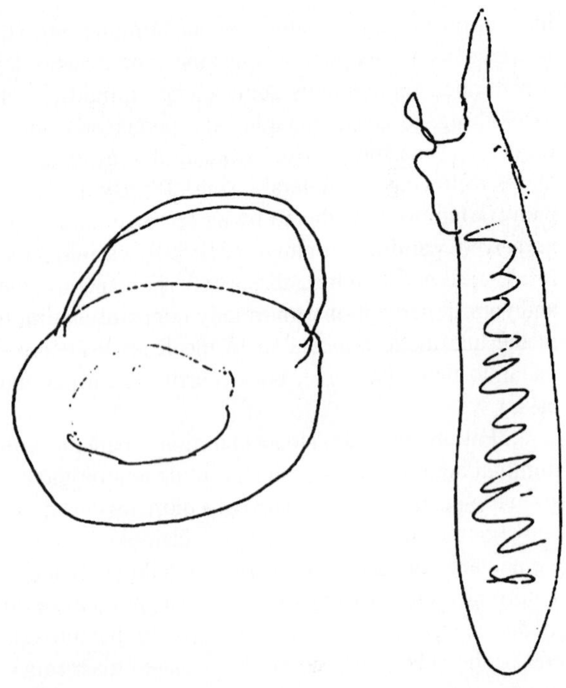

Figure 22-2
Drawings of a combination lock and a can opener made by a tactile agnosic after feeling but not seeing these objects. She was unable to identify these objects tactually. (Reproduced with permission from Caselli.[73])

It should be noted parenthetically that, to date, there has not been a patient studied with normal development who, as an adult, developed selective bilateral damage to ventrolateral association cortices. Before our knowledge of tactile agnosia can be considered complete, such a patient will need to be studied. The resulting somesthetic disorder in such a patient might prove far more revealing than the nondisabling unilateral disorder described above.

Mechanisms Based upon lesion studies in monkeys, Mishkin posited a role for the posterior insula in tactile learning and object recognition in which it served to connect SII to mesial temporal limbic structures.[75] From this perspective, tactile agnosia

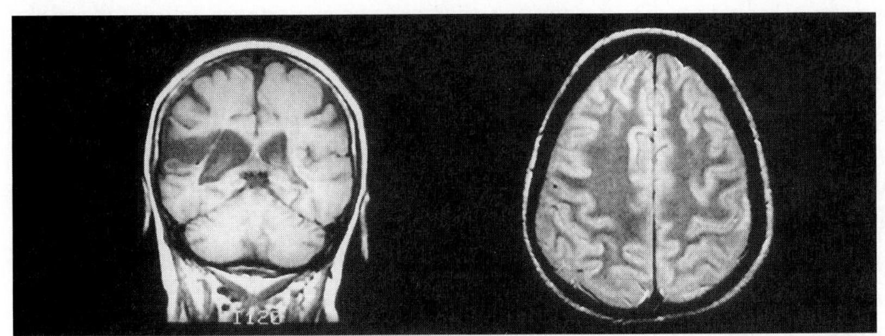

Figure 22-3
MRI sections of two patients with tactile agnosia. The patient to the left (T1-weighted coronal section) had infarction of both the parietal operculum and posterior insula of the right hemisphere. The patient to the right (proton density weighted transverse section) had a tiny infarction confined to the left inferior parietal lobule.

results from an interruption in the flow of information between the somatosensory and memory systems. Behavioral evidence favoring such a role for the anatomically defined somesthetic-limbic pathway includes the finding that amnesic subjects have difficulty learning a tactually mediated task (maze-learning).[76] However, on the basis of more recent demonstrations that amnesics have no difficulty tactually recognizing familiar objects, impaired memory alone is not sufficient to impair TOR in humans.[53]

Tactile agnosia seems to reflect a faulty high-level perceptual process. This conclusion stems from two observations: (1) tactile agnosia is a unilateral disorder (it affects only the left or only the right hand)[53,63–65] and (2) tactile agnosics have impaired haptic mental rotation.[63] With regard to the first observation, patients with unilateral damage to ventrolateral SAC have contralateral tactile agnosia but normal TOR with their ipsilateral hand.[53,63–65] Although lesion studies in monkeys have shown bilateral impairment of shape recognition following unilateral SII ablation,[77–79] the overwhelming majority of instances of bilaterally impaired TOR in human subjects have followed massive right hemispheric lesions in the setting of left hemineglect.[77] These patients had severe astereognosis in the left hand and tactile agnosia in their right hand.[77] The finding of right-sided tactile agnosia was unexpected but may have reflected transcallosal diaschisis, since the right hemisphere is dominant for cortical arousal mechanisms and was clinically impaired in these patients.[77,80] One patient has also been described who had mild, bilateral impairment of TOR following extensive damage to dorsomedial somatosensory association cortices[65] (see "Dorsomedial Syndrome," below). With regard to the second observation, tactile agnosics have difficulty tactually recognizing a letter that has been rotated in space, or its mirror image. Yet they can tactually recognize the letter in its normal orientation, can tactually judge simple line orientation, and have normal haptic mental imagery,[63] the three conditions that would seem to be sufficient to accomplish the very task they fail. However, an additional step must be inferred which involves the mental rotation of an object not in its normal orientation, so that the mental image becomes recognizable.[81]

Anatomic Considerations Tactile agnosia results from lesions involving inferior parietal cortices (Fig. 22-3), including Brodmann area 40 and probably area 39.[53,63,65] (SII is an inferior parietal cortical region, but it is defined physiologically.) However, the posterior insula may also play a role: positron emission tomography (PET) studies have shown a somatotopic representation in humans,[20] and lesions causing tactile agnosia have included but were not restricted to the posterior insula.[53,65] The observation that tactile agnosia results from damage to the inferior parietal lobule supports the idea that certain parts of the human inferior parietal lobule are homologous to simian area 7b (area 7 is located in the superior parietal lobule of humans but is inferior to the intraparietal sulcus of monkeys).[63,65]

Based upon behavioral[76] and anatomic[82] studies in monkeys and behavioral-anatomic correlation studies in humans,[65] it has been posited that there are dual streams of somesthetic information processing including a ventral stream concerned with object recognition, tactual learning and memory, and a dorsal stream possibly concerned with sensorimotor integration and somesthetic spatiotemporal functions. Lesions of the ventral object recognition pathway result in tactile agnosia, and lesions of the dorsal sensorimotor integration pathway result in severe apraxia and a type of astereognosis. Neither somatosensory association cortex syndrome reflects damage to SI.

The Dorsomedial Somatosensory Association Cortex Syndrome: Apraxia-Astereognosis Syndrome

An unusual type of astereognosis results from damage to the dorsomedial somatosensory association cortices,[65] though more cases need to be studied. Patients with extensive damage to SMA and SSA (Fig. 22-4) have moderate to severe impairment of basic, intermediate, and complex somesthetic functions. They have severe limb apraxia with an exteremly disordered tactile search strategy. In addition to the faulty spatial and temporal control of movements that characterizes the apraxia, they have an analogous spatiotemporal defect of somesthetic perception: they have difficulty localizing a stimulus within a limb or telling if they have been touched once or twice. Finally, they show surprisingly good recovery in the chronic stages.

Somesthetic Results of Other Behavioral Disorders

Cerebral Commissurotomy Studies of patients with complete separation of the cerebral hemispheres have shown that the somesthetic representation of the limbs is more highly lateralized than that of the trunk.[83] Stimuli presented to the right hand can be described by the perceiving and linguistically eloquent left hemisphere. Objects presented to the left hand are equally well recognized, but cannot be named by the linguistically deprived right hemisphere. The right hemisphere is superior on some perceptual and tactile-memory

Figure 22-4
MRI (T1-weighted sagittal top row, coronal middle row, and transverse bottom row) of a patient with infarction of left mesial frontal and parietal cortices who had the "dorsomedial syndrome" (see text).

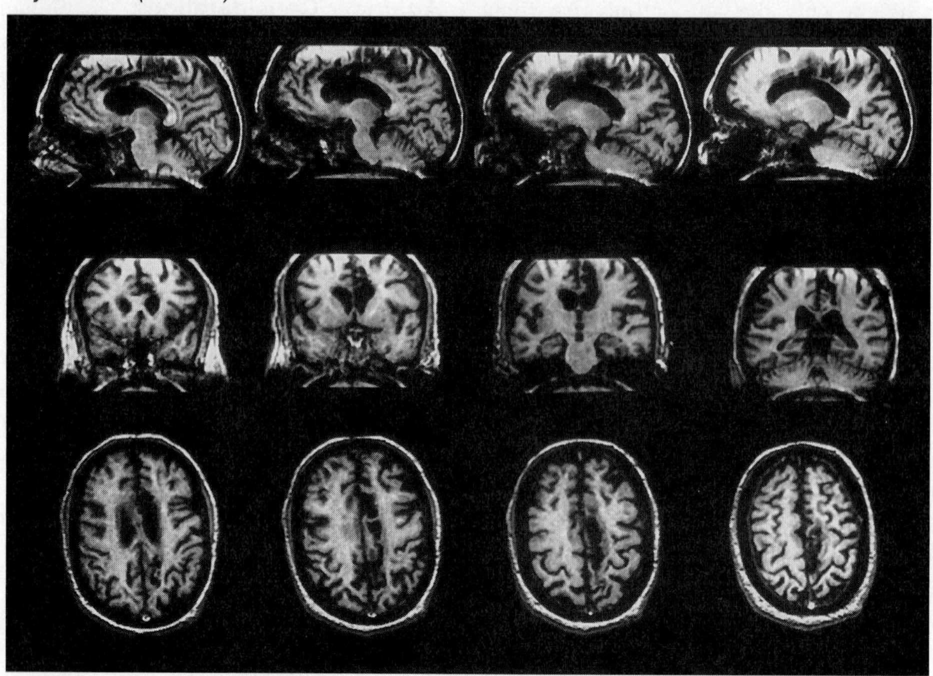

tasks,[84,85] and children have better left than right hand ability in learning braille.[86]

Amnesia Patients have difficulty with new learning in somatosensory[76] and other[87] modalities.

Tactile Aphasia This is a somatosensory modality-specific naming impairment[72] which should not be confused with tactile agnosia (see Chap. 39).

Asymboly for Pain As Critchley states, "there is nothing symbolic about a pain stimulus, or the patient's reaction thereto,"[57] so the term itself is unfortunate. Nonetheless, PET studies have demonstrated that painful thermal stimuli activate not only somatosensory cortices but also anterior cingulate cortex,[88] an area thought to play a role in emotion. Anosognosia (unawareness of illness) and anosodiaphoria (unconcern about illness) lend further credence to the concept of pathologic disregard for the painful nature of a stimulus. Lesion studies of patients with asymboly for pain, however, have implicated the posterior insula as the critical substrate,[89] and such findings have been thought to support Geschwind's theory[90] that asymbolia for pain is a disconnection syndrome between the ventrolateral somatosensory cortices and mesial temporal limbic structures.[89]

Anosognosia The denial of illness that is a frequent accompaniment of right hemispheric lesions may reflect damage to a body schema system in which right hemisphere somatosensory cortices—including SI, SII, and the posterior insula—play a pivotal role.[91]

DEGENERATIVE DISEASES AS A CAUSE OF CORTICAL SENSORY LOSS

Any lesion affecting somatosensory cortices can result in cortical patterns of sensory loss, but the severe cortical somatosensory impairments caused by certain degenerative brain diseases are underrecognized.

Degeneration of primary sensorimotor cortices or of more posteriorly situated parietal cortices (which includes mesial hemispheric cortices) causes gradually progressive apraxic disorders (including limb, constructional, dressing, and writing apraxia) as well as astereognosis,[92,93] consistent with the dorsomedial somatosensory association cortex syndrome (Fig. 22-5). Tactile object recognition occasionally is more severely affected than more basic somesthetic functions, reminiscent of tactile agnosia, though it is rarely pure when it occurs in a degenerative context. Although a tumor or other structural lesion should be sought, severe sensorimotor impairment evolving over a few years in an elderly patient is commonly degenerative. Several pathologic patterns have been described, including corticobasal degeneration with neuronal achromasia, nonspecific degenerative changes, Alzheimer's disease, and Pick's disease.[94] Clinical features and kinesiological patterns overlap extensively between these varied histologies.[95]

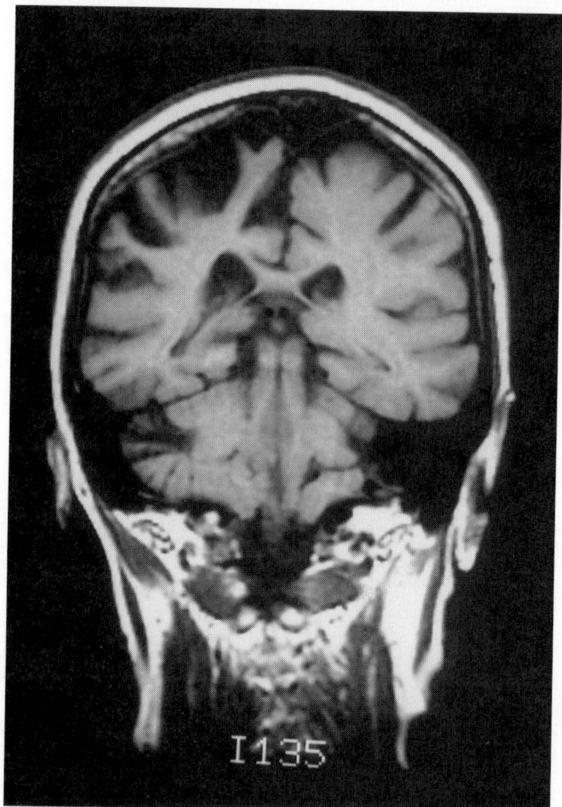

Figure 22-5
MRI (T1-weighted coronal section) of a patient with corticobasal degeneration primarily involving the right hemisphere who had severe apraxia and astereognosis affecting the left arm.

REFERENCES

1. Darian-Smith I: The sense of touch: performance and peripheral neural processes, in *Handbook of Physiology—The Nervous System III.* Bethesda, MD: American Physiological Society, 1984, pp 739–788.
2. Johansson RS, Vallbo AB: Tactile sensibility in the human hand: relative and absolute densities of four types of mechanoreceptive units in glabrous skin. *J Physiol (Lond)* 286:283–300, 1979.
3. Johnson KO, Phillips JR: A rotating drum stimulator for scanning embossed patterns and textures across skin. *J Neurosci Methods* 22:221–231, 1988.
4. Phillips JR, Johansson RS, Johnson KO: Representation of braille characters in human nerve fibres. *Exp Brain Res* 81:589–592, 1990.
5. Johnson KO, Hsiao SS: Neural mechanisms of tactual form and texture perception. *Annu Rev Neurosci* 15:227–250, 1992.
6. Phillips JR, Johnson KO, Hsiao SS: Spatial pattern representation and transformation in monkey somatosensory cortex. *Proc Natl Acad Sci U S A* 85:1317–1321, 1988.
7. Torebjork HE, Ochoa JL: Specific sensations evoked by activity in single identified sensory units in man. *Acta Physiol Scand* 110:445–447, 1980.
8. Vega-Bermudez F, Johnson KO, Hsiao SS: Human tactile pattern recognition: active versus passive touch, velocity effects, and patterns of confusion. *J Neurophysiol* 65:531–546, 1991.
9. Klatzky RL, McCloskey B, Doherty S, et al: Knowledge about hand shaping and knowledge about objects. *J Mot Behav* 19:187–213, 1987.
10. Lederman SJ, Klatzky RL: Hand movements: A window into haptic object recognition. *Cogn Psychol* 19:342–368, 1987.
11. Marshall WH, Woolsey CN, Bard R: Cortical representation of tactile sensibility as indicated by cortical potentials. *Science* 85:388–390, 1937.
12. Woolsey CN, Fairman D: Contralateral, ipsilateral, and bilateral representation of cutaneous receptors in somatic areas I and II of cerebral cortex of pig, sheep, and other animals. *Surgery* 19:684–702, 1946.
13. Penfield W, Jasper H: *Epilepsy and the Functional Anatomy of the Human Brain.* Boston: Little, Brown, 1954.
14. Kaas JH, Sur M, Nelson RJ, Merzenich MM: The postcentral somatosensory cortex: Multiple representations of the body in primates, in Woolsey CN (ed): *Cortical Sensory Organization.* Clifton, NJ: Humana Press, 1981, vol 1, pp 29–45.
15. Kaas JH: The segregation of function in the nervous system: Why do sensory systems have so many subdivisions? in Neff WD (ed): *Contributions to Sensory Physiology.* New York: Academic Press,1982, vol 7, pp 201–240.
16. Kaas JH: What, if anything, is SI? Organization of first somatosensory area of cortex. *Physiol Rev* 63:206–231, 1983.
17. Robinson CJ, Burton H: Somatotopographic organization in the second somatosensory area of *M. fascicularis*. *J Comp Neurol* 192:43–67, 1980.
18. Lueders H, Lesser RP, Dinner DS, et al: The second sensory area in humans: Evoked potential and electrical stimulation studies. *Ann Neurol* 17:177–184, 1985.
19. Hari R, Karhu J, Hamalainen M, et al: Functional organization of human first and second somatosensory cortices: a neuromagnetic study. *Eur J Neurosci* 5:724–734, 1993.
20. Burton H, Videen TO, Raichle ME: Tactile-vibration-activated foci in insular and parietal-opercular cortex studied with positron emission tomography: Mapping the second somatosensory area in humans. *Somat Mot Res* 10:297–308, 1993.
21. Darian-Smith I, Isbister J, Mok H, Yokota T: Somatic sensory cortical projection areas excited by tactile stimulation of the cat: a triple representation. *J Physiol (Lond)* 182:671–689, 1966.
22. Clemo HR, Stein BE: Somatosensory cortex: a "new" somatotopic representation. *Brain Res* 235:162–168, 1982.
23. Clemo HR, Stein BE: Organization of a fourth somatosensory area of cortex in cat. *J Neurophysiol* 50:910–925, 1983.
24. Burton H, Robinson CJ: Organization of the SII parietal cortex: multiple somatic sensory representations within and near the second somatic sensory area of cynomolgus monkeys, in Woolsey CN (ed): *Cortical Sensory Organization.* Clifton, NJ: Humana Press, 1981, vol 1, pp 67–119.
25. Friedman DP: Body topography in the second somatic sensory area: Monkey SII somatotopy, in Woolsey CN (ed): *Cortical Sensory Organization.* Clifton, NJ: Humana Press, 1981, vol 1, pp 121–165.
26. Rijntjes M, Dettmers C, Buchel C, et al: A blueprint for movement: functional and anatomical representations in the human motor system. *J Neurosci* 19: 8043–8048, 1999.
27. Isnard J, Guenot M, Ostrowsky K, et al: The role of the insular cortex in temporal lobe epilepsy. *Ann Neurol* 48:614–623, 2000.
28. Blomquist AJ, Lorenzini CA: Projection of dorsal roots and sensory nerves to cortical sensory motor regions of squirrel monkey. *J Neurophysiol* 28:1195–1205, 1965.

29. Bowker RM, Coulter JD: Intracortical connectivities of somatic sensory and motor areas: Multiple cortical pathways in monkeys, in Woolsey CN (ed): *Cortical Sensory Organization*. Clifton, NJ: Humana Press, 1981, vol 1, pp 205–242.
30. Murray EA, Coulter JD: Supplementary sensory area: the medial parietal cortex in the monkey, in Woolsey CN (ed): *Cortical Sensory Organization.* Clifton, NJ: Humana Press, 1981, vol 1 pp 167–195.
31. Penfield W, Welch K: The supplementary motor area of the cerebral cortex: A clinical and experimental study. *AMA Arch Neurol Psychiatry* 66:289–317, 1951.
32. Van Buren JM, Fedio P: Functional representation on the medial aspect of the frontal lobe in man. *J Neurosurg* 44:275–289, 1976.
33. Fried I, Katz A, McCarthy G, et al: Functional organization of human supplementary motor cortex studied by electrical stimulation. *J Neurosci* 11:3656–3666, 1991.
34. Laplane D, Talairach J, Meininger V, et al: Clinical consequences of corticectomies involving the supplementary motor area in humans. *J Neurol Sci* 34:301–314, 1977.
35. Sanides F: Functional architecture of motor and sensory cortices in primates in the light of a new concept of neocortex evolution, in Noback CR, Montagna W (eds): *The Primate Brain: Advances in Primatology.* New York: Appleton-Century-Crofts, 1970, vol I, pp 137–208.
36. Burton H: Second somatosensory cortex and related areas, in Jones EG, Peters A (eds): *Cerebral Cortex.* New York: Plenum Press, 1985, vol 5, pp 31–98.
37. Cavada C, Goldman-Rakic PS: Posterior parietal cortex in rhesus monkey: I. Parcellation of areas based on distinctive limbic and sensory corticocortical connections. *J Comp Neurol* 287:393–421, 1989.
38. Pons TP, Garraghty PE, Friedman DP, Mishkin M: Physiological evidence for serial processing in somatosensory cortex. *Science* 237:417–420, 1987.
39. Johansson RS, LaMotte RH: Tactile detection of a single asperity on an otherwise smooth surface. *Somat Res* 1:21–31, 1983.
40. Srinivasan MA, Whitehouse JM, LaMotte RH: Tactile detection of slip: surface microgeometry and peripheral neural codes. *J Neurophysiol* 63:1323–1332, 1990.
41. Johnson KO, Phillips JR: Tactile spatial resolution: I. Two-point discrimination, gap detection, grating resolution, and letter recognition. *J Neurophysiol* 46:1177–1191, 1981.
42. Verrillo RT, Fraioli AJ, Smith RL: Sensation magnitude of vibrotactile stimuli. *Percept Psychophys* 6:366–372, 1969.
43. Mountcastle VB, LaMotte RH, Carli G: Detection thresholds for stimuli in humans and monkeys: Comparisons with threshold events in mechanoreceptive afferent nerve fibers innervating the monkey hand. *J Neurophysiol* 35:122–136, 1972.
44. Mountcastle VB, Steinmetz MA, Romo R: Frequency discrimination in the sense of flutter: psychophysical measurements correlated with postcentral events in behaving monkeys. *J Neurosci* 10:3032–3044, 1990.
45. Loomis JM: Tactile recognition of raised letters: A parametric study. *Bull Psychosom Soc* 23:18–20, 1985.
46. Lederman SJ: Tactile roughness of grooved surfaces: The touching process and effects of macro- and micro-surface structure. *Percept Psychophys* 16:385–395, 1974.
47. Sathian K, Goodwin AW, Darian-Smith I: Perceived roughness of a grating: Correlation with responses of mechanoreceptive afferents innervating the monkey's fingerpad. *J Neurosci* 9:1273–1279, 1989.
48. Lamb G: Tactile discrimination of textured surfaces: Psychophysical performance measurements in humans. *J Physiol* 338:551–565, 1983.
49. Klatzky RL, Lederman S, Reed C: Haptic integration of object properties: Texture, hardness, and planar contour. *J Exp Psychol Hum Percept Perf* 15:45–57, 1989.
50. Reed CL, Lederman SJ, Klatzky RL: Haptic integration of planar size with hardness, texture, and planar contour. *Can J Psychol* 44:522–545, 1990.
51. Members of the Department of Neurology Mayo Clinic and Mayo Foundation for Medical Education and Research: *Clinical Examinations in Neurology,* 6th ed. St Louis: Mosby–Year Book, 1991, pp 255–275.
52. Lezak MD: *Neuropsychological Assessment,* 2d ed. New York: Oxford University Press, 1983.
53. Caselli RJ: Rediscovering tactile agnosia. *Mayo Clin Proc* 66:129–142, 1991.
54. Klatzky RL, Lederman SJ, Metzger VA: Identifying objects by touch: An "expert system." *Percept Psychophys* 37:299–302, 1985.
55. Craig JC: Tactile pattern perception and its perturbations. *J Acoust Soc Am* 77:238–246, 1985.
56. Dyck PJ, Karnes J, O'Brien PC, Zimmerman IR: Detection threshold of cutaneous sensation in humans, in Dyck PJ, Thomas PK, Griffin JW, et al (eds): *Peripheral Neuropathy,* 3d ed. Philadelphia: Saunders, 1993, pp 706–728.
57. Critchley M: *The Parietal Lobes.* New York: Hafner, 1971, pp 86–155.
58. Head H, Holmes G: Sensory disturbances from cerebral lesions. *Brain* 34:102–254, 1911–1912.

59. Bassetti C, Bogousslavsky J, Regli F: Sensory syndromes in parietal stroke. *Neurology* 43:1942–1949, 1993.
60. McHenry LC: *Garrison's History of Neurology.* Springfield, IL: Charles C Thomas, 1969, pp 297.
61. Delay JPL: *Les Asterognosies, Pathologie du Toucher, Clinique, Physiologique, Topographie.* Paris: Masson, 1935.
62. Teuber HL: Postscript: some needed revisions of the clinical views of agnosia. *Neuropsychologia* 3:371–378, 1965.
63. Reed CL, Caselli RJ: The nature of tactile agnosia: A case study. *Neuropsychologia* 32:527–539, 1994.
64. Reed CL, Caselli RJ, Farah MJ: Tactile agnosia: Underlying impairment and implications for normal tactile object recognition. *Brain* 119:875–888, 1996.
65. Caselli RJ: Ventrolateral and dorsomedial somatosensory association cortex infarctions produce distinct somesthetic syndromes. *Neurology* 43:762–771, 1993.
66. Halpern L: Astereognosis not of cortical origin. *J Neurol Sci* 7:245–250, 1968.
67. Norrsell U: Behavioral studies of the somatosensory system. *Psychol Rev* 60:327–354, 1980.
68. Byl NN, Merzenich MM, Jenkins WM: A primate genesis model of focal dystonia and repetitive strain injury: I. Learning-induced dedifferentiation of the representation of the hand in the primary somatosensory cortex in adult monkeys. *Neurology* 47:508–520,1996.
69. Bara-Jimenez W, Catalan MJ, Hallett M, Gerloff C: Abnormal somatosensory homunculus in dystonia of the hand. *Ann Neurol* 44:828–831, 1998.
70. Tempel LW, Perlmutter JS: Abnormal cortical responses in patients with writers' cramp. *Neurology* 43:2252–2257, 1993.
71. Bara-Jimenez W, Shelton P, Hallett M: Spatial discrimination is abnormal in focal hand dystonia. *Neurology* 55:1869–1873, 2000.
72. Beauvois MF, Saillant B, Meininger V, Lhermitte F: Bilateral tactile aphasia: a tactoverbal dysfunction. *Brain* 101:381–401, 1978.
73. Caselli RJ: Somesthetic syndrome (letter). *Neurology* 43:2423–2424, 1993
74. Caselli RJ: Bilateral impairment of somesthetically mediated object recognition in humans. *Mayo Clin Proc* 66:357–364, 1991.
75. Mishkin M: Analogous neural models for tactual and visual learning. *Neuropsychologia* 17:139–150, 1979.
76. Corkin S: Tactually guided maze-learning in man: effects of unilateral cortical excisions and bilateral hippocampal lesions. *Neuropsychologia* 3:339–351, 1965.
77. Garcha HS, Ettlinger G: The effects of unilateral or bilateral removals of the second somatosensory cortex (area SII): A profound tactile disorder in monkeys. *Cortex* 14:319–326, 1978.
78. Garcha HS, Ettlinger G: Tactile discrimination learning in the monkey: the effects of unilateral or bilateral removals of the second somatosensory cortex (area SII). *Cortex* 16:397–412, 1980.
79. Garcha HS, Ettlinger G, Maccabe JJ: Unilateral removal of the second somatosensory projection cortex in the monkey: Evidence for cerebral predominance? *Brain* 105:787–810, 1982.
80. Meyer JS: Does diaschisis have clinical correlates? *Mayo Clin Proc* 66:430–432, 1991.
81. Warrington EK, Taylor AM: The contribution of the right parietal lobe to object recognition. *Cortex* 9:152–164, 1973.
82. Friedman DP, Murray EA, O'Neill JB, Mishkin M: Cortical connections of the somatosensory fields of the lateral sulcus of macaques: Evidence for a corticolimbic pathway for touch. *J Comp Neurol* 252:323–347, 1986.
83. Gazzaniga MS, Bogen JE, Sperry RW: Laterality effects following cerebral commissurotomy in man. *Neuropsychologia* 1:209–215, 1963.
84. Milner B, Taylor L: Right-hemisphere superiority in tactile pattern-recognition after cerebral commissurotomy: evidence for nonverbal memory. *Neuropsychologia* 10:1–15, 1972.
85. Sperry RW: Cerebral organization and behavior. *Science* 133:1749–1757, 1981.
86. Rudel RG, Denckla MB, Spalten E: The functional asymmetry of Braille letter learning in normal, sighted children. *Neurology* 24:733–738, 1974.
87. Milner B: Visually-guided maze learning in man: effects of bilateral hippocampal, bilateral frontal, and unilateral cerebral lesions. *Neuropsychologia* 3:317–338, 1965.
88. Talbot JD, Marrett S, Evans AC, et al: Multiple representations of pain in human cerebral cortex. *Science* 251:1355–1358, 1991.
89. Berthier M, Starkstein S, Leiguarda R: Asymbolia for pain: a sensory-limbic disconnection syndrome. *Ann Neurol* 24:41–49, 1988.
90. Geschwind N: Disconnexion syndromes in animals and man. *Brain* 88:237–294, 1965.
91. Damasio AR: *Descartes' Error.* New York: Putnam, 1994, pp 65–66.

92. Caselli RJ, Jack CR Jr: Asymmetric cortical degeneration syndromes: a proposed clinical classification. *Arch Neurol* 49:770–780, 1992.
93. Caselli RJ, Jack CR Jr, Petersen RC, et al: Asymmetric cortical degenerative syndromes: clinical, planar MRI, MRI-based surface rendering, and SPECT correlations. *Neurology* 42:1462–1468, 1992.
94. Boeve BF, Maraganore DM, Parisi JE, et al: Pathologic heterogeneity in clinically diagnosed corticobasal degeneration. *Neurology* 53:795–800, 1999.
95. Caselli RJ, Stelmach GE, Caviness JN, et al: A kinematic study of progressive apraxia with and without dementia. *Mov Disord* 14:276–287, 1999.

Chapter 23

DISORDERS OF BODY PERCEPTION AND REPRESENTATION

Georg Goldenberg

In classic neuropsychology, disorders of the perception and of the mental representation of one's body have been conceptualized as being due to the breakdown of a mental "body schema." The body schema has been a central concept to neuropsychological thinking for many years (see reviews in Refs. 1 to 3). It has been attacked as being ill-defined and as narrowing the view to isolated aspects of more general disorders of language and spatial perception, respectively.[4] However, recent research in normal psychology and physiology has brought forward experimental evidence for the contention that perception and representation of one's body are distinct psychological functions[5–8] and has revived interest in their neuropsychological disturbances.

LEVELS OF INFORMATION ABOUT ONE'S BODY

In this chapter, three levels are distinguished at which information about one's body is processed and represented in the cognitive architecture of the human:

A Body-Centered Reference System for Motor Actions Information about the current configuration and position of one's body is a necessary prerequisite for the planning and execution of most movements aimed at external targets. Muscles move limbs relative to the body and hence within a body-centered frame of reference. The simple motor act of reaching with the hand for a visually presented object requires that the retinotopic coordinates of the perceived object are transformed into body-centered coordinates. This transformation has to take into account the current position of the eyes relative to the head and of the head relative to the trunk. In addition to the representation of the target in body-centered coordinates, the brain must also represent the initial arm configuration in order to plan the trajectory. Single-cell recordings in monkeys have provided evidence that cells in the intraparietal sulcus and adjacent areas 7 and 5 of the posterior parietal lobe are informed about the current position and configuration of the eyes, the head, the body, and the limbs and perform the computations necessary for transforming visually perceived locations into body-centered coordinates.[9,10]

Reaching for an object is a highly automatized task. One need not pay attention to the position and configuration of one's body in order to accurately reach for a seen object. Assessement of the body-centered reference frame and computation of the target's location in body-centered coordinates take place automatically and without necessitating conscious awareness of one's body. The body-centered reference frames used for the planning of movements are implicitly involved in movement planning but do not regularly enter into explicit awareness.

Awareness of One's Own Body One can pay attention to the position and configuration of one's own body. One can use vestibular, kinesthetic, tactile, and to a limited degree also visual perceptions for inferring the actual position and configuration of one's body. Even in the absence of distinct afferents from these channels, one has a basic "feeling" of where one's body parts are. One can point to the tip of one's nose without a mirror even if the nose does not itch. It is this basic awareness of the limits and of the spatial layout of one's own body which has originally been conceptualized as the "body schema."[11]

General Knowledge about the Human Body General knowledge about the human body and body parts can have two basically different forms.[12] On the one hand, there is lexical and semantic knowledge, which defines the names, categories, and functions of body parts. This knowledge base specifies, for example, that the wrist and ankle are both articulations, or that the mouth is for speaking and the ear for hearing. On the other hand, there is knowledge about the spatial structure of body parts. This knowledge base specifies the position of individual body parts, the proximity relations that exist between them, and the boundaries that define each body part. For example, it specifies that the nose is in the middle of the face and that its upper end is contiguous to the forehead, with the line of the eyebrows marking the border between them. Furthermore, it defines the back of the nose as an entity that is different from the tip or from the flanks. Hence, the small spatial distance between back and flank is significant, whereas larger distances within the back are not significant for the definition of these body parts.

This knowledge applies equally to one's own or another person's body as well as to sculptural and pictorial representations of the human body. It may also be needed for successful performance of tasks intended to test awareness of one's own body. When given the order "point to the back of your nose," one must have a general concept of what and where the back of the nose is before one can search for it.

With this schematic division of the "body schema" in mind, seven neuropsychological symptoms are treated here: optic ataxia, body-part phantoms, unilateral neglect, awareness of one's own body, autotopagnosia, finger agnosia, and impaired imitation of gestures.

OPTIC ATAXIA

Optic ataxia was originally described in association with apraxia of gaze and simultanagnosia,[13] but it has since then been recognized as an independent symptom that can occur without the other elements of Balint's syndrome.[14–18] Patients with optic ataxia cannot accurately reach for visually perceived external targets. They move their hands into the approximate vicinity of the target and then start searching movements with the widely opened hand. By contrast, they can reach without hesitation or error to parts of their own body. Asked to touch the tip of the nose, they do so as fast and accurately as do controls. A patient who was unable to grasp the outstretched finger of the examiner could accurately touch her own finger placed passively in the same location.[14] Pointing to auditorily perceived locations can be preserved as well.[15] Misreaching may be confined to the periphery of the visual field, leaving patients able to reach accurately for external targets when they are allowed to fixate them visually before moving the hand.[18]

Many patients with optic ataxia also have difficulties when asked to explore, compare, and estimate spatial positions without reaching for them, but there is no correlation between the severity of this general visuospatial disorder and the severity of visual misreaching. Single patients with optic ataxia pass all tests of visuospatial estimation and exploration perfectly,[14,15] and many patients with severe visuospatial problems can accurately reach for visually presented targets.[19–21]

One interpretation of optic ataxia is that the basic disorder concerns the transformation of retinotopic locations into a body-centered reference frame necessary for movement planning. The patients can accurately reach for parts of their own bodies because body parts are a priori coded in body-centered coordinates. At the same time, successful pointing to body parts indicates that awareness of the patient's own body is preserved as well as general conceptual knowledge about the human body.

Single-cell recordings in monkeys have provided ample evidence that neuronal networks in parietal area 5 and 7 are capable of transcoding visual locations from retinotopic to body-centered reference frames.[9,10,22] The lesions causing optic ataxia are centered around the intraparietal sulcus too and regularly affect area 5 or 7.[15]

With unilateral lesions, optic ataxia can be restricted to the hand or the hemifield opposite the lesioned hemisphere or even only to their combination.[15,16] As already mentioned, manual misreaching may contrast with accurate fixation by saccades.[18] These dissociations indicate that transformations from retinotopic to body-centered coordinates are made by mechanisms dedicated to single body parts and restricted sectors of the visual field.

BODY-PART PHANTOMS

The occurrence of phantom limbs has been among the first[11] and continues to be among the most impressive arguments for the contention that the brain houses a mental body schema that underlies and modifies the way in which we experience our own bodies. After amputations, about 90 percent of adults experience a phantom of lost limbs.[23–25] Phantom experiences have also been reported after loss of eyes, teeth, external genitalia, and the female breast.[24] Phantoms of the amputated breast occur less regularly than phantoms of amputated limbs; still, they occur in about 40 percent of women after mastectomy.[26,27]

Limb phantoms occur not only after amputation but can also be caused by nervous system lesions provided that all afferents from the affected body part are interrupted. This may be the case with lesions of the peripheral nerves, the plexus, and the spinal cord but also with subcortical cerebral lesions.[23,24,28] If the deafferented limb is still present and visible, the phantom may be experienced as an additional, supernumerary limb,[24,28] thus violating the anatomic constraints of the normal body.

Initially, most limb phantoms are experienced in the same way as the true limb was experienced before amputation, but over time the experience may become less natural. Particularly in upper limb phantoms, the representation of the proximal portions may become weaker and eventually vanish, leading to the strange sensation of a hand belonging to one's own body but being disconnected from it. Alternatively, a shrinking of the proximal portions may lead to "telescoping" and give rise to the belief that the phantom arm is shorter than the other arm. Telescoping causes a severe deformation of size and shape of phantoms and may result in the anatomically impossible location of fingers inside the stump.[11,24,29] Full-sized phantoms may be in unnatural positions, violating anatomic constraints. For example, the hand of a phantom arm may penetrate into the chest.[30]

Visual and Somatosensory Influences on Phantom Sensation

Although the very existence of a phantom contradicts the visual evidence for absence of the limb, the phantom experience can be shaped by visual experience. In patients fitted with prostheses, phantoms frequently adapt to their shape.[31,32] Some amputated patients integrate the prosthesis into their body and identify it with the phantom. They feel touch directly at the surface of the prosthesis rather than deducing it from the prosthesis's pressure on the stump.[33] Visual influence on phantom sensations has also been demonstrated in a series of elegant experiments on patients with upper limb phantoms by Ramachandran and coworkers.[25,34] They "resurrected" vision of the phantom arm by means of a mirror reflecting the patient's opposite arm. Movement of the mirror image induced a feeling of phantom movement and touch of the intact arm a sensation at the mirror location on the phantom.

It has been established for about 50 years that touch of the stump can evoke referred sensations in phantoms of amputated limbs,[29,35] but only recently has it been shown that referred sensations can originate in body parts that have no anatomic proximity to the amputated body part. In patients with upper limb amputations, referred sensations have been evoked from both sides of the chest, both sides of the face, and the contralateral arm.[25,36–40] Sensations in phantoms of amputated breasts have been evoked by touch of both sides of the back and the ipsilateral pinna.[41] The presence, extent, and localization of referred sensations vary greatly between patients. In some an exact and reproducible topographic remapping from stimulated to referred locations has been demonstrated, which remained stable for up to several weeks. Reexaminations after longer delays, however, have documented radical changes or even complete breakdown of topographic referral without accompanying changes of the phantom's size and shape.[6,36,38]

Phantoms in Congenital Absence of Limbs

The possibility of phantom limbs in persons with congenital absence or very early amputation of limbs has been reliably established,[31–33,42–46] but their frequency is substantially lower than after later amputation. Permanent phantoms are reported by some 10 percent of persons with congenital absence or very early amputation of limbs as compared to about 90 percent of persons amputated after the age of 10 years.[31,33] The incidence rises to some 20 percent when temporary phantom sensations are considered.[32,42] Some persons report to have had phantoms as long as they can remember,[46,47] but in the majority phantoms occur only after a delay. The mean time to phantom onset has been calculated to be 9 years in congenital absence and 2.3 years in early amputation.[32] The emergence of the phantom may be triggered by minor trauma to the stump.[31]

As the affected children had no or only rudimentary opportunity to experience the presence of the now missing limb, the phantom has been said to testify a genetic prefiguration of the mental representation of body shape.[32,43] There is, however, evidence that experience does shape phantoms in children. In children with early amputation of congenitally deformed limbs, the phantom may replicate the initial deformation rather than a normal limb.[32,42] This shaping by early experience may contrast with an inability to consciously remember the deformation. Like phantoms of adult patients, those of children may be triggered or shaped by prostheses: phantoms of congenitally absent or early lost limbs are more frequent in children who had been fitted with prostheses than in those without,[31,42] and they usually adapt their size and shape to the prosthesis.[31,44,47]

The Cerebral Substrate of Phantom Experience

Plasticity of somatotopic organization of primary sensory cortex in patients with phantoms after amputation of the lower arm and hand has been demonstrated by functional imaging with magnetoencephalography.[38,39,45,48,49] The receptive fields of adjacent regions, devoted to the face on one side and to the upper arm on the other, invade the receptive field originally devoted to the hand. The parallel to remapping of sensations from face and stump to the phantom is striking, but a longitudinal study found that the topography of referred sensations can change without correlated changes in cortical remapping.[38] This finding would suggest that some factor other than cortical remapping must contribute to remapping of sensation. Possibly this factor is to be sought in an interpretative activity of higher brain centers that integrate information from sensory cortex with other sensory afferents to produce a coherent body image.

There are a few cases on record where a cerebral lesion abolished a phantom limb. In all of them the clinical evidence pointed to lesion in the parietal lobe of the opposite hemisphere,[30,50,51] and one autopsy confirmed a metastasis in the supramarginal gyrus. In a further case, clinical evidence strongly suggested sparing of primary sensory cortex.[51] A recent study by functional magnetic resonance imaging [46] found activations in inferior parietal and premotor but not in primary motor or sensory cortex of a patient with phantoms of congenitally absent limbs when she moved her phantom arms. Taken together, these findings suggest that the phantom experience is constructed in the parietal lobe.

NEGLECT OF ONE-HALF OF THE BODY

Patients with hemineglect may neglect not only one-half of external space but also one-half of their own body. They behave as if they had lost one-half of the body. When combing, washing, shaving, and dressing, they restrict grooming to the nonneglected half of their body. When asked to indicate with their normal hand the midline of their body, they deviate to the healthy side[52,53] as if they would bisect only the nonneglected half of their body. When asked to reach with their normal hand to the neglected one, their reaching movement may end at the shoulder or even at the midline of the trunk.[54]

Studies looking for the possibility that neglect of one-half of the body may dissociate from neglect of one-half of external space have yielded inconsistent results. One found personal hemineglect without extrapersonal hemineglect in only 1 out of 97 right brain–damaged patients, while the reverse dissociation occurred in 9 patients.[54] Another study with a smaller sample of patients and more sensitive tests of personal neglect found that one-third of the patients had predominantly extrapersonal, one-third predominantly personal, and one-third combined hemineglect[55]; there also is one report of a patient showing severe personal neglect in testing as well as in spontaneous behavior but no extrapersonal hemineglect at all.[56] On the other hand, there are experimental demonstrations of intricate interactions between personal and extrapersonal neglect in patients who display both. In patients with left hemineglect, blindfolded detection of touch of the left hand improves when the hand is placed across the body midline into the right hemispace.[57] When the ulnar and radial sides of the left hand are touched simultaneously, neglect will affect the side that happens to lie on the left side. Ulnar touch will be neglected when the hand is pronated and radial touch when the hand is supinated.[58,59] The dependence of tactile sensation on hand position suggests an influence of position in peripersonal space on sensations arising from intrapersonal space.

In view of the paucity of systematic observation, it would be premature to offer any speculation as to the location of lesions responsible for personal neglect. It is not even clear whether the preponderance of left-sided hemineglect applies to personal neglect. The large studies that established this hemispheric asymmetry were all restricted to measures of extrapersonal neglect, and the above-mentioned studies that systematically compared personal and extrapersonal neglect were restricted to patients with right brain damage. In clinical practice, right-sided personal neglect following left brain damage may escape observation when there is right-sided hemiplegia and apraxia of the left limbs, as this constellation renders patients unable to groom and dress themselves and thus prevents dramatic manifestations of personal neglect—as, for example, the shaving or dressing of only one-half of the body.

AWARENESS OF ONE'S OWN BODY

Body-part phantoms and neglect of one-half of the body are both disorders that involve the awareness of the patient's own body. In a way, they mirror each other: in body-part phantoms there is awareness of body parts that in reality are absent, while in neglect, body parts that in reality are present are excluded from awareness.

Kinematic analyses revealed abnormalities of reaching in patients with left hemineglect,[19,20,52] but they are different from those shown by patients with optic ataxia. Movements toward targets in the neglected half of space are slowed down and the movement path may deviate toward the nonaffected side of space, but the patients ultimately reach visible targets accurately and without insecurity or searching. Defective awareness of one's own body is usually associated with normal general knowledge about the human body. Patients with phantom limbs or with hemineglect are able to point on command to single parts of their own body provided that these parts are not amputated or, respectively, neglected.[60]

AUTOTOPAGNOSIA

Taken literally, the term *autotopagnosia* would indicate an inablity to recognize locations on one's own body, but it is generally understood as designating the inability to localize body parts on one's own body as well as on another person's body or on a model of the human body. The term *somatotopagnosia*[61] would be more appropriate but has not found wide acceptance.

Earlier case reports of autotopagnosia have been criticized as demonstrating nothing more than the effects of general mental deterioration or of aphasia on the task of pointing to body parts on verbal command; since then, however, several carefully conducted single-case studies have established the independence of autotopagnosia from aphasia and dementia and have drawn a consistent clinical picture of "pure" autotopagnosia.[12,62–68] When asked to point to body parts on themselves, another person, or a model of the human body, these patients commit errors. The majority of these errors are "contiguity" errors: the patients search in the vicinity of the designated body part. Less frequent are "semantic" errors that confuse body parts of the same category, as, for example, the elbow and the knee. These errors occur not only when the body parts are designated by verbal command but also when they are shown on pictures or even when the examiner demonstrates correct pointing and the patient tries to imitate. Most of the patients were able to name the body parts when they were pointed at by someone else or shown on pictures, and although they invariably had left-sided brain lesions (see below), several of them were not aphasic at all.[12,62,63,65,68] Some patients were asked to give verbal descriptions of body parts. They could describe the function and the individual visual appearance of body parts but got lost when asked to describe their location.[12,62,65]

The inability to locate a body part need not affect all body parts nor must it be restricted to the human body. There are patients with autotopagnosia in whom localizing of individual fingers was found to be preserved,[62–64] while some patients had problems not only with pointing to body parts but also with pointing to single parts of other multipart objects like bicycles.[62,63,69] There are, however, other patients with autotopagnosia who could locate the parts of bicycles or animals.[65–67] The conclusion that their disturbance is restricted to the topography of only the human body remains nonetheless arguable. It may be questioned whether the structure of other multipart objects involves, to a similar degree, subtle distinctions between easily confusable and adjacent parts as the structure of the human body. If such distinctions exist, their cognizance is reserved to experts and falls outside the scope of neuropsychological examination. By contrast, subtle distinctions between easily confusable parts of the human body are tested in autotopagnosia and account for the majority of errors. Knowledge about the structure of the human body may be more vulnerable to brain damage because it is more fine-grained and diversified than knowledge about other multipart objects. Few persons have expert knowledge about bicycles but all have expert knowledge about the human body.

Awareness of the patient's own body seems to be preserved in autotopagnosia: Such patients can reach body parts accurately when asked to indicate the typical location of accessories (e.g., a wristwatch) or the location of objects which had been temporarily fixed to a body part.[12,66,67] Apparently they can orient themselves on their own body, and their autotopagnosia stems from the inability to link preserved spatial orientation on their own body with conceptual knowledge about the human body.

The lesions in "pure" cases of autotopagnosia are remarkably uniform and always affect the posterior parietal lobe of the left hemisphere.[62–68] In a group study of patients with left or right brain damage, errors in pointing to body parts occurred only in left brain–damaged patients.[70] In this unselected sample there were no "pure" cases of autotopagnosia. The patients who committed errors in localizing body parts were all aphasic and had on average larger lesions than patients who performed without error.

FINGER AGNOSIA

Finger agnosia was originally described as part of the "Gerstmann syndrome,"[71] which is a combination of finger agnosia with right-left confusion, acalculia, and agraphia, but it has been demonstrated that these symptoms can occur independently of each other.[72]

The value of verbal tasks of finger identification has been called in question because they may be more sensitive to language disorders than to defective orientation on the body.[70,73] However, a considerable number of brain-damaged patients fail on nonverbal tasks of finger localization such as pointing on a drawing of a hand to fingers touched on the own hand[70,73–75] or indicating how many fingers lie between two fingers touched simultaneously by the examiner.[76]

Finger agnosia has been considered as a minor form of autotopagnosia,[71] but we have already mentioned that there are patients with autotopagnosia in whom identification of fingers is preserved. Whereas autotopagnosia has been observed exclusively in patients with left brain damage, finger agnosia occurs with approximately equal frequency in patients with left and right brain damage.[70,73,74,76] There is thus no regular association of finger agnosia with autotopagnosia. Another association has hitherto been examined only in a few patients and may turn out to be more regular: these patients had similar difficulties with selection of toes as with selection of fingers.[75,77]

IMITATION OF MEANINGLESS GESTURES

Defective imitation of meaningless gestures has been recognized as a symptom of apraxia following left brain damage.[78–80] Other symptoms of apraxia are disturbed production and imitation of meaningful gestures, like waving good-bye or miming the use of a hammer, and disturbed use of real objects. There are, however, patients with pure "visuoimitative apraxia" in whom defective imitation of meaningless gestures contrasts with preservation of production and imitation of meaningful gestures and object use.[81,82] It thus seems justified to discuss defective imitation of meaningless gestures as a disorder on its own.

Defective imitation of meaningless gestures affects not only the translation of gestures from a model to the patient's own body but also translation to other instances of human bodies. Patients who commit errors when imitating with their own bodies also commit errors when asked to replicate the demonstrated gesture on a mannikin[83] or to select the gesture from an array of photographs showing gestures performed by different persons and seen under different angles of view.[84]

Like the dissociation between autotopagnosia and finger agnosia, defective imitation of meaningless gestures can affect imitation of gestures defined by

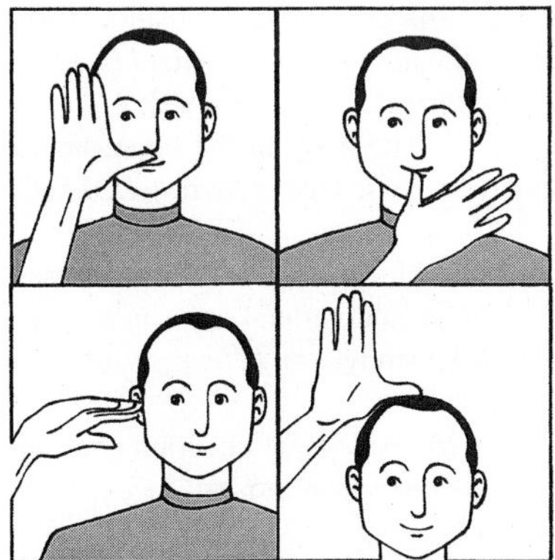
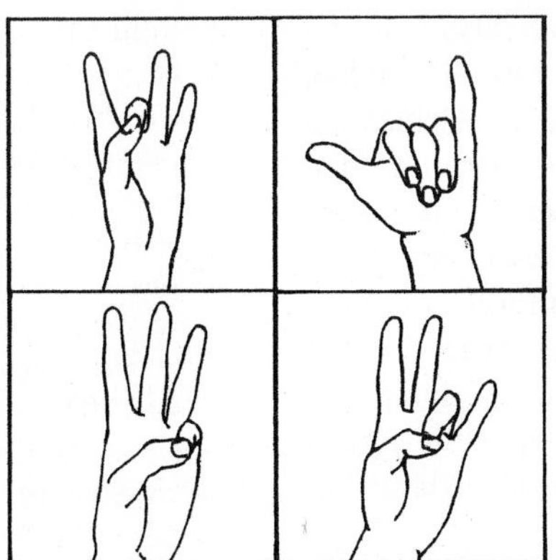
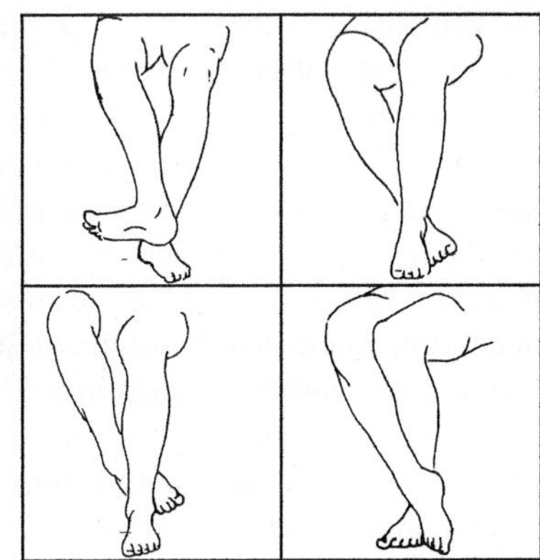

Figure 23-1
Examples of hand, finger, and foot posture used for assessing imitation of meaningless gestures.

proximal body parts differently from finger configurations. Figure 23-1 shows three types of meaningless gestures that have been used to explore these differences: Hand postures specify a position of the hand relative to face and head while the internal configuration of the hand remains invariant. Finger postures specify different configurations of the fingers while the position of the hand is not considered for scoring. Foot postures specify a position of one foot relative to the other foot and leg.[85] Patients with left brain damage have problems with all kind of gestures, but the impairment is distinctly less severe for finger than for hand and foot postures. There are even single apraxic patients in whom defective imitation of hand postures contrasts with completely normal imitation of finger configurations.[82] By contrast, patients with right brain damage have the most difficulties with finger postures and imitate hand postures nearly as perfectly as controls.[84–86]

The dissociation between imitation of hand and finger postures is very similar to the dissociation between autotopagnosia and finger agnosia. Indeed, nonverbal testing for autotopagnosia and finger agnosia may be conceptualized as being a variant of imitation of hand positions and finger configurations.

BODY-PART SPECIFICITY OF KNOWLEDGE ABOUT THE HUMAN BODY

A possible explanation for body-part specificity of disturbed imitation starts from the assumption that imitation of meaningless gestures is accomplished by body-part coding based on general knowledge about the human body.[82,84,85,87] Body-part coding reduces the multiple visual details of the demonstrated gesture to simple relationships between a limited number of well-defined body parts and produces an equivalence between demonstration and imitation that is independent of the different modalities and perspectives of perceiving one's own and other persons' bodies. It accommodates novel and meaningless gestures to combinations of familiar elements. Demands on body-part coding increase with increasing number and diversity of body parts involved in the gesture.

The body-part specificity of autotopagnosia, finger agnosia, and disturbed imitation of meaningless gestures could be accommodated by the assumption that access to knowledge needed for body-part coding is bound to integrity of the left hemisphere but that an additional right hemisphere contribution is needed when demands on perceptual discrimination of body parts increase. Finger configurations pose exceptionally low demands on access to knowledge because they are constituted by one set of uniform elements that differ only in their serial position; however, for the same reasons, their perceptual discrimination is difficult. By contrast, hand postures demand consideration of a variety of different body parts—like forehead, eyebrows, eyes, nose, cheeks, lips and chin on the face, or shoulder, upper arm, elbow, lower arm, wrist, back, and palm of the hand on the upper extremity. Most of them are, however, perceptually salient and hence easy to discriminate. Imitation of foot postures also involves a number of conceptually different parts—like ankle, heel, calf, big toe, and little toe—several of which are perceptually less salient than the parts of the face that have been used to determine hand postures. The different distribution of demands on body-part coding and perceptual discrimination can account for the predominant affection of hand postures in left brain damage and of finger postures in right brain damage and possibly also for disturbed pointing to proximal body parts in autotopagnosia and disturbed selection of single fingers in finger agnosia.

CONCLUSION

We have postulated that information about one's body is represented at three levels. The review of clinical disorders of body perception confirmed the validity of the classification by demonstrating that distinct disorders arise from disturbances at each level. It did not yield evidence for the existence of a unitary "body schema" underlying all forms of body perception. Body perception for different purposes employs different representations. It is questionable whether some of these representations are specifically dedicated to body perception or are applications of more general mechanisms and representations to perception of that highly familiar but intricate mechanical device that is the human body.

REFERENCES

1. Frederiks JAM: Disorders of the body schema, in Frederiks JAM (ed): *Handbook of Clinical Neurology*. Amsterdam: Elsevier, 1985, vol 1, pp 373–393.
2. Denes G: Disorders of body awareness and body knowledge, in Boller F, Grafman J (eds): *Handbook of Neuropsychology*. Amsterdam, New York, Oxford: Elsevier, 1990, vol 2, pp 207–228.
3. Goldenberg G: Body perception disorders, in Ramachandran VS (ed): *Encyclopedia of the Human Brain*. San Diego, CA: Academic Press; 2002, vol 1, pp 443–458.
4. Poeck K, Orgass B: The concept of the body schema: A critical review and some experimental results. *Cortex* 7:254–277, 1971.
5. Reed CL, Farah MJ: The psychological reality of the body schema: A test with normal participants. *J Exp Psychol Hum Percept Perform* 21:334–343, 1995.
6. Berlucchi G, Aglioti S: The body in the brain: neural bases of corporeal awareness. *Trends Neurosci* 20:560–564, 1997.
7. Buccino G, Binkowski F, Fink GR, et al: Action observation activates premotor and parietal areas in a somatotopic manner: an fMRI study. *Eur J Neurosci* 13:400–404, 2001.
8. Grossman E, Donelly M, Price R, et al: Brain areas involved in perception of biological motion. *J Cogn Neurosci* 12:711–720, 2000.
9. Stein JF: The representation of egocentric space in the posterior parietal cortex. *Behav Brain Sci* 15:691–700, 1992.
10. Milner AD, Goodale MA: *The Visual Brain in Action*. Oxford, New York, Tokyo: Oxford University Press; 1995.
11. Pick A: Zur Pathologie des Bewuβtseins vom eigenen Körper—Ein Beitrag aus der Kriegsmedizin. *Neurol Zentralbl* 34:257–265, 1915.
12. Sirigu A, Grafman J, Bressler K, Sunderland T: Multiple representations contribute to body knowledge processing. *Brain* 114:629–642, 1991.
13. Balint R: Seelenlaehmung des "Schauens," optische Ataxie, raeumlice Stoerung der Aufmerksamkeit. *Monatschr Psychiatr Neurol* 25:51–81, 1909.
14. Rondot P, De Recondo J, Dumas JLR: Visuomotor ataxia. *Brain* 100:355–376, 1977.
15. Perenin MT, Vighetto A: Optic ataxia; a specific disruption in visuomotor mechanisms: I. Different aspects of the deficit in reaching for objects. *Brain* 111:643–674, 1988.
16. Rizzo M, Rotella D, Darling W: Troubled reaching after right occipito-temporal damage. *Neuropsychologia* 30:711–722, 1992.
17. Jeannerod M, Decety J, Michel F: Impairment of grasping movements following a bilateral posterior parietal lesion. *Neuropsychologia* 32:369–380, 1994.
18. Buxbaum LJ, Coslett HB: Subtypes of optic ataxia: Reframing the disconnection account. *Neurocase* 3:159–166, 1997.
19. Chieffi S, Gentilucci M, Allport A, et al: Study of selective reaching and grasping in a patient with unilateral parietal lesion. *Brain* 116:1119–1137, 1993.
20. Mattingley JB, Phillips JG, Bradshaw JL: Impairment of movement execution in unilateral neglect: A kinematic analysis of directional bradykinesia. *Neuropsychologia* 32:1111–1134, 1994.

21. Hermsdörfer J, Ulrich S, Marquardt C, et al: Prehension with the ipsilesional hand after unilateral brain damage. *Cortex* 35:139–162, 1999.
22. Andersen RA: Visual and eye movement functions of the posterior parietal cortex. *Annu Rev Neurosci* 12:377–403, 1989.
23. Poeck K: Zur Psychophysiologie der Phantomerlebnisse. *Nervenarzt* 34:241–256, 1963.
24. Frederiks JAM: Phantom limb and phantom limb pain, in Frederiks JAM (ed): *Handbook of Neurology*. Amsterdam: Elsevier, 1985, vol 1, pp 395–404.
25. Ramachandran VS, Hirstein W: The perception of phantom limbs—the D.O. Hebb lecture. *Brain* 121:1603–1630, 1998.
26. Kroner K, Krebs B, Skov J, Jorgensen HJ: Immediate and long-term phantom breast syndrome after mastectomy: Incidence, clinical characteristics and relationship to premastectomy breast pain. *Pain* 36:327–334, 1989.
27. Christensen K, Blichert-Toft M, Giersing U, et al: Phantom breast syndrome in young women after mastectomy for breast cancer. *Acta Chir Scand* 148:351–354, 1982.
28. Halligan PW, Marshall JC, Wade DT: Three arms: a case study of supernumerary phantom limb after right hemisphere stroke. *J Neurol Neurosurg Psychiatry* 56:159–166, 1993.
29. Haber WE: Observations on phantom-limb phenomena. *Arch Neurol Psychiatry* 75:624–636, 1956.
30. Bornstein B: Sur le phénomène du membre fantome. *Encéphale* 38:32–46, 1949.
31. Saadah ESM, Melzack R: Phantom limb experiences in congenital limb-deficient adults. *Cortex* 30:469–478, 1994.
32. Melzack R, Israel R, Lacroix R, Schultz G: Phantom limbs in people with congenital limb deficiency or amputation in early childhood. *Brain* 120:1603–1620, 1997.
33. Poeck K: Phantome nach Amputation und bei angeborenen Gliedmaβenmangel. *Dtsch Med Wochenschr* 46:2367–2374, 1969.
34. Ramachandran VS, Rogers-Ramachandran D: Synaesthesia in phantom limbs induced with mirrors. *Proc R Soc Lond B* 263:377–386, 1996.
35. Cronholm B: Phantom limbs in amputees: Study of changes in integration of centripetal impulses with special reference to referred sensation. *Acta Psychiatr Neurol Scand Suppl* 72:1–310, 1951.
36. Halligan PJ, Marshall JC, Wade DT: Sensory disorganization and perceptual plasticity after limb amputation: A follow-up study. *Neuroreport* 5:1341–1345, 1994.
37. Halligan PJ, Marshall JC, Wade DT, et al: Thumb in cheek? Sensory reorganization and perceptual plasticity after limb amputation. *Neuroreport* 4:233–236, 1993.
38. Knecht S, Henningsen H, Höhling C, et al: Plasticity of plasticity? Changes in the pattern of perceptual correlates of reorganization after amputation. *Brain* 121:717–724, 1998.
39. Knecht S, Henningsen H, Elbert T, et al: Reorganizational and perceptional changes after amputation. *Brain* 119:1213–1219, 1996.
40. Kew JJM, Halligan PW, Marshall JC, et al: Abnormal access of axial vibrotactile input to deafferented somatosensory cortex in human upper limb amputees. *J Neurophysiol* 77:2753–2764, 1997.
41. Aglioti S, Cortese F, Franchini C: Rapid sensory remapping in the adult human brain as inferred from phantom breast sensation. *Neuroreport* 5:473–476, 1994.
42. Weinstein S, Sersen EA, Vetter RJ: Phantom and somatic sensation in cases of congenital aplasia. *Cortex* 1:276–290, 1964.
43. Melzack R: Phantom limbs and the concept of a neuromatrix. *Trends Neurosci* 13:88–92, 1990.
44. Lacroix R, Melzack R, Smith D, Mitchell N: Multiple phantom limbs in a child. *Cortex* 28:503–508, 1992.
45. Ramachandran VS: Behavioral and magnetoencephalographic correlates of plasticity in the adult human brain. *Proc Natl Acad Sci U S A* 90:10413–10420, 1993.
46. Brugger P, Kollias S, Müri RM, et al: Beyond remembering: Phantom sensations of congenitally absent limbs. *Proc Natl Acad Sci U S A* 97:6167–6172, 2000.
47. Poeck K: Phantoms following amputation in early childhood and in congenital absence of limbs. *Cortex* 1:269–275, 1964.
48. Flor H, Elbert T, Knecht S, et al: Phantom-limb pain as a perceptual correlate of cortical reorganization following arm amputation. *Nature* 375:482–484, 1995.
49. Pascual-Leone A, Peris M, Pascual AP, Catalá MD: Reorganization of human cortical motor output maps following traumatic forearm amptutation. *Neuroreport* 7:2068–2070, 1996.
50. Head H, Holmes G: Sensory disturbances from cerebral lesions. *Brain* 34:102–254, 1911.
51. Appenzeller O, Bicknell JM: Effects of nervous system lesions on phantom experience in amputees. *Neurology* 19:141–146, 1969.
52. Jeannerod M: *The Neural and Behavioural Organization of Goal-Directed Movements*. Oxford: Clarendon Press, 1988.
53. Karnath HO: Subjective body orientation in neglect and the interactive contribution of neck muscle proprioception and vestibular stimulation. *Brain* 117:1001–1012, 1994.

54. Bisiach E, Perani D, Vallar G, Berti A: Unilateral neglect: personal and extrapersonal. *Neuropsychologia* 24:759–767, 1986.
55. Beschin N, Robertson IH: Personal versus extrapersonal neglect: A group study of their dissociation using a reliable clinical test. *Cortex* 33:379–384, 1997.
56. Guariglia C, Padovani A, Pantano P, Pizzamiglio L: Unilateral neglect restricted to visual imagery. *Nature* 364:235–237, 1993.
57. Aglioti S, Smania N, Manfredi M, Berlucchi G: Disownership of left hand and objects related to it in a patient with right brain damage. *Neuroreport* 8:293–296, 1996.
58. Moscovitch M, Behrmann M: Coding of spatial information in the somatosensory system: Evidence from patients with neglect following parietal lobe damage. *J Cogn Neurosci* 6:151–155, 1994.
59. Mattingley JB, Bradshaw JL: Can tactile neglect occur at an intra-limb level? Vibrotactile reaction times in patients with right hemisphere damage. *Behav Neurol* 7:67–77, 1994.
60. Guariglia C, Antonucci G: Personal and extrapersonal space: A case of neglect dissociation. *Neuropsychologia* 30:1001–1010, 1992.
61. Gerstmann J: Problems of imperception of disease and of impaired body territories with organic lesions. Relation to body scheme and its disorders. *Arch Neurol Psychiatry* 48:890–913, 1942.
62. De Renzi E, Scotti G: Autotopagnosia: fiction or reality? *Arch Neurol* 23:221–227, 1970.
63. Poncet M, Pellissier JF, Sebahoun M, Nasser CJ: A propos d'un cas d'autotopagnosie secondaire à une lésion pariéto-occipitale de l'hémisphère majeur. *Encéphale* 61:1–14, 1971.
64. Assal G, Butters J: Troubles du schéma corporel lors des atteintes hémisphériques gauches. *Schweiz Med Rundsch* 62:172–179, 1973.
65. Ogden JA: Autotopagnosia. Occurence in a patient without nominal aphasia and with an intact ability to point to parts of animals and objects. *Brain* 108:1009–1022, 1985.
66. Semenza C: Impairment of localization of body parts following brain damage. *Cortex* 24:443–450, 1988.
67. Denes G, Cappelletti JY, Zilli T, et al: A category-specific deficit of spatial representation: the case of autotopagnosia. *Neuropsychologia* 38:345–350, 2000.
68. Buxbaum LJ, Coslett HB: Specialised structural descriptions for human body parts: Evidence from autotopagnosia. *Cogn Neuropsychol* 18:289–306, 2001.
69. Denes G, Caviezel F, Semenza C: Difficulty in reaching objects and body parts: A sensory motor disconnection syndrome. *Cortex* 18:165–173, 1982.
70. Sauguet J, Benton AL, Hecaen H: Disturbances of the body schema in relation to language impairment and hemispheric locus of lesion. *J Neurol Neurosurg Psychiatry* 34:496–501, 1971.
71. Gerstmann J: Zur Symptomatologie der Hirnläsionen im Übergangsgebiet der unteren Parietal- und mittleren Occipitalwindung. *Nervenarzt* 3:691–696, 1930.
72. Benton AL: The fiction of the "Gerstmann syndrome." *J Neurol Neurosurg Psychiatry* 24:176–181, 1961.
73. Poeck K, Orgass B: An experimental investigation of finger agnosia. *Neurology* 19:801–807, 1969.
74. Gainotti G, Cianchetti C, Tiacci C: The influence of the hemispheric side of lesion on nonverbal tasks of finger localization. *Cortex* 8:364–381, 1972.
75. Mayer E, Martory MD, Pegna AJ, et al: A pure case of Gerstmann syndrome with a subangular lesion. *Brain* 122:1107–1120, 1999.
76. Kinsbourne M, Warrington EK: A study of finger agnosia. *Brain* 85:47–66, 1962.
77. Tucha O, Steup O, Smely C, Lange KW: Toe agnosia in Gerstmann syndrome. *J Neurol Neurosurg Psychiatry* 63:399–403, 1997.
78. De Renzi E, Motti F, Nichelli P: Imitating gestures—a quantitative approach to ideomotor apraxia. *Arch Neurol* 37:6–10, 1980.
79. De Renzi E: Apraxia, in Boller F, Grafman J (eds): *Handbook of Clinical Neuropsychology*. Amsterdam, New York, Oxford: Elsevier, 1990, vol 2, pp 245–263.
80. Rothi LJG, Ochipa C, Heilman KM: A cognitive neuropsychological model of limb praxis. *Cogn Neuropsychol* 8:443–458, 1991.
81. Mehler MF: Visuo-imitative apraxia. *Neurology* 37(suppl):129, 1987.
82. Goldenberg G, Hagmann S: The meaning of meaningless gestures: A study of visuo-imitative apraxia. *Neuropsychologia* 35:333–341, 1997.
83. Goldenberg G: Imitating gestures and manipulating a mannikin—the representation of the human body in ideomotor apraxia. *Neuropsychologia* 33:63–72, 1995.
84. Goldenberg G: Matching and imitation of hand and finger postures in patients with damage in the left or right hemisphere. *Neuropsychologia* 37:559–366, 1999.
85. Goldenberg G, Strauss S: Hemisphere asymmetries for imitation of novel gestures. *Neurology* 59:893–897, 2002.
86. Goldenberg G: Defective imitation of gestures in patients with damage in the left or right hemisphere. *J Neurol Neurosurg Psychiatry* 61:176–180, 1996.
87. Meltzoff AN, Moore MK: Explaining facial imitation: A theoretical model. *Early Dev Parent* 6:179–192, 1997.

Chapter 24

VISUOSPATIAL FUNCTION

Martha J. Farah

The integrality of vision and action has recently come to be recognized in vision research (e.g., Milner and Goodale 1995) and is starkly apparent in the behavior of patients with damage to posterior parietal cortex and certain other visual areas. Whereas they may be able to read, recognize faces, perceive colors, and so on, their ability to move through space, reach for objects, or assemble an object from spatially separated parts may be severely impaired. Humans have a constant need to move through space and manipulate the spatial disposition of objects and have evolved a complex system of spatial vision. Damage to any part of this system will result in a visuospatial disorder, the precise nature of which depends on the location of the lesion.

For purposes of organizing a review of these disorders, it is helpful to divide them into two general categories: disorders relating to the space visible at a given moment, in which all relevant stimuli can be perceived from one vantage point given free eye movement, and disorders relating to the topography of an environment, in which multiple views must be integrated into a large-scale spatial representation. These are distinct abilities, although they can, of course, influence one another. For example, certain impairments of the first type of ability will impact a person's ability to learn or navigate a larger-scale environment. The major subtypes of each of these disorders are reviewed in this chapter, including their main features, associated lesion sites, and implications for our understanding of normal vision.

VISIBLE (SMALL-SCALE) SPACE

Impaired Attention to Space

Hemispatial neglect is the most common disorder of visuospatial perception and is mentioned only in passing here because it is the subject of Chaps. 25 and 26. In its most typical manifestation, a patient with neglect will be unaware of the locations and objects contralateral to the brain lesion, which most often affects right posterior parietal cortex. Most authors discuss neglect as a disorder of spatial attention, whereby information from the contralateral hemispace is not fully encoded due to insufficient spatial attention (e.g., Heilman and Valenstein, 1979). Other authors prefer to view it as a disorder of spatial representation, whereby the brain fails to construct a full internal representation of the affected side of space (e.g., Bisiach and Luzzatti, 1978). Still others fail to see the distinction, as one cannot attend to a stimulus without representing it, and one cannot represent it without attending to it (Farah, 2000). Balint's syndrome, which is the subject of Chap. 27, affects processing of stimuli on both sides of space and is sometimes considered a bilateral neglect syndrome.

Impaired Perception of Location and Orientation

It is difficult to conceive of a person having vision with preserved color and form perception but the inability to perceive location. Yet just such a dissociation, known as *visual disorientation,* exists. Patients with visual disorientation are not only inaccurate in pointing or reaching to an object but also fail at describing its location verbally. For example, they will have difficulty answering whether a pen is above or below a pair of eyeglasses held in front of them by the examiner. Not surprisingly, such patients are severely handicapped in their everyday lives, being effectively blind as far as most visual interactions with the world go. It has been known for many decades that the critical lesion site is the occipitoparietal junction, and in some cases a unilateral form of the disorder is observed after damage to either the left or right hemisphere alone (Riddoch, 1935). Along with visual object agnosia (see Chap. 18), this is probably the strongest evidence for the hypothesis of "two cortical visual systems" in human vision, as it demonstrates the mutual independence (i.e., one can function without the other) of object recognition and spatial localization.

In rare cases, patients may develop an *orientation agnosia,* the selective impairment of orientation perception. Such cases have been described by Turnbull and colleagues (e.g., Turnbull, Beschin, and Della Salla, 1997). One patient's orientation perception was sufficiently compromised that he had hung pictures upside down on the wall of his home.

A subtler impairment of spatial perception, generally brought out by testing, is the impaired perception of line orientation. A widely used test of orientation perception is that of Benton, Varney, and Hamsher (1978), in which diagonal lines of varying orientation are presented and the patient must indicate the identical orientations in an array of oriented lines. The spatial nature of the judgment and the minimal nature of the shape information involved suggests that this ability would depend strongly on parietal cortex, and indeed that is the case. There is also a pronounced asymmetry in favor of greater right hemisphere involvement in this ability (De Renzi, 1982).

Impaired Visually Guided Reaching

Although it can be difficult to disentangle impairments of visual localization from impairments of visually guided reaching, a number of careful studies have done so (DeRenzi, 1982). The latter impairment, also known as optic ataxia, is usually observed in unilateral form, but this generality covers a surprising array of variants. The unilateral aspect may pertain to the hemispace, as when either limb is inaccurate reaching for objects in, for example, the left hemispace. Alternatively, it may pertain to the limb, as when one limb—for example, the left—is inaccurate in reaching for objects at any location. It may even combine these two forms of unilateral selectivity, as when one arm (e.g., the left) is disproportionately inaccurate reaching to the same (left) hemispace compared to other limb-space combinations. Some patients with unilateral lesions show a milder level of optic ataxia on the ipsilateral side of space. Optic ataxia usually follows damage high in the parietal lobe, anterior to the regions most likely to cause visual disorientation. The precise scope of the impairment presumably depends on what parts of parietal gray and underlying white matter are damaged.

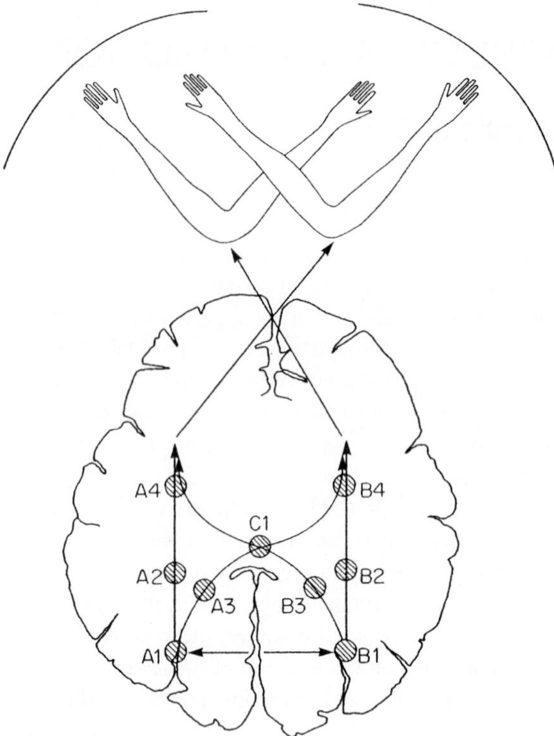

Figure 24-1
Schematic diagram of different possible lesions interrupting visuomotor control, which would result in different patterns of limb and visual field differences in visually guided reaching. Lesions at points marked 1 and 4 would result in pure field selectivity and limb selectivity, respectively. Lesions at points marked 2 and 3 would result in both field and limb selectivity, contralateral and ipsilateral, respectively. A lesion at C would result in a different pattern of field and limb selectivity, with contralateral combinations of limb and field, on either side, impaired (as in callosotomy patients). (From De Renzi E: Disorders of Space Exploration and Cognition, New York: John Wiley, 1982.)

Figure 24-1 shows how different combinations of hemispace and limb selectivity could result from interruption of the pathways from visual to motor cortex at different points.

Impaired Construction: Drawing and Building

Before the days when laptop computers could be carried to patients' bedsides, clinicians relied heavily on construction tasks to assess visuospatial function. These included copying meaningful drawings and arbitrary geometric figures as well as recreating a pattern made from sticks or blocks (the latter either in two or three dimensions). Impairments in construction, known as *constructional apraxia,* were therefore an important topic of study in the neuropsychology of the 1970s and 1980s and continue to be assessed in most mental status exams to this day (see Chap. 2).

Constructional apraxia differs in two important ways from the other impairments reviewed here. Whereas the perception of object location, navigation through the environment, and so on are basic spatial abilities for which our brains may have evolved specific systems over the course of the millennia, the scope of abilities classified together by the category of constructional apraxia does not seem to instantiate the same kind of basic category. To be sure, the ability to construct complex objects from simple ones would have great adaptive value. What is in doubt is that a single system is responsible for the ability to draw arbitrary geometric figures, meaningful line drawings, and build block or stick structures.

It seems likely, therefore, that the disorder known as constructional apraxia is many disorders, most of which are secondary to other, more fundamental impairments, including visuospatial perception, visually guided action, and executive function. Sometimes the underlying cause of the constructional impairment is fairly obvious, as when a patient with prefrontal damage and disorganization evident in other tasks produces a disorganized construction. Other times, it is difficult to characterize the underlying impairment. For example, the bicycles shown in Fig. 24-2 were drawn by patients with unilateral posterior brain damage. There is a clear trend for patients with left-sided injuries to produce spare, impoverished constructions and those with right-sided injuries to produce abundantly detailed

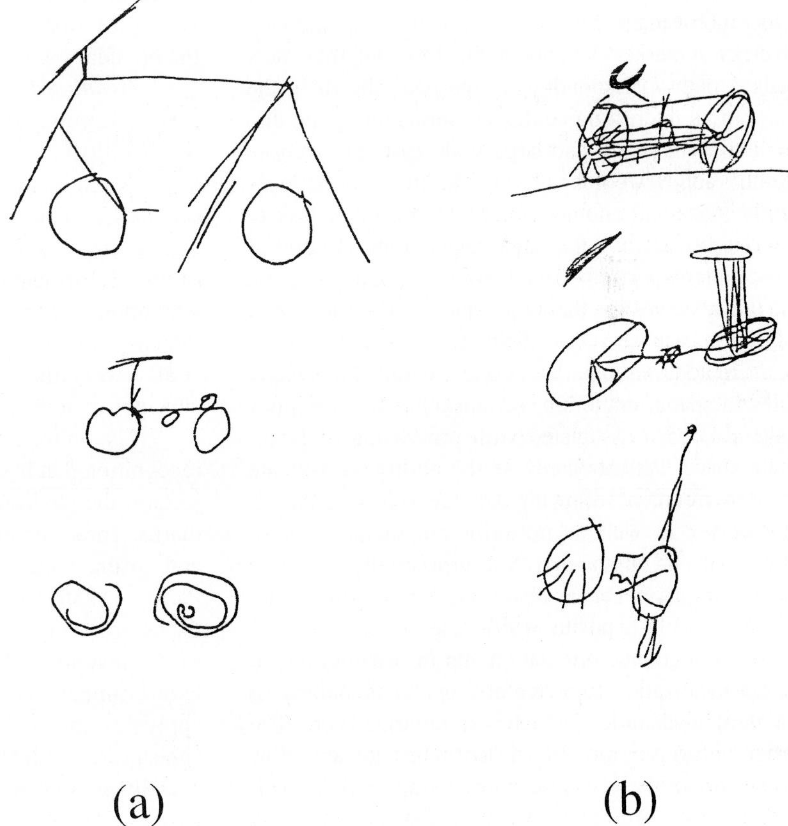

Figure 24-2
Examples of constructional apraxia in a bicycle drawing task following (a) left and (b) right hemisphere lesions. (From McFie J, Zangwill OL: Visual-constructive disabilities associated with lesions of the left cerebral hemisphere. Brain 83:243–261, 1960.)

but spatially disorganized constructions. However, the underlying impairment in each case is not clear.

ENVIRONMENTAL (LARGE-SCALE) SPACE

There is relatively little experimental literature on disorders of large-scale spatial cognition. This is undoubtedly due to the practical difficulties of designing "test materials" the size of rooms, houses, or city blocks. Most of what we know about topographic orientation comes from individual case reports of patients with clinically significant topographic disorders. In some of the more recent reports, patients were studied using experimental designs tailored to the patients' own environments.

The one exception to the rule that the neuropsychology of large-scale space has not been studied in any systematic way using experimental tasks originates with the work of Semmes et al. (1955), who developed a locomotor maze. Subjects are given a map showing an array of markers laid out on the floor, and they must walk a path corresponding to the path shown in the map. In an interesting contrast demonstrating the dissociability of small- and large-scale spatial cognition, Ratcliff and Newcombe (1973) administered the locomotor maze and another small tabletop maze task to a group of focally brain-damaged patients. Several of these patients performed well on one task and poorly on the other, suggesting that large- and small-scale spatial cognition is subserved by distinct neural systems.

In addition to parietal cortex, which plays many roles in spatial cognition, certain other brain regions have also been associated with processing of large-scale space. Patients can lose the ability to navigate their environment following damage to posterior parietal cortex as well as posterior cingulate, parahippocampal, and lingual gyri. Not surprisingly, the nature of their impairments can also vary. A recent review by Aguirre and D'Esposito (1999) used cognitive theories of topographic orientation and information about lesion localization to arrive at a useful taxonomy of topographic disorders, which is summarized here. The different forms of topographic disorientation are informative about the organization of topographic knowledge in the normal brain. The patterns of preserved and impaired abilities described below suggest that spatial orientation in the environment involves both specialized topographic representations and more general spatial abilities, that spatial and landmark knowledge of the environment are subserved by different systems, and that the acquisition of topographic knowledge may be carried out by a specialized learning system.

Egocentric disorientation is the term used to describe patients whose topographic disorientation is secondary to visual disorientation, discussed earlier. Not surprisingly, patients who cannot localize seen objects in space are severely handicapped in navigating both familiar and unfamiliar terrain. Of course, this form of topographic impairment is not specific to topographic knowledge. A representative patient, described by Levine, Warach, and Farah (1985), was unable to find his way even around his own home, despite intact recognition of objects and landmarks, and showed spatial impairment on even the simplest small-scale spatial tasks. The critical lesion site, as noted earlier, is the posterior parietal cortex bilaterally, often right at the boundary with occipital cortex.

Heading disorientation is a more specific impairment in large-scale spatial representation, consisting of the inability to perceive and remember the spatial relations among landmarks in the environment and one's orientation relative to them. These patients, who are rare in the literature, do not have a more global form of visual disorientation but are selectively impaired at way finding, map use, and other tests of orientation in the environment. Three cases described by Takahashi et al. (1997) illustrate this disorder. The critical lesion site appears to be the posterior cingulate gyrus.

Landmark agnosia is an impairment of visual recognition that is selective or disproportionate for objects in the environment that normally serve as landmarks. These include buildings, monuments, squares, and so on. Patients with landmark agnosia, such as Pallis's (1955) case, retain their spatial knowledge of the environment, as evidenced by good descriptions of routes, layouts, and maps. However, without the ability to discriminate one building from another, they cannot apply this knowledge. The typical lesions in landmark agnosia are similar to those of other visual agnosias, especially prosopagnosia—that is, the inferior surface of

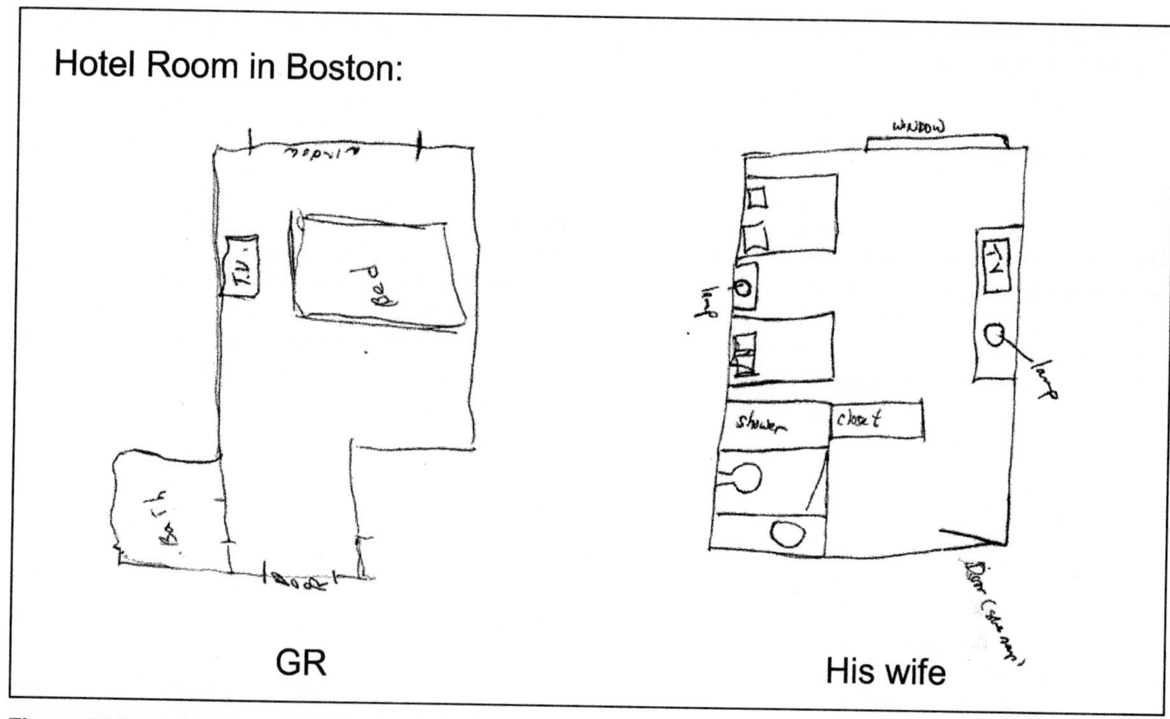

Figure 24-3
Maps of a hotel room drawn by a patient with anterograde topographic disorientation and by his neurologically normal wife.

the occipitotemporal regions, either bilateral or right-sided.

Anterograde disorientation refers to a topographic impairment that encompasses both spatial and landmark knowledge and is selective for the acquisition of this knowledge. Such patients show normal topographic abilities for environments that were familiar before their brain injury, but cannot learn to navigate new environments. The critical lesion site for anterograde disorientation appears to be the right parahippocampal gyrus. Epstein et al. (2001) describe a patient who provides a dramatic example of a selective impairment in learning new environments. Although able to draw an accurate map of the house in which he lived years earlier, the map of his current house was drawn with great difficulty and some inaccuracy, and, as shown in Fig. 24-3, he was completely unable to draw a map of the hotel room in which he had just spent 2 days. He was also unable to learn new landmarks despite good recognition of famous landmarks. Such cases suggest a heretofore unsuspected form of specialization within memory systems for learning the spatial environment.

REFERENCES

Aguirre GK, D'Esposito M: Topographical disorientation: A synthesis and taxonomy. *Brain* 122:1613–1628, 1999.

Benton AL, Varney NR, Hamsher KD: Visuospatial judgement: A clinical test. *Arch Neurol* 35:364–367, 1978.

Bisiach E, Luzzatti C: Unilateral neglect of representational space. *Cortex* 14:129–133, 1978.

De Renzi E: *Disorders of Space Exploration and Cognition*. New York: John Wiley, 1982.

Epstein R, DeYoe EA, Press DZ, et al: Neuropsychological evidence for a topographical learning mechanism in parahippocampal cortex. *Cognit Neuropsychol* 18: 481–508, 2001.

Farah MJ: *The Cognitive Neuroscience of Vision*. Oxford: Blackwell, 2000.

Heilman KM, Valenstein E: Mechanisms underlying hemispatial neglect. *Ann Neurol* 5:166–170, 1979.

Levine DN, Warach J, Farah MJ: Two visual systems in mental imagery: Dissociation of "What" and "Where" in imagery disorders due to bilateral posterior cerebral lesions. *Neurology* 35:1010–1018, 1985.

Milner AD, Goodale MA (eds): *The Visual Brain in Action*. Oxford, UK: Oxford Science Publications, 1995.

Pallis CA: Impaired identification of faces and places with agnosia for colors. *J Neurol Neurosurg Psychiatry* 18:218–224, 1955.

Ratcliff G, Newcombe F: Spatial orientation in man: Effects of left, right, and bilateral posterior cerebral lesions. *J Neurol Neurosurg Psychiatry* 36:448–454, 1973.

Riddoch G: Visual disorientation in homonymous half-fields. *Brain* 58:376–382, 1935.

Semmes J, Weinstein S, Ghent L, Teuber HL: Spatial orientation in man: I. Analyses by locus of lesion. *J Psychol* 39:227–244, 1955.

Takahashi N, Kawamura MKS, Kasahata N, Hirayama K: Pure topographic disorientation due to right retrosplenial lesion. *Neurology* 49:464–469, 1997.

Turnbull OH, Beschin N, Della Sala S: Agnosia for object orientation: Implications for theories of object recognition. *Neuropsychologia* 35:153–163, 1997.

Part 4

DISORDERS OF ATTENTION AND AWARENESS

Chapter 25

NEGLECT: CLINICAL AND ANATOMIC ISSUES

Kenneth M. Heilman
Robert T. Watson
Edward Valenstein

Neglect is a failure to report, respond, or orient to stimuli that are presented contralateral to a brain lesion when this failure is not due to elementary sensory or motor disorders.[1] Many subtypes of neglect have been described. A major distinction is between neglect of perceptual input, termed *sensory neglect* or *inattention,* and neglect affecting response outputs, termed *motor* or *intentional neglect*. Some further distinctions are outlined below.

Sensory neglect involves a selective deficit in awareness, which may apply to all stimuli on the affected side of space (*spatial neglect*) or be confined to stimuli impinging on the patient's body (*personal neglect*). It may even effect awareness of one side of internal mental images (*representational neglect*). The perceptual modalities affected by neglect may also vary: subtypes of sensory neglect exist for the visual, auditory, and tactile modalities. The deficit in awareness is accompanied by an abnormal attentional bias. Attention is usually biased toward the ipsilesional side (*contralateral neglect*) but in rare cases may be contralesional (*ipsilateral neglect*). Once attention is engaged on an ipsilesional stimulus, subjects may have difficulty disengaging their attention to move it to the contralesional side. If the lack of awareness and attentional bias are present only when there is a competing stimulus at a more ipsilateral location, the disorder is termed *extinction*. Many patients with neglect recover and become able to detect isolated contralesional stimuli, but they continue to manifest extinction.

Motor or *intentional neglect* involves a response failure that cannot be explained by weakness, sensory loss, or unawareness. There may be a failure to move a limb (*limb akinesia*), or the limb can be moved but only after a long delay and strong encouragement (*hypokinesia*). Patients with intentional neglect who can move may make movements of decreased amplitude (*hypometria*). They may also have an inability to maintain posture or movements (*impersistence*). Patients with motor neglect who can move their contralesional limb may fail to move this limb (or have a delay) when they are also required to move their ipsilateral limb (*motor extinction*). Limb akinesia, hypokinesia, hypometria, and motor impersistence can affect some or all parts of the body, including limbs, eyes, or head. The elements of intentional neglect discussed above can be *directional* (toward the contralesional hemispace) or *spatial* (within the contralesional hemispace). Patients with motor neglect may have intentional biases such that there is a propensity to move toward ipsilesional space. There may also be impaired ability to disengage from motor activities (*motor perseveration*).

TESTING FOR NEGLECT

In this brief review we cannot address all aspects of testing; therefore, for a complete discussion and list of references, the reader is referred to Heilman and coworkers.[1]

Inattention or Sensory Neglect

To test for inattention, the patient is presented with unilateral stimuli on either the ipsilesional or contralesional side in random order. If a patient fails to detect more stimuli on the contralesional side than the ipsilesional side, it would suggest that the patient is suffering from inattention. However, if the patient totally fails to detect any stimuli on the contralesional side, it is often difficult to tell whether or not the patient has inattention or a sensory loss. The auditory modality is the least difficult in which to dissociate inattention and sensory loss, because sounds made on one side of the head project to both ears, and each ear projects to both the ipsilateral and the contralateral hemisphere. Therefore, if a patient is unaware of noises made on one side of his or her head, this unawareness cannot be explained by a sensory defect and suggests that the patient has inattention. In the visual modality, because unawareness may be hemispatial (body-centered) rather than retinotopic, having the patient deviate the eyes toward ipsilateral hemispace may allow him or her to become aware of stimuli projected to the contralesional portion of the retina. In regard to tactile neglect, one may have to use caloric stimulation of the ear to see if the patient can detect stimuli during such stimulation. One may also use psychophysiologic techniques such as evoked potentials or galvanic skin responses to see whether patients who are unaware of stimuli demonstrate autonomic signs of stimulus detection.[2]

Extinction

To test for extinction, one may randomly intermix the unilateral stimuli described above with bilateral simultaneous stimuli. The stimuli can be given in any modality (e.g., visual, auditory, tactile). When a subject has hemianopia, extinction may occur even within the ipsilesional visual field.

Intentional or Motor Neglect

Patients who have severe limb akinesia may appear to have a hemiparesis. An arm may flaccidly hang off the bed or wheelchair. Sometimes, with strong encouragement from the examiner, it can be demonstrated that such a patient has normal strength. Some patients, however, will still not move, and one may have to rely on brain imaging to learn whether the corticospinal tract is involved. In patients with motor neglect, the lesion should not involve the corticospinal system. Magnetic stimulation may also be helpful in demonstrating that the corticospinal tract is normal.[3] As discussed, patients with hypokinesia are reluctant to move the affected arm or only move it after delay. However, once they have moved, their strength may be normal. To test for hypometria, the arm is passively moved or the patient is shown a line and asked to make a movement of the same length. Patients with hypometria will undershoot the target. To test for impersistence, the patient is asked to sustain a posture. Patients with impersistence cannot maintain postures. As mentioned, patients can be tested for forms of motor neglect by using the limbs, eyes, or even head. They can be tested in ipsilateral versus contralateral hemispace and in an ipsilesional versus contralesional direction. For example, patients with right hemisphere lesions might have trouble spontaneously looking leftward (directional akinesia) and even have their eyes deviate to the right (gaze palsy). Other patients might be able to look leftward but make small (hypometric) saccades (directional hypometria). Patients with right hemisphere lesions who are able to look to the left might be unable to sustain gaze in this direction (directional impersistence).

Further Assessments of Spatial Neglect

A more complete assessment of neglect involves additional tests, which require the patient to perform simple tasks that go beyond the reporting of a stimulus or the movement of eyes or limbs toward a target. These tasks can nevertheless be performed at bedside without special equipment. The four most commonly used tests are described here.

In the *line bisection task,* the patient is given a long line and asked to indicate its midpoint (Fig. 25-1). Although horizontal lines are most commonly used (intersection of the coronal and axial planes), neglect has been reported in the vertical dimension (both up neglect and down neglect) and in the radial dimension (near neglect and far neglect). In general, the longer the line, the greater the percentage of error. Placing the line in contralesional hemispace can also increase the severity of the error, as can putting cues on the ipsilesional side.

In performing the *cancellation task,* a sheet of paper that contains targets is placed before the patient and the patient is asked to mark out (cancel) all the targets (Fig. 25-2). Increasing the number of targets can increase the sensitivity of this test. Increasing the difficulty with which one discriminates targets from distractors can also increase the sensitivity of this task.

In testing *drawing,* the patient should be asked to draw spontaneously as well as to copy figures (Figs. 25-3 and 25-4). Copying asymmetrical nonsense figures may be more difficult than copying well-known symmetrical figures.

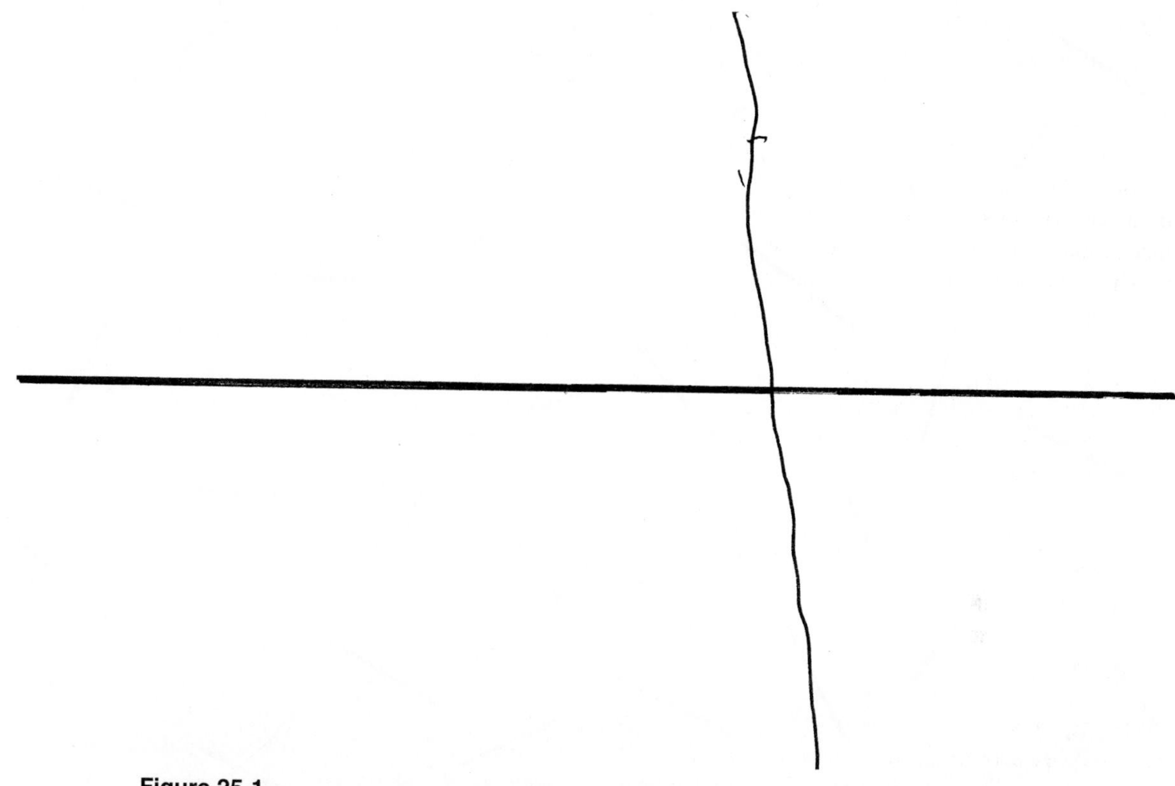

Figure 25-1
Line bisection task performed by a patient with a right hemisphere infarction and left hemispatial neglect. (Courtesy of Dr. Todd E. Feinberg.)

In testing for representational neglect, one should ask a subject to *image a familar scene* and then report what he or she sees. A patient with representational neglect will recall more objects from the ipsilesional than the contralesional part of the image.

Further testing can elucidate the underlying systems of spatial representation, attention, and intention that are affected. For example, it may be difficult to dissociate sensory attentional disorders from motor intentional disorders. In general, the best means of doing this is by performing cross-response tasks where the subject responds in one side of space to a stimulus presented on the opposite side. Video cameras, strings and pulleys, or mirrors can be used in the performance of a cross response task.

To dissociate intentional from representational defects, one can use a fixed-aperture technique. To do this, an opaque sheet with a fixed window is placed over a sheet with targets so that only one target can be seen at a time, thereby reducing attentional demands. In one-half the trials, the subject moves the top sheet; in the other trials, the subject moves the target sheet. A failure to explore one portion of the target sheet in both conditions suggests a representational defect, and a failure to explore opposite sides of the target sheet in direct and indirect conditions suggests a motor intentional deficit.[4]

To dissociate spatial neglect of one side of the environment from neglect of one side of the person, one can ask the patient to lie down on his or her side. This decouples the environmental left and right from the body's left and right. If the patient has a right hemispheric lesion, is lying on the right side, and now fails to detect targets toward the ceiling, the neglect is body-centered. However, if the patient continues to neglect targets on the left side of the room, the neglect is environmentally centered (see Chap. 26).[5,6]

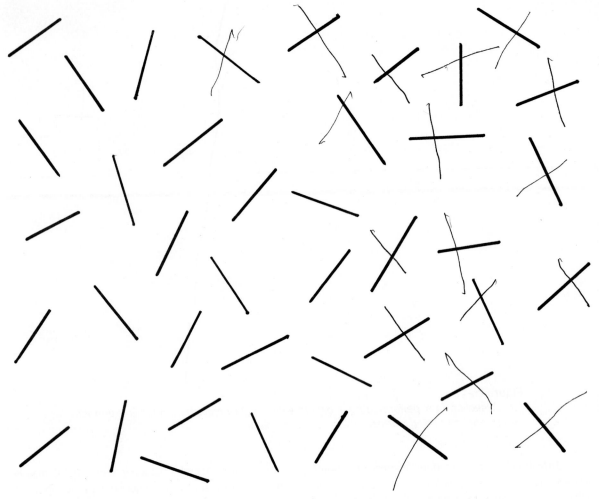

Figure 25-2
Cancellation task of same patient as in Fig. 25-1. (Courtesy of Dr. Todd E. Feinberg.)

PATHOPHYSIOLOGY

As the foregoing review suggests, neglect is not a homogeneous syndrome. The neglect syndrome has not only many manifestations but also many levels of explanation. For a more complete discussion, see Heilman and coworkers.[1] The heterogeneity of neglect is apparent on an anatomic level as well.

In humans, neglect is most often associated with lesions of the inferior parietal lobe (IPL), which includes Brodmann's areas 40 and 39. However, neglect has also been reported from dorsolateral frontal lesions, medial frontal lesions that include the cingulate gyrus, thalamic-mesencephalic lesions, basal ganglia, and white matter lesions. Because there is a limit on the anatomic, physiologic, and behavioral research that can be done in humans, much of what we know about the pathophysiology of the neglect syndrome comes from research on Old World monkeys. Monkeys also have an IPL; however, their IPL is Brodmann's area 7. In humans, the intraparietal sulcus separates the superior parietal area, Brodmann's area 7, from the inferior parietal lobule, Brodmann's areas 40 and 39. Some have thought that the IPL of monkeys is a homologue of the IPL in humans. Others, however, have thought that both banks of the superior temporal sulcus (STS)

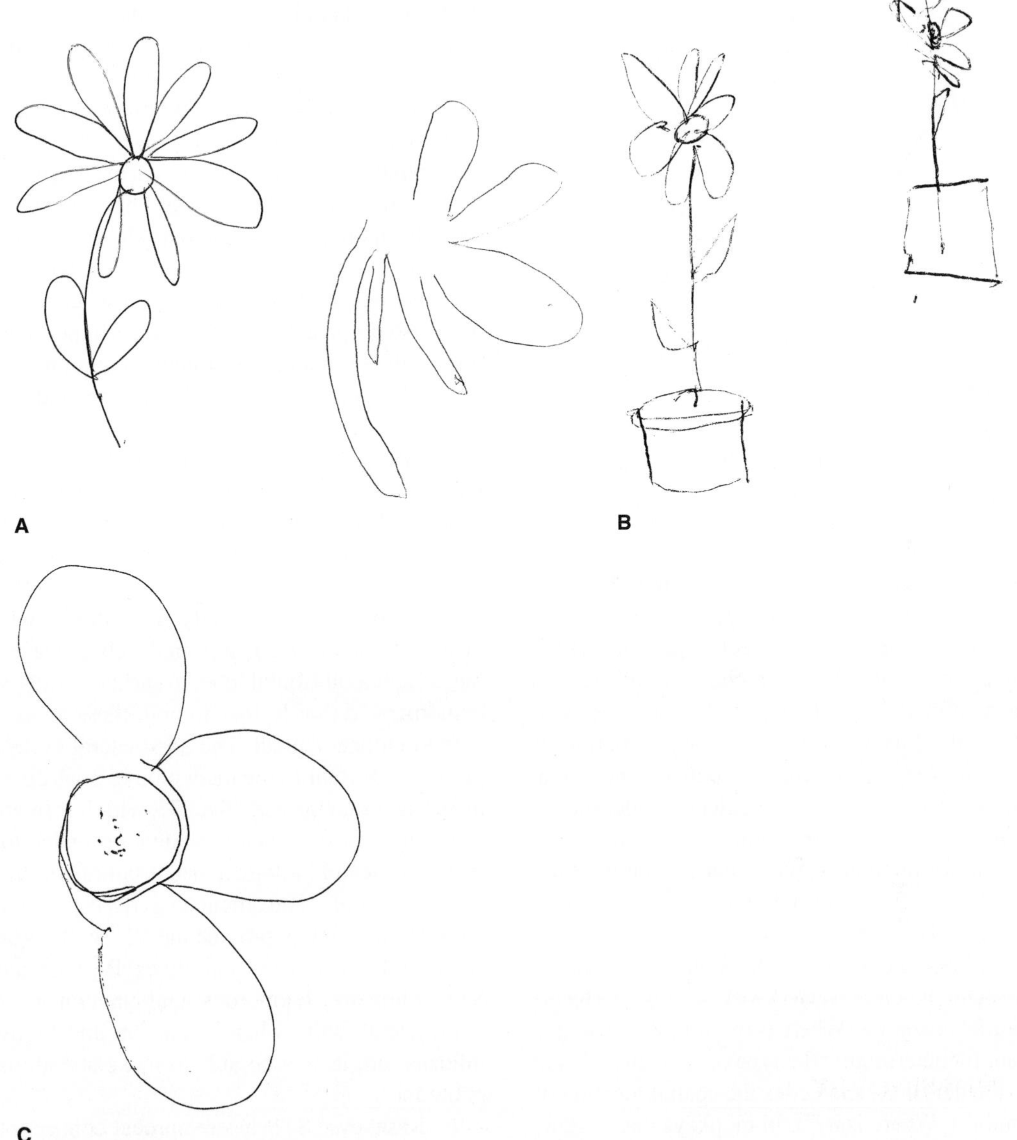

Figure 25-3
Copies of flower demonstrate left hemispatial neglect. A *and* B *provide models on left, patient production on right. (Parts* A *and* B *courtesy of Dr. Todd E. Feinberg; part* C *courtesy of Dr. Robert Rafal.)*

are the homologue of the inferior parietal lobule in humans. We[7] have demonstrated that spatial neglect in monkeys is primarily associated with ablation of the STS region and not the IPL. These results suggest that, in regard to neglect, it is the monkeys' STS that is the homologue of the temporoparietal junction of humans.

Anatomic studies of the STS of monkeys have provided some information as to why this area produces neglect when ablated. The STS is composed of

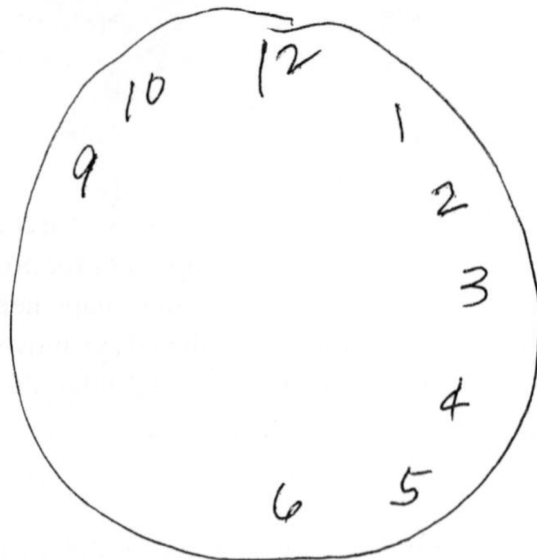

Figure 25-4
Clock drawn by a patient with left hemispatial neglect. (Courtesy of Dr. Robert Rafal.)

multiple subareas and is one of the sites of multimodal sensory convergence. Visual, auditory, and somatosensory association cortices all project to portions of the STS. In addition, the STS has reciprocal connections to other multimodal convergence areas, such as monkeys' IPL (Brodmann's area 7). Because ablation of area 7 in monkeys, a multimodal convergence area, was not associated with spatial neglect, we do not believe that ablation of a sensory convergence area alone can account for the unawareness that is seen with neglect syndrome. Therefore, we[7] have proposed a role for monkeys' STS in awareness.

Mishkin and colleagues[8] have suggested that the visual system, when presented with stimuli, performs dual parallel processes. Whereas the ventral division is important for determining the type of stimulus ("What is it?"), the dorsal system codes the spatial location of the stimulus ("Where is it?"). In monkeys the "where" system is in part mediated by the posterior portion of Brodmann's area 7 or the monkey's IPL, and the "what" system is in part being mediated by the inferior visual association cortex found in the ventral temporal lobe. It has long been recognized that bilateral ventral temporal lesions in humans and monkeys induce visual object agnosia, a deficit in the "what" system. In contrast, biparietal lesions in monkeys induce deficits of visual spatial localization but not object discrimination. We[7] have posited that these "where" and "what" systems integrate in the banks of monkeys' STS or in the inferior parietal lobule of humans. According to our research,[7] lesions of monkeys' STS and humans' temporoparietal junction induce unawareness or neglect not only because this is the area that receives polymodal sensory input but also because it is a convergence site of these perceptual-cognitive systems that deal with both the "what" and "where" aspects of environmental awareness. Both anatomic and electrophysiologic data substantiate the hypothesis that monkeys' STS is an area of convergence of these two systems (see Ref. 7). We[7] have also proposed that similar areas important for spatial localization and object identification may also exist in the auditory and tactile systems and that these modalities may also converge in the STS.

Although there is anatomic and physiologic evidence that there is convergence from the Brodmann's area 7 "where" system and the ventral temporal lobes' "what" system, this cannot account for the observation that ablation of the STS induces unawareness. The STS receives input not only from these "what" and "where" systems but also from the cingulate gyrus and the dorsolateral frontal lobe. In earlier studies, we have demonstrated that lesions in both these areas are also able to induce neglect. The dorsolateral prefrontal region is important in the mediation of goal-directed behavior and may provide the STS with information that is not directly stimulus-dependent or related to immediate drives and biological needs but rather directed at long-term goals. The cingulate gyrus is part of the limbic system and may provide the STS with information about biological needs and drives. Because monkeys' STS or humans' temporoparietal junction are supplied with "what" and "where" conative and motivational information, it may be able to make attentional computations.

Monkeys' STS has reciprocal connections with the ventral temporal "what" region and the parietal "where" region. Therefore, after the STS region performs an attentional computation, it may reciprocally influence the neurons in the ventral temporal lobe and Brodmann's area 7 regions.

Electrical stimulation of the STS is capable of activating the midbrain reticular formation more than stimulation of surrounding posterior regions. Therefore, the superior temporal sulcus appears to be important in the cortical control of arousal, and the supermodal synthesis discussed above may also lead to neuronal activation in the ventral temporal "what" and dorsal area 7 "where" systems. Therefore, if the STS in monkeys or the temporoparietal junction in humans is dysfunctional, it not only fails to make attentional computations but also cannot arouse or activate directly or indirectly those areas that determine both location of objects and their identity. This failure of activation may prevent the monkey or human from being aware that there is a stimulus in the space opposite the lesion.

Bisiach and Luzzati[9] have demonstrated that subjects with neglect may have an inability to image those objects in scenes that would fall into contralesional hemispace, and Heilman and coworkers[10] have demonstrated a hemispatial antegrade memory deficit associated with neglect. Therefore, lesions of the IPL in humans may be associated with the inability to activate old memories or form new memories of objects that are located in contralesional hemispace. In monkeys, the STS has strong reciprocal connections with the hippocampus and the hippocampus has been posited to be important in retroactivation of sensory association areas.[11] Thus, a partial (spatial) failure of retroactivation may account for the imagery-memory deficits.

In monkeys and humans, spatial neglect can often be distinguished from deafferentation by observing exploratory behaviors. Deafferented subjects fully explore their environment. However, patients with neglect often fail to fully explore the neglected portion of space. Theoretically, if we ablated both area 7 (the "where" system) and the ventral temporal cortex (the "what" system in monkeys), we suspect that these animals would continue to be able to explore their contralateral hemispace. The failure to explore contralesional space that we observed in animals with STS lesions and humans with IPL lesions may be related to the reciprocal connections that the STS has with the frontal arcuate gyrus region. The frontal arcuate gyrus region or frontal eye field is important for the initiation of purposeful saccades to important visual targets. The periarcuate region is important for the initiation of voluntary arm movements to important visual stimuli. It has been demonstrated that lesions of this region, as well as the basal ganglia and thalamus, which are all part of an intentional functional network, may induce motor intentional neglect. However, exploratory defects may be also seen with posterior STS lesions in monkeys or IPL lesions in humans. In monkeys, the frontal arcuate area and periarcuate regions have strong connections with both area 7 and the STS. Whereas the STS may be critical in activating both periarcuate and arcuate regions, area 7 may be important for providing these frontal regions with the spatial maps needed to make purposeful exploratory limb and eye movements. In addition to the dorsolateral frontal lobe, the motor intentional network also includes the medial frontal lobes, the cingulate gyrus, the basal ganglia, and the thalamic cortical loops as well as input from the STS or IPL. Whereas the attentional and intentional networks are highly interactive, they do not entirely overlap. Therefore one may, as discussed, see neglect fractionate into motor intentional and sensory attentional components.

In humans, neglect can be associated with both right and left hemispheric lesions, but neglect is in general more severe and frequent with right than left hemispheric lesions. These asymmetries appear to be related to asymmetrical representations of space and the body. For example, whereas the left hemisphere primarily attends to the right side, the right hemisphere attends to both sides.[12,13] Similarly, while the left hemisphere prepares for right-side action, the right prepares for both.[12]

TREATMENT AND MANAGEMENT OF NEGLECT

Neglect is a sign and symptom of cerebral disease and thus it is critical to treat the underlying disease and to prevent further insults. Because patients with neglect may be unaware of stimuli, they should avoid both driving and working with tools or machines that might cause injury to themselves or others.

Many patients with neglect have anosognosia; during the acute stages when patients have anosognosia, rehabilitation is often difficult. In most patients, anosognosia is transient; but because patients with neglect remain inattentive to their left side and in general are poorly motivated, training is laborious and in many cases unrewarding. There are, however, some rehabilitation strategies that might be helpful. Diller and Weinberg[14] were able to train patients with neglect to look to their neglected side; however, it was not clear that these top-down attentional-exploratory treatments generalized to other situations. In contrast to this top-down treatment, Butter et al.[15] used a bottom-up treatment, where they used flashing lights to attract attention to the left side and demonstrated that dynamic stimuli presented on the contralesional (left) side reduced neglect. Even patients with hemianopia improved, suggesting that these dynamic stimuli influenced brainstem structures. Robertson and North[16] demonstrated that having patients move their contralesional hand in contralesional hemispace can also reduce the severity of hemispatial neglect.

Rubens[17] induced asymmetrical vestibular activation in patients with left-sided neglect by injecting cold water into the left ear and noting that unilateral spatial neglect abated. Vestibular stimulation can also help sensory inattention.[18] Optokinetic nystagmus and cervical vibration can also reduce neglect.[19,20] Unfortunately, these procedures produce only temporary relief. Rossi et al.[21] used prisms to shift images from the neglected side toward the normal side. Although the treated group performed better than the control group in tasks such as line bisection and cancelation, activities of daily living did not improve. Rossetti et al.[22] had subjects with neglect repeatedly point straight ahead while wearing the prisms. Thereafter, on tests of neglect, these treated patients showed a reduction of their ipsilesional bias, which lasted for 2 h after the prisms had been removed, but it is uncertain how much longer this effect can last.

Some investigators have found that an ipsilesional patching procedure reduces neglect,[23] but others have found that it can make neglect more severe.[24] Thus, when using patching, each eye should be tested before deciding which eye should be patched. Neglect in rats was treated with apomorphine, a dopamine agonist; this treatment significantly reduced neglect in these animals.[25] Fleet et al.[26] treated two neglect patients with bromocriptine, a dopamine agonist. Both showed dramatic improvements. Subsequently, other investigators have also shown that dopamine agonist therapy may be helpful in the treatment of both sensory and motor neglect.[27] Barrett et al.[28] and Grujic et al.[29] found, however, that in some patients, dopamine agonist therapy increased rather than decreased the severity of neglect. Barrett et al.'s patient had striatal injury and suggested that the paradoxical effect seen in their patient may be related to involvement of the basal ganglia. In patients with striatal injury, dopamine agonists may be unable to activate the striatum on the injured side but instead activate the striatum on the uninjured side, thereby increasing the ipsilesional orientation bias.

REFERENCES

1. Heilman KM, Watson RT, Valenstein E: Neglect and related disorders, in Heilman KM, Valenstein E (eds): *Clinical Neuropsychology*. New York: Oxford University Press, 2003.
2. Valler G, Sandroni P, Rusconi ML, Barberi S: Hemianopia, hemianesthesia, and spatial neglect: A study with evoked potentials. *Neurology* 41:1918–1922, 1991.
3. Triggs WJ, Gold M, Gerstle G, et al: Motor neglect associated with a discrete parietal lesion. *Neurology* 44:1164–1166, 1994.
4. Gold M, Shuren J, Heilman KM: Proximal intentional neglect: A case study. *J Neurol Neurosurg Psychiatry* 57:1395–1400, 1994.
5. Mennemeier MS, Wertman E, Heilman KM: Neglect of near peripersonal space: Evidence for multidirectional attentional systems in humans. *Brain* 115:37–50, 1992.
6. Ladavas E: Is the hemispatial deficit produced by right parietal damage associated with retinal or gravitational coordinates. *Brain* 110:167–180, 1987.
7. Watson RT, Valenstein E, Day A, Heilman KM: Posterior neocortical systems subserving awareness and neglect: Neglect after superior temporal sulcus but not area 7 lesions. *Arch Neurol* 51:1014–1021, 1994.
8. Mishkin M, Ungerleider LG, Macko KA: Object vision and spatial vision: Two cortical pathways. *Trends Neurosci* 6:414–417, 1983.
9. Bisiach E, Luzzati C: Unilateral neglect of representational space. *Cortex* 14:129–133, 1978.
10. Heilman KM, Watson RT, Schulman H: A unilateral memory deficit. *J Neurol Neurosurg Psychiatry* 37:790–793, 1974.
11. Damasio AR: Time locked multiregional retroactivation: A systems-level proposal for the neural substrates of recall and recognition. *Cognition* 33:25–62, 1989.
12. Heilman KM, Van Den Abell T: Right hemisphere dominance for attention: The mechanisms underlying

hemispheric asymmetries of inattention (neglect). *Neurology* 30:327–330, 1980.

13. Pardo JV, Fox PT, Raichle ME: Localization of a human system for sustained attention by positron emission tomography. *Nature* 349:61–64, 1991.
14. Diller L, Weinberg J: Hemi-inattention in rehabilitation: The evolution of a rational remediation program, in Weinstein EA, Friedland RR (eds): *Advances in Neurology*. New York: Raven Press, 1977, vol 18.
15. Butter CM, Kirsch NL, Reeves G: The effect of lateralized dynamic stimuli on unilateral neglect following right hemisphere lesions. *Restor Neurol Neurosci* 2:39–46, 1990.
16. Robertson IH, North NT: Spatio-motor cueing in unilateral left neglect: the role of hemispace, hand and motor activiation. *Neuropsychologia* 30:553–563, 1992.
17. Rubens AB: Caloric stimulation and unilateral visual neglect. *Neurology* 35(7):1019–1024, 1985.
18. Vallar G, Papagno C, Rusconi ML, Bisiach E: Vestibular stimulation, spatial hemineglect and dysphasia, selective effects. *Cortex* 31(3):589–593, 1995.
19. Pizzamiglio L, Frasca R, Guariglia C, et al: Effect of optokinetic stimulation in patients with visual neglect. *Cortex* 26(4):535–540, 1990.
20. Karnath HO: Transcutaneous electrical stimulation and vibration of neck muscles in neglect. *Exp Brain Res* 105(2):321–324, 1995.
21. Rossi PW, Kheyfets S, Reding MJ: Fresnel prisms improve visual perception in stroke patients with homonymous hemianopia unilateral visual neglect. *Neurology* 40:1597–1599, 1990.
22. Rossetti Y, Rode, G, Pisella L, et al: Prism adaptation to a rightward optical deviation rehabilitates left hemispatial neglect. *Nature* 395:166–169, 1998.
23. Butter CM, Kirsch N: Combined and separate effects of eye patching and visual stimulation on unilateral neglect following stroke. *Arch Phys Med Rehabil* 73(12):1133–1139, 1992.
24. Barrett AM, Crucian GP, Beversdorf DQ, Heilman KM: Monocular patching worsens sensory attentional neglect. *Arch Phys Med Rehabil* 82:516–518, 2001.
25. Corwin JV, Kanter S, Watson RT, et al: Apomorphine has a therapeutic effect on neglect produced by unilateral dorsomedial prefrontal cortex lesions in rats. *Exp Neurol* 36:683–698, 1986.
26. Fleet WS, Valenstein E, Watson RT, Heilman KM: Dopamine agonist therapy for neglect in humans. *Neurology* 37:1765–1771, 1987.
27. Geminiani G, Bottini G, Sterzi R: Dopaminergic stimulation in unilateral neglect. *J Neurol Neurosurg Psychiatry* 65(3):344–347, 1998.
28. Barrett AM, Crucian GP, Schwartz RL, Heilman KM: Adverse effect of dopamine agonist therapy in a patient with motor-intentional neglect. *Arch Phys Med Rehabil* 80(5):600–603, 1999.
29. Grujic Z, Mapstone M, Gitelman DR, et al: Dopamine agonists reorient visual exploration away from the neglected hemispace. *Neurology* 51(5):1395–1398, 1998.

Chapter 26

NEGLECT: COGNITIVE NEUROPSYCHOLOGICAL ISSUES*

Anjan Chatterjee
H. Branch Coslett

As the previous chapter makes clear, unilateral spatial neglect is a fascinating clinical syndrome in which patients are unaware of entire sectors of space on the side opposite to their lesion. These patients may neglect parts of their own body, parts of their environment, and even parts of scenes in their imagination. This clinical syndrome raises several questions, which this chapter addresses. How do humans direct spatial attention? How do humans represent space, and what is meant by a mental representation of space? How do humans direct actions in the environment? Is attention related to perception? Can information be processed without attention? Can information be processed without awareness?

GENERAL THEORIES OF NEGLECT

Spatial Attention

Attention is the process by which some stimuli are selected for privileged processing, presumably because the nervous system has a limited capacity and cannot process all things at all times. Stimuli compete for limited resources and some stimuli may be selected over others for a variety of reasons,[1] among which spatial location seems to be important. Neglect is most often viewed as a disorder of spatial attention. In neglect, spatial attention is biased ipsilesionally so that patients preferentially process stimuli in ipsilesional space over those in contralesional space.

Neglect is more common and severe with right than with left brain damage. Attentional accounts of neglect attempt to explain this hemispheric asymmetry. Kinsbourne postulated that each hemisphere generates a vector of spatial attention toward contralateral space, and these attentional vectors are inhibited by the opposite hemisphere.[2,3] The left hemisphere's vector of spatial attention is more strongly biased than that of the right hemisphere and, after right brain damage, the left hemisphere's unfettered vector of attention is powerfully oriented to the right. Since the right hemisphere's intrinsic vector of attention is only weakly directed, left brain damage does not produce a similar orientation bias to the left. Thus, neglect of the left side is more common and severe than neglect of the right side.

Heilman and coworkers[4,5] and Mesulam,[6,7] in contrast to Kinsbourne, proposed that the right hemisphere is dominant for arousal and spatial attention. Right brain damage produces greater electroencephalographic slowing than left brain damage. These patients also have decreased galvanic skin responses compared to normal subjects or patients with left hemisphere damage.[8] Behaviorally, they also show a markedly diminished capacity to perform more that one task at a time.[9] Thus, right hemisphere damage diminishes arousal and cognitive capacity, which, combined with hemispheric biases in directing attention, produces the manifestations of left-neglect.[10] The right hemisphere is capable of directing attention into both hemispaces, while the left hemisphere directs attention only into contralateral space. Thus, after right brain damage, the left hemisphere is ill equipped to direct attention into the left hemispace. However, after left brain damage, the right is capable of directing attention in both directions and neglect does not occur with the same severity as after right brain damage.

Posner and colleagues proposed a different model of spatial attention in which spatial attention is decomposed into elementary operations, such as "engage," "disengage," and "shift."[11] They reported that patients with right superior parietal damage are

* **ACKNOWLEDGMENT:** We would like to thank Lisa Santer for helpful editorial suggestions on this chapter.

selectively impaired at disengaging attention from right-sided stimuli before they shift and engage left-sided stimuli. This disengage deficit may contribute to some of the symptoms associated with neglect, most notably visual extinction.

The clearest evidence that these patients have a restricted attentional capacity comes from the phenomenon of extinction. Patients may be aware of single left-sided stimuli but then "extinguish" these stimuli when left-sided stimuli are presented simultaneously with right-sided stimuli.[12] Extinction can occur for visual, auditory, or tactile stimuli[13] and even when patients assess weights placed in their hands simultaneously.[14] Extinction may also be observed with multiple stimuli in ipsilesional space,[15,16] suggesting that the pathologic restriction in processing stimuli is not limited to stimuli competing for processing resources across hemispaces.

Spatial Intention

Spatial intention refers to the cognitive processes by which one selects spatial locations for actions. The selection of locations for action contrasts with their selection for perception[17,18]—a distinction that underlies the notions of intentional and attentional neglect. Some time ago, Watson and colleagues advanced the idea that neglect patients may have an intentional deficit, or a disinclination to initiate movements toward or into contralesional hemispace.[19,20] Similarly, Posner and colleagues proposed an "anterior attentional network" involved in selecting locations for actions. Rizzolatti and coworkers have extended this idea even further by arguing that preparations for actions might be critical to perception.[21]

In most situations, attention and intention are inextricably linked, since attention is naturally directed to objects on which one intends to act. Several experiments have tried to dissociate attention from intention using cameras, pulleys, and mirrors.[22–27] The general strategy in these studies is to disentangle where patients are looking (or attending) from where their limbs are acting (or intending). When patients perform tasks in which attentional and intentional selection are in conflict, some patients' neglect is determined by where they look (attentional neglect) and that of others by where they move their limb (intentional neglect).

Using a different approach, Milner and colleagues[25] introduced the "landmark task." Subjects are asked to point to the end of a pretransected line they think is shorter. Patients with attentional left neglect are biased to think that the left side is shorter for transections close to the objective midpoint and therefore point to the left end of the line. By contrast, patients with intentional neglect are disinclined to move their hand to the left and therefore are more likely to point to the right end of the line. Several studies using the landmark task and its variations have reported dissociations between attentional and intentional neglect.[28,29]

Neglect accompanied by ipsilesional biases in limb movements is sometimes associated with frontal lesions.[22,26,30] However, patients with lesions restricted to the posterior parietal cortex can also have intentional neglect.[31–33] Most patients with neglect probably have combinations of attentional and intentional neglect.[34]

Attention and Intention or Different Perceptual-Motor Systems?

One problem with framing these tasks as probing attentional or intentional systems may be that the attention/intention distinction is not the critical difference being assessed. Instead, the "attention" experimental conditions may reflect the link of visual attention to eye gaze, while the "intention" conditions may reflect the link of visual attention to limb movements.[24,35] The relevant distinction may actually be between two perceptual-motor systems, one driven by direction of gaze and the other by direction of limb movements. Such an interpretation would be consonant with single cell neurophysiologic data from monkeys, which show that visual attentional neurons in the posterior parietal cortex are selectively linked to eye or to limb movements.[36,37]

Spatial Representation

Representational theories of neglect propose that the inability to form adequate contralateral mental representations of space underlies the clinical phenomena.[38] In a classic observation, Bisiach and Luzzatti asked two patients to imagine the Piazza del Duomo in Milan, Italy, from two perspectives: looking across the square toward the cathedral, and looking from the cathedral across the square.[39] In each condition, the patients reported landmarks only to the right of their imagined position in the piazza. In addition to their difficulties with evoking contralateral representations from memory, patients with neglect may also have difficulties with forming new contralateral representations.[40] In sleeping patients with neglect, rapid eye movements are restricted ipsilaterally,[41] raising the intriguing possibility that these patients' dreams are also spatially biased. Neglect for images evoked from memory may dissociate from neglect of stimuli in extrapersonal space.[42,43] Thus, the processes by which spatial representations are formed by memory and those that are derived on line from perception may be selectively damaged.

REGIONS OF SPACE

Brain[44] introduced the idea that space could be viewed as concentric shells around the body's trunk—an idea echoed more recently by Previc.[45] Personal space is the space occupied by the body, peripersonal space is the space surrounding the body but within reach of the limbs, and extrapersonal space is the space beyond that reach. The notion that the nervous system treats these forms of space differently is supported by the observation that neglect in personal space dissociates from neglect in peripersonal and extrapersonal space[46] and that left neglect in peripersonal space also dissociates from neglect in and extrapersonal space.[47]

Personal Neglect

The observation of patients provides a rough indication of personal neglect. They ignore the left side of their body and might not use a comb, use make-up, or shave the left side of their face[48] Patients with personal neglect often deny ownership of their left arm even after this limb is brought into their view. When asked to touch their left arm with their right hand, patients with left personal neglect fail to reach over and touch their left side.[46] They may also fail to explore the left side of their body. Patients may be aware of their contralesional limb but not that it is paralyzed.[38] This phenomenon, called *anosognosia for hemiplegia,* is not an all-or-none phenomenon, with some patients having partial awareness of their contralesional weakness.[49]

Peripersonal and Extrapersonal Neglect

Peripersonal neglect is evident in commonly used bedside tests for neglect, such as line bisection, cancellation, and drawing tasks. On line bisection tasks, patients with left neglect typically place their mark to the right of the true midposition, demonstrating a bias to rightward orientation.[50] When the entire line is placed contralateral to their lesion, patients make larger errors with longer lines.[51,52]

On cancelation tasks, patients demonstrate reluctance to explore contralesional peripersonal space. When asked to "cancel" targets presented in an array, patients typically start at the top right of the display and often search in a vertical pattern.[53] They neglect left-sided targets.[54] Sometimes patients cancel right-sided targets repeatedly. The sensitivity of cancelation tasks can be enhanced by increasing the number of targets[55,56] and presenting arrays in which targets are difficult to discriminate from distracter stimuli.[57]

On drawing tasks, patients copy or draw objects and scenes from memory. When asked to copy drawings with multiple objects or complex objects with multiple parts, patients may omit left-sided objects in the array and/or omit the left side of individual objects.[58,59] In all these tasks, patients demonstrate a lack of awareness of contralesional stimuli located in peripersonal space.

The idea that peripersonal and extrapersonal space are considered different regions by the nervous system is supported by behavioral double dissociations in neglect patients. Halligan and Marshall[47] reported a patient whose severe left neglect for stimuli in peripersonal space was abolished or attenuated for similar stimuli in extrapersonal space. The opposite dissociation of patients with neglect for stimuli in far but not near space has been reported[60,61]

SPATIAL COORDINATES BEYOND LEFT AND RIGHT

Neglect is usually described along the horizontal (left-right) axis. However, our spatial environment also includes radial (near/far) and vertical (up/down) axes. Neglect may be evident in these coordinate systems. Patients with typical left neglect often have subtle neglect for near space. On cancelation tasks, they are most likely to omit targets in the left lower/nearer quadrant.[56,62] Dramatic vertical and radial neglect can occur in patients with bilateral lesions.[63–66] Bilateral lesions to temporoparietal areas may produce neglect for lower and near personal space, whereas bilateral lesions to the ventral temporal structures are associated with neglect for upper and far extrapersonal space. Neglect in the vertical axis probably represents complex interactions of the visual and vestibular influences on spatial attention.[67,68]

ATTENTION AND PERCEPTION

Spatial Anisometry

In patients with neglect, the pathologic capacity limitations and ipsilesional attentional bias result in left-right distortions or "anisometries" of space.[29,69–73] The nature of this anisometry, or distorted perception of spatial extent, can be explored by investigating the relationship between the magnitude of stimuli and the magnitude of patients' representations of these stimuli.[74] It turns out that patients' awareness of stimuli is systematically related to the quantity of stimuli presented.

The evidence that neglect patients are systematically influenced by the magnitude of the stimuli with which they are confronted has been studied most extensively in line bisection tasks.[75] Patients make greater errors on longer lines. Marshall and Halligan[76] described the systematic nature of these performances in psychophysical terms. Following this reasoning, Chatterjee and colleagues showed that patients' performances on a variety of tasks including line bisection, cancellation, single-word reading tasks, and weight judgments can be described mathematically by power functions.[14,51,55,77,78] In these functions, expressed mathematically as $\psi = K\phi^{\beta}$, ψ represents subjective magnitude of the stimuli and ϕ represents the objective magnitude. The constant K and exponent β are derived empirically. Power–function relationships appear to represent a fundamental organizational principle by which the nervous system estimates magnitude across different sensory stimuli.[79] An exponent of 1 suggests that changes in mental representations remain proportionate to changes in physical stimuli. Exponents less than 1, as occur in normal judgments of luminance magnitudes, suggest that mental representations are compressed in relation to the range of the physical stimulus.

The power functions derived from neglect patients' judgments of stimuli across various tasks have exponents that are diminished compared to functions derived from such judgments by normal subjects. Thus, while patients remain sensitive to changes in sensory magnitudes, their awareness of the magnitude of these changes is blunted.[74] For example, the exponent for normal judgments of linear extension is very close to 1. By contrast, neglect patients have diminished exponents suggesting that they, unlike normal subjects, experience horizontal lines of increasing lengths as increasing less than proportionately.[51,77] These observations also mean that magnitude transformations of sensations to mental representations occur nonlinearly within the central nervous system and not simply at sensory receptors, as implied by some psychophysicists.[80]

Representational Instability

Halligan and Marshall[81,82] discovered that patients with neglect tended to bisect short lines to the left of the objective midpoint and seemed to demonstrate ipsilesional neglect of these stimuli. This crossover behavior is found in most patients with neglect[51] and is not explained easily by most neglect theories. In fact, Bisiach referred to it as "a repressed pain in the neck for neglect theorists."[83] Using performance on single-word reading tasks, Chatterjee[78] showed that neglect patients sometimes confabulate letters to the left side of short words and thus read short words as longer than their objective length. He argued that this crossover behavior represented a contralesional release of mental representations—an idea found plausible in a formal computational model.[84]

The crossover in line bisection is influenced by the context in which these lines are seen. Thus, patients are more likely to cross over and bisect to the left of a true midpoint if these bisections are preceded by a longer line.[85,86] A phenomenon like crossover also occurs with weight judgments.[14,87] Patients with left neglect are likely to judge right-sided weights as heavier than left-sided weights. However, with lighter-weight pairs, this bias may reverse to where they judge the left side to be heavier than the right. Crossover seems to be a general perceptual phenomenon not restricted to vision. It also suggests that patients with left neglect are more susceptible to contextual biases when apprehending stimuli on the left than on the right.

SPATIAL REFERENCE FRAMES

Humans have the intuition and experience of a coherent sense of space in which we perceive and act on objects.[88] However, this coherent sense of space harbors different representations anchored to distinct reference frames.[89] These reference frames may be centered on the viewer, the object, or the environment. For example, we can locate a chair in a room in each of these frames. A viewer-centered frame would locate the chair to the left or right of the viewer. An object-centered frame refers to the intrinsic spatial coordinates of the object itself, its top or bottom or right and left. The object-centered reference frames is not altered by changes in the position of the viewer. The top of the chair remains its top regardless of where the viewer is located. An environment-centered reference frame refers to the location of the object in relation to its surroundings, also independent of the location of the viewer. The chair would be coded with respect to other objects in the room and its relation to gravitational coordinates.

Viewer-centered reference frames can be divided further into retinal, head-centered or body-centered coordinates. For example, Nadeau and Heilman[90] described a patient with a "gaze-dependent hemianopia." This patient seemed to have a left visual field defect when his eyes gazed straight ahead but not when he gazed 30 degrees to his right. His neglect of left-sided stimuli was determined by "left" with respect to his head or trunk and not his eyes. Others have described dissociations of neglect within different viewer-centered reference frames.[91] Karnath[92,93] showed that, in many patients, neglect is determined by the trunk or body-centered coordinates.

In object-centered neglect, patients are unaware of parts of objects in ways that cannot be explained by viewer-centered reference frames (although for some descriptions of object-centered neglect, this claim is disputed [94,95]). Low-level mechanisms by which objects are perceptually distinguished, such as figure-ground segmentation or principal axes, can influence which parts of a stimulus are neglected.[96,97] Forms of object-centered neglect have been demonstrated when patients draw pictures,[58] take photographs,[98] perceive rotated objects,[99] and read single words.[100] In one striking case,[101] a well-known sculptor sculpted a head that was grossly deformed on the left side despite the fact that the sculpture was done on a turntable and could be rotated!

Environment-centered coordinates may influence neglect in two ways. First, gravitational influences and the vestibular system help to anchor this reference frame.[67] Some patients' performance on search tasks and line-bisection tasks is influenced by changes in the patients' body position, which alter vestibular input and can disentangle the environmental axis from viewer and object axes. The lateralized biases in some patients are modulated by these changes in body position.[67,68,102–104] Second, environmental coordinates are also established by appreciating stable spatial relationships between objects that exist independent of the viewer's position. When searching for hidden objects, some patients are insensitive to cues provided by other objects in the environment.[105]

CROSS-MODAL AND SENSORIMOTOR INTEGRATION

Different sensory and motor systems interact to give rise to our sense of space. Cross-modal links between interoceptive sensations (vestibular and proprioceptive) with exteroceptive sensations (vision, audition, and touch) modulate neglect. Rubens and colleagues,[106] following an early observation by Silberfennig,[107] demonstrated that left-sided vestibular input with cold water caloric stimulation improves left-neglect. Such vestibular stimulation can also improve contralesional somatosensory awareness[108] and may transiently improve anosognosia.[109] The deployment of spatial attention may also be influenced by changes in posture, which are presumably mediated by otolith vestibular inputs.[67,68] Proprioceptive input from neck muscles can also modify neglect.[92,110]

Recent studies have also focused on cross-modal links between exteroceptive sensory modalities such as links between vision and touch. Visual input close to the location of tactile stimulation may improve contralesional tactile awareness.[111–113]

Movement may also modulate sensory awareness in these patients. Patients with tactile extinction are more likely to be aware of contralesional tactile stimuli when they actively move their limbs than when they apprehend these stimuli passively.[113] The fact that patients with neglect can have personal neglect and deficits of contralesional body representations[46,114] raises the question of how personal space is integrated with extrapersonal space. Tactile sensations are experienced as being produced by objects on the body, the surface of personal space. Visual sensations are experienced as being produced by objects at a distance from the body, in extrapersonal space. The integration of these two sources of information may contribute to bringing personal and peripersonal space into register.[115]

The manipulation of sensorimotor links may be helpful in rehabilitating patients with neglect. Reaching or pointing to objects involves coordinating vision and movement. This visuomotor mapping can be altered if a subject wears prisms that displace stimuli to the left or right of his or her field of view. Recent work suggests that forcing patients to remap ballistic movements leftward by having them wear prisms that displace visual stimuli to their right can improve neglect.[116] These preliminary data suggest that the improvement persists for some time even after the prisms are removed.

LEVELS OF PROCESSING

Processing without Attention

Visual information is processed in stages.[117] First, simple visual elements such as color and movement are extracted from the visual scene. This level of processing is followed by preattentive processing in that the figure is initially segmented from the background and the visual elements are grouped together. Thus, preattentive processing parses the visual scene into regions and possible objects, which are then subject to detailed scrutiny. Preattentive processing is generally automatic and operates in parallel across different locations. Brain damage can produce selective deficits at the preattentive level with relatively preserved visual-spatial attention.[118,119] These patients view the world in a piecemeal fashion, since visual elements are not grouped together automatically.

If neglect is an attentional disorder, then preattentive processing might still be preserved. Neglect patients are able to segment figure from ground even when the relevant aspect of the object to be segmented is on the left.[120,121] They also perform better on extinction and bisection tasks when left-sided stimuli can be grouped with right-sided stimuli than when they are not so linked.[122,123] Finally, neglect patients are susceptible to various visual illusions, such as the Müller-Lyer and Oppel-Kundt illusions,[124–127] which are presumed to be processed preattentively. Together, these observations support the idea that preattentive processing of contralesional stimuli is often preserved in neglect patients.

Processing without Awareness

Are stimuli that are neglected processed at all? Volpe and colleagues[128] found that patients with visual extinction had some awareness of stimuli that were extinguished. They were able to judge if two pictures were the same or different more accurately than would be expected by chance, even though they claimed to be unaware that there was even a left-sided stimulus present. Marshall and Halligan[129] reported, curiously enough, a patient who could not distinguish between two pictures of a house in which one had flames emanating out a window on the left. However, when asked which house she would live in, she consistently chose the house without the flames. The implication was that she processed "neglected" stimuli sufficiently to make logical judgments despite not seeming to be aware of the basis for making these judgments. The interpretation of these findings has been questioned by Bisiach and colleagues,[130] who find that although patients may have consistent biases in the pictures they choose, their choices do not always make sense. Other reports confirm that some patients process neglected stimuli to quite high levels. For example, neglected pictures on the left can facilitate processing of words centrally located (and not neglected) if the pictures and words belong to the same semantic category, such as animals.[131] Similarly, when patients with neglect are asked to decide if a string of letters on the right form a real word, they perform better if the neglected contralesional string is a word that is associated with the target word.[132]

CONCLUSION

The syndrome of unilateral neglect has contributed greatly to our understanding of the general organizational principles of spatial attention, intention, and representation. However, neglect is also quite heterogeneous. Despite broad similarity of symptoms, the specific details vary considerably across patients.[35,133] Some theorists wonder if it is meaningful to consider neglect a coherent entity.[134] However, rather than a cause for alarm, this heterogeneity itself has been critical to investigations of the organization of spatial attention and representation. Widely distributed neural networks mediate spatial attention, intention, and representation. Damage to parts of these networks can produce subtle differences in deficits of these complex functions. These differences themselves offer insight into how space is organized into different regions and reference frames, how different sensory modalities and perceptual motor systems interact, and how information processing, attention, and awareness are related.

REFERENCES

1. Desimone R, Duncan J: Neural mechanisms of selective visual attention. *Annu Rev Neurosci* 18:193–222, 1995.
2. Kinsbourne M: A model for the mechanisms of unilateral neglect of space. *Trans Am Neurol Assoc* 95:143–147, 1970.
3. Kinsbourne M: Mechanisms of unilateral neglect, in Jeannerod M (ed): *Neurophysiological and Neuropsychological Aspects of Spatial Neglect*. New York: North Holland, 1987, pp 69–86.
4. Heilman KM: Neglect and related disorders, in Heilman KM, Valenstein E (eds): *Clinical Neuropsychology*. New York: Oxford University Press, 1979, pp 268–307.
5. Heilman KM, Van Den Abell T: Right hemisphere dominance for attention: the mechanisms underlying hemispheric asymmetries of inattention (neglect). *Neurology* 30:327–330, 1980.
6. Mesulam M-M: A cortical network for directed attention and unilateral neglect. *Ann Neurol* 10:309–325, 1981.
7. Mesulam M-M: Large-scale neurocognitive networks and distributed processing for attention, language and memory. *Ann Neurol* 28:597–613, 1990.
8. Heilman KM, Schwartz HD, Watson RT: Hypoarousal in patients with the neglect syndrome and emotional indifference. *Neurology* 28:229–232, 1978.
9. Coslett H, Bowers D, Heilman K: Reduction in cognitive activation after right hemisphere stroke. *Neurology* 37:957–962, 1987.
10. Duncan J, Olson A, Humphreys G, et al: Systematic analysis of deficits in visual attention. *J Exp Psychol Gen* 128:450–478, 1999.
11. Posner M, Walker J, Friedrich F, et al: Effects of parietal injury on covert orienting of attention. *J Neurosci* 4:1863–1874, 1984.
12. Bender MB, Furlow CT: Phenomenon of visual extinction and homonomous fields and psychological principles involved. *Arch Neurol Psychiatry* 53:29–33, 945.
13. Heilman KM, Pandya DN, Geschwind N: Trimodal inattention following parietal lobe ablations. *Trans Am Neurol Assoc* 95:259–261, 1970.
14. Chatterjee A, Thompson KA: Weigh(t)ing for awareness. *Brain Cogn* 37:477–490, 1998.
15. Rapcsak SZ, Watson RT, Heilman KM: Hemispace-visual field interactions in visual extinction. *J Neurol Neurosurg Psychiatry* 50:1117–1124, 1987.
16. Feinberg T, Haber L, Stacy C: Ipsilateral extinction in the hemineglect syndrome. *Arch Neurol* 47:802–804, 1990.
17. Rizzolatti G, Berti A: Neural mechanisms in spatial neglect, in Robertson IH Marshall JC (eds): *Unilateral Neglect: Clinical and Experimental Studies*. Hillsdale, NJ: Erlbaum, 1993, pp 87–105.
18. Milner A, Goodale M: *The Visual Brain in Action*. New York: Oxford University Press, 1995.
19. Watson RT, Valenstein E, Heilman KM: Nonsensory neglect. *Ann Neurol* 3:505–508, 1978.
20. Heilman K, Bowers D, Coslett H, et al: Directional hypokinesia: prolonged reaction times for leftward movements in patients with right hemisphere lesions and neglect. *Neurology* 35:855–859, 1985.
21. Rizzolatti G, Matelli M, Pavesi G: Deficits in attention and movement following the removal of postarcuate (area 6) and prearcuate (area 8) cortex in macaque monkeys. *Brain* 106:655–673, 1983.
22. Coslett HB, Bowers D, Fitzpatrick E, et al: Directional hypokinesia and hemispatial inattention in neglect. *Brain* 113:475–486, 1990.

23. Bisiach E, Geminiani G, Berti A, et al: Perceptual and premotor factors of unilateral neglect. *Neurology* 40:1278–1281, 1990.
24. Bisiach E, Tegnér R, Làdavas E, et al : Dissociation of ophthalmokinetic and melokinetic attention in unilateral neglect. *Cereb Cortex* 5:439–447, 1995.
25. Milner AD, Harvey M, Roberts RC, et al: Line bisection error in visual neglect: Misguided action or size distortion? *Neuropsychologia* 31:39–49, 1993.
26. Tegner R, Levander M: Through the looking glass. A new technique to demonstrate directional hypokinesia in unilateral neglect. *Brain* 114:1943–1951, 1991.
27. Na DL, Adair JD, Williamson DJG, et al: Dissociation of sensory-attentional from motor-intentional neglect. *J Neurol Neurosurg Psychiatry* 64:331–338, 1998.
28. Bisiach E, Ricci R, Lualdi M, et al: Perceptual and response bias in unilateral neglect: Two modified versions of the Milner landmark task. *Brain Cogn* 37:369–386, 1998.
29. Milner AD, Harvey M: Distortion of size perception in visuospatial neglect. *Curr Biol* 5:85–89, 1995.
30. Binder J, Marshall R, Lazar R, et al: Distinct syndromes of hemineglect. *Arch Neurol* 49:1187–1194, 1992.
31. Triggs WJ, Gold M, Gerstle G, et al: Motor neglect associated with a discrete parietal lesion. *Neurology* 44:1164–1166, 1994.
32. Mattingley JB, Bradshaw JL, Phillips JG: Impairments of movement initiation and execution in unilateral neglect. *Brain* 115:1849–1874, 1992.
33. Mattingley J, Husain M, Rorden C, et al: Motor role of the human inferior parietal lobe in unilateral neglect patients. *Nature* 392:179–182, 1998.
34. Adair JC, Na DL, Schwartz RL, et al: Analysis of primary and secondary influences on spatial neglect. *Brain Cogn* 37:419–440, 1998.
35. Chatterjee A: Motor minds and mental models in neglect. *Brain Cogn* 37:339–349, 1998.
36. Colby CL: Action oriented spatial reference frames in cortex. *Neuron* 20:15–24, 1998.
37. Graziano MSA, Gross CG: The representation of extrapersonal space: a possible role for biomodal, visual-tactile neurons, in Gazzaniga MS (ed): *The Cognitive Neurosciences*. Cambridge, MA: MIT Press, 1995, pp 1021–1034.
38. Bisiach E: Mental representation in unilateral neglect and related disorders: The twentieth Bartlett Memorial lecture. *Q J Exp Psychol* 46A:435–461, 1993.
39. Bisiach E, Luzzatti C: Unilateral neglect of representational space. *Cortex* 14:129–133, 1978.
40. Bisiach E, Luzzatti C, Perani D: Unilateral neglect, representational schema and consciousness. *Brain* 102:609–618, 1979.
41. Doricchi F, Guariglia C, Paolucci S, et al: Disturbance of the rapid eye movements (REM) of REM sleep in patients with unilateral attentional neglect: Clue for the understanding of the functional meaning of REMs. *Electroencephalogr Clin Neurophysiol* 87:105–116, 1993.
42. Anderson B: Spared awareness for the left side of internal visual images in patients with left-sided extrapersonal neglect. *Neurology* 43:213–216, 1993.
43. Coslett HB: Neglect in vision and visual imagery: A double dissociation. *Brain* 120:1163–1171, 1997.
44. Brain WR: Visual disorientation with special reference to lesions of the right hemisphere. *Brain* 64:224–272, 1941.
45. Previc FH: The neuropsychology of 3–D space. *Psychol Bull* 124:123–163, 1998.
46. Bisiach E, Perani D, Vallar G, et al: Unilateral neglect: Personal and extrapersonal. *Neuropsychologia* 24:759–767, 1986.
47. Halligan PW, Marshall JC: Left neglect for near but not for far space in man. *Nature* 350:498–500, 1991.
48. Beschin N, Robertson IH: Personal versus extrapersonal neglect: a group study of their dissociation using a reliable clinical test. *Cortex* 33:379–384, 1997.
49. Chatterjee A, Mennemeier M: Anosognosia for hemiplegia: Patient retrospections. *Cogn Neuropsychiatry*, 1:221–237, 1996.
50. Schenkenberg T, Bradford DC, Ajax ET: Line bisection and unilateral visual neglect in patients with neurologic impairment. *Neurology* 30:509–517, 1980.
51. Chatterjee A, Dajani BM, Gage RJ: Psychophysical constraints on behavior in unilateral spatial neglect. *Neuropsychiatr Neuropsychol Behav Neurol* 7:267–274, 1994.
52. Heilman KM, Valenstein E: Mechanisms underlying hemispatial neglect. *Ann Neurol* 5:166–170, 1979.
53. Chatterjee A, Mennemeier M, Heilman KM: Search patterns and neglect: A case study. *Neuropsychologia* 30(7):657–672, 1992.
54. Albert ML: A simple test of visual neglect. *Neurology* 23:658–664, 1973.
55. Chatterjee A, Mennemeier M, Heilman KM: A stimulus-response relationship in unilateral neglect: The power function. *Neuropsychologia* 30:1101–1108, 1992.
56. Chatterjee A, Thompson KA, Ricci R: Quantitative analysis of cancellation tasks in neglect. *Cortex* 35:253–262, 1999.

57. Rapcsak S, Verfaellie M, Fleet W, et al: Selective attention in hemispatial neglect. *Arch Neurol* 46:172–178, 1989.
58. Marshall JC, Halligan PW: Visuo-spatial neglect: A new copying test to assess perceptual parsing. *J Neurol* 240:37–40, 1993.
59. Seki K, Ishiai S: Diverse patterns of performance in copying and severity of unilateral spatial neglect. *J Neurol* 243:1–8, 1996.
60. Cowey A, Small M, Ellis S: Left visuo-spatial neglect can be worse in far than in near space. *Neuropsychologia* 32:1059–1066, 1994.
61. Vuilleumier P, Valenza N, Mayer E, et al: Near and far visual space in unilateral neglect. *Ann Neurol* 43:406–410, 1998.
62. Mark VW, Heilman KM: Diagonal neglect on cancellation. *Neuropsychologia* 35:1425–1436, 1997.
63. Rapcsak SZ, Fleet WS, Verfaellie M, et al: Altitudinal neglect. *Neurology* 38:277–281, 1988.
64. Butter CM, Evans J, Kirsch N, et al: Altitudinal neglect following traumatic brain injury. *Cortex* 25:135–146, 1989.
65. Shelton PA, Bowers D, Heilman KM: Peripersonal and vertical neglect. *Brain* 113:191–205, 1990.
66. Mennemeier M, Wertman E, Heilman KM: Neglect of near peripersonal space: Evidence for multidirectional attentional systems in humans. *Brain* 115:37–50, 1992.
67. Mennemeier M, Chatterjee A, Heilman KM: A comparison of the influences of body and environment centred references on neglect. *Brain* 117:1013–1021, 1994.
68. Pizzamiglio L, Vallar G, Doricchi F: Gravitational inputs modulate visuospatial neglect. *Exp Brain Res* 117:341–345, 1997.
69. Werth R, Poppel E: Compression and lateral shift of mental coordinate systems in a line bisection task. *Neuropsychologia* 26:741–745, 1988.
70. Anderson B: A mathematical model of line bisection behaviour in neglect. *Brain* 119:841–850, 1996.
71. Karnath H-O, Ferber S: Is space representation distorted in neglect? *Neuropsychologia* 37:7–15, 1999.
72. Bisiach E, Ricci R, Modona MN: Visual awareness and anisometry of space representation in unilateral neglect: A panoramic investigation by means of a line extension task. *Consc Cogn* 7:327–355, 1998.
73. Mennemeier M, Rapcsak SZ, Dillon M, et al: A search for the optimal stimulus. *Brain Cogn* 37:439–459, 1998.
74. Chatterjee A: Spatial anisometry and representational release in neglect, in Karnath H-O, Milner D, Vallar G (eds): *The Cognitive and Neural Bases of Spatial Neglect*. Oxford, England: Oxford University Press, In press.
75. Bisiach E, Bulgarelli C, Sterzi R, et al: Line bisection and cognitive plasticity of unilateral neglect of space. *Brain Cogn* 2:32–38, 1983.
76. Marshall JC, Halligan PW: Line bisection in a case of visual neglect: psychophysical studies with implications for theory. *Cogn Neuropsychol* 7(2):107–130, 1990.
77. Chatterjee A, Mennemeier M, Heilman KM: The psychophysical power law and unilateral spatial neglect. *Brain Cogn* 25:92–107, 1994.
78. Chatterjee A: Cross over, completion and confabulation in unilateral spatial neglect. *Brain* 118:455–465, 1995.
79. Stevens SS: Neural events and the psychophysical power law. *Science* 170(3962):1043–1050, 1970.
80. Stevens SS: A neural quantum in sensory discrimination. *Science* 177(4051):749–762, 1972.
81. Halligan PW, Marshall JC: How long is a piece of string? A study of line bisection in a case of visual neglect. *Cortex* 24:321–328, 1988.
82. Marshall JC, Halligan PW: When right goes left: An investigation of line bisection in a case of visual neglect. *Cortex* 25:503–515, 1989.
83. Bisiach E, Rusconi ML, Peretti VA, et al: Challenging current accounts of unilateral neglect. *Neuropsychologia* 32:1431–1434, 1994.
84. Monaghan P, Shillcock R: The cross-over effect in unilateral neglect. Modelling detailed data in the line-bisection task. *Brain* 121:907–921, 1998.
85. Marshall RS, Lazar RM, Krakauer JW, et al: Stimulus context in hemineglect. *Brain* 121:2003–2010, 1998.
86. Ricci R, Chatterjee A: Context and crossover in unilateral neglect. *Neuropsychologia* 39:1138–1143, 2001.
87. Chatterjee A, Ricci R, Calhoun J: Weighing the evidence for cross over in neglect. *Neuropsychologia* 38(10):1390–1397, 2000.
88. Driver J, Spence C: Cross-modal links in spatial attention. *Philos Trans R Soc Lond B* 353:1319–1331, 1998.
89. Feldman JA: Four frames suffice: a provisional model of vision and space. *Behav Brain Sci* 8:265–289, 1985.
90. Nadeau SE, Heilman KM: Gaze-dependent hemianopia without hemispatial neglect. *Neurology* 41:1244–1250, 1991.
91. Hillis AE, Rapp B, Benzing L, et al: Dissociable coordinate frames of unilateral spatial neglect: "Viewer-centered" neglect. *Brain Cogn* 37:491–526, 1998.
92. Karnath HO, Schenkel P, Fischer B: Trunk orientation as the determining factor of the "contralateral" deficit in the neglect syndrome and as the physical anchor of the internal representation of body orientation in space. *Brain* 114:1997–2014, 1991.

93. Karnath HO, Christ K, Hartje W: Decrease of contralateral neglect by neck muscle vibration and spatial orientation of trunk midline. *Brain* 116:383–396, 1993.
94. Buxbaum L, Coslett H, Montgomery M, et al: Mental rotation may underlie apparent object-based neglect. *Neuropsychologia* 34:113–126, 1996.
95. Mozer M: Explaining deficits in unilateral neglect with object-based frames of reference. *Prog Brain Res* 121:99–119, 1999.
96. Driver J, Halligan PW: Can visual neglect operate in object-centered coordinates? An affirmative single-case study. *Cogn Neuropsychol* 8:475–496, 1991.
97. Driver J: Object segmentation and visual neglect. *Behav Brain Res* 71:135–146, 1995.
98. Chatterjee A: Picturing unilateral spatial neglect: Viewer versus object centred reference frames. *J Neurol Neurosurg Psychiatry* 57:1236–1240, 1994.
99. Behrmann M, Moscovitch M, Black SE, et al: Object-centered neglect in patients with unilateral neglect: Effects of left-right coordinates of objects. *J Cogn Neurosci* 6:1–16, 1994.
100. Caramazza A, Hillis AE: Levels of representation, coordinate frames, and unilateral neglect. *Cogn Neuropsychol* 7:391–445, 1990.
101. Halligan PW, Marshall JC: The art of visual neglect. *Lancet* 350:139–140, 1997.
102. Calvanio R, Petrone PN, Levine DN: Left visual spatial neglect is both environment-centered and body-centered. *Neurology* 37:1179–1183, 1987.
103. Farah MJ, Brun JL, Wong AB, et al: Frames of reference for allocating attention to space: Evidence from the neglect syndrome. *Neuropsychologia* 28(4):335–347, 1990.
104. Ladavas E: Is the hemispatial damage produced by right parietal lobe damage associated with retinal or gravitational coordinates. *Brain* 110:167–180, 1987.
105. Pizzamiglio L, Guariglia C, Cosentino T: Evidence for seperate allocentric and egocentric space processing in neglect patients. *Cortex* 34:719–730, 1998.
106. Rubens A: Caloric stimulation and unilateral neglect. *Neurology* 35:1019–1024, 1985.
107. Silberfennig J: Contributions to the problem of eye movements. III. Disturbances of ocular movements with pseudohemianopsia in frontal lobe tumors. *Confin Neurol* 4:1–13, 1941.
108. Vallar G, Bottini G, Rusconi ML, et al: Exploring somatosensory hemineglect by vestibular stimulation. *Brain* 116:71–86, 1993.
109. Cappa S, Sterzi R, Guiseppe V, et al: Remission of hemineglect and anosagnosia during vestibular stimulation. *Neuropsychologia* 25:775–782, 1987.
110. Karnath H-O, Sievering D, Fetter M: The interactive contribution of neck muscle proprioception and vestibular stimulation to subjective "straight ahead" orientation in man. *Brain Res* 101:140–146, 1994.
111. di Pellegrino G, Basso G, Frassinetti F: Visual extinction as a spatio-temporal disorder of selective attention. *Neuroreport* 9:835–839, 1998.
112. Ladavas E, Di Pellegrino G, Farne A, et al: Neuropsychological evidence of an integrated visuotactile representation of peripersonal space in humans. *J Cogn Neurosci* 10:581–589, 1998.
113. Vaishnavi S, Calhoun J, Chatterjee A: Crossmodal and sensorimotor integration in tactile awareness. *Neurology* 53:1596–1598, 1999.
114. Coslett HB: Evidence for a disturbance of the body schema in neglect. *Brain Cogn* 37:529–544, 1998.
115. Vaishnavi S, Calhoun J, Chatterjee A: Binding personal and peripersonal space: Evidence from tactile extinction. *J Cogn Neurosci* 13(2):181–189, 2001.
116. Rossetti Y, GR, Pisella L, et al.: Prism adaptation to a rightward optical deviation rehabilitates left spatial neglect. *Nature* 395:166–169, 1998.
117. Farah M: *The Cognitive Neuroscience of Vision*. Malden, MA: Blackwell, 2000.
118. Vecera S, Behrmann M: Spatial attention does not require preattentive grouping. *Neuropsychology* 11:30–43, 1997.
119. Ricci R, Vaishnavi S, Chatterjee A: A deficit of preattentive vision: experimental observations and theoretical implications. *Neurocase* 5(1):1–12, 1999.
120. Driver J, Baylis G, Rafal R: Preserved figure-ground segregation and symmetry perception in visual neglect. *Nature* 360:73–75, 1992.
121. Marshall JC, Halligan PW: The yin and the yang of visuo-spatial neglect: A case study. *Neuropsychologia* 32:1037–1057, 1994.
122. Mattingley JB, Davis G, Driver J: Preattentive filling-in of visual surfaces in parietal extinction. *Science* 275:671–674, 1997.
123. Vuilleumier P, Landis T: Illusory contours and spatial neglect. *Neuroreport* 9:2481–2484, 1998.
124. Mattingley J, Bradshaw J, Bradshaw J: The effect of unilateral visuospatial neglect on perception of Muller-Lyer illusory figures. *Perception* 24:415–433, 1995.
125. Ricci R, Calhoun J, Chatterjee A: Orientation bias in unilateral neglect: Representational contributions. *Cortex* 36:671–677, 2000.
126. Ro T, Rafal R: Perception of geometric illusions in hemispatial neglect. *Neuropsychologia* 34:973–978, 1995.

127. Vallar G, Daini R, Antonucci G: Processing of illusion of length in spatial hemineglect: A study of line bisection. *Neuropsychologia* 38:1087–1097, 2000.
128. Volpe BT, Ledoux JE, Gazzaniga MS: Information processing of visual stimuli in an "extinguished" field. *Nature* 282:722–724, 1979.
129. Marshall JC, Halligan PW: Blindsight and insight in visuospatial neglect. *Nature* 336:766–767, 1988.
130. Bisiach E, Rusconi ML: Breakdown of perceptual awareness in unilateral neglect. *Cortex* 26:643–649, 1990.
131. McGlinchey-Berroth R, Milberg WP, Verfaellie M, et al: Semantic processing in the neglected visual field: evidence from a lexical decision task. *Cogn Neuropsychol* 10:79–108, 1993.
132. Ladavas E, Paladini R, Cubelli R: Implicit associative priming in a patient with left visual neglect. *Neuropsychologia* 31:1307–1320, 1993.
133. Halligan PW, Marshall JC: Visuo-spatial neglect: The ultimate deconstruction. *Brain Cogn* 37:419–438, 1998.
134. Halligan PW, Marshall JC: Left visuo-spatial neglect: a meaningless entity? *Cortex* 28:525–535, 1992.
135. Chatterjee A: Neglect, in D'Esposito M (ed): *Neurological Foundations of Cognitive Neuroscience*. Cambridge, MA: MIT Press. In press.

Chapter 27

BÁLINT'S SYNDROME AND RELATED DISORDERS

H. Branch Coslett
Anjan Chatterjee

There are few neurologic conditions more arresting than the disorders associated with bilateral lesions of the posterior parietal and occipital lobes. One such disorder was described by the Hungarian neurologist Rezsö Bálint in 1909[1] (translated by Harvey and Milner[2]). A similar syndrome was subsequently described by Holmes and colleagues.[3,4] This chapter reviews the clinical and pathoanatomic bases of these disorders and considers the implications of these conditions for accounts of the role of the parietal lobe in visuospatial processing.

BÁLINT'S SYNDROME

In 1903, Bálint evaluated a middle-aged engineer who complained of an inability to use his hands to write and draw despite the fact that he was not weak or incoordinated. He also noted difficulty reading both single words and text.

In spite of these disabling deficits, Bálint's patient was normal in many respects. Although his intellectual abilities were described as "a little blunted," cognition was at least relatively preserved and spoken language was apparently normal. He exhibited normal visual fields and, in contrast to patients later reported by Holmes and colleagues,[3,4] ocular movements were conjugate with a full range of excursion. He recognized single objects quite well and read short words, but longer words were not consistently identified; when he failed to recognize a word he often reported single letters; he was sometimes able to piece together the word by serially identifying letters. Even when reading short words in a text format, the patient often got lost on the page.

Bálint's patient was not weak or clumsy; although unable to read music, he played several simple pieces on the piano from memory. Sensation was normal. Finally, his gait was neither ataxic nor unsteady, but he walked slowly and cautiously to avoid bumping into stationary objects in his path.

Bálint concluded that his patient's difficulties were neither purely sensory nor motor but appeared to be caused by a disruption of the linkage between sensation and movement. Furthermore, he suggested that the patient exhibited three primary deficits: a disorder of spatial attention causing an inability to identify more than one object at a time (termed *simultanagnosia* by Wolpert[5]), optic ataxia, and psychic paralysis of gaze. Below we consider Bálint's account of these disorders that, collectively, were designated "Bálint's syndrome" by Hecaen and Ajuriaguerra,[6] as well as more recent contributions to their understanding.

OPTIC ATAXIA

Bálint coined the term *optic ataxia* to refer to misreaching to visualized targets that could not be attributed to a primary motor deficit. Bálint reported that even after visualizing and naming objects, his patient was unable to reliably touch them. For example, when attempting to light a cigarette, the patient often lit it in the middle; similarly, he could not use a knife to cut his food as he was unable to reliably direct his hand to his plate. He could, however, reach to targets defined by proprioceptive information. For example, he could touch parts of his own body to command or after the target location was indicated by a touch of the patient's body. Additionally, he was able to bring his hands together in front of him with his eyes closed. Unlike many subsequently reported patients[7–9] who exhibit deficits in reaching with both hands, inaccurate reaching was observed only with the right hand.

Bálint's interpretation of this disorder was framed in the prevailing "disconnection" model of his day. He suggested that visuospatial information was adequately represented in the brain but that motor systems controlling the hands were disconnected from this visual center. He persuasively argued that his patient's reaching deficit could not be attributed to motor or sensory deficits for several reasons. First, Bálint argued that the asymmetry in performance with the right and left hands demonstrated that a visuospatial deficit could not explain the impairment as this would give rise to poor performance with both hands. Second, the patient's accurate reaching with the right hand to body parts demonstrated that motor systems were at least relatively preserved. Bálint attributed the greater impairment in the right hand to the fact that the left parietal lesion interrupted more of the underlying white matter tracts than the right hemisphere lesion.

Optic ataxia has been reported in many instances since Bálint's report. As noted by DeRenzi,[7] a variety of variants of the disorder have been reported. Some patients exhibit misreaching with only one hand whereas other patients exhibit the deficit in only one side of space. Occasionally, the disorder may affect only one hand in one side of space. Finally, patients may be impaired with both hands in both sides of space (see Chap. 24, Fig. 24-1).

Although controversy persists regarding some aspects of the disconnection account of optic ataxia (e.g., whether the relevant disconnection is from the dorsolateral frontal cortex as has often been assumed[7] or from the lateral cerebellar cortex[10]), most investigators have continued to support the disconnection model of optic ataxia. Holmes[3,4] argued that misreaching under visual guidance was attributable to an impairment in localizing objects in space. On this account, then, optic ataxia reflected an imprecision in the visual system.

One of the puzzling features of optic ataxia, however, is the fact that most human subjects with this disorder reach accurately when gazing directly at the target but may misreach by centimeters or more when reaching to targets in the periphery of the visual field.[9] If optic ataxia is simply attributable to a disconnection of spatial and motor systems or an inability to map the location of the limbs in space, then conveying the limb to the target should be equally inaccurate whether or not the target is foveated.

We[11] have recently reported data from a patient with optic ataxia that suggest an alternative account of this disorder. We found that one patient, D.P., was utterly unable to reach to targets unless he gazed directly at them. For example, D.P. was asked to identify a laterally presented target while gazing at a fixation point. He consistently named the targets. When asked to continue to gaze at the fixation point while reaching to touch the target, D.P. reached to the fixation point while verbally indicating that his response was incorrect. Additionally, D.P. was asked to identify an object reflected in a mirror. He was unable to reach to the target but instead touched the reflection of the object in the mirror; when the mirror was removed, he reached quickly and accurately to the target. Finally, D.P. was unable to touch named body parts unless he was able to visualize them; thus, he reached accurately to his knee and elbow but was unable to touch his ear. In light of the extensive evidence demonstrating that the parietal lobes are critical for coding the location of visualized targets in motor coordinates (e.g., see Ref. 12), we suggested that D.P.'s extensive bilateral parietal lesions rendered him unable to program movements in shoulder- and hand-centered spatio-motor coordinates; instead, D.P. appeared to rely on oculocentric coding; that is, we argued that for D.P. both the arm and eyes were driven by spatial information coded in oculocentric coordinates.

These data suggest that a simple "disconnection" model of optic ataxia is not adequate but that a full account of the disorder must appeal to differences in the frames of reference [e.g., retinotopic, oculocentric, shoulder-centered, etc. (see Ref. 13)], in which location information must be coded.

Optic ataxia may be identified by asking patients to reach to visualized targets. Reaching should be assessed with both the right and left hands in the right and left hemispaces. As many patients with optic ataxia will exhibit a greater impairment in reaching to targets to which they are not permitted to foveate,[9,11] patients should be tested while gazing directly at the target as well as while viewing the target in the periphery of the visual field. Optic ataxia is differentiated from motor or cerebellar disturbances by the fact that reaching to targets for which the location is defined by proprioceptive or auditory cues is normal (or nearly so).

PSYCHIC PARALYSIS OF GAZE

Psychic paralysis of gaze, or as the phenomenon was later termed by Cogan and Adams,[14] *oculomotor apraxia,* is characterized by an impairment of the ability to direct gaze volitionally; the deficit cannot be attributed to an impairment in the brainstem mechanisms controlling eye movements because these subjects exhibit normal oculocephalic reflexes and preserved reflex (that is, exogenously cued) saccadic eye movements.

Psychic paralysis of gaze was reported but not emphasized by Bálint in his description of his patient. Indeed, as has been noted by others,[7,10] Bálint provided little information about the eye movements of his patient and may not have fully assessed saccadic eye movements, smooth pursuit, and vergence movements. Bálint attributed this symptom to the lesions of the posterior parietal cortex, which he considered to be critical for the voluntary control of eye movements. Interestingly, more recent evidence in monkeys has confirmed the role of neurons in the region of the intraparietal sulcus in the control of eye movements.[15]

The disorder is identified by assessing conjugate eye movements under a variety of conditions. Patients with this disorder will typically perform well on pursuit tasks (both "smooth" and "saccadic"); although there is variability between patients, saccadic eye movements to exogenously cued stimuli such as a moving hand or rattling keys may be well executed. Eye movements to verbal command or gesture are typically impaired; for example, when asked to look to the ceiling or the door, patients with psychic paralysis of gaze are often unable to shift their gaze to the targeted location. In some instances, patients may be able to point to the location to which they are unable to direct their gaze. Disorders of the voluntary control of eye movement are the least common of Bálint's triad and are frequently evanescent, lasting days to a week before resolving.

SIMULTANAGNOSIA

Bálint's patient exhibited a striking impairment in the processing of visual arrays: he reported seeing only one "object" at a time. For example, even when shown an overlapping letter and triangle, this patient reported seeing only the letter; when cued to look for something else, he reported the triangle but no longer saw the letter. Furthermore, as the deficit appeared to spare auditory and tactile processing, Bálint argued that the deficit was caused by a disconnection between preserved visual cortices and the association cortex that might mediate attentional processes.

Bálint attributed this to impaired visual attention rather than a low level visual deficit for several reasons. First, he emphasized that the patient's visual fields were full with repeated testing. Second, and perhaps, most significantly, Bálint noted that object recognition was generally preserved and that performance was not influenced by object size; that is, his patient successfully identified single large objects, suggesting that he could integrate information over a large visual domain. He failed, however, to identify two small objects separated only by a small distance; for example, when asked to name a needle, he failed to see a candle only 5 cm away.

Simultanagnosia has subsequently been reported by a number of investigators.[6,16–21] The core feature of the disorder is a "piecemeal" perception of the visual environment. In severe cases, patients appear to "see" only one object in the environment despite being told that multiple items are present and being given ample time for inspection. We have observed one patient, for example, who reported seeing only a spoon when shown a table laden with food and eating utensils; he continued to report only this object until it was removed by the examiner, at which point, he reported seeing only a plate.[17] Patients with this disorder often behave as though they were blind; despite full visual fields and normal visual acuity, they may, for example, bump into stationary objects or even walk into a wall while directing their gaze elsewhere.

In more subtle forms, the disorder may be appreciated by asking a patient to describe a complex scene such as the Cookie Theft Picture from the Boston Diagnostic Aphasia Examination.[22] In this instance, patients often report items in the array in a slow and sometimes random fashion. As reported by Bálint, many patients with simultanagnosia read familiar single words accurately but are impaired in text reading because they lose their place on the page. Reflecting the tendency to report the largest, single coherent or meaningful "object" in the array, patients with simultanagnosia often report words but are unable to report the constituent letters of nonwords.[23] We[19] reported a patient who read the word "flag," but when shown the letter string "flig," reported seeing only an "l."

Testing for simultanagnosia should include not only assessment of visual fields and visual acuity but also the ability to identify single objects and visual arrays. Complex scenes such as that depicted by Cookie Theft Picture are of particular interest. Simultanagnosic subjects will typically correctly report seeing elements of the array in a serial and laborious fashion and may be unable to derive an understanding of the scene even with unlimited time. These subjects may be particularly impaired at counting dots, stars, or other stimuli as they often fail to count a number of the stimuli and count others repeatedly.

HOLMES'S CONTRIBUTION: DISTURBANCES OF VISUAL ORIENTATION

Shortly after Bálint's contribution, a number of patients were reported whose deficits were similar to Bálint's patient. As discussed below, impairments in the analysis of complex visual scenes (e.g., simultanagnosia) and disorders involving reaching and eye movements are commonly observed in patients with posterior brain lesions. Careful assessment of these disorders, however, reveals substantial variability between patients.

This heterogeneity is illustrated by the elegant descriptions by Holmes[3] and Holmes and Horrax[4] of patients with penetrating missile injuries. Holmes's patients differed from the patient described by Bálint, however, with respect to ocular movements. As previously noted, Bálint's patient exhibited a "psychic paralysis of gaze" or an inability to voluntarily direct his gaze in response to verbal commands. In contrast, the gaze deficits described by Holmes and coworkers[4] were far more profound. As with Bálint's patients, their eye movements were full and conjugate, but the patients were unable to maintain fixation on a target or follow a moving target, an impairment termed *gaze aproxia* by DeRenzi,[7] and also failed to blink in response to threat. Interestingly, at least some of the patients were able to direct their gaze accurately to auditory (Ref. 3, case 1)[4,18] or tactile (Ref. 3, case 5) stimuli.

A number of other features were described by Holmes. His patients exhibited difficulty in estimating the size and shape of objects as well as the distance of the object relative to other objects or themselves. These patients exhibited prominent spatial deficits while navigating familiar environments. For example, Holmes[3] reported that when instructed to walk to a bed to which he had just pointed, one patient veered sharply and walked into a wall.

Although the disorders described by Holmes and Bálint are similar in many respects, the accounts offered by the two investigators differed substantially. Whereas Bálint attributed simultanagnosia and "psychic paralysis of gaze" to an impairment in visual attention and optic ataxia to a disconnection between visual and motor systems, Holmes argued that the syndrome was best characterized as an inability to construct an adequate representation of the visual environment.

Emphasizing the similarity between the disorders described by Holmes and Bálint as well as the fact that patients with bilateral posterior parietooccipital lesions often exhibit combinations of the deficits reported by Holmes and Bálint, some investigators have argued that these "syndromes" are not distinct but represent variations on a common theme.[8] Proponents of this view have suggested that the clinical picture associated with bilateral parietooccipital lesions be designated the *Bálint-Holmes syndrome.*

Subtypes of Simultanagnosia

Although the core feature of simultanagnosia—impaired ability to "see" more than one object at a time—appears to be similar across patients, careful assessment of simultanagnosics reveals important differences in their visual impairment. We believe, in fact, that simultanagnosia may be caused by different types of impairment in visual processing; furthermore, as will be discussed below, we suggest that these deficits have different pathologic substrates.

Ventral Simultanagnosia The first systematic attempt to distinguish between distinct subtypes of simultanagnosia was offered by Farah's[24] distinction between "dorsal" and "ventral" simultanagnosia. Ventral simultanagnosia, which is associated with inferior occipitotemporal lesions on the left,[25,26] is generally less severe and disabling than dorsal simultanagnosia. These subjects, for example, appear to operate efficiently in the world, rarely bumping into people or objects, and they usually exhibit less dramatic deficits in reports of complicated arrays. Other features of Bálint's syndrome, such as optic ataxia, "psychic" paralysis of gaze, or spatial disorientation are not normally present.

The first detailed report of this disorder was provided by Wolpert,[5] who described a 58-year-old man who performed well in naming single objects but was quite impaired in describing a complex scene; he identified the constituent elements slowly and was impaired in appreciating the relationships between the elements. Wolpert's patient also exhibited letter-by-letter reading (see Chap. 14), which is highly characteristic of ventral simultanagnosia. Similar patients have been described by Kinsbourne and Warrington[25,27] and Levine and Calvanio,[26] who attribute the disorder to a "prolonged refractory period" in visual processing.

Dorsal Simultanagnosia The deficit in "dorsal" simultanagnosia is often far more profound. As noted, subjects with dorsal simultanagnosia may be impaired in the interpretation of visual arrays in the everyday environment and often appear to be blind. We observed such patients, for example, who fail to see more than one item in the Cookie Theft Picture; when the picture was removed and later shown again, a single but different person or object may be reported. Like ventral simultanagnosics, the size of stimuli does not usually affect the performance of dorsal simultanagnosics. Luria et al.,[28] reported that a simultanagnosic patient recognized objects that extended across a 16- to 20-degree of visual angle but failed to recognize two objects that occupied a far smaller area.

In contrast to ventral simultanagnosics, patients with this disorder tend to report a meaningful unit or "object" that incorporates the constituents that may be included in a more complex "object". Thus, when confronted with the letter string CAT, these subjects may say "cat" rather than name a single letter.[19] Similarly, when shown a picture of a face, dorsal simultanagnosics usually do not report seeing a component "object" such as an eye, mouth, nose, or cheek but "see" a face. If the integrity of the face is disrupted by shifting the positions of the features, subjects may report seeing one of the constituent parts rather than the face. Another difference is that at least some subjects with this disorder do not exhibit a slowing of the rate of visual processing.[19]

We suggest that "dorsal" simultanagnosia may be further subdivided on the basis of the nature of the processing deficit and, as discussed below, lesion locus. One variant of dorsal simultanagnosia may be characterized primarily by impaired visual attention. As one might expect given the diversity of the processes subsumed under this construct, a number of variants of this "attention deficit" account have been offered.

Simultanagnosia as a Disengage Deficit Several investigators have suggested that the disorder is attributable to a bilateral "disengage" deficit.[24,29] Posner and colleagues[30,31] have shown that parietal lobe damage can result in a specific difficulty with disengaging attention from a correctly attended object to another. Farah[24] suggested that simultanagnosia is attributable to a failure to disengage attention or a pathologic "stickiness" of attention. Verfaellie et al.[29] reported data from a simultanagnosic patient that are consistent with this account.

We investigated a patient with simultanagnosia resulting from bilateral parietooccipital lesions whose performance provides strong support for the claim that simultanagnosia may be associated with a disengage deficit.[17] I.C. was a 65-year-old right-handed man who after cardiac surgery was noted to be "confused" and to appear blind. The confusion abated over the next week. I.C. also exhibited optic ataxia, particularly in the right hemispace. I.C. exhibited simultanagnosia; when shown the Cookie Theft Picture, for example, I.C. reported seeing only a stool and, after a considerable delay, a girl. He performed poorly on visual search tasks.

The critical data in this context come from a series of investigations in which I.C. was asked to name two vertically arrayed stimuli on a computer screen. In these experiments the timing of stimulus onset and offset was systematically manipulated. As expected, I.C. named both stimuli on only 6 percent of trials. Critically, when two stimuli were presented initially but one stimulus was extinguished, early, helping to "release" attention, he named both stimuli significantly more frequently (55 percent). These data suggest that, at least in some instances, simultanagnosia may be attributable to impaired disengagement of attention.

Simultanagnosia as a Deficit in Visual Feature Integration or Spatial Registration A second variant of the attentional deficit of simultanagnosia attributes the disorder to a failure to integrate visual features. Several models of high-level visual processing argue that visual attention is critical to the recognition of objects and processing of arrays. Treisman and colleagues, for example, have argued that visual attention serves as the "glue" that links visual features to a common site in the "master map of locations,"[33] thereby permitting the visual features (e.g., color, shape, angle, etc.) to be integrated. A number of investigators have demonstrated that when attention is overloaded, subjects produce "illusory conjunctions" reflecting the miscombination of visual feature information.[34,35] For example, with brief display of arrays containing green X's and red O's, normal subjects may report seeing green O's, presumably reflecting the failure to bind the color and identity information to the correct spatial locations.

If simultanagnosia is attributable to a deficit in visual attention, one might expect patients with this disorder to exhibit illusory conjunctions. Consistent with this prediction, several simultanagnosic subjects who produce illusory conjunctions have been reported.[16,17] Additionally, we have investigated one subject, E.D., for example, who produced frequent illusory conjunctions when confronted with arrays containing two letters. For example, when shown PQ, E.D. reported seeing RO, a response that could be generated by transposing the oblique line from the Q to the P. Support for this feature transposition account comes from control conditions. E.D. made significantly fewer errors in reporting letters in arrays such as SO. in which there was no discrete letter component that could "migrate" to generate a letter not in the display. Similarly, errors were less likely to occur when the attentional demands were reduced by introducing information that served to segregate the stimuli; thus, E.D. produced significantly fewer illusory conjunction errors in trials in which the two letters were different colors (e.g., red P, black Q). This finding is reminiscent of Luria's observation that a simultanagnosic reported seeing a Star of David when shown overlapping triangles of the same color but "saw" only a triangle when the overlapping triangles wave blue and red.[21]

Robertson and colleagues have reported an extensive series of investigations of a simultanagnosic patient, E.M., who also produced illusory conjunctions on a variety of tasks involving the features of color, shape and motion.[16,36,37] In conjunction with other lines of evidence, such as his inability to explicitly report the location of a single stimulus in relation to the boundaries of the spatial array, Robertson et al. argued that R.M.'s primary deficit was the loss of spatial information normally provided by the parietal lobes.[16]

Simultanagnosia as a "What-where Binding" Deficit In contradistinction to the "attentional deficit" conceptualization of simultanagnosia discussed above, we have proposed that, at least in some instances, simultanagnosia is attributable to impaired "binding" of information computed in the dorsal and ventral stream. On this account, processing in the ventral stream is assumed to be normal or nearly so; the fact that object identification is at least relatively preserved for many simultanagnosics is consistent with this claim. Processing in the dorsal visual stream is also assumed to be at least relatively preserved. The inability to "see" more than one object is attributed to a failure to link object representations and their location in egocentric space.

Support for the binding deficit account comes from the evaluation of a simultanagnosic (B.P.) with bilateral lesions involving the posterior parietal and superior temporal lobes.[19] B.P. performed well on "preattentive" tasks in which she was asked to determine whether a specific visual feature (e.g., the color red) was present in the array; in contrast, she performed quite poorly on attention-requiring serial search tasks. On no task, however, did she produce illusory conjunctions. B.P. exhibited a normal pattern of performance on tests sensitive to the "disengage" deficit. As she was able to categorize words presented in a rapid serial visual presentation paradigm, her deficit could not be attributed to a slowing of visual information processing. Perhaps of greatest relevance in the present context is that her report of two item arrays (both line drawings and words) was influenced by the semantic relationship between the stimuli. For example, she reported both items correctly significantly more frequently on trials on which the items were drawn from the same semantic category (e.g., tools, animals, etc.) as compared to trials on which the items were drawn from different semantic categories (e.g., clothes and fruit). The fact that performance was significantly influenced by semantic factors, we suggest, argues that B.P.'s deficit is not attributable to "early" visual processing deficits (e.g., the precise registration of visual feature information). Rather, we suggest that the fact that B.P.'s performance is influenced by stimuli that she was unable to "see" argues for an inability to link information regarding object identity to an egocentrically defined location. Similar results have been obtained with a second simultanagnosic patient, J.J.D. (manuscript in preparation).

We note here that the binding deficit account of dorsal simultanagnosia attributes the disorder to an impairment in a limited-capacity operation that integrates information and therefore, may itself be regarded as a variant of the attentional deficit account of simultanagnosia. We suggest, however, that the "attentional" and "ventral-dorsal binding deficit" models differ in one important respect. In the former the deficit impairs the integration of visual feature information at an earlier level of the representation of visual information, whereas in the latter, the impairment is in the binding of information computed in the ventral stream to an egocentric map of space.

A final point in this context is that the putative subtypes of dorsal simultanagnosia described above are conceptually distinct but are similar in many respects. In light of the variability in the lesion sites and phenomenology characteristic of dorsal simultanagnosia, it would appear likely that some simultanagnosics may exhibit features of both putative subtypes. R.M., the extensively investigated subject reported by Robertson and colleagues,[16,36,37] may be such a patient. R.M. exhibits phenomena that we consider to be typical of both "attention deficit" simultanagnosia (e.g., illusory conjunctions) as well as implicit processing of unreported information that we have suggested is attributable to an impairment in binding dorsal and ventral visual streams.

Anatomic Basis of Simultanagnosia

Ventral simultanagnosia is typically associated with lesions involving the occipital lobe or inferior temporooccipital region on the left.[25,26] Dorsal simultanagnosia, in contrast, is associated with bilateral posterior parietal or parietooccipital regions. If, as we have suggested, dorsal simultanagnosia may be further subdivided into disorders that disrupt visual attention as well as variants that impair the linking of information in the ventral and dorsal visual pathways, one might expect to observe different lesion loci for the two subtypes of dorsal simultanagnosia. More specifically, one would expect simultanagnosia characterized by visual attentional deficits to be associated with lesions involving (but not necessarily restricted to) the superior parietal lobe and visual association cortex; in contrast, simultanagnosia associated with an impairment in "binding" what and where/how to information would be expected to be associated with lesions involving (but not necessarily restricted to) the inferior parietal lobes, a structure that has been claimed by some to be important for linking the dorsal and ventral streams.[38,39] Structural imaging data from four dorsal simultanagnosics evaluated in our laboratories are consistent with this claim. I.C.[17] and E.D. (see above) exhibited prominent deficits in visual attention and/or feature registration; as demonstrated in Figs. 27-1 and 27-2, both patients exhibited lesions that involved BA 19 bilaterally; neither exhibited bilateral lesions in BA 39 to 40. In contrast, for B.P.[19] and J.J.D. the lesions overlapped in the bilateral posterior parietal cortex; neither suffered bilateral BA 19 lesions (see Figs. 27-3 and 27-4).

The generality of this anatomic account is difficult to assess because of the lack of relevant behavioral data and reliable information about lesion localization for most patients. We suggest, however, that the limited data available from other patients are consistent with this claim. For example, as previously noted, R.M.[16,36,37] exhibited findings consistent with both the "attentional deficit" and "binding deficit" accounts. As noted by Robertson et al.,[16] R.M.'s lesions involved both the superior parietal lobe and visual association cortex as well as the inferior parietal lobe bilaterally.

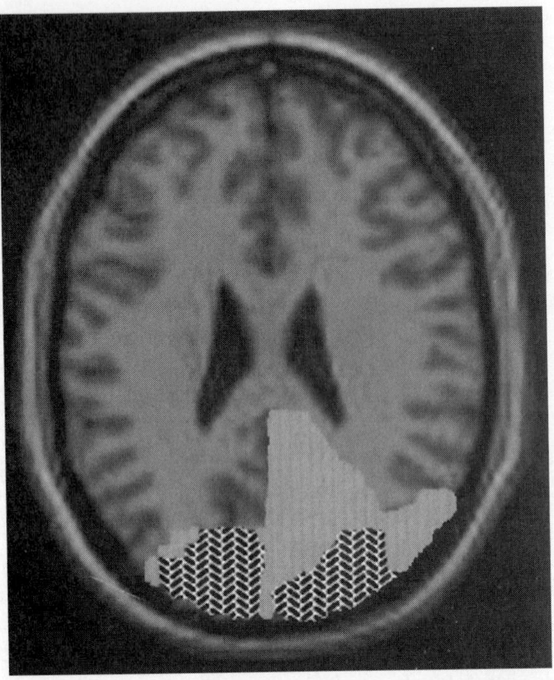

Figure 27-1
A high-ventricular section of CT scans from I.C. and E.D. demonstrating areas of infarction common to both patients (stippled) in BA 19. For this and subsequent images, areas of infarction not common to both subjects are gray.

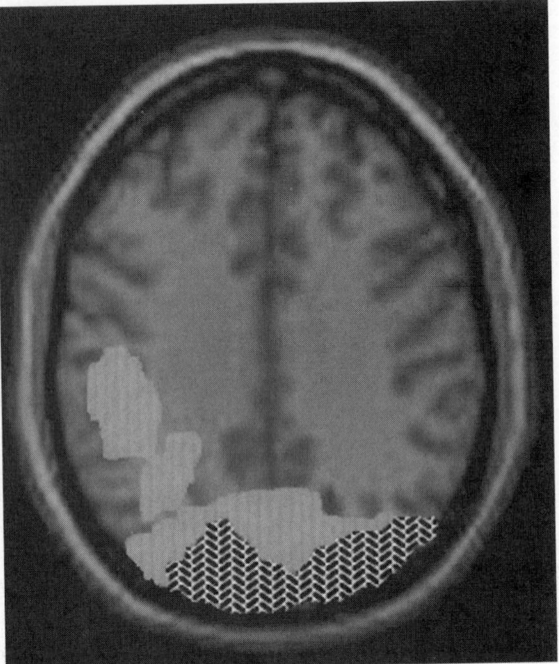

Figure 27-2
A supraventricular section demonstrating areas of infarction for both I.C. and E.D. (stippled) in BA 19.

"SIMULTANAGNOSIA-LIKE" VISUAL IMPAIRMENTS

A number of disorders that differ in important ways from the syndromes described above but are characterized by "piecemeal" recognition of visual arrays may also be identified. The most common of these is the impairment-associated degenerative disorders involving posterior brain regions. This pathologically heterogeneous group of disorders, designated *posterior cortical atrophies* by Benson and colleagues, is often characterized by a size effect in object recognition such that small objects are identified more reliably than large objects. We[40] reported a patient with presumed Alzheimer's disease, who reported seeing "a T" when shown the letter string CAT in letters 1 in. high but named the word when the letters were 1/2 in. high; as her disease progressed, the size of the word that she could name gradually decreased. On the basis of these and other observations, we argued that these subjects exhibit a restriction in the "spotlight" of attention, characterized by a decrease in the region from which visual feature information could be integrated.

Laeng et al.[42] reported a patient with alexia and piecemeal visual perception after head injury with bilateral temporal lobe damage who performed well on tasks on which the target appeared at expected locations. They argued that the patient's impairment reflected an inability to index stimulus location as well as an impairment in pattern analysis. The latter impairment was emphasized in Humphrey and Price's account[43] of two patients with piecemeal visual perception.

Another group of patients that have piecemeal perception and superficially resemble patients with dorsal simultanagnosia are those with intermediate vision deficits. *Intermediate vision* refers to the level of visual processing at which elementary visual attributes are grouped together based on similarity of visual

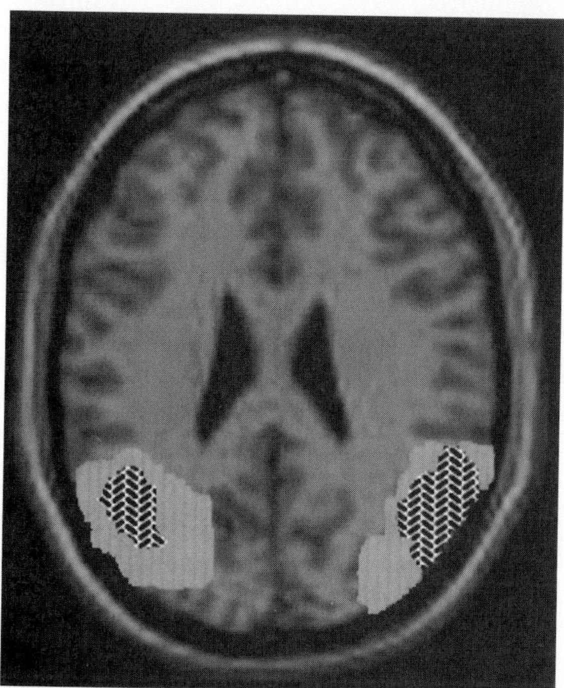

Figure 27-3
A high-ventricular section of CT scans from J.J.D. and B.P. demonstrating areas of infarction common to both patients (stippled) in BA 39 on the left.

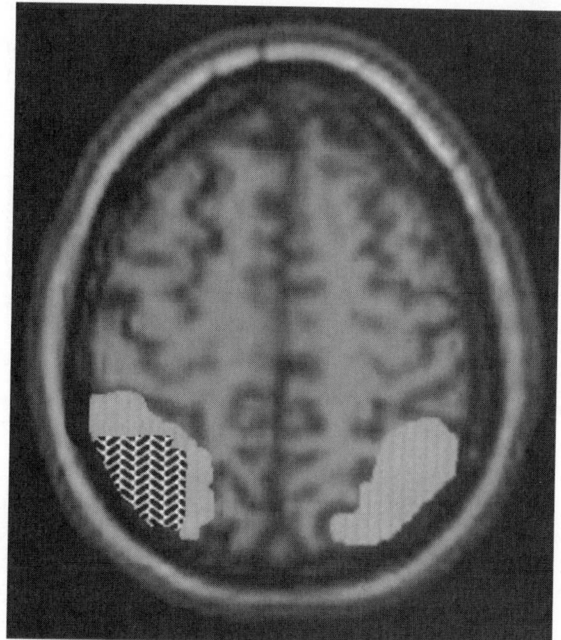

Figure 27-4
A supraventricular section demonstrating areas of infarction for both J.J.D. and B.P. (stippled) in BAs 39 and 40.

attributes, such as color, texture, or colinearity. These processes, studied extensively by Gestalt psychologists, generally occur automatically and effortlessly.[44] We reported a patient, N.M., with a relatively selective intermediate vision deficit following head trauma.[45] She could not perceive illusory contours or automatically group visual attributes of color, luminance, or orientation. Her recognition of simple objects did not deteriorate with increasing size, suggesting that she did not have an attentional restriction agnosia. In her case, mechanisms that automatically or preattentively parse the visual scene into candidate regions were not operational. Rather, she used effortful shifts of attention to scrutinize a myriad of details, from which she laboriously built up a representation of the visual scene. As a consequence, she experienced everyday activities, such as looking for cereal in the grocery store, as extremely laborious, since she had to inspect each box individually. Crossing a street was impossible for her, because she could not select the important relevant candidate objects (such as moving cars) efficiently. Vecera and Behrmann reported a similar patient with a selective preattentive deficit following anoxic brain injury.[46] The anatomic substrate of these disorders is not known; however, perceiving illusory contours and linking low-level visual attributes are thought to involve coordinated activity in early striate and extrastriate cortex.

CONCLUSION

A patient with Bálint's syndrome may have normal visual fields and visual acuity yet walk into a wall while looking at his watch. He may also be unable to eat soup as he cannot compute the location of the spoon and bowl at the same time or, succeeding in that effort, accurately direct the spoon to the bowl. We have attempted to provide a systematic account of the clinical aspects of this variable and often confusing disorder. Additionally, we have offered a new nosology of "dorsal" simultanagnosia that postulates that the disorder may arise from deficits at different levels of visual processing. Future investigations will serve to evaluate the validity of this classification as data from these patients speak to accounts of visual processing.

REFERENCES

1. Bálint R: Seelenlähmung des "Schauens," optische Ataxie, raümliche Störung der Aufmerksamkeit. *Monatschr Psychiatrie Neurol* 25:51–81, 1909.
2. Harvey M, Milner AD: Bálint's patient. *Cogn Neuropsychol* 12:261–281, 1995.
3. Holmes G: Disturbances of visual orientation. *Br J Ophthalmol* 2:449–468, 506–516, 1918.
4. Holmes G, Horrax G: Disturbances of spatial orientation and visual attention with loss of stereoscopic vision. *Arch Neurol Psychiatry* 1:385–407, 1919.
5. Wolpert I: Die Simultanagnosie: Storung der Gesamtauffassung. *Z Gesamte Neurol Psychiatrie* 93:397–413, 1924.
6. Hecaen H, de Ajuriaguerra J: Bálint's syndrome (psychic paralysis of visual fixation) and its minor forms. *Brain* 77:373–400, 1954.
7. DeRenzi E: *Disorders of Space Exploration and Cognition*. Chichester, UK: Wiley, 1982.
8. DeRenzi E: Bálint-Holmes' syndrome, in Code C, Wallesch C-W, Joanette Y, Lecours AR (eds): *Classic Cases in Neuropsychology*. Hove, East Sussex, UK: Psychology Press, 1996, pp 123–143.
9. Perenin MT, Vighetto A: Optic ataxia: A specific disruption in visuomotor mechanisms: I. Different aspects of the deficit in reaching for objects. *Brain* 111:643–674, 1988.
10. Husain M, Stein J: Rezsö Bálint and his most celebrated case. *Arch Neurol* 45:89–93, 1988.
11. Buxbaum L, Coslett HB: Subtypes of optic ataxia: Reframing the disconnection account. *Neurocase* 3:159–166, 1997.
12. Goodale M, Milner A: Separate visual pathways for perception and action. *Trends Neurosci* 15:20–25.
13. Andersen RA, Snyder LH, Li CS, Strieanne B: Coordinate transformations in the representation of spatial information. *Curr Opin Neurobiol* 3:171–176, 1993.
14. Cogan DG, Adams RD: A type of paralysis of conjugate gaze (ocular motor apraxia). *Arch Ophthalmol* 50:434–442, 1953.
15. Colby NT, Duhamel J, Goldberg ME: Oculocentric spatial representation in parietal cortex. *Cereb Cortex* 5:470–481, 1995.
16. Robertson L, Treisman A, Friedman-Hill S, Grabowecky M: The interaction of spatial and object pathways: Evidence from Bálint's syndrome. *J Cogn Neurosci* 9:295–317, 1997.
17. Pavese A, Coslett HB, Saffran EM, Buxbaum L: Limitations of attentional orienting: Effects of abrupt visual onsets and offsets on naming two objects in a patient with simultanagnosia. *Neuropsychologia* 40:1097–1103, 2002.
18. Kase CS, Troncoso JF, Court JR, et al: Global spatial disorientation. *J Neurol Sci* 34:453–458, 1977.
19. Coslett HB, Saffran EM: Simultanagnosia: To see but not two see. *Brain* 114:1523–1545, 1991.
20. Tyler HH: Abnormalities of perception with defective eye movements (Bálint's syndrome). *Cortex* 4:154–171, 1968.
21. Luria AR: Disorders of "simultaneous perception" in a case of bilateral occipitoparietal brain injury. *Brain* 83:437–449, 1959.
22. Goodglass H, Kaplan E: *Assessment of Aphasia and Related Disorders*. Philadelphia: Lea & Febiger, 1972.
23. Baylis GC, Driver J, Baylis LL, Rafal RD: Perception of letters and words in Bálint's syndrome: Evidence for the unity of words. *Neuropsychologia* 32:1273–1286, 1994.
24. Farah MJ: *Visual Agnosia*. Cambridge, MA: MIT Press, 1990.
25. Kinsbourne M, Warrington EK: The localizing significance of limited simultaneous form perception. *Brain* 86:697–702, 1963.
26. Levine DN, Calvanio R: A study of the visual defect in verbal alexia-simultanagnosia. *Brain* 101:65–81, 1978.
27. Kinsbourne M, Warrington EK: A disorder of simultaneous form perception. *Brain* 85:461–486, 1962.
28. Luria AR, Praudina-Vinarskaya EN, Yarbus AL: Disorders of ocular movement in a case of simultanagnosia. *Brain* 86:219–228, 1963.
29. Verfaellie M, Rapcsak SZ, Heilman KM: Impaired shifting of attention in Bálint's syndrome. *Brain Cogn* 12:195–204, 1990.
30. Posner MI, Walker JA, Friedrich EJ, Rafal RD: Effects of parietal injury on covert orienting of visual attention. *J Neurosci* 4:1863–1874, 1984.
31. Posner MI, Petersen SE: The attention system of the human brain. *Annu Rev Neurosci* 13:25–42, 1990.
32. Navon D: Forest before trees: The precedence of global features in visual perception. *Cogn Psychol* 9:353–383, 1977.
33. Treisman A, Gormican S: Feature analysis in early vision: Evidence for search asymmetries. *Psychol Rev* 95:15–48, 1988.

34. Treisman A, Schmidt N: Illusory conjunctions in the perception of objects. *Cogn Psychol* 14:107–141, 1982.
35. Prinzmetal W, Henderson D, Ivry R: Loosening the constraints on illusory conjunctions: Assessing the roles of exposure duration and attention. *J Exp Psychol Perform: HPP* 21:1362–1375, 1995.
36. Friedman-Hill SR, Robertson LC, Treisman A: Parietal contributions to visual feature binding: Evidence from a patient with bilateral lesions. *Science* 269:853–855, 1995.
37. Bernstein LJ, Robertson LC: Illusory conjunctions of color and motion with shape following bilateral parietal lesions. *Psychol Sci* 9:167–175, 1998.
38. Watson RT, Valenstein E, Day A, Heilman KM: Posterior neocortical systems subserving awareness and neglect. Neglect associated with superior temporal sulcus but not area 7 lesions. *Arch Neurol* 51:1014–1021, 1994.
39. Kanwisher N: Neural events and perceptual awareness. *Cognition* 79:89–113, 2001.
40. Benson DF, Davis J, Snyder BD: Posterior cortical atrophy. *Arch Neurol* 45:789–793, 1988.
41. Coslett HB, Starke M, Rajaram S, Saffran EM: Narrowing the spotlight: A visual attentional disorder in Alzheimer's disease. *Neurocase* 1:305–318, 1995.
42. Laeng B, Kosslyn SM, Caviness VS, Bates J: Can deficits in spatial indexing contribute to simultanagnosia? *Cogn Neuropsychol* 16:81–114, 1999.
43. Humphreys GW, Price CJ: Visual feature discrimination in simultanagnosia. A study of two cases. *Cogn Neuropsychol* 11:393–434, 1994.
44. Grossberg S, Mingolla E, Ros WD: Visual brain and visual perception: How does the cortex do perceptual grouping? *Trends Neurosci* 20:106–111, 1997.
45. Ricci R, Vaishnavi S, Chatterjee A: A deficit of intermediate vision: Experimental observations and theoretical implications. *Neurocase* 5:1–12, 1999.
46. Vecera S, Behrmann M: Spatial attention does not require preattentive grouping. *Neuropsychology* 11(1): 30–43, 1997.

Chapter 28

DISORDERS OF CONSCIOUSNESS IN COMA, STUPOR, AND MINIMALLY RESPONSIVE STATES

Joseph T. Giacino

Borrowing from William James,[1] one could admit with confidence that "everyone knows what *consciousness* is, until he tries to define it." A recent literature review by the author revealed approximately 20 terms shown in Table 28-1 that have been used to describe states of altered consciousness, few of which have been operationalized. Since the limits of consciousness have not been well defined,[2] it should come as no surprise that disorders of consciousness (DOCs) also remain enigmatic. Recent estimates of the rate of misdiagnosis of coma and the vegetative state (VS) range from 18 to 43 percent.[3–5] Clinical variables thought to cloud diagnostic accuracy include neuromuscular dysfunction, sensory impairment, slow processing speed, and inadequate assessment tools.[5]

In response to these problems, professional organizations in neurology and rehabilitation have recently published position statements concerning the diagnostic and prognostic parameters associated with specific DOCs.[6–9] Unfortunately, there are significant differences in the recommendations proposed by these groups relative to the assessment and management of individuals with DOC. Recognizing the potential detrimental effects of these conflicting recommendations, the Aspen Neurobehavioral Conference Workgroup on the vegetative and minimally conscious states was convened.[10] This work group, comprising individuals involved in development of the prior position statements, was charged with establishing consensus-based recommendations for clinical management of patients with DOC. This chapter provides a basic overview of the neural substrate underlying consciousness and summarizes the recommendations proposed by the Aspen Workgroup for establishing differential diagnosis and prognosis among patients with DOCs.

THE FUNCTIONAL NEUROANATOMY OF CONSCIOUSNESS

Consciousness is dependent upon the coherent integration of interdependent neural subsystems. Alterations in consciousness may arise from focal lesions to specific mesencephalic and diencephalic structures or from mesodiencephalic-cortical disconnection. Consciousness is primarily regulated by the reticular formation, which comprises two subsystems, one responsible for arousal and the other for gating of attention. These activities have been referred to as *tonic* and *phasic* arousal, respectively.[11]

Arousal System

Tonic arousal relates to diurnal fluctuations in wakefulness that are not contingent upon sensory events. Structures contained in the caudal portion of the reticular formation (RF)—including the medulla, raphe nuclei, pontine tegmentum, locus ceruleus, and midbrain—modulate wakefulness. Cholinergic, serotoninergic, noradrenergic, and dopaminergic input from these widely distributed structures influences cortical activation.[12,13] The RF also receives feedback from cortical regions, allowing for bidirectional regulation of arousal. Disruption of this system produces global reductions in wakefulness ranging from drowsiness to coma.[14]

Gating System

While tonic arousal can be viewed as a steady-state mechanism, phasic arousal involves rapid changes in alertness triggered by novel, unexpected, or otherwise

Table 28-1
Terms used to refer to disorders of consciousness

Akinetic mutism	Obtundation
Anoetic state	Parasomnia
Apallic syndrome	Permanent vegetative state
Coma	Persistent vegetative state
Coma vigil	Post-coma unawareness
Cognitive death	Prolonged coma
Decerebrate state	Prolonged post-traumatic unconsciousness
Low level	Stupor
Minimally conscious state	Vegetative state
Minimally responsive state	

salient environmental stimuli. Phasic arousal is primarily mediated by thalamic nuclei located in the rostral RF. The reticular thalamic nucleus appears to selectively gate sensorimotor input to the thalamus through neural inhibition.[15,16] This process allows for immediate execution of discrete attentional shifts necessitated by environmental events.

The second component of this system, termed the ascending reticular activating system (ARAS), was originally thought to represent a nonspecific cortical activating system capable of transmitting diffuse physiologic arousal independent of sensory stimulation.[17] More recent investigations have shown that the intralaminar nuclei (ILN) of the ARAS have discernible subdivisions that project to particular cortical and subcortical targets. Three groups of thalamic nuclei have been identified that project to discrete cortical targets.[18,19] The posterior division of the ILN projects to premotor, prefrontal, and parietal association cortex. The anterior ILN contains projections to prefrontal cortex, frontal eye fields, anterior cingulate, and anterior parietotemporal cortices. The centromedial ILN projects to limbic structures including orbitofrontal cortex, amygdala, and hippocampus. The neural architecture and topography of the ILN are central to their pivotal role in cerebral neuromodulation. The regional specificity of the ILN allows them to selectively influence specific cognitive subsystems involved in sensorimotor integration, visual scanning, attentional allocation, working memory, and behavioral initiation and control.

Disorders of consciousness are caused by structural or functional lesions that disrupt the arousal and gating systems. Because consciousness is dually mediated by these systems, distinguishable behavioral syndromes can be identified that are characterized by various permutations of impaired wakefulness, behavioral responsiveness, and cognitive control.

DISORDERS OF CONSCIOUSNESS

Disorders of consciousness range in severity from those that result in mild, transient diminution of awareness of self or environment (e.g., delirium) to disorders characterized by complete and persistent loss of cognitive awareness (e.g., vegetative state). In evaluating individuals with DOCs, it is important to recognize the distinction between arousal and awareness. Arousal pertains to level of wakefulness and can be operationally defined as the intensity of sensory stimulation required to interrupt sleep.[20] Arousal level largely determines the capacity to detect environmental events. Awareness is contingent upon arousal and reflects the capacity to sustain vigilance toward the environment in order to extract meaning from the stimuli apprehended.[21]

Coma

Coma is perhaps the best-recognized disorder of consciousness. The behavioral and electrophysiologic features of coma have been comprehensively characterized by Plum and Posner[2] and are well accepted. Descriptively, coma represents a state of unarousable unresponsiveness in which there is no evidence of awareness of self or environment.

Diagnostic Criteria for Coma The clinical syndrome of coma consists of the following:

Absence of sleep-wake cycles on EEG

No evidence of purposeful motor activity

No response to command

No evidence of language comprehension or expression

Inability to discretely localize noxious stimuli

Prognosis and Outcome from Coma The eyes remain continuously closed during coma and fail to open in response to vigorous sensory stimulation. Eye-opening signals emergence from coma and almost always occurs within 2 to 4 weeks of onset.[22] The prognosis for recovery of consciousness is largely dependent upon injury severity[23–25] and duration of unconsciousness.[26,27] Katz found that 50 percent of 119 patients who remained comatose for 2 weeks or more were severely disabled or vegetative at 1 year.[28] Moreover, none of these patients achieved a rating of good recovery on the Glasgow Outcome Scale.[29] Conversely, 80 percent of those with less than 2 weeks of posttraumatic amnesia (PTA) achieved good recovery at 1 year, as compared to none with more than 4 weeks of PTA. In a large multicenter study, Whyte and colleagues reported that duration of unconsciousness, measured by time to command-following, was a highly significant predictor of functional outcome on 10 different indices.[26]

Vegetative State

The least understood and most controversial DOC is the vegetative state (VS). The clinical features of VS were first outlined by Jennett and Plum in 1972.[30] They noted that after a period of coma, the eyes open first to pain and then to less arousing stimuli. Stimulation-induced arousal is subsequently followed by periods of spontaneous eye-opening. The patient may blink to menace but appears to be inattentive. There may be roving eye movements or brief orienting toward moving objects. Slow, dystonic, reflexive posturing may occur spontaneously or following application of nociceptive stimuli. There may be fragments of coordinated movement and the upper extremities may move toward noxious stimuli but discrete localization does not occur. Release of oromotor reflexes (e.g., chewing, bruxism) is frequently observed, although solids or liquids placed in the mouth may be swallowed. Grunting and moaning may be provoked by environmental or noxious stimuli, but there is no indication of preserved receptive or expressive language function.

Diagnostic Criteria for VS In 1995, the Quality Standards Subcommittee of the American Academy of Neurology (AAN) published guidelines for diagnosing VS.[6] These were based on a comprehensive review of the world literature on VS conducted by the Multi-Society Task Force on PVS (MSTF).[22] The following criteria were recommended for diagnosing VS and have been widely incorporated into clinical practice:

No evidence of awareness of self or environment and an inability to interact with others

No evidence of sustained, reproducible, purposeful or voluntary behavioral responses to visual, auditory, tactile or noxious stimuli

No evidence of language comprehension or expression

Intermittent wakefulness manifested by the presence of sleep-wake cycles

Sufficiently preserved hypothalamic and brain stem functions to permit survival with medical and nursing care

Bowel and bladder incontinence

Variable preservation of cranial nerve and spinal reflexes

Prognosis and Outcome of VS The prognosis for recovery of consciousness in both adults and children is highly dependent upon the cause of injury and the duration of unconsciousness. Data provided by the MSTF[22] indicate that approximately 30 percent of patients who are in VS at 3 months following a traumatic brain injury will recover consciousness by 1 year. Another 30 percent will remain in VS after 1 year, and the remaining 30 percent will die. After 6 months in traumatic VS, the recovery rate at 1 year declines to 15 percent. In sharp contrast, fewer than 10 percent of patients diagnosed with VS at 3 months following hypoxic-ischemic, metabolic, and other types of nontraumatic brain injury will recover consciousness by 1 year. Of the remaining 90 percent, approximately one-half will remain in VS and the other half will die within 12 months. After 6 months in nontraumatic VS, the probability of recovery at 1 year appears to be less than 5 percent.

The MSTF arbitrarily defined the *persistent vegetative state* as a VS present at 1 month after acute traumatic and nontraumatic brain injury and present for a minimum of 1 month in degenerative, metabolic, and developmental disorders. Based on the available data from their review, the MSTF coined the term *permanent vegetative state* to denote the point at which VS can be considered irreversible. With rare exception, VS is judged to be permanent 12 months after traumatic brain injury and after 3 months following nontraumatic causes. It is important to note that the temporal guidelines for establishing permanent VS are based on empiric data extracted from fewer than 30 cases, with the length of follow-up on these cases ranging from 14 months to 10 years.

Although neuroimaging studies are inadequte to establish prognosis in the absence of clinical data, there is recent evidence that specific lesion profiles may be associated with failure to recover consciousness from VS. Kampfl and others completed cerebral MRI studies on 80 consecutive patients with closed head injury admitted to a trauma and rehabilitation center.[31] Patients were categorized into two groups, those who met diagnostic criteria for persistent VS according to the MSTF and those who were conscious but remained disabled. Lesions were characterized by number, location, size, and signal intensity by three independent neuroradiologists. Adjusted odds ratios indicated that patients with lesions involving the corpus callosum (214:1) and dorsolateral brainstem (7:1) were significantly less likely to recover consciousness relative to patients with lesions in other regions. A logistic regression model incorporating lesion locus correctly classified 87 percent of patients by group membership after accounting for age, GCS score, pupillary abnormalities, and total number of lesions.

Minimally Conscious State

The minimally conscious state (MCS) is a newly defined condition described by the Aspen Workgroup.[10] MCS refers to a condition of severely altered consciousness in which minimal but definite behavioral evidence of self or environmental awareness is demonstrated. MCS usually exists as a transitional state reflecting either neurologic improvement from coma or VS or neurologic decline, as in progressive neurodegenerative conditions such as Alzheimer's disease. A primary objective of the Aspen Workgroup in recommending this term was to clearly distinguish individuals with some evidence of consciousness from those who demonstrate no evidence of cognition or purposeful behavior (e.g., vegetative state). The detection of consciousness mandates aggressive management of medical complications (including pain), consideration of rehabilitative treatment, and long-term follow-up.

Diagnostic Criteria for MCS The diagnosis of MCS is based on the presence of one or more behavioral responses discernible on bedside assessment. These responses are characteristically inconsistent in MCS but must be shown to occur on a reproducible or sustained basis. Serial assessment is often required before the diagnosis of MCS can be made because of the degree of response inconsistency associated with this condition. The diagnosis of MCS rests on clear demonstration of one or more of the following behaviors:

Simple command-following

Gestural or verbal yes/no responses

Intelligible verbalization

Movements or affective behaviors that occur in contingent relation to relevant environmental stimuli and are not attributable to reflexive activity

Any of the following examples provides sufficient evidence for the last of these criteria:

Episodes of crying, smiling, or laughter in response to the linguistic or visual content of emotional but not neutral topics or stimuli

Vocalizations or gestures that occur in direct response to the linguistic content of comments or questions

Reaching for objects that demonstrates a clear relationship between object location and direction of reach

Touching or holding objects in a manner that accommodates the size and shape of the object

Pursuit eye movement or sustained fixation that occurs in direct response to moving or salient stimuli

Criteria for Emergence from MCS The lower boundary of MCS is dichotomously demarcated by the presence or absence of consciousness. The upper boundary is obviously less clear and necessarily arbitrary. Nevertheless, it is important to establish behaviorally referenced criteria that correspond to the upper boundary to serve as benchmarks for measuring progress and to inform clinical management. In many cases, recovery of the capacity to communicate or interact consistently with the environment marks the transition to a higher level of consciousness and signals the need to modify existing assessment and treatment methods. In this context, the Aspen Workgroup operationally defined emergence from MCS as the *reliable and consistent* demonstration of either (1) interactive communication or (2) functional use of at least two objects.

Interactive communication may occur through verbalization, writing, yes/no signals, or using augmentative communication devices. Functional object use requires discrimination and appropriate use of common articles (e.g., cup, hairbrush). Disturbances of higher cognitive function, particularly aphasia and apraxia, may confound assessment of these criteria and should be considered before establishing a diagnosis.

Clinician ratings of consciousness are inherently constrained by the need to rely on behavioral indicators. Thus, consciousness is inferred based on behavior. Judgments concerning level of consciousness are typically considered with regard to the frequency and complexity of observed behavior. The limitations of this approach are illustrated in the two-dimensional matrix shown in Fig. 28-1 and are especially relevant to the distinction between MCS and emergence from MCS. Patients who frequently demonstrate highly complex behavior (cell A) clearly meet the criteria for emergence from MCS. This situation is exemplified by patients who are intermittently capable of conversational speech. Patients who show exclusively low-complexity behavior (cells C and D) and evidence rudimentary signs of cognition only fall well within the boundaries of MCS. Patients who demonstrate sustained visual pursuit but no other sign of intentional behavior would fall within cell C or D. But what can be concluded about those patients who infrequently demonstrate complex behavior (cell B)? These individuals clearly demonstrate cognitively complex behaviors (e.g., intelligible verbalizations) but do so so infrequently that it is not possible to discern their cognitive status reliably over time. Do these complex behaviors occur infrequently because of fluctuations in level of consciousness, or is the low response rate simply attributable to limitations in the capacity to express behavior?

This problem is best illustrated by patients with akinetic mutism, a condition first described by Cairns in 1941[32] to describe the dramatic diminution of speech and movement caused by drive-reducing lesions in diencephalic and basal frontal structures. Cairns and others[33,34] have shown, however, that individuals with akinetic mutism are capable of generating cognitively complex behavior when they are exposed to external sources of stimulation. Fisher[35] has described patients who do not speak or respond to motor commands but, when called on the telephone, readily engage in conversation, only to fall mute again upon termination of the phone call. This raises questions about the degree to which cognition is correlated with behavioral responsiveness and challenges the reliability of commonly employed assessment procedures. In this context, patients with akinetic mutism represent a specific subgroup of MCS.

Prognosis and Outcome of MCS The natural history and long-term outcome of MCS have not been adequately investigated, largely because this condition has only recently been defined.[10]

Strauss and colleagues[36] determined mortality rates for children included in a large state registry with

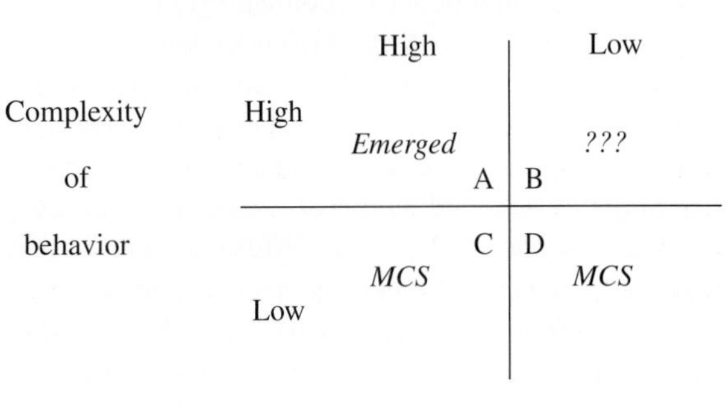

Complexity of behavior	Frequency of behavior: High	Frequency of behavior: Low
High	*Emerged* (A)	*???* (B)
Low	*MCS* (C)	*MCS* (D)

Figure 28-1
Two-dimensional matrix depicting the relationship of behavioral frequency and complexity to judgments concerning level of consciousness.

diagnoses of traumatic and nontraumatic MCS and VS. The MCS group was divided into two subgroups based on degree of preserved mobility. Mobility was operationally defined as the presence of one or more spontaneous or elicited movements of the head, trunk, or extremities. Patients in mobile MCS survived significantly longer than did immobile MCS and VS patients (81 percent versus 65 percent and 63 percent, respectively at 8 years postinjury). In addition, mortality rates were found to be lowest in patients with traumatic VS and MCS relative to those with nontraumatic etiologies.

There is some evidence to suggest that morbidity may generally be more favorable following MCS as compared to VS. Giacino and Kalmar[37] obtained functional outcome ratings on the Disability Rating Scale (DRS)[38] at 1, 3, 6, and 12 months postinjury for 104 patients diagnosed with VS or MCS on admission to rehabilitation. While both diagnostic groups received DRS scores in the severe to vegetative range at 1 month postinjury, the MCS group improved more rapidly, showed a longer course of recovery, and had significantly better mean DRS scores at 12 months. Patients in the traumatic MCS group achieved the best outcomes at 1 year. Fifty percent of the traumatic MCS group were found to have no disability to moderate disability at 1 year, while only 3 percent of the VS group and none of the nontraumatic MCS patients received DRS scores within these outcome categories. Two other recent studies have reported similar findings.[39,40]

INTO THE FUTURE

Neuroimaging technology is poised to dramatically influence the way we think about disorders of consciousness. As reviewed in Chaps. 6–8, advances in structural and functional neuroimaging have already begun to yield important clues to understanding pathophysiology, neural circuits for cognition, probability of recovery, and prerequisites for effective treatment interventions. A structural imaging method known as *diffusion-weighted magnetic resonance imaging* (DWI), capable of detecting diffuse axonal injury, will improve the acute management of patients with alterations in consciousness. DWI may help predict recovery of consciousness and response to early clinical interventions when correlated with changes in intracranial pressure.[41]

Resting metabolic brain mapping provides a means of identifying viable cortical function in patients with minimal behavioral output. Positron emission tomography (PET) has been used in VS patients to identify regions of preserved cerebral metabolism in auditory,[42] motor,[43] and language[43] cortex. These studies show a close relationship between preserved fragments of behavior and corresponding regions of cortical and subcortical activation in otherwise unconscious patients.

Activation studies employing functional PET and magnetic resonance imaging will likely assume a primary role in outcome prediction, given the expected link between inducible changes in cerebral metabolism and recovery of function. Functional PET has been used to identify "covert cortical processing" in patients diagnosed with persistent VS. In one case study,[44] significant activation of visual association cortex was noted following presentation of photographs of faces but not after presenting the same photographs in repixellated form. The authors reported that the patient recovered consciousness and demonstrated clear evidence of face recognition 2 months after this finding was observed.

There has also been renewed interest in developing effective treatment interventions for patients with disorders of consciousness. Neuromodulation strategies utilizing pharmacologic interventions,[45–47] deep brain stimulation,[19] and hyperbaric oxygen treatment[48] hold promise for reducing mortality and morbidity associated with catastrophic brain injury.

REFERENCES

1. James W: *The Principles of Psychology*. New York: Holt, 1890.
2. Plum F, Posner J: *The Diagnosis of Stupor and Coma*, 3d ed. Philadelphia: Davis, 1982.
3. Tresch DD, Sims FH, Duthie EH, et al: Clinical characteristics of patients in the persistent vegetative state. *Arch Intern Med* 151:930, 1991.
4. Childs NL, Mercer WN, Childs HW: Accuracy of diagnosis of persistent vegetative state. *Neurology* 43:1465, 1993.

5. Andrews K, Murphy L, Munday R, et al: Misdiagnosis of the vegetative state: Retrospective study in a rehabilitation unit. *BMJ* 313:13, 1996.
6. The Quality Standards Subcommittee: Practice parameter: Assessment and management of persons in the persistent vegetative state. *Neurology* 45:1015, 1995.
7. American Congress of Rehabilitation Medicine: Recommendations for use of uniform nomenclature pertinent to persons with severe alterations in consciousness. *Arch Phys Med Rehabil* 76:205, 1995.
8. Andrews K: International working party on the management of the vegetative state: Summary report. *Brain Inj* 10(11):797, 1996.
9. Royal College of Physicians Working Group: The permanent vegetative state. *J R Coll Phys (Lond)* 30:119, 1996.
10. Giacino JT, Zasler ND, Katz DI, et al: Development of practice guidelines for assessment and management of the vegetative and minimally conscious states. *J Head Trauma Rehabil* 12(4):79, 1997.
11. Posner MI, Rafal RD: Cognitive theories of attention and the rehabilitation of attentional deficits, in Meier M, Benton A, Diller L (eds): *Neuropsychological Rehabilitation*. New York: Guilford Press, 1987, p 182.
12. Steriade M: Thalamic substrates of disturbances in states of vigilance and consciousness in humans, in Steriade M, Jones E, McCormick D (eds): *Thalamus*. New York: Elsevier, 1997.
13. McCormick DA: Neurotransmitter actions in the thalamus and cerebral cortex and their role in neuromodulation of thalamocortical activity. *Prog Neurobiol* 39(4):337, 1992.
14. Plum F: Coma and related global disturbances of the human conscious state, in Peters A (ed): *Cerebral Cortex*. New York: Plenum, 1991.
15. Schiebel AB: Anatomical and physiological substrates of arousal, in Hobson JA, Brazier MA (eds): *The Reticular Formation Revisited*. New York: Raven Press, 1980.
16. Yingling CD, Skinner JE: Regulation of unit activity in nucleus reticularis thalami by the mesencephalic reticular formation and frontal granular cortex. *EEG Clin Neurophysiol* 39:635, 1975.
17. Moruzzi G, Magoun HW: Brain stem reticular formation and activation of the EEG. *EEG Clin Neurophysiol* 1:455, 1949.
18. Gronewegen H, Berendse H: The specificity of the nonspecific midline and intralaminar thalamic nuclei. *Trends Neurosci* 17:52, 1994.
19. Shiff ND, Rezai AR, Plum FP: A neuromodulation strategy for rational therapy of complex brain injury states. *Neurol Res* 22:267, 2000.
20. Benson DF: *The Neurology of Thinking*. New York: Oxford University Press, 1994.
21. Young GB, Pigott SE: Neurobiological basis of consciousness. *Arch Neurol* 56:153, 1999.
22. The Multi-Society Task Force Report on PVS: Medical aspects of the persistent vegetative state. *N Engl J Med* 330:1499–1572, 1994.
23. Katz DI, Alexander MP: Predicting outcome and course of recovery in patients admitted to rehabilitation. *Arch Neurol* 51:661, 1994.
24. Levin HS, Gary HE, Eisenberg HM, et al: Neurobehavioral outcome 1 year after severe head injury. *J Neurosurg* 73:699, 1990.
25. Marshall LF, Gautille T, Klauber MR, et al: The outcome of severe closed head injury. *J Neurosurg* 75:S28, 1991.
26. Whyte J, Cifu D, Dikmen S, et al: Prediction of functional outcomes after traumatic brain injury: A comparison of two measures of duration of unconsciousness. *Arch Phys Med Rehabil* 82:1355, 2001.
27. Choi SC, Barnes TY, Bullock R, et al: Temporal profile of outcomes in severe head injury. *J Neurosurg* 81:169, 1994.
28. Katz DI : Neuropathology and neurobehavioral recovery from closed head injury. *J Head Trauma Rehabil* 7(2):1, 1992.
29. Jennett B, Bond M: Assessment of outcome after severe brain damage: A practical scale. *Lancet* 1:480, 1975.
30. Jennett B, Plum F: Persistent vegetative state after brain damage: A syndrome in search of a name. *Lancet* 1:734, 1972.
31. Kampfl A, Schmutzhard E, Franz G, et al: Prediction of recovery from post-traumatic vegetative state with cerebral magnetic-resonance imaging. *Lancet* 351:1763, 1998.
32. Cairns H, Oldfield RC, Pennybacker JB, Whitteridge D: Akinetic mutism with an epidermoid cyst of the third ventricle. *Brain* 64:273, 1941.
33. Burruss JW, Chacko RC: Episodically remitting akinetic mutism following subarachnoid hemorrhage. *J Neuropsychiatry Clin Neurosci* 11(1):100, 1999.
34. Brooke MM, Andary MT, Mitsuda PM, et al: Telephone use to elicit voice or speech in brain injured subjects. *Arch Phys Med Rehabil* 72:106, 1991.
35. Fisher CM: Honored guest presentation: Abulia minor vs agitated behavior. *Clin Neurosurg* 9:1983.

36. Strauss DJ, Ashwal S, Day SM, Shavelle RM: Life expectancy of children in vegetative and minimally conscious states. *Pediatr Neurol* 23(4):1, 2000.
37. Giacino JT, Kalmar K: The vegetative and minimally conscious states: A comparison of clinical features and functional outcome. *J Head Trauma Rehabil* 12(4):36, 1997.
38. Rappaport M, Hall KM, Hopkins K, et al: Disability rating scale for severe head trauma: coma to community. *Arch Phys Med Rehabil* 73:628, 1992.
39. Francisco GE, Yablon SA, Ivanhoe CB, et al: Outcome among vegetative and minimally responsive patients with severe acquired brain injury (abstr). *Am J Phys Med Rehabil* 75:158, 1996.
40. Whyte J, DiPasquale MC, Childs N, et al: Recovery from the vegetative and minimally conscious states: Preparation for a multi-center clinical trial (abstr). *Am J Phys Med Rehabil* 78(2):181, 1999.
41. Ashwal S, Holshouser BA: New neuroimaging techniques and their potential role in patients with acute brain injury. *J Head Trauma Rehabil* 12(4):13, 1997.
42. Laureys S, Faymonville ME, Degueldre C, et al: Auditory processing in vegetative state. *Brain* 123:1589, 2000.
43. Plum FP, Schiff N, Ribary U, et al.: Coordinated expression in chronically unconscious persons. *Phil Trans R Soc (Lond)* 353:1929, 1998.
44. Menon DK, Owen AM, Williams EJ, et al: Cortical processing in persistent vegetative state. *Lancet* 352:200, 1998.
45. Zafonte R: Amantadine: A potential treatment for the minimally conscious state. *Brain Injury* 12(7):617, 1998.
46. Rhinehard DL, Whyte J, Sandel ME: Improved arousal and initiation following tricyclic antidepressant use in severe brain injury. *Arch Phys Med Rehabil* 77:80, 1996.
47. Elovic E: Pharmacology of attention and arousal in the low level patient. *Neurorehabilitation* 6:97, 1996.
48. Rockswold GL, Ford SE, Anderson DC, et al: Results of a prospective randomized trial for treatment of severely brain-injured patients with hyperbaric oxygen. *J Neurosurg* 76:929, 1992.

Chapter 29

ANOSOGNOSIA

Todd E. Feinberg
David M. Roane

Unawareness of neurologic defects or illness, also referred to as anosognosia, has many aspects, and consideration of the nature and origin of this complex symptom has engendered many theories. In this chapter we focus on a few seemingly diverse conditions that entail unawareness of a neurologic defect—namely, unawareness of visual defects including the blind spot, scotomas, hemianopias, and cerebral blindness; issues of unawareness after callosal disconnection; unawareness of hemiplegia; and unawareness of memory defects.

UNAWARENESS OF VISUAL DEFECTS

Unawareness of the Blind Spot

The physiologic blind spot in the temporal field of each eye is caused by the lack of retinal ganglion cells at the optic disk, located 3 to 4 mm nasal to the fovea. Unawareness of the blind spot was first described by Mariotte in 1668.[1] It is well known that even when viewing with one eye closed, we are generally unaware of our own blind spot unless its presence is specifically sought. Gassel and Williams[2] reviewed Helmholtz's explanation for unawareness of the blind spot; namely, that the blind spot was discovered only negatively by careful observation of the absent aspects of the stimulus. When these absences were recognized, the gap could be deduced. They suggested that "The discovery is therefore a judgment rather than a direct sensation."

Fuchs[3] explained unawareness of the blind spot on the basis of perceptual completion for certain stimuli such as evenly colored surfaces, printed pages, and continuous lines and circles. This completion is not total, however. For example, as Fuchs points out, if a line enters and ends within the blind spot, it will not be completed. He explained these findings on the basis of gestalt principles, suggesting "completion can and does occur only if the 'seen' part implies a whole of which it is a part—i.e., whose law it already contains. . . . The tendency towards wholeness exhibited by an incomplete part is a tendency towards simplicity or *Prägnanz*." Only when the missing part enters into a "totalized whole-apprehension" will the stimulus be completed and the blind spot pass unnoticed. Ramachandran[4] has also provided evidence that the filling in of the blind spot is perceptual as opposed to conceptual and is a perceptually "primitive" process, occurring at an early stage of visual processing.

Some preliminary physiologic evidence regarding completion of the blind spot has been provided by Gattass and coworkers.[5] They performed unit recordings on neurons in layer 4C of V1 in the area of the representation of the contralateral blind spot. A line stimulus, which exceeded in diameter the blind spot, was swept across it. They found a significant potentiation of the response when both sides of the blind spot were stimulated in this manner as compared with unilateral stimulation of either side alone. The authors suggest that through this process, these cells "interpolated" the area across the blind spot and completed this region of blindness. Based on their review of the literature, Walker and Mattingly[6] concluded that unawareness of the blind spot may not require active "filling in" because the blind spot may simply be ignored.

Unawareness of Acquired Scotomata and Hemianopias

Unawareness of acquired scotomata and hemianopias has been reported by most investigators to be the rule rather than the exception. Critchley[7] noted that anterior lesions were more likely to be noticed by patients than posterior lesions and that lack of awareness did not correlate with mental confusion. Bender[8] noted that patients with homonymous visual field defects usually do not see the surrounding space as split in the middle, though they may notice blurring of vision. Both of these authors suggested that macula-sparing lesions were more likely to remain unnoticed than those in which the macular was split.

Critchley described two types of experience associated with hemianopia. "Positive hemianopias," in which objects appear bisected with one half obscured, occur rarely in posteriorly situated cerebral lesions. Alternatively, patients may have a "negative hemianopia," in which no obscurity is experienced, though there is the experience of something missing on the impaired side. Critchley terms this the *hémianopsie nulle of Dufour.*[9] Teuber and coworkers[10] found that of 46 persons with visual field defects due to penetrating gunshot wounds of the brain, only 2 experienced positive scotomata, while 44 experienced negative scotomata such as a "blank" or "void." If they were aware of the problems, most patients attributed their visual difficulties to deficits in their eyes—typically the eye contralateral to the occipital lesion. Patients were generally unaware of the ipsilateral (nasal field) defect. Teuber and colleagues[10] suggested that the functional dominance of the crossed temporal field over the uncrossed nasal field accounted for greater subjective awareness of the disordered temporal field of the contralateral eye.

Another factor related to unawareness of visual defects cited by Bender and Teuber[11] and Critchley[7] is the development of the "pseudofovea." Originally described by Fuchs,[3] the pseudofovea arises as an adaptation to hemianopia, in which the patient develops a functional shift in "central" fixation toward the hemianopic side, with the development of a new center of maximal acuity. In this manner, the patient somewhat "automatically" decreases the functional significance of the hemianopia, thus facilitating unawareness of the visual defect.[12]

Another factor undoubtedly significant in unawareness of hemianopias is the presence of perceptual completion. Poppelreuter in 1917[13] reported that if a figure, such as a circle or square, was presented such that a portion of it fell into a hemianopic field, the patient would nonetheless report seeing the whole figure. He also found that even if objectively incomplete figures were presented such that the gap fell within the hemianopic field, perceptual completion would nonetheless occur.

Fuchs[3] found that patients who experience visual blackness in the defective region do not report completion. In those few patients reporting completion, Fuchs found that (1) "simple" geometric figures such as circles and squares could be completed but complex though highly familiar figures such as a dog, face, or bottle—or even symmetrical but complex figures such as a butterfly—would not be completed; (2) simple figures objectively incomplete in the area of visual defect would nonetheless be completed; (3) figures presented in defective fields might be *extinguished* (disappear from awareness) if presented simultaneously with a stimulus in the normal field to which it bore no relation but might enter into completion with the normal field if an appropriate "gestalt" were formed.

Bender and Teuber[11] suggested that completion resulted from residual visual perception occurring in a damaged area of the brain. Completion of a stimulus in an area of perimetric blindness could occur if stimuli were presented briefly enough to prevent the occurrence of extinction. Completion in their view was the "absence of extinction"; it would occur only with objectively intact objects and could not be the result of a "psychological filling in" of a missing part. In agreement, Torjussen[14] demonstrated completion in hemianopic subjects only when using objectively complete stimuli. He suggested that completion resulted from an interaction between the normal and impaired visual areas, in which the normal field facilitated perception in the abnormal field.

It has been suggested by many investigators over the years that insight into hemianopic defects is inversely related to perceptual completion.[2,3,11,12] Fuchs found he could eliminate the completion effect if the patient was encouraged to adopt a "critical attitude" toward his or her perceptual experience. Fuchs[3] and Bender and Teuber[11] found the subjective fields to vary with the extent of completion. Gassel and Williams[2] tested 35 hemianopic patients for perceptual completion. In one condition, patients fixated either to the examiner's nose or to the eye opposite the lesion and were asked whether the whole face was seen. They were tested with and without a black object covering the portion of the face falling in the defective field. The investigators found completion of the face in 28 of the 35 patients. Most important for present purposes, Gassel and Williams made the following observations: (1) completion would occur even when a black object was slowly interposed to cover the completed side of the face, thus making residual perception of that side impossible; (2) encouraging an "analytic attitude" toward perceptions tended to decrease the degree of completion; and (3) completion and awareness of defects were inversely related. An additional important issue emphasized by these authors is that gaps in the visual fields have no direct sensory effect but rather are *deduced* when the missing aspects of a stimulus are recognized. In their words: "The hemianopic field is an area of absence which is discovered rather than sensed; it is a negative area whose presence is *judged* from some specific failure in function, rather than directly perceived."

Warrington[15] reported her observations on 20 patients with homonymous hemianopic defects from various etiologies. She observed completion of both whole and half figures and found that of the 20 patients, the 11 who were unaware of their visual defects all showed visual completion, while none of those patients who were aware of their defects demonstrated completion. Completion was found to be associated with parietal lobe damage and tended to be associated with unilateral neglect but not mental deterioration.

In the presence of neglect, therefore, incomplete stimuli may be completed, and this phenomenon cannot be explained by latent perception made explicit via a process of facilitation. Rather, it is more appropriate to describe these patients as having *confabulated* the missing aspects of the stimulus. Significantly, Warrington[15] found this type of completion to be inversely related to awareness of defect and Zangwill[16] surmised that "completion, far from being a compensatory reaction to hemianopia (as Poppelreuter supposed), is in fact a variety of visual confabulation constrained by unawareness or denial of defect." Zangwill attributed this "anosognosic misperception" to parietal lobe pathology.

More recently Celesia and coworkers[17] have concluded that "filling in" could be only one of several factors resulting in anosognosia for hemianopia. They posit that the unawareness of visual defects may be dissociable from both hemispatial neglect and parietal lobe involvement.

Unawareness of Divided Visual Fields in Split-Brain Patients

The corpus callosum, anterior commissure, and hippocampal commissure provide the only direct pathways connecting the neocortices of the left and right hemispheres. It is through these connections that unilateral neocortical contributions to sensorimotor functions, learning, and cognition are unified.[18–28] After cerebral commissurotomy, the patient essentially has a fovea-splitting "double hemianopia"[22] with regard to the two hemispheres. As a result, stimuli requiring detailed visual discrimination cannot be compared across the vertical meridian.[21,22,28] In spite of this, it has been repeatedly and somewhat surprisingly noted that these patients may appear (and apparently feel) in most respects quite normal after the acute postoperative period has elapsed.[24,29] Except in cases where intermanual conflict and the alien hand syndrome arise,[30] patients appear to be largely unaware of any change in themselves.

Many mechanisms are available to these patients that allow them to compensate for their deficits and remain subjectively unaware (anosognosic) of any alteration in brain function. Sperry[29,31] points out that a number of sensory projection systems—including tactile representation of the face, crude representation of pain, temperature, and position sense as well as audition—provide bilateral cortical projections, therefore enabling each hemisphere to develop some degree of independent sensory representation. A certain degree of bilateral motor control,[31] including ipsilateral control of eye movements, also provides some unification of action. The emotional tone in response to a unilateral stimulus may spread to the contralateral hemisphere via an intact anterior commissure[18] or remaining brainstem connections[29,31] and provide unification or double representation of an emotional experience.[32,33] Functional adaptations such as exploratory head and eye movements and cross-cueing strategies[26] also provide the disconnected hemispheres with a shared experience. While the split hemispheres are functionally disconnected for detailed visual perception involving foveal geniculostriate vision, Trevarthen has pointed out that ambient nongeniculostriate vision remains undivided after callosal division.[21,27] The speaking left hemisphere may still be able to detect and report the presence of an ipsilaterally presented flash of light or movement and some direction information of a stimulus while also attending to and dealing with ipsilaterally positioned targets. This is particularly true for high-contrast, low-spatial-resolution stimuli.[21] It is also possible that transfer via the anterior commissure may account for the lack of disconnection in some cases.[21,22]

Other factors are important in the lack of divided self-awareness in these patients, however. Levy and colleagues[33–36] presented to callosally sectioned patients visual "chimeric" figures composed of two different halves joined at the midline. With the patient's gaze fixated centrally, each hemisphere would receive different visual input. In these investigations it was demonstrated that when a single response was called for, patients typically responded to either the left or right side of the chimeric stimulus, and the side they responded to was to a large extent determined by task requirements.[33,37] Thus, if a verbal response or a match based on semantic knowledge was required, the right half of the chimera presented to the subject's left hemisphere determined the response. If a visual match based on the object's appearance was required, the left half of the chimera presented to the subject's right hemisphere determined the response.

From the standpoint of unawareness, a number of points are pertinent here. First, patients are not aware that they have seen chimeric figures, though both hemispheres have processed, at least partially, the contralateral aspects of the chimeras. Trevarthen pointed out that one of his patients (L.B.), though able to respond to *both* sides of the chimera simultaneously, never became aware that the stimuli were chimeras.[34] Levy noted that when the patient's left hemisphere responded verbally and even *confabulated* a response to a stimulus that only the right hemisphere knew, the right hemisphere never indicated that it knew via a "frown or head shake" whether the response was in error. Likewise, the patient's left hemisphere did not verbally object to a right hemisphere response.

Second, "completion" of the conflicting or absent aspects of the stimulus probably contributes to this unawareness. Trevarthen noted that when a verbal response was called for, split-brain patients completed the missing left side of objectively partial figures[34] and reported a whole face when shown chimeras with only the right half of a drawing of a face.[18] When shown a chimera with the left side of a tree, the patient's left hand drew a whole tree when instructed to draw what it "saw." Thus, each hemisphere was capable of experiencing a "whole" stimulus, though each actually saw only half.

Third, I suggest that this phenomenon occurs as a result of *confabulatory completion*. As noted previously, the conception of completion developed by Bender and Teuber[11] and Torjussen[14] was that completion resulted from residual visual perception occurring in a damaged area of the brain. According to this view, completion would occur only with objectively intact objects and could not be the result of a "psychological filling in" of a missing part. In split-brain patients, however, the completed aspects of the stimulus that these patients claim to see in the ipsilateral field do not need to be objectively present. This phenomenon, which does not rely on the presence of the actual stimulus in the impaired field, is thus an example of *confabulatory completion* and should be distinguished from the *veridical completion* (a term suggested by Weizkrantz[38]) of objectively complete figures as described by Bender and Teuber[11] and Torjussen.[14,39] It thus may be concluded that the unawareness of defect in split-brain patients depends in part upon the presence of this form of perceptual confabulation.

Unawareness of Blindness

Von Monakow is credited with the first scientific report of unawareness of cortical blindness in patients with bilateral posterior cortical pathology.[40–45] Subsequently, similar cases were described by Müller[46] and Dèjerine and Vialet.[47] Gabriel Anton, in a series of papers between 1893 and 1899, presented the first systematic treatment and theoretical discussion of personal unawareness of neurologic signs including visual loss, cortical deafness, and hemiparesis.[44]

Anton is best known for his description of unawareness of cortical blindness, a particular condition that Albrecht[48] suggested be grouped under the rubric "Anton's symptom" in 1918. It is now known as Anton's syndrome. Anton's most widely cited case[49] was a 56-year-old seamstress named Ursula Mercz who, in spite of complete amaurosis of central origin, was unaware of her visual loss.[42,44,45] Neuropathologic findings on autopsy revealed bilateral cystic necrosis of the white matter of the occipital lobes. Though Anton found generalized cognitive impairment in many of his patients with unawareness of deficits, he maintained that these patients lacked sufficient dementia to explain their unawareness. He proposed that they were mentally blind (seelenblind) to their neurologic defects.[44] Anton suggested that the destruction of association tracts between primary sensory areas and the remaining brain was necessary to produce unawareness of neurologic deficits.

Neuropathologic Features of Anton's Syndrome

The causes of Anton's syndrome are diverse. The blindness most commonly originates in bilateral occipital lobe infarctions.[42,50,51] For instance, Redlich and Dorsey[42] found that 4 of 6 patients with Anton's had bilateral hemianopias. However, they suggested that the cause of the blindness was actually not important for the appearance of the Anton's syndrome. In a more recent review of the syndrome,[50] it was also concluded that the blindness may be caused by lesions at any point along the visual pathways. Geschwind[52] suggested that blindness caused by peripheral lesions is much less likely to cause unawareness of deficit in the absence of significant dementia, while patients with occipital infarctions may manifest unawareness without clouding of consciousness.

Previous authors have observed clinical similarities between Anton's and Korsakoff's syndromes.[51] Stuss and Benson[53] noted that bilateral infarction in the distribution of the posterior cerebral artery is a frequent cause of Anton's syndrome and can produce damage to the hippocampus and limbic structures, which may result in a Korsakoff-like syndrome. In this circumstance, the two syndromes, which involve both unawareness of defects and confabulation, may share a common limbic neuropathology.[54]

Other lines of evidence point to the importance of frontal pathology. Stengel and Steele[55] reported a patient with bilateral optic atrophy and frontal lobe tumors with denial of blindness. Stuss and Benson[53] described a patient with bilateral traumatic optic neuropathy and frontal damage sustained as a result of a motor vehicle accident. The patient was described as alert, oriented, and without other neurologic deficits. While he readily admitted his blindness, he stated that with the proper illumination he could see perfectly. McDaniel and McDaniel[51] described a similar case of a patient with monocular blindness due to optic nerve pathology and bifrontal encephalomalacia. This patient denied her visual defect and her illness in general. She exhibited visual as well as generalized confabulation. The anosognosia and confabulation persisted after the resolution of an acute confusional state. These authors suggest that a memory defect coupled with a failure of self-monitoring due to frontal pathology produced the denial of blindness and further offered that Bychowski may have been the first to make this suggestion.[56]

Relationship to Cognitive Impairment

The presence of generalized cognitive impairment has been noted in many instances of Anton's syndrome,[13,42,45,50,57,58] particularly, as noted above, when the visual loss is due to peripheral pathology.[52] However, the presence of total denial of blindness in the absence of significant (or presence of only mild) cognitive impairment has suggested to many investigators that cognitive impairment alone does not explain Anton's syndrome.[42,51,52,59]

Relationship to Confabulation

Visual and other forms of confabulation appear frequently if not universally in patients with Anton's syndrome. Redlich and Dorsey[42] found prominent confabulation in their patients, leading them to suggest that "'Anton's syndrome may be said to consist of a Korsakoff psychosis in a blind person." Brockman and von Hagen also noted prominent confabulation in patients with Anton's.[60] McDaniel and McDaniel[51] suggested that in virtually all cases of Anton's syndrome, whether due to peripheral or central pathology, confabulation is present in relation to both the visual defect itself as well as to other aspects of the patient's clinical state. They also found confabulation and anosognosia to be closely allied conditions and considered confabulation to be a necessary accompaniment to Anton's syndrome regardless of the site of damage to the visual system. Finally, in a case description of Anton's syndrome,[61] confabulation of visual experience was associated with intact visual imagery.

UNAWARENESS OF HEMIPLEGIA

Gabriel Anton, in 1893, probably provided the first descriptions of unawareness of hemiplegia.[62] One patient, Wilhelmy H., was reportedly unaware of a left hemiparesis,[45] and a second, Johann K., expressed the belief that his daughter (not his hemiplegic arm) was lying to his left.[43,44] Pick provided an additional report of denial of left hemiparesis in 1898.[63] Babinski, in 1914[64] and 1918,[65] provided additional clinical examples of unawareness of left hemiplegia and coined the term *anosognosia*.

While the diagnosis of anosognosia for hemiplegia (AHP) requires only a simple unawareness of hemiplegia, the actual clinical syndrome is far more complex. While some patients may appear simply unaware of their paralysis, frequently the belief in the normalcy of the limb is quite refractory to correction. In severe AHP, repeated efforts by the examiner to demonstrate the weakness are futile. In these cases, even when the paralyzed limb is dropped limply in the hemispace ipsilateral to the lesion, still no admission of paralysis is obtained. For this reason, anosognosia often appears to be delusional in nature.[66] Even when the patient admits that the limb does not move upon request, excuses such as "laziness" or "tiredness"[67] may be offered as explanations. Alternatively, the patient may *confabulate* that the limb has indeed moved,[64,68–73] as in Babinski's 1914 case, who, when asked to move the arm responded "Voilá, c'est fait."[63,70]

A host of rather unique and colorful clinical findings not directly related to limb movement per se often accompany the anosognosia. Patients may reject the limb entirely, a condition called *asomatognosia,*[74] and attribute its ownership to someone else.[68–70,74] Such was the case with a patient of ours who described her limb as belonging to her deceased husband. The limb may be personified with designations such as "Silly Jimmy" or "Floppy Joe," as described by Critchley.[77,80] Patients may admit the paralysis but appear indifferent to it, a condition first described by Babinski[64] and termed *anosodiaphoria.*[70] Patients may also display hostility toward and hatred of the limb, called *misoplegia.*[80]

Frequency and Laterality of Anosognosia for Hemiplegia

Nathanson and coworkers[81] found that 28 of 100 hemiplegic patients had "denial of illness," 48 had full awareness, and 24 had left hemispheric lesions with severe aphasia that prevented adequate assessment. In the anosognosia group, 69 percent (19 patients) had left hemiplegia, 21 percent (6 patients) had right hemiplegia with aphasia, and 11 percent (3 patients) had right hemiplegia without aphasia. In Cutting's[82] investigation of a series of 100 acute hemiplegics from presumed "cerebrovascular accidents," 30 right hemiplegics were eliminated due to severe aphasia. Of 48 left hemiplegics, 28 (58 percent) demonstrated anosognosia for hemiplegia (AHP); 3 of 52 right hemiplegic patients (14 percent of the testable right hemiplegic group) demonstrated anosognosia. Willanger and coworkers[83] found AHP in 25 percent (14 of 55) and Hier and associates[84] in 36 percent (15 of 41) of right hemispheric stroke patients with varying degrees of weakness, and Bisiach and colleagues[85] found moderate or severe AHP in 12 (33 percent) of 36 patients with severe left hemiplegia.

Starkstein and coworkers[86] reported on 80 patients who had acute cerebrovascular accidents (CVAs) and found that 8 (10 percent) showed mild, 9 (11 percent) moderate, and 10 (13 percent) severe AHP. Fifty-three (66 percent) showed no anosognosia. The AHP was significantly more common with right hemispheric lesions even when aphasic patients were arbitrarily included as "anosognosic." Of 17 moderately or severely anosognosic patients with positive scans, 12 had right hemispheric lesions compared to 3 with left hemispheric lesions (2 had bilateral lesions). Finally, Stone and colleagues[87] studied 171 acute stroke patients (69 right, 102 left) and found AHP in 28 percent of right hemispheric strokes and in 5 percent of left hemispheric strokes, but 45 percent with left hemispheric strokes could not be assessed, compared with only 13 percent with right hemispheric strokes.

The collective impression of these studies is that while AHP is more commonly associated with right hemispheric lesions, some of this difference may be due to the large number of patients with left hemispheric stroke excluded from analysis because the presence of aphasia made their examination impossible or unreliable. In order to circumvent to some extent the issue of aphasia, investigators have employed the Wada test and asked patients if they recall the contralateral paralysis after the effects of the injection have passed and speech recovery has occurred.[88–93] Using amobarbital, Terzian[88] found that patients had poor recall of paralysis regardless of the site of injection. Gilmore and coworkers,[89] using the shorter-acting barbiturate methohexital, found recall of paralysis only after left hemispheric injection. Durkin and coworkers,[90] using amobarbital, found only a small difference in recall favoring the left hemispheric injections (4 percent recall right; 9 percent recall left) and noted that 85 percent did not recall weakness after either injection. However, Adair and colleagues,[91] using methohexital, found failure to recall paralysis in 97 percent of right hemispheric injections compared with 48 percent of those in the left hemispheres. Similar results were reported by Breier and coworkers[92] using methohexital and by Carpenter and associates[93] using amobarbital. Taken together, the data from Wada testing corroborate the clinical studies and suggest that AHP is more common after right hemispheric lesions, but some of this difference is likely due to the presence of aphasia in the subjects with left hemispheric lesions. Based on this right hemisphere predominance, Heilman[94] has proposed that AHP could be due to the failure of a hypothetical comparator or monitor to detect a mismatch between intention and movement. The failure of expectation is "related to dysfunction in the intentional/premotor stems, which are asymmetrically distributed between the hemispheres."[95]

Anatomic Considerations in Anosognosia for Hemiplegia

Although the various forms of anosognosia may have different anatomic bases, be they focal or diffuse, AHP has traditionally been reported in association with lesions of the nondominant parietal lobe, the thalamus, or their connections to other sites or each other.[7,41,96–99]

Hier and coworkers[84] found anosognosia associated with right hemispheric strokes only after larger strokes involving the frontal, parietal, and temporal lobes in addition to subcortical involvement. Levine and coworkers[73] also reported AHP associated with large strokes that involved either the cerebral gyri or adjacent corona radiata. Insular and opercular cortex were the most common cortical structures involved. Levine[73] suggested that no particular focal pathology was required to produce AHP beyond that which was necessary to produce severe sensorimotor loss. Feinberg and coworkers reported verbal asomatognosia associated with lesions of the supramarginal gyrus and posterior corona radiata[74] and AHP associated with lesions of the posterior corona radiata, posterior limb of the internal capsule, and the central gyri and insula, but they found that involvement of these structures did not distinguish patients with and without AHP.[100] Finally, Starkstein and colleagues[86] found AHP associated with lesions of the right thalamus, temporoparietal cortex, and basal ganglia as well as with bilateral subcortical atrophy.

Sensory Loss

Babinski noted that sensory loss appeared to be a necessary prerequisite for AHP.[65] This is not surprising, since the lesions associated with paralysis are likely to involve primary somatosensory areas as well, were the latter directly related or not. Barré[101] emphasized the proprioceptive loss often seen in AHP, and authors including Barkman,[97] Gerstmann,[41] Schilder,[102] Weinstein and Kahn,[103] and Critchley[7] noted the common association between AHP and sensory loss.

Cutting[82] reported sensory loss in 87 percent of 31 patients with AHP, compared with its presence in only 38 percent of 16 patients without either AHP or other anosognosia-related phenomena. Bisiach and associates[85] found that of 12 patients with moderate or severe AHP, 11 had impairments in light touch to unilateral stimuli. Many cases with severe sensory impairments did not display AHP; one case of moderate AHP had no sensory impairment within the limited testing performed. Levine and coworkers[73] found severe left sensory impairment in all modalities in cases of persistent AHP and to a greater extent than in those cases without AHP. They concluded that severe hemisensory impairment is necessary but not sufficient to produce AHP.

Relationship to Hemispatial Neglect

While the manifestations of personal and extrapersonal neglect in a certain sense resemble AHP and these conditions frequently co-occur, they are at least partially dissociable and cannot be reduced one to the other. As Table 29-1 demonstrates, however, these conditions appear related. Some 50 to 100 percent (mean 74 percent) of patients with AHP demonstrated extrapersonal neglect; the percentage of patients with personal neglect has not been extensively studied, but numbers have varied from 32 to 72 percent. In those patients without AHP, extrapersonal neglect may occur, though significantly less frequently (average 21 percent), and this includes many more cases with mild neglect. Cutting[82] found no cases of personal neglect in patients without AHP. Although Bisiach and colleagues[85] reported incidence of personal neglect in 6 of 8 (33 percent)

Table 29-1
Occurrence of left neglect in right-hemisphere-lesioned patients with and without anosognosia for hemiplegia (AHP)

	With AHP		*Without AHP*	
Author	*Extrapersonal neglect, No. (%)*	*Personal neglect, No. (%)*	*Extrapersonal neglect, No. (%)*	*Personal neglect, No. (%)*
Cutting[82]	16/31 (52%)	10/31 (32%)	1/16 (6%)	0/16 (0%)
Hier et al.[84]	13/15 (87%)	—	6/26 (23%)	—
Bisiach et al.[85]	14/18 (78%)	—		
Levine et al.[73]	6/6 (100%) (100% severe)		4/7 (57%) (14% severe)	—
Starkstein et al.[86]	15/22 (55%)	—	2/53 (4%)	—

Occurrence of AHP in patients with and without left neglect

	With neglect		*Without neglect*	
	Extrapersonal	*Personal*	*Extrapersonal*	*Personal*
Hier et al.[84]	13/19 (68%)	—	2/22 (9%)	—
Bisiach et al.[85]	14/17 (82%)	13/19 (68%)	4/19 (21%)	5/17 (29% overall) (18% moderate; 12% mild)

non-AHP patients, they found no severe cases and only 1 moderate case of personal neglect in this group. Bisiach found 3 cases of moderate AHP with no personal neglect at all. This finding is compatible with the observation that AHP may persist if the paralysis is demonstrated to the patient in both the abnormal as well as normal hemispace.

Conversely, AHP occurs in 68 to 82 percent of hemineglect patients (Table 29-1) and much less commonly in those without neglect. This overall relationship between AHP and hemineglect is corroborated by the observation of Cappa and coworkers,[104] who reported reversal of AHP in 2 of 4 right hemispheric hemineglect patients, with remission of personal and extrapersonal neglect during vestibular stimulation.

Relationship to General Intellectual Functioning

It has long been noted that many anosognosic patients may appear impaired in general intellectual functions. Nathanson and coworkers[81] reported a series of 100 hemiplegic patients among whom all 28 with AHP showed disorientation; however, only 15 of 40 (31 percent) patients without AHP had an organic mental syndrome. Weinstein and Kahn[103] noted that patients with various forms of anosognosia for a variety of defects including AHP had a high incidence of cognitive and memory impairment. The investigators felt that these defects were an insufficient explanation for the anosognosia. Cutting[82] reported that 71 percent of AHP patients showed disorientation and 86 percent showed visuoperceptual defects, compared with a frequency of 6 percent for both of these disorders in hemiplegic patients without AHP. Levine and colleagues also found a greater incidence of impairments in multiple neuropsychological domains in patients with AHP than in those with right hemispheric lesions without AHP, which they suggest prevented the AHP patients from discovering their hemiplegia.[73]

Anosognosia for Hemiplegia and Confabulation

Confabulation and AHP are frequently if not universally associated.[7,81,100,103] Critchley[7] and others[71,73,105] noted that when some patients with AHP were told to raise their arms and then asked why no movement occurred, these patients might insist that the limb really had moved or moved "less quickly" than the normal limb. The aforementioned phenomena are generally interpreted as instances of "phantom supernumerary limb" or "phantom third hand,"[7,106] as suggested by Critchley, who coined these terms and likened the phenomenon to other instances of phantom limb following amputation or deafferentation from plexus or spinal cord lesions.[107–109] However, the patient with phantom limb from the latter conditions recognizes the unreality of the phantom sensation and will try to clarify his or her perceptions by touching or looking at the limb, while the anosognosic patient claims to be able to move the limb, though he or she may never attempt to do so. In phantom limb from amputation and deafferentation,[107] the physical location of the phantom—as experienced by the patient—extends from the remaining stump in a position where the limb would be normally; the two dissociate only when the patient does not visually observe the limb and the actual limb is moved.

In contrast, in patients with AHP, the illusory limbs and imagined limb movements are delusional in nature. The patient experiences a partial or complete dissociation between the real limb and the "limb" that performs the "movements"; visual inspection of the actual limb in the AHP patient does not correct the misperception. Indeed, these patients typically deny ownership of the real limb.[74] The supernumerary limb is experienced as healthy by the AHP patient and as intact and possessing normal strength, while phantom limbs are often felt to be missing parts or to be "telescoped" and to possess limited mobility. Based upon these differences, the phenomenon of illusory limb movements and supernumerary limbs in AHP should not be equated with phantom limbs (Table 29-2).

The question naturally arises whether the occurrence of illusory limb movements and supernumerary limbs in AHP can be explained on the basis of perceptual completion.[12] Bender and Teuber[11] and Torjussen[39] suggested that completion resulted from residual perception occurring in a damaged area of the brain. For amputated limbs, it is clearly not possible for

Table 29-2
Comparison of phantom and supernumerary limbs

Characteristics of illusory limb	*Phantom limb after amputation*	*Phantom limb after deafferentation*	*Supernumerary limb after (nondominant) central lesion*
Time of onset	Acute and tends to diminish with time	Frequency increases with time after injury	Acute and tends to resolve rapidly
Duration	Months or years	Typically weeks to months	Rapid resolution usually within weeks
Physical and functional status	Over time becomes incomplete, shrunken, or telescoped	Telescoping may occur but generally does not	Intact and healthy
Willed movements	Limited, effortful	Limited, effortful	Equal or nearly so to intact limb
Effect of visual inspection	Merges with stump	Merges with limb	Remains dissociated from actual limb
Relation to actual limb	Projected from stump Moves in appropriate relation to the body May dissociate if stump deafferented	Usually located within limb; dissociation may occur acutely but typically fades	Always dissociated from actual limb: actual limb denied (asomatognosia)
Confabulation	Absent	Absent	Usually present
Delusional	Typically absent	Typically absent	Usually present
Anosognosia	Absent	Absent	Usually present

there to be actual perception of the missing part. Even if phantom limbs did derive in part from movements of the stump, this form of projective hallucination would not warrant the designation "perceptual completion" in this sense, since it is not produced by the facilitation of veridical perception in damaged areas of the brain via the activation of intact regions. These considerations also make perceptual completion an unlikely explanation for phantoms occurring after deafferentation.

However, in the presence of right hemispheric damage and especially left hemispatial neglect, the presence of an actual stimulus on the completed side may not be necessary. As noted, Warrington[15] reported that patients with hemispatial neglect who had objectively incomplete figures shown tachistoscopically to their normal field would indeed report whole figures, while hemianopics without neglect reported half figures under these circumstances. This phenomenon, which does not depend on the sensory representation of an actual stimulus being present in the impaired field, is another example of *confabulatory completion*, a term suggested in this context by Geschwind.[52] This suggests that the supernumerary limbs and illusory limb movements in AHP represent a form of confabulatory completion in which the patients confabulate normal limbs. The presence of hemispatial neglect could contribute to this tendency toward the confabulatory completion of the left side of the body.

Taken together with the previously described findings, we conclude that the syndromes of unawareness of visual defects in hemianopia, neglect, and split-brain patients and of paralysis in AHP patients all involve confabulation or confabulatory completion. This point of view is supported by the study of Feinberg and coworkers,[100] who found that when patients with right hemisphere lesions with neglect and AHP were compared with patients without AHP, those with AHP showed a significantly greater tendency toward visuoverbal confabulation for visual objects in the left hemispace that were not perceived. In other words, the presence of AHP was associated with the occurrence of confabulation in the visual domain as well as with reference to the hemiplegia. In a separate study of right hemisphere patients designed to look specifically at confabulations related to the hemiplegia, Feinberg et al.[110] tested for the presence of illusory limb movements where the patient claims movement of the paralyzed limb. They found a highly significant association between illusory limb movements and anosognosia. Additionally, all patients with unequivocal illusory limb movements had asomatognosia.

The relationship between anosognosia and confabulation has also been studied with the Wada test, used in the presurgical evaluation of epilepsy patients. Examining patients during right hemisphere inactivation, Meador et al.[111] reported a positive correlation between AHP and both verbal and nonverbal forms of confabulation. Lu et al.[112] were unable to show an association between AHP and confabulations concerning tactile stimulation in patients undergoing Wada. This could be explained by the fact that their procedure produced high rates of confabulations in patients with and without AHP. A more recent Wada study by Lu et al.[113] failed to show an association between AHP and confabulated or "phantom" movements except in the presence of proprioceptive loss.

In understanding these findings, it is necessary to compare evaluations performed during the Wada with the examination of patients after stroke. As noted above, clinical studies have shown that between 25 and 58 percent of patients with left hemiplegia after a cerebrovascular accident (CVA) manifest AHP. The rate of AHP with right hemisphere inactivation during Wada is much higher, ranging from 80 to 97 percent in the larger studies.[91,111,112] This discrepancy could result from the simple inability of the Wada patients to "discover"[73] their paralysis during the brief period of cerebral inactivation. Whereas virtually all anosognosic stroke patients with AHP have sensory loss, Lu et al.[113] found intact proprioception in 2 of 5 patients with AHP and 2 of 3 patients with confabulated movements during Wada testing. Finally, assessments with Wada must be completed within 3 min, while a thorough examination of AHP in a stroke patient can last an hour. Thus, the findings obtained with the Wada procedure are not directly comparable to the studies examining AHP after stroke.

UNAWARENESS OF AMNESIA

In general, insight into amnesia and confabulation are inversely related; although Talland[114] noted that the chronic Wernicke-Korsakoff amnestic might stop confabulating without return of insight, Williams and Rupp[115] noted that with the return of insight, confabulation cleared. Weinstein and Kahn noted prominent confabulation in patients with denial of their impairments in general.[69] Alexander and Freedman[116] reported that in recovery from amnesia following rupture of an aneurysm of the anterior communicating artery (ACoA), there was a co-occurrence of recovery from confabulation and denial of memory impairment, and Mercer and coworkers[117] also proposed that return of insight related inversely to confabulation. Zangwill[118] and Parkin[119] suggested that the constellation of amnesia, confabulation, and lack of insight was typical of diencephalic amnesia, yet amnesics of temporal lobe origin did not display these additional features. It should be noted, however, that many of the confabulatory "diencephalic" cases had lesions that also involved the inferior frontal regions either by compression, direct invasion, postsurgical changes, or possibly acute hydrocephalus.

Other Forms of Unawareness

Numerous other varieties of conditions producing unawareness have been described. These include unawareness of disability in such neuropsychiatric conditions as Alzheimer's disease,[45,120–127] Huntington's disease,[128] auditory agnosia,[129] aphasia,[130–132] schizophrenia,[123] and many nonneurologic conditions including cardiac disease, cancer, acquired immunodeficiency syndrome, and many others.[133,134] Interestingly, two studies have found that frontal impairment correlates with unawareness in Alzheimer's disease[125,126] and that patients with Pick's disease associated with severe and early frontal lobe pathology have an earlier loss of insight than patients with Alzheimer's disease.[45] Another investigation has found, on single photon emission tomography (PET), evidence for right frontal involvement in Alzheimer's disease associated with anosognosia.[127]

UNAWARENESS AND DENIAL

The role of psychological defense, particularly denial, in the production of unawareness syndromes remains unresolved. Schilder[102] was among the first to emphasize motivational factors and coined the term *organic repression* to describe the tendency of hemiplegic patients unconsciously to suppress knowledge of their paralysis. Goldstein[135] interpreted the unawareness of brain-damaged patients in terms of adaptation to deficits and avoidance of the "catastrophic reaction"; a position also favored by Sandifer.[66] More recently, Giacino and Cicerone[136] have argued that psychological denial of deficit is one of several possible factors, along with diffuse cognitive impairment and focal impairment in the ability to recognize functional loss, which can contribute to unawareness of disease.

Paterson and Zangwill[137] made many astute observations relevant to this subject when they considered the patterns of disorientation and confabulation in the posttraumatic confusional state. They noted that patients in the early postacute periods would claim they were located in their home town when they were actually many miles away. During the course of recovering, the patients would simultaneously maintain that they were located in both the correct *and* incorrect locations, a condition termed *reduplicative paramnesia*[138] by Pick and linked by Weinstein and Kahn[69] to anosognosia. Paterson and Zangwill noted that patients in large part were oblivious to the conflict presented by their dual orientation and would confabulate explanations when confronted with the disparity. The investigators observed that patients might accept the correct orientation in an "abstract geographical" sense, such as knowing the correct locale "according to the map," but still maintain they "felt" they were located in a different locale (usually closer to home) based more upon "concrete experience." Thus one patient originally from Grimsby but hospitalized in Scotland reported "If it comes to the map this part is the north of Scotland . . . but if people say 'Do you live here?' I say 'yes, Grimsby!' I feel I'm right . . . I know by my own language, by my own town streets." This patient was confabulatory, had left-hemispatial neglect, and was anosognosic for his left hemiparesis. Although amnesia was initially present, the "retention deficit cleared rapidly" and memory was adequate to recall the day's events a full week before correct orientation returned. This suggested to the investigators that affective motivational factors played a role in the persistent disorientation. This particular patient verbally expressed a strong desire to return home (a feature noted in other reduplicative patients).[139] Paterson and Zangwill suggested that, under the conditions of brain damage, this desire was "actively inhibiting the cognitive mechanisms which normally subserve orientation" and accounted for the persistent disorientation when "cognitive recovery had proceeded far enough to permit and sustain proper orientation." They interpreted the disorientation on the basis of both the *negative* features (in a Jacksonian sense[140]) of anterograde and retrograde amnesia, restriction of perception, and a defect in judgment in which there is a failure to correct incompatible interpretations as well as the *positive* features of affect and motivation. Thus, motivation and affect could play a determining role in what patients might say about their situation.

The above quote of Paterson and Zangwill's patient is astonishingly similar to that of a patient of Olsen's cited by Nielsen.[141] This patient had asomatognosia of her left hemiplegic arm and claimed that the examiner's or another's arm was in bed with her. When confronted with the connection between her left arm and her own body, she stated "But my eyes and my feelings don't agree, and I must believe my feelings. I know they look like mine [referring to her arm], but I can feel they are not, and I can't believe my eyes." These two patients have in common anosognosia for hemiplegia and confabulation; both patients in different domains (orientation versus limb ownership) were able in one sense to recognize the actual circumstances (correct orientation versus the real arm) yet maintain their false beliefs in spite of this conflict. These patients seem motivated to hold to a personal, idiosyncratic, concrete belief even when the correct information is supplied and even partially admitted.

It is this sort of observation, among others, that led Weinstein, Kahn, and coworkers[67,69,79,103,126,130] to emphasize the positive motivational and adaptive features of anosognosia and to emphasize the role of *denial* in producing unawareness of any of a variety of neurologic defects. Indeed, Weinstein suggested that these patients tended to deny any of their current personal problems. Weinstein and coworkers also noted the refractoriness of these beliefs to correction and argued that cognitive defects alone could not explain the unawareness. They also pointed out that patients appeared implicitly aware of their defects.[79] For instance, they described how a patient with AHP, when asked to raise the left arm, might raise the right arm but perform normally on other tests of right-left orientation. In the course of our investigations, we have frequently noted the tendency for patients with AHP, while denying left limb paralysis, when asked to raise the hemiplegic left arm, to lift it with the right arm, suggesting they are implicitly aware that they cannot move the left arm normally. In a similar fashion, a patient of ours with Anton's syndrome due to peripheral blindness and frontal lobe lesions, in spite of denying his blindness and confabulating visual experience, would never attempt to read or walk without the help of his companion and even obtained and used a blind cane.

Finally, Weinstein and coworkers have provided evidence that many of the reduplications and confabulations produced by these patients are "metaphorical or symbolic representations" of the patients' neurologic disabilities or other problems.[79,142] These fictitious accounts or reduplications are accepted over reality because they provide a greater sense of identity and relatedness, create order and unity, and "provide a more vivid *feeling* of reality than a more referential veridical statement."[79]

Striking examples of these confabulatory reduplications can be found throughout the literature and the neurologic wards if one is attuned to see them. Weinstein and Kahn reported the case of a patient with papilledema, bilateral slowing of the EEG, and enlarged ventricals who underwent resection of a right cerebellar lung metastasis. She stated that she had two sons, Bill (her actual son) and "Willie" (a fictitious son). While she denied any illness or operations on herself, she confabulated that Willie was "recuperating from an illness." Weinstein and Kahn suggested the reduplication expressed her own feelings about herself. Another good example of this type of reduplicative confabulation is provided in a case described by Baddeley and Wilson,[143] as follows: R.J., a 42-year-old man who sustained a severe closed head injury, bilateral frontal hematomas, prominent anterograde and retrograde memory impairment, perseveration, and confabulation. He admitted being in a car accident and being "hurt" but "not badly." He also confabulated, supposedly verbatim, light-hearted conversations, which purportedly took place after the accident and tended to minimize the seriousness of the event. He produced a reduplicative confabulation claiming that he had two brothers, both named "Martin" (he actually had one living brother named Martin) and that one "Martin" had been "killed in a car accident." We examined a 65-year-old woman who sustained bifrontal infarcts after repair of a ruptured ACoA aneurysm. She displayed retrograde and anterograde amnesia and initially denied surgery or illness in herself but confabulated that she was visiting her niece who had an aneurysm. Subsequently she would occasionally admit she had surgery for the aneurysm but confabulated that she had an aunt who "couldn't think straight" because of an aneurysm and a "couple of cousins" who "all came for the same reason, aneurysm on top of the heads." In all these cases we see a constellation of amnesia (both retrograde and anterograde), unawareness, minimization or denial of illness, and confabulations that in a certain sense describe many of the problems of which the patient is seemingly unaware. Like confabulations in AHP and Anton's syndrome, these confabulations and beliefs are refractory to correction and are produced not only *within* a domain of neurologic dysfunction, but are often *about* the defect or illness in question.

TWO TYPES OF CONFABULATION AND UNAWARENESS

The studies reviewed above suggest that there are actually two major varieties of unawareness and that both are linked to different types of completion and confabulation[144] (Table 29-3). One form we suggest be called *neutral* unawareness and confabulation, which may occur in any domain, (e.g., visual, somatosensory, memory) but is usually confined to that domain and represents an exaggerated tendency of the normal sort of "gap-filling" that occurs in normal perception or memory processes in general. Its occurrence is facilitated by impaired self-monitoring, but it is nondelusional and the material is not self-referential. Hence the designation *neutral*. Visual completion in hemianopics, split-brain patients, and neglect patients, some aspects of AHP, and some varieties of "provoked" confabulation in amnesia are examples.

The second variety is somewhat more complex and difficult to define. We suggest *personal* unawareness and confabulation as a term to describe this type. Weinstein and coworkers provided the best description of this variety. It may occur with or without the first type, and hence the two are potentially dissociable. The content of the confabulation is personal in the sense that the material is about the patient and the patient's defects or problems, not about particular stimuli or word associations that have no personal relevance for the patient. As described by Weinstein and coworkers, Paterson and Zangwill, and others, the confabulations are motivated in the sense that they appear to serve a role in the adaptation to the defect(s) of which the patient is seemingly explicitly unaware. While patients with neutral forms may show implicit knowledge within their sensory or memory defects,[145] patients with personal forms may show implicit awareness of the defects themselves.[79] The confabulations are delusional beliefs that cut across sensory domains and are refractory to correction; impaired self-monitoring may be

Table 29-3
Two types of unawareness and confabulation

Neutral unawareness and confabulation	*Personal unawareness and confabulation*
Gap filling	± Gap filling
Impersonal	Self-referential/autobiographical
Unimodal (tied to defect)	Polymodal
Nondelusional (may be corrected)	Often delusional (impervious to correction)
Impaired self-monitoring	Impaired self-monitoring
Personality and motivation not important	Personality and motivation important
Nonsymbolic	May be symbolic/metaphoric
Exaggeration of normal gap filling	Pathologic gap filling
Associated with completion/confabulatory completion	Associated with dissociation/denial
± Implicit knowledge of stimulus	± Implicit knowledge of defect itself

important in both varieties. Orbital and ventromedial frontal damage, particularly of the right hemisphere, may contribute to this impairment in the personal form.

The tendency for right hemispheric lesions to produce neglect and disorders of attention and intention may account for the tendency of the right hemisphere to produce some of the neutral aspects of AHP and confabulation; this in some way might actually facilitate the expression of personal forms of confabulation, which are more dependent on verbal behaviors and hence preserved language mechanisms. The observation that requiring split-brain patients to produce a verbal response facilitates the extinction of the left half of stimuli may also help explain some of the laterality seen in AHP. As far as the personal forms of confabulation and unawareness are concerned, it has been suggested that the greater limbic connections of the right hemisphere may play a role.[79]

CONCLUSIONS

This chapter has surveyed some varieties of anosognosia. It is apparent that multiple forms of anosognosia exist, and an effort has been made to classify these according to the extent that perceptual, memory, and personal and adaptive features are important. While it is suggested that there are two types, they are not mutually exclusive. In fact, both may coexist and may even interact. This dichotomy is offered in the hope that it might provide a framework within which the various issues in unawareness and confabulation may be organized.

REFERENCES

1. Finger S: *Origins of Neuroscience: A History of Explorations into Brain Function*. New York: Oxford University Press, 1994.
2. Gassel MM, Williams D: Visual function in patients with homonymous hemianopia. III. The completion phenomenon; insight and attitude to the defect; and visual functional efficiency. *Brain* 86:229–260, 1963.
3. Fuchs W: Completion phenomena in hemianopic vision, in Ellis WD (ed): *A Source Book of Gestalt Psychology*. London: Routledge, 1955.
4. Ramachandran VS: Filling in gaps in perception: Part I. *Curr Dir Psychol Sci* 1:199–205, 1992.
5. Gattass R, Fiorani M Jr, Rosa MGP, et al: Visual responses outside the classical receptive field in primate striate cortex: A possible correlate of perceptual completion, in Lent R (ed): *The Visual System from Genesis to Maturity*. Boston, Birkhauser, 1992.
6. Walker R, Mattingly JB: Ghosts in the machine? Pathological visual completion phenomena in the damaged brain. *Neurocase* 3:313–315, 1997.
7. Critchley M: *The Parietal Lobes*. New York: Hafner, 1953.
8. Bender MB: Disorders in visual perception, in Halpern L (ed): *Problems of Dynamic Neurology*. Jerusalem, Jerusalem Post Press, 1963, pp 319–375.
9. Dufour M: Sur la vision nulle dans i'hémianopsie. *Rev Med Suisse Romande* 9:445–451, 1889.
10. Teuber HL, Battersby WS, Bender MB: *Visual Field Defects after Penetrating Missile Wounds of the Brain*. Cambridge, MA: Harvard University Press, 1960, p 87.
11. Bender MB, Teuber HL: Phenomena of fluctuation, extinction and completion in visual perception. *Arch Neurol Psychiatry* 55:627–658, 1946.
12. Levine DH: Unawareness of visual and sensorimotor defects: A hypothesis. *Brain Cogn* 13:233–281, 1990.
13. Poppelreuter W: *Die Psychischem Schadigungen durch Kopfschuss im Kriege*. Leipzig: Leopold Voss, 1917.
14. Torjussen T: Visual processing in cortially blind hemifields. *Neuropsychologia* 16:15–21, 1978.
15. Warrington EK: The completion of visual forms across hemianopic field defects. *Neurol Neurosurg Psychiatry* 25:208–217, 1962.
16. Zangwill OL: The completion effect in hemianopia and its relation to anosognosia, in Halpern L (ed): *Problems of Dynamic Neurology*. Jerusalem: Jerusalem Post Press, 1963, pp 274–282.
17. Celesia DG, Brigell MG, Vaphiades MS: Hemianopic anosognosia. *Neurology* 49:88–97, 1997.
18. Myers RE, Sperry RW: Interocular transfer of a visual form discrimination habit in cats after section of the optic chiasm and corpus callosum. *Anat Rec* 115:351, 1953.
19. Myers RE: Function of corpus callosum in interocular transfer. *Brain* 79:358–363, 1956.
20. Sperry RW: Cerebral organizations and behavior. *Science* 1749–1757, 1961.
21. Trevarthen C: Integrative functions of the cerebral commissures, in Nebes RD, Corkin S (eds): *Handbook of Neuropsychology*. New York, Elsevier, 1991, pp 49–83.

22. Bogen JE: The callosal syndromes, in Heilman KM, Valenstein E (eds): *Clinical Neuropsychology*. New York, Oxford University Press, 1993, pp 337–407.
23. Gazzaniga MS, Bogen JE, Sperry RW: Some functional effects of sectioning the cerebral commissures in man. *Proc Natl Acad Sci U S A* 48:1765–1769, 1962.
24. Sperry RW, Gazzaniga MS, Bogen JE: Interhemispheric relationships: The neocortical commissures; syndromes of hemispheric disconnection, in Vinken PJ, Bruyn GW (eds): *Handbook of Clinical Neurology*. Amsterdam: North-Holland, 1969, pp 273–290.
25. Gazzaniga MS: *The Bisected Brain*. New York: Appleton-Century-Crofts, 1970.
26. Gazzaniga MS, Le Doux JE: *The Integrated Mind*. New York: Plenum Press, 1978.
27. Trevarthen C, Sperry RW: Perceptual unity of the ambient visual field in human commissurotomy patients. *Brain* 96:547–570, 1973.
28. Frendrich R, Gazzaniga MS: Evidence for foveal splitting in a commissurotomy patient. *Neuropsychologia* 27:273–281, 1989.
29. Sperry RW: Consciousness, personal identity and the divided brain. *Neuropsychology* 22:661–673, 1984.
30. Feinberg TE, Schindler RJ, Flanagan NG, Haber LD: Two alien hand syndromes. *Neurology* 42:19–24, 1992.
31. Sperry RW: Forebrain commissurotomy and conscious awareness, in Trevarthen C (ed): *Brain Circuits and Functions of the Mind*. New York: Cambridge University Press, 1990, pp 371–388.
32. Sperry RW, Zaidel E, Zaidel D: Self-recognition and social awareness in the disconnected minor hemisphere. *Neuropsychologia* 17:153–166, 1979.
33. Levy J, Trevarthen C, Sperry RW: Perception of bilateral chimeric figures following hemispheric disconnection. *Brain* 95:60–78, 1972.
34. Trevarthen C: Functional relations of disconnected hemispheres with the brain stem and with each other: Monkey and man, in Kinsbourne M, Smith WL (eds): *Hemispheric Disconnection and Cerebral Function*. Springfield, IL: Charles C Thomas, 1974, pp 187–207.
35. Levy J, Trevarthen C: Metacontrol of hemispheric function in human split-brain patients. *J Exp Psychol Hum Percept Perform* 2:299–312, 1976.
36. Levy J: Manifestations and implications of shifting hemi-inattention in commissurotomy patients, in Weinstein EA, Friedland RP (eds): *Advances in Neurology*. New York: Raven Press, 1977.
37. Levy J: Regulation and generation of perception in the asymmetric brain, in Trevarthen C (ed): *Brain Circuits and Functions of the Mind*. New York: Cambridge University Press, 1990, pp 231–248.
38. Weizkrantz L: *Blindsight—A Case Study and Implications*. New York: Oxford University Press, 1986.
39. Torjussen T: Residual function in cortically blind hemifields. *Scand J Psychol* 17:320–322, 1976.
40. von Monakow C: Experimentelle und pathlolgisch-anatomische Untersuchungen über die Beziehungen der sogenannten Sehsphäre zu den infracorticalen Opticus-centren und zum N opticus. *Arch Psychiatrie* 16:151–199, 317–352, 1885.
41. Gerstmann J: Problem of imperception of disease and of impaired body territories with organic lesions. *Arch Neurol Psychiatry* 48:890–913, 1942.
42. Redlich FC, Dorsey JF: Denial of blindness by patients with cerebral disease. *Arch Neurol Psychiatry* 53:407–417, 1945.
43. Bisiach E, Geminiani G: Anosognosia related to hemiplegia and hemianopia, in Prigatano GP, Schacter DL (eds): *Awareness of Deficit after Brain Injury: Clinical and Theoretical Issues*. New York: Oxford University Press, 1991.
44. Förstl H, Owen AM, David AS: Gabriel Anton and "Anton's symptom": on focal diseases of the brain which are not perceived by the patient (1898). *Neuropsychiatr Neuropsychol Behav Neurol* 1:1–8, 1993.
45. McGlynn SM, Schacter DL: Unawareness of deficits in neuropsychological syndromes. *J Clin Exp Neuropsychol* 11:143–205, 1989.
46. Müller F: Ein Beitrag zur Kenntnis der Seelenblindhert. *Arch Psychiatrie* 24:857–917, 1918.
47. Dèjerine J, Vialet N: Sur un cas de cécitécorticale. *Compt Rend Soc Biol* 11:983–997, 1893.
48. Albrecht O: Drei Fälle mit Anton's symptom. *Arch Psychiatrie* 59:883–941, 1918.
49. Anton G: Über die Selbstwahrnehmung der Herderkrankungen des Gehirns durch den Kranken bein Rindenblindheit und Rindentaubheit. *Arch Psychiatrie* 32:86–127, 1899.
50. Swartz BE, Brust JCM: Anton's syndrome accompanying withdrawal hallucinosis in a blind alcoholic. *Neurology (Cleveland)* 34:969–973, 1984.
51. McDaniel KD, McDaniel LD: Anton's syndrome in a patient with posttraumatic optic neuropathy and bifrontal contusions. *Arch Neurol* 48:101–105, 1991.
52. Geschwind N: Disconnexion syndromes in animals and man. *Brain* 88:237–294, 585–643, 1965.
53. Stuss DT, Benson DF: *The Frontal Lobes*. New York: Raven Press, 1986, p 144.
54. Benson DF, Marsden DC, Meadows JC: The amnesic syndrome of posterior cerebral artery occlusion. *Acta Neurol Scand* 50:133–145, 1974.

55. Stengel E, Steele GDF: Unawareness of physical disability (anosognosia). *Br J Psychiatry* 92:379–388, 1946.
56. Bychowski Z: Über das fehlen der Wahrnehmung der eigen Blindheit bei zwei Kriegsverletzen. *Neurol Centralbl* 106:354–357, 1920.
57. Hemphill RE, Klein R: Contribution to the dressing disability as a focal sign and to the imperception phenomena. *J Ment Sci* 94:611–622, 1948.
58. Bergman PS: Cerebral blindness. *Arch Neurol Psychiatry* 78:568–584, 1957.
59. Redlich E, Bonvicini G: Über mangelnde Wahrnehmung (Autoanä autoanästhesie) der Blindheit bei cerebralen Erkrankugen. *Neurol Centralbl* 20:945–951, 1907.
60. Brockman NW, von Hagen KO: Denial of own blindness (Anton's syndrome). *Bull LA Neurol Soc* 11:178–180, 1946.
61. Goldenberg G, Mulbacher W, Nowak A: Imagery without perception—a case study of anosognosia for cortical blindness. *Neuropsychologia* 33:1373–1382, 1995.
62. Anton G: Beiträge zur klinischen Beurthelung und zur Localisation der Muskelsinnstorungen im Grosshirne. *Zeitschr Heilk* 14:313–348, 1893.
63. Pick A: *Beiträge zur Pathologie und Pathologischen Anatomie des Centralnervensystes unit Bemerkungen zur Normalen Anatomie Desselben*. Berlin: Karger, 1898.
64. Babinski J: Contribution a l'étude des troubles mantaux dans l'hémiplégie organique cérébrale (anosognosie). *Rev Neurol (Paris)* 27:845–848, 1914.
65. Babinski J: Anosognosie. *Rev Neurol (Paris)* 31:365–367, 1918.
66. Sandifer PH: Anosognosia and disorders of body scheme. *Brain* 69:122–137, 1946.
67. Weinstein EA, Cole M: Concepts of anosognosia, in Halpern LE (ed): *Dynamic Neurology*. Jerusalem: Jerusalem Post Press, 1964.
68. Fisher CM: Neurologic fragment: II. Remarks on anosognosia, confabulation, memory, and other topics; and an appendix on self-observation. *Neurology* 39:127–132, 1989.
69. Weinstein EA, Kahn RL: *Denial of Illness*. Springfield, IL: Charles C Thomas, 1955.
70. Friedland RP, Weinstein EA: Hemi-inattention and hemisphere specialization: Introduction and historical review, in Weinstein EA, Friedland RP (eds): *Advances in Neurology*. New York: Raven Press, 1977, pp 1–31.
71. Nielsen JM: *Agnosia, Apraxia, Aphasia: Their Value in Cerebral Localization*. New York: Hoeber, 1936, p 84.
72. Hécaen H, Albert ML: *Human Neuropsychology*. New York: Wiley, 1978, pp 678–682.
73. Levine DH, Calvanio R, Rinn WE: The pathogenesis of anosognosia for hemiplegia. *Neurology* 41:1770–1781, 1991.
74. Feinberg TE, Haber LD, Leeds NE: Verbal asomatognosia. *Neurology* 40:1391–1394, 1990.
75. Ives ER, Nielsen JM: Disturbance of body scheme: Delusion of the absence of part of body in two cases with autopsy verification of lesion. *Bull LA Neurol Soc* 2:120–125, 1937.
76. Wortis H, Datner B: An analysis of a somatic delusion: A case report. *Psychosom Med* 4:319–323, 1942.
77. Critchley M: Personification of paralyzed limbs in hemiplegics. *Br Med J* 30:284, 1955.
78. Ullman M: Motivational and structural factors in denial of hemiplegia. *Arch Neurol* 3:306–318, 1960.
79. Weinstein EA: Anosognosia and denial of illness, in Prigatano GP, Schacter DL (eds): *Awareness of Deficit after Brain Injury: Clinical and Theoretical Issues*. New York: Oxford University Press, 1991, pp 240–257.
80. Critchley M: Misoplegia or hatred of hemiplegia. *Mt Sinai J Med* 41:82–87, 1974.
81. Nathanson M, Bergman PS, Gordon GG: Denial of illness: Its occurrence in one hundred consecutive cases of hemiplegia. *Arch Neurol Psychiatry* 68:380–387, 1952.
82. Cutting J: Study of anosognosia. *Neurol Neurosurg Psychiatry* 41:548–555, 1978.
83. Willanger R, Danielsen VT, Ankerbus J: Denial and neglect of hemiparesis in right-sided apoplectic lesions. *Acta Neurol Scand* 64:310–326, 1981.
84. Hier DB, Mondlock J, Caplan LR: Behavioural abnormalities after right hemisphere stroke. *Neurology* 33:337–344, 1983.
85. Bisiach E, Vallar G, Perani D, et al: Unawareness of disease following lesions of the right hemisphere: Anosognosia for hemiplegia and anosognosia for hemianopia. *Neuropsychologia* 24:471–482, 1986.
86. Starkstein SE, Fedoroff JP, Price TR, et al: Anosognosia in patients with cerebrovascular lesions: A study of causative factors. *Stroke* 23:1446–1453, 1992.
87. Stone SP, Halligan PW, Greenwood RJ: The incidence of neglect phenomena and related disorders in patients with an acute right or left hemisphere stroke. *Age Aging* 22:46–52, 1993.
88. Terzian H: Behavioral and EEG effects of intracarotid sodium amytal injection. *Acta Neurochir (Wein)* 12:230–239, 1964.
89. Gilmore RL, Heilman KM, Schmidt RP, et al: Anosognosia during Wada testing. *Neurology* 42:925–927, 1992.

90. Durkin MW, Meador KJ, Nichols ME, et al: Anosognosia and the intracarotid amobarbital procedure (Wada test). *Neurology* 44:978–979, 1994.
91. Adair JC, Gilmore RL, Fennell EB, et al: Anosognosia during intracarotid barbiturate anesthesia: Unawareness or amnesia for weakness. *Neurology* 45:241–243, 1995.
92. Breier JI, Adair JC, Gold M, et al: Dissociation of anosognosia for hemiplegia and aphasia during left-hemisphere anesthesia. *Neurology* 45:65–67, 1995.
93. Carpenter K, Berti A, Oxbury S, et al: Awareness of and memory for arm weakness during intracarotid sodium amytal testing. *Brain* 118:243–251, 1995.
94. Heilman, KM: Anosognosia, possible neuropsychological mechanisms, in Prigatano GP, Schachter DL (eds): *Awareness Of Deficit after Brain Injury, Clinical and Theoretical Issues*. New York: Oxford University Press, 1991, pp 52–62.
95. Gold M, Adair JC, Jacobs DH, Heilman KM: Anosognosia for hemiplegia: An electrophysiologic investigation of the feed-forward hypothesis. *Neurology* 44:1804–1808, 1994.
96. Pötzl O: Über störungen der Selbstwahrnehmung bei linksseitiger Hemiplegie. *Zeitschr Neurol Psychiatry* 93:117–168, 1925.
97. Barkman A: De l'anosognosie dans l'hémiplégie cérébrale: contribution clinique a l'étude de ce symptome. *Acta Med Scand* 62:235–254, 1925.
98. Von Hagen K, Ives FR: Two autopsied cases of anosognosia. *Bull LA Neurol Soc* 4:41–44, 1939.
99. Nielsen JM: Disturbances of the body scheme: their physiological mechanism. *Bull LA Neurol Soc* 3:127–135, 1938.
100. Feinberg TE, Roane DM, Kwan PC, et al: Anosognosia and visuoverbal confabulation. *Arch Neurol* 51:468–473, 1994.
101. Barré JA, Morin L, Kaiser: Étude clinique d'un nouveau cas d'anosognosie de Babinski. *Rev Neurol (Paris)* 39:500–503, 1923.
102. Schilder P: *The Image and Appearance of the Human Body*. London: Kegan Paul, 1935.
103. Weinstein EA, Kahn RL: The syndrome of anosognosia. *Arch Neurol Psychiatry* 64:772–791, 1950.
104. Cappa S, Sterzi R, Giuseppe V, Bisiach E: Remission of hemineglect and anosognosia during vestibular stimulation. *Neuropsychologia* 5:775–782, 1987.
105. Von Hagen KO, Ives ER: Anosognosia (Babinski), imperception of hemiplegia. *Bull LA Neurol Soc* 2:95–103, 1937.
106. Critchley M: A phantom supernumerary limb after a cervical root lesion. *Arch Neuropsic São Paulo* 10:269–275, 1952.
107. Riddoch G: Phantom limbs and body shape. *Brain* 64:197–222, 1941.
108. Bors E: Phantom limbs of patients with spinal cord injury. *AMA Arch Neurol Psychiatry* 66:610–631, 1951.
109. Frederiks JAM: Occurrence and nature of phantom limb phenomena following amputation of body parts and following lesions of the central and peripheral nervous system. *Psychiatr Neurol Neurochir* 66:73–97, 1963.
110. Feinberg TE, Roane DM, Ali J: Illusory limb movements in anosognosia for hemiplegia. *J Neurol Neurosurg Psychiatry* 68:511–513, 2000.
111. Meador KJ, Loring DW, Feinberg TE, Lee GP, Nichols ME: Anosognosia and asomatognosia during intracarotid amobarbital inactivation. *Neurology* 55:816–820, 2000.
112. Lu LH, Barrett AM, Schwartz RL, Cibula JE, et al: Anosognosia and confabulation during the Wada test. *Neurology* 49:1316–1322, 1997.
113. Lu LH, Barrett AM, Cibula JE, et al: Dissociation of anosognosia and phantom movements during the Wada test. *J Neurol Neurosurg Psychiatry* 69:820–823, 2000.
114. Talland GA: Confabulation in the Wernicke-Korsakoff syndrome. *Nerv Ment Dis* 132:361–381, 1961.
115. Williams HW, Rupp C: Observations on confabulation. *Am J Psychiatry* 95:395–405, 1938.
116. Alexander MR, Freedman M: Amnesia after anterior communicating artery aneurysm rupture. *Neurology* 34:752–757, 1984.
117. Mercer B, Wapner W, Gardner H, Benson P: A study of confabulation. *Arch Neurol* 34:429–433, 1977.
118. Zangwill OL: The amnesic syndrome, in Whitty CWM, Zangwill OL (eds): *Amnesia*. London: Butterworth, 1966.
119. Parkin AJ: Amnesic syndrome: A lesion-specific disorder? *Cortex* 20:479–508, 1984.
120. Gainotti G: Confabulation of denial in senile dementia: An experimental study. *Psychiatr Clin North Am* 8:99–108, 1975.
121. Gustafson I, Nilsson L: Differential diagnosis of presenile dementia on clinical grounds. *Acta Psychiatr Scand* 65:194–209, 1982.
122. Reisberg B, Gordon B, McCarthy M: Insight and denial accompanying progressive cognitive decline in normal aging and Alzheimer's disease, in Stanley B (ed): *Geriatric Psychiatry: Ethical and Legal Issues*. Washington, DC: American Psychiatric Press, 1985, pp 19–39.
123. McGlynn SM, Kaszniak AW: Unawareness of deficits in dementia and schizophrenia, in Prigatano GP, Schachter DL (eds): *Awareness of Deficit after Brain*

Injury: Clinical and Theoretical Issues. New York: Oxford University Press, 1991, pp 84–110.

124. Sevush S, Leve N: Denial of memory deficit in Alzheimer's disease. *Am J Psychiatry* 150:748–751, 1993.
125. Michon A, Deweer B, Pillon B, et al: Relation of anosognosia to frontal lobe dysfunction in Alzheimer's disease. *Neurol Neurosurg Psychiatry* 57:805–809, 1994.
126. Weinstein EA, Friedland RP, Wagner EE: Denial/unawareness of impairment and symbolic behavior in Alzheimer's disease. *Neuropsychiatry Neuropsychol Behav Neurol* 7:176–184, 1994.
127. Starkstein SE, Vazquez S, Migliorelli R, et al: A single-photon emission computed tomographic study of anosognosia in Alzheimer's disease. *Arch Neurol* 52:415–420, 1995.
128. Caine ED, Shoulson I: Psychiatric syndromes in Huntington's disease. *Am J Psychiatry* 140:728–733, 1983.
129. Roth N: Unusual types of anosognosia and their relation to the body image. *Nerv Ment Dis* 100:35–43, 1944.
130. Weinstein EA, Cole M, Mitchell MS, Lyerly O: Anosognosia and aphasia. *Arch Neurol Psychiatry* 10:376–386, 1964.
131. Lebrun Y: Anosognosia in aphasics. *Cortex* 23:251–263, 1987.
132. Rubens AB, Garrett MF: Anosognosia of linguistic deficits in patients with neurological deficits, in Prigatano GP, Schachter DL (eds): *Awareness of Deficits after Brain Injury: Clinical and Theoretical Issues*. New York: Oxford University Press, 1991.
133. Lewis L: Role of psychological factors in disordered awareness, in Prigatano GP, Schachter DL (eds): *Awareness of Deficit after Brain Injury: Clinical and Theoretical Issues*. New York: Oxford University Press, 1991.
134. Levine J, Warrenburg S, Kerns R, et al: The role of denial in recovery from coronary artery disease. *Psychosom Med* 49:109–117.
135. Goldstein K: *The Organism: A Holistic Approach to Biology Derived from Pathological Data on Man*. New York: American Book, 1939.
136. Giacino JT, Cicerone KD: Varieties of deficit awareness after brain injury. *J Head Trauma Rehabil* 5:1–15, 1998.
137. Paterson A, Zangwill OL: Recovery of spatial orientation in the post-traumatic confusional state. *Brain* 67:54–68, 1944.
138. Pick A: On reduplication paramnesia. *Brain* 26:260–267, 1903.
139. Ruff RL, Volpe BT: Environmental reduplication associated with right frontal and parietal lobe injury. *Neurol Neurosurg Psychiatry* 44:382–386, 1981.
140. Taylor J: *Selected Writings of John Hughlings Jackson*. New York: Basic Books, 1958.
141. Nielsen JM: Gerstmann syndrome: finger agnosia, agraphia, confusion of right and left and acalculia: Comparison of this syndrome with disturbance of body scheme resulting from lesions of the right side of the brain. *Arch Neurol Psychiatry* 39:536–559, 1938.
142. Weinstein EA, Friedland RP: Behavioral disorders associated with hemi-inattention, in Weinstein EA, Friedland RP (eds): *Advances in Neurology*. New York: Raven Press, 1977, pp 51–62.
143. Baddeley AD, Wilson B: Amnesia, autobiographical memory and confabulation, in Rubin DC (ed): *Autobiographical Memory.* Cambridge, England: Cambridge University Press, 1986.
144. Feinberg TE, Roane DM: Anosognosia, completion and confabulation: The neutral-personal dichotomy. *Neurocase* 3:73–85, 1997.
145. Schachter DL, McAndrews MP, Moscovitch M: Access to consciousness: dissociations between implicit and explicit knowledge in neuropsychological syndromes, in Weskranz L (ed): *Thought without Language*. Oxford, England: Clarendon Press, 1988.

Chapter 30

CONFABULATION

Todd E. Feinberg
Joseph T. Giacino

Although no single definition of the term *confabulation* is universally agreed upon, confabulation can be broadly defined as an erroneous statement that is made without a conscious effort to deceive.[1] Korsakoff[2,3] first observed the tendency of patients with what is now known as Wernicke-Korsakoff syndrome to display both amnesia and confabulation ("pseudoreminiscences"). This syndrome was subsequently labeled *confabulation* by Kraepelin,[4] and many authors subsequently confirmed confabulation in Korsakoff's syndrome.[5–10] Although confabulation is usually associated with amnesia, the symptom occurs in a wide variety of neurologic and psychiatric conditions. This chapter addresses mainly confabulation associated with memory loss.

VARIETIES OF CONFABULATION

Kraeplin[11–13] distinguished two subtypes of confabulation. One variety, which he designated as *simple confabulation,* consisted in minor errors in content or temporal order. The other type, termed *fantastic confabulation,* comprised bizarre and patently impossible statements.[4] In a similar fashion, Bonhoeffer[5,6] distinguished between *momentary confabulation* due to the patient's efforts to cover a gap in memory and *fantastic confabulations,* which appeared to exceed the need to conceal or excuse such a gap. Berlyne[1] also found this distinction useful and suggested that momentary confabulation had to be provoked by questions from the examiner and that the content of such confabulations consisted of true memories that were temporally displaced. Van der Horst,[7] Williams and Rupp,[8] and Talland[9,10] previously suggested the notion that confabulations consisted of temporally displaced but veridical memories. Berlyne[1] suggested that fantastic confabulations were not rooted in true memory and that their content was grandiose and wish-fulfilling.

Kopelman[14] reframed the two major catagories of confabulation while retaining the essential characteristics of the two types, and this terminology is in widest usage today. He distinguished *provoked confabulations* that were elicited specifically in response to questions that probed memory from *spontaneous confabulations* that were more grandiose, were more florid, and occurred without provocation. Kopelman found that provoked confabulatory errors of patients with Korsakoff's and Alzheimer's syndromes resembled those of healthy subjects whose memory was tested at prolonged retention intervals.

Feinberg[15] and Feinberg and Roane[16] suggested an alternative dichotomy within confabulatory subtypes. They suggest that there are two major varieties of confabulation. One form, which they called *neutral confabulation,* may occur in any domain (e.g., visual, somatosensory, memory) but is usually confined to that domain. This form of confabulation in part represents an exaggerated tendency of the sort of completion and filling in that occurs in normal perception or memory processes. Its occurrence is facilitated by impaired self-monitoring, but it is nondelusional and the material is not self-referential. Hence the designation *neutral*. Examples of neutral confabulation are visual completion in hemianopic, split-brain, and neglect patients (see Chap. 29). Some varieties of provoked confabulation in amnesic patients are also examples of neutral confabulation. The second variety is termed *personal confabulation.* The content of these confabulations is personal in the sense that the material is about the patient and the patient's defects or problems, not about particular stimuli or word associations that have no personal relevance for the patient. The confabulations are delusional beliefs that cut across sensory domains and are refractory to correction. In the final analysis, these designations for the varieties of confabulation are to a certain extent overlapping but emphasize different aspects of common underlying symptoms.

NEUROPSYCHOLOGICAL MECHANISMS OF CONFABULATION ASSOCIATED WITH AMNESIA

Over the last 30 years, various neuropsychological mechanisms have been proposed to account for confabulatory symptoms, although none have been universally accepted. Putative mechanisms underlying confabulation can generally be broken down into three categories: (1) amnestic-dysexecutive syndrome, (2) temporal/contextual displacement, and (3) deficient strategic retrieval.

While amnesia and confabulation frequently co-occur, amnesia and confabulation are partially dissociable symptoms. Both Talland[9] and Victor and coworkers[3] noted that in patients with Wernicke-Korsakoff syndrome, confabulation occurred most notably in the early stages of the disease, and Talland[9] described how, in the chronic phase of the illness, confabulation may recede from the clinical picture while notable memory impairment persists. Similarly, Alexander and Freedman[17] found that in patients who developed amnesia after rupture of an aneurysm of the anterior communicating artery (ACoA), confabulation cleared after recovery of weeks or months but amnesia might remain; Vilkki[18] also reported that only some of such patients with amnesia confabulate. The study of Mercer and associates[19] also found a lack of correlation between the degrees of amnesia and confabulation in a group of mixed etiologies.

While it is clear that amnesia in general and amnesia due to frontal lesions can occur without confabulation, whether confabulation occurs in the absence of memory impairment is more controversial. Some authors have suggested that confabulation does not require amnesia. Wyke and Warrington[20] made this argument with reference to a Korsakoff patient who showed visual completion to tachistoscopic stimuli in a fashion not attributable to memory impairment. They interpreted their findings as suggesting that confabulation per se was a primary symptom of Korsakoff's and not a consequence of amnesia. Kapur and Coughlan[21] also reported, of their postaneurysm frontally damaged patient, that while memory was impaired, confabulation was prominent in spite of normal or near normal scores on tests of verbal and nonverbal recognition and paired-associate learning.

Deluca[4,22] argues that studies purporting to show that confabulation can occur without memory impairment,[23] particularly those studies that address this issue in patients with a ruptured ACoA aneurysm, did not sufficiently assess delayed recall. In support of this view, Deluca found that among six ACoA patients, only those with amnesia confabulated.[22]

Amnestic-Dysexecutive Syndrome

The majority of published studies concerning mechanisms of confabulation implicate some *combination* of memory impairment and executive dysfunction.[14,22,24–26] Stuss and coworkers,[24] in a series of five confabulatory patients, found evidence of frontal dysfunction superimposed upon a memory deficit, and Kopelman[14] also suggested that spontaneous confabulation was the result of the superimposition of frontal dysfunction on amnesia. Deluca[22] compared amnesic to nonamnesic patients after ACoA aneurysmal rupture. He found that confabulation occurred only in those patients with combined frontal and amnesic impairments.

Joseph[27] proposed that confabulated responses may arise from ideational disinhibition caused by injury to the frontal lobes. In this account, frontal disinhibition and behavioral overresponsiveness result in flooding and amplification of tangential and irrelevant associations. Consequently, pertinent information is overwhelmed and indiscriminate response selection produces confabulation. Among other shortcomings, this account does not explain why all patients with behavioral disinhibition do not confabulate or why some confabulatory patients do not evidence other signs of behavioral disinhibition.

Based on their analysis of 9 patients with confabulation following ACoA rupture, Fischer et al.[25] suggested that a common profile of executive deficits underlies confabulatory tendencies. These investigators reported that the 5 cases with severe spontaneous confabulation (i.e., unprovoked and persistent) had significantly greater perseveration and set-shifting deficits than the remaining 4 cases with provoked confabulation (i.e., reactive, transient). No significant between-group difference was found in the severity of memory encoding or retrieval deficits. The authors concluded that confabulation is dependent on the severity of executive dysfunction, particularly those functions involved in self-monitoring, and is not caused by memory impairment alone.

Deficient self-monitoring has also been causally linked to confabulation by Benson and colleagues.[28] Serial neuropsychological assessment and single photon emission computed tomography (SPECT) were performed across a 4-month period to monitor the resolution of confabulation in a 32-year-old woman who presented with acute Wernicke-Kosakoff's syndrome. On initial evaluation, basic attentional functions were intact, but performance was severely impaired on tests of simple and complex processing speed, free and cued recall, and verbal and design fluency. The initial SPECT scan showed focal hypoperfusion in the cingulate gyrus, orbitofrontal cortex, and mesial diencephalic region. On reevaluation 4 months later, the patient remained amnestic, but there were no further episodes of confabulation. Neuropsychometric findings were indicative of significant improvement on the executive measures but not on tests of memory. The change in executive functions occurred in association with recovery of perfusion of the cingulum to near normal levels on SPECT. The absence of improvement in memory was correlated with persistent mesial diencephalic hypoperfusion. In light of the simultaneous resolution of the confabulation and executive disturbance, the authors suggested that the confabulation was due to loss of self-monitoring, which, in turn, was secondary to hypoperfusion of the mesial and orbitofrontal regions.

Box and coworkers[29] also conducted longitudinal assessment of confabulation relative to cognitive functions but reported results that challenge the conclusions reached by Benson et al.[28] A 27-year-old woman presented with spontaneous confabulation and delusional misidentification following a traumatic brain injury. Cognitive assessment was completed on three occasions over a 4-month period. There was no consistent relationship between the presence of executive, memory, or visuoperceptual deficits and the emergence *or* disappearance of confabulation. Specifically, confabulation emerged in the setting of severe impairments in executive (i.e., cognitive estimation, perseveration), memory (i.e., recall and recognition), and visuoperceptual (i.e., object recognition) functions but resolved on reevaluation 4 months later, despite significant, persistent cognitive deficits.

O'Connor and coworkers[30] completed neuropsychological assessment of a 74-year-old woman with a 10-year history of amnesia of unknown origin who developed Capgras' syndrome following a traumatic brain injury. Prior to the brain injury, neuropsychological evaluations showed global amnesia in the setting of superior intellectual and reasoning abilities. Subsequent to the injury, the patient presented with confabulatory delusions and there was dramatic decline on tests of mental flexibility and problem solving. Memory assessment was consistent with preinjury performance except that confabulated responses were noted for the first time. In view of the long-standing history of amnesia without confabulation and the simultaneous onset of reasoning deficits and confabulatory delusions, the authors argued that the confabulation was attributable to the convergence of impairments in reasoning (i.e., loss of critical attitude) and memory.

Although confabulation has frequently been shown to accompany combined deficits in memory and executive abilities, not all executive functions play a role. Cunningham and associates[31] reported that confabulation ratios (i.e., the number of confabulatory responses on formal tests of verbal and visuospatial recall divided by the total number of responses) were significantly greater in a group of high confabulators relative to low- and nonconfabulating groups. The high-confabulator group also performed significantly worse on tests of executive function involving sustained attention, set-shifting, and mental tracking. There was, however, no difference between groups on measures of concept formation, problem solving, and verbal fluency. These findings were construed as support for the combined-deficit model, which holds that memory and executive functions must be impaired for confabulation to develop, although specific components of the executive system must be implicated.

Lack of support for the combined-deficit model has been reported in a number of case studies. Kopelman and coworkers[32] investigated the nature of confabulatory erotic delusions in a 47-year-old woman who was diagnosed with schizophrenia. Neuropsychological test findings indicated superior intelligence and normal performance on tests assessing anterograde and retrograde memory and on all of the measures of executive function administered, including tests of verbal fluency, mental flexibility, and cognitive estimation. Based on these findings, the authors rejected the notion that executive dysfunction is a necessary component of confabulation.

Papagno and Baddeley[23] proposed that confabulation is contingent upon disruption of a particular component of the executive system. They described a 29-year-old patient who presented with florid confabulation and anosognosia following resection of a ruptured right subcortical frontoparietal arteriovenous malformation. Interestingly, the patient perfomed normally on four of six standardized memory tests. On interview, he was able to answer factual questions correctly but typically went on to embellish his responses with confabulated material. The authors characterized the underlying problem as a failure to discontinue the search process. The patient generally provided the correct information when it was requested but continued to supplement his initial answer with erroneous responses after exhausting his supply of valid information. This tendency was attributed to a specific aspect of self-monitoring responsible for evaluating the retrieval process and determining when it should be discontinued.

Temporal/Contextual Displacement

The temporal/contextual displacement model holds that confabulation results from inaccurate identification of the temporal order in which information is stored. Schnider and colleagues have completed a series of studies showing that confabulatory recall occurs when discrete elements of information become disconnected from their corresponding spatial and temporal contexts. Schnider et al.[33] described a 62-year-old woman who presented with global anterograde amnesia and confabulation on neuropsychometric assessment. Despite her amnesia, her test-induced confabulations almost exclusively represented actual or semantically related intrusions of material from prior evaluations conducted 4 months earlier. A series of experiments using recall and recognition paradigms were designed to determine whether the patient's memory failures stemmed from an inability to store new information or were due to lack of access to knowledge about where and when the information was acquired. Results indicated that despite very poor performance on free recognition tasks related to a high rate of false-positive errors, recognition discriminability improved significantly when an active information search strategy was imposed (i.e., use of a forced-choice response format). In addition, judgments concerning the personal (tester), temporal (order of presentation of stimuli), and spatial (place of testing) contexts in which the information was acquired were found to approximate chance level. The patient was also noted to perform normally on a recognition task that was not dependent upon contextual information (i.e., stimuli consisting of novel nonwords and nonsense designs). These findings support the premise that confabulation reflects an inability to label information contextually, thus producing pathologic fusion of unrelated memory elements.

In a second study using experimental paradigms similar to those described above, Schnider et al.[33] found a double dissociation in the memory profiles of spontaneous and provoked confabulators. When spontaneous confabulators were compared to amnesics with and without provoked confabulation, only the spontaneous confabulators failed to recognize the temporal order of stored information. Further, no correlation was found between the failure of temporal order recognition and provoked confabulation. Interestingly, there was no consistent relationship between performance on measures of executive function and confabulation. There were no significant differences in performance between spontaneous confabulators and other amnesics on six indices associated with executive dysfunction. The authors concluded that confabulation is based on a specific form of frontal dysfunction that causes impairment in temporal order discrimination and suggested that this disturbance is due to disconnection of the orbitofrontal cortex from the amygdala.

Further support for the premise that traditional symptoms of executive dysfunction do not account for confabulation was provided in a case report by Ptak and Schnider.[34] The authors described a 49-year-old male who became amnestic with spontaneous confabulation after sustaining rupture of the ACoA. Contrary to previous findings reported by these investigators, this patient did not demonstrate failure of temporal order recognition. In this study, the patient was given two runs of a recognition task for pictures. In the second run, administered 1 h after the first, the patient was required to distinguish between target stimuli from the first and second runs. Although target identification was low, there were no false-positive errors during either run, providing no evidence for temporal context confusion. The authors speculated that the absence of false-positive errors was related to the application of a very conservative recognition criterion, implicating strong reliance on self-monitoring strategies. This hypothesis was tested by repeating the same test with the admonition to avoid missing too many target items. In this condition, the number of false-positive errors exceeded the number of hits. It was concluded that the disturbance in temporal context order was masked by the patient's well-preserved capacity for self-monitoring. When monitoring processes were externally suppressed, temporal context confusion was released. These findings call into question the contribution of self-monitoring deficits to confabulation.

Additional evidence for a dissociation between confabulation and memory and executive functions comes from a longitudinal study of the evolution of spontaneous confabulation. Schnider et al.[35] performed neuropsychological reevaluations of 8 spontaneous confabulators 18 months after initial onset. Of these 8 patients, 3 stopped confabulating within 3 months, while 2 patients continued to confabulate for 2 or more years. Test results indicated that temporal context confusion, but not memory or executive performance, perfectly paralleled resolution of the confabulation. The duration of confabulation was also found to be related to the severity of orbitofrontal injury in this group.

Deficient Strategic Retrieval

In recent studies, confabulation has been directly tied to disruption of strategic retrieval processes.[26,36,37] These processes constitute problem-solving routines that are triggered when proximal cues are inadequate to retrieve the required information. Under normal conditions, memory demands initially engage automatic "associative" processes. During the associative process, proximal cues interact with previously stored memories to produce memory traces. If the recovered trace is insufficient, a second retrieval process is activated to guide continuation of the search process. In opposition to the automatic associative retrieval process, strategic retrieval is conscious, effortful, and self-directed. This process is designed to locate the desired information or identify other appropriate cues that facilitate associative retrieval operations. Once the memory trace is retrieved, strategic processes evaluate the fit between the trace and the intended information. In this model, confabulation is presumed to be the result of a breakdown in strategic retrieval processes involved in memory search, temporal ordering, and output monitoring. The predisposition to confabulation increases when a particular cognitive subsystem (e.g., memory) is damaged and produces faulty output (e.g., failure to remember) in addition to impaired output monitoring (e.g., unawareness of response discrepancies).

While the strategic retrieval mechanism may appear similar to the temporal/contextual displacement model in explaining confabulation, there are important differences. Given its emphasis on temporal order and context-specific stimuli, the temporal/contextual displacement model predicts that confabulation should involve episodic but not semantic material. Dalla Barba has indeed shown that confabulation can be confined to the episodic memory system.[36] Using a questionnaire designed to elicit confabulation in a 75-year-old male diagnosed with Binswanger's encephalopathy, Dalla Barba found that confabulated responses occurred exclusively on questions related to episodic memory and not on items dependent upon the semantic system. He concluded that disruption of the episodic system causes faulty reporting of events, although the manner in which the event is reported depends upon the integrity of the semantic system. The greater the degree of semantic degradation, the more fantastic the confabulation. Conversely, Sandson and colleagues[38] described a 66-year-old male who sustained a left intracerebral hematoma. The patient presented with two distinct forms of confabulation. In addition to typical event-based confabulations, episodes of confabulation were also directly precipitated by semantic memory prompts. The latter occurred in response to questions concerning attributes of common objects and "definitions" of nonsense words. These confabulations occurred in the setting of literal and verbal paraphasic errors. The link between semantic confabulation and language disturbance in this case supports the premise that the probability of confabulation increases when specific cognitive subsystems are damaged along with strategic retrieval processes.

Laws and colleagues[39] argue that confabulation arises from imbalance or miscommunication between the autobiographical, semantic, and episodic components of the memory system rather than lack of access to these systems. This view also holds that the autobiographical system is organized around thematic frameworks that serve to index and reconstruct personally relevant information. Under normal circumstances, activation of a thematic framework (e.g., thinking about work) coactivates the semantic knowledge base to generate distinct memories (e.g., characteristics of individual coworkers), which concurrently activate the episodic system to retrieve past events associated with these individuals (e.g., "The day John and I got stuck in the airport in Boston"). When one of these components is damaged, an imbalance develops and the other components attempt to compensate for the deficiency. The remaining intact systems attempt to match the desired information requirements against preserved knowledge that is available within these systems. Personally relevant themes readily attract attention during the search process. Confabulation emerges from inappropriate binding of information from the three systems.

To illustrate the interrelationship among the three systems, Laws et al.[39] completed extensive neuropsychological assessment of a 39-year-old schizophrenic male who presented with multiple episodes of self-referential confabulation, including the belief that he was "Baron Caernarvon." This particular belief emerged following a dinner held at Caernarvon Castle that was attended by the patient. Assessment findings indicated that episodes of confabulation occurred (1) in response to names but not to faces, (2) primarily when the patient was acquainted with the topic but not when he was unfamiliar with it, and (3) more frequently for names of specific categories of people (e.g., politicians versus nonpoliticians). Of particular interest, the content of the confabulation was typically of personal and autobiographical relevance. These findings were interpreted as evidence that the confabulatory misidentification was not secondary to perceptual disturbance but rather that it was based largely on *preserved* knowledge and was the result of compensatory albeit aberrant overreliance on specific personally relevant thematic frameworks. The authors suggest that repeated coactivation of information from these interdependent systems ultimately results in reinforcement of erroneously reconstructed events and acts to sustain the confabulation.

NEUROANATOMY OF AMNESIC CONFABULATION

The pathology of alcoholic patients with Wernicke-Korsakoff syndrome involves primarily the dorsomedial nucleus of the thalamus,[3] mamillary bodies,[40] both of these in combination,[41] or other thalamic nuclei.[42,43] Stuss and coworkers[24] found spontaneous confabulation of the "fantastical" variety in five patients with either head trauma, subarachnoid hemorrhage, or infarcts and found that this form of confabulation correlated with frontal dysfunction as judged by neurologic examination, computed tomography (CT)/electroencephalography (EEG), and neuropsychological test data.

As noted above, rupture of aneurysms of the ACoA have been noted to produce an amnestic syndrome that in some cases is accompanied by confabulation.[17,18,22,25,44–49] In the ACoA series of Alexander and Freedman,[17] 5 of 11 patients had the most marked and persistent confabulation. Of these 5 patients, 3 had right anterior cerebral artery (ACA) infarcts, a fourth had bilateral ACA territory infarcts (right greater than left), and the fifth had a right parietal infarct. Thus frontal and particularly right hemispheric regions were implicated. All patients had anterograde and retrograde amnesia. It was suggested that damage to basal forebrain, particularly the septal nuclei (which provide widespread cholinergic projections to cortical sites including hippocampus), might produce the amnesia. Vilkki's series[18] of ACoA patients also provided links between confabulation and frontal lobe damage; of 5 amnesic ACoA patients, 2 had profound confabulation; of these, 1 had bilateral frontobasal infarctions and the other had a right frontobasal subdural empyema treated surgically.

Damasio and coworkers[46] reported on several patients with spontaneous, "dreamlike" confabulations, all of whom had basal forebrain lesions including septal nuclei, nucleus accumbens, diagonal band, and medial substantia innominata. It was felt that the nucleus basalis was also probably involved. All patients had unilateral orbitofrontal lesions as well. The septal lesions were believed to be responsible for the amnesia due to interruption of connections with the hippocampus, amygdala, and parahippocampal gyrus. The anatomy of confabulation was not explored in this series. In another series of amnesic patients of mixed etiology, Baddeley and Wilson[47] found that among the 10 amnesics, there were 2 with confabulation. One had an ACoA and the other a head injury; both had bilateral frontal lesions. Interestingly, while neither of these patients differed from nonconfabulators on measures of delayed recall, both did significantly worse on measures of retrograde autobiographical memory. They attributed the confabulation to a dysexecutive syndrome due to frontal pathology.

Deluca and coworkers[4,22,48,49] provided additional support for the role of combined basal forebrain and frontal damage in producing confabulation in ACoA patients. Fischer and associates[25] reported on 9 ACoA patients divided into spontaneous (extended, grandiose) and provoked (limited, plausible) groups. While both groups had lesions of basal forebrain and anterograde amnesia, the spontaneous group had more extensive medial frontal and striatal pathology. They also showed more extensive retrograde amnesia and "executive deficits" on frontal-type tasks.

Finally, Schnider and Ptak[50] compared 6 patients with spontaneous confabulation to 12 nonconfabulatory amnesic patients. These authors found extensive overlap in the lesions of the confabulatory patients in the anterior limbic system, including medial orbitofrontal cortex, basal forebrain, amygdala, and perirhinal cortex or medial hypothalamus (Fig. 30-1).

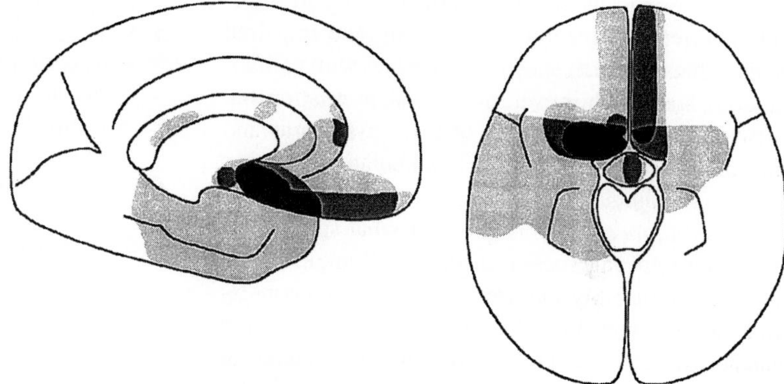

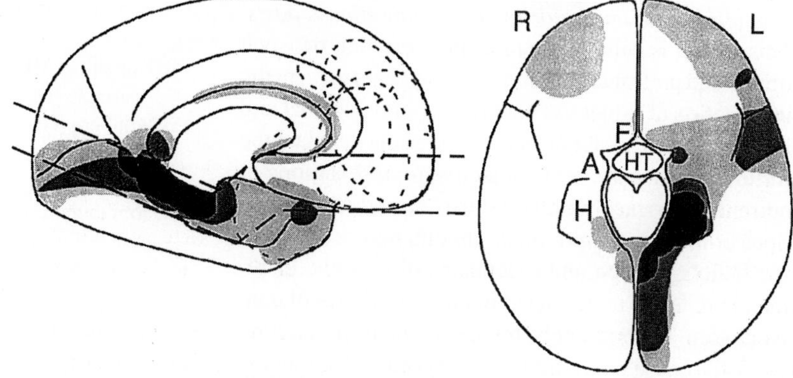

Figure 30-1
Lesion analysis of (a) *spontaneous confabulators and* (b) *nonconfabulatory amnesics. Shaded areas represent paramedian lesions, dashed lines indicate lateral lesions. Straight parallel dashed lines in the lower part of the sagittal view in* (b) *indicate the composite axial slice used in the right column to indicate lesions of the (A) amygdala, (F) basal forebrain, (H) hippocampus, (HT) hypothalamus, and orbitofrontal cortex. (From Schnider and Ptak,[50] with permission.)*

CONCLUSIONS

Most of the empiric evidence concerning neuropsychological mechanisms of confabulation is based on single case studies. Consequently, it is difficult to compare findings across studies because of significant differences in the operational definition of confabulation and variability in the design and procedures employed. Notwithstanding these differences, there appears to be some convergence among published findings:

1. *Memory impairment commonly but not necessarily accompanies confabulation.* This conclusion is tempered by the fact that most neuropsychometric measures tap episodic but not semantic memory processes. This leaves open the possibility that semantic memory impairment or disruption of the interface between the semantic and episodic systems is a prerequisite for confabulation.

2. *Executive dysfunction is a common but variable component of confabulatory syndromes.* Deficient self-monitoring, disinhibition, susceptibility to intrusive interference, inability to shift set, and impaired fluency have all been shown to correlate with confabulation. There is, however, no consistent relationship between the presence of any of these symptoms and the emergence or resolution of confabulation.

3. *Confabulation primarily involves disruption of retrieval processes.* It is not clear what specific aspect of the retrieval process is disturbed. Some evidence suggests an inability to retrieve temporal and contextual "tags" (versus difficulty retrieving the information itself), while other data support failure to regulate or disengage the search process.

4. *Direct damage or functional disconnection involving the ventromesial and orbitofrontal cortices is implicated in the majority of confabulation reports.* This region is believed to mediate cross-talk between limbic and prefrontal structures and appears to form the intersection of subjective experience with personal and social reasoning.[51] Lesions in this area may explain the fortuitous association of subjective representations of current experience with previously stored representations or imagined approximations and may account for the faulty selection and acceptance of episodic or semantic memory traces noted in empiric studies of confabulation. Unfortunately, traditional neuropsychological measures are relatively insensitive to the functional sequelae of ventromesial and orbitofrontal lesions.

REFERENCES

1. Berlyne N: Confabulation. *Br J Psychiatry* 120:31–39, 1972.
2. Victor M, Yakovlev PI: SS Korsakoff's psychic disorder in conjunction with peripheral neuritis: A translation of Korsakoff's original article with brief comments on the author and his contribution to clinical medicine. *Neurology* 5:394–406, 1955.
3. Victor M, Adams RD, Collins GH: *The Wernicke-Korsakoff Syndrome and Related Neurologic Disorders Due to Alcoholism and Malnutrition,* 2d ed. Philadelphia: Davis, 1989.
4. Deluca J: A cognitive neuroscience perspective on confabulation. *Neuropsychoanalysis* 3:3–16, 2001.
5. Bonhoeffer K: *Die akuten Geisteskrankheiten der Gewohnheitstrinker*. Jena: Gustav Fischer, 1901.
6. Bonhoeffer K: Der Korsakowsche Symptomenkomplex in seinen Beziehungen zu den verschiedenen Krankheitsformen. *Allg Z Psychiatry* 61:744–752, 1904.
7. Van der Horst L: Über die Psychologie des Korsakowsyndroms. *Monatschr Psychiatry Neurol* 83: 65–84, 1932.
8. Williams HW, Rupp C: Observations on confabulation. *Am J Psychiatry* 95:395–405, 1938.
9. Talland GA: Confabulation in the Wernicke-Korsakoff syndrome. *Nerv Ment Dis* 132:361–381, 1961.
10. Talland GA: *Deranged Memory*. New York: Academic Press, 1965.
11. Kraepelin E: *Lectures on Clinical Psychiatry*. Johnson T, transl. London: Baillière Tindall, 1904.
12. Kraepelin E: *Clinical Psychiatry: A Textbook for Students and Physicians*. Diefendorf AR, transl. New York: Macmillan, 1907.
13. Kraepelin E: *Dementia Praecox and Paraphrenia*. Barclay RM, transl. Edinburgh: E and S Livingstone, 1919.
14. Kopelman MD: Two types of confabulation. *Neurol Neurosurg Psychiatry* 43:461–463, 1980.
15. Feinberg TE: *Altered Egos: How the Brain Creates the Self*. New York: Oxford University Press, 2001.
16. Feinberg TE, Roane DM: Anosognosia, completion and confabulation: The neutral-personal dichotomy. *Neurocase* 3:73–85, 1997.
17. Alexander MR, Freedman M: Amnesia after anterior communicating artery aneurysm rupture. *Neurology* 34:752–757, 1984.

18. Vilkki J: Amnesic syndromes after surgery of anterior communicating artery aneurysms. *Cortex* 21:431–444, 1985.
19. Mercer B, Wapner W, Gardner H, Benson P: A study of confabulation. *Arch Neurol* 34:429–433, 1977.
20. Wyke M, Warrington E: An experimental analysis of confabulation in a case of Korsakoff's syndrome using a tachistoscopic method. *J Neurol Neurosurg Psychiatry* 23:327–333, 1960.
21. Kapur N, Coughlan AK: Confabulation and frontal lobe dysfunction. *Neurol Neurosurg Psychiatry* 43:461–463, 1980.
22. Deluca J: Predicting neurobehavioral patterns following anterior communicating artery aneurysm. *Cortex* 29:639–647, 1993.
23. Papagno C, Baddeley A: Confabulation in a dysexecutive patient: Implication for models of retrieval. *Cortex* 33:743–752, 1997.
24. Stuss DT, Alexander MP, Lieberman A, Levine H: An extraordinary form of confabulation. *Neurology* 28:1166–1172, 1978.
25. Fischer RS, Alexander MP, D'Esposito M, Otto R: Neuropsychological and neuroanatomical correlates of confabulation. *Clin Exp Neuropsychol* 17:20–28, 1995.
26. Moscovitch M, Melo B: Strategic retrieval and the frontal lobes: evidence from confabulation and amnesia. *Neuropsychologia* 35:1017–1034, 1997.
27. Joseph R: Confabulation and delusional denial: Frontal lobe and lateralized influences. *J Clin Psychol* 42:507–519, 1986.
28. Benson DF, Djenderedjian A, Miller BL, et al: Neural basis of confabulation. *Neurology* 46:1239–1243, 1996.
29. Box O, Laing H, Kopelman K: The evolution of spontaneous confabulation, delusional misidentification and a related delusion in a case of severe head injury. *Neurocase* 5:251–262, 1999.
30. O'Connor M, Walbridge M, Sandson T, et al: A neuropsychological analysis of Capgras syndrome. *Neuropsychiatry Neuropsychol Behav Neurol* 9(4):265–271, 1996.
31. Cunningham JM, Pliskin NH, Cassisi JE, et al: Relationship between confabulation and measures of memory and executive function. *J Clin Exp Neuropsychol* 19(6):867–877, 1997.
32. Kopelman MD, Guinan EM, Lewis PDR: Delusional memory, confabulation and frontal lobe dysfunction: A case study in De Clerambault's syndrome. *Neurocase* 1:71–77, 1995.
33. Schnider A, Gutbrod K, Hess CW, et al: Memory without context: Amnesia with confabulations after infarction of the right capsular genu. *J Neurol Neurosurg Psychiatry* 61:186–193, 1996.
34. Ptak R, Schnider A: Spontaneous confabulations after orbitofrontal damage: The role of temporal context confusion and self-monitoring. *Neurocase* 5:243–250, 1999.
35. Schnider A, Ptak R, von Daniken C, et al: Recovery from spontaneous confabulations parallels recovery of temporal confusion in memory. *Neurology* 55:74–83, 2000.
36. Dalla Barba G: Confabulation: knowledge and recollective experience. *Cogn Neuropsychol* 10(1):1–20, 1993.
37. Moscovitch M: Confabulation, in Schachter DL (ed): *Memory Distortion: How Minds, Brains and Societies Reconstruct the Past*. Cambridge, MA: Harvard University Press, 1995; p226–251.
38. Sandson J, Albert ML, Alexander MP: Confabulation in aphasia. *Cortex* 22:621–626, 1986.
39. Laws KR, McKenna PJ, McCarthy RA: Delusions about people. *Neurocase* 1:3439–362, 1995.
40. Barbizet J: Defect of memorizing of hippocampal-mammillary origin: A review. *Neurol Neurosurg Psychiatry* 26:127–135, 1963.
41. Weiskrantz L: Neuroanatomy of memory and amnesia: A case for multiple memory systems. *Human Neurobiol* 6:93–105, 1987.
42. Mair WGP, Warrington EK, Weiskrantz L: Memory disorder in Korsakoff's psychosis: A neuropathological and neuropsychological investigation of two cases. *Brain* 102:749–783, 1979.
43. Mayes AR, Meudell PR, Mann D, Pickering A: Location of lesions in Korsakoff's syndrome: Neuropsychological and neuropathological data on two patients. *Cortex* 24:367–388, 1988.
44. Talland GA, Sweet WH, Ballantine HT: Amnesic syndrome with anterior communicating artery aneurysm. *Nerv Ment Dis* 145:179–192, 1967.
45. Lindqvist G, Norlen G: Korsakoff's syndrome after operation on ruptured aneurysm of the anterior communicating artery. *Acta Psychiatr Scand* 42:24–34, 1966.
46. Damasio AR, Graff-Radford NR, Eslinger PJ, et al: Amnesia following basal forebrain lesions. *Arch Neurol* 42:263–271, 1985.
47. Baddeley AD, Wilson B: Amnesia, autobiographical memory, and confabulation, in Rubin DC (ed): *Autobiographical Memory*. Cambridge, England: Cambridge University Press, 1986.
48. Deluca J, Cicerone KD: Confabulation following aneurysm of the anterior communicating artery. *Cortex* 27:417–424, 1991.
49. Deluca J, Diamond BJ: Aneurysm of the anterior communicating artery: A review of neuroanatomical and

neuropsychologic sequelae. *Clin Exp Neuropsychol* 17:100–121, 1995.

50. Schnider A, Ptak R: Spontaneous confabulators fail to suppress currently irrelevant memory traces. *Nat Neurosci* 2:677–681, 1999.
51. Damasio A, Tranel D, Damasio H: Somatic markers and the guidance of behavior: Theory and preliminary testing, in Levin HS, Eisenberg HM, Benton AL (eds): *Frontal Lobe Function and Dysfunction*. New York: Oxford University Press, 1991, pp 217–229.

Chapter 31

MISIDENTIFICATION SYNDROMES

Todd E. Feinberg
David M. Roane

Misidentification syndromes, sometimes referred to as delusional misidentification syndromes (DMS), are conditions in which a patient incorrectly identifies and reduplicates persons, places, objects, or events. The most commonly reported form of misidentification for persons is known as *Capgras' syndrome.* The syndrome was first reported in 1923 by Capgras and Reboul-Lachaux,[1] who described a 53-year-old woman with a chronic paranoid psychosis who became convinced that multiple persons, including members of her family, had been replaced by imposters. She also asserted that there were several duplicates of herself. Since that time, hundreds of cases of Capgras' syndrome have been reported. The essence of the disorder lies in the delusional belief that a person or persons, generally close to the patient, have been replaced by "doubles" or imposters.[2]

A related type of DMS is the Frégoli syndrome.[3] First reported in 1927, the syndrome is named after the famous Italian actor Leopoldo Frégoli, who was extremely adept at impersonation. This condition involves the belief that a person who is well known to the patient is really impersonating, and hence taking on the appearance of, a stranger in the patient's environment. Several authors have commented on the relationship between Capgras' and Frégoli syndromes.[4–6] Christodoulou[6] suggested that Capgras' syndrome is characterized by a "hypoidentification" of a person known by the patient who is felt to be an imposter, while Frégoli syndrome was the manifestation of a "hyperidentification" in which a known person could be seen in the guise of others. The syndrome of *intermetamorphosis,* described by Courbon and Tusques,[7] is a related condition in which persons known to the patient are believed to have exchanged identities with each other. In the delusion of subjective doubles,[8] the patients believe they themselves have been replaced. Other varieties of delusional misidentification syndromes exist, and different varieties may co-occur in any given patient.

The delusional misidentification syndromes are related to the syndrome of reduplicative paramnesia (see Chap. 29). For instance, Alexander and colleagues[9] described a case of Capgras' syndrome following a head injury that resulted in a large right frontal subdural hematoma. The patient stated that his wife and five children had been replaced by a nearly identical family, and he persisted in his conviction even when challenged by his examiners. Alexander and associates suggested a similarity between their case and *reduplicative paramnesia,* a syndrome originally described by Pick[10] in 1903. Pick's patient was a 67-year-old woman who confabulated the existence of two clinics, both headed by Professor Pick. While Capgras' syndrome had traditionally been considered a psychiatric condition, reduplicative paramnesia had generally been felt to be a neurologic disorder, since it was usually seen in the setting of brain disorders and was often associated with confusion and memory loss. It differed as well from Capgras' syndrome in that it typically involved misidentification of places rather than persons. However, the distinction between the two conditions is not entirely clear. Cases of reduplication reported by Weinstein[11] in the setting of brain disease involved duplication of persons, events, body parts, and even the self (see Chap. 29). Furthermore, Weinstein's cases of reduplication were frequently associated with other psychiatric symptoms including other delusions, hallucinations, and mood changes. It has therefore become customary to group DMS and reduplicative paramnesia together.

The Capgras' delusion is most commonly associated with psychiatric illness and is often accompanied by derealization, depersonalization,[12,13] and other paranoid symptomatology.[14,15] Literature reviews of patients with the Capgras' delusion have demonstrated the diagnostic heterogeneity of this condition.[14,16,17] Schizophrenia, mood disorders, and organic conditions, including Alzheimer's disease,[18] have all been associated with Capgras' syndrome.

Misidentification and reduplication in general have been associated with a wide variety of medical and neurologic conditions.[19,20] In a large literature review of cases of reduplication, Signer[19] found cases due to drug intoxication or withdrawal, infectious and inflammatory disease, and endocrine disorders. Neurologic conditions included seizures, cerebral infarction, and head injury. Diffuse brain syndromes including delirium, dementia, and mental retardation accounted for over 40 percent of patients with diagnosable organic conditions. More recently, DMS has been reported in association with parkinsonism in general[21] and Lewy body dementia in particular.[22] Ballard[23] has found that DMS occurs significantly more frequently in Lewy body dementia than in Alzheimer's dementia. Electroconvulsive therapy has also been implicated in cases of misidentification.[24,25]

NEUROANATOMIC CORRELATES

In a report of 29 personally examined patients with misidentification for person, Joseph[26] found that 16 patients with abnormal computed tomography (CT) scans had bilateral cortical atrophy, including bifrontal atrophy (88 percent), bitemporal atrophy (73 percent), and biparietal atrophy (60 percent). A subsequent study by the same author and coworkers[27] showed CT evidence for bilateral anterior cortical atrophy and subcortical atrophy in psychiatric patients with reduplicative amnesia. Weinstein and Burnham suggested that bilateral and diffuse brain involvement with right-hemispheric predominance were the most common neurologic findings.[28] Along these lines, Feinberg and Shapiro[29] reviewed the anatomic correlates on a selected series of case reports of patients with misidentification-reduplication. They found that bilateral cortical involvement occurred frequently (62 percent of Capgras' patients and 41 percent of reduplication cases). In considering those cases where cerebral dysfunction was unilateral, they found that right hemispheric predominance in reduplication was highly significant (52 percent right versus 7 percent left), with a statistical trend for more frequent right hemispheric damage in the smaller number of Capgras' cases (32 percent right versus 7 percent left). Förstl and coworkers[20] grouped together a wide range of misidentification cases and found that 19 of 20 patients with focal lesions on brain CT scans showed right-sided abnormalities. In a subsequent study, Förstland colleagues[30] focused on patients with dementia of the Alzheimer's type and found that patients with misidentification had significantly greater atrophy in the right frontal lobe than did demented controls. Positron emission tomography (PET) has demonstrated significant hypometabolism in bilateral orbitofrontal and cingulate regions of Alzheimer's patients with DMS in comparison to Alzheimer's patients with no DMS.[31] Based on three cases of head trauma, Benson and associates[32] suggested that reduplicative paramnesia occurred in the setting of bifrontal impairment in concert with damage to the posterior portion of the right hemisphere. Hakim and coworkers,[33] in a prospective study of 50 patients with alcoholism, found that 3 of 4 reduplicators had acute right hemispheric lesions. They presumed all patients to have chronic bifrontal damage on the basis of their chronic alcohol use and neuropsychological test results. Finally, Fleminger and Burns[34] compared right versus left hemispheric asymmetries in CT scans of patients with misidentification. In one selected group, asymmetry was found, with greater right hemispheric damage in the occipitoparietal area. In the analysis of a second group of patients, greater right hemispheric damage could be detected in frontal, temporal, and parietal lobes.

At present, while some evidence suggests that a right hemispheric lesion (particularly right frontal impairment[35]) can be both necessary and sufficient to produce misidentification, the bulk of cases support the argument that a right hemispheric lesion is much more likely to be associated with misidentification in the context of bifrontal or diffuse cortical disturbance. This finding may reflect the greater tendency in these patients to demonstrate confabulation in general (see Chap. 30).

REPRESENTATIVE THEORIES

It has been suggested that delusional misidentification is a symptom, rather than a distinct syndrome, associated with various psychiatric and neurologic diagnoses.[36] Nonetheless, several explanations have attempted to account for a broad range of misidentification phenomena. Anatomic disconnection has been offered as a mechanism by several authors. Joseph[26] theorized that misidentification could result from hemispheric disconnection of cortical areas responsible for orientation. This could result in each hemisphere's maintaining an independent "image" of person, place, and time, which might lead to reduplication of entities in the environment. However, Ellis and colleagues[37] showed that patients with Capgras' syndrome could judge face stimuli more rapidly with bilateral than with unilateral presentation, a finding that they suggested was inconsistent with the hemispheric disconnection hypothesis. Based on PET data, Mentis and others[31] state that DMS could reflect impaired connectivity between multimodal cortical association areas and paralimbic areas whereby patients fail to appreciate the "emotional significance and relevance" of intact perceptions. Staton and coworkers[38] suggested that reduplication could be a failure to integrate previously stored memories and new information resulting from disconnection of the right hippocampus. Alexander and associates[9] considered that a disconnection of the right temporal and limbic area from the frontal lobes could alter the patients' familiarity for people and places and prevent them from utilizing available information appropriately.

Staton and associates[38] and Alexander and colleagues[9] attribute misidentification particularly to the loss of functions subsumed by the right hemisphere. Several investigators have emphasized other nondominant hemispheric functions, such as disorders of visuospatial orientation,[33,35] problem solving,[35] and the ability to determine the exact identity and uniqueness of stimuli[39] in the origin of delusional misidentification syndromes and reduplication. A study by Ellis and coworkers[37] confirmed that three Capgras' patients lacked the normal right hemispheric superiority for visual processing of faces.

A final disconnectionist account, formulated by Ellis and Young,[40] is based on the suggestion that there are two anatomically independent pathways for facial recognition: a "ventral route" subserving explicit recognition and a "dorsal route" responsible for recognition of the emotional significance of faces but not sufficient to allow for conscious identification.[41] While Capgras' syndrome has been linked with prosopagnosia,[42–44] Ellis and Young[40] argue that the two are dissociable because they result from separate lesions. The ventral route disconnection causes prosopagnosia, while the dorsal route interruption yields Capgras' syndrome. Ellis and coworkers[45] have shown that Capgras' patients who fail to distinguish familiar from unfamiliar faces on the basis of autonomic response, measured by skin conductance, can still demonstrate overt recognition of familiar faces.

The role of perceptual disturbance and impaired face processing in the production of DMS has been debated. Sellal and associates[46] attribute misidentification for place to visual-perceptual impairment in the context of a defect in self-awareness. In their case report, neuropsychological testing showed that their patient consistently misused visual details in the process of orienting herself. While face-processing deficits short of full-fledged prosopagnosia have been demonstrated in Capgras' syndrome,[47,48] Edelstyn and Oyebode[49] have concluded that the various studies of face processing in Capgras' have not shown any consistent pattern of impairment. With regard to Frégoli-like misidentifications, Rapcsak et al.[50] have divided patients with right hemisphere pathology who falsely recognized unfamiliar faces into two categories. Patients with both false recognition and prosopagnosia presented with posterior lesions and impaired face perception or face recognition on neuropsychological testing. False recognition without prosopagnosia was associated with prefrontal damage and confabulation and no evidence of perceptual impairment. Consistent with this latter mechanism, Feinberg et al.,[51] describing a case of multiple Frégoli delusions following head trauma to right frontal and left temporoparietal areas, attributed the DMS to a combination of executive and memory deficits. This pattern of neuropsychological deficits is similar to what is typically seen in confabulators with Korsakoff's syndrome. Box et al.[52] and Mattioli et al.[53] have also described cases of DMS associated with frontal impairment and confabulation. However, both note that DMS and confabulation can follow a different course in the same patient depending on the evolution of a number of neuropsychological deficits. Discussing a case of Frégoli which did involve both a right posterior temporoparietal infarct and significant face-processing deficits, Ellis and Szulecka[54] conclude that perceptual impairment alone cannot account for delusional misidentification. They support the view that the delusional nature of this symptom requires "a failure at a higher level where self-beliefs are monitored."

The position of Ellis and Szulecka[54] and of Sellal et al.[46] is consistent with the notion that the *interaction* of neurologic and psychiatric factors is critical in the production of DMS. Early important work emphasizing the link between neurologic and psychiatric factors in DMS can be found in the writings of Jacques Vié,[4,55–57] who noted that the diverse DMS (*méconnaissance systématique*) such as Capgras' and Frégoli syndromes were related to the neurologic syndromes of anosognosia of Babinski (unawareness of hemiplegia) (see Chap. 29) and asomatognosia[58] (denial of ownership of limb). Vié pointed out that in all these conditions, systematic and selective misidentifications occurred that could not be explained solely on the basis of factors such as generalized confusion.

The position of Weinstein and Kahn,[11,28,59] because of its emphasis on psychological denial, is usually taken to represent a psychological theory. In actuality these authors also suggested that DMS occurred through an interaction of neurologic and psychiatric factors. They suggested that misidentification and reduplication were facilitated by brain alteration and that they represented a denial, representation of, or solution to the patient's problems. More recent analysis by other investigators has also suggested an interaction between neurologic and psychiatric factors.[60,61]

An additional link between neurologic and psychiatric causation of delusional misidentification syndromes is provided by the fact that dissociative symptoms occur in delusional misidentification syndromes associated with both neurologic and psychiatric disorders.[28] Capgras, in the original report,[1] emphasized the importance of the *sentiment d'étrangeté* in the production of the syndrome in his chronic paranoid patient. Many authors have provided additional support for the association of depersonalization/derealization with delusional misidentification syndromes (see Christodoulou[5,6,12]). Christodoulou has suggested that depersonalization/derealization symptoms, under certain circumstances (paranoia, cerebral dysfunction, charged emotional circumstances), may evolve into delusional misidentification syndromes. Weinstein and coworkers have noted that patients with retrograde amnesia after head injury may also display elements of depersonalization and derealization.[28,62] Feelings of altered familiarity also occur during psychomotor seizures and with temporal lobe stimulation (see Feinberg and Shapiro[29] for review).

A PROPOSED FRAMEWORK FOR DELUSIONAL MISIDENTIFICATION SYNDROMES

As noted by prior authors, we agree that DMS can be viewed as being especially related to, and perhaps a special instance of, dissociative disorders, and we regard the origin of these symptoms as a perturbation, as opposed to a loss, of personal relatedness. We suggest that DMS cleaves along the dimension of personal relatedness into three basic groups based upon the pattern of relatedness between the object (person, event, or experience) and the self. The various subtypes of DMS and reduplication can thus be characterized as showing a pattern of decreased (withdrawal) or increased (insertion of) personal relatedness (or both) between the self and the misidentified object or event.

Our basic dichotomization into patterns of withdrawal or insertion of personal relatedness corresponds in part to several previously suggested dichotomies (Table 31-1) and is consistent with the viewpoint that Capgras' syndrome may be similar to jamais vu phenomena[29,63–66] and that Frégoli[64] and environmental reduplication[29,64–67] are similar to déjà vu phenomena. Our model (Table 31-1), however, differs in two fundamental ways from previously proposed models (see, for example, de Pauw[66]). First of all, as to the basic means of distinguishing Capgras' from Frégoli, these syndromes have previously been categorized on the basis of physical versus psychological substitution or hypoidentification versus hyperidentification. In contrast, we view the distinguishing feature to be alteration of personal relatedness or significance. Those syndromes exemplified by decreased relatedness may be said to represent a disavowal, estrangement, or alienation from persons, objects, or events, while those with increased relatedness are manifestations of an overrelatedness with elements in the environment.

We prefer the concept of an alteration in relatedness as opposed to an alteration in familiarity because

Table 31-1
Prior formulations of basic dichotomization of Capgras and Frégoli syndromes

Author		
Vié[4]	Illusion of negative doubles (Capgras)	Illusion of positive doubles (Frégoli)
Christodoulou[6]	Delusional hypoidentification	Delusional hyperidentification
Christoldoulou[5]	Physically identical, psychologically different	Physically different, psychologically identical
de Pauw[64–66]	Hypoidentification, denial of familiarity, jamais vu (Capgras)	Hyperidentification, affirmation of familiarity, déjà vu (environmental reduplication)
Feinberg and Shapiro[29]	Pathologic unfamiliarity, jamais vu, substitute familiar for unfamiliar (Capgras)	Pathologic familiarity, déjà vu, substitute unfamiliar for familiar (environmental reduplication)

many stimuli that the patient misidentifies, such as hospitals and aneurysms, are not particularly "familiar" in any sense of the word. Rather they are significant and actually do pertain to the self, though the patient rejects them in spite of this.

As Edelstyn and colleagues[68] have argued, this approach is particularly useful in explaining instances where Capgras' and Frégoli-type misidentifications co-occur within a single misidentification (Table 31-2, column 4). This occurs, for instance, in asomatognosia

Table 31-2
Proposed model of common DMS

Examples of misidentified entities	*Mechanism supporting misidentification/reduplication and clinical examples*		
	Withdrawal of personal relatedness	Insertion of personal relatedness	Combined withdrawal/insertion of personal relatedness
Persons	Misidentifies wife as "impostor" (Capgras–jamais vu)	Misidentifies stranger as son (Frégoli–déjà vu)	Misidentifies personal physician as a friend from home[59,69] (Capgras/Frégoli–jamais vu/déjà vu)
Hemiplegic arm[55,58,59,69] (asomatognosia)	Denies ownership of arm[65,66]		Misidentifies own arm as belonging to close friend[58,59,69]
Hospital[11,28,59,69,70] (environmental reduplication)	Calls the hospital a "branch" or "annex" of actual hospital[59]	Mislocates actual hospital closer to patient's own neighborhood[59,64–66]	Misidentifies hospital as "annex" of actual hospital and locates it closer to patient's own neighborhood[59]
Traumatic events[11,28,69,70] (temporal reduplication) i.e., car accident	Denies accident occurred to patient (jamais vécu)	Claims similar accident happened previously to patient (déjà vécu)	Minimizes own accident but claims reduplicated brother "Martin" killed in (fictitious) car accident[70]
Illness[11,28,59,69]	Denial of illness	Had similar illness previously	Patient denies illness but claims reduplicated child Bill called "Willie" had same illness as patient[59] Patient with aneurysm minimizes it and claims her relatives have aneurysms

where the patient simultaneously denies ownership of the arm[58,59,69] (withdrawal of personal relatedness) while identifying the arm as belonging to a friend or relative (insertion of personal relatedness). In a similar fashion, when a patient with environmental reduplication claims he is located in a hospital "annex" in his own neighborhood, he is *both* denying the actual identity of his current location as well as inserting an element of personal relatedness.

The same pattern of withdrawal and insertion of relatedness occurs in reduplication of illness in the context of anosognosia. Thus a patient of Weinstein did not recognize her own illness but claimed she had two children, Bill (real) and "Willie" (fictitious), and that Willie had an illness similar to hers.[59,69] We saw a patient who minimized the problems posed by her own aneurysm but claimed that several of her relatives had aneurysms. Finally, with regard to misidentification of a traumatic event, Baddeley and Wilson[70] described their patient R.J., who denied that he was seriously injured in a car accident, yet simultaneously claimed to have two brothers named Martin. There was one Martin who actually existed and a second, fictitious "Martin" who, the patient stated, was killed in a car accident (see Chap. 29 for further discussion of these cases). In these cases we hypothesize that the neurologic impairment facilitates the derealization/depersonalization (dissociation) of an actual person, place, or event, which is then replaced by some other personally significant relationship. Motivational factors appear important in determining both the withdrawal and insertion of significance.

CONCLUDING REMARKS

If a perturbation in personal relatedness to oneself or one's environment is an essential ingredient in delusional misidentification syndromes, one may ask whether this distortion is primarily a result of a neurologic lesion, a psychiatric mechanism linked with motivational variables, or both. Many theories emphasizing a neurologic etiology for Capgras' syndrome[9,38,61] assert a limbic disconnection of current perceptions from past experience. This causes a reduced feeling of familiarity with environmental stimuli and a confabulation of "doubleness" to explain the disparity between current and past experience. These theories do not account for the selectivity of many cases of Capgras', their delusional nature, the lack of gross neuropathologic lesions in most cases, the occurrence of misidentification of relatively unfamiliar persons in many cases, the occurrence of misidentifications of the hyperfamiliar type, and the role of motivation. For instance, in regard to the last of these, it has been pointed out that in environmental reduplication, while abnormal spatial perception, poor visual memory, and other neuropsychological defects are evident, these patients often show, in addition, a pronounced desire to return home.[71]

Other theories express the viewpoint that derealization/depersonalization is the result of psychological defense mechanisms. As noted by Nemiah,[72] "From the earliest period of the development of psychoanalytic concepts, the experience of estrangement that is central to depersonalization phenomena has been viewed as a psychological defense." In this scenario, derealization/depersonalization occurs as a defense against irreconcilable affects or unacceptable and conflicting motivations. The ambivalence produces the delusion of "doubleness" through mechanisms such as "splitting."[36,73] While these theories can account for selectivity, delusional nature, and the possibility of hypo- and hyperfamiliar misidentifications, they do not account for delusional misidentification syndromes occurring in the context of neurologic disease.

A mediating point of view is that the neurologic lesion, and certain neurologic lesions in particular, cause a distortion of normal sensation, memory, and awareness. The response to this distortion, particularly when it involves personally significant objects or events, creates the circumstances which, in the susceptible individual, results in derealization/depersonalization. It is upon this substrate that motivational variables may become evident.

REFERENCES

1. Capgras J, Reboul-Lachaux J: L'illusion des "sosies" dans un délire systématisé. *Bull Soc Clin Med Ment* 11: 6–16, 1923.
2. Christodoulou GN: The delusional misidentification syndromes. *Br J Psychiatry* 14:65–69, 1991.
3. Courbon P, Fail G: Syndrome "d'illusion de Frégoli" et schizophrenie. *Ann Med Psychol* 85:289–290, 1927.

4. Vié J: Un trouble de l'identification des personnes: l'illusion des sosies. *Ann Med Psychol* 88:214–237, 1930.
5. Christodoulou GN: Delusional hyper-identifications of the Frégoli type. *Acta Psychiatr Scand* 54:305–314, 1976.
6. Christodoulou GN: The syndrome of Capgras: *Br J Psychiatry* 130:556–564, 1977.
7. Courbon P, Tusques J: L'illusion d'intermetamorphose et de charme. *Ann Med Psychol* 90:401–406, 1932.
8. Christodoulou GN: Syndrome of subjective doubles. *Am J Psychiatry* 135:249–251, 1978.
9. Alexander MP, Stuss DT, Benson DF: Capgras syndrome: A reduplicative phenomenon. *Neurology* 29:334–339, 1979.
10. Pick A: Clinical studies. *Brain* 26:242–267, 1903.
11. Weinstein EA, Kahn RL, Sugarman LA: Phenomenon of reduplication. *AMA Arch Neurol Psychiatry* 67:808–814, 1952.
12. Christodoulou GN: Role of depersonalization-derealization phenomena in the delusional misidentification syndromes, in Christodoulou GN (ed): *The Delusional Misidentification Syndromes.* Basel: Karger, 1986.
13. Spier SA: Capgras' syndrome and the delusions of misidentification. *Psychiatr Ann* 22:279–285, 1992.
14. Kimura S: Review of 106 cases with the syndrome of Capgras. *Bibl Psychiatry* 164:121–130, 1986.
15. Todd J, Dewhurst K, Wallis G: The syndrome of Capgras. *Br J Psychiatry* 139:319–327, 1981.
16. Merrin EL, Silberfarb PM: The Capgras phenomenon. *Arch Gen Psychiatry* 33:965, 1970.
17. Signer SF: Capgras' syndrome: The delusion of substitution. *Clin Psychiatry* 48:147–150, 1987.
18. Mendez MF, Martin RJ, Symth KA, Whitehouse PJ: Disturbances of person identification in Alzheimer's disease: a retrospective study. *J Nerv Ment Dis* 180:94, 1992.
19. Signer SF: Psychosis in neurologic disease: Capgras symptom and delusions of reduplication in neurologic disorders. *Neuropsychiatr Neuropsychol Behav Neurol* 5:138–143, 1992.
20. Förstl H, Almeida OP, Owen A, et al: Psychiatric, neurological and medical aspects of misidentification syndromes: A review of 260 cases. *Psychol Med* 21:905–950, 1991.
21. Roane DM, Rogers JD, Robinson JH, Feinberg TE: Delusional misidentification in association with parkinsonism. *J Neuropsychiatry Clin Neurosci* 10:194–198, 1998.
22. Ballard CG, O'Brien J, Lowery K, et al: A prospective study of dementia with Lewy bodies. *Age Ageing* 27: 631–636, 1998.
23. Ballard C: Psychiatric morbidity in dementia with Lewy bodies: A prospective clinical and neuropathological comparative study with Alzheimer's disease. *Am J Psychiatry* 156:1039–1045, 1999.
24. Weinstein EA, Linn L, Kahn RL: Psychosis during electroshock therapy: Its relation to the theory of shock therapy. *Am J Psychiatry* 109:22–26, 1952.
25. Hay GG: Electroconvulsive therapy as a contributor to the production of delusional misidentification. *Br J Psychiatry* 148:667–669, 1986.
26. Joseph AB: Focal central nervous system abnormalities in patients with misidentification syndromes, in Christodoulou GN (ed): *The Delusional Misidentification Syndromes.* Basel: Karger, 1986, p 68.
27. Joseph AB, O'Leary DH, Kurland R, Ellis HD: Bilateral anterior cortical atrophy and subcortical atrophy in reduplicative paramnesia: A case-control study of computed tomography in 10 patients. *Can J Psychiatry* 44:685–689, 1999.
28. Weinstein EA, Burnham DL: Reduplication and the syndrome of Capgras. *Psychiatry* 54:78, 1991.
29. Feinberg TE, Shapiro RM: Misidentification-reduplication and the right hemisphere. *Neuropsychiatr Neuropsychol Behav Neurol* 2:39–48, 1989.
30. Förstl H, Burns A, Jacoby R, Levy R: Neuroanatomical correlates of clinical misidentification and misperception in senile dementia of the Alzheimer type. *Clin Psychiatry* 52:268, 1991.
31. Mentis MJ, Weinstein EA, Horwitz B, et al: Abnormal brain glucose metabolism in the delusional misidentification syndromes: A positron emission tomography study in Alzheimer disease. *Biol Psychiatry* 38:438–449, 1995.
32. Benson DF, Gardner H, Meadows JC: Reduplicative paramnesia. *Neurology* 26:147–151, 1978.
33. Hakim H, Verma NP, Greiffenstein MF: Pathogenesis of reduplicative paramnesia. *Neurol Neurosurg Psychiatry* 51:839–841, 1988.
34. Fleminger S, Burns A: The delusional misidentification syndromes in patients with and without evidence of organic cerebral disorder: A structured review of case reports. *Biol Psychiatry* 33:22–32, 1993.
35. Kapur N, Turner A, King C: Reduplicative paramnesia: Possible anatomical and neuropsychological mechanisms. *Neurol Neurosurg Psychiatry* 51:579–581, 1988.
36. Enoch MD, Trethowan WH: *Uncommon Psychiatric Syndromes.* Bristol: John Wright, 1979.
37. Ellis HD, de Pauw KW, Christodoulou GN, et al: Responses to facial and non-facial stimuli presented tachistoscopically in either or both visual fields by patients with the Capgras delusion and paranoid schizophrenics. *Neurol Neurosurg Psychiatry* 56:215–219, 1993.

38. Staton RD, Brumback RA, Wilson H: Reduplicative paramnesia: A disconnection syndrome of memory. *Cortex* 18:23–36, 1982.
39. Cutting J: Delusional misidentification and the role of the right hemisphere in the appreciation of identity. *Br J Psychiatry* 159:70–74, 1991.
40. Ellis HD, Young AW: Accounting for delusional misidentifications. *Br J Psychiatry* 147:239–248, 1900.
41. Bauer RM: The cognitive psychophysiology of prosopagnosia, in Ellis H, Felves M, Newcombe F, et al (eds): *Aspects of Face Processing.* Dordrecht: Nijhoff, 1986.
42. Shraberg D, Weitzel WD: Prosopagnosia and the Capgras syndrome. *Clin Psychiatry* 40:313–316, 1979.
43. Bidault E, Luaute JP, Tzavaras A: Prosopagnosia and the delusional misidentification syndromes. *Bibl Psychiatry* 164:80–91, 1986.
44. Lewis SW: Brain imaging in a case of Capgras' syndrome. *Br J Psychiatry* 150:117–120, 1987.
45. Ellis HD, Young AW, Quayle AH, de Pauw KW: Reduced autonomic responses to faces in Capgras delusion. *Proc R Soc Lond* 264:1085–1092, 1997.
46. Sellal F, Fontaine SF, Van Der Linden M, et al: To be or not to be at home? A neuropsychological approach to delusion for place. *J Clin Exp Neuropsychol* 18(2):234–248, 1996.
47. Young AW, Reid I, Wright S, et al: Face-processing impairments and the Capgras delusion. *Br J Psychiatry* 162:695–698, 1993.
48. Silva JA, Leong GB: Visual-perceptual abnormalities in delusional misidentification. *Can J Psychiatry* 40:6–8, 1995.
49. Edelstyn NMJ, Oyebode F: A review of the phenomenology and cognitive neuropsychological origins of the Capgras syndrome. *Int J Geriat Psychiatry* 14:48–59, 1999.
50. Rapcsak SZ, Polster MR, Glisky ML, Comer JF: False recognition of unfamiliar faces following right hemisphere damage: Neuropsychological and anatomical observations. *Cortex* 32:593–611, 1996.
51. Feinberg TE, Eaton LA, Roane DM, Giacino JT: Multiple Frégoli delusions after traumatic brain injury. *Cortex* 35:373–387, 1999.
52. Box O, Laing H, Kopelman M: The evolution of spontaneous confabulation, delusional misidentification, and a related delusion in a case of severe head injury. *Neurocase* 5:251–262, 1999.
53. Mattioli F, Miozzo A, Vignoto LA: Confabulation and delusional misidentification: A four year follow-up study. *Cortex* 35:413–422, 1999.
54. Ellis HD, Szulecka TK: The disguised lover: A case of Frégoli delusion. in Halligan PW, Marshall JC (eds): *Method in Madness: Case Studies in Cognitive Neuropsychiatry.* East Sussex: Psychology Press, 1996, pp 37–50.
55. Vié J: Les méconnaissances systématiques. *Ann Med Psychol (Paris)* 102:410–455, 1944.
56. Vié J: Le substratum morbide et les stades évolutifs des méconnaissances systématiques. *Ann Med Psychol (Paris)* 102:410–455, 1944.
57. Vié J: Étude psychopathologique des méconnaissances systématiques. *Ann Med Psychol (Paris)* 102:1–15, 1944.
58. Feinberg TE, Haber LD, Leeds NE: Verbal asomatognosia. *Neurology* 40:1391–1394, 1990.
59. Weinstein EA, Kahn RL: *Denial of Illness: Symbolic and Physiological Aspects.* Springfield, IL: Charles C Thomas, 1955.
60. Gordon MacCallum WA: The interplay of organic and psychological factors in the delusional misidentification syndrome. *Bibl Psychiatry* 164:92–98, 1986.
61. Fleminger S: Delusional misidentification: An exemplary symptom illustrating an interaction between organic brain disease and psychological processes. *Psychopathology* 27:161–167, 1994.
62. Weinstein EA, Marvin SL, Keller NJA: Amnesia as a language pattern. *Arch Gen Psychiatry* 6:269–270, 1962.
63. Todd J, Dewhurst K, Wallis G: The syndrome of Capgras. *Br J Psychiatry* 139:319–327, 1981.
64. de Pauw KW, Szulecka TK, Poltock TL: Frégoli syndrome after cerebral infarction. *J Nerv Ment Dis* 175:433–438, 1987.
65. de Pauw KW: Delusional misidentification syndromes, in Bizon Z, Szyszkowski W (eds): *Proceedings of the 35th Congress Polish Psychiatrists.* Warsaw: Polish Psychiatric Association, 1989.
66. de Pauw KW: Delusional misidentification: A plea for an agreed terminology and classification. *Psychopathology* 27:123–129, 1994.
67. Sno HN, Linszen DH, DeJonghe F: Déjà vu experiences and reduplicative paramnesia. *Br J Psychiatry* 161:565–568, 1992.
68. Edelstyn NMJ, Oyebode F, Barrett K: Delusional misidentification: A neuropsychological case study in dementia associated with Parkinson's disease. *Neurocase* 4:181–187, 1998.
69. Weinstein EA: Patterns of reduplication in organic brain disease, in Vinken PJ, Bruyn GW (eds): *Handbook of Clinical Neurology.* Amsterdam: North Holland, 1969.
70. Baddeley AD, Wilson B: Amnesia, autobiographical memory, and confabulation, in Rubin DC (ed):

Autobiographical Memory. Cambridge, England: Cambridge University Press, 1986.

71. Ruff RL, Volpe BT: Environmental reduplication associated with right frontal and parietal lobe injury. *Neurol Neurosurg Psychiatry* 44:382–386, 1981.
72. Nemiah J: Dissociative disorders, in Kaplan HI, Sadock BJ (eds): *Comprehensive Textbook of Psychiatry.* Baltimore: Williams & Wilkins, 1989, vol 5.
73. Benson RJ: Capgras' syndrome. *Am J Psychiatry* 140: 969–978, 1983.

Part 5

FRONTAL, CALLOSAL, AND SUBCORTICAL SYNDROMES

Chapter 32

FRONTAL LOBES: CLINICAL AND ANATOMIC ISSUES

Bruce L. Miller
D. Frank Benson
Julene K. Johnson

For over a century, the frontal lobes have been an enigma to brain scientists. Significant progress has been made in the past several decades, but many anatomic and functional aspects remain mysterious. The frontal lobes, particularly in humans, are massive in relation to other, better-understood cortical areas, and it was long considered that the frontal lobes were the seat of human intelligence. This proved overly simple, at least as intelligence is defined by psychometric testing. A better generalization is that prefrontal cortex is concerned with the regulation of mental activities[1] and thus stands in a superordinate relation to the activities of posterior cortical areas.[2] As this chapter and the next will attest, our understanding the functions of the frontal lobes in human behavior is still at an early stage.

Classic neuroanatomy divides the cortical surface of the frontal lobes into three major segments: (1) motor–the narrow strip of cortical tissue located just anterior to the rolandic fissure; (2) premotor–the larger area of frontal tissue anterior to the motor strip that acts as a motor association cortex (Brodmann areas 6 and 8); and (3) prefrontal–the vast amount of frontal cortex anterior to the premotor cortex, including a significant amount of the anterior/lateral cortex, most of the medial frontal cortex, and the entire orbital frontal cortex. In the classification suggested by Luria, the motor and premotor areas of the frontal lobes would be included in the sensorimotor division and the prefrontal cortex would carry out the regulatory activities. The motor functions of the frontal lobes are adequately reviewed in many neuroanatomy texts. The prefrontal regulatory functions are important for psychology and are the topic of this chapter.

Of considerable significance in discussion of the neural basis of prefrontal psychological functions are the connections of frontal cortex with other brain areas. The prefrontal cortex receives direct or indirect input from most ipsilateral cortical areas and from the opposite hemisphere via callosal connections. In addition, prefrontal cortex receives strong input from a number of significant subcortical sources: (1) the limbic system, (2) the reticular system, (3) the hypothalamus, and (4) neurotransmitter systems. Prefrontal cortex is the only cortical area that receives strong sensorimotor, limbic, and reticular input. Additional input of hypothalamic and autonomic information and the effects of the cholinergic, serotoninergic, noradrenergic, and glutamatergic neurotransmitter systems arriving from subcortical regions place prefrontal cortex in a strong position to monitor both intrinsic and extrinsic stimuli and to exert regulatory control of brain functions.

PREFRONTAL FUNCTION: INSIGHTS FROM THE CLINIC

The precise contribution of prefrontal cortex to behavior has proven difficult to delineate. To date, most information has been derived from the study of behavioral aberrations that develop following frontal brain damage. In the past several decades some psychological tests aimed directly at the assessment of prefrontal function have been devised (see Chap. 33), and more recently psychological testing has been combined with functional brain imaging techniques to provide valuable insights into the dynamic functions of prefrontal cortex. In general, however, psychological tests of prefrontal function demand inferences from data obtained through primary sensorimotor functions, which themselves may be impaired.[3]

A second problem in studying prefrontal function is a lack of cleanly delineated clinical/neuropathologic correlations. Frontal brain tumors tend to become massive, affecting both posterior ipsilateral tissues and tissues in the opposite frontal lobe, before diagnosis can be made. The only vascular lesion confined to prefrontal cortex involves the anterior cerebral artery, a vessel with considerable collaterals; consistent vascular lesions are rare. Prefrontal leukotomies provided clean, relatively precise prefrontal lesions but were performed only in individuals with significant behavioral abnormality prior to the operation; postsurgical testing was often frustrated by the inherent mental disorder. Finally, degenerative disorders, particularly frontotemporal dementia, offer insights into the functions of the frontal lobes, but patients tend to be recognized by physicians only after massive loss of function has occurred.

Perhaps because of these problems, the underlying impairment in frontally damaged patients has yet to be satisfactorily established. A review of current attempts at characterizing prefrontal function and its impairment is presented in the following chapter. Here we note some of the more common effects of prefrontal damage in terms of their clinical manifestations.

Personality changes following frontal lobe lesions are of two main types. One type could be called pseudoretarded or pseudodepressed, and is characterized by apathy, lethargy, little spontaneity of behavior, unconcern, reduced sexual interest, little overt emotion, and reduced ability to plan ahead. Although such patients appear retarded, their IQs may be normal or near normal. The other type could be called pseudopsychopathic and is characterized by inappropriate social behavior, lack of concern for others, increased motor activity, sexual disinhibition, and "Witzelsucht," an inappropriately puerile, jocular attitude. There is some suggestion of differential localization for these two types of personality change, the former being associated with dorsolateral lesions and the latter with orbitofrontal lesions. However, because of the nonfocal effects of many frontal lesions, mentioned above, patients will frequently manifest an almost paradoxical mixture of both personality types.

The right and left frontal lobes have differing contributions to behavior. Injury to the right frontal lobe is more likely to cause gross social impairment than is injury to the left side. Loss of insight, verbal and behavioral disinhibition, loss of respect for the interpersonal space of others, and changes in personality are common features of patients with asymmetric injury to the right frontal injury.

The cognitive impairments of patients with prefrontal damage are apparent in a variety of tasks, some of which are reviewed in the following chapter. The domains affected include complex motor behavior (see also Chap. 16), planning and sequencing, attention, memory, and language (see discussions of Broca's aphasia and transcortical motor aphasia in Chap. 11). Often patients can perform well on standard tests of intelligence but fail miserably in less constrained real-life situations calling for planning and flexibility.

MAJOR ETIOLOGIES OF PREFRONTAL DYSFUNCTION

Vascular

Ischemic Infarction The vascular territory for the frontal lobes comes from the anterior cerebral artery (ACA) and middle cerebral artery (MCA), both of which are branches of the internal carotid artery.[4] The anterior and medial portions of the frontal lobes are supplied by the ACA, while the anterior branch of the MCA supplies most of the lateral dorsal frontal cortex. With ACA infarctions (see Fig. 32-1), the eyes tend to deviate toward the injured hemisphere. This conjugate eye deviation occurs following injury to the frontal eye fields in Brodmann area 8 and is accompanied by frontal neglect. Conjugate deviation following injury to area 8 tends to disappear after a few days, while the frontal neglect often persists. Neglect from frontal injury is not always easily differentiated from neglect due to parietal injury but is characterized motor akinesia rather than visual or sensory neglect on formal testing. Because the medial portion of the motor strip of the frontal cortex contains fibers for the leg, weakness and sensory loss associated with these infarctions is greatest in the leg, with relative sparing of motor and sensory function in the arm and face. Involvement of the supplementary motor area leads to a forced grasp of the contralateral hand. Transcortical motor aphasia is the most common aphasia syndrome seen with ACA occlusion of the dominant hemisphere.[5] Following ACA infarcts, common behavioral abnormalities include profound apathy and loss of executive control. A manic

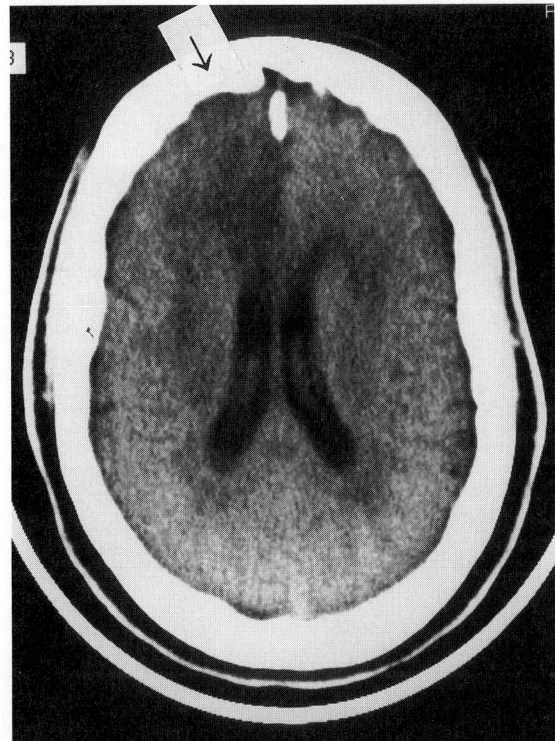

Figure 32-1
Computed tomography scan showing findings of a large anterior cerebral artery infarction involving the medial frontal cortex.

syndrome sometimes follows acute injury, particularly when the infarction involves the right hemisphere. Depression can occur with injury to either side. Rarely, a single ACA supplies both medial frontal lobes; ACA occlusion can produce bifrontal infarction leading to an akinetic mute state.

Strokes of the dominant MCA lead to paralysis of the face and arm on the contralateral side, with the eyes deviated toward the side of infarction (away from the paralysis). When the stroke is restricted to the anterior MCA branch of the dominant hemisphere, Broca's aphasia occurs; in contrast, complete MCA strokes lead to global aphasia. Loss of sequencing ability and disturbed executive control may be persistent problems. Forced grasp is not a feature of MCA stroke. Neglect occurs following either right- or left-sided MCA occlusion, but denial of illness is more common with right-sided lesions.

Other Vascular Lesions Other types of vascular injury can also produce frontal dysfunction. A common site for aneurysms is the ACA; following rupture, ischemia or infarction within the territory of the ACA often occurs. The sagittal sinus lies adjacent to the medial portions of the frontal lobes, and thrombus formation in this sinus can produce variations on anterior artery syndromes, although seizures and alterations in consciousness are more common with sinus thrombosis than with simple arterial infarction. This disease is often idiopathic, although hypercoagulable states such as pregnancy, dehydration, and sickle cell anemia are known to cause this disorder.[6]

Trauma

The poles of the frontal lobes lie adjacent to frontal bone, while the basal (orbital) frontal regions sit on the skull's cribriform plate. The frontal lobe's intimate association with bone makes this area particularly prone to injury following trauma (see Fig. 32-2). Patients often recover from the motor and sensory deficits that follow a head injury only to be left with profound behavioral abnormalities such as disinhibition, apathy, and loss of executive control. Disinhibition associated with head trauma is often associated with injury of frontal orbitobasal regions. Loss of executive control is a sequela of injury involving dorsolateral cortex.[3] Neuropsychological tests of executive function can help to identify a frontal injury. When the injury affects orbitofrontal regions, test results may be normal, even when there is profound behavioral disinhibition.[7] In these patients, careful questioning and recording of the insights of the family, along with systematic observations by the physician, help delineate the presence and severity of the frontal syndrome.

Documentation of the severity of frontal dysfunction associated with head injury is important, as therapy for these patients is difficult. A rigidly structured environment can help patients with frontal injury cope with routine daily activities. Unfortunately, current therapies and management of apathy and loss of executive control have only limited efficacy. Antidepressant medications may help to relieve the depressions that follow frontal injury; divalproex sodium (Depakote) and atypical antipsychotics have some efficacy for disinhibition, violence, and irritability.

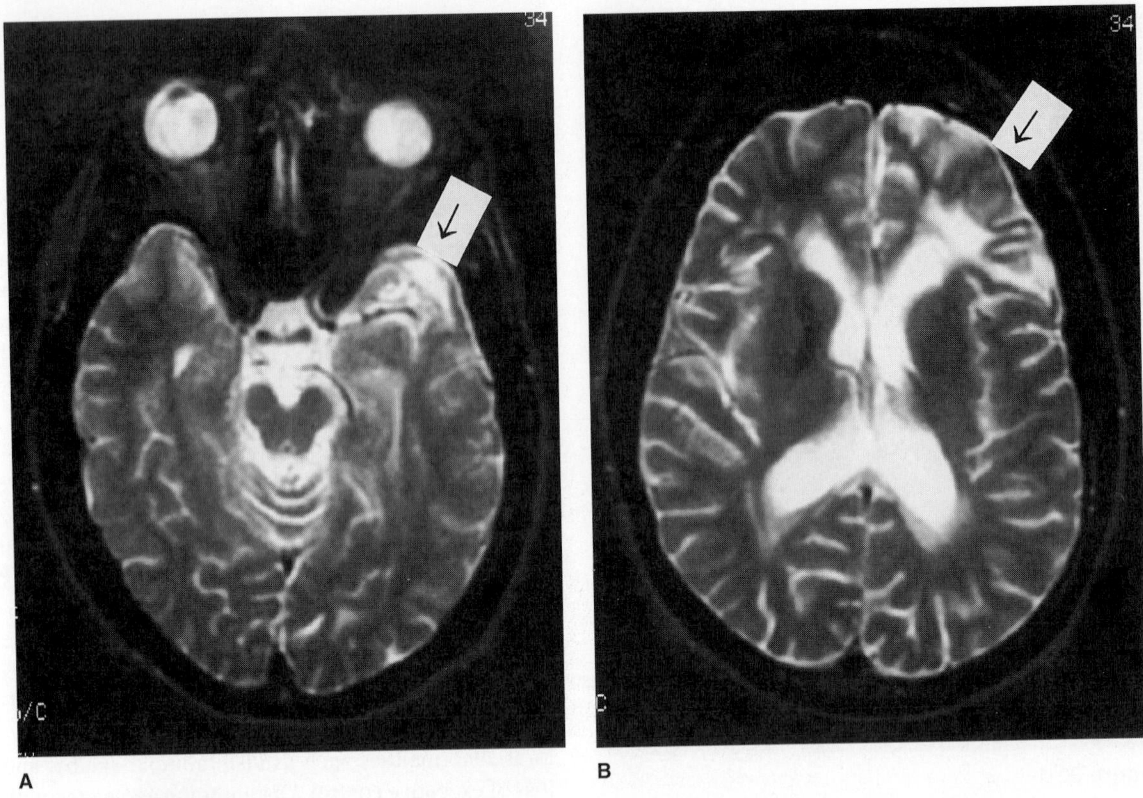

Figure 32-2
These T2-weighted MRI scans from the anterior temporal (A) and anterior frontal (B) lobes demonstrate loss of tissue secondary to trauma. The patient was a sexually and verbally disinhibited male with profound frontal systems deficits on neuropsychological testing.

Tumors

Tumors—either intrinsic or extrinsic to the frontal lobes—can produce frontal lobe symptomatology. The most common extrinsic tumors are meningiomas, which typically compress the frontal lobes in either the parasagittal (see Fig. 32-3) or cribriform plate regions.[8] Parasagittal meningiomas affect the medial aspects of the frontal lobes, so that bilateral leg weakness is a common finding. Once these tumors become sufficiently large, apathy, loss of executive control, or disinhibition can occur. Loss of the sense of smell is a common finding because of the close association of midline frontal tumors to the olfactory nerves. Cribriform plate meningiomas affect the basofrontal lobes, and behavioral disinhibition is common.

Primary brain tumors (gliomas, oligodendrogliomas, etc.) and metastases that involve the frontal lobes also alter frontal function. In current practice, these lesions are easily detected with computed tomography (CT) or magnetic resonance imaging (MRI), and effective surgical and medical therapies can be administered. However, diagnosis is often preceded by vague behavioral alterations that, in retrospect, are found to have been caused by frontal dysfunction.

Hydrocephalus

Abnormal absorption of cerebrospinal fluid (CSF) via the arachnoid granulation can cause "normal-pressure hydrocephalus" (NPH; see Chap. 53). The classic triad of hydrocephalus includes memory disturbance,

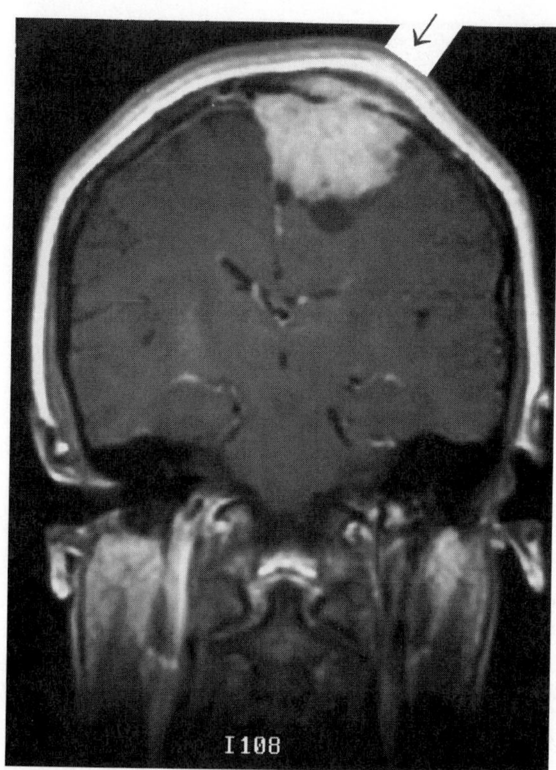

Figure 32-3
This T1-weighted gadolinium-enhanced MRI scan demonstrates a large parasagittal frontal meningioma.

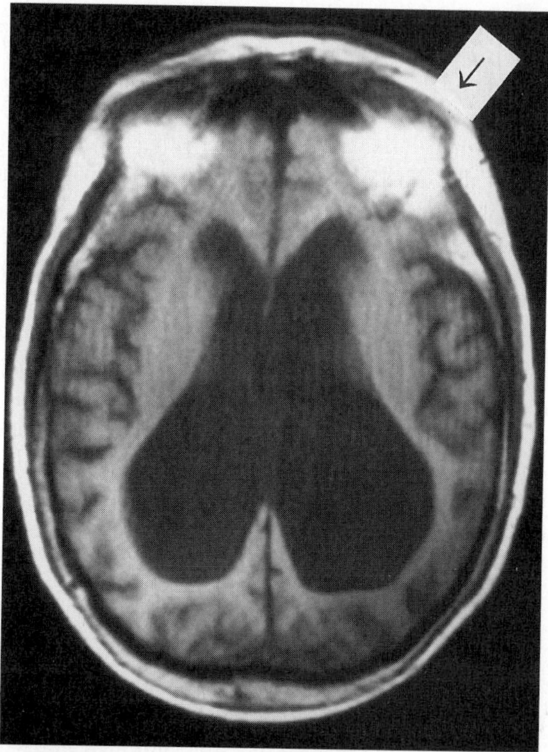

Figure 32-4
A T1-weighted MRI scan demonstrating hydrocephalus with enlarged frontal and posterior ventricles. There is no periventricular extravasation of fluid.

urinary incontinence, and gait apraxia. Other common findings are profound apathy and even akinetic states.[9] MRI typically shows the panventricular dilatation (see Fig. 32-4) as well as extravasated periventricular fluid. The treatment of obstructive hydrocephalus (including NPH) is shunting CSF from the ventricles to a distant area for absorption. Unfortunately, this therapy is effective in only a minority of cases, and complications of shunt therapy can be troublesome.

Infections

Many infectious processes can involve frontal cerebral tissues (see Chap. 50). Bacterial, tuberculous, fungal, cysticercal, and toxoplasmal abscesses can selectively penetrate the frontal regions. Tertiary syphilis, or "general paresis of the insane" (GPI), now rare, showed a predilection to involve the frontal regions.[10] One of the clinical syndromes associated with GPI was characterized by disinhibition and grandiose manic syndromes. Another was characterized by disinterest and slowed cognitive processing. An apathetic frontal lobe syndrome is the most typical clinical feature of dementia due to human immunodeficiency virus (HIV). This is probably based on involvement of both subcortical and frontal structures.[11] Often, HIV dementia responds at least transiently to antiviral therapy. Creutzfeldt-Jakob disease can begin in the frontal lobes.

Degenerative Dementias

Frontotemporal Dementia As reviewed in greater detail in Chap. 47, frontotemporal dementia (FTD) is a neurodegenerative disorder that involves progressive degeneration of the frontal and/or temporal lobes. It is probably the second most common presenile neurodegenerative disorder, ranking second only to early-onset Alzheimer's disease. Onset of FTD typically occurs in the fifth and sixth decade.[12] Neurodegeneration in FTD can be either symmetrical or asymmetrical, involving one or both frontal or temporal lobes. The clinical presentation of FTD, therefore, can be heterogeneous and reflects the relative pathologic involvement of the frontal and/or temporal cortices.[13]

The initial symptoms of FTD most commonly involve behavioral abnormalities and/or language impairments. Disinhibition, apathy, social withdrawal, loss of insight and social awareness, emotional blunting, and compulsive behaviors are common manifestations of FTD and relate to alterations in the frontal lobes. Additional impairments in executive functioning—such as planning, organizing, and shifting attention—are also common on neuropsychological testing.[14] Language is also affected by FTD. In a variant of FTD known as "primary progressive aphasia," there is a progressive nonfluent language presentation, with difficulties with speech output, grammar, and paraphasias (e.g., incorrect substitution of words or phonemes). Other individuals can present with a fluent-type aphasia and exhibit a progressive loss of semantic knowledge known as "semantic dementia," resulting in empty speech (e.g., "Show me the thing. I went to that place.").[15] Those symptoms are secondary to temporal, not frontal involvement (see also Chap. 39). The striking frontal and language impairments in FTD often contrast with a preservation of visuospatial abilities (e.g., copying designs, navigating around a neighborhood) and calculations, thereby reflecting the relative preservation of the parietal cortex. Memory abilities are also often preserved. This constellation of impaired and preserved symptoms in FTD and its variants contrasts with Alzheimer's disease, in which memory and word-finding impairments are most commonly the prominent early symptoms.

Focal presentations of FTD occur; patients with predominantly left-sided degeneration usually show progressive aphasia, while those with right-sided degeneration exhibit profound alterations of social skills. FTD invariably progresses; in the later stages, parkinsonian features and eye-movement abnormalities are common, reflecting degeneration in the basal ganglia.

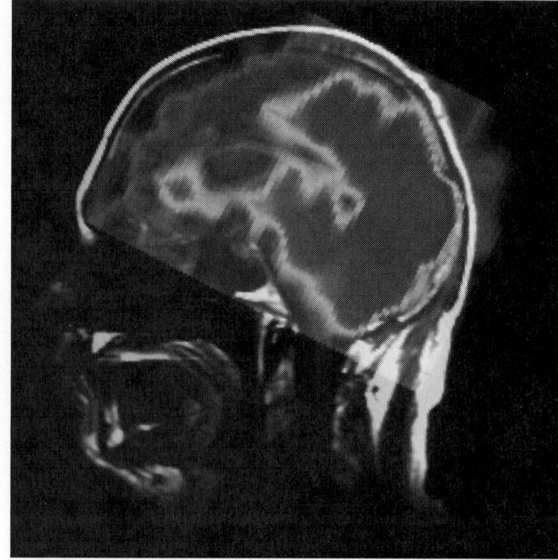

Figure 32-5
This is a xenon-133–corrected HMPAO SPECT coregistered upon a T2-weighted MRI scan from a patient with frontotemporal dementia. There is profound frontal hypoperfusion.

Eventually, profound apathy supervenes and most subjects enter a mute, akinetic state.[16] Recently, an international group of investigators proposed consensus criteria for three clinical subgroups of frontotemporal lobar degeneration: (1) frontotemporal dementia (FTD proper), (2) progressive nonfluent aphasia, and (3) semantic dementia.[17] Clinical misdiagnosis of FTD is common, but recent studies suggest that the combination of clinical data, behavioral questionnaires, and neuroimaging tools can yield a more accurate diagnosis. In most FTD patients, MRI shows atrophy of the frontal lobe and anterior temporal lobes (see Fig. 32-5), but generalized atrophy or even normal MRIs may be seen. Functional studies [e.g., single photon emission tomography (SPECT) or positron emission tomography (PET)] invariably show focal frontal or temporal deficits.

Histopathologic studies of FTD reveal severe neuronal loss and gliosis that is most prominent in the frontal and anterior temporal regions. In approximately 20 percent of FTD patients, cellular inclusions called Pick bodies are also found. Gliosis in the thalamus and basal ganglia can also be evident. Severe deficiencies in serotonin may correlate with clinical findings of weight gain and compulsions. Mutations in the tau gene on chromosome 17 have been linked to some kindreds with FTD and are associated with tau-positive neuronal or glial inclusions.[18]

Other Degenerative Dementias Most of the degenerative dementias eventually involve the frontal lobes, even though primary pathology is elsewhere. A few disorders appear to have a selective influence upon frontal lobe function.

Alzheimer's Disease Alzheimer's disease typically begins in the medial temporal cortex; frontal deficits rarely herald this dementia. However, a frontal variant of Alzheimer's disease has been described, and in these patients the syndrome is characterized by apathy, behavioral disorder, and loss of executive function. Their pathology is localized to frontal cortex.

Progressive Supranuclear Palsy In this degenerative disorder the primary pathology is located in the midbrain. Extensive frontal connections with midbrain may explain the combination of midbrain and frontal lobe findings. Primary frontal degeneration occurs in some of these patients. The classic clinical findings in progressive supranuclear palsy (PSP) include frequent falls, axial rigidity, pseudobulbar palsy, apathy, and loss of both executive function, and vertical gaze. On functional imaging, dorsolateral and mediofrontal hypoperfusion is seen.[19]

Metachromatic Leukodystrophy This degenerative disorder selectively injures white matter underlying the frontal cortex. A progressive frontal dementia occurs; diagnosis is made by demonstration of an enzymatic abnormality in arylsulfatase A. Although most cases occur in childhood and early adolescence, late-life onset can occur.[20]

Alcohol Many toxins can affect cerebral cortex, but the symptom picture most often suggests diffuse (toxic) rather than focal abnormalities. The concept of alcohol-induced dementia remains somewhat controversial; in some individuals, chronic alcohol abuse appears to be associated with selective dysfunction of the frontal lobes (apathy and cognitive slowing). In some instances, the frontal symptoms disappear or are considerably improved following abstinence from alcohol; in other cases, permanent dementia seems to develop.[21] The pathology of this dementia is poorly understood, but the presence of frontal symptoms is consistent.

REFERENCES

1. Luria AR: *The Working Brain: An Introduction to Neuropsychology.* Haig B, trans. New York: Basic Books, 1973.
2. Albert ML: Subcortical dementia, in Katzman R, Terry RD, Bick KI (eds): *Alzheimer's Disease, Senile Dementia and Related Disorders.* New York: Raven Press, 1978, pp 173–180.
3. Stuss DT, Benson DF: *The Frontal Lobes.* New York: Raven Press, 1986.
4. Gauthier JC, Mohr JP: Intracranial internal carotid artery disease, in Barnett HJM, Mohr JP, Stein BM, Yatsu FM (eds): *Stroke.* New York: Churchill Livingstone, 1986, pp 337–350.
5. Benson DF: *Aphasia, Alexia, and Agraphia.* New York: Churchill Livingstone, 1979.
6. Tsai FY, Higashida RT, Matovich V, Alrieri K: Acute thrombosis of the intracranial dural sinus: Direct thrombolytic treatment. *Am J Neuroradiol* 13:1137–1141, 1992.
7. Damasio AR: The frontal lobes, in Heilman KM, Valenstein E (eds): *Clinical Neuropsychology.* New York: Oxford University Press, 1979, pp 360–412.
8. Adams RD, Victor M: *Principles of Neurology*, 5th ed. New York: McGraw-Hill, 1993.
9. Hakim S: Biomechanics of hydrocephalus, in Harbert JC (ed): *Cisternography and Hydrocephalus.* Springfield, IL: Charles C Thomas, 1972, pp 22–25.
10. Cummings JL, Benson DF: *Dementia: A Clinical Approach.* Boston: Butterworth-Heinemann, 1992.
11. Price RW, Brew B, Sidtis J, et al: The brain in AIDS: Central nervous system HIV-1 infection and AIDS dementia complex. *Science* 239:286–292, 1988.
12. Brun A: Frontal lobe degeneration of non-Alzheimer type: I. Neuropathology. *Arch Gerontol Geriatr* 6:193–208, 1987.
13. Neary D, Snowden JS, Northen B, Goulding PJ: Dementia of frontal lobe type. *J Neurol Neurosurg Psychiatry* 51:353–361, 1988.
14. Miller BL, Cummings JL, Villanueva-Meyer J, et al: Frontal lobe degeneration: Clinical, neuropsychological

and SPECT characteristics. *Neurology* 41:1374–1382, 1991.

15. Hodges JR, Patterson K: Nonfluent progressive aphasia and semantic dementia: A comparative neuropsychological study. *J Int Neuropsychol Soc* 1996;6:511–524.
16. Miller BL, Chang L, Mena I, et al: Progressive right frontotemporal degeneration: clinical, neuropsychological and SPECT characteristics. *Dementia* 4:204–213, 1993.
17. Neary D, Snowden JS, Gustafson L, et al: Frontotemporal lobar degeneration: A consensus on clinical diagnostic criteria. *Neurology* 51:1546–1552, 1998.
18. Hutton M, Lendon C, Rizzu P, et al. Association of missense and 5′splicesite mutations in tau with the inherited dementia FTDP-17. *Nature* 393:702–705, 1998.
19. Johnson KA, Sperling RA, Holman BL, et al: Cerebral perfusion in progressive supranuclear palsy. *J Nucl Med* 33:704–709, 1992.
20. Austin J, Armstrong D, Fouch S, et al: Metachromatic leukodystrophy (MLD). *Arch Neurol* 18:225–240, 1968.
21. Lishman WA: Cerebral disorder in alcoholism: syndromes of impairment. *Brain* 104:1–20, 1981.

Chapter 33

FRONTAL LOBES: COGNITIVE NEUROPSYCHOLOGICAL ISSUES

Martha J. Farah

Behavioral neurology has long recognized the crucial importance of prefrontal cortex in human behavior; the previous chapter summarizes much of what has been learned clinically about the effects of damage to this part of the brain from disease or injury. The goal of the present chapter is to review the current state of scientific understanding of prefrontal function. The emphasis is on those scientific findings and theories that help illuminate the role of prefrontal cortex (PFC) in normal human behavior and the underlying cognitive changes responsible for changes in behavior following PFC damage.

EFFECTS OF PREFRONTAL DAMAGE IN CLINICAL AND LABORATORY TASKS

The previous chapter described some of the behavioral changes seen following damage to PFC, which are typically observed (with concern) by family members, medical staff, and sometimes the patients themselves. These changes involve cognitive, social, and emotional functioning in patients' everyday lives. A complementary approach to characterizing the effects of PFC lesions is with relatively simple tasks that are either standardized relative to the performance of other people or designed to isolate specific cognitive abilities underlying task performance. Countless such tasks have been administered to PFC-damaged patients in the context of systematic research programs. The tasks and results described here are a small but representative sample.

Sequencing Tasks

A variety of clinical tests assess the ability to sequence items, from simple hand motions to strategic games such as the Towers of Hanoi. Penfield and Evans (1935) describe the difficulty that Penfield's sister had in preparing a meal after surgery to remove a frontal brain tumor. She could perform all the individual actions necessary to cook dinner but could not actually prepare the meal without someone to tell her the order in which to do things. Most clinical tests of sequencing involve simple gestures or stimuli; it is typically found that PFC-damaged patients are the most impaired (e.g., Kimura, 1982). Although the well-known tendency of PFC-damaged patients to perseverate would be expected to interfere with sequencing tasks, the errors made by such patients include nonperseverative errors. However, even more abstract sequencing tasks, such as the classic Towers of Hanoi game, reveal impairments in PFC-damaged patients (Morris et al., 1997; Shallice, 1982).

Fluency Tasks

"Fluency" tasks might be better named *generation* or *continuous generation* tasks. They require patients to generate as many exemplars of a category as possible within a time limit. Commonly used clinical tests of verbal fluency include *category fluency* tasks, in which a semantic category is used, for example naming as many animals as possible in 60 s, and *letter fluency* tasks, in which words beginning with a particular letter must be generated. Such tasks are particularly dependent on left PFC. *Design fluency,* which is most often compromised after right PFC damage, requires patients to draw a series of unique nonsense shapes to a certain specification, such as all having three sides (Jones-Gotman and Milner, 1977). As with sequencing performance, fluency is somewhat compromised by the occurrence of perseveration, but patients' output is generally impoverished beyond the "crowding out" of new items by perseverative responses.

Tests of Response Inhibition

Although important differences exist among the tasks used to assess response inhibition, they all share the following property: there are stimuli to which the subject must respond, certain stimulus-response pairings are "stronger" than others, and the tasks require that subjects override these stronger pairings in producing a correct response. Perhaps the best-known such task is the Stroop task (Stroop, 1935), in which subjects must name the ink color in which words are written, but the words themselves are color names (e.g., the word "red" written in blue ink). A lifetime of reading has automatized the process enough that effort is required to suppress the incorrect word-reading response and produce the correct color-naming response. A number of researchers report that left PFC–damaged patients have difficulty in so doing and are prone to frequent word-reading intrusion errors (Perret, 1974; Stuss and Benson, 1984).

The Go-No-Go task also taxes the testee's ability to restrain a strongly established response. There are many versions of this task, in which one stimulus-response pairing is strengthened by practice (e.g., "always tap twice when I tap once," or "always push the button when you see a letter") and then becomes the incorrect response (e.g., "now don't tap when I tap once," or "keep pushing for all the letters except for M"). Go-No-Go performance has long been recognized to depend on PFC (Drewe, 1975). Yet another test of inhibitory control is the Anti-Saccade Task, in which subjects strengthen the already potent tendency to look toward a sudden salient stimulus by performing a number of such saccades toward such stimuli but must then carry out the opposite action: saccading away from the sudden salient stimulus. This ability depends crucially on PFC (Roberts et al., 1994).

The Wisconsin Card Sorting Test (WCST) is often used as a test of prefrontal function and does require the inhibition of a recently rewarded response, although it also requires other abilities, some with nonfrontal localizations (e.g., Stuss et al., 2000; Monchi et al., 2001). The patient's task is to sort cards—on which are sets of geometric shapes that can vary in their color, shape, and numerosity—into piles according to one of these variables (e.g., blue cards together, red cards together, etc.). The task begins with the patient being given one card at a time and discovering the correct sorting rule by placing each card on a pile and being told "right" or "wrong." At some point after the patient has discovered the rule, the rule is changed (e.g., from sorting on the basis of color to sorting on the basis of shape). Thus the patient is required to shift his or her responding away from the recently used successful sorting rule. It is at this stage of the task, rather than the initial rule discovery, that PFC-damaged patients fail (e.g., Milner, 1963; Nelson, 1976).

Delayed Response and Span Tasks

Although not usually classified together under a single heading, both Delayed Response and Span tasks test the ability to maintain information in working memory. The Delayed Response task was first used in the animal literature many decades ago (Jacobsen, 1936) and has been adapted for humans more recently (Freedman and Oscar-Berman, 1986). In a typical simple version of the task, a stimulus object is shown and then hidden in one of a small number of locations. A delay interval of some number of seconds ensues, during which the subject cannot see the locations (to prevent simply fixating the correct location for the duration of the delay). The locations are then revealed and the subject must locate the hidden object, providing a measure of how accurately the location was maintained in spatial working memory. Both the animal and human lesion literature indicates prefrontal involvement in Delayed Response tasks (D'Esposito and Postle, 1999; Freedman and Oscar-Berman, 1986).

Whereas the limiting factor on performance in Delayed Response is the length of time over which information must be maintained, in Span tasks the limiting factor is the number of items. In a typical Span task, multiple items are presented to the subject, who must retain them in working memory just long enough to repeat or reproduce them. The most familiar version of this task is the forward Digit Span task (see Chaps. 2 and 3), although spatial span is also frequently assessed by clinicians. In their literature review on Span-lesion correlations, D'Esposito and Postle (1999) found a weak trend toward decreased span in patients with focal damage to the lateral PFC.

Decision-Making Tasks

One of the most noticeable effects of PFC damage is personality change. The social-emotional dysfunction and poor judgment in such cases have recently become topics of study in cognitive neuropsychology. A number of researchers have attempted to capture these changes in relatively simple and controlled laboratory tasks, which can be grouped under the general rubric of Decision-Making tasks. The best known of these, the Iowa Gambling task (Bechara et al., 1997), requires patients to choose cards from among decks with different likelihoods and magnitudes of wins and losses. Patients with ventromedial PFC damage tend to persist in choosing from decks with large rewards, ignoring the intermittent losses from those decks, which more than wipe out their gains. Rogers and colleagues (Mavaddat et al., 2000; Rogers et al., 1999) developed a simpler type of gambling task that enables various aspects of decision making to be assessed and thus allows a more specific characterization of ventromedial PFC-damaged patients' impairment. In an even simpler decision-making task, choosing among alternative stimuli to obtain rewards, Rolls and colleagues (1994) demonstrated that socially dysfunctional PFC-damaged patients have difficulty avoiding a punishment-associated stimulus if that stimulus was once rewarding for them.

PFC-Damaged Patients in the Cognitive Neuropsychology Lab: Diversity and Commonality

The abilities tested by these tasks have a certain "family resemblance," which hints at underlying commonalities. For example, one could view perseveration on the WCST as the result of inadequate inhibition of previously successful sorting responses. Sequencing a set of pictures to tell a story requires an adequate working memory span, because the sequential position of each picture can be assessed only by comparing its temporal and causal relations with those of all the other pictures. Verbal fluency performance depends in part on a strategic search through alternative candidate words, not unlike the search through alternative candidate sorting criteria in the WCST. And most of the decision-making tasks involve the integration of positive and negative feedback over multiple trials, requiring working memory over delays.

In view of these interrelations among many of the PFC tasks, it is not surprising that patients may display impairments on many or all of the tasks described above. Yet dissociations are also frequently observed, implying that the different processing systems may in fact underlie this network of similarities and calling into question the concept of a "frontal syndrome." Patients may have normal working memory spans but profound impairments in decision making (Bechara et al., 1998) or normal fluency but severely impaired problem solving (Goldstein et al., 1993). The recent burgeoning of functional neuroimaging studies of PFC function have also highlighted the likely multiplicity of underlying cognitive systems within PFC. Well-designed experiments with normal subjects can isolate systems whose anatomic boundaries would likely be crossed by naturally occurring lesions.

CURRENT THEORIES OF PREFRONTAL FUNCTION

Given the range of impairments found after PFC damage and their dissociability, is it foolish to seek "a theory of prefrontal function"? Is this as ill conceived as, for example, a search for "a theory of temporal lobe function," when we already know that the temporal lobe subserves such diverse abilities as vision, hearing, and memory? The answer is no, and the reason highlights a difference between the organization of prefrontal and temporal cortex. Whereas vision, hearing, and memory are sufficiently independent systems that they can operate normally without one another, the function of PFC is highly integrated. For example, damage to auditory parts of temporal cortex has no effect on the function of visual parts or on a patient's visual ability. In contrast, even though the subsystems of PFC have distinct functions, these functions normally dovetail. The major functional distinctions and their interrelations are summarized here.

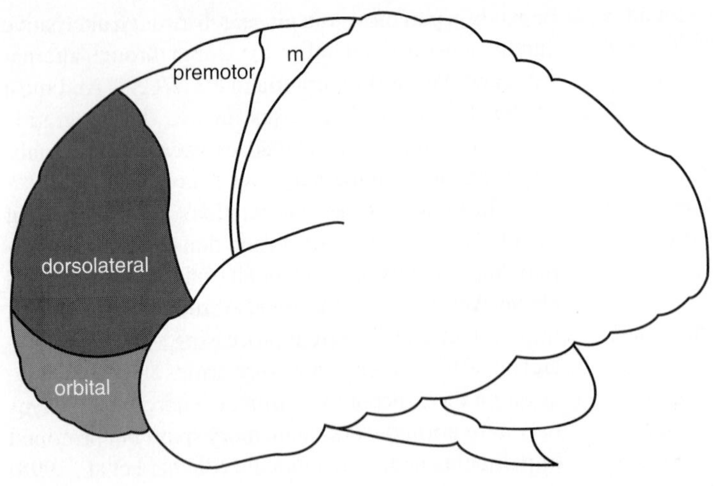

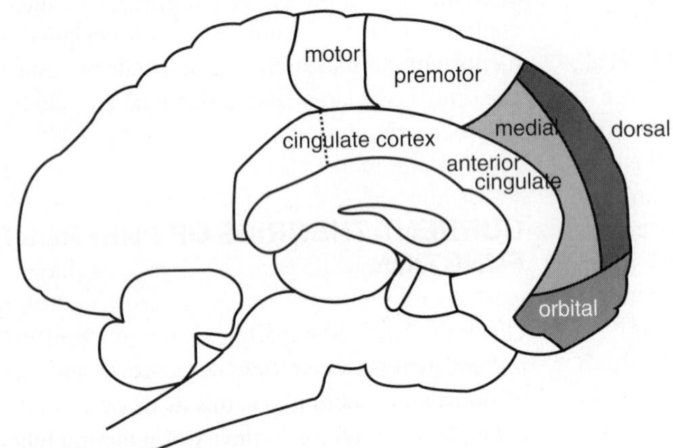

Figure 33-1
Areas of prefrontal cortex and neighboring brain regions.

The clinical observation, described in the previous chapter, of different behaviors following dorsolateral and orbital PFC damage, combined with laboratory tasks used with patients and in neuroimaging studies, leads to the following generalization about the organization PFC function. Lateral regions of PFC are essential for working memory and hence for a multitude of cognitive tasks that depend on working memory, including working memory for task instructions that run counter to prepotent response tendencies (e.g., in the Stroop task). Ventral and medial regions, including orbital cortex, play an important role in reward-related cognition and hence in tasks that require learning about, or making decisions about, reward- and punishment-related stimuli. In addition, the anterior cingulate cortex, which is not strictly speaking part of PFC but is closely related both spatially and functionally, is an integral part of this system. Its function has been characterized as "conflict monitoring"—in other words assessing the degree to which one's actual or planned response conflicts with the desired outcome (Botvinick et al., 2001). Figure 33-1 shows the locations of these areas.

These simple generalizations have been elaborated in various ways by different scientists, some of whom focus their interest on one particular component

Table 33-1
Representative current theories of prefrontal function

Theory: specific to a region	*Representative reference*
Somatic marker hypothesis (ventromedial PFC)	Damasio (1995)
Reversal learning (ventromedial PFC)	Rolls (2000)
Domain-specific working memory (lateral PFC)	Smith and Jonides (1999)
Process-specific working memory (lateral PFC)	Owen (1997)
Working memory and inhibition combined (dorsolateral PFC)	Diamond (1989)
Selection (inferolateral PFC)	Thompson-Schill (1997)
Theory: Unified	
Supervisory attentional system	Shallice and Burgess (1991)
Working memory	Kimberg and Farah (2000)
Adaptive coding	Duncan (2001)

of PFC and others of whom attempt a unification. Table 33-1 lists a number of these theories. A well-known theory of relatively narrow scope is Damasio's (1994) *somatic marker hypothesis,* which assigns ventromedial PFC a role in mediating intuitive "hunches" based on (literally) gut and other bodily reactions. An alternative conception of this area is offered by Rolls (2000), who emphasizes the importance of this area in the updating of *reversal of stimulus-reward associations*. There are also different theories of the organization of working memory within lateral PFC, with some authors suggesting a stimulus domain or *modality-specific organization* (e.g., Smith and Jonides, 1999) or alternatively a *process-specific organization,* whereby the nature of the processing to be performed on working memory governs the functional anatomy (e.g., Owen, 1997). Diamond (1989) has hypothesized that dorsolateral PFC is essential only for the *joint use of working memory and inhibitory control*. The *selection hypothesis* of Thompson-Schill (1997) concerns the role of inferior lateral PFC in memory and language tasks; she suggests that this region of PFC is needed when task-relevant information must be selected from competing irrelevant information. Finally, the *conflict-monitoring hypothesis* of anterior cingulate function (Botvinick et al., 2001) asserts that this region measures conflict between task goals and performance in order to control attentional allocation.

Unified theories of PFC function are less common now than in previous decades. This may be the result of our increasing awareness of dissociations among "PFC tasks," thanks to a shift in neuropsychology research from large group studies of patients' performance on one task to single case studies of patients' performance on many tasks, which can reveal dissociations (see Chap. 1), as well as the proliferation of functional imaging studies capable of isolating small foci of activation. Some of the unified theories described in the previous edition of this book are now of more historical than scientific interest. Three unified theories with some currency are summarized here.

Supervisory Attentional System

This theory is based on an information processing model developed by Norman and Shallice (1986), which distinguishes between routine, automatic actions, and more novel actions requiring attentional control. Shallice and Burgess (1991) have proposed that the supervisory attentional system (SAS) is implemented in PFC, and argue that a wide variety of behavioral impairments following PFC damage can be attributed to the weakening or loss of this system. The sensitivity of PFC-damaged patients' performance to the familiarity of the task and the degree of constraint provided by the task, as well as the tendency of routinized actions to intrude when inappropriate (e.g., word-reading in the Stroop task), are among the characteristics consistent with an impaired SAS.

Working Memory

Although only a subset of the laboratory tasks described earlier are considered tests of working memory per se, cognitive psychologists have long hypothesized that working memory plays a crucial role in the performance of a wide variety of verbal and visuospatial tasks (Miyake and Shah, 1999). On the basis of extensive single-cell recording and lesion data linking PFC to working memory (e.g., Goldman-Rakic, 1987), Kimberg and Farah (1993, 2000) used computer simulation to determine whether the wider array of cognitive impairments following PFC damage could result from an underlying impairment in working memory. The simulations demonstrated that the weakening of working memory associations was in itself sufficient to evoke perseveration in the WCST, word-reading intrusions in the Stroop task, perseverative and nonperseverative errors in a sequencing task, and disinhibited responses in the antisaccade task, among other signs of PFC damage. The possibility that different domains of working memory might have different anatomic loci makes it possible for this hypothesis to account for dissociations among tasks. The extension of this idea to the domain of emotional or reward-related working memory (see Davidson and Sutton, 1995) suggests its applicability to even those tasks associated with orbital cortex.

Adaptive Coding

A related proposal concerning prefrontal function explains many aspects of patient behavior after PFC damage, as well as the results of neuroimaging experiments, in terms of the flexible response properties of PFC neurons. Drawing on the results of single cell recording in monkeys, John Duncan (2001) notes that many PFC neurons represent different information in different task contexts. This must be so, he points out, given the large proportion of neurons found to be responsive to the particular stimuli used in any given task. For example, in a dog-cat discrimination task 20 percent of neurons are selective for pictures of dogs versus cats. This seems more likely to be the result of adaptive coding in response to task demands than a reflection of the permanent response properties of these neurons prior to the task, particularly when one considers that the sum of just a few such experiments' responsive neurons exceeds 100 percent! According to Duncan, PFC neurons have the capacity to respond selectively to a wide range of input information, thanks to the extensive connectivity of PFC and posterior cortices and within the PFC itself. The dynamic reassignment of PFC representations functions as a kind of working memory, which is used to guide processing, as described in the previous section.

The more recent hypotheses concerning PFC function make contact, to varying degrees, with our growing knowledge of individual neuron behavior and of the computational properties of ensembles of neurons. Such evidence entered to a degree in the formulation of Kimberg and Farah's (1993, 2000) working memory hypothesis, and it plays a central role in Duncan's (2001) adaptive coding hypothesis. Future development in this field will undoubtedly continue to integrate evidence from animal studies, including neurochemical studies of many cortical-cortical and cortical-subcortical circuits through which PFC function influences behavior. (Robbins, 2000).

REFERENCES

Bechara A, Damasio H, Tranel D, Damasio AR: Deciding advantageously before knowing the advantageous strategy. *Science* 275:1293–1295, 1997.

Bechara A, Damasio H, Tranel D, Anderson SW: Dissociation of working memory from decision making within the human prefrontal cortex. *J Neurosci* 18:428–437, 1998.

Botvinick M, Braver TS, Barch DM, et al: Conflict monitoring and cognitive control. *Psychol Rev* 108:624–652, 2001.

Cohen JD, Servan-Schreiber D: Context, cortex, and dopamine: A connectionist approach to behavior and biology in schizophrenia. *Psychol Rev* 99:45–77, 1992.

Damasio AR: *Descartes' Error*. New York: Grosset, Putnam, 1994.

Diamond A: Developmental progression in human infants and infant monkeys, and the neural bases of inhibitory control of reaching, in Diamond A (ed): The *Development and Neural Bases of Higher Cognitive Functions*. New York: New York Academy of Science Press, 1989.

Drewe EA: The effect of type and area of brain lesion on Wisconsin Card Sorting Test performance. *Cortex*, 10:159–170, 1974.

Drewe EA: Go-no go learning after frontal lobe lesions in humans. *Cortex* 11:8–16, 1975.

Freedman M, Oscar-Berman M: Bilateral frontal lobe disease and selective delayed response deficits in humans. *Behav Neurosci* 100:337–342, 1986.

Goldman-Rakic PS: Circuitry of primate prefrontal cortex and regulation of behavior by representational memory, in Plum F, Mountcastle V (eds): *Handbook of Physiology, The Nervous System V.* Bethesda, MD: American Physiological Society, 1987.

Jacobsen CF: Studies of cerebral functions in primates. I. The function of the frontal association areas in monkeys. *Comp Psychol Monogr* 13:1–60, 1936.

Jones-Gotman M, Milner B: Design fluency: The invention of nonsense drawings after focal cortical lesions. *Neuropsychologia* 15:653–674, 1977.

Kimberg DY, Farah MJ: A unified account of cognitive impairments following frontal lobe damage: The role of working memory in complex, organized behavior. *J Exp Psychol Gen* 122:411–428, 1993.

Kimberg DY, Farah MJ: Is there an inhibitory module in prefrontal cortex? Working memory and the mechanisms of cognitive control, in Monsell S, Driver J (eds): *Control of Cognitive Processes: Attention and Performance XVIII.* Cambridge, MA: MIT Press, 2000.

Kimura D: Left-hemisphere control of oral and brachial movements and their relation to communication. *Philos Trans R Soc Lond B* 298:135–149, 1982.

Mavaddat N, Kirkpatrick PJ, Rogers RD, Sahakian BJ: Deficits in decision-making in patients with aneurysms of the anterior communicating artery. *Brain* 123:2109–2117, 2000.

Milner B: Effects of different brain lesions on card sorting. *Arch Neurol* 9:90–100, 1963.

Miyake A, Shah P (eds). *Models of Working Memory: Mechanisms of Maintenance and Executive Control.* New York: Cambridge University Press, 1999.

Nelson HE: A modified card sorting test sensitive to frontal lobe defects. *Cortex* 12:313–324, 1976.

Owen AM: Memory: Dissociating multiple memory processes. *Curr Biol* 8:850–852, 1998.

Penfield W, Evans J: The frontal lobe in man: a clinical study of maximum removals. *Brain* 58:115–133, 1935.

Perret E: The left frontal lobe of man and the suppression of habitual responses in verbal categorical behavior. *Neuropsychologia* 12:323–330, 1914.

Roberts RJ, Hager LD, Heron C: Prefrontal cognitive processes: Working memory and inhibition in the antisaccade task. *J Exp Psychol Gen* 123:374–393, 1994.

Robbins TW: Chemical modulation of frontal-executive functions in humans and other animals. *Exp Brain Res* 133:130–138, 2000.

Rogers RD, Owen AM, Middleton HC, et al: Choosing between small, likely rewards and large, unlikely rewards activates inferior and orbital prefrontal cortex. *J Neurosci* 20:9029–9038, 1999.

Rolls ET: The orbitofrontal cortex and reward. *Cereb Cortex* 10:284–294, 2000.

Rolls ET, Hornak J, Wade D, McGrath J: Emotion-related learning in patients with social and emotional changes associated with frontal lobe damage. *J Neurol Neurosurg Psychiatry* 57:1518–1524, 1994.

Shallice T: Specific impairments of planning. *Philos Trans R Soc Lond B* 298:199–209, 1982.

Shallice T, Burgess P: Higher-order cognitive impairments and frontal lobe lesions in man, in Levin HS, Eisenberg HM, Benton AL (eds): *Frontal Lobe Function and Dysfunction.* New York: Oxford University Press, 1991.

Smith EE, Jonides J: Storage and executive processes in the frontal lobes. *Science* 283:1657–1661, 1999.

Stroop JR: Studies of interference in serial verbal reactions. *J Exp Psychol* 18:643–662, 1935.

Stuss DT, Benson DF: Neuropsychological studies of the frontal lobes. *Psychol Bull* 95:3–28, 1984.

Thompson-Schill S, D'Esposito M, Aguirre GK, Farah MJ: The role of left prefrontal cortex in semantic retrieval: A re-evaluation. *Proc Natl Acad Sci U S A* 94:14792–14797, 1997.

Chapter 34

CALLOSAL DISCONNECTION*

Kathleen Baynes
Michael S. Gazzaniga

BRIEF HISTORICAL BACKGROUND

Appropriate Techniques Required to Demonstrate Disconnection Phenomena

Although the anatomic prominence of the corpus callosum suggested to early neuroanatomists that it played a key role in human cognition, actual demonstration of its function was difficult to accomplish. The first attempts to surgically separate the two hemispheres were undertaken by Van Wagenen in the 1940s.[1] The hope was that patients with debilitating epileptic seizures would have some relief if electric activity could not spread from one hemisphere to the other via the callosum. In this series of patients, unfortunately, there was inconsistent evidence of improved seizure control. Moreover, despite administration of a battery of standard neuropsychological tests before and after surgery, no consistent cognitive effects were observed.[2,3] The enormous band of fibers connecting the two hemispheres seemed to have an insignificant functional role, and section of the corpus callosum as a treatment for epilepsy was abandoned.

During the 1950s, Sperry and Meyers discovered in animals that it was necessary to use special techniques that isolated the acquisition of new information to a single hemisphere to see the radical behavioral effects of callosal section.[4,5] Although their work was accomplished with cats, the lessons learned there were applied to the evaluation of a new series of surgeries initiated by Bogen and Vogel in the 1960s.[6,7] In addition, Geschwind's work on disconnection syndromes indicated that more profound changes should result from the interruption of fiber tracts than had been observed in the earlier series.[8] Bogen and Vogel surmised that perhaps the early callosotomies had been ineffective because they failed to include the other cerebral commissures; therefore a new series of commissurotomies was planned that included the anterior commissure. In light of the work of Sperry and Geschwind, a more sophisticated investigation of cognitive changes was included.

When the new series was initiated, careful evaluation of cognitive function of each hemisphere was undertaken using brief (tachistoscopic) presentations to assure that stimuli were displayed to only one hemisphere.[8] Once the callosum is completely sectioned, information cannot be easily shared between the two hemispheres. Eye movements, however, can cause a loss of lateralization. The work in the 1970s eliminated this possibility by displaying words and pictures for 150 ms or less, faster than the eye can move from the central fixation point to the display.[9] Later, special contact lenses, eye-tracking techniques, and lateral fixation techniques would be used as well.[10,11]

These initial studies confirmed assertions that the left hemisphere (LH) was dominant for language whereas the right could neither name nor describe objects presented to it visually or tactually, although it could perform certain visuospatial tasks. Current eye-tracking techniques permit visual displays with extended durations, thus allowing more precise observations.[11] Theoretical and methodologic advances continue to develop our understanding of perceptual, cognitive, mnemonic, and linguistic processes and their integration into coherent thought and behavior. Such techniques provide unique means of testing hemispheric hypotheses and enriching our understanding of neurologic and neuropsychological symptoms, from alexia to alien-hand sign, as well as yielding insights to the evolution of lateralized processing and the understanding of consciousness.

* **ACKNOWLEDGMENTS:** Supported in part by NIH/NIDCD grant R01 DC04442 to KB and NIH/NINDS grant P01 NS17778 to MSG and the John S. McDonnell Foundation.

LANGUAGE

One of the most striking of the split-brain observations was the ability of the mute right hemisphere (RH) to understand spoken language and read single words. It was apparent that the right hemisphere could respond to some simple verbal commands and read single words as long as a verbal response was not required. This ability facilitated the demonstration of two hemispheres responding independently to stimuli and generated excitement in fields from neurology to philosophy. The demonstration of this basic phenomenon required as little as a blindfold or screen to keep the dominant LH in the dark and a response method to permit the nondominant right hemisphere a nonverbal means of expression.

Basic language skills appeared to be present in the RH of all of the Bogen and Vogel series of splits, suggesting that the RH might play a larger role in language than had been expected.[7,12,13] Theories implicating the RH in errors made by dyslexic and aphasic patients abounded,[14,15] but the RH was given little credit for being more than an error generator when the LH was weakened or damaged or when developmental lateralization processes had gone awry. However, in the larger Wilson-Roberts series initiated in the 1970s, the presence of even rudimentary RH language was much less frequent. By 1983, of the 28 completed callosotomies, only 3 patients had documented RH language. Today the series stands at about 40 callosotomies (Roberts DW: Personal communication, 2001), but those three remain the only ones with sufficient RH language to participate in tachistoscopic experiments. Over time, the population from which the callosotomy candidates are drawn has changed, which may influence the frequency with which RH language occurs. Increased ability to identify and remove focal areas that initiate seizure activity has led to a greater number of focal surgeries, with only a few patients with very severe and often diffuse seizure activity being considered for split-brain surgery. Such severe illness often leaves the patients with decreased mental capacity and limited reading ability prior to surgery. Only one new patient with robust RH reading has been added to the active testing group since the mid-1980s.[16–18] Hence, most of these observations regarding RH language are based on a small but well-studied group of patients. The degree to which they generalize to the neurologically normal population remains a matter of speculation. However many functional magnetic resonance imaging (fMRI) studies have demonstrated RH activation during some language tasks in normal subjects, and RH activation appears to be important during some stage of recovery from LH stroke.[19,20]

In those patients with RH language capacity, semantic and conceptual information appears to be more adequately represented in the RH than is phonological and syntactic information. The lexicon or vocabulary of the RH appears to be similar to, albeit somewhat smaller than, the corresponding LH lexicon.[21] Both hemispheres can make a variety of semantic judgments, recognizing categorical, functional, and associative relations among words. The ability to discriminate word from nonword letter strings is limited but possible,[22,23] which suggests that the visual word form is represented in the RH of these patients. One way to conceptualize the right/left difference is in terms of a static lexicon and a productive grammar.[24] The lexicon stores information about the meaning and associations of words and is present in both hemispheres. In contrast, the grammar that contains rules for generating new sentences which communicate meaning is present only in the LH.

Limited Control of Speech and Grammar in the Isolated Right Hemisphere

In the same way as grammar allows the combination of words into sentences, phonology allows the combination of the sounds of a language in a meaningful way to create words or lexical items. Both processes present difficulties for the RH. Although the RH possesses some limited phonological competence and can both generate and understand limited speech, it shows very little ability to perform any of the letter-to-sound tasks used to test phonological competence. It has difficulty with the identification of written rhymes or even selecting pictures with rhyming names.[25,26] There is better evidence for some ability to discriminate auditory phonemes,[27] but this would be the minimal competence expected to support auditory comprehension in the RH. Moreover, some higher-level influences on perception of auditory sounds can be demonstrated using manipulations like the McGurk effect, in which the perception of an auditory sound is altered by viewing a speaker pronouncing a different sound.[27] These basic perceptual integrations can be accomplished by the RH, whereas those required to decode sound from written language do not appear to be possible.

Nor does the linguistic prowess of the RH extend to the use of grammatical rules for the comprehension and production of sentences. Although the RH can distinguish between grammatical and ungrammatical sentences, the ability to use grammatical information is limited in other tasks such as sentence/ picture matching.[21,28] Hence, it appears that a rapid, almost reflexive judgment about grammar is possible, but a decision that requires decoding of the meaning carried by grammar is not. Likewise, although the RH can sometimes make single-word verbal responses to words and pictures, there is no evidence of the ability to use grammar to combine words to generate more complex, sentence length responses. Passive use of both phonological and grammatical knowledge in the RH in the absence of generative use may indicate that both phonology and grammar depend upon LH output mechanisms to be used productively.

Right Hemisphere Reading

Right hemisphere reading proceeds more slowly than LH reading and may use a different mode of processing.[29] A right hemisphere lexicon has been suggested as the source of certain reading errors in deep dyslexic[14,30] and pure dyslexic patients[31,32] (see Chaps. 12 and 14). Although insensitivity to grammar and poor print-to-sound skills in the RH of these patients is consistent with some aspects of these claims, both left and right hemispheres appear to be capable of generating the range of errors found in deep dyslexia.[33] The language profile seen in callosotomy patients is more consistent with the profile reported by Coslett and Saffran[31,32] for the preserved reading of their pure alexic patients than with that reported for deep dyslexic patients.

Perhaps more interesting are the claims that the RH lexicon is needed to support a variety of metalinguistic tasks, from interpretation of humor to metaphor to indirect requests.[34–37] One source for these problems might be RH differences in semantic representation and/or processing.[38,39] Lateralized presentations to normal readers show that whereas the right visual field/left hemisphere (RVF/LH) shows priming for a variety of relations between words after reading short paragraphs, the left visual field/right hemisphere (LVF/RH) shows priming only for primarily lexical relations, not those that are dependent on grammatical information.[40] Moreover, the LH of split-brain patients shows priming for all of these relations as well. It is possible that the spreading of lexical activation without grammar is sufficient to facilitate some discourse-level processes and may support some other metalinguistic functions as well.

MEMORY

Recall and Recognition Memory Following Callosotomy

Changes in mnemonic capacity after callosotomy may reflect discrete processing capacities in the isolated hemispheres. Loss of general memory capacity as measured by standardized tests has been reported for some patients,[41,42] whereas Clark and Geffen[43] suggested that discrepancies in memory function reported after callosotomy might be due to involvement of the hippocampal commissure. Phelps and coworkers[44] have observed a decrement in both visual and verbal recall following posterior callosal section, which may damage the hippocampal commissure, but preserved or even improved memory after anterior callosal section, which does not. Recognition memory was relatively intact in both groups. Kroll and colleagues[45,46] reported that complete callosotomy interferes with the binding of visual and verbal material, yielding error patterns similar to those of hippocampally lesioned patients.

There appear to be hemisphere-specific changes in the accuracy of memory processses that may be useful in understanding the behavior of some neurologically impaired patients. The LH appears to make greater use of general knowledge schemas to explain perceptions and experiences and to use them to "interpret" events[47] than does the RH, and this predilection has an impact on the accuracy of memory.[44] When subjects were presented with a series of pictures that represented common events (i.e., getting up in the morning or making cookies) and were then asked, several hours later, to identify whether pictures in another series had appeared in the original series, both hemispheres were equally accurate in recognizing previously viewed pictures and rejecting novel, unrelated ones. Only the RH, however, correctly rejected pictures in the second set that were not previously viewed but were semantically congruent with pictures from the first set. The LH incorrectly "recalled" significantly more of these semantically congruent lures as having occurred in the first set, presumably because they fit into the schema it had constructed regarding the event. This finding is consistent with the hypothesis that there is an LH "interpreter" that constructs theories to assimilate perceived information into a comprehensible whole.[48,49] As a result, however, the elaborative processing involved has a deleterious effect on the accuracy of perceptual recognition. This has been confirmed by Metcalfe and colleagues and extended to include verbal material.[50]

HEMISPHERIC DOMINANCE

The Left Hemisphere as Interpreter

The LH is considered to be the "dominant" hemisphere in most right-handed people. The term *dominant* is usually taken to mean language-dominant, but Gazzaniga has suggested that the LH is not only superior in terms of language function but also in the ability to make simple inferences and to interpret its own behavior and emotions.[51] It is, in fact, the "intelligent" hemisphere. It is unclear whether these functions are dependent upon the development of generative language skills or if they arise independently. Nonetheless, such observations strongly indicate that the LH is not only more able than the RH to express itself verbally but that it plays a dominant role in interpreting behavior and providing a rationale for events in the world. Taking the evolutionary view, Gazzaniga and colleagues suggest that the corpus callosum allowed the evolution of these lateralized skills to occur and enabled the development of consciousness.[49,52]

Evolution of Dominance

One of the most perplexing and recalcitrant questions about the neural representation of cognition is the basis for hemispheric lateralization. Although the split-brain model confirmed that the LH is language dominant and the RH is better at many visuospatial tasks, it is clear that both hemispheres share many capacities and possess at least rudimentary skills in both verbal and nonverbal domains. One insightful approach to this problem is under investigation by Paul Corballis and colleagues.[52–56]

Corballis suggests that the corpus callosum has played a role in the evolution of lateralized skills in what was previously a symmetrical system.[52] The inhibitory power of the corpus callosum allowed new skills associated with language to develop in the LH, while prior visuospatial abilities were maintained in the RH. Hence, certain low-level visual effects are common to both hemispheres (i.e., luminance[56,57] and binocular rivalry[58]), whereas other visual processes that require spatial localization are present only in the RH (i.e., size and orientation discrimination[56] and perceptual matching[59]). Corballis further suggests that this division may reflect the what/where system's association with the dorsal and ventral pathways.[56] Although still under investigation, such a view provides an interesting perspective from which to examine visuospatial function.

Visuospatial Functions

The expected right hemispheric superiority in visuospatial function has been demonstrated in callosotomy patients,[6,60] but the LH has some visuospatial skills as well. In fact, superior use of visual imagery using a letter-based task has been demonstrated in the LH.[61] Although the use of tactile information to build spatial representations of abstract shapes also appears to be better developed in the RH,[60] tasks such as block design from the Wechsler Adult Intelligence Scale (WAIS), which are typically associated with the right parietal lobe, appear to require integration between hemispheres in some patients.[62] This observation is compatible with neuropsychological observations that document different types of visuospatial errors associated with lesions to the right and left hemispheres.

As noted above, Corballis and colleagues have tried to explain the distribution of skills in the two hemispheres by comparing visual tasks that vary in their dependence on high-level spatial processing for completion. The RH shows competence for all of the tested visual tasks, regardless of whether there is a strong need for spatial processing. In contrast, the LH shows competence only for those tasks and effects that depend upon luminance, timing, or some other lower-level perceptual information. Hence, this line of investigation is finding increasing support for the view that the hemispheres share the capacity for basic perceptual processing, whereas the RH dominance becomes more apparent as higher-level spatial information is required.

INTERHEMISPHERIC INTEGRATION OF PERCEPTION AND ATTENTION

Hemispheric Isolation of Visual and Tactile Information

When appropriate lateralization procedures are followed (see Fig. 34-1), visual and tactile perception can be isolated to each hemisphere. Although split subjects can make accurate same/different judgments about visual material that has been isolated to one hemisphere or the other, they cannot make comparisons between the two hemifields. Performance is at or near chance levels when words or pictures are presented in different visual fields for same/different judgments.[63–65] Despite reports of integration of higher-order information following callosotomy,[66,67] such reports have not always proved replicable or explicable through the patient's strategic maneuvers.[65,68,69] At present, it appears that if visual or tactile information is presented so that it is initially perceived by only one hemisphere, the perception remains isolated within that hemisphere.

The animal literature, however, has documented that information from areas close to the visual midline is shared by both hemispheres.[70,71] It appears that this observation is also true for the human species in an area no more than 2 degrees from the vertical meridian.[72] Although represented, the visual information in this area has little utility, as neither detailed shape comparisons nor brief displays could be reliably compared across the meridian.[73]

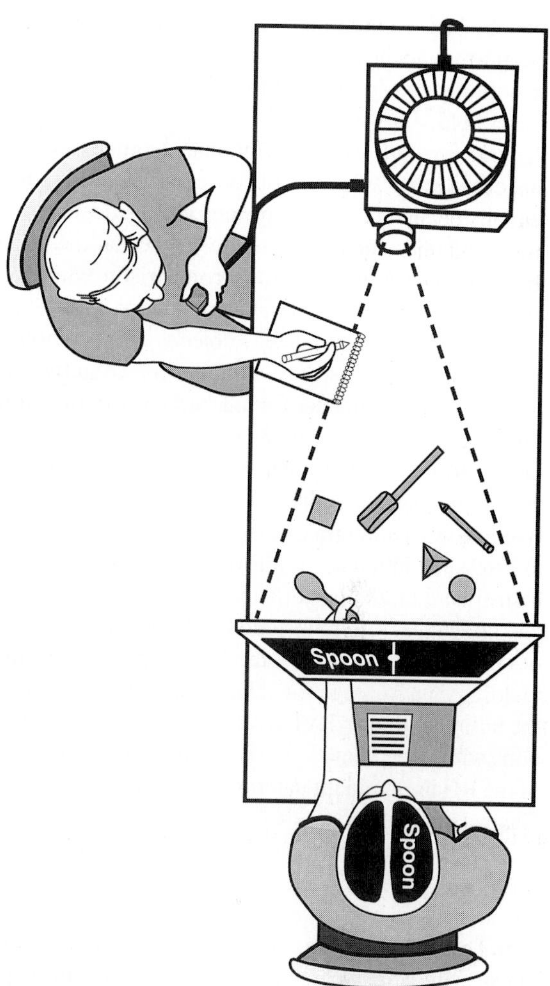

Figure 34-1
Tachistoscopic method of data collection from split-brain patients used in original studies. Current studies use computers and eye-tracking technology to control display and timing of lateralized stimuli.

Sharing of Attentional Control

Although both higher cognitive function and basic perceptual information appear to be isolated within each hemisphere, there is some evidence for sharing control of visual attention. The hemispheres appear to share control of the "attentional spotlight" via their subcortical connections. That is, if attention is directed to a particular position in the visual field by a cue in one field, that information can be used by both hemispheres.[64,74]

Nonetheless, explicit interfield comparisons of spatial location cannot be made accurately,[64] nor can attention be simultaneously directed to different points in each visual field.[75]

It also appears that attentional resources are limited despite the "splitting" of consciousness. Holtzman demonstrated that increasing processing demands in one hemisphere had a deleterious effect on the other hemisphere.[76] Nonetheless, in comparison with normal subjects, there was less decrement in a dual-task condition for callosotomized subjects.[77] Thus, though the two hemispheres may compete for cognitive resources, there is evidence for independence of function. This latter finding is consistent with the observation of Luck and coworkers[78] that visual search is independently mediated by both hemispheres. Using a standard spatial cuing paradigm that incorporated a bilateral cue to assess the influence of information presented to one hemisphere on the performance of the other, Mangun and colleagues[79] demonstrated differential processing of spatial cues, with only the LVF (right-hand) trials yielding an advantage for validly cued trials. Although the failure to find an RVF advantage for valid trials is at odds with other results,[74,80] it is consistent with a view of the RH as dominant in terms of spatial attention (see Chaps. 25 and 26).

Apparent inconsistencies uncovered in untangling the ways in which the hemispheres compete for attentional resources has suggested to some researchers that there are different types of attention that engage the hemispheres differently at different levels of processing. Kingstone and colleagues[81,82] have suggested that reflexive or exogenous orienting engages each hemisphere independently but that voluntary (or endogenous) orienting involves competition between the hemispheres for a single resource pool. Luck and Hillyard[83] emphasize that differences in mechanisms utilized at different processing stages determine the ways in which attentional resources are used.

SPECIFICITY OF CALLOSAL FIBERS

In human studies, observations regarding functional specificity of callosal fibers arise from three different sources. First, callosal sections are completed in two different stages, usually anterior first, allowing for observation of functional differences in partially resected patients. Second, development of high-resolution imaging techniques like MRI has permitted verification of the fibers resected during callosotomy and identification of inadvertently spared fibers. Finally, some strokes leave patients with clearly defined lesions of parts of the callosum. Examination of differences in transfer ability in these three groups allows better understanding of specificity of transfer.

It has long been observed that separating up to two-thirds of the anterior callosum leads to little if any change in abilities.[84] If the anterior split continues far enough, disruption of the ability to transfer sensory and position information from hand to hand will be observed. In contrast, the section of the splenium disrupts the transfer of visual information between the hemispheres, which isolates lateralized visual input in a single hemisphere. After posterior section, although explicit identification and naming of LVF stimuli is not possible, some transfer of higher order information may occur.[85]

CONCLUSIONS

Although the behaving being is remarkably intact following callosotomy, investigation reveals hemispheric capacities that refine and confirm hypotheses based on normal subjects and patients with focal lesions. The isolated RH usually cannot read, write, or speak, despite displaying a variety of cognitive behaviors. Dissociations like left-handed tactile anomia or agraphia may be an indication of less competence in language output in the RH. However, the ability to comprehend auditory and visual language may be present in the RH and may contribute to the presentation of aphasic and alexic patients. Recent observations indicate that the RH may participate in long-term recovery from aphasia.[19] Perhaps of greater interest, however, is the study of callosotomy patients to investigate the hemispheric bases of cognition and the integration of diverse perceptual, sensory, and emotional information into a single behavioral plan. The important role played by the LH in allowing the organism to observe and interpret its own actions and emotional states was first recognized in this population. Insights regarding the components of perception, attention, and language continue to arise from this population and to inform our models of normal perceptual and cognitive processing.

REFERENCES

1. Van Wagenen WP, Herren RY: Surgical division of commissural pathways in the corpus callosum: Relation to spread of an epileptic attack. *Arch Neurol Psychiatry* 44:740–759, 1940.
2. Akelaitis AJ: Studies on the corpus callosum: Higher visual functions in each homonymous field following complete section of corpus callosum. *Arch Neurol Psychiatry* 45:788–796, 1941.
3. Akelaitis AJ: A study of gnosis, praxis, and language following section of the corpus callosum and anterior commissure. *J Neurosurg* 7:94–102, 1944.
4. Meyers RE: Function of the corpus callosum in intraocular transfer. *Brain* 79:358, 1956.
5. Meyers RE, Sperry RW: Interhemisperic communication through the corpus callosum: Mnemonic carry-over between the hemispheres. *Arch Neurol Psychiatry* 80:298–303, 1958.
6. Bogen, JE, Gazzaniga MS: Cerebral commissurotomy in man: Minor hemisphere dominance for certain visuospatial functions. *J Neurosurg* 23:394–399, 1965.
7. Sperry RW et al: Interhemispheric relationships: The neocortical commissures; syndromes of hemisphere disconnection, in Vinken PJ, Bruyn GW (eds): *Handbook of Clinical Neurology.* New York: Wiley, 1969, vol 4, pp 273–290.
8. Geschwind N: Disconnection syndromes in animals and man. Part I. *Brain* 88:237–294, 1965.
9. Gazzaniga MS: *The Bisected Brain.* New York: Appleton-Century-Crofts, 1970.
10. Zaidel E: A technique for presenting lateralized visual input with prolonged exposure. *Vision Res* 15:283–289, 1974.
11. Gazzaniga MS: Principles of human brain organization derived from split-brain studies. *Neuron* 14:217–288, 1995.
12. Gazzaniga MS et al: Some functional effects of sectioning the cerebral commissures in man. *Proc Natl Acad Sci U S A* 48:1765–1769, 1962.
13. Levy J et al: Expressive language in the surgically separated minor hemisphere. *Cortex* 7:49–58, 1971.
14. Coltheart M: Deep dyslexia: A right-hemisphere hypothesis, in Coltheart M et al (eds): *Deep Dyslexia.* London: Routledge, 1980.
15. Coltheart M: Disorders of reading and their implications for models of normal reading. *Vis Lang* 15:246–286, 1981.
16. Baynes K et al: Modular organization of cognitive systems masked by interhemispheric integration. *Science* 280:902–905, 1998.
17. Eliassen JC et al: Direction information coordinated via the posterior third of the corpus callosum during bimanual movements. *Exp Brain Res* 128:573–577, 1999.
18. Eliassen JC et al: Anterior and posterior callosal contributions to simultaneous bimanual movements of the hands and fingers. *Brain* 123:2501–2511, 2000.
19. Weiller C: Imaging recovery from stroke. *Exp Brain Res* 123:13–17, 1998.
20. Weiller C et al: Recovery from Wernicke's aphasia: A positron emission tomographic study. *Ann Neurol* 37:723–732, 1995.
21. Gazzaniga MS et al: Profiles of right hemisphere language and speech following brain bisection. *Brain Lang* 22:206–220, 1984.
22. Baynes K, Eliassen JC: The visual lexicon: Its access and organization in commissurotomy patients, in Beeman M, Chiarello C (eds): *Right Hemisphere Language Comprehension.* Hillsdale NJ: Erlbaum, 1998, pp 79–104.
23. Eviatar Z, Zaidel E: The effects of word length and emotionality on hemispheric contributions to lexical decision. *Neuropsychologia* 29:415–428, 1991.
24. Pinker S: *The Language Instinct.* New York: Morrow, 1994.
25. Sidtis JJ et al: Variability in right hemisphere language function after callosal section: Evidence for a continuum of generative capacity. *J Neurosci* 1:323–331, 1981.
26. Zaidel E, Peters AM: Phonological encoding and ideographic reading by the disconnected right hemisphere: Two case studies. *Brain Lang* 14:205–234, 1981.
27. Baynes K et al: Hemispheric contributions to the integration of visual and auditory information in speech perception. *Percept Psychophys* 55:633–641, 1994.
28. Baynes K, Gazzaniga MS: Right hemisphere language: Insights into normal language mechanisms? in Plum F (ed): *Language, Communication, and the Brain.* New York: Raven Press, 1988.
29. Reuter-Lorenz PA, Baynes K: Modes of lexical access in the callosotomized brain. *J Cogn Neurosci* 4(2):155–164, 1992.
30. Schweiger A et al: Right hemisphere contribution to lexical access in an aphasic with deep dyslexia. *Brain Lang* 37:73–89, 1989.
31. Coslett HB, Saffran E: Evidence for preserved reading in "pure alexia." *Brain* 112:327–359, 1989.

32. Coslett HB, Saffran EM: Reading and the right hemisphere: Evidence from acquired dyslexia, in Beeman M, Chiarello C. (eds): *Right Hemisphere Language Comprehension: Perspectives from Cognitive Neuroscience.* Hillsdale, NJ: Erlbaum, 1998, pp 105–132.
33. Baynes K et al: Emergence of access to speech in a disconnected right hemisphere. *Soc Neurosci Abstr* 19: 1809, 1993.
34. Brownell HH: Appreciation of metaphoric and connotative word meaning by brain-damaged patients, in Chiarello C (ed): *Right Hemisphere Contributions to Lexical-Semantics.* New York: Springer-Verlag, 1988, pp 18–31.
35. Brownell HH et al: Inference deficits in right brain-damage. *Brain Lang* 22:310–321, 1986.
36. Gardner H, Denes G: Connotative judgments by aphasic patients on a pictorial adaptation of the semantic differential. *Cortex* 9:183–196, 1973.
37. Hirst W et al: Constraints on the processing of indirect speech acts: Evidence from aphasiology. *Brain Lang* 23:26–33, 1984.
38. Beeman M: Course semantic coding and discourse comprehension, in Beeman M, Chiarello C (eds): *Right Hemisphere Language Comprehension.* Hillsdale, NJ: Erlbaum, 1998, pp 255–284.
39. Chiarello C: On codes of meaning and the meaning of codes: Semantic access and retrieval within and between hemispheres, in Beeman M, Chiarello C (eds): *Right Hemisphere Language Comprehension.* Hillsdale, NJ: Erlbaum, 1998, pp 141–160.
40. Long DL, Baynes K: Discourse representation in the two cerebral hemispheres. *J Cogn Neurosci* 14(2):228–242, 2002.
41. Zaidel D, Sperry RW: Memory impairment after commissurotomy in man. *Brain* 97:263–272, 1974.
42. Zaidel E: Language functions in the two hemispheres following complete cerebral commissurotomy and hemispherectomy, in Boller F, Grafman G (eds): *Handbook of Neuropsychology.* Amsterdam: Elsevier, 1990, vol 4, pp 115–150.
43. Clark CR, Geffen GM: Corpus callosum surgery and recent memory. *Brain* 112:165–175, 1989.
44. Phelps EA, Gazzaniga MS: Hemispheric differences in mnemonic processing: The effects of left hemisphere interpretation. *Neuropsychologia* 30:293–297, 1992.
45. Kroll NEA et al: Cohesion failure as a source of memory illusions. *Mem Lang* 35:176–196, 1996.
46. Jha AP et al: Memory encoding following commissurotomy. *J Cogn Neurosci* 9:143–159, 1997.
47. Gazzaniga MS: *The Social Brain.* New York: Basic Books, 1985.
48. Funnell MG et al (eds): *Hemispheric Interactions and Specializations: Insights From the Split Brain.* Amsterdam: Elsevier, 2000.
49. Gazzaniga MS: Cerebral specialization and interhemispheric communication: Does the corpus callosum enable the human condition? *Brain* 123:1293–1326, 2000.
50. Metcalfe J et al: Right hemisphere memory superiority: studies of a split-brain patient. *Psychol Sci* 6(3):157–164, 1995.
51. Gazzaniga MS: Consciousness and the cerebral hemispheres, in Gazzaniga MS (ed): *The Cognitive Neurosciences.* Cambridge, MA: MIT Press, 1995, pp 1391–1400.
52. Corballis PM et al: An evolutionary perspective on hemispheric asymmetries. *Brain Cogn* 43:112–117, 2000.
53. Corballis PM et al: Illusory contour perception and amodal boundary completion: Evidence of a dissociation following callosotomy. *J Cogn Neurosci* 11:459–466, 1999.
54. Corballis PM et al: A dissociation between spatial and identity matching in callosotomy patients. *Neuroreport* 10(10):2183–2187, 1999.
55. Corballis PM et al: An investigation of the line motion effect in a callosotomy patient. *Brain Cogn* 48(2–3):327–332, 2002.
56. Corballis PM et al: Hemispheric asymmetries for simple visual judgments in the split brain. *Neuropsychologia* 40(4):401–410, 2002.
57. Forster B et al: Effect of luminance on successive discrimination in the absence of the corpus callosum. *Neuropsychologia* 38:441–450, 2000.
58. O'Shea RP, Corballis PM: Binocular rivalry between complex stimuli in split-brain observers. *Brain Mind.* In press.
59. Funnell MG et al: A deficit in perceptual matching in the left hemisphere of a callosotomy patient. *Neuropsychologia* 37:1143–1154, 1999.
60. Milner B, Taylor L: Right hemisphere superiority in tactile pattern recognition after cerebral commissurotomy: Evidence for non-verbal memory. *Neuropsychologia* 10:1–15, 1972.
61. Farah MJ et al: A left hemisphere basis for visual mental imagery? *Neuropsychologia* 23:115–118, 1985.
62. Gazzaniga MS: Organization of the human brain. *Science* 245:947–952, 1989.
63. Baynes K et al: The emergence of the capacity to name left visual field stimuli in a callosotomy patient:

Implications for functional plasticity. *Neuropsychologia* 33(10):1225–1242, 1995.

64. Holtzman JD et al: Dissociation of spatial information for stimulus localization and the control of attention. *Brain* 104:861–872, 1981.
65. Seymour S et al: The disconnection syndrome: Basic findings reaffirmed. *Brain* 117:105–115, 1994.
66. Sergent J: Unified response to bilateral hemispheric stimulation by a split-brain patient. *Nature* 305(27):800–802, 1983.
67. Sergent J: Furtive incursions into bicameral minds. *Brain* 113:537–568, 1990.
68. Corballis MC: Can commissurotomized subjects compare digits between the visual fields? *Neuropsychologia* 32:1475–1486, 1994.
69. Kingstone A, Gazzaniga MS: Subcortical transfer of higher order information in the split-brain patient: More illusory than real? *Neuropsychology* 9:321–328, 1995.
70. Fukuda Y et al: Nasotemporal overlap of crossed and uncrossed retinal ganglion cell projections in the Japanese monkey (*Macaca fuscata*). *J Neurosci* 9:2353–2373, 1989.
71. Stone J: The naso-temporal division of the monkey retina. *J Comp Neurol* 135:585–600, 1966.
72. Fendrich R et al: Naso-temporal overlap at the retinal vertical meridian: Investigations with a callosotomy patient. *Neuropsychologia* 34:637–646, 1996.
73. Fendrich R, Gazzaniga MS: Evidence of foveal splitting in a commissurotomy patient. *Neuropsychologia* 27(3):273–281, 1989.
74. Holtzman JD et al: Spatial orientation following commissural section, in Parasuraman R, Davies DR (eds): *Varieties of Attention.* New York: Academic Press, 1984, pp 375–394.
75. Holtzman JD: Interactions between cortical and subcortical visual areas: Evidence from human commissurotomy patients. *Vis Res* 24:801–813, 1984.
76. Holtzman JD, Gazzaniga MS: Dual task interactions due exclusively to limits in processing resources. *Science* 218:1325–1327, 1982.
77. Holtzman JD, Gazzaniga MS: Enhanced dual task performance following callosal commissurotomy in humans. *Neuropsychologia* 23:315–321, 1985.
78. Luck SJ et al: Independent hemispheric attentional systems mediate visual search in split-brain patients. *Nature* 342:543–545, 1989.
79. Mangun GR et al: Monitoring the visual world: Hemispheric asymmetries and subcortical processes in attention. *J Cogn Neurosci* 6:265–273, 1994.
80. Reuter-Lorenz PA, Fendrich R: Orienting attention across the vertical meridian: Evidence from callosotomy patients. *J Cogn Neurosci* 2:232–238, 1990.
81. Enns J, Kingstone A: Hemispheric cooperation in visual search: Evidence from normal and split-brain observers, in Christman S (ed): *Cerebral Asymmetries in Sensory and Perceptual Processes.* Amsterdam: North-Holland, 1997, pp 197–231.
82. Kingstone A et al: Paying attention to the brain: The study of selective visual attention in cognitive neuroscience, in Burak J, Enns J (eds): *Attention, Development, and Psychopathology.* New York: Guilford, 1997, pp 263–287.
83. Luck SJ, Hillyard SA: The operation of selective attention at multiple stages of processing: Evidence from human and monkey electrophysiology, in Gazzaniga MS (ed): *The Cognitive Neurosciences.* Cambridge, MA: MIT Press, 1999, pp 687–700.
84. Risse GL et al: Interhemispheric transfer in patients with incomplete section of the corpus callosum: Anatomic verification with magnetic resonance imaging. *Arch Neurol* 46:437–443, 1989.
85. Sidtis JJ et al: Cognitive interaction after staged callosal section: Evidence for transfer of semantic activation. *Science* 212:344–346, 1981.

Chapter 35

SYNDROMES DUE TO ACQUIRED BASAL GANGLIA DAMAGE

Bruce Crosson
Anna Bacon Moore
Christina E. Wierenga

Outside of dementias that may occur with degenerative diseases of the basal ganglia (e.g., Parkinson's disease, Huntington's disease), the most commonly studied clinical entities involving the basal ganglia are vascular lesions. Because dementias involving degeneration of the basal ganglia are covered in Chap. 48 of this volume, the current chapter concentrates primarily on the effects of vascular lesions. Prior to doing so, however, we must briefly address mechanisms of vascular lesions to the basal ganglia. The lenticulostriate arteries, supplying a large portion of the basal ganglia and surrounding white matter, originate from the M1 segment of the middle cerebral artery (MCA; see schematic diagram in Fig. 35-1). Large ischemic lesions of the basal ganglia are often the result of occlusion of the MCA, from blockage at the bifurcation of the internal carotid artery or blockage of the M1 segment of the MCA. Less often, blockage of the internal carotid artery may be the culprit. In such cases, the function and integrity of cortices supplied by the MCA depend on anastomotic circulation[1,2] (Fig. 35–1). These anastomoses may vary widely in patency; in many cases, circulation is adequate to prevent cystic infarction though not other changes. Although cortical damage may not be identified on computed tomography (CT) or magnetic resonance imaging (MRI) in cases of large infarcts of the basal ganglia, inadequate anastomotic circulation may cause structural (ischemic neuronal loss) or functional changes (inadequate neuronal function without cell death) in inadequately supplied cortical areas. When these circumstances are present, the symptoms may be determined more by which cortical areas experience unidentified structural or functional changes than by which subcortical structures demonstrate damage on CT or MRI.[1–3]

Cerebral blood flow images from single photon emission computed tomography (SPECT) or positron emission tomography (PET) may be useful in determining the full extent of cortical and subcortical dysfunction.[2] It is worth noting as an exception to these vascular dynamics that, since lacunar infarctions frequently result from small-vessel as opposed to large-vessel disease,[4] cortical dysfunction is not necessarily expected to accompany subcortical lacunar infarction. Thus, these smaller lesions may be more useful in exploring structural-functional relationships.

Hemorrhagic lesions can be complicated in a slightly different fashion by ischemic effects not seen on CT or MRI. Large hemorrhagic lesions of the basal ganglia will produce a hematoma that radiates pressure effects. In such cases, pressure may cause temporary or permanent ischemic effects in surrounding areas, including perisylvian language cortex and the thalamus.[1,3] Other space-occupying lesions, such as tumors, may also cause pressure ischemia, resulting in temporary functional effects or permanent structural changes. Again, in such cases the location of cortical or subcortical ischemia may affect symptom presentation. Keeping these thoughts in mind, we can explore symptom complexes seen after lesions of the basal ganglia identified by CT or MRI.

APHASIA AFTER LESION OF THE BASAL GANGLIA

Although outside the classical language areas of the brain (see Chap. 11), the incidence of aphasia in larger lesions including the dominant basal ganglia can be substantial. Crosson[5] found the rates of aphasia in vascular lesions involving the dominant basal ganglia to

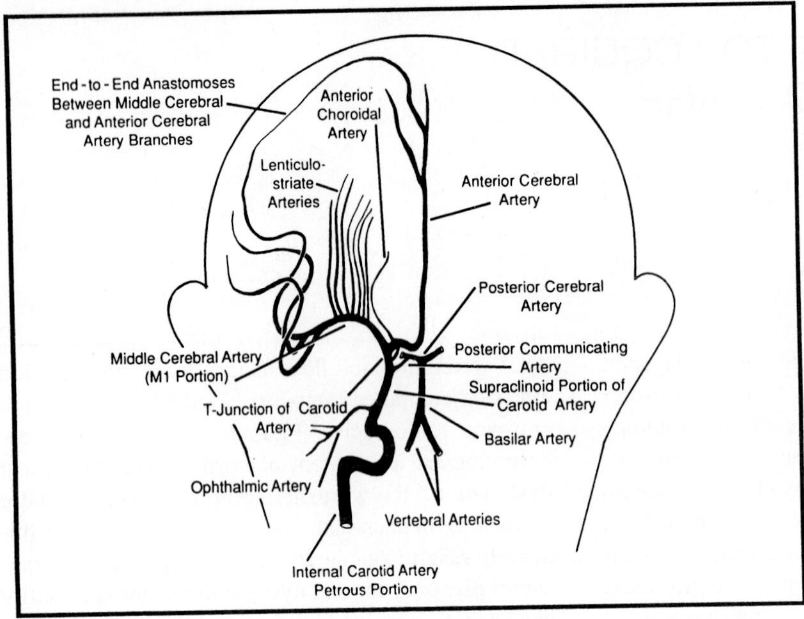

Figure 35-1
Schematic diagram showing the internal carotid artery branching into the middle and anterior cerebral arteries. The lenticulostriate arteries, which supply much of the basal ganglia and surrounding white matter, emerge from the M1 segment of the middle cerebral artery. End-to-end anastomoses between branches of the middle and anterior cerebral arteries are also depicted. (From Nadeau and Crosson,[1] with permission.)

vary between 20 and 83 percent; however, Nadeau and Crosson[1] have noted that the rate of aphasia in cases of smaller lesions confined to the caudate head may be negligible.

When aphasia is present after a lesion of the dominant basal ganglia, the symptoms vary considerably. Crosson[5] reviewed the literature on aphasia after vascular lesion of the dominant basal ganglia and rated reported cases on four dimensions: fluent versus nonfluent output, severity of comprehension deficit, severity of repetition deficit, and predominance of phonemic versus semantic paraphasias. The picture was rather different for hemorrhagic lesions versus infarcts. For aphasia after hemorrhage, the dominant putamen was most frequently involved and aphasia was primarily of a fluent variety. Repetition and comprehension were usually impaired to some degree, often severely. Paraphasias were predominantly semantic as opposed to phonemic. While hemorrhagic cases seemed, at least loosely, to fit a syndrome, cases of infarction did not cohere into a syndrome. Speech/language output could be fluent or nonfluent. Comprehension was usually impaired to at least some degree, but repetition ranged from unimpaired to severely impaired. When one type of paraphasia predominated for an individual case, it could be phonemic or semantic. No syndrome emerged whether the infarct included the putamen, caudate head, or globus pallidus. The weakness in this analysis was that lesions frequently included multiple structures, and it was difficult to parcel out the effects on one structure versus another.

For this reason, Nadeau and Crosson[1] reviewed a single type of lesion, dominant striatocapsular infarcts. These lesions have a characteristic comma shape (Fig. 35-2) and most often include the putamen, anterior limb of the internal capsule, and caudate head. Since the structures included are fairly consistent, this type of lesion should produce a characteristic syndrome if the basal ganglia are involved in language. According to this review, patients with dominant striatocapsular infarcts may ($n = 33$) or may not ($n = 17$) have aphasia. When aphasia is reported, levels of impairment are quite variable for fluency, comprehension, repetition, naming, and paraphasia. Articulation is most often moderately impaired. Similarly, Weiller and colleagues[2] studied 57 consecutive cases of striatocapsular infarction. When the lesion involved the dominant hemisphere, patients might or might not be aphasic. Of 15 cases with aphasia, the initial syndrome was Broca's aphasia in 4, Wernicke's aphasia in 3, amnesic aphasia in 4, global aphasia in 2, residual symptoms in 1, and unclassifiable in 1. Thus,

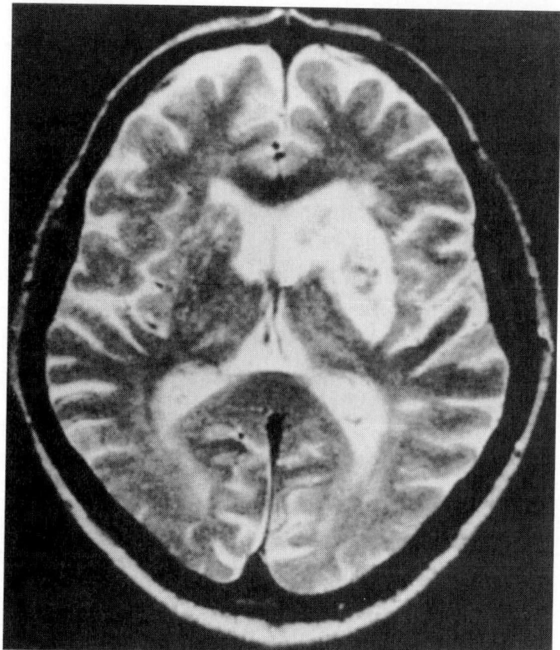

Figure 35-2
T2-weighted MRI of striatocapsular infarction. Note the comma-shaped appearance. (From Weiller et al.,[2] with permission.)

consistent with the review of Nadeau and Crosson,[1] no coherent syndrome emerged. For the aphasic patients of Weiller and coworkers,[2] the prognosis was generally good: 9 of 14 patients seen at 1-year follow-up had no or minor language symptoms. Recanalization of the MCA (or internal carotid) occurred later if at all in patients with aphasia as opposed to those without aphasia; patients with aphasia as opposed to those without aphasia had poor anastomotic circulation.

Although classic symptoms of aphasia after a lesion of the dominant basal ganglia may be due to concomitant effects on perisylvian cortex, as noted above, recent work indicates that such lesions may affect generative aspects of language and word finding to some degree.[6,7] Consistent with these findings, Copland and colleagues[8] found that patients with lesions of the dominant basal ganglia and/or surrounding white matter demonstrated normal performance on tests of aphasia except for impaired word-list generation. On the other hand, these patients demonstrated impairment in higher-order language tasks—for example, the ability to generate two meanings for semantically ambiguous sentences. These investigators further found deficits in semantic priming tasks that suggested impairment in controlled as opposed to automatic processing of words with lexical-semantic ambiguities.[9] Thus, consensus is growing that the dominant basal ganglia are involved in executive language functions. This involvement is attributed to participation of the basal ganglia in cortico-striato-pallido-thalamo-cortical loops.[10]

In summary, patients with sizable hemorrhages in the dominant basal ganglia tend to have fluent aphasias with semantic paraphasias and at least some impairment of comprehension and repetition. Patients with infarction of the dominant basal ganglia, including those with characteristic striatocapsular lesions, may or may not demonstrate aphasia. When aphasia is present, it may be of almost any variety. Available evidence suggests that in cases of large infarction of the dominant basal ganglia, the adequacy of anastomotic circulation to the cortex may determine whether aphasia is seen, and the type of aphasia will depend on which cortical regions cannot function properly.[1,2] For hemorrhagic lesions of the dominant basal ganglia, symptoms may be related to compressive ischemia of the cortex, the thalamus, or the connections between them.[1] However, more subtle effects on language may be obscured after large vascular lesion of the dominant basal ganglia by ischemic effects on these other structures. Evidence is mounting that the dominant basal ganglia are involved in executive language functions.[6–9] These effects may be evident in the generative aspects of language (e.g., word-list generation) or when language is used in reasoning processes.

APRAXIA AFTER LESION OF THE BASAL GANGLIA

As reviewed in Chap. 16, apraxia involves deficits in the execution of learned, skilled movements.[11] A useful distinction is between ideational apraxia in which conceptual knowledge of such movements is disrupted and ideomotor apraxia in which the action plan for such movements seems to be disrupted. Most frequently, ideomotor apraxia has been the target of investigations after subcortical lesion. In one review, Crosson[12] described the literature on acquired basal ganglia lesions and praxis as problematic. As with aphasia, ischemic phenomena accompanying cystic infarction or large hemorrhages may cause cortical dysfunction, and the cortical dysfunction, in turn, could cause deficits in praxis. A second problem is that different investigators have used different definitions of praxis, with some testing already learned, skilled movements and others testing novel movements or postures that have not been learned. The presence of preexisting representations of the movements for the already *learned,* skilled movements could make a large difference in the performance of the appropriate actions. In his review of cortical and subcortical functions in praxis, Leiguarda[13] noted a third variable complicating cross-study comparisons: the cognitive demands of the action that patients must perform (e.g., working memory, attention, auditory comprehension). Finally, Maeshima and colleagues[14] indicated that time postlesion can impact the presence of both ideomotor and ideational apraxia after basal ganglia lesion, with deficits remitting in many cases after 6 months. These caveats must be kept in mind in examining the literature on apraxia after acquired lesion of the basal ganglia.

Some studies suggest that apraxia after lesion to the dominant basal ganglia and/or surrounding white matter is less frequent than after lesions to the cortex.[15] Most commonly, apraxia with basal ganglia lesion occurs after dominant hemisphere lesion, though apraxia has been reported after nondominant hemisphere lesion as well. In his review, Leiguarda[13] suggested that ideomotor apraxia is most severe and persistent when lesions interrupt both cortical and basal ganglia mechanisms, or the connections between them. This conclusion is generally consistent with the meta-analysis of Pramstaller and Marsden[16] who indicated that apraxia rarely occurs with lesions confined to the basal ganglia but instead with lesions extending into surrounding association fibers, the internal capsule, and/or the thalamus.

As with aphasia, the pattern of apraxia that accompanies basal ganglia lesions can be examined to determine whether it coheres into a consistent syndrome and whether the pattern of deficits is unique. A consistent pattern of deficits with at least some unique features relative to cortical apraxia would argue in favor of a role for the basal ganglia in praxis. Unfortunately, such studies have barely begun. Rothi and coworkers[17] reported three cases of striatocapsular infarction, two of which had severe ideomotor apraxia. In general, these patients made spatial errors on a praxis task similar to those made by patients with cortical apraxias. One patient made perseverative errors that were generally not made by patients with apraxia after cortical lesions. Thus, in this small sample, no consistent syndrome with unique features was found.

In summary, the case for the involvement of the basal ganglia in praxis is not definitive at this time. Isolated lesions of the basal ganglia are less likely to cause apraxia than lesions involving surrounding white matter, nearby cortex, and/or the thalamus.[13,16] It is likely that the existence, severity, and character of apraxia after basal ganglia lesion is largely determined by the extent of dysfunction in other structures. The lack of unique symptoms for apraxia with basal ganglia lesions makes it difficult to distinguish a specific role for the basal ganglia in praxis. As with aphasia, structural changes or dysfunction in the cortex that impact the clinical presentation of apraxia may not be seen on structural images. It is of some interest that Leiguarda[13] maintained that ideomotor apraxia is most severe when both cortical and basal ganglia structures are implicated. Perhaps the disruption of executive functions with basal ganglia lesions (see below) exacerbates apraxia.

NEGLECT AFTER LESION OF THE BASAL GANGLIA

As explained in Chaps. 25 and 26, *neglect* can affect sensory-perceptual phenomena or movement-related phenomena.[18] On the sensory-perceptual side, *neglect* refers to a tendency, not attributable to primary sensory deficit, to ignore or neglect visual, auditory, and/or tactile stimuli contralateral to a brain lesion. It may be unimodal or multimodal. In addition to affecting the ability to process incoming sensory information, neglect may also affect internal representations of space.[19] Although sensory neglect is more common with right hemisphere lesions in right-handed patients, more subtle forms of neglect can appear after left hemisphere lesion in dextrals.[20] On the movement-related side, *neglect* refers to disorders of the intention to act; the term *akinesia* has been used to describe these disorders.

With respect to unilateral lesions affecting intention, patients can have a defect in initiating movement with a limb on one side of the body (limb akinesia), a defect initiating movement in one hemispace (hemispatial akinesia), or a defect initiating movement toward one side of space (directional akinesia).[21] The analysis of Watson and colleagues[22] suggests that dysfunction of the basal ganglia is more likely to produce akinesia than sensory-perceptual neglect (see also Ref. 18).

Case reports suggest that neglect is frequently found in cases where scans have identified structural lesions in the basal ganglia and surrounding white matter. As with cortical lesions, neglect appears to be more common with lesions of the basal ganglia in the right than in the left hemisphere. Unfortunately, some reports have not distinguished sensory-perceptual from intentional neglect.[23] In addressing neglect after vascular lesion of the basal ganglia, it is useful to distinguish between infarction caused by small vessel versus large vessel disease. The former is more likely to be limited to subcortical structures, while the latter is more likely to include damage or dysfunction of cortical structures that is not seen on routine clinical structural CT or MR images.[1,2] Kumral and colleagues[24] studied motor-intentional neglect as one symptom of caudate nucleus lesions caused primarily by small vessel disease or embolism as opposed to large vessel disease. When lesions of the right caudate head were in the territory of the right lateral lenticulostriate arteries, these investigators found that roughly half of the patients experienced motor-intentional neglect. In cases of large striatocapsular infarcts, sensory-perceptual neglect is common.[2,25] Such infarcts are caused by large vessel disease.[2] In specifically addressing this phenomenon, Weiller and colleagues[2] found that striatocapsular infarct patients with neglect or aphasia showed later or lesser recanalization of the middle cerebral artery and poorer anastomotic circulation than striatocapsular infarct patients without aphasia or neglect. They concluded that when sensory-perceptual neglect occurred in cases of large striatocapsular infarcts, cortical dysfunction accounted for it.

In summary, neglect after vascular lesion of the basal ganglia occurs primarily in right hemisphere locations. There is some support in the literature for the position of Watson and coworkers,[22] whose analyses suggested that lesions confined to the basal ganglia should result in primarily motor-intentional as opposed to sensory-perceptual neglect. With smaller infarcts caused by small vessel disease or embolism, motor-intentional neglect may be found with basal ganglia lesion.[24] This symptom may be sensitive to lesion location, as it was found with lesions in the territory of the lateral lenticulostriate arteries but not in other areas of the right caudate head. Sensory-perceptual neglect can be found after basal ganglia infarcts caused by large vessel disease—i.e., striatocapsular infarcts.[2,25] In such cases, the sensory-perceptual neglect is most likely caused by cortical dysfunction accompanying the basal ganglia lesions even when cortical damage is not evident on routine clinical imaging.[2]

EMOTIONAL CHANGES AFTER LESION OF THE BASAL GANGLIA

Cummings[26] reviewed much of the literature regarding emotional changes that accompany subcortical lesions, including those of the basal ganglia. Such alterations are apparently common. One report by Mendez and associates[27] is of particular interest, because the vast majority of the 12 cases reported had unilateral lacunar infarcts of the caudate head, suggesting that concomitant cortical ischemia was not a factor in all of them. Emotional changes were dependent on location of the infarct within the caudate head. Lesions of the dorsolateral caudate head resulted in apathy with decreased spontaneous verbal and motor behavior. This area of the caudate head is involved in a cortico-striato-pallido-thalamo-cortical loop that terminates in the dorsolateral frontal cortex.[10] Patients with lesions of the ventromedial caudate head demonstrate disinhibition, impulsivity, and inappropriate behavior.[27] This area of the caudate head is in a cortico-striato-pallido-thalamo-cortical loop that terminates in the orbitofrontal cortex,[10] thus the resemblance to behavior resulting from orbitofrontal lesions. Lesions involving most of the caudate head plus surrounding white matter produced affective symptoms with psychotic features. Mendez and colleagues[27] indicated that emotional effects of lesions did not depend upon lateralization and occurred with both left and right caudate lesions, as confirmed by Kumral and colleagues.[24] A study by

Starkstein and coworkers[28] indicated that lesions of the left basal ganglia (hemorrhage or infarction) resulted in significantly greater depression than lesions of the right basal ganglia or of the left or right thalamus. The heterogeneity of lesions and the inclusion of larger lesions in this latter study suggest that many patients may have had cortical dysfunction, as detailed above. However, in a study of bilateral calcification of the basal ganglia without other radiologic defect, López-Villegas and associates[29] noted depression in some cases; obsessive-compulsive disorder was also present in others of these cases.

Thus, lesion of the basal ganglia causes a variety of emotional symptoms. Many of these symptoms, unlike some cognitive symptoms, do not depend on lateralization of the lesion. Location within the caudate nucleus may be important, most likely because of the specific frontobasal ganglia loops in which the various basal ganglia regions are involved.

EXECUTIVE FUNCTION, FRONTAL, AND MOTOR DEFICITS

The term *executive functions* refers to a constellation of abilities necessary to formulate and project action into internal and external environments (see Chaps. 32 and 33). Executive functions have sometimes been defined as abilities affected by frontal lesions. However, the latter definition can become circular, does little to elucidate the relevant set of abilities, and does not do justice to the diversity of functions of the frontal lobes. Organization and planning, reasoning, shifting of cognitive sets, initiation, and response suppression are among the abilities often included under the rubric of *executive functions*. As reviewed elsewhere in this volume, most of these abilities are strongly influenced by various regions of the prefrontal cortex.

The basal ganglia are in a position to strongly influence frontal functions. In 1986, Alexander and colleagues[10] described multiple cortico-striato-pallido-thalamo-cortical loops whose output targeted specific regions of the frontal cortex. While these frontal-basal ganglia circuits originally were thought to be partially open, more recent data indicate that their structure is better conceptualized as closed—i.e., they start and terminate in the same area of frontal cortex.[30] Further, there are similar loops outside the frontal cortex. The current conceptualization of the relationship between cognitive functions and frontal basal ganglia loops is that separate loops may be fairly specific for different cognitive activities—e.g., spatial working memory, object working memory, or planning.[30]

Evidence is mounting that vascular lesions of the basal ganglia cause executive function and frontal deficits. It was noted above that dominant basal ganglia lesions cause deficits in generative aspects of language[7] and verbal reasoning,[8] which can be classified as executive language deficits. Because motor-intentional neglect involves initiation deficits, this deficit also can be considered an executive function deficit. As discussed above, this type of initiation problem may occur with right caudate lesion.[24] Also discussed above were specific relationships between emotional deficits after caudate head lesions and the specific cortico-striato-pallido-thalamo-cortical loop implicated.[27] In cases of isolated bilateral calcification of the basal ganglia, psychometric measures indicate that patients show deficits in a variety of executive functions.[29] Because executive function deficits clearly occur in such cases and in cases of small vessel disease causing caudate infarcts,[24] it can be concluded that damage of the basal ganglia per se contributes to these deficits.

The basal ganglia have long been considered to play a role in motor functions, primarily because of the motor symptoms that occur in degenerative diseases of the basal ganglia—i.e., tremor, rigidity, gait disturbance, akinesia in Parkinson's disease. Motor functions are related to executive functions in that motor functions can be considered the endpoint of executive functions—i.e., the means by which action is projected into an external environment. The so-called extrapyramidal symptoms seen in degenerative diseases of the basal ganglia are often absent after vascular lesion. Hemiplegia often occurs after vascular lesion of the basal ganglia, but it is frequently difficult to determine whether it is the basal ganglia lesion or lesion of the adjacent internal capsule that causes this symptom.

To summarize, while there is some doubt that basal ganglia lesions directly cause classic aphasias or sensory-perceptual neglect, evidence is mounting that basal ganglia lesions may cause executive function deficits. The nature of the executive function deficit may depend on the location of the lesion within the basal ganglia and the particular frontal-basal ganglia circuit implicated.

SUMMARY AND CONCLUSIONS

For large lesions of the basal ganglia, such as striatocapsular infarction, significant dysfunction may occur because of reduced blood flow to various areas of the cortex. This dynamic relates to blockage of the proximal MCA and the adequacy of anastomotic circulation to the various cortical regions supplied by the MCA. In such lesions, many cognitive symptoms may be determined by which areas of the cortex are functionally or structurally compromised in a way that is not detectable by routine structural imaging. This phenomenon most likely accounts for the classic symptoms of aphasia in striatocapsular infarction, sensory-perceptual neglect in striatocapsular infarction, and the similarity of apraxic symptoms in lesions of the cortex and basal ganglia. Further, any function that depends upon cortex in the distribution of the MCA might be affected after large striatocapsular infarction. Hemorrhage of the basal ganglia, because of the pressure effects surrounding an intracerebral hematoma, and tumors of the basal ganglia, for similar reasons, are likely to cause some pressure ischemia, which will affect the cortex. However, recent studies indicate that cognitive deficits do occur in patients with lesions of the basal ganglia due to small vessel disease. In such lesions, effects are more likely to be confined to the damage seen on structural imaging. In these instances, deficits of executive and frontal functions are common. These symptoms can be attributed to the existence of closed cortico-striato-pallido-thalamo-cortical circuits. It is unclear if the function of the basal ganglia in these loops is simply to enhance the relevant frontal functions or if the basal ganglia serve a unique function in these loops. Further research on this question would be a welcome addition to the literature.

REFERENCES

1. Nadeau SE, Crosson B: Subcortical aphasia. *Brain Lang* 58:355–402, 1997.
2. Weiller C, Willmes K, Reiche W, et al: The case of aphasia or neglect after striatocapsular infarction. *Brain* 116:1509–1525, 1993.
3. Skyhoj Olsen T, Bruhn P, Oberg RGW: Cortical hypoperfusion as a possible cause of "subcortical aphasia." *Brain* 109:393–410, 1986.
4. Poirier J, Gray F, Escourolle R: *Manual of Basic Neuropathology*. Philadelphia: Saunders, 1990.
5. Crosson B: *Subcortical Functions in Language and Memory*. New York: Guilford Press, 1992.
6. D'Esposito M, Alexander MP: Subcortical aphasia: Distinct profiles following left putaminal hemorrhage. *Neurology* 45:38–41, 1995.
7. Mega MS, Alexander MP: Subcortical aphasia: The core profile of capsulostriatal infarction. *Neurology* 44:1824–1829, 1994.
8. Copland DA, Chenery HJ, Murdoch BE: Persistent deficits in complex language function following dominant nonthalamic subcortical lesions. *J Med Speech Lang Pathol* 8:1–15, 2000.
9. Copland DA, Chenery HJ, Murdoch BE: Processing lexical ambiguities in word triplets: Evidence of lexical-semantic deficits following dominant nonthalamic subcortical lesions. *Neuropsychology* 14:379–390, 2000.
10. Alexander GE, DeLong MR, Strick PL: Parallel organization of functionally segregated circuits linking basal ganglia and cortex. *Annu Rev Neurosci* 9:357–381, 1986.
11. Heilman KM, Rothi LJG: Apraxia, in Heilman KM, Valenstein E (eds): *Clinical Neuropsychology,* 4th ed. New York: Oxford, 2003.
12. Crosson B: Subcortical limb apraxia, in Rothi LJG, Heilman KM (eds): *Apraxia*. East Sussex, UK: Erlbaum (UK), 1997, pp 207–243.
13. Leiguarda R: Limb apraxia: Cortical or subcortical. *Neuroimage* 14:S137–S141, 2001.
14. Maeshima S, Truman G, Smith DS, et al: Apraxia and cerebral haemorrhage: The relationship between haematoma volume and prognosis. *J Clin Neurosci* 7: 309–311, 2000.
15. Basso A, Luzzatti C, Spinnler H: Is ideomotor apraxia the outcome of damage of well-defined regions of the left hemisphere? *J Neurol Neurosurg Psychiatry* 43:118–126, 1980.
16. Pramstaller PP, Marsden CD: The basal ganglia and apraxia. *Brain* 119:319–340, 1996.
17. Rothi LJG, Kooistra C, Heilman KM, Mack L: Subcortical ideomotor apraxia. *J Clin Exp Neuropsychol* 10:48, 1988.
18. Heilman KM, Watson RT, Valenstein E: Neglect and related disorders, in Heilman KM, Valenstein E (eds): *Clinical Neuropsychology,* 3d ed. New York: Oxford University Press, 1993, pp 279–336.
19. Bisiach E, Luzzatti C: Unilateral neglect of representational space. *Cortex* 14:129–133, 1978.

20. Maeshima S, Shigeno K, Dohi N, et al: A study of right unilateral spatial neglect in left hemispheric lesions: The difference between right-handed and non-right-handed post-stroke patients. *Acta Neurol Scand* 85:418–424, 1992.
21. Heilman KM, Bowers D, Valenstein E, Watson RT: Hemispace and hemispatial neglect, in Jeannerod M (ed): *Neurophysiological and Neuropsychological Aspects of Spatial Neglect*. Amsterdam: Elsevier, pp 115–150.
22. Watson RT, Valenstein E, Heilman KM: Thalamic neglect: possible role of the medial thalamus and nucleus reticularis in behavior. *Arch Neurol* 38:501–506, 1981.
23. Fromm D, Holland AL, Swindell CS, Reinmuth OM: Various consequences of subcortical stroke: Prospective study of 16 consecutive cases. *Arch Neurol* 42:943–950, 1985.
24. Kumral E, Evyapan D, Balkir K: Acute caudate vascular lesions. *Stroke* 30:1734–1735, 1999.
25. Bladin PF, Berkovik SF: Straitocapsular infarction: Large infarcts in the lenticulostriate arterial territory. *Neurology* 34:1423–1430, 1984.
26. Cummings JL: Frontal-subcortical circuits and human behavior. *Arch Neurol* 50:873–880, 1993.
27. Mendez MF, Adams NL, Lewandowski KS: Neurobehavioral changes associated with caudate lesions. *Neurology* 39:349–354, 1989.
28. Starkstein SS, Robinson RG, Berthier ML, et al: Differential mood changes following basal ganglia vs thalamic lesions. *Arch Neurol* 45:725–730, 1988.
29. López-Villegas D, Kulisevsky J, Deus J, et al: Neuropsychological alterations in patients with computed tomography-detected basal ganglia calcification. *Arch Neurol* 53:251–256, 1996.
30. Middleton FA, Strick PL: Basal ganglia and cerebellar loops: Motor and cognitive circuits. *Brain Res Rev* 31:236–250, 2000.

Chapter 36

SYNDROMES DUE TO ACQUIRED THALAMIC DAMAGE*

Neill R. Graff-Radford

When the thalamus is damaged, the resulting types of deficits can be thought of in terms of the afferent and efferent connections of the affected thalamic nuclei (Table 36-1).[1] Certain nuclei have both afferent input from primary sense organs and efferent output to primary cortices. Damage to these nuclei causes primary sensory deficits. The best clinical examples are damage to the ventroposterolateral (VPL) and ventroposteromedial (VPM) thalamic nuclei, resulting in sensory loss on the opposite side of the body, and damage to the lateral geniculate, causing a contralateral visual field cut. The motor-related thalamic nuclei receive afferent input from the basal ganglia, the substantia nigra, and the cerebellum and give efferent projections to the primary motor and premotor cortices. Damage to these nuclei causes contralateral motor deficits such as an emotional facial weakness and, in the dominant thalamus, a language difficulty. Limbic-related thalamic nuclei receive input from the hippocampus via the fornix and the medial temporal cortex and amygdala via the inferior thalamic peduncle. The output is to the cingulate gyrus and frontal lobes. Damage to these pathways may cause a permanent amnesia. Damage to nuclei with connections to cortical association areas may conceivably result in deficits of higher cortical functions; examples described include neglect[2] and aphasia,[3] but these abnormalities are less well characterized as to their anatomic basis.

A further constraint in understanding disorders related to thalamic damage is the blood supply of the thalamus. There are 16 named arteries that supply blood to the thalamus, most of which are not end arteries, and the nuclei supplied by one artery differ in different individuals.[4] Thus, knowing both the nuclei that these arteries commonly supply and the arterial territory affected does not necessarily translate into deducing which nuclei are damaged. To establish this, one has to analyze the lesion and plot it in three-dimensional space, using an atlas such as that of Schaltenbrand and Wahren.[5] Infarctions in four arterial territories commonly occur, can be recognized, and are described in this chapter. The anatomic basis of amnesia and aphasia following thalamic damage will also be addressed.[3,6,7]

SYNDROMES RELATED TO INFARCTION IN DIFFERENT ARTERIAL TERRITORIES

Infarction in the Territory of the Geniculothalamic Artery

The geniculothalamic artery is a branch of the posterior cerebral artery and may be affected by posterior cerebral occlusion.[8] Figure 36-1*A* shows a typical infarction in this territory. It commonly supplies part of the following thalamic nuclei: dorsomedial, posterolateral, reticular, parafascicular, and lateral geniculate (Fig. 36-1*B*). Infarction in this territory may cause the Dejerine-Roussy syndrome,[9] characterized by a fleeting hemiparesis, persistent hemianesthesia to touch, hyperesthesia and paroxysmal pain, slight ataxia, astereognosis, and choreoathetosis. Development of this syndrome does not invariably result from infarction in this territory; some may develop this syndrome and some may not. The Dejerine-Roussy syndrome is more common with right- than with left-sided thalamic infarction. The hallmark of geniculothalamic infarction is loss of sensation in all primary modalities on the contralateral side. Cognitive deficits do not characteristically

* **ACKNOWLEDGMENTS:** This work was supported in part by a National Institute of Aging grant AG08031-06S1 and the State of Florida Alzheimer's Disease Initiative.

Table 36-1
Thalamic connections[a]

Afferent connections	*Thalamic nucleus*	*Efferent connections*
Mammillothalamic tract Fornix	Anterior group (AV)	Cingulate gyrus
Globus pallidus Substantia nigra	Anterior ventral (VA)	Area 6 Diffuse frontal
Dentate nucleus Globus pallidus Substantia nigra	Ventrolateral (VL)	Area 4
Medial lemniscus	Ventroposterolateral (VPL)	Areas 1, 2, and 3
Spinothalamic tract	Ventroposteromedial (VPM)	
Trigeminothalamic tract	Lateral dorsal (LD)	Cingulate Medial parietal
	Lateral posterior	Superior parietal
Areas 18 and 19 Inferior parietal lobule	Pulvinar	Areas 18 and 19 Inferior parietal lobule
Optic tract	Lateral geniculate	Area 17
Inferior colliculus Lateral lemniscus	Medial geniculate	Areas 41 and 42
Amygdaloid complex Temporal neocortex	Dorsomedial nucleus Midline nuclei	Prefrontal cortex Amygdaloid nuclei Anterior cingulate cortex
Reticular formation Spinothalamic tract Dentate nucleus Areas 4, 6, 8, and 9 Globus pallidus Substantia reticulata	Intralaminar nuclei	Putamen Caudate nucleus

[a]Numbers in table refer to Brodmann's cortical areas.

occur with infarction in this territory unless there is associated posterior cerebral artery infarction. Sensory evoked potentials show absence of all waves after the positive wave at about 14 ms when the contralateral arm is stimulated.[7]

A geniculothalamic lacune (Fig. 36-1*C*) in the primary sensory nuclei causes the so-called pure hemisensory loss syndrome with contralateral pain and touch loss but no proprioception or vibration sense deficit.[7,10] There may be some dysesthesia but there is no concomitant neuropsychological deficit.

INFARCTION IN THE TERRITORY OF THE TUBEROTHALAMIC ARTERY

The tuberothalamic artery (also called the polar artery, the anterior internal optic artery, and the premammillary pedicle) is a branch of the posterior communicating artery. It supplies the anterolateral quadrant of the thalamus. Figure 36-2*A* shows a typical infarction in this territory, and the nuclei it typically supplies are seen in Fig. 36-2*B*. Circumstances in which there is infarction in this arterial territory include clipping of a posterior communicating aneurysm and a watershed

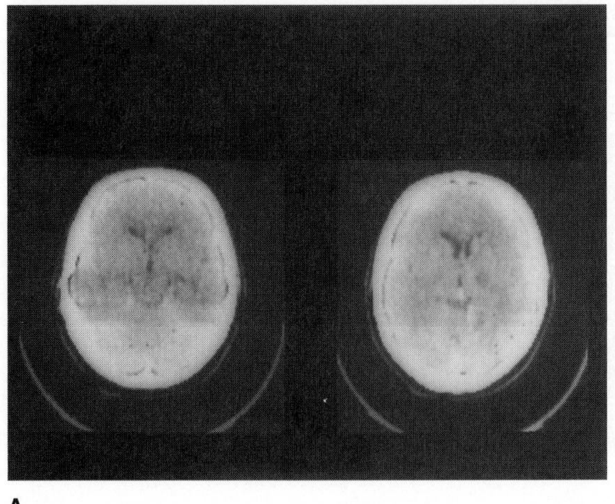
A

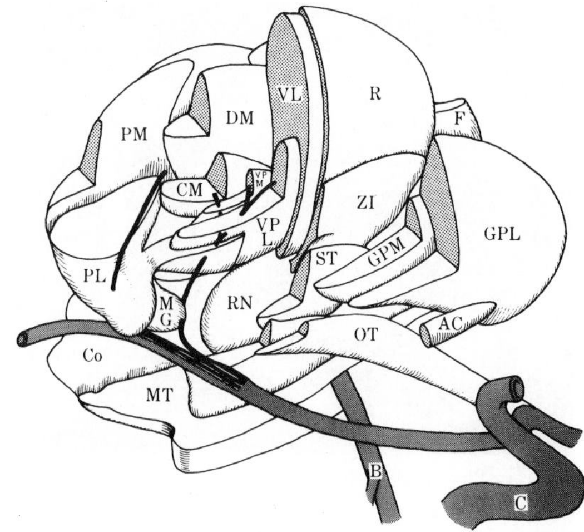

B

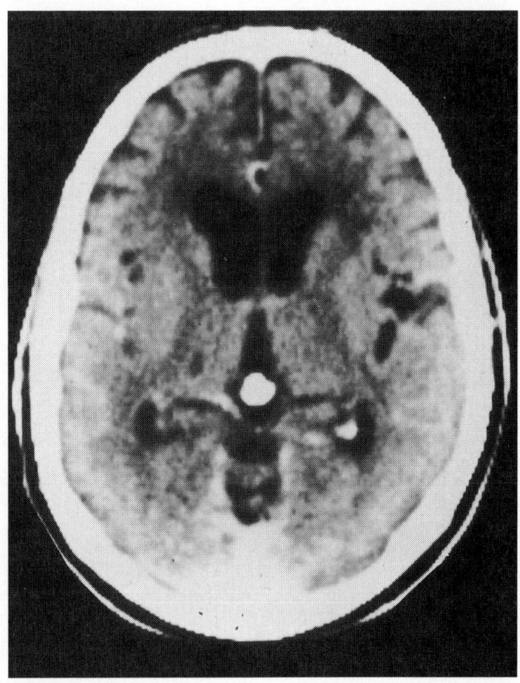
C

Figure 36-1
A. *Computed tomography scan showing infarction in the geniculothalamic arterial territory.* B. *Territory of the geniculothalamic artery. This is based upon Figs. 27-4 and 27-5 in the Schlesinger atlas.*[4] C. *Lacune in the geniculothalamic territory. This patient had contralateral hemisensory loss to pinprick and light touch sensations. A = anterior nucleus; AC = anterior commissure; AV = anterior ventral nucleus; B = basilar artery; C = carotid artery; CM = centrum medianum; Co = colliculi; DM = dorsomedial nucleus; DP = deep interpeduncular profundus artery; F = fornix; GPL = globus pallidus (lateral); GPM = globus pallidus (medial); LG = lateral geniculate; LP = lateral posterior nucleus; MG = medial geniculate; MAM = mammillary bodies; MT = midbrain tegmentum; MTT = mammillothalamic tract; OT = optic tract; PCe = posterior cerebral artery; PCo = posterior communicating artery; PL = pulvinar (lateral); PM = pulvinar (medial); R = reticular nucleus; RN = red nucleus; ST = subthalamic nucleus; Tt = tuberothalamic artery; VL = ventrolateral nucleus; VPL = ventral posterolateral nucleus; VPM = ventral posteromedial nucleus; ZI = zona inceta. (From Graff-Radford et al.,*[7] *with permission.)*

infarction. As a branch of the posterior communicating artery, this artery is between the anterior and posterior circulations, possibly making it vulnerable during the circumstances of a watershed infarction, such as a cardiac arrest. Patients with infarction in this territory often have an emotional facial paresis and sometimes have a hemiparesis if the infarction extends into the internal capsule, but they do not have sensory loss. In those with left-sided lesions, aphasia is frequent, along with impaired intellect, visuospatial abilities, memory, and temporal orientation. Patients with right-sided lesions have impaired nonverbal intellect,

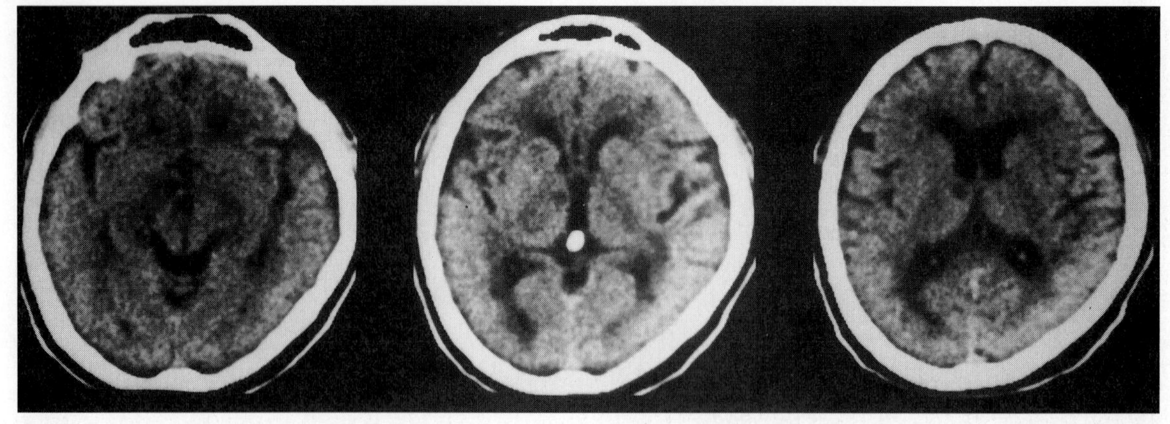

A

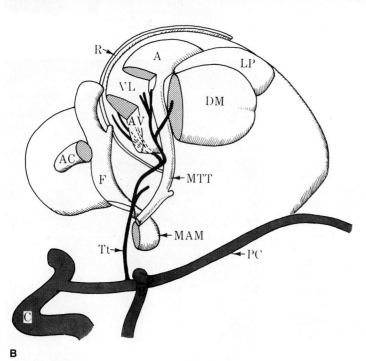

B

Figure 36-2
A. *Computed tomography showing a typical infarction in the tuberothalamic arterial territory.* B. *Territory of the tuberothalamic artery. This is based on Fig. 28-4 of the Schlesinger atlas.*[4] *Abbreviations as in Fig. 34-1. (From Graff-Radford et al.,*[7] *with permission.)*

visual perceptual discrimination, spatial judgment, visual memory, and constructional praxis. In contrast, they have preserved verbal intellect, verbal memory, and speech and language. Over time, patients improve substantially, but the pattern of deficits remains. Figure 36-2*A* shows the brain of a patient with infarction in this territory.

INFARCTION IN THE TERRITORY OF THE INTERPEDUNCULAR PROFUNDA ARTERY

This artery (also called the paramedian thalamic, the internal optic, and thalamoperforating pedicle) is a branch of the basilar portion of the posterior cerebral

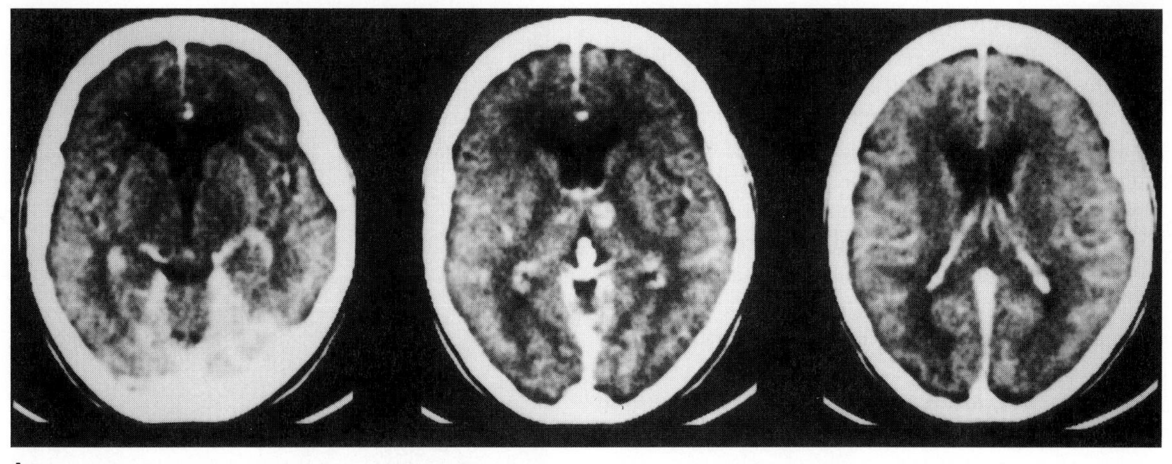

A

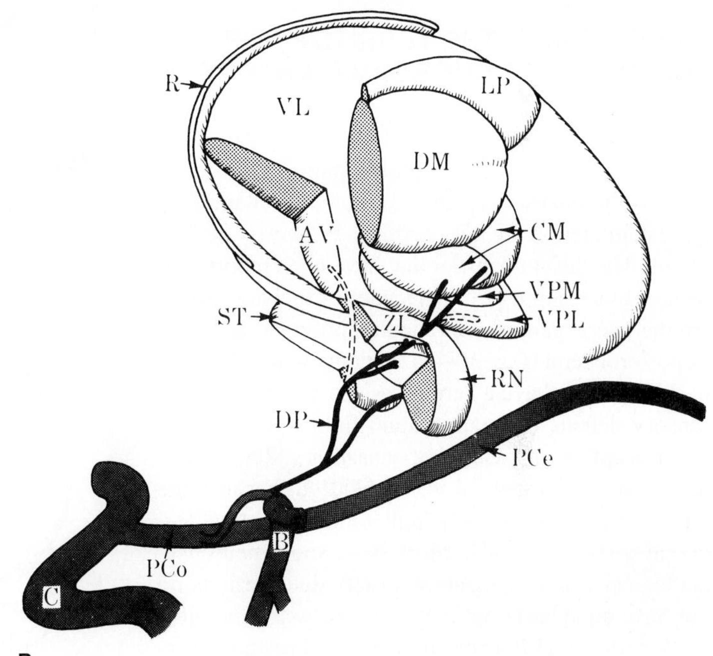

B

Figure 36-3
A. *Computed tomography showing bilateral infarction in the interpeduncular arterial territory.* B. *Territory of the interpeduncular profundus artery. The dotted line indicates other areas that may be supplied by this artery. Based on Figs. 28-6 and 28-7 of the Schlesinger atlas.*[4] *Abbreviations as in Fig. 34-1. (From Graff-Radford et al.,*[7] *with permission.)*

artery. It originates soon after the basilar artery bifurcates and may come off as one branch supplying both sides of the medial thalamus or as two separate branches. A typical infarction in this territory is seen in Fig. 36-3*A*. The typical nuclei it supplies can be seen in Fig. 36-3*B*. As the tuberothalamic artery may be small or even absent, the interpeduncular profunda may supply the dorsomedial, ventrolateral, and anteroventral thalamic nuclei; in addition, it has been described as supplying the dorsolateral, posterolateral, ventroposteromedial, and ventroposterolateral thalamic nuclei. In the majority of cases, part of the dorsomedial, the centrum medianum, and parafascicular nuclei make up its main territory of supply. The clinical picture of patients with infarction in this territory includes drowsiness in the early stages after the infarction and a vertical supranuclear gaze paresis.[11] At this stage, clinicians have difficulty diagnosing patients with infarction in this territory because there are usually no motor or sensory deficits and acute computed tomography (CT) is often normal. The vertical gaze paresis is probably related to infarction in the rostral part of the medial longitudinal fasciculus. As the patient improves, deficits can be found in intellect, memory, visuospatial processing, and orientation. Following these patients over time reveals that they either recover fairly well or have a permanent amnesia. The anatomic basis of this is discussed below.

INFARCTION IN THE TERRITORY OF THE ANTERIOR CHOROIDAL ARTERY

The anterior choroidal artery supplies part of the amygdala, medial temporal lobe, globus pallidus, posterior limb of the internal capsule, and lateral thalamus. A typical infarction in this territory is shown in Fig. 36-4*A*. The thalamic nuclei that have been reported to receive blood supply from the anterior thalamic artery are the lateral geniculate, reticular, pulvinar, and ventroposterolateral (Fig. 36-4*B*). Patients with infarction in this territory have a hemiparesis; a few have minor sensory deficits (to pinprick and light touch but not proprioception and vibration sensation). Rarely they may have a contralateral visual field cut because the artery does provide some supply to the optic tract and lateral geniculate body. Most have some neuropsychological deficit. Patients with left-sided lesions do not have an aphasia but may have a dysarthria, difficulty with verbal fluency, and impaired reading comprehension. Upon testing, there might be a mild verbal memory deficit, but this does not translate into a clinically significant amnesia. Visual memory may also be defective despite normal visual perception. Right-sided lesions impair visual perception, visual memory, and nonverbal intellect. Patients with infarction in this territory are often left with a significant hemiparesis.[12]

Figure 36-5 summarizes the sections of the thalamus where infarction in the above four arterial territories occurs.

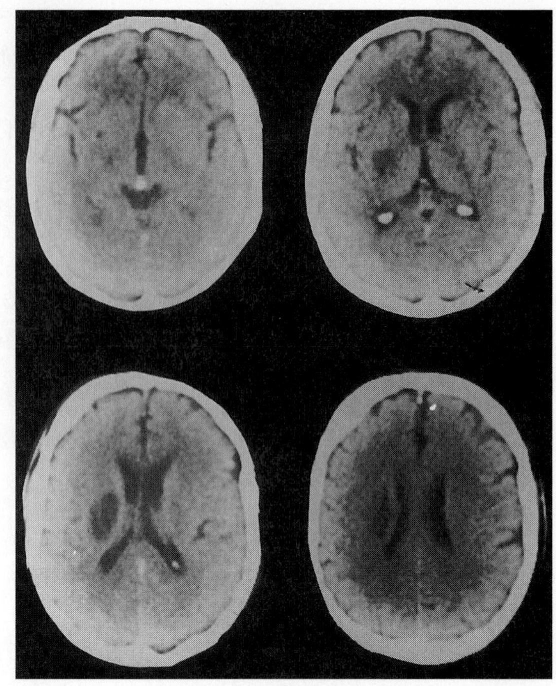

A

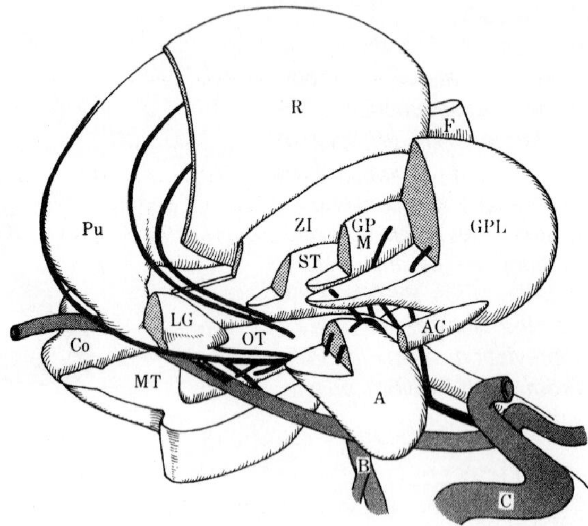

B

Figure 36-4
A. *Computed tomography showing infarction in the anterior choroidal territory. B. The territory of the anterior choroid is based on Fig. 27-2 of the Schlesinger atlas.*[4] *Abbreviations as in Fig. 34-1. (From Graff-Radford et al.,*[7] *with permission.)*

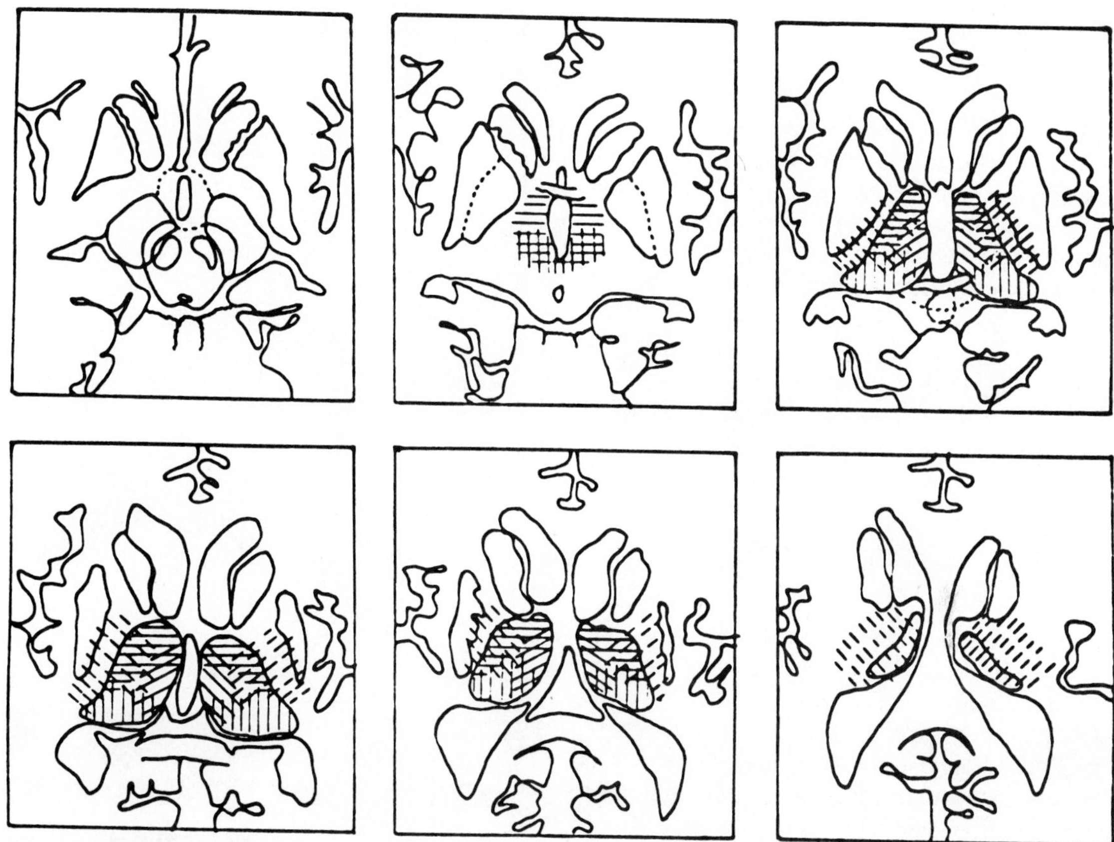

Figure 36-5
Templates (4 mm) through the thalamus depicting the following four arterial territories: Vertical hatching = geniculothalamic territory; horizontal hatching = tuberothalamic territory; unbroken diagonal hatching = interpeduncular profundus territory; broken diagonal hatching = anterior choroidal territory. (From Graff-Radford et al.,[7] with permission.)

DIENCEPHALIC AMNESIA

Anatomic Basis

From the classic case of H.M., it became clear that the medial temporal lobes are important in memory[13] (see Chap. 37). After numerous experiments in the primate, Mishkin[14] proposed that the structures involved in medial temporal lobe amnesia were the amygdala and hippocampus, and combined damage to these structures or their connections resulted in a severe amnesia. This work was further refined by Zola-Morgan and coworkers,[15,16] who have shown that the crucial areas in the medial temporal lobe which, when damaged, result in a severe amnesia are the hippocampus and the perirhinal cortex. Lesions to both these areas together increase the severity of the amnesia. Keeping this in mind, let us now look at the anatomy of the diencephalic lesions that result in amnesia.

Patients with bilateral infarction in the interpeduncular territory may be left with a permanent disabling amnesia. Lesions situated anteriorly cause an amnesia, whereas those situated posteriorly do not.[17] We believe that the crucial locus of the lesion that results in amnesia is where the mammillothalamic artery is adjacent to the ventroamygdalofugal pathway[6] (also called the inferior thalamic peduncle) (Fig. 36-6). A major hippocampal pathway to the thalamus is the fornix, which goes to the mammillary bodies from

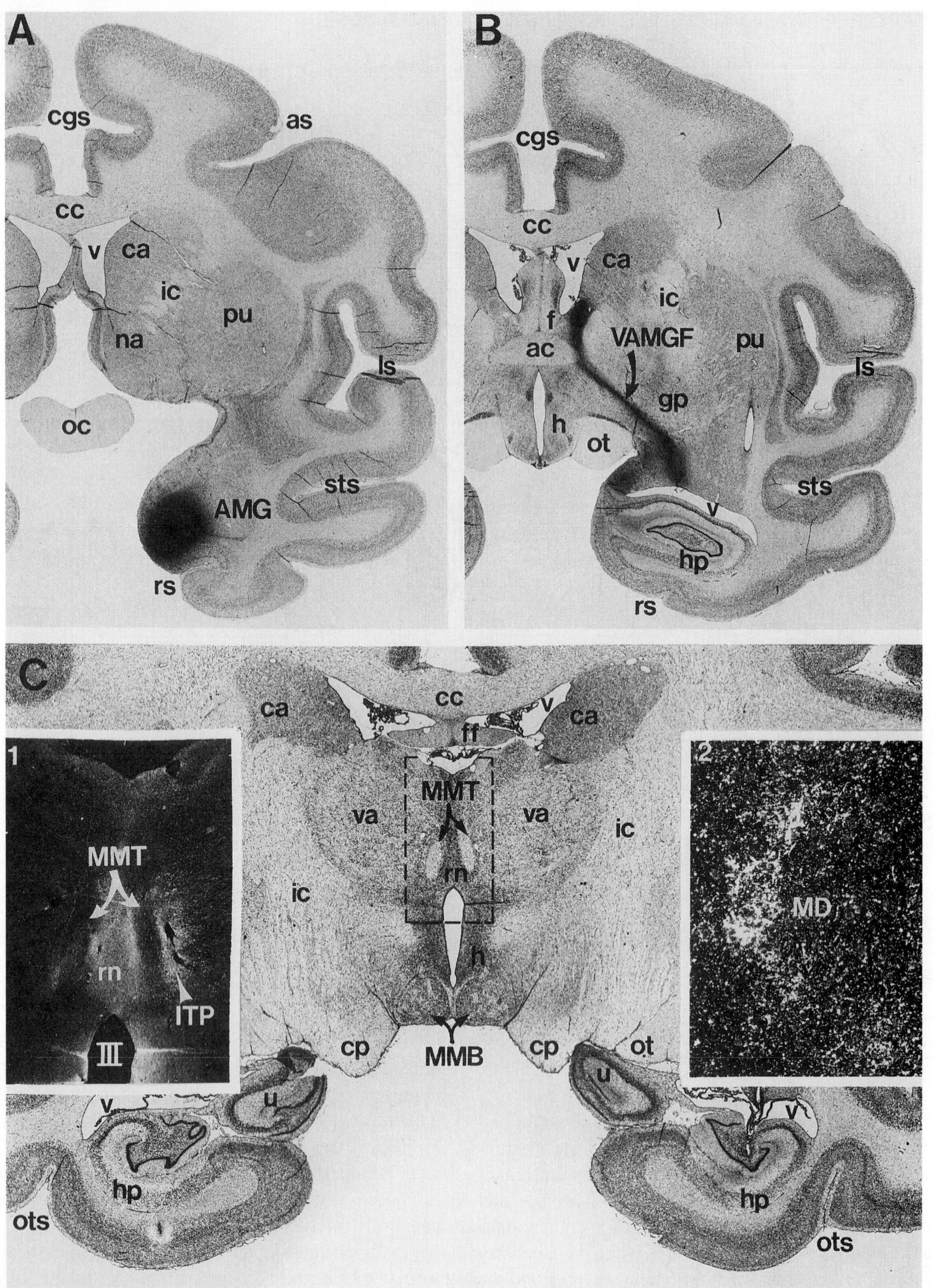

A
cgs
as
cc
v
ca
ic
pu
na
ls
oc
sts
AMG
rs
B
cgs
cc
v
ca
ic
f
VAMGF
pu
ac
ls
gp
h
ot
sts
v
hp
rs
C
cc
ca
v
ca
ff
1
2
MMT
va
va
ic
MMT
rn
ic
MD
rn
h
ITP
III
cp
MMB
cp
ot
u
u
v
v
hp
hp
ots
ots

which the mammillothalamic tract arises and then goes to the anterior thalamic nucleus. We also know that the amygdala sends a pathway through the ventroamygdalofugal pathway to the dorsomedial nucleus.[6] Although it has not yet been proved, it is likely that the ventroamygdalofugal pathway contains a pathway connecting the perirhinal cortex and the dorsomedial thalamic nucleus. Thus damage in the anterior thalamus may affect both hippocampal (mammillothalamic tract) and perirhinal (ventroamygdalofugal) pathways with small, strategically located bilateral lesions. This is analogous to the work of Zola-Morgan and colleagues, mentioned above. Further, there is an experimental primate model of this combination of lesions. Bachevalier and colleagues[18] reported on the effects of separate versus combined transection lesions of the fornix and amygdalofugal pathway. They found that the combined but not the separate lesions resulted in a severe recognition deficit in monkeys. We believe that this is analogous to the anatomic damage in our amnestic patients.

Other thalamic nuclei that, by their connections, may be involved in memory, are the midline thalamic nuclei, such as nucleus reunions. These nuclei have both afferent and efferent projections to the hippocampus and other medial temporal lobe structures.[1]

Neuropsychological Features

As with most amnesic patients (see Chaps. 37 and 38), the amnesia in these patients is characterized by severe anterograde memory loss, preservation of motor learning, and—in some patients—impaired retrograde memory.[6] In one of our patients whom we followed for 8 years, there was a temporal gradient to the memory loss.[6] Malamut and colleagues[19] reported a young postman who developed a disabling amnesia from bilateral thalamic infarction but was still able to sort the mail for the people and addresses on his route (except for the new persons added since his stroke). It is unclear if this represents preservation of retrograde memory or preservation of overlearned retrograde memories. Further patients should be studied in this regard.

DISTURBANCES OF SPEECH AND LANGUAGE ASSOCIATED WITH THALAMIC DYSFUNCTION

In an analysis of reported cases, we found that there were probably two kinds of thalamic language disturbance.[3] The first is associated with damage to the ventrolateral and anteroventral nuclei and is

Figure 36-6
A. *Nissl-stained transverse section from the rhesus monkey brain, developed from autoradiography showing the location of tritiated amino acids injected into the medial parts of the basolateral amygdaloid nuclei and the deep layers of the entorhinal cortex.* B. *Transverse section from the same animal demonstrating the ventroamygdalofugal pathway (VAMGF) in its course from the posterior amygdala beneath the globus pallidus (gp) to the bed nucleus of the stria terminalis at the base of the body of the lateral ventricle (v).* C. *Nissl-stained transverse section from the same case at the level of the uncus (u) and mammillary bodies (MMB). Note the midline region of the thalamus* (outlined rectangle) *and the position of the mammillothalamic tracts (MMT). Inset 1 is a dark-field photomicrograph of the rectangular area that demonstrates tritium-labeled axons in the inferior thalamic peduncle (ITP), immediately lateral to the mammillothalamic tract ipsilateral to the amygdaloid injection. As shown in inset 2, these axons follow a posterior intrathalamic course where they terminate in the dorsomedial thalamic nucleus. Note that a selective vascular lesion at the level of inset 1 would disrupt both the mammillothalamic tract and the inferior thalamic peduncle. Other abbreviations: ac = anterior commissure; as = arcuate sulcus; ca = caudate nucleus; cc = corpus callosum; cgs = cingulate sulcus; cp = cerebral peduncle; h = hypothalamus; hp = hippocampal formation; ic = internal capsule; ls = lateral sulcus; na = nucleus accumbens; oc = optic chiasm; ot = optic tract; ots = occipitotemporal sulcus; pu = putamen; rn = nucleus reunions; rs = rhinal sulcus; sts = superior temporal sulcus. (From Graff-Radford et al.,[7] with permission.)*

characterized by decreased but fluent speech output with paraphasias but no neologisms (see Chap. 9). An alternative anatomic explanation is that damage in this area might affect the reticular nucleus, which could influence the frontal lobes' input to the thalamus and in this way affect language.[20] The second type is characterized by normal or increased speech output and neologisms. The anatomic correlate is possibly damage in the pulvinar and posterolateral thalamic nucleus, but the anatomic evidence for this is not as convincing as that for the first hypothesis.

Whether or not these disturbances should be called aphasia is a matter of opinion. The fact that there are nonlinguistic disturbances in most of these patients distinguishes them from other aphasic patients in whom attention and memory are intact. However, these disturbances contain all the symptomatology of an aphasia and occur exclusively with lesions in the dominant thalamus in a set of nuclei that is closely interconnected with the language cortices. The similarity with transcortical aphasia is striking. Many of these patients have a good prognosis, improving considerably over time.[3]

REFERENCES

1. Carpenter BM, Sutin J: *Human Neuroanatomy,* 8th ed. Baltimore: Williams & Wilkins, 1983.
2. Watson RT, Valenstein E, Heilman KM: Thalamic neglect: Possible role of the medial thalamus and nucleus reticularis in behavior. *Arch Neurol* 38:501–506, 1981.
3. Graff-Radford N, Damasio A: Disturbances of speech and language associated with thalamic dysfunction. *Semin Neurol* 4:162–168, 1984.
4. Schlesinger B: *The Upper Brainstem in the Human.* Berlin: Springer-Verlag, 1976.
5. Schaltenbrand G, Wahren W: *Atlas for Stereotaxy of the Human Brain.* Stuttgart, Germany: Thieme, 1977.
6. Graff-Radford N, Tranel D, Van Hoesen G, Brandt J: Diencephalic amnesia. *Brain* 113:1–25, 1990.
7. Graff-Radford N, Damasio H, Yamada T, et al: Nonhemorrhagic thalamic infarctions: Clinical, neuropsychological and electrophysiological findings in four anatomical groups defined by CT. *Brain* 108:485–516, 1985.
8. Goto K, Tagawa K, Uemura K, et al: Posterior cerebral artery occlusion: Clinical, computed tomographic, and angiographic correlation. *Radiology* 132:357–368, 1979.
9. Dejerine J, Roussy G: Le syndrome thalamique. *Rev Neurol* 14:521–532, 1906.
10. Fisher CM: Thalamic pure sensory stroke: A pathological study. *Neurology* 32:871–876, 1978.
11. Buttner-Ennever JA, Buttner U, Cohen B, Baumgartner G: Vertical gaze paralysis and the rostral interstitial nucleus of the medial longitudinal fasciculus. *Brain* 105:125–149, 1982.
12. Bruno A, Graff-Radford N, Biller J, Adams H: Anterior choroidal artery territory infarction: A small vessel disease. *Stroke* 20:616–619, 1989.
13. Corkin S: Lasting consequences of bilateral medial temporal lobectomy: Clinical course and experimental findings in H.M. *Semin Neurol* 4:249–259, 1984.
14. Mishkin M: A memory system in the monkey. *Philos Trans R Soc Lond B Biol Sci* 298:85–95, 1982.
15. Zola-Morgan S, Squire LR, Amaral DG: Human amnesia and the medial temporal region: Enduring memory impairments following a bilateral lesion limited to field CA1 of the hippocampus. *J Neurosci* 6:2950–2967, 1986.
16. Zola-Morgan S, Squire LR, Amaral DG, Suzuki WA: Lesions of perirhinal and parahippocampal cortex that spare the amygdala and hippocampal formation produce severe memory impairment. *J Neurosci* 9:4355–4370, 1989.
17. Cramon DYV, Hebel N, Schuri U: A contribution to the anatomical basis of thalamic amnesia. *Brain* 108:993–1008, 1985.
18. Bachevalier J, Parkinson JK, Mishkin M: Visual recognition in monkeys: Effects of separate vs combined transection of fornix and amygdalofugal pathways. *Exp Brain Res* 57:554–561, 1985.
19. Malamut B, Graff-Radford N, Chawluk J, Gur R: Preserved and impaired memory function in a case of bilateral thalamic infarction. *Neurology* 42:163–169, 1992.
20. Nadeau SE, Crosson B: Subcortical aphasia. *Brain Lang.* In press.

Part 6

MEMORY AND AMNESIA

Chapter 37

AMNESIA: NEUROANATOMIC AND CLINICAL ISSUES

Matthias Brand
Hans J. Markowitsch

Memory is one of the most important and complex human brain functions and disturbances of memory processes can result in disastrous restrictions of life quality. Amnesic syndromes can occur as a consequence of widespread brain damage, as in Alzheimer's disease, as well as following tiny lesions of specific structures (e.g., in amnesics with diencephalic or mediotemporal lobe damage), or functional alterations of the brain (e.g., in psychogenic amnesia). Our knowledge of brain and memory interactions has increased greatly in recent years. The expansion of various methods to study brain-behavior interactions—primarily modern static and functional neuroimaging methods but also refined techniques in studying brain-lesioned animals—has substantiated our knowledge of interactions between different brain structures, neural nets, and specific memory processes. Detailed descriptions and neuropsychological examinations of brain-damaged patients complete the multifarious spectrum of methods used in neuroscientific reasearch and have considerably advanced our theoretical framework with respect to brain-memory relations.

CLASSIFICATION OF MEMORY

Memory can be subdivided along the dimensions of time (e.g., short- and long-term memory)[1] and content (e.g., episodic and semantic memory). Along the content-based distinction of memory, the division of four long-term memory systems—originally postulated by Tulving[2]—is widely accepted: episodic memory, semantic memory, procedural memory, and priming[3] (see also Chap. 38). The *episodic memory* system represents episodes of a person's life with respect to time and locus (e.g. "my first trip to New York in summer 1990"). The *semantic memory* system, discussed in Chap. 39, comprises facts without a personal reference (e.g., arithmetical rules, world knowledge). *Procedural memory* comprises motor, sensory, and cognitive skills (e.g., knowing how to play cards), and *priming* describes the improved reproduction or recognition of information that has already been experienced. Retrieval of episodic memories occurs explicitly or intentionally, while retrieval of information of the other memory systems is implicit or incidental.[2]

Furthermore, memory can be classified according to the stages of information processing, whereby the *encoding* (initial entry into memory), *consolidation* (gradually increasing durability of the memory) as well as, *storage,* and *retrieval* of information are established. Regarding this subdivision, it is assumed that specific brain structures, so-called bottleneck structures (e.g., Refs. 4 and 5), are primarily involved in different memory processes (see Table 37-1).

Memory depends on a wide range of sensory, perceptual, attentive, emotional, and motivational processes and their neuroanatomic correlates. As discussed in Chap. 8, the role of a brain area cannot be understood either through isolated lesion studies or functional imaging studies in normal subjects. Specifically in the domain of memory, Chow[7] has pointed out that if a brain lesion does not affect a learning task, it cannot be concluded that this brain region is not involved in that function. And further, if the lesion influences the performance of a task, it does not unconditionally mean that it is the only structure engaged. The aim of ablation methods to clarify the functions of damaged brain structures is effectively never attainable, for it is based on observations in patients without the region of interest. It is important to take these statements into account in interpreting and integrating results from descriptions of brain-damaged patients as well as from neuroimaging studies.

Table 37-1
Structures relevant for the four long-term memory systems and the different memory processes

	Episodic memory	*Semantic memory*	*Procedural memory*	*Priming*
Encoding and consolidation	Limbic system, prefrontal cortex?*	Limbic system/ cerebral cortex	Basal ganglia, cerebellar structures	Cerebral cortex (uni- and polymodal areas)
Storage	Cerebral cortex (mainly association areas), limbic regions?*	Cerebral cortex (mainly association areas)	Basal ganglia, cerebellar structures	Cerebral cortex (uni- and polymodal areas)
Retrieval	Temporofrontal cortex (right)	Temporofrontal cortex (left)	Basal ganglia, cerebellar structures	Cerebral cortex (uni- and polymodal areas)

*No consistent evidence.
Source: Modified from Markowitsch.[6]

AMNESIC SYNDROMES

In describing patients' amnesic symptoms, the distinction between anterograde and retrograde amnesia is of crucial importance. Patients with anterograde amnesia are unable to form new memories, whereas patients with retrograde amnesia are impaired in retrieving "old" memories stored in the long-term memory system. Figure 37-1 shows relations between the point of a critical incident and possible amnesic states.

The term *amnesia* comprises various amnesic types, which differ in the severity and specificity of their symptoms as well as in their origins. The most extensive type is global amnesia, consisting of both anterograde and retrograde memory impairments. Global amnesia can occur following different etiologies with various lesion sites of brain damage. In Table 37-2, common etiologies of global amnesia and affected brain regions are listed. Examples of different amnesic states are given in Table 37-3.

The following sections contain examples of typical amnesic syndromes and their neuroanatomic and functional aspects.

H.M.: The Classic Case of Mediotemporal Lobe Amnesia

H.M. is probably the most extensively studied patient of this type and represents one of the milestones in the history of neuropsychological research. H.M., a 23-year-old right-handed man of average intelligence, was suffering from pharmacologically intractable epilepsy when his doctor decided to perform a bilateral resection of major portions of his mediotemporal lobes in order to reduce the frequency of H.M.'s attacks.[10] Magnetic resonance imaging (MRI), done several decades later, showed brain lesions comprising the amygdala, the parahippocampal-entorhinal cortex, and the anterior hippocampus bilaterally.[11] After surgery, H.M. became persistently anterograde amnesic. He lost his ability to store new information long-term, so that

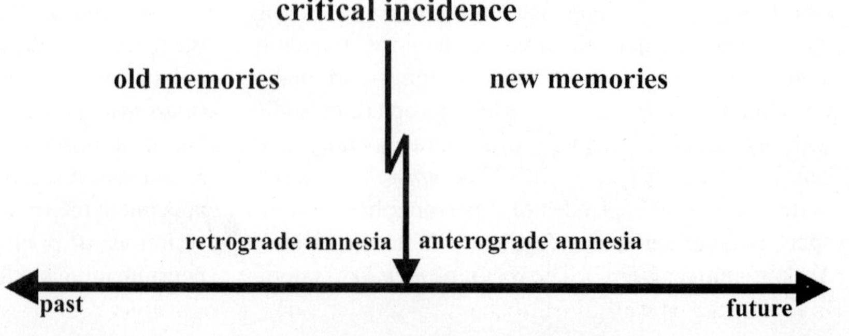

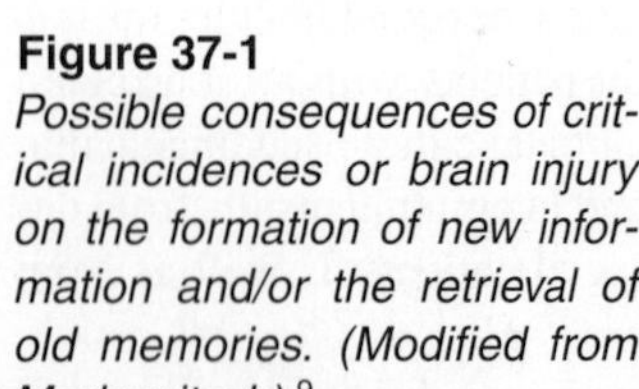
Figure 37-1
Possible consequences of critical incidences or brain injury on the formation of new information and/or the retrieval of old memories. (Modified from Markowitsch).[9]

Table 37-2
Overview of patient groups in whom global amnesic syndromes may be prominent

Etiology	*Most common lesion sites*
Intracranial tumors	Limbic thalamus, medial temporal lobe, posterior cingulate gyrus, fornix, orbitofrontal cortex
Cerebral infarctions, ruptured aneurysms, aneurysm surgery	Limbic nuclei of the thalamus (paramedian, polar artery), orbitofrontal cortex and basal forebrain (anterior communicating artery)
Closed head injury	Orbitofrontal cortex, temporal pole
Viral infections (e.g., herpes simplex encephalitis)	Limbic and paralimbic cortex
Avitaminoses (e.g., B_1 deficiency)	Limbic thalamus, mammillary bodies (as in Korsakoff's syndrome)
Neurotoxin exposure	Hippocampus
Temporal lobe epilepsy	Temporal lobe
Degenerative diseases of the CNS (e.g., Alzheimer's or Pick's disease)	Entorhinal cortex, hippocampal formation, amygdala, prefrontal and inferotemporal cortex
Anoxia or hypoxia (e.g., after a heart attack or drowning)	Hippocampus (CA1 sector)
Drugs	Limbic system
Electroconvulsive therapy	Probably limbic system

Source: Modified from Markowitsch.[8]

time appeared to have stopped for him. Intellectual functions as well as emotional, behavioral, and social skills were not disturbed. Furthermore, impairments in short-term memory, working memory, and other cognitive abilities like reading, writing, and calculating were not observed. Recall of remote autobiographic memories was also unaffected. H.M. was extensively examined from 1955 to the present, and the reports on H.M. have pointed out the importance of the mediotemporal lobes for forming new memories.

The Korsakoff's Syndrome: A Classic Disease Related to Medial Diencephalic Lesions

Also discussed in Chap. 51, Korsakoff's syndrome results from long-term alcohol addiction or abuse. Brain damage as well as neurochemical dysfunctions in Korsakoff's patients are probably due to thiamine (vitamin B_1) deficiency and/or additional neurotoxic effects of ethanol. The damage presumably resulting in memory deficits in Korsakoff's syndrome comprises medial diencephalic structures such as the mammillary bodies, the mediodorsal and anterior thalamic nuclei, as well as nonspecific medial thalamic nuclei and the medial pulvinar.

Clinical symptoms of Korsakoff's patients consist of remarkable memory impairments, largely comparable to those after mediotemporal lobe damage, while intelligence may remain unchanged. Besides the mnestic deficits, disorientation and a tendency to confabulate are traditionally associated with Korsakoff's syndrome.[12]

The main symptom, the inability to store new information, includes both verbal and figural memory. Figure 37-2 shows an example for the deficient

Table 37-3
Examples of different types of amnesia and amnesic states

Amnesia type or state	*Amnesic symptoms*
Anterograde amnesia	The failure to store new memories long-term
Retrograde amnesia	The failure to retrieve (or ecphorize) old memories
Transient global amnesia	Anterograde (and possibly, although to a lesser degree, retrograde) amnesia for a time period of 1 day or less
Psychogenic amnesia	Retrograde (and in rare instances, also anterograde) amnesia without (obvious) brain damage, usually as a consequence of strong psychic pressure(s)
Functional amnesia	Retrograde (and in rare instances, also anterograde) amnesia of differing, but at least partly psychic, origin
Material- and modality-specific amnesias	Inability to retrieve specific material (e.g., common names) or to process within a specific modality (e.g., to remember or retrieve colors)
Reduplicative paramnesia	The phenomenon of being convinced that a person, place, or object exists twice

Source: Modified from Markowitsch.[9]

Figure 37-2
A. The nearly perfect copy of the Rey-Osterrieth complex figure (R-O-F) made by a 45-year-old male Korsakoff's patient.
B. Drawing of the R-O-F from memory after a 30-min delay by the same patient.

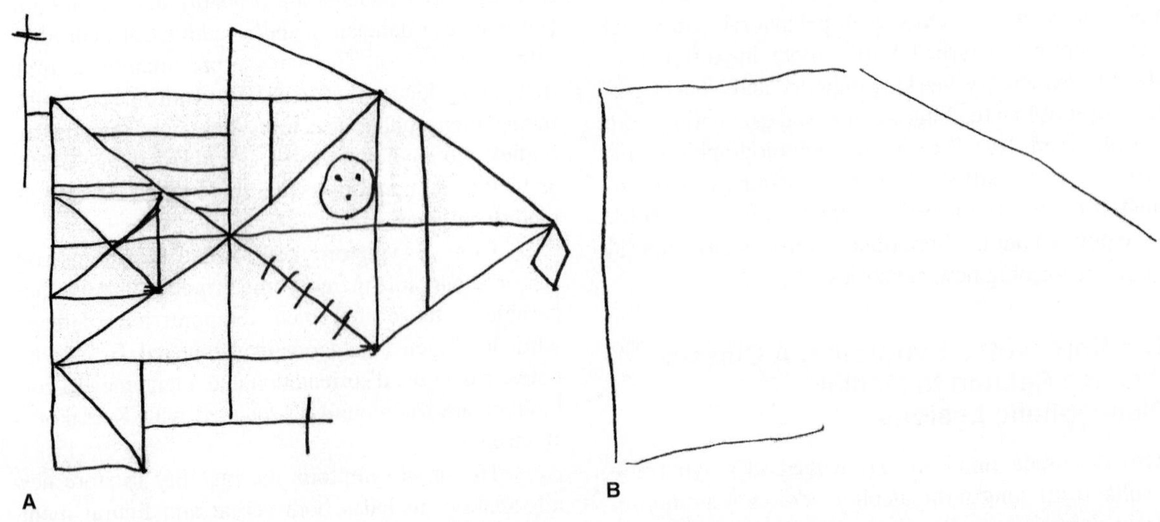

figural memory of a patient with Korsakoff's symptomatology.

Retrograde amnesia can also be observed in Korsakoff's patients, but to a more variable degree.[13–15] Furthermore, recent studies have revealed additional impairments of other cognitive domains in Korsakoff's patients, primarily of functions associated with the frontal lobes.[16]

The relevance of individual diencephalic structures for the memory deficits of Korsakoff's patients has been controversial. Mair et al.[17] described in detail neuropsychological changes and pathological alterations of the brain after postmortem analyses of two cases and concluded that the mammillary bodies and anterior and midline thalamic nuclei (e.g., the paratenial nuclei) are involved in the amnesic symptoms of Korsakoff's syndrome, whereas the medial dorsal nuclei play a minor role only. To work out structures involved in Korsakoff's syndrome, more recent reports differentiate between the Wernicke's encephalopathy, the first, transient phase of the Wernicke-Korsakoff syndrome, and the later and chronic Korsakoff's state. In this context, Harding et al.[18] revealed that the anterior thalamic nuclei are probably specifically affected in the Korsakoff's state but not in the Wernicke's phase and therefore might be relevant for the amnesic symptoms.

Although Korsakoff's syndrome is one of the most common etiologies for diencephalic amnesia, other causes for damage of diencephalic structures such as thalamic infarctions (e.g., Refs. 19 and 20) can also result in memory disturbances.

Given these examples of classic amnesic syndromes, we come back to the main subject of this chapter: the anatomic bases of memory and amnesia.

THE BRAIN SITES OF MEMORY PROCESSES AND THEIR DISTURBANCES

Encoding and Consolidation

The different memory systems described above are probably represented in specific agglomerates of brain regions. For the episodic memory system the medial temporal lobes, the medial diencephalon, and the basal forebrain as well as prefrontal regions act as so-called "bottleneck structures"[4,5] and their involvement in encoding and consolidation of (episodic and semantic) information is described consistently.[8] For encoding and consolidation of information, two interconnected but separable limbic circuits are proposed to act: the Papez circuit and the amygdaloid (basolateral limbic) circuit (Figs. 37-3 and 37-4).

Papez himself[21] viewed the circuit named after him as principally relevant for emotional analyses, but more recent studies have revealed a strong engagement of these structures and fiber connections in the

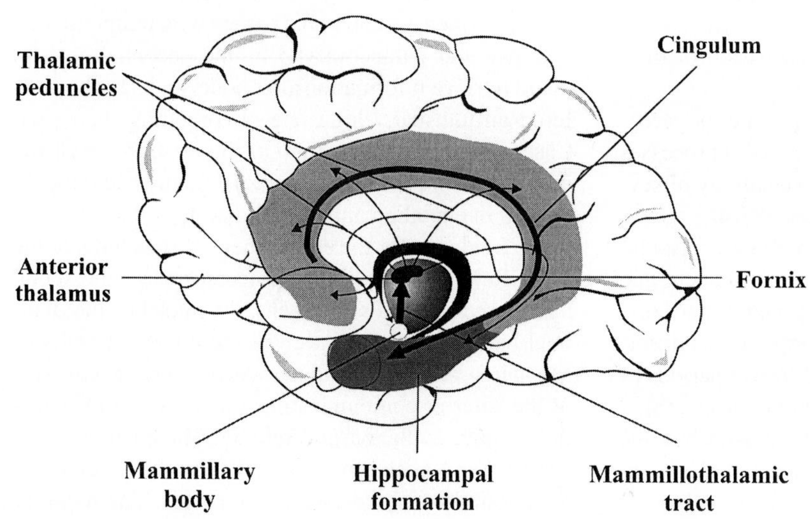

Figure 37-3
The Papez circuit.

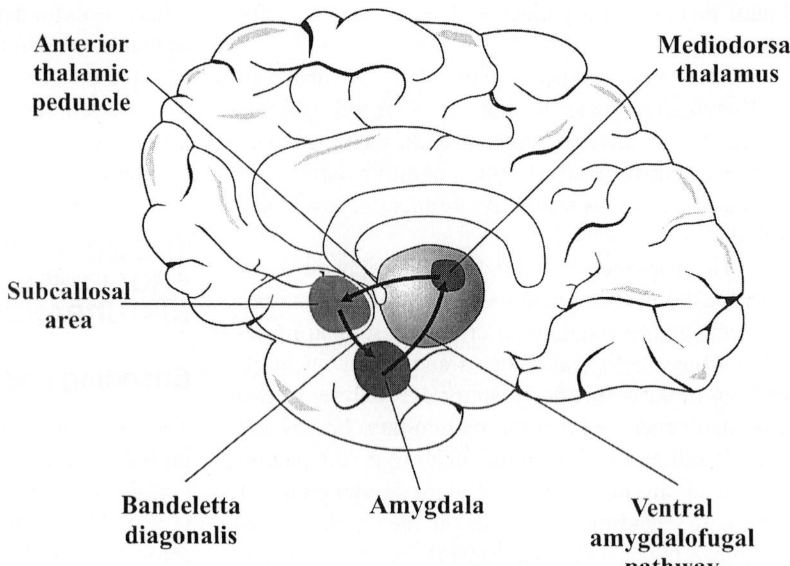

Figure 37-4
The basolateral limbic circuit comprising the amygdala, the mediodorsal nucleus of the thalamus, and portions of the basal forebrain as well as various interconnecting fibers such as the bandeletta diagonalis.

transfer of all kinds of information from short- to long-term memory.[22] The amygdaloid or basolateral limbic circuit, on the other hand, seems to be predominantly engaged in emotional processing and in encoding the emotional valence of experiences.

The hippocampal-entorhinal complex and the limbic thalamic nuclei, especially, are most closely related to the encoding and consolidation of information of the episodic memory system. Damage to these regions usually causes severe memory impairments. Vargha-Khadem and coworkers[23] have suggested that the hippocampus proper is of crucial importance for episodic memory encoding (for a discussion of their findings).[24]

Different cortical and subcortical limbic structures are involved in memory and emotional processes to a variable degree. The functional specificity of several limbic structures is shown in Table 37-4.

Various clinical observations suggest a dissociation between initial encoding and the subsequent and more stable consolidation of information. Furthermore, various case reports lead to the assumption that different brain structures are engaged at different periods of the memory process. For instance, Markowitsch et al.[26] described a 30-year-old female patient who became amnesic after a whiplash trauma. Neuroradiologic investigations revealed no specific brain damage, but she had sustained hearing deficits and a tunnel view after her injury. She lost her ability to retrieve newly acquired information within 30 min to a few hours, whereas non-memory-related verbal and nonverbal functions remained unchanged and her intelligence was quite superior.

Another patient, reported by Kapur et al.,[27] suffering from temporal lobe epilepsy, showed remarkable impairments to remember information 40 days after learning, although he was able to encode and recall information for hours and days. O'Connor et al.[28] described a comparable patient with temporal lobe epilepsy and paraneoplastic limbic encephalitis who could retrieve information after hours and days but suffered an unusually high rate of forgetting thereafter. Case reports like these support the assumption of the involvement of different (limbic) structures and mechanisms in encoding and consolidation.

Evidence for the engagement of structures of the basal forebrain in memory processes (e.g., the septal nuclei, the nucleus accumbens, the nuclei of the diagonal band of Broca, as well as the nucleus basalis of Meynert) comes from patients with ruptured aneurysms of the anterior communicating artery (ACoA),[29] causing damage to the basal forebrain. The eventually resulting AcoA syndrome consists of amnesia, a tendency to confabulate, and personality changes. The memory

Table 37-4
Structures of the limbic system and their principal functional involvements

Structure	*Functional implication(s)*
Telencephalon, cortical	
Cingulate gyrus	Attention, drive, pain reception
Hippocampal formation	Memory, spatiotemporal integration
Entorhinal region	Memory
Telencephalon, subcortical	
Amygdala	Emotional evaluation, motivations, olfaction
Basal forebrain	Emotional evaluation, memory
Diencephalon	
Mammillary bodies	Memory, emotion?*
Anterior thalamic nucleus	Memory, emotion, attention
Mediodorsal thalamic nucleus	Memory, consciousness?*/sleep, emotion
Nonspecific thalamic nuclei	Consciousness?*
Associated regions ("paralimbic cortex"; expanded limbic system)	
Medial and orbitofrontal cortex	Emotional evaluation, social behavior, initiative (initiation of retrieval)
Insula	Sensory-motivational integration?*
Temporal pole (area 38)	Memory-related sensory integration, initiation of recall

*No consistent evidence.
Source: Modified from Markowitsch.[25]

impairments comprise both recall and recognition, with a disproportionate deficit in recall probably caused by additional frontal lobe lesions. Furthermore, septal lesions or damage of interconnecting fibers between the septum and hippocampal formation can lead to anterograde and retrograde amnesia.[30]

Storage

Long-term storage of information is presumed to involve widespread cortical regions— primarily association cortices—with alterations in synaptic conjunctions.[31] For binding information, limbic regions seem to play a critical role.[8]

The role of both cortical and limbic regions for long-term storage is shown, for instance, in patients with Alzheimer's disease. Alzheimer's patients are known to have persistent and severe memory impairments comprising episodic (e.g., Refs. 32 and 33) as well as semantic memory (e.g., Refs. 34 and 36). Furthermore, priming deficits and procedural memory impairments can occur.[37–39] Short-term and working memory functions may also be affected,[40,41] just like attention and executive functions.[42,43] Further possible symptoms of Alzheimer's disease are agnosia, apraxia, and aphasia. Though Alzheimer's disease is discussed as being a "cortical dementia," it must be mentioned that noncortical limbic and other subcortical structures are affected as well.[44] Therefore the various memory deficits observed in Alzheimer's patients may not be caused by damage of cortical and limbic structures alone. For instance, procedural memory deficits of Alzheimer's patients are found similarly as in patients with Huntington's or Parkinson's disease. As mentioned above, the third long-term memory system—procedural memory—depends significantly on basal ganglial structures. Therefore it is not unexpected that patients with damage of these regions are impaired in procedural memory.

Support for the major role of uni- and polymodal neocortical areas for priming—the fourth long-term memory system—came, for instance, from the study of Nielsen-Bohlman et al.[45] They found that patients with temporooccipital lesions are impaired in an implicit memory task (word-stem completion task). Though their patients suffered from lesions extending to mediotemporal lobe structures, these investigators argued that priming deficits are not typical in patients with mediotemporal lobe amnesia; they therefore concluded that the deficits of their patients were caused by the temporooccipital lesions (cf. also Refs. 46 and 47).

The important role of neocortical regions for the storage and retrieval of information can also be seen in material- and modality-restricted forms of amnesia (cf. Table 37-3); as an example, Reinkemeier et al.[48] reported the case of a patient who, following neocortical damage, was unable to remember names and faces.

Retrieval

For retrieval of information, a right-left distinction is assumed: the right hemisphere is viewed as to be primarily engaged in retrieval of episodic memories, while the left hemisphere seems to play a critical role in retrieval of semantic memories.[8,49] The brain region most strongly associated with retrieval is the prefrontal cortex of both hemispheres, following the content-based distinction (right-left) mentioned previously. Additionally, anterior temporal and limbic structures of the medial diencephalon and mediotemporal lobe regions support the retrieval especially of emotionally flavored information.[5]

The role of the hippocampal formation in episodic memory retrieval has been controversial. While Conway et al.[50] did not find substantial differences between hippocampal activation in recent and remote memory, Haist et al.[51] revealed a probable time-limited engagement of the hippocampal formation in human memory. They argued that the entorhinal cortex would be more involved than the hippocampus in remote memory functions. Similarly, Piefke et al.,[52] in a study with functional magnetic resonance imaging, demonstrated a time-limited engagement of the hippocampal formation for the retrieval of autobiographical events.

Lepage et al.[53] proposed that there is a distinction between different portions of the hippocampal formation and suggested that encoding is associated with activation of rostral portions of the hippocampal formation, whereas retrieval is related to activation of the caudal portions of this region. Dolan and Fletcher[54] confirmed this anterior-posterior functional segregation of the mediotemporal lobe (which had been questioned by Schacter and Wagner[55]).

Case reports of patients with more or less isolated retrograde amnesia support the involvement of mediotemporal regions in retrieval of memories.[56] In line with the mentioned right-left distinction of prefrontal activation in retrieval in healthy subjects, left-sided damage to the anterior temporal regions is related to semantic remote memory impairments,[57,58] whereas right-sided lesions tend to produce autobiographical memory disturbances.[59,60]

To summarize, the neural correlate of memory is not a single brain structure but a distributed network of structures and fiber connections. Figure 37-5 provides an overview of structures and circuits assumed to be centrally engaged in memory processes.

MEMORY AND EMOTION

The affective connotation of information is of crucial importance for its encoding and consolidation as well as for storage and retrieval. The most widely mentioned brain structure for an evaluation of the affective valence of information is the amygdala.[61] The amygdala, located in the anterior medial portion of the temporal lobe, consists of various nuclei and is connected with the hippocampal formation and further cortical and subcortical structures.[62] Various studies have revealed an amygdalar activity–dependent modulation of long-term memory storage and retrieval,[63] with an unequal participation of the two amygdalae.[64] Research on the functions of the amygdala in memory have revealed that gender is a major factor influencing the right-left distinction, with increased activity of the right amygdala in men related to emotion-induced improved recall of material and increased activity of the left amygdala in female subjects linked to better recall of emotional stimuli.[65] In addition to the amygdala, the septum plays an important role in emotional processing.[66]

The emotional valence of information can affect both increasing and decreasing storage. It has long been known that bilateral damage of the amygdaloid complex may lead to the Klüver-Bucy syndrome.[67]

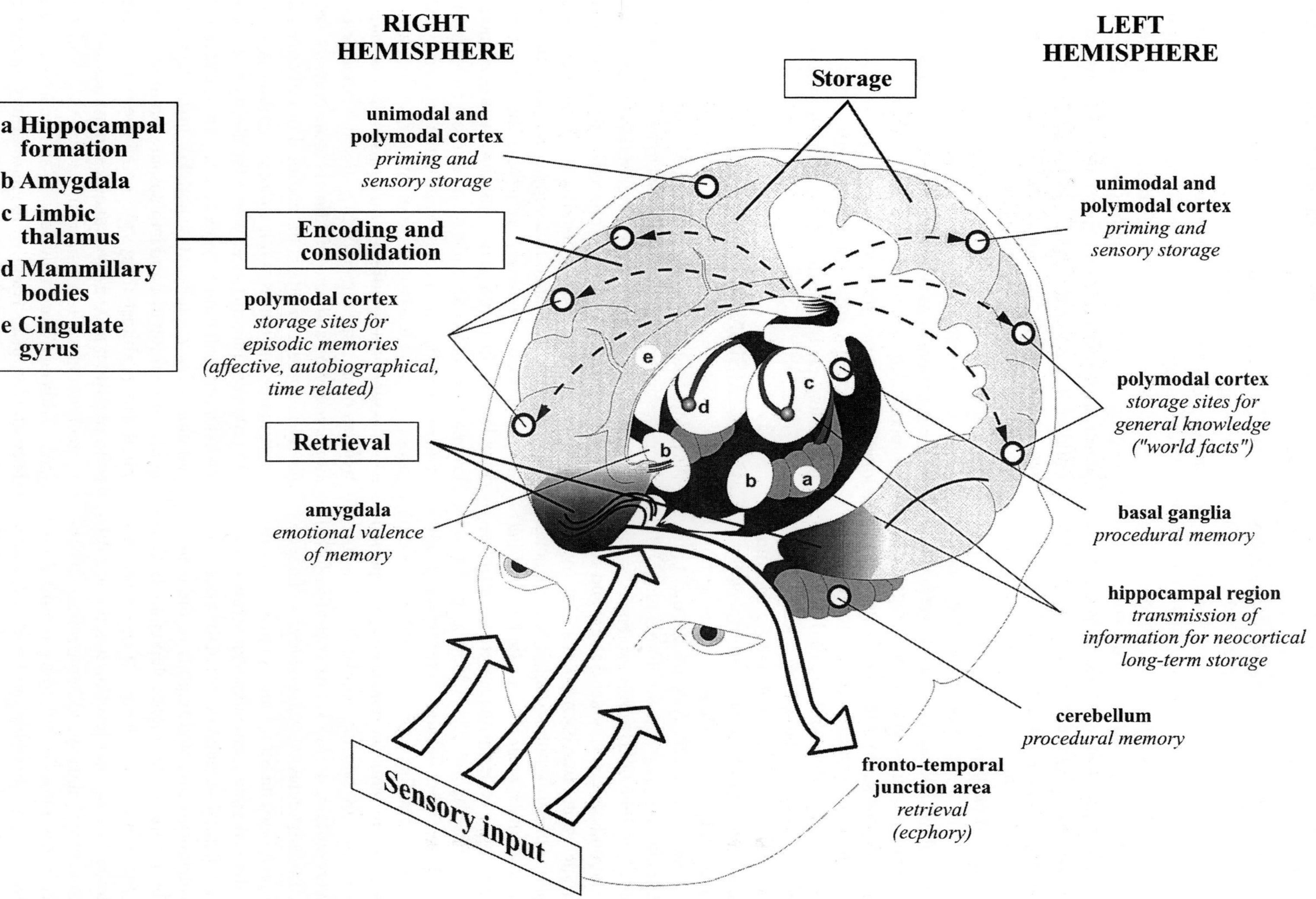

Figure 37-5
Overview of the brain structures engaged in long-term memory encoding and consolidation, storage, and retrieval. (Modified from Markowitsch.[8])

The Klüver-Bucy syndrome is composed of a complex symptomatology that includes (anterograde) amnesia and emotional disturbances as well as agnosia, hypersexuality, hyperorality, hyperphagia, tameness, and hypermetamorphosis. More recently, descriptions of patients with a selective mineralization of the amygdaloid complex due to Urbach-Wiethe disease (UWD)[68] have supported the assumption of the relevance of this limbic structure for the enhancement of memory for emotionally arousing information.[69,70]

Besides the reduced memory performance for emotional material because of brain damage (primarily damage to limbic regions), emotional overflow can also result in memory impairments. For instance, traumatic stress accompanied by improper coping strategies may lead to remarkable encoding and retrieval disturbances, probably due to increased release of stress-related hormones.[71] The intense release of such glucocorticoids may result in morphologic and functional alterations of limbic structures, especially in mediotemporal regions.[72,73] These can cause broad changes in neurotransmitter systems of the brain, such as of the cholinergic,[74] the serotoninergic,[75] the dopaminergic,[76] and the GABAergic systems.[77]

The relation between traumatic stress and functional brain alterations has been pointed out by recent descriptions of cases with so called "psychogenic amnesia." Markowitsch et al.[78] described a male patient (A.M.N.) who, at age 4, had seen a man burning to death. At the age of 23, A.M.N. experienced a fire in his house and became anterogradely amnesic immediately after that event. Additionally, he developed a retrograde amnesia concerning the period of the last 6 years of his life. Conventional neurologic and neuroradiologic (MRI) investigations failed to reveal clinically relevant morphologic changes. However, a positron emission tomography (PET) investigation showed functional alterations (decreased regional cerebral glucose metabolism) of the brain, particularly in memory-associated regions of the mediotemporal lobe and the medial diencephalon. In the case of A.M.N., these functional changes were temporary, and he returned to a normal level of functioning following pharmacologic and psychotherapeutic interventions. Similarly, his amnesic symptoms improved.

Another case of probable stress-related amnesia is that of F.A., also reported by Markowitsch et al.[79] F.A., a 46-year-old male patient, showed severe and persistent anterograde amnesia and short-term memory deficits with otherwise largely preserved intellectual capacities. He was diagnosed as being depressed, but different forms of drug treatment as well as psychotherapeutic interventions were ineffective. Exploration revealed a complicated, stressful life since childhood (e.g., severe conflicts with his authoritarian father). Neurologic investigations including static and dynamic neuroimaging did not reveal any pathologic brain alteration. The authors concluded that stress- or depression-related prolonged glucosteroid release can cause functional changes in memory-associated brain structures and introduced the term of *mnestic block syndrome* to describe memory impairments without clear organic or explicit psychogenic origin and including the various characteristics of functional amnesia.

CONCLUSION

As pointed out above, amnesia can be due to various etiologies and therefore by alterations to various and very divergent structures of the brain as well as by functional alterations of neuronal nets, induced by stress-hormone releases. Major mnestic disturbances can occur as a consequence of damage to a single brain structure, as has been seen in patients with focal mediotemporal lobe lesions, or they can be caused by neurodegenerative diseases affecting widespread cortical and subcortical regions. Psychic pressure and enduring or massive stress may also lead to severe memory impairments.

Amnesia also differs in quantitive and qualitative aspects of its appearance. While in some amnesic patients encoding and consolidation is more or less selectively disturbed, in others the retrieval of old episodic or semantic memories is impaired. Nevertheless, there are only very rare instances where the ability to encode and store information long-term as well as the recall of old memories is totally abolished. For instance, riding a bike or learning to avoid unpleasant stimuli in an implicit way is almost always preserved even in patients with persistent and severe amnesic syndromes such as in mediotemporal lobe amnesia.

Although our knowledge of the neuroanatomic bases and clinical features of amnesia has increased in recent years, mainly due to the expanded and refined methodologic repertoire of neuroscientic research, many questions remain unsettled. For example, the specific contribution of individual structures to specific memory processes is still a subject of controversy. In this context, for example, the specific engagement of the hippocampal formation in recent and/or remote memory and the importance of further limbic regions for storage and retrieval are still being debated. Likewise, the mechanisms of recovery from amnesic states, as in the case of patient A.M.N., described above, have not been unraveled in a satisfactory way. However, studies of such patients stress a dynamic view of the brain and suggest a potential for neural plasticity even in severely brain-damaged patients.

REFERENCES

1. Rosenzweig MR, Bennett EL, Colombo PJ, et al: Short-term, intermediate-term, and long-term memories. *Behav Brain Res* 57:193–198, 1993.
2. Tulving E: Organization of memory: Quo vadis? in Gazzaniga MS (ed): *The Cognitive Neurosciences.* Cambridge, MA: MIT Press, 1995, pp 839–847.
3. Markowitsch HJ: Anatomical basis of memory disorders, in Gazzaniga MS (ed): *The Cognitive Neurosciences.* Cambridge, MA: MIT Press, 1995, pp 947–967.
4. Brand M, Markowitsch HJ: The principle of bottleneck structures, in Kluwe RH, Lüer G, Rösler F (eds): *Principles of Learning and Memory.* Basel: Birkhäuser. In press.
5. Markowitsch HJ: Which brain regions are critically involved in the retrieval of old episodic memory? *Brain Res Rev* 21:117–127, 1995.
6. Markowitsch HJ: *Gedächtnisstörungen.* Stuttgart: Kohlhammer, 1999.
7. Chow KL: Effects of ablation, in Quarton GC, Melnechuk T, Schmitt FO (eds): *The Neurosciences.* New York: Rockefeller University Press, 1967, pp 705–713.
8. Markowitsch HJ: Memory and amnesia, in Mesulam M-M (ed): *Principles of Behavioral and Cognitive Neurology.* New York: Oxford University Press, 2000, pp 257–293.
9. Markowitsch HJ: The anatomical bases of memory, in Gazzaniga MS (ed): *The New Cognitive Neurosciences.* 2nd ed. Cambridge, MA: MIT Press, 2000, pp 781–795.
10. Scoville WB, Milner B: Loss of recent memory after bilateral hippocampal lesions. *J Neurol Neurosurg Psychiatry* 20:11–21, 1957.
11. Corkin S, Amaral DG, Gonzalez RG, et al: H.M.'s medial temporal lobe lesion: Findings from magnetic resonance imaging. *J Neurosci* 17:3964–3979, 1997.
12. Bonhoeffer K: Der Korsakowsche Symptomenkomplex in seinen Beziehungen zu den verschiedenen Krankheitsformen. *Allgem Zeitsch Psychiatrie* 61:744–752, 1904.
13. Kopelman MD, Stanhope N, Kingsley D: Retrograde amnesia in patients with diencephalic, temporal lobe or frontal lesions. *Neuropsychologia* 37:939–958, 1999.
14. Mayes AR, Daum I, Markowitsch HJ, et al: The relationship between retrograde and anterograde amnesia in patients with typical global amnesia. *Cortex* 33:197–217, 1997.
15. Shimamura A, Squire LR: Korsakoff's syndrome: A study of the relation between anterograde amnesia and remote memory impairment. *Behav Neurosci* 100:165–170, 1991.
16. Joyce EM, Robbins TW: Frontal lobe function in Korsakoff and non-Korsakoff alcoholics: Planning and spatial working memory. *Neuropsychologia* 29:709–723, 1991.
17. Mair WGP, Warrington EK, Weiskrantz L: Memory disorder in Korsakoff's psychosis. *Brain* 102:749–783, 1979.
18. Harding A, Halliday G, Caine D, et al: Degeneration of anterior thalamic nuclei differentiates alcoholics with amnesia. *Brain* 123:141–154, 2000.
19. Graff-Radford NR, Tranel D, Van Hoesen GW, et al: Diencephalic amnesia. *Brain* 113:1–25, 1990.
20. Markowitsch HJ, von Cramon DY, Schuri U: Mnestic performance profile of a bilateral diencephalic infarct patient with preserved intelligence and severe amnesic disturbances. *J Clin Exp Neuropsychol* 15:627–652, 1993.
21. Papez JW: A proposed mechanism of emotion. *Arch Neurol Psychiatry* 38:725–743, 1937.
22. Markowitsch HJ: The biological basis of memory, in Tröster AI (ed): *Memory in Neurodegenerative Disease: Biological, Cognitive and Clinical Perspective.* New York: Cambridge University Press, 1998, pp 140–153.
23. Vargha-Khadem F, Gadian DG, Watkins KE, et al: Differential effects of early hippocampal pathology on episodic and semantic memory. *Science* 277:376–380, 1997.
24. Tulving E, Markowitsch HJ: Episodic and declarative memory: Role of the hippocampus. *Hippocampus* 8:198–204, 1998.
25. Markowitsch HJ: Cognitive neuroscience of memory. *Neurocase* 4:429–435, 1998.
26. Markowitsch HJ, Kessler J, Kalbe E, et al: Functional amnesia and memory consolidation. A case of persistent anterograde amnesia with rapid forgetting following whiplash injury. *Neurocase* 5:189–200, 1999.

27. Kapur N, Millar J, Colbourn C, et al: Very long-term amnesia in association with temporal lobe epilepsy: Evidence for multiple-stage consolidation process. *Brain Cogn* 35:58–70, 1997.
28. O'Connor M, Sieggreen MA, Ahern G, et al: Accelerated forgetting in association with temporal lobe epilepsy and paraneoplastic encephalitis. *Brain Cogn* 35:71–84, 1997.
29. De Luca J, Diamond BJ: Aneurysm of the anterior communicating artery: A review of neuroanatomical and neuropsychological sequelae. *J Clin Exp Psychol* 17:100–121, 1995.
30. Von Cramon DY, Markowitsch HJ: The septum and human memory, in Numan R (ed): *The Behavioral Neuroscience of the Septal Region.* Berlin: Springer-Verlag, 2000, pp 380–413.
31. Baily CH, Kandel ER: Molecular and structural mechanisms underlying long-term memory, in Gazzaniga MS (ed): *The Cognitive Neurosciences.* Cambridge, MA: MIT Press, 1995, pp 19–36.
32. Beatty WW, Salmon DP, Butters N, et al: Retrograde amnesia in patients with Alzheimer's disease or Huntington's disease. *Neurobiol Aging* 8:181–186, 1988.
33. Bondi MW, Salmon DP, Butters N: Neuropsychological features of memory disorders in Alzheimer disease, in Terry RD, Katzman R, Bick KL (eds): *Alzheimer Disease.* New York: Raven Press, 1994, pp 41–63.
34. Hodges JR, Salmon DP, Butters N: Semantic memory impairment in Alzheimer's disease: Failure of access of degraded knowledge. *Neuropsychologia* 30:301–304, 1992.
35. Lambon Ralph MA, Patterson K, Hodges JR: The relationship between naming and semantic knowledge for different categories in dementia of Alzheimer's type. *Neuropsychologia* 35:1251–1260, 1997.
36. Nebes RD: Semantic memory in Alzheimer's disease. *Psychol Bull* 106:377–394, 1989.
37. Salmon DP, Shimamura AP, Butters N, et al: Lexical and semantic priming deficits in patients with Alzheimer's disease. *J Clin Exp Neuropsychol* 10:477–494, 1988.
38. Shimamura AP, Salmon DP, Squire LR, et al: Memory dysfunction and word priming in dementia and amnesia. *Behav Neurosci* 101:347–351, 1987.
39. Starkstein SE, Sabe L, Cuerva AG, et al.: Anosognosia and procedural learning in Alzheimer's disease. *Neuropsychiatry Neuropsychol Behav Neurol* 10:96–101, 1997.
40. Collette F, Van der Linden M, Bechet S, et al: Phonological loop and central executive functioning in Alzheimer's disease. *Neuropsychologia* 37:905–918, 1999.
41. White DA, Murphy CF: Working memory for nonverbal auditory information in dementia of the Alzheimer type. *Arch Clin Neuropsychol* 13:339–347, 1998.
42. Perry RJ, Hodges JR: Attention and executive deficits in Alzheimer's disease. A critical review. *Brain* 122:383–404, 1999.
43. Perry RJ, Watson P, Hodges JR: The nature and staging of attention dysfunction in early (minimal an mild) Alzheimer's disease: Relationship to episodic and semantic memory impairment. *Neuropsychologia* 38:252–271, 2000.
44. Braak H, Braak E: Frequency of stages of Alzheimer-related lesions in different age categories. *Neurobiol Aging* 18:351–357, 1997.
45. Nielsen-Bohlman L, Ciranni M, Shimamura AP, et al: Impaired word-stem priming in patients with temporal-occipital lesions. *Neuropsychologia* 35:1087–1092, 1997.
46. Schacter DL, Buckner RL: Priming and the brain. *Neuron* 20:185–195, 1998.
47. Buckner RL, Koutstaal W, Schacter DL, et al: Functional MRI evidence for a role of frontal and inferior temporal cortex in amodal components of priming. *Brain* 123:620–640, 2000.
48. Reinkemeier M, Markowitsch HJ, Rauch B, et al: Memory systems for people's names: A case study of a patient with deficits in recalling, but not learning people's names. *Neuropsychologia* 35:677–684, 1997.
49. Tulving E, Kapur S, Craik FIM, et al: Hemispheric encoding/retrieval asymmetry in episodic memory: Positron emission tomography findings. *Proc Natl Acad Sci U S A* 91:2016–2020, 1994.
50. Conway MA, Turk DJ, Miller SL, et al: A positron emission tomography (PET) study of autobiographical memory retrieval. *Memory* 7:679–702, 1999.
51. Haist F, Bowden Gore J, Mao H: Consolidation of human memory over decades revealed by functional magnetic resonance imaging. *Nature* 4:1139–1145, 2001.
52. Piefke M, Weiss PH, Zilles K, et al: Differential remoteness and emotional tone modulate the neural correlates of autobiographical memory. *Brain.* In press.
53. Lepage M, Habib R, Tulving E: Hippocampal PET activations of memory encoding and retrieval: The HIPER model. *Hippocampus* 8:313–322, 1998.
54. Dolan RJ, Fletcher PC: Encoding and retrieval in human medial temporal lobes: An empirical investigation using functional magnetic resonance imaging (MRI). *Hippocampus* 9:25–34, 1999.
55. Schacter DL, Wagner AD: Medial temporal lobe activations in fMRI and PET studies of episodic encoding and retrieval. *Hippocampus* 9:7–24, 1999.
56. Kopelman MD, Kapur N: The loss of episodic memories in retrograde amnesia: single case and group studies. *Philos Trans R Soc Lond Ser B: Biol Sci* 356:1409–1421, 2001.

57. De Renzi E, Liotti M, Nichelli P: Semantic amnesia with preservation of autobiographic memory. A case report. *Cortex* 23:575–597, 1987.
58. Markowitsch HJ, Calabrese P, Neufeld H, et al: Retrograde amnesia for famous events and faces after left fronto-temporal brain damage. *Cortex* 35:243–252, 1999.
59. O'Connor M, Butters N, Miliotis P, et al: The dissociation of anterograde and retrograde amnesia in a patient with herpes encephalitis. *J Clin Exp Neuropsychol* 14:159–178, 1992.
60. Kroll N, Markowitsch HJ, Knight R, et al: Retrieval of old memories—the temporo-frontal hypothesis. *Brain* 120:1377–1399, 1997.
61. LeDoux JE: The amygdala and emotion: a view through fear, in Aggleton JP (ed): *The Amygdala,* 2d ed. Oxford, UK: Oxford University Press, 2000, pp 289–310.
62. Sarter M, Markowitsch HJ: Involvement of the amygdala in learning and memory: A critical review, with emphasis on anatomical relations. *Behav Neurosci* 99:342–380, 1985.
63. Cahill L: Modulation of long-term memory storage in humans by emotional arousal: Adrenergic activation and the amygdala, in Aggleton JP (ed): *The Amygdala: A Functional Analysis.* Oxford, UK: Oxford University Press, 2000, pp 425–446.
64. Markowitsch HJ: Differential contribution of right and left amygdala to affective information processing. *Behavioural Neurology* 11:233–244, 1998/1999.
65. Cahill L, Haier RJ, White NS, et al: Sex-related differences in amygdala activity during emotionally influenced memory storage. *Neurobiol Learn Mem* 75:1–9, 2001.
66. Von Cramon DY, Markowitsch HJ, Schuri U: The possible contribution of the septal region to memory. *Neuropsychologia* 31:1159–1180, 1993.
67. Klüver H, Bucy PC: "Psychic blindness" and other symptoms following bilateral temporal lobectomy in rhesus monkeys. *Am J Physiol* 119:352–353, 1937.
68. Urbach E, Wiethe C: Lipoidosis cutis et mucosae. *Virchows Arch* 273:285–319, 1929.
69. Tranel D, Hyman BT: Neuropsychological correlates of bilateral amygdala damage. *Arch Neurol* 47:349–355, 1990.
70. Markowitsch HJ, Calabrese P, Würker M, et al: The amygdala's contribution to memory—a study on two patients with Urbach-Wiethe disease. *Neuroreport* 5:1349–1352, 1994.
71. Markowitsch HJ: Stress-related memory disorders, in Nilsson L-G, Markowitsch HJ (eds): *Cognitive Neuroscience of Memory.* Göttingen, Germany: Hogrefe, 1999, pp 193–211.
72. Sapolsky RM: Stress, glucocorticoids, and damage to the nervous system: The current state of confusion. *Stress* 1:1–19, 1996.
73. Lupien SJ, McEwen BS: The acute effects of corticosteroids on cognition: Intergration of animal and human model studies. *Brain Res Rev* 24:1–27, 1997.
74. Kaufer D, Friedman A, Seldman S, et al: Acute stress facilitates long-lasting changes in cholinergic gene expression. *Nature* 393:373–377, 1998.
75. Davis LL, Suris A, Lambert MT, et al: Post-traumatic stress disorder and serotonin: New directions for research and treatment. *J Psychiatry Neurosci* 22:318–326, 1997.
76. Arnsten AFT, Goldman-Rakic PS: Noise stress impairs prefrontal cortical cognitive function in monkeys. *Arch Gen Psychiatry* 55:362–368, 1998.
77. Rupprecht R: The neuropsychopharmacological potential of neuroactive steroids. *J Psychiatr Res* 31:297–314, 1997.
78. Markowitsch HJ, Kessler J, Van der Ven C, et al: Psychic trauma causing grossly reduced brain metabolism and cognitive deterioration. *Neuropsychologia* 36:77–82, 1998.
79. Markowitsch HJ, Kessler J, Russ MO, et al: Mnestic block syndrome. *Cortex* 35:219–230, 1999.

Chapter 38

AMNESIA: COGNITIVE NEUROPSYCHOLOGICAL ISSUES*

Margaret M. Keane
Mieke Verfaellie

The hallmark of the amnesic syndrome is a severe deficit in new learning (anterograde amnesia) coupled with a variable impairment in the ability to retrieve memories formed prior to the onset of the amnesia (retrograde amnesia). As reviewed in the previous chapter, amnesia is typically associated with lesions of the hippocampus and/or related structures in the mediotemporal lobe and diencephalon[1] and can have a variety of etiologies including Korsakoff's disease, anoxia, herpes simplex encephalitis, and vascular accident.

Over the past several decades, studies of human amnesia have yielded crucial insights into the functional role of the hippocampus and related structures in human memory. In this chapter, we review three important behavioral phenomena in amnesia. We first review patterns of retrograde memory loss in amnesia and consider their implications for the role of the hippocampus in memory consolidation. We then turn to anterograde memory. First we consider the distinction between episodic and semantic memory and evaluate the role of the hippocampus in the acquisition of new semantic knowledge. Then we discuss the distinction between explicit and implicit memory and consider the differential role of the hippocampus in memory tasks that vary in terms of their underlying processing demands. Research within each of these domains has enhanced our understanding of the nature and neural bases of distinct memory processes.

* **ACKNOWLEDGMENTS:** Writing of this chapter was supported by NINDS Program Project Grant NS 26985 and NIMH Grant 57681 to Boston University and by the Medical Research Service of the VA Healthcare system.

RETROGRADE AMNESIA

An influential theory about the role of the mediotemporal lobe in memory function[2–4] came from the observation that the retrograde memory impairment in amnesia is typically temporally limited, such that very remote memories are spared. Clear examples of this pattern are provided by patients with documented damage to the hippocampal region. In one patient whose damage was limited to the CA1 field of the hippocampus, retrograde amnesia was limited to 1 or 2 years before the onset of amnesia.[5] In several other patients with more extensive damage, retrograde amnesia covered as much as 15 years but did not extend to earlier time periods.[6] In a patient with virtually complete damage to the hippocampus as well as extensive damage to adjacent structures, spatial memories acquired many years before the onset of amnesia were nonetheless preserved.[7]

These findings have been taken as evidence for the view that the hippocampus and related mediotemporal-lobe structures have a time-limited role in the *consolidation* (stabilization) of new memories, which are ultimately stored in neocortex. Anatomically, this process is enabled by the extensive and reciprocal connections that exist between the medial temporal lobe (particularly the hippocampus and related cortices) and distributed neocortical sites. During initial learning, such connections allow the hippocampus to bind together the various neocortical sites that represent the memorial event. Subsequently, when the memory is partially reactivated, the hippocampus serves as a "pointer," enabling activation of the full complement of neocortical sites associated with that memory. During consolidation, repeated (hippocampally mediated) coactivation of these neocortical components facilitates the establishment of corticocortical connections, which bind these components together directly. Thus, when consolidation is complete, the hippocampus is no longer necessary for memory retrieval.

By this view, retrograde amnesia reflects the disruption of memories that are in the process of consolidation (and thus still dependent on the hippocampus). The preservation of very remote memories is attributed to the fact that the consolidation process for those memories is complete, so that the hippocampus is no longer necessary for retrieval. Importantly, the theory postulates that the mediotemporal lobe has a similar role in the consolidation of episodic memory (memory for personally experienced events that occurred in a particular temporospatial context) and of semantic memory (i.e., memory for facts and general world knowledge).[8] Several computational models have been developed that successfully simulate the findings in amnesia and shed light on the reasons why such consolidation mechanisms might have evolved.[4,9,10]

Nadel and colleagues[11–13] have recently challenged consolidation theory, arguing instead that the hippocampal complex has a permanent role in the storage and retrieval of autobiographical (episodic) memories regardless of the age of those memories. This theory (known as "multiple memory trace" or MMT theory[11]) agrees with consolidation theory that memories are initially encoded by the hippocampus and stored as hippocampal-neocortical ensembles. According to MMT theory, each time a memory is retrieved, the hippocampus engages in a new encoding event, yielding a new (hippocampal-neocortical) memory trace, wherein the hippocampal component provides the spatial contextual framework for the memory.[14] Semantic memories (which are context-free) are believed to become stabilized over time in neocortex and thus ultimately independent of the hippocampus (a point on which MMT and consolidation theory agree). Episodic memories, by contrast, are thought to depend permanently on the hippocampus for the "spatial scaffold" that is essential to such memories.[14] By this view, in contrast to the consolidation view, extensive damage to the hippocampal complex should produce retrograde amnesia for episodes covering all time periods prior to the onset of the disorder.

Indeed, Nadel and Moscovitch[11,15] have challenged common notions about the nature of retrograde amnesia following damage to the mediotemporal lobe, pointing to evidence that the retrograde memory loss is often extensive, sometimes covering an entire lifetime. MMT theory attributes the apparent sparing of very remote memories to the greater accumulation of memory traces associated with those memories compared to more recent memories.[16] Importantly, however, MMT theory predicts that even remote memories in individuals with hippocampal damage should differ in quality from remote memories retrieved by neurologically intact individuals, whose retrieval of such memories would benefit from the availability of the hippocampal storage system. By contrast, consolidation theory predicts that very remote memories should be qualitatively and quantitatively equivalent in individuals with and without hippocampal damage, because such memories are thought to be independent of the hippocampus.[2,3]

Thus, consolidation theory and MMT theory differ in how they characterize retrograde amnesia following damage to the hippocampal complex: as a temporally limited phenomenon, applying equally to episodic and semantic memory, with complete sparing of very remote memories, or as a temporally extensive phenomenon, applying primarily to episodic memory and covering very remote as well as more recent time periods. Empiric evidence from human and animal studies has been marshaled in support of each viewpoint (Refs. 3, 13, and 15 to 18), and the debate awaits resolution.

The distinction between episodic and semantic memory drawn by MMT theory, but not by consolidation theory, echoes a long-standing debate about the relative status of semantic and episodic memory in amnesia. In the next section, we consider this debate in the context of findings concerning the acquisition of new semantic memories following hippocampal damage.

SEMANTIC MEMORY IN AMNESIA

One of the early theoretical accounts of amnesia borrowed from a distinction between episodic and semantic memory that was first developed by Tulving[19,20] in the context of normal cognition. *Episodic memory* refers to memory for personally experienced events that occurred in a particular spatiotemporal context, whereas *semantic memory* refers to general knowledge of the world (including knowledge of words and their meanings), which is abstracted from the specific time and place in which the knowledge was acquired (see Chap. 39). The episodic/semantic distinction seemed to account well for the observation that amnesic individuals are severely impaired in remembering personally experienced events (including, for example, recalling or recognizing stimuli in a recently presented list) but nonetheless retain their fund of general world knowledge, including "the vocabulary and syntax of the language, the social amenities, or other much rehearsed skills."[21] (See also Refs. 20, 22, and 23.) As the basis for an episodic/semantic theory of impaired and intact memory in amnesia, however, such observations were flawed insofar as they confounded the type of memory (episodic or semantic) with the time period in which the memory was acquired (post- or premorbidly). Subsequent tests of the episodic/semantic account remedied this flaw by holding constant the time period of acquisition, either evaluating remote memory for both kinds of information or examining new (anterograde) learning for both kinds of information.

We focus below on studies that assessed new learning of episodic and semantic information in adult- and childhood-onset amnesia. It is noncontroversial that new episodic learning is impaired in amnesia, so the critical question addressed in these studies concerns the status of new semantic learning in amnesia.

Studies of new semantic learning in individuals with adult-onset amnesia vary markedly in the theoretical conclusions they elicit. Some researchers emphasize the fact that amnesic patients can acquire *some* semantic knowledge (a finding taken as support for the episodic/semantic account), while others highlight the fact that the amount of semantic knowledge acquired in amnesia is far below that of normal individuals (a finding taken as counterevidence to the episodic/semantic account). Thus, for example, several studies report that amnesic individuals can acquire some semantic information in the form of factual statements[24,25] or simple computer commands and vocabulary.[26,27] On the other hand, studies of new vocabulary learning have reported severe impairments in amnesia in the acquisition of knowledge about words new to the language since the onset of amnesia.[28,29]

In studies of childhood-onset amnesia, the status of new semantic learning is typically evaluated by examining the child's academic progress in school or performance on standardized tests that tap semantic knowledge. The assumption in these studies is that, prior to the onset of amnesia, a semantic knowledge base had not yet been well established. Thus, demonstrations of good semantic knowledge must be due to postmorbid acquisition (new learning). The evidence from two initial case studies was mixed, with one study demonstrating good academic progress in a child with amnesia secondary to encephalitis[30,31] and another demonstrating poor academic progress and impaired performance on several laboratory tests of semantic knowledge in a child with amnesia consequent to anoxia.[32]

More recently, Vargha-Khadem and coworkers[33–35] described as many as 11 cases of childhood-onset amnesia resulting from hypoxic-ischemic damage occurring at time points ranging from birth to 14 years. Magnetic resonance imaging data in these individuals revealed clear, bilateral damage to the hippocampus and apparent sparing of underlying cortices, including the entorhinal, perirhinal, and parahippocampal cortices. Across these cases, the investigators report a pattern of spared new semantic learning as measured by progress in school, performance on IQ tests, and/or performance on standardized tests of reading, spelling, and reading comprehension, coupled with marked impairments on standardized tests of episodic memory.

Thus, the behavioral evidence, from studies of both adult-onset amnesia and childhood-onset amnesia, is mixed, with some studies reporting marked semantic learning and others reporting little or no such learning in amnesic individuals. These findings have been interpreted in two different ways. On the one hand, Tulving and colleagues[25] have argued that these data favor an episodic/semantic memory account of amnesia insofar as they demonstrate that amnesic individuals can acquire an impressive amount of new semantic knowledge despite profound impairments in episodic memory. Such results are taken as evidence that semantic knowledge can be acquired independently of the mediotemporal-lobe structures that are damaged in amnesia. According to this view, that such knowledge is acquired quite slowly and does not reach normal levels is attributable to the fact that healthy individuals may draw on intact episodic memory abilities to enhance their semantic learning, putting amnesic individuals at a disadvantage.

On the other hand, Squire and colleagues[8,36,37] have argued that these results do not provide compelling evidence in support of an episodic/semantic account of amnesia because, in those instances in which semantic learning was significant, there was no evidence that such learning went beyond what would be expected on the basis of residual episodic memory. According to this view, episodic and semantic memory are similarly dependent on the mediotemporal-lobe structures that are damaged in amnesia. In support of this view, Hamann and Squire[37] directly compared memory for facts (semantic information) and events (episodic information) to which amnesic and control participants had been exposed during the course of an experiment. Although the amnesic group acquired some factual information, such knowledge was proportional to their level of episodic memory. More specifically, when the performance of the amnesic group was compared to that of a control group tested after a longer delay, the two groups showed similar levels of episodic memory performance and similar levels of semantic memory performance, indicating that semantic memory was not disproportionately spared in amnesia.

An alternative suggestion put forward by Vargha-Khadem and colleagues[33–35] offers a neuroanatomic account of spared semantic learning in their studies of childhood-onset amnesia and provides a possible way to reconcile conflicting results on this question across other studies. Specifically, based on their combined behavioral and neuroimaging findings (described above), Vargha-Khadem and colleagues have proposed that subhippocampal cortices (entorhinal, perirhinal, and parahippocampal) may be sufficient to support the acquisition of semantic memories, whereas the hippocampus may be additionally necessary for the acquisition of episodic memories. By this view, both forms of memory (episodic and semantic) depend on the integrity of the mediotemporal-lobe system, but each depends upon a distinct component of that system. Thus, the variable findings across studies concerning the status of new semantic learning in amnesia could be accounted for by the variable involvement of subhippocampal cortices in the amnesic individuals under study (for review, see Ref. 38).

This neuroanatomic hypothesis could be considered a neurally specified variation of Tulving's theory concerning the separability of episodic and semantic memory in amnesia.[20,25] Both accounts stand in contrast to Squire and colleagues' view that episodic and semantic memory are equivalently impaired in amnesia and similarly dependent on all components of the mediotemporal/diencephalic system implicated in amnesia.[8,37] A clear resolution to this debate will require precise and detailed information about the nature and extent of the brain lesions in each amnesic individual under study as well as a consensus about what kind of evidence is necessary to demonstrate a disproportionate sparing of semantic memory in amnesia (see Ref. 8).

EXPLICIT AND IMPLICIT MEMORY

Whereas the distinction between episodic and semantic memory is based on the kind of information to be remembered (personally experienced episodes versus general world knowledge), the distinction between explicit and implicit memory (first introduced by Graf and Schacter[39]) is based upon the way in which memory is tested. In explicit memory tasks, subjects are asked to make deliberate (explicit) reference to a prior episode. In the laboratory, for example, subjects might be exposed to a list of words or pictures in a "study" phase and then asked to recall those stimuli in a subsequent "test" phase. By contrast, in implicit memory tasks, subjects are not required to make deliberate reference to a prior episode; memory for that episode is "implicit" in performance on a subsequent task. For example, subjects might be exposed to a list of stimuli in a study phase and, in a subsequent test phase, asked to perform a seemingly unrelated task, such as identifying stimuli flashed very briefly on a computer screen or generating exemplars from particular semantic categories. Half of the stimuli in the test phase correspond to stimuli from the prior study phase and half correspond to new, unstudied stimuli. (The unstudied items are included to provide a measure of baseline or "chance" performance.) Implicit memory for the study episode is reflected in subjects' enhanced performance in identifying or generating studied compared to unstudied stimuli (an effect known as *priming*). Thus, explicit memory tasks require conscious and deliberate reference to a prior experience, whereas implicit memory tasks measure the influence of prior experience without requiring conscious reference to it. In the following sections, we review some major theoretical issues regarding the status of explicit and implicit memory in amnesia.

Explicit Memory in Amnesia

Explicit memory is typically tested using either recall or recognition tasks. In free recall tasks, subjects are asked to remember and generate (without cues) previously encountered stimuli, whereas in recognition tasks, subjects are presented with a stimulus and asked to judge whether it was encountered previously. Dual-process models[40,41] have postulated that performance on such tasks is the product of two distinct processes: (1) recollection—an effortful process by which information from a prior experience is deliberately brought to mind, and (2) familiarity—a facility or fluency in stimulus processing that is attributed to prior experience with the stimulus. Free recall performance is thought to depend primarily on recollection, whereas recognition performance may be mediated both by recollection and by familiarity.

Amnesic individuals typically show impaired performance both on recall and on recognition tasks. There is debate, however, about the *relative* impairment of recall and recognition memory performance in amnesia, and this debate is closely linked to the question of whether recollection and familiarity are differentially affected in amnesia. Some studies demonstrate a disproportionate deficit in recall compared to recognition in amnesia,[42,43] and such results are taken as evidence that amnesia is associated with a greater impairment in recollection than in familiarity. Other studies demonstrate that recall and recognition are equivalently (proportionately) impaired in amnesia,[44–47] suggesting that recollection and familiarity are similarly affected.

Because the measurement scales in recall and recognition tasks are so different, most studies comparing the status of these two kinds of memory in amnesia do so by equating performance in amnesic and control subjects on a recognition task (either by providing additional study exposure to amnesic subjects or by delaying the memory test for control subjects) and then comparing the performance of the two groups on a recall task under the same experimental conditions. Equivalent performance in the two groups on the recall task suggests a proportionate recall deficit in amnesia, whereas impaired recall performance in the amnesic group suggests a disproportionate recall deficit in amnesia.

Giovanello and Verfaellie[48] suggested that the discrepancies in the literature concerning the relative status of recall and recognition in amnesia may be due to variability across studies in the method used to equate recognition performance in amnesic and control subjects. They tested this hypothesis by comparing two different methods within their own study: they equated recognition performance in amnesic and control groups in experiment 1 by administering six study presentations to the amnesic group and one to the control group and in experiment 2 by testing the amnesic group after a 1-min study-test delay and the control group after a 24-h delay. Their results showed that recall performance was impaired in the amnesic group in experiment 1 but not in experiment 2.

Giovanello and Verfaellie[48] suggested that these results could be understood in the context of two assumptions: (1) that familiarity is less impaired than is recollection in amnesia and forms the basis of explicit memory performance in amnesia and (2) that equating recognition memory performance in amnesic and control groups does not necessarily equate the processes underlying performance in the two groups. Thus, when recognition memory performance is equated by providing additional study exposures to the amnesic patients (experiment 1), performance in amnesia is nonetheless mediated solely by familiarity (albeit enhanced familiarity), whereas performance in control subjects is mediated both by familiarity and by recollection. Under these conditions, control subjects showed an advantage over amnesic subjects in recall performance because of their ability to use recollection. On the other hand, increasing the delay between study and test has been shown to have a larger detrimental effect on recollection than on familiarity.[49,50] Thus, when recognition performance in amnesic and control groups is equated by delaying the test for the control group, performance in both groups is likely mediated by familiarity. Under these conditions, recall performance is similar in amnesic and control subjects. In sum, Giovanello and Verfaellie[48] argue that the recall and recognition data from amnesic patients are consistent with the notion that the impairment in amnesia in recollection is more severe than the impairment in familiarity. Yonelinas[51] reached a similar conclusion in a comprehensive review of studies using a variety of techniques to assess the integrity of recollection and familiarity in amnesia.

Based on an extensive review of findings in animals as well as in humans, Aggleton and Brown[52,53] have recently suggested that recollection and familiarity are mediated by two distinct memory circuits, a hippocampal anterior thalamic system mediating recollection, and a perirhinal dorsal mediothalamic system mediating familiarity. Thus, the relative preservation of familiarity in amnesic patients may be accounted for by the fact that the hippocampus is typically more severely compromised than are the surrounding subhippocampal (i.e., entorhinal, perirhinal, and parahippocampal) cortices. This proposal can also account for the recent observation that recognition memory can be fully preserved in patients with lesions limited to the hippocampus proper.[33,54,55]

Arguing against the foregoing account, Squire and colleagues have demonstrated that recognition memory can be markedly impaired even when lesions are restricted to the hippocampus.[56,57] At present, the reason for the inconsistent results across studies is unclear, but such discrepancies highlight the importance of precise neuroanatomic characterization of the patients under study. Clearly, further work will be needed to reach firmer conclusions about the role of specific neuroanatomic structures in the mediation of different processes that contribute to explicit memory.

Implicit Memory in Amnesia

Perceptual and Conceptual Priming Numerous studies have demonstrated that, despite impaired performance on explicit memory tasks, amnesic patients can show normal performance on implicit memory or priming tasks (for review, see Refs. 58 and 59). It is useful to draw a distinction between priming tasks that draw primarily on perceptual processes and those that draw primarily on conceptual processes.[60,61] In perceptual priming paradigms, the test-phase task requires subjects to identify a stimulus under speeded conditions, or given incomplete or degraded perceptual information (e.g., words or pictures presented very briefly or in fragmented form). In conceptual priming paradigms, by contrast, subjects must retrieve a word that satisfies a particular semantic constraint (e.g., is a member of a specified semantic category or is semantically related to a cue word), or must evaluate a semantic property of a stimulus (e.g., decide whether it denotes an abstract or concrete concept). Operationally, perceptual and conceptual priming effects can be distinguished in terms of their sensitivity to various experimental manipulations. Manipulations of the surface similarity of stimuli in the study and test phases (e.g., study-test changes in sensory modality) influence the magnitude of perceptual priming effects[62–65] but not conceptual priming effects.[66,67] On the other hand, variations in the level of semantic processing of stimuli during the study phase have little effect on perceptual priming[63] but have a marked effect on conceptual priming.[66,68]

Amnesic patients have shown normal performance both on perceptual[69–72] and conceptual[73–76] priming tasks. These findings indicate that perceptual and conceptual priming effects do not depend upon the integrity of the mediotemporal-lobe and diencephalic brain structures that are damaged in amnesia. However, such findings fail to reveal which of the brain structures spared in amnesia support normal priming in this group and leave open the question of whether perceptual and conceptual priming depend on a unitary neural system or on dissociable neural systems.

Answers to such questions have been yielded by studies examining perceptual priming in individuals with brain lesions outside of the mediotemporal/diencephalic system. Important insights have come from studies of priming in patients with Alzheimer's disease (AD). AD resembles amnesia in that it is associated with lesions of the hippocampal formation,[77] but it differs from amnesia in that it is also associated with neocortical lesions of temporal, parietal, and frontal cortices.[78–80] Importantly for the present discussion, primary sensory cortices are relatively spared in AD.[80–82] The hippocampal lesions that are common to amnesia and AD account for the explicit memory deficits that are observed in AD patients.[83] However, because priming survives the hippocampal lesions in amnesia, we can infer that priming deficits observed in AD reflect pathology outside of that region.

A wide range of studies have shown that the status of priming in AD varies depending on the particular priming task. AD patients have shown normal priming in visual identification of briefly presented words,[84,85] auditory identification of words presented in white noise,[86] speeded lexical decision (deciding whether a string of letters constitutes a real word),[87,88] speeded picture identification,[89,90] and visual pattern completion.[91] In contrast, they have shown impaired priming in category exemplar production (generating exemplars in response to category cues)[90,92] and in word-association tasks (generating the first word that comes to mind in response to a word cue).[93–95] This pattern of results may be understood with reference to the distinction between perceptual and conceptual priming: AD patients appear to show normal priming on perceptual tasks but impaired priming on conceptual tasks. These findings suggest that conceptual priming is mediated by neocortical association areas that are compromised in AD, whereas perceptual priming may be mediated by sensory cortices that are relatively preserved in AD.

To address this neuroanatomic hypothesis, researchers have examined both forms of priming in individuals with focal occipital lobe lesions. Such individuals would be expected to exhibit impaired performance on visual perceptual priming tasks but normal performance on conceptual priming tasks. Consistent with this hypothesis, these patients have shown impaired priming on visual word identification but normal priming in category exemplar production.[67,96]

Converging evidence regarding the neural separability and localization of perceptual and conceptual priming comes from neuroimaging studies in healthy individuals. These studies have shown that priming is typically accompanied by reductions in brain activity. Such reductions are thought to reflect the decreased processing demands associated with processing of primed (compared to nonprimed) stimuli. A number of studies have demonstrated that perceptual priming is associated with reduced activity in extrastriate visual areas,[97–101] whereas conceptual priming is associated with reduced activation in left inferior prefrontal cortex.[102–104]

Taken together, the findings from behavioral studies of patients with neocortical lesions and neuroimaging studies in healthy individuals suggest that visuoperceptual priming is supported by occipital cortex and conceptual priming is supported by left inferior prefrontal cortex. Intact perceptual and conceptual priming in amnesic patients is likely due to the preservation of these brain regions in amnesia.

Priming of Novel Information in Amnesia

Most of the priming tasks described thus far have used stimuli that are represented in long-term knowledge, i.e., words or drawings of objects that are familiar to participants. There has been a great deal of interest, however, in whether amnesic patients can show priming for novel stimuli, i.e., stimuli that lack preexisting representations in long-term knowledge. The motivation for this interest is a theory positing that spared priming in amnesia is due to activation mechanisms operating on premorbidly acquired knowledge representations.[69,105] According to this theory, when a stimulus is encountered in the study phase of a priming task, its representation in long-term knowledge is activated. During the test phase, such activation renders the stimulus more accessible and increases the likelihood (compared to nonprimed stimuli) that the stimulus will be identified or generated. By this view, amnesic patients should not show priming for novel stimuli because such stimuli do not have preexisting representations to be activated. Contrary to this prediction, amnesic patients have shown normal priming for novel stimuli such as pseudowords,[67,70,72,106] novel geometric patterns,[107,108] drawings of novel three-dimensional objects,[109] and photographs of unfamiliar faces.[110]

In a different approach to this question, Graf and Schacter[39] and Moscovitch and colleagues[111] developed paradigms to examine priming of novel word pairs (e.g., *anger-pattern*) in amnesia. Even though the constituent parts of such pairs are represented in long-term knowledge, the link between them is not. Thus, any priming that can be attributed to implicit memory for that link would constitute priming for novel information (or "new-associative priming"). In this sort of paradigm, subjects are exposed in the study phase to normatively unrelated word pairs (e.g., *anger-pattern, merchant-tribute*). In the subsequent test phase, subjects are exposed to pairs that had appeared in the study phase ("old" pairs, e.g., *anger-patterns*), to pairs formed by recombining words from the study phase ("recombined" pairs, e.g., *anger-tribute*), and to new, unstudied word pairs (e.g., *crying-topic*). The test phase might require word-stem completion (in which case the second item of each pair would consist of the three-letter beginning of a word), speeded reading, identification on very brief presentation, or speeded lexical decision. The measure of performance is the accuracy or speed of the response. For the present purposes, the critical comparison is between performance in the old condition and performance in the recombined condition. In both of these conditions, the constituents of each pair had appeared in the prior study phase; the conditions differ in that the novel pairing established in the study phase is preserved in the old condition but not in the recombined condition. Thus, any enhancement in performance in the old compared to the recombined condition would reflect new associative priming.

Studies that have used this paradigm with amnesic patients have yielded mixed results, with some studies reporting intact new-associative priming[111–113] and others reporting impaired new-associative priming in amnesia.[114–116] One way to reconcile these apparently contradictory findings is to consider the nature of the task on which amnesic patients have shown intact or impaired performance. Amnesic patients appear to show intact new-associative priming on tasks that require identification of briefly presented word pairs[112] (but see Ref. 117) or speeded identification (reading or lexical decision) of word pairs.[111,113] In at least one of these tasks (lexical decision), new-associative priming has been shown to be sensitive to study-test shifts in perceptual modality but insensitive to variations in level of semantic processing at study,[118,119] suggesting that the effect is perceptually based. Amnesic patients have shown impaired new-associative priming in word-stem completion,[114–116] an effect that appears to require semantic processing of word pairs in the study phase.[120] Thus, the status of new-associative priming in amnesia may depend upon the nature of the association to be primed, such that priming of new *perceptual* associations is intact in amnesia but priming of new *conceptual* associations is impaired.[121] Understanding the conditions under which amnesic patients can show implicit memory for novel associations may also be relevant to theories that assign a critical role to the hippocampus in binding together unrelated items in memory.[122]

In summary, the studies described above provide strong counterevidence to an activation account of spared priming in amnesia: amnesic patients show normal priming with pseudowords, orthographically illegal nonwords, novel patterns and objects, and at least some kinds of novel associations. Thus, it appears as though priming in amnesia is not limited to material that is premorbidly represented in long-term knowledge. Rather, amnesic patients can establish novel representations, and these representations can support normal priming effects.

CONCLUSION

Studies of spared and impaired memory function in amnesia have provided the empiric foundation for many of the theories that frame contemporary thinking about human memory. Evidence concerning the nature and extent of retrograde memory loss in amnesia elucidates the role of the hippocampus in the formation, maintenance, and retrieval of long-term memories. Examination of the relative integrity of episodic and semantic memory in amnesia sheds light on the potential neural separability of memory for personally experienced events and memory for facts about the world. Comparisons of recall and recognition performance in amnesia highlight the distinct contributions of recollection and familiarity to explicit memory performance and the distinct neural bases of those processes. Finally, the study of implicit memory effects in amnesia reveals the nature and localization of memory processes that operate outside of conscious awareness. In sum, behavioral studies in amnesia provide a powerful means to deepen our understanding of the nature and organization of normal human memory capacities.

REFERENCES

1. Zola-Morgan S, Squire LR: Neuroanatomy of memory. *Ann Rev Neurosci* 16:547–563, 1993.
2. Squire LR, Cohen NJ, Nadel L: The medial temporal region and memory consolidation: A new hypothesis, in Weingartner H, Parker ES (eds): *Memory Consolidation: Psychobiology of Cognition.* Hillsdale, NJ: Erlbaum, 1984, pp 185–210.
3. Squire LR, Alvarez P: Retrograde amnesia and memory consolidation: A neurobiological perspective. *Curr Opin Neurobiol* 5:169–177, 1995.
4. McClelland JL, McNaughton BL, O'Reilly RC: Why there are complementary learning systems in

the hippocampus and neocortex: Insights from the successes and failures of connectionist models of learning and memory. *Psychol Rev* 102:419–457, 1995.

5. Zola-Morgan S, Squire LR, Amaral DG: Human amnesia and the medial temporal region: Enduring memory impairment following a bilateral lesion limited to field CA1 of the hippocampus. *J Neurosci* 6:2950–2967, 1986.
6. Rempel-Clower NL, Zola SM, Squire LR, et al: Three cases of enduring memory impairment after bilateral damage limited to the hippocampal formation. *J Neurosci* 16:5233–5255, 1996.
7. Teng E, Squire LR: Memory for places learned long ago is intact after hippocampal damage. *Nature* 400:675–677, 1999.
8. Squire LR, Zola SM: Episodic memory, semantic memory, and amnesia. *Hippocampus* 8:205–211, 1998.
9. Alvarez P, Squire LR: Memory consolidation and the medial temporal lobe: A simple network model. *Proc Natl Acad Sci USA* 91:7041–7045, 1994.
10. Murre JMJ: TraceLink: A model of amnesia and consolidation of memory. *Hippocampus* 6:675–684, 1996.
11. Nadel L, Moscovitch M: Memory consolidation, retrograde amnesia and the hippocampal complex. *Curr Opin Neurobiol* 7:217–227, 1997.
12. Moscovitch M, Nadel L: Consolidation and the hippocampal complex revisited: In defense of the multiple-trace model. *Curr Opin Neurobiol* 8:297–300, 1998.
13. Nadel L, Samsonovich A, Ryan L, et al: Multiple trace theory of human memory: Computational, neuroimaging, and neuropsychological results. *Hippocampus* 10:352–368, 2000.
14. Nadel L, Moscovitch M: Hippocampal contributions to cortical plasticity. *Neuropharmacology* 37:431–439, 1998.
15. Nadel L, Moscovitch M: The hippocampal complex and long-term memory revisited. *Trends Cogn Sci* 5:228–230, 2001.
16. Nadel L, Bohbot V: Consolidation of memory. *Hippocampus* 11:56–60, 2001.
17. Squire LR, Clark RE, Knowlton BJ: Retrograde amnesia. *Hippocampus* 11:50–55, 2001.
18. Eichenbaum H, Cohen NJ: *From Conditioning to Conscious Recollection.* Oxford, UK: Oxford University Press, 2001.
19. Tulving E: Episodic and semantic memory, in Tulving E, Donaldson W (eds): *Organization of Memory.* New York: Academic Press, 1972, pp 381–403.
20. Tulving E: *Elements of Episodic Memory.* Oxford, UK: Oxford University Press, 1983.
21. Kinsbourne M, Wood F: Short-term memory processes and the amnesic syndrome, in Deutsch DD, Deutsch JA (eds): *Short-Term Memory.* New York: Academic Press, 1975, pp 258–291.
22. Warrington EK: The selective impairment of semantic memory. *Q J Exp Psychol* 27:635–657, 1975.
23. Shallice T: *From Neuropsychology to Mental Structure.* Cambridge, UK: Cambridge University Press, 1988.
24. Shimamura AP, Squire LR: A neuropsychological study of fact memory and source amnesia. *J Exp Psychol Learn Mem Cogn* 13:464–473, 1987.
25. Tulving E, Hayman CAG, MacDonald CA: Long-lasting perceptual priming and semantic learning in amnesia: A case experiment. *J Exp Psychol Learn Mem Cogn* 17:595–617, 1991.
26. Glisky EL, Schacter DL, Tulving E: Computer learning by memory-impaired patients: Acquisition and retention of complex knowledge. *Neuropsychologia* 24:313–328, 1986.
27. Glisky EL, Schacter DL: Long-term retention of computer learning by patients with memory disorders. *Neuropsychologia* 26:173–178, 1988.
28. Gabrieli JDE, Cohen NJ, Corkin S: The impaired learning of semantic knowledge following bilateral medial temporal-lobe resection. *Brain Cogn* 7:157–177, 1988.
29. Verfaellie M, Croce P, Milberg WP: The role of episodic memory in semantic learning: An examination of vocabulary acquisition in a patient with amnesia due to encephalitis. *Neurocase* 1:291–304, 1995.
30. Wood F, Ebert V, Kinsbourne M: The episodic-semantic memory distinction in memory and amnesia: Clinical and experimental observations, in Cermak LS (ed): *Human Memory and Amnesia.* Hillsdale, NJ: Erlbaum, 1982, pp 167–193.
31. Wood FB, Brown IS, Felton RH: Long-term follow-up of a childhood amnesic syndrome. *Brain Cogn* 10:76–86, 1989.
32. Ostergaard AL: Episodic, semantic and procedural memory in a case of amnesia at an early age. *Neuropsychologia* 25:341–357, 1987.
33. Vargha-Khadem F, Gadian DG, Watkins KE, et al: Differential effects of early hippocampal pathology on episodic and semantic memory. *Science* 277:376–380, 1997.
34. Gadian DG, Aicardi J, Watkins KE, et al: Developmental amnesia associated with early hypoxic-ischaemic injury. *Brain* 123:499–507, 2000.
35. Vargha-Khadem F, Gadian DG, Mishkin M: Dissociations in cognitive memory: The syndrome of developmental amnesia. *Philos Trans R Soc Lond* 356:1435–1440, 2001.

36. Ostergaard AL, Squire LR: Childhood amnesia and distinctions between forms of memory: A comment on Wood, Brown, and Felton. *Brain Cogn* 14:127–133, 1990.
37. Hamann SB, Squire LR: On the acquisition of new declarative knowledge in amnesia. *Behav Neurosci* 109: 1027–1044, 1995.
38. Verfaellie M: Semantic learning in amnesia, in Boller F, Grafman J (eds): *Handbook of Neuropsychology,* 2d ed. Amsterdam: Elsevier, 2000, pp 335–354.
39. Graf P, Schacter DL: Implicit and explicit memory for new associations in normal and amnesic subjects. *J Exp Psychol Learn Mem Cogn* 11(3):501–518, 1985.
40. Mandler G: Recognizing: The judgment of previous occurrence. *Psychol Rev* 87:252–271, 1980.
41. Jacoby LL: Remembering the data: Analyzing interactive processes in reading. *J Verb Learn Verb Behav* 22:485–508, 1983.
42. Hirst W, Johnson MK, Kim JK, et al: Recognition and recall in amnesics. *J Exp Psychol Learn Mem Cogn* 12:445–451, 1986.
43. Hirst W, Johnson MK, Phelps AE, et al: More on recognition and recall in amnesics. *J Exp Psychol Learn Mem Cogn* 14:758–762, 1988.
44. Shimamura AP, Squire LR: Long-term memory in amnesia: Cued recall, recognition memory and confidence ratings. *J Exp Psychol Learn Mem Cogn* 14:763–770, 1988.
45. Haist F, Shimamura AP, Squire LR: On the relationship between recall and recognition memory. *J Exp Psychol Learn Mem Cogn* 18:691–702, 1992.
46. MacAndrew SBG, Jones GV, Mayes AR: No selective deficit in recall in amnesia. *Memory* 2:241–254, 1994.
47. Kopelman MD, Stanhope N: Recall and recognition memory in patients with focal frontal, temporal lobe and diencephalic lesions. *Neuropsychologia* 36:785–796, 1998.
48. Giovanello KS, Verfaellie M: The relationship between recall and recognition in amnesia: Effects of matching recognition between patients with amnesia and controls. *Neuropsychology* 15:444–451, 2001.
49. Hockley WA, Consoli A: Familiarity and recollection in item and associative recognition. *Mem Cogn* 27:657–664, 1999.
50. Gardiner JM, Java RJ: Forgetting in recognition memory with and without recollective experience. *Mem Cogn* 19:617–623, 1991.
51. Yonelinas AP, Kroll NEA, Dobbins I, et al: Recollection and familiarity deficits in amnesia: Convergence of remember-know, process dissociation, and receiver operating characteristic data. *Neuropsychology* 12:323–339, 1998.
52. Aggleton JP, Brown MW: Episodic memory, amnesia, and the hippocampal-anterior thalamic axis. *Behav Brain Sci* 425–489, 1999.
53. Brown MW, Aggleton JP: Recognition memory: What are the roles of the perirhinal cortex and hippocampus? *Nature Rev Neurosci* 2:51–61, 2001.
54. Mayes AR, Holdstock JS, Isaac CL, et al: Relative sparing of item recognition memory in a patient with adult-onset damage limited to the hippocampus. *Hippocampus.* 12:325–340, 2002.
55. Henke K, Kroll NEA, Hamraz B, et al: Memory lost and regained following bilateral hippocampal damage. *J Cogn Neurosci* 11:682–697, 1999.
56. Reed JM, Squire LR: Impaired recognition memory in patients with lesions limited to the hippocampal formation. *Behav Neurosci* 111:667–675, 1997.
57. Manns JR, Squire LR: Impaired recognition memory on the doors and people test after damage limited to the hippocampal region. *Hippocampus* 9:495–499, 1999.
58. Moscovitch M, Vriezen E, Goshen-Gottstein Y: Implicit tests of memory in patients with focal lesions and degenerative brain disorders, in Spinnler H, Boller F (eds): *Handbook of Neuropsychology.* Amsterdam: Elsevier, 1993, pp 133–173.
59. Schacter DL, Chiu C-YP, Ochsner KN: Implicit memory: A selective review. *Ann Rev Neurosci* 16:159–182, 1993.
60. Roediger HL, Weldon MS, Challis BH: Explaining dissociations between implicit and explicit measures of retention: A processing account, in Roediger HL, Craik FIM (eds): *Varieties of Memory and Consciousness: Essays in Honour of Endel Tulving.* Hillsdale, NJ: Erlbaum, 1989, pp 3–41.
61. Blaxton TA: Investigating dissociations among memory measures: Support for a transfer-appropriate processing framework. *J Exp Psychol Learn Mem Cogn* 15(4):657–668, 1989.
62. Clarke R, Morton J: Cross modality facilitation in tachistoscopic word recognition. *Q J Exp Psychol* 35A: 79–96, 1983.
63. Jacoby LL, Dallas M: On the relationship between autobiographical memory and perceptual learning. *J Exp Psychol Genl* 110(3):306–340, 1981.
64. Rajaram S, Roediger HL: Direct comparison of four implicit memory tests. *J Exp Psychol Learn Mem Cogn* 19(19):765–776, 1993.
65. Blum D, Yonelinas AP: Transfer across modality in perceptual implicit memory. *Psychonom Bull Rev* 8:147–154, 2001.

66. Srinivas K, Roediger HL: Classifying implicit memory tests: Category association and anagram solution. *J Mem Lang* 29:389–412, 1990.
67. Keane MM, Gabrieli JDE, Mapstone HC, et al: Double dissociation of memory capacities after bilateral occipital-lobe or medial temporal-lobe lesions. *Brain* 118:1129–1148, 1995.
68. Hamann SB: Level-of-processing effects in conceptually driven implicit tasks. *J Exp Psychol Learn Mem Cogn* 16(6):970–977, 1990.
69. Cermak LS, Talbot N, Chandler K, et al: The perceptual priming phenomenon in amnesia. *Neuropsychologia* 23(5):615–622, 1985.
70. Haist F, Musen G, Squire LR: Intact priming of words and nonwords in amnesia. *Psychobiology* 19(4):275–285, 1991.
71. Hamann SB, Squire LR, Schacter DL: Perceptual thresholds and priming in amnesia. *Neuropsychology* 9:3–15, 1995.
72. Hamann SB, Squire LR: Intact priming for novel perceptual representations in amnesia. *J Cogn Neurosci* 9:699–713, 1997.
73. Graf P, Shimamura AP, Squire LR: Priming across modalities and priming across category levels: Extending the domain of preserved function in amnesia. *J Exp Psychol Learn Mem Cogn* 11:386–396, 1985.
74. Cermak LS, Verfaellie M, Chase KA: Implicit and explicit memory in amnesia: An analysis of data-driven and conceptually driven processes. *Neuropsychology* 9:281–290, 1995.
75. Vaidya CJ, Gabrieli JDE, Keane MM, et al: Perceptual and conceptual memory processes in global amnesia. *Neuropsychology* 9:580–591, 1995.
76. Keane MM, Gabrieli JDE, Monti LA, et al: Intact and impaired conceptual memory processes in amnesia. *Neuropsychology* 11:59–69, 1997.
77. Hyman BT, Van Hoesen GW, Damasio AR, et al: Alzheimer's disease: Cell-specific pathology isolates the hippocampal formation. *Science* 225:1168–1170, 1984.
78. Brun A, Englund E: Regional pattern of degeneration in Alzheimer's disease: Neuronal loss and histopathological grading. *Histopathology* 5:549–564, 1981.
79. Rogers J, Morrison JH: Quantitative morphology and regional and laminar distributions of senile plaques in Alzheimer's disease. *J Neurosci* 5(10):2801–2808, 1985.
80. Arnold SE, Hyman BT, Flory J, et al: The topographical and neuroanatomical distribution of neurofibrillary tangles and neuritic plaques in the cerebral cortex of patients with Alzheimer's disease. *Cereb Cortex* 1:1–6, 1991.
81. Esiri MM, Pearson RCA, Powell TPS: The cortex of the primary auditory area in Alzheimer's disease. *Brain Res* 366:385–387, 1986.
82. Lewis DA, Campbell MJ, Terry RD, et al: Laminar and regional distributions of neurofibrillary tangles and neuritic plaques in Alzheimer's disease: A quantitative study of visual and auditory cortices. *J Neurosci* 7(6):1799–1808, 1987.
83. Wilson RS, Sullivan M, deToledo-Morrell, et al: Association of memory and cognition in Alzheimer's disease with volumetric estimates of temporal lobe structures. *Neuropsychology* 10:459–463, 1996.
84. Keane MM, Gabrieli JDE, Fennema AC, et al: Evidence for a dissociation between perceptual and conceptual priming in Alzheimer's disease. *Behav Neurosci* 105(2):326–342, 1991.
85. Fleischman DA, Gabrieli JDE, Reminger S, et al: Conceptual priming in perceptual identification for patients with Alzheimer's disease and a patient with right occipital lobectomy. *Neuropsychology* 9:187–197, 1995.
86. Verfaellie M, Keane MM, Johnson G: Preserved priming in auditory perceptual identification in Alzheimer's disease. *Neuropsychologia* 38:1581–1592, 2000.
87. Moscovitch M: A neuropsychological approach to perception and memory in normal and pathological aging, in Craik FIM, Trehub S (eds): *Aging and Cognitive Processes.* New York: Plenum Press, 1982, pp 55–78.
88. Ober BA, Shenaut GK: Lexical decision and priming in Alzheimer's disease. *Neuropsychologia* 26(2):273–286, 1988.
89. Park SM, Gabrieli JDE, Reminger SL, et al: Preserved priming across study-test picture transformations in patients with Alzheimer's disease. *Neuropsychology* 12:340–352, 1998.
90. Gabrieli JDE, Vaidya CJ, Stone M, et al: Convergent behavioral and neuropsychological evidence for a distinction between identification and production forms of repetition priming. *J Exp Psychol Genl* 128:479–498, 1999.
91. Postle BR, Corkin S, Growdon JH: Intact implicit memory for novel patterns in Alzheimer's disease. *Learn Mem* 3:305–312, 1996.
92. Monti LA, Gabrieli JDE, Reminger SL, et al: Differential effects of aging and Alzheimer's disease upon conceptual implicit and explicit memory. *Neuropsychology* 10:101–112, 1996.
93. Brandt J, Spencer M, McSorley P, et al: Semantic activation and implicit memory in Alzheimer disease. *Alzheimer Dis Assoc Disord* 2:112–119, 1988.

94. Huff FJ, Mack L, Mahlmann J, et al: A comparison of lexical-semantic impairments in left hemisphere stroke and Alzheimer's disease. *Brain Lang* 34:262–278, 1988.
95. Salmon DP, Shimamura AP, Butters N, et al: Lexical and semantic priming deficits in patients with Alzheimer's disease. *J Clin Exp Neuropsychol* 10(4):477–494, 1988.
96. Gabrieli JDE, Fleischman DA, Keane MM, et al: Double dissociation between memory systems underlying explicit and implicit memory in the human brain. *Psychol Sci* 6:76–82, 1995.
97. Squire LR, Ojemann JG, Miezin FM, et al: Activation of the hippocampus in normal humans: A functional anatomical study of memory. *Proc Natl Acad Sci U S A* 89:1837–1841, 1992.
98. Buckner RL, Petersen SE, Ojemann JG, et al: Functional anatomical studies of explicit and implicit memory retrieval tasks. *J Neurosci* 15:12–29, 1995.
99. Schacter DL, Alpert NM, Savage CR, et al: Conscious recollection and the human hippocampal formation: Evidence from positron emission tomography. *Proc Natl Acad Sci USA* 93:321–325, 1996.
100. Badgaiyan RD, Posner MI: Time course of cortical activations in implicit and explicit recall. *J Neurosci* 17:4904–4913, 1997.
101. Lebreton K, Desgranges B, Landeau B, et al: Visual priming within and across symbolic format using a tachistoscopic picture identification task: A PET study. *J Cogn Neurosci* 13:670–686, 2001.
102. Demb JB, Desmond JE, Wagner AD, et al: Semantic encoding and retrieval in the left inferior prefrontal cortex: A functional MRI study of task difficulty and process specificity. *J Neurosci* 15:5870–5878, 1995.
103. Gabrieli JDE, Desmond JE, Demb JB, et al: Functional magnetic resonance imaging of semantic memory processes in the frontal lobes. *Psychol Sci* 7:278–283, 1996.
104. Wagner AD, Desmond JE, Demb JB, et al: Semantic repetition priming for verbal and pictorial knowledge: A functional MRI study of left inferior prefrontal cortex. *J Cogn Neurosci* 9:714–726, 1997.
105. Diamond R, Rozin P: Activation of existing memories in the amnesic syndromes. *J Abnorm Psychol* 93:98–105, 1984.
106. Keane MM, Gabrieli JDE, Noland JS, et al: Normal perceptual priming of orthographically illegal nonwords in amnesia. *J Int Neuropsychol Soc* 1:425–433, 1995.
107. Gabrieli JDE, Milberg W, Keane MM, et al: Intact priming of patterns despite impaired memory. *Neuropsychologia* 28(5):417–427, 1990.
108. Musen G, Squire LR: Nonverbal priming in amnesia. *Mem Cogn* 20:441–448, 1992.
109. Schacter DL, Cooper LA, Tharan M, et al: Preserved priming of novel objects in patients with memory disorders. *J Cogn Neurosci* 3:117–130, 1991.
110. Paller KA, Mayes AR, Thompson KM, et al: Priming of face matching in amnesia. *Brain Cogn* 18:46–59, 1992.
111. Moscovitch M, Winocur G, McLachlan D: Memory as assessed by recognition and reading time in normal and memory-impaired people with Alzheimer's disease and other neurological disorders. *J Exp Psychol Genl* 115:331–347, 1986.
112. Gabrieli JDE, Keane MM, Zarella MM, et al: Preservation of implicit memory for new associations in global amnesia. *Psychol Sci* 7:326–329, 1997.
113. Goshen-Gottstein Y, Moscovitch M, Melo B: Intact implicit memory for newly formed verbal associations in amnesic patients following single study trials. *Neuropsychology* 14:570–578, 2000.
114. Schacter DL, Graf P: Preserved learning in amnesic patients: Perspectives from research on direct priming. *J Clin Exp Neuropsychol* 8:727–743, 1986.
115. Mayes AR, Gooding P: Enhancement of word completion priming in amnesics by cueing with previously novel associates. *Neuropsychologia* 27(8):1057–1072, 1989.
116. Shimamura AP, Squire LR: Impaired priming of new associations in amnesia. *J Exp Psychol Learn Mem Cogn* 15:721–728, 1989.
117. Musen G, Squire LR: On the implicit learning of novel associations by amnesic patients and normal subjects. *Neuropsychology* 7(2):119–135, 1993.
118. Goshen-Gottstein Y, Moscovitch M: Repetition priming for newly formed and preexisting associations: Perceptual and conceptual influences. *J Exp Psychol Learn Mem Cogn* 21:1229–1248, 1995.
119. Goshen-Gottstein Y, Moscovitch M: Repetition priming effects for newly formed associations are perceptually based: Evidence from shallow encoding and format specificity. *J Exp Psychol Learn Mem Cogn* 21:1249–1262, 1995.
120. Schacter DL, Graf P: Effects of elaborative processing on implicit and explicit memory for new associations. *J Exp Psychol Learn Mem Cogn* 12(3):432–444, 1986.
121. Verfaellie M, Keane MM: Scope and limits of implicit memory in amnesia, in De Gelder B, De Haan EHF, Heywood CA (eds): *Out of Mind: Varieties of Unconscious Processes.* Oxford, UK: Oxford University Press, 2001.
122. Cohen NJ, Poldrack RA, Eichenbaum H: Memory for items and memory for relations in the procedural/declarative memory framework. *Memory* 5:131–178, 1997.

Chapter 39

SEMANTIC MEMORY IMPAIRMENTS

Martha J. Farah
Murray Grossman

Semantic memory refers to our general knowledge of the objects, people, and events of the world (Tulving, 1972). The knowledge that Paris is the capital of France, that birds have feathers, and that a desk is a piece of furniture exemplifies semantic memory. More particular knowledge, tied to an individual's personal experience, is considered *episodic memory* rather than semantic memory. Examples of the latter include the knowledge that you bought this book at a certain store or ate a certain food for breakfast this morning.

Neurologic disease and damage can affect semantic memory disproportionately. In this chapter the different forms of semantic memory impairment are reviewed, with attention to their etiologies, major behavioral features, and implications for the neural substrates and functional organization of semantic memory in the normal brain.

GENERALIZED IMPAIRMENT OF SEMANTIC MEMORY

Warrington (1975) first documented a pattern of preserved and impaired performance indicative of semantic memory impairment in a series of three patients suffering from progressive degenerative brain disease. Her subjects were relatively preserved on most measures of language and cognitive function but did poorly on tasks dependent on semantic memory, including confrontation naming, word-picture matching, and a verification task in which subjects were shown pictures or words and asked questions such as "Is it a bird?" or "Is it heavy?" In subsequent years a number of similar cases were reported, and the term *semantic dementia* was coined in the context of one such report (Snowden et al., 1989). Hodges and coworkers (1992) presented a wide-ranging study of five new cases of semantic dementia, reviewed the literature, and drew a number of useful generalizations concerning the condition. A summary of their conclusions is presented here.

Semantic dementia may present initially as a language disorder whose most prominent feature is vocabulary loss, both expressive and receptive. Naming is minimally aided by phonemic cues, and naming errors tend to share a semantic relation with the correct name (e.g., "violin" for accordion, or "animal" for fox). In production, category fluency is severely impaired, and word definitions are improverished or wrong. Such patients have sometimes been described as having a fluent form of primary progressive aphasia (see Chaps. 11 and 12), but additional language testing and nonverbal semantic memory testing suggests that the underlying impairment is one of semantic memory knowledge rather than language. Syntax and phonology tend to be preserved, whereas entirely pictorial tasks that depend on knowledge of the depicted objects, such as sorting together semantically related objects or distinguishing real from imaginary objects, are failed. Although the formal assessment of episodic memory is difficult because of the loss of knowledge of word and picture meanings, Hodges and coworkers (Hodges et al., 1992) observe that at least some patients show significant preservation of autobiographical memories and practical day-to-day memory. The neuropathologic changes in semantic dementia are focused in the temporal lobes, often affecting the left more than the right, and semantic dementia has come to be regarded as a variant of frontotemporal lobar degeneration (see Chap. 47).

Another degenerative disease affecting semantic memory is Alzheimer's disease (AD) (Martin and Fedio, 1983; Bayles and coworkers, 1990; Chertkow and Bub, 1990; Hodges et al., 1992; Nebes, 1992; Grossman and Mickanin, 1994) although semantic memory is just one of many aspects of cognition impaired in AD (see Chap. 45), and initially some cases may present with only episodic memory impairment.

To the extent that semantic memory is impaired in AD, pathologic changes in temporal cortex are responsible.

In recent years the study of semantic memory in neurologic patients has been complemented by a growing literature on semantic memory studied with functional neuroimaging in normal subjects (see Thompson-Schill, 2003, for a review). The temporal localization inferred from the cases of generalized semantic memory impairment, in degenerative conditions such as semantic dementia and AD, accords well with the conclusions emerging from the neuroimaging literature. For example, when Vandenberghe et al. (1996) mapped the regions active during different types of semantic tasks and presented via different modalities, regions in left temporal cortex were invariably activated. Using semantic priming as a marker for regions subserving semantics, Thompson-Schill et al. (1999) also found temporal activation.

In sum, semantic memory is at least partially dissociable from other forms of memory, language and cognition, and the dissociation is generally seen in the context of degenerative diseases. The neuropathology in these cases implicates temporal cortex, with some degree of lateralization to the left—a conclusion that finds growing support within the functional neuroimaging literature.

SELECTIVE IMPAIRMENTS OF SEMANTIC MEMORY

In addition to the generalized impairments of semantic memory described above, particular aspects of semanatic memory can be disproportionately impaired. These disorders suggest that semantic memory has an internal organization, with different components of semantics localized in different brain regions.

Category-Specific Semantic Memory Impairment

In some cases it appears that knowledge from certain semantic categories is disproportionately impaired, suggesting that the neural bases of semantic memory are subdivided by semantic category. The most common category-specific semantic memory impairment affects knowledge of living things.

The first report of impaired knowledge of living things was made by Warrington and Shallice (1984), who described three postencephalitic patients. Although the patients were generally impaired at tasks such as picture naming and defining words, they were dramatically worse when the pictures or words represented animals and plants than when they represented artifacts. In subsequent years numerous other reports appeared of similar patients, generally suffering damage to temporal cortex from herpes encephalitis, closed head injury, or, less frequently, cerebrovascular or degenerative disease. Category-specific disorders of semantic memory are distinct from the disorders described in the previous section, despite the implication of temporal brain regions in both, as neither semantic dementia (Hodges et al., 1992) nor AD (Tippett et al., 1996) routinely affects knowledge of living things more than nonliving.

The idea that certain brain regions are specialized for representing knowledge about living things has naturally aroused some skepticism and prompted a search for alternative explanations of apparently impaired knowledge of living things. The simplest alternative explanation is that the impairment is an artifact of the greater difficulty of retrieving knowledge about living things. It has been suggested that when difficulty is equated across living and nonliving test items, the selectivity of the semantic memory impairment disappears (Funnell and Sheridan, 1992; Stewart et al., 1992). However, the selectivity has been shown to persist in two cases when multiple measures of difficulty are accounted for (Farah et al., 1991), and the null results in other controlled studies are likely due to insufficient statistical power, as our reliable findings disappeared when we reduced our data set to the size of the other studies (Farah et al., 1996).

Cases of impaired knowledge of nonliving things with relatively spared knowledge of living things are rarer but have also been described (Warrington and McCarthy, 1983, 1987; Hillis and Caramazza, 1991; Sacchett and Humphreys, 1992). The lesions in these cases are confined to the left hemisphere. A precise intrahemispheric localization is not possible, as the lesions are typically large and relatively few cases have been reported, although the left temporal region again seems involved (Tippett et al., 1996). These patients provide the other half of a double dissociation with impaired knowledge of living things, thus adding further support to the hypothesis that category-specific semantic memory impairments are not simply due to the differential difficulty of particular categories.

Building on the hypothesis of Allport (1985), that semantic memory is subdivided into different sensorimotor modalities (e.g., visual knowledge, tactile knowledge, motor knowledge), Warrington and Shallice (1984) proposed a different kind of alternative explanation for category-specific knowledge deficits. They suggested that living and nonliving things may differ from one another in their reliance on knowledge from different sensorimotor modalities, with living things being known predominantly by their visual and other sensory attributes. Impaired knowledge of living things could result from an impairment of visual knowledge. Similarly, nonliving things might be known predominantly by their function, an abstract form of motoric representation, and impaired knowledge of nonliving things could result from an impairment of functional knowledge. This interpretation has the advantage of parsimony, in that it invokes a type of organization already known to exist in the brain—modality-specific organization—rather than invoking an organization based on semantic categories such as aliveness.

A computer simulation of semantic memory and its impairments has shown that a modality-specific organization can account for category-specific impairments, even the finding that functional knowledge of living things is impaired after visual semantic damage (Farah and McClelland, 1991). The latter finding is explained by the need for a certain "critical mass" of associated knowledge to help activate collaterally any one part of a distributed representation; if most of the representation of living things is visual and visual knowledge is damaged, then the remaining functional knowledge cannot be activated. The finding that visual knowledge of living things is the most impaired type of knowledge, with nonvisual knowledge of nonliving things the least impaired and visual nonliving and nonvisual living intermediate (Farah et al., 1989), is consistent with this fundamentally modality-specific view of semantic memory organization.

Nevertheless, the semantic impairment in some cases seems equally severe for visual and nonvisual knowledge of living things, while knowledge of even the visual attributes of nonliving things is relatively preserved, implying that semantic memory is organized by category rather than, or in addition to, by modality of knowledge (Caramazza and Shelton, 1998; Farah and Rabinowitz, 2003). Findings from functional neuroimaging of normal subjects also offer evidence of both modality specificity in knowledge of living things (Thompson-Schill et al., 1999) and segregation of living things within the visual modality-specific semantic system (Chao and Martin, 1999). It now seems likely that the organization of semantic memory involves multiple levels of representation, some more closely related to the modality of the information represented and some more closely related to the semantic category.

A final point concerning category-specific impairments is that semantic memory is not the only functional system with a categorical internal structure, and this fact has led to some confusion. Within vision, the dissociability of face, object, and printed word recognition suggests the existence of subsystems whose specialization might be considered categorical. These subsystems differ crucially from those for living and nonliving things, however, in that they are required for visual recognition but not for more general knowledge retrieval. A visual object agnosic knows what a horse is and is simply unable to recognize it by sight. A patient with semantic memory impairment, in contrast, can neither recognize a horse by sight nor provide information of any kind about horses. Category-specific semantic memory impairments are also sometimes confused with category-specific impairments in name retrieval. The "fruit and vegetable" impairment observed in two cases (Hart et al., 1985; Farah and Wallace, 1992) affects naming only. As with more general anomias, the names are recognized when seen or heard, the objects themselves are recognized, and semantic information appears intact.

Modality-Specific Semantic Memory Impairment

There is a second way in which the phrase *modality-specific semantic memory* has been used in neuropsychology, and that is for components of semantic memory that are accessed *through* a particular input or output modality. According to this usage, visual semantics refers not to semantic knowledge of the visual appearance of objects but to the semantic knowledge of appearance, function, and so on that is accessed when an object is seen. The puzzling syndrome of "optic aphasia" has led some to conclude that semantic memory must have a modality-specific organization in this input-defined sense.

Optic aphasia consists of an impairment in naming visually presented stimuli in the face of relatively preserved naming of nonvisual stimuli and relatively preserved nonverbal demonstrations of visual recognition. It seems reasonable to assume that visual confrontation naming requires three major stages of processing: vision, semantics, and lexical retrieval. That is, it requires seeing the object clearly enough to access semantic knowledge of it and using that semantic knowledge of what the object is to retrieve its name. Paradoxically, the preserved nonvisual naming and nonverbal recognition performance of optic aphasics seem to exonerate all three stages.

A variety of attempts have been made to explain how an anomia could exist for visual stimuli only. An early and influential account takes the dissociations at face value and invokes separate modality-specific semantic memory systems for interpreting visual input and other modality inputs, so that optic aphasia can be explained as a disconnection between visual semantics (i.e., the semantic knowledge accessed by visual inputs) and verbal semantics (i.e., the semantic knowledge necessary to access a verbal output) (Beauvois, 1982). In recent years, more parsimonious alternative explanations of optic aphasia have been proposed (Plaut and Shallice, 1993; Sitton et al., 2000; see Chap. 10), thereby diminishing the need to hypothesize semantic systems specific for each input modality.

REFERENCES

Allport DA: Distributed memory, modular subsystems and dysphasia, in Newmans, Epstein R (eds): *Current Perspectives in Dysphasia*. Edinburgh: Churchill Livingstone, 1985.

Bayles KA, Tomoeda CK, Trosset MW: Naming and categorical knowledge in Alzheimer's disease: The process of semantic memory deterioration. *Brain Lang* 39:498–510, 1990.

Beauvois MF: Optic aphasia: A process of interaction between vision and language. *Philos Trans R Soc Lond* B 298:35–47, 1982.

Caramazza A, Shelton JR: Domain specific knowledge systems in the brain: The animate-inanimate distinction. *J Cogn Neurosci* 10:1–34, 1998.

Chao LL, Martin A: Cortical representation of perception, naming and knowledge of color. *J Cogn Neurosci* 11:25–35, 1999.

Chertkow H, Bub D: Semantic memory loss in dementia of Alzheimer's type: What do various measures measure? *Brain* 113:397–417, 1990.

Epstein R, DeYoe EA, Press DZ, et al: Neuropsychological evidence for a topographical learning mechanism in parahippocampal cortex. *Cogn Neuropsychol* 18:481–508, 2001.

Farah MJ: *Visual Agnosia: Disorders of Object Recognition and What They Tell Us About Normal Vision*. Cambridge, MA: MIT Press/Bradford Books, 1990.

Farah MJ, Hammon KH, Mehta Z, Ratcliff G: Category-specificity and modality-specificity in semantic memory. *Neuropsychologia* 27:193–200, 1989.

Farah MJ, McClelland JL: A computational model of semantic memory impairment: Modality-specificity and emergent category-specificity. *J Exp Psychol Genl* 120:339–357, 1991.

Farah MJ, McMullen PA, Meyer MM: Can recognition of living things be selectively impaired? *Neuropsychologia* 29:185–193, 1991.

Farah MJ, Meyer MM, McMullen PA: The living/nonliving dissociation is not an artifact: Giving an a priori implausible hypothesis a strong test. *Cogn Neuropsychol* 13:152–154, 1996.

Farah M, Rabinowitz C: Genetic and environmental influences on the organization of semantic memory in the brain: Is "living things" an innate category?" *Cogn Neuropsychol* 2003.

Farah MJ, Wallace MA: Semantically-bounded anomia: Implications for the neural implementation of naming. *Neuropsychologia* 30:609–621, 1992.

Funnell E, Sheridan J: Categories of knowledge? Unfamiliar aspects of living and non-living things. *Cogn Neuropsychol* 9:135–154, 1992.

Grossman M, Mickanin J: Picture comprehension and probable Alzheimer's disease. *Brain Cogn* 26:43–64, 1994.

Hart J, Berndt RS, Caramazza A: Category-specific naming deficit following cerebral infarction. *Nature* 316:439–440, 1985.

Hillis A, Caramazza C: Category-specific naming and comprehension impairment: A double dissociation. *Brain* 114:2081–2094, 1991.

Hodges JR, Patterson K, Oxbury S, Funnell E: Semantic dementia. *Brain* 115:1783–1806, 1992.

Hodges JR, Salmon DP, Butters N: Semantic memory impairment in Alzheimer's disease: Failure of access of degraded knowledge? *Neuropsychologia* 30:301–314, 1992.

Martin A, Fedio P: Word production and comprehension in Alzheimer's disease: The breakdown of semantic knowledge. *Brain Lang* 19:124–141, 1983.

Nebes RD: Cognitive dysfunction in Alzheimer's disease, in Craik FIM, Salthouse A (eds): *The Handbook of Aging and Cognition*. Hillsdale, NJ: Erlbaum, 1992.

Plaut DC, Shallice T: Perseverative and semantic influences on visual object naming errors in optic aphasia: A connectionist account. *J Cogn Neurosci* 5:89-117, 1993.

Sacchett C, Humphreys GW: Calling a squirrel a squirrel but a canoe a wigwam: A category-specific deficit for artifactual objects and body parts. *Cogn Neuropsychol* 9:73-86, 1992.

Shallice T: Impairments of semantic processing: Multiple dissociations, in Coltheart M, Sartori G, Job R (eds): *The Cognitive Neuropsychology of Language*. London: Erlbaum, 1987.

Sitton M, Mozer MC, Farah MJ: Superadditive effects of multiple lesions in a connectionist architecture: Implications for the neuropsychology of optic aphasia. *Psychol Rev* 709–734, 2000.

Snowden JS, Goulding PJ, Neary D: Semantic dementia: A form of circumscribed cerebral atrophy. *Behav Neurol* 2:167–182, 1989.

Stewart F, Parkin AJ, Hunkin NM: Naming impairments following recovery from herpes simplex encephalitis: Category specific? *Q J Exp Psychol* 44A:261–284, 1992.

Thompson-Schill SL: Neuroimaging studies of semantic memory: inferring "how" from "where." *Neuropsychologia*, 41:280–292, 2003.

Thompson-Schill SL, Aguirre GK, D'Esposito M, Farah MJ: A neural basis for category and modality specificity of semantic knowledge. *Neuropsychologia* 37:671–676, 1999.

Thompson-Schill SL, D'Esposito M, Kan IP: Effects of repetition and competition on prefrontal activity during word generation. *Neuron* 23:513–522, 1999.

Thompson-Schill SL, Gabrieli JD: Priming of visual and functional knowledge on a semantic classification task. *J Exp Psychol Learn Mem Cogn* 25:41–53, 1999.

Tippett LJ, Glosser G, Farah MJ: A category-specific naming deficit after temporal lobectomy. *Neuropsychologia*. 34:139–146, 1996.

Tippett LJ, Grossman M, Farah MJ: The semantic memory deficit of Alzheimer's disease: category-specific? *Cortex* 32:143–153, 1996.

Tulving E: Episodic and semantic memory, in Tulving E, Donaldson W (eds): *Organization of Memory*. New York: Academic Press, 1972.

Vandenberghe R, Price C, Wise R, et al: Functional anatomy of a common semantic system for words and pictures. *Nature* 383:254–256, 1996.

Warrington EK: The selective impairment of semantic memory. *Q J Exp Psychol* 27:635–657, 1975.

Warrington EK, McCarthy R: Category specific access dysphasia. *Brain* 106:859–878, 1983.

Warrington EK, McCarthy R: Categories of knowledge: Further fractionations and an attempted explanation. *Brain* 110:1273–1296, 1987.

Warrington EK, Shallice T: Category specific semantic impairments. *Brain* 107:829–854, 1984.

Chapter 40

LEARNING AND MEMORY DYSFUNCTION FOLLOWING TRAUMATIC BRAIN INJURY*

Frank G. Hillary
John DeLuca

Traumatic brain injury (TBI) has been defined as an injury to the brain resulting from an external source, which may lead to significant impairment in the individual's physical, cognitive, and psychosocial functioning.[1] Each year approximately 1.5 to 2 million people sustain TBI in the United States.[1] According to the Centers for Disease Control and Prevention (CDC), each year 1 million people are treated and released from hospital emergency rooms,[2] 230,000 people are hospitalized and survive,[3]and 50,000 people die from traumatic brain injury.[4]

Memory dysfunction following TBI is the most common cognitive symptom reported by patients.[5] It has been documented that between 54 and 84 percent of individuals sustaining severe TBI experience significant memory impairment.[6] This high incidence of memory dysfunction is important because memory problems have been linked to an inability to return to work[6] and to success rates in rehabilitation and vocational training.[7] Moreover, in cases of severe TBI, residual memory impairment has been reported 5 and 10 years after the initial injury,[8,9] forcing individuals with TBI to adjust to long-term deficits in learning and memory.

MEMORY PROCESSES IN THE BRAIN

Memory is not a unitary construct. This was a central idea in each of the preceding three chapters on memory, which reviewed the dissociable subsystems and processes of memory revealed by brain damage. The relation between memory dysfunction and memory subsystems will be reviewed here first, followed by a similar analysis of memory dysfunction and memory processes. While some debate the benefits of a "systems" versus "processing" approach to the study of learning and memory, these approaches are likely more complementary than incompatible.[10]

One major distinction in the human memory system is between declarative (i.e., knowing that) and procedural (i.e., knowing how).[11] This distinction between the declarative and procedural memory systems is important because each may be differentially affected following TBI. Typically, aspects of declarative memory are significantly impaired following TBI, and procedural memory typically remains intact. The declarative and procedural memory systems can be further decomposed into specific subsystems (see Fig. 40-1).

Procedural memory refers to the acquisition of motor and cognitive skills or routines. Examples include learning to ride a bike, read, or drive a car. Figure 40-1 lists several major subdivisions of procedural memory. Procedural memory skills are usually characterized by gradual and incremental learning.

The declarative memory system can be divided into the episodic and semantic memory systems. *Episodic memory* refers to the recollection of facts, or episodes—the reflection of personal experiences. For example, remembering what you ate for lunch or recalling the name of a person you knew in college are examples of episodic memories. Episodic memory is the primary memory system impaired following TBI. *Semantic memory* refers to the acquisition of general knowledge about the world that is not tied to personal

* **ACKNOWLEDGMENTS:** This chapter was supported in part by NIH grant HD07522. We would like to thank Scott Millis, Ph.D., for his comments on an earlier version of this manuscript, and Cassandra Racasi for preparing the manuscript for publication.

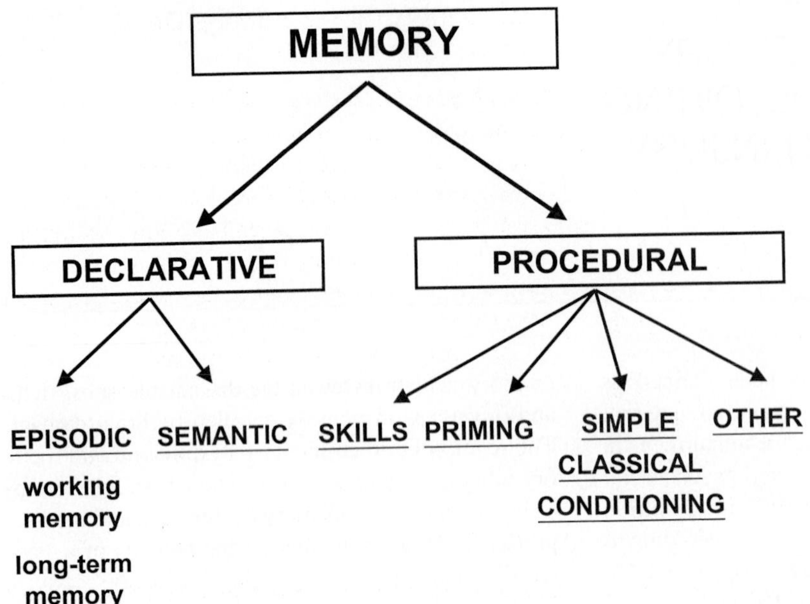

Figure 40-1 *Schematic diagram of the human memory system and its various subdivisions. (Adapted from Squire,[98] with permission.)*

experience. For example, semantic memory is required to understand the meaning of words or concepts. In general, semantic memory remains relatively intact following TBI,[10] although, as discussed below, there may be rare instances of semantic memory disruption in such individuals.

Learning and memory can be viewed not only as a multidimensional, modular system but also in terms of an information processing framework.[11] Within this framework, learning and memory can be conceptualized in terms of "stages" or "processes." For instance, in episodic memory, in order for information to move from temporary to long-term storage, several processes must take place. Specifically, the processes within the episodic memory system can be discussed in terms of *working memory, encoding, consolidation,* and *retrieval. Working memory* (WM) refers to the temporary storage and active maintenance and manipulation of internal representations for on-line use (e.g., maintaining an address or phone number while searching for a pen to write it down).[12] WM is considered the first step in the encoding of information into episodic memory.[13] Although well established, the concept of WM is not without controversy.[14] For instance, some investigators feel that WM (particularly the central executive component) is composed of previously established cognitive constructs such as attention, concentration, and "executive functions" and is therefore not unique to "memory" processes. Nonetheless, the cognitive functions occurring at this early stage in information processing directly impact later memory processes, are particularly vulnerable to disruption following TBI, and are therefore critical when discussing learning and memory following TBI.

Encoding refers to the process of acquiring information. For instance, while information is rehearsed in WM, memory traces are developed. The process by which this encoded memory trace is transferred from short-term temporary storage to more enduring (or long-term) storage is called *consolidation* or *elaboration.*[15] *Retrieval* refers to the process of accessing previously encoded information from long-term storage so that it can be processed within the working memory system.[15] There remains some debate regarding the stages and fluidity of these processes, but these basic operating definitions will serve for the purposes of this chapter. As will be discussed later, knowing where in this process learning and memory break down can have significant implications for rehabilitation.

ACUTE MEMORY DYSFUNCTION FOLLOWING TBI

In the acute stages following moderate and severe TBI, the trauma often induces a transient confusional state that was originally recognized as a distinct clinical syndrome by Symonds and colleagues over 70 years ago.[16] These investigators drew a clinical distinction between the "cloudiness" of this time period and the preceding period of unconsciousness. Later, the term *posttraumatic amnesia* (PTA) was used by Russell and Nathan to describe this transient period following TBI, where new learning and memory are significantly disrupted.[17] PTA is characterized by dense declarative memory deficits resulting in confusion and disorientation. In addition to the memory loss for information after the trauma (anterograde amnesia), there is often memory loss for information prior to the trauma (retrograde amnesia), and the nature of these memory deficits has a temporal gradient (i.e., older memories are more resistant to disruption).[18] In addition to memory deficits, other cognitive difficulties common during PTA include reduced information processing speed, significantly impaired attention, and impaired higher cognitive functioning.[19] Not surprisingly, the cognitive deficits observed during PTA are often accompanied by significant behavioral problems, including agitation, restlessness, confabulation, lethargy, and disinhibition.[20]

Predicting Outcome Based on PTA Duration

As early as 1932, PTA was determined to be an important predictor of patient prognosis.[21] More recent data have verified the close relationship between duration of PTA and TBI severity[22,23] and the relationship between PTA and recovery potential.[24] The relationship between PTA duration and outcome is illustrated in Fig. 40-2. In fact, PTA has proven to be the best predictor of cognitive outcome compared to other injury severity markers such as the Glasgow Coma Scale (GCS)[25] and duration of loss of consciousness.[26] Because PTA duration is such an important prognostic tool, assessment of PTA is widely emphasized in acute and subacute rehabilitation facilities.

Assessment of PTA

Bedside evaluations of PTA are typically brief and geared toward the assessment of episodic memory and orientation. The first instrument designed for prospective measurement of PTA was the Galveston Orientation and Amnesia Test (GOAT).[27] Other measures used for prospective determination of PTA include the Westmead PTA scale[28] and, more recently, the Wessex Head Injury Matrix (WHIM).[29] The WHIM was designed to categorize the early recovery patterns typically observed following severe TBI. These instruments are typically administered serially over the course of days

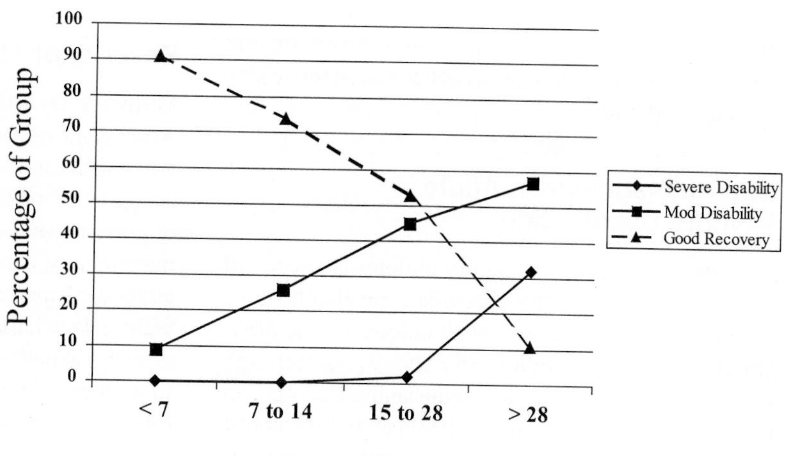

Figure 40-2
The relationship between duration of PTA and recovery based on Glasgow Outcome Scale scores. (Adapted from Jennet,[99] with permission.)

to weeks following injury. A patient is considered to be emerging from PTA once scores of 75 or greater (out of a total of 108) are achieved on consecutive days on the GOAT[27] or 3 consecutive days with perfect scores are achieved on the Westmead PTA scale.

There has been some debate regarding the method of determining PTA duration. While some investigators have included the period of unconsciousness preceding PTA in the assessment, others have defined PTA as beginning once the patient has emerged from coma.[26,30] Assessment can be difficult because emergence from PTA is a gradual process that may include "islands" of orientation or intact memory amid periods of significant confusion and disorientation.[19] In one study of severe TBI, 94 percent of the time (or in 29 of 31 patients), recovery from PTA involved reorientation to person first, followed by place (e.g., name of hospital) and then time (i.e., date, month, year).[31]

PTA assessment is also complicated by the fact that patients who have emerged from PTA may continue to experience significant episodic memory dysfunction that may be difficult to distinguish from the disorientation that characterizes it.[32] Furthermore, while a chief clinical feature of PTA is disorientation, seminal work by Gronwall and Wrightson[33] determined that 5 of their 13 patients were oriented but remained in PTA. For this reason, investigators have emphasized that cognitive functions other than orientation and episodic memory—such as information processing speed, attention, and executive functions—be assessed in order to accurately determine when patients have emerged from PTA.[19] Some examiners have even proposed redefining PTA as a period of posttraumatic "confusional state" in order to better characterize this clinical syndrome.[34]

Neurometabolism in Acute Memory Dysfunction

In cases of severe TBI the injury initiates a cascade of neurochemical events that exacerbate the effects of the primary injury, which may result in long-lasting alterations in cellular functioning (for review, see Ref. 35). Recent research (particularly with animals) suggests that many of these early neurochemical and metabolic changes significantly affect learning and memory performance (see Ref. 36 for a review).

In humans, neuroimaging advances such as magnetic resonance spectroscopy (MRS) have allowed researchers to track acute neurometabolic changes in individuals sustaining TBI. For example, reductions in *N*-acetylaspartate (a marker for axonal integrity) and elevations in choline (a neurometabolite that increases at sites of local tissue breakdown) have been documented during the acute recovery period following TBI.[37] These changes in neurometabolism have been shown to correlate significantly with learning and memory performance at the time of injury[38] and with general cognitive performance at 3 months postinjury.[39] Figure 40-3 illustrates the relationship between specific neurometabolic markers and learning and memory performance. Further application of advanced neuroimaging techniques, such as MRS, will improve our understanding of the neurophysiologic and neurometabolic conditions responsible for PTA.

CHRONIC MEMORY DYSFUNCTION FOLLOWING TBI

Once patients have emerged from PTA, they often experience episodic memory impairments of varying severity. These decrements in new learning and memory may last for months or years and in many cases are permanent. Because of this, investigating the mechanism responsible for memory impairment and the nature of these impairments has received considerable attention.

Severity of TBI and Memory Dysfunction

Memory Dysfunction in Mild TBI In 1993 the American Congress of Rehabilitation Medicine[40] provided a definition of mild TBI (mTBI) consisting of at least one of the following: (1) any period of loss of consciousness, (2) any loss of memory for events immediately before or after the accident, (3) any alteration of mental state at the time of accident (e.g., feeling dazed, disoriented, or confused), and (4) focal neurologic deficit(s) that may or may not be transient. In addition, TBI is not considered mild if any of the following occurs: (1) loss of consciousness exceeding approximately 30 min; (2) after 30 min, a GCS falling below 13; (3) PTA persisting longer than 24 h.

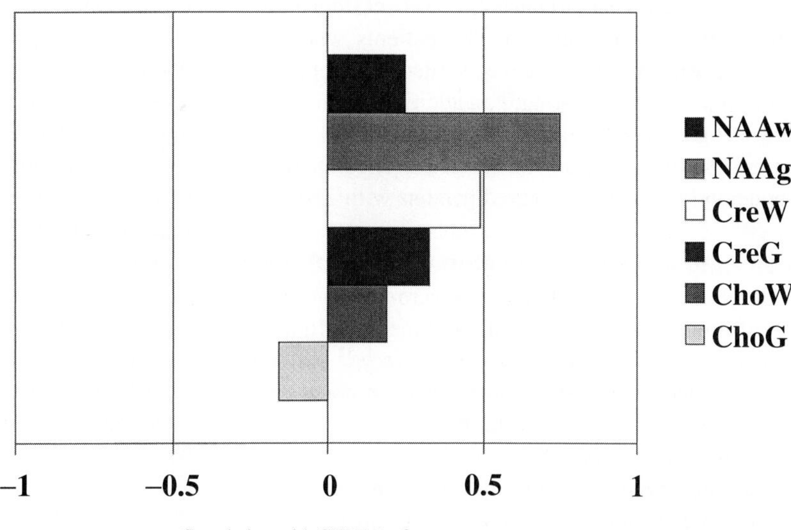

Figure 40-3
The relationship between acute neurometabolic functioning and memory scores on the California Verbal Learning Test (CVLT). For the neurometabolites, gray matter N-acetylaspartate is NAAg, white matter N-acetylaspartate is NAAw, gray matter creatinine is CreG, white matter creatinine is CreW, gray matter choline is ChoG, and white matter choline is ChoW. (Adapted from Friedman et al.,[100] with permission from the author.)

Investigation of mTBI came to the forefront in the 1970s and early 1980s, when cases of very mild brain injury were being linked to difficulty in returning to work and concomitant cognitive deficits, including memory impairment.[33,41,42] This early research noted that memory dysfunction is one of the most common consequences of mTBI and that, in some individuals, these symptoms remained for months following the injury.

Since that time, investigators have examined the factors contributing to recovery of memory functions following mTBI. In a study combining the findings across three treatment facilities, the results indicated that individuals sustaining a single mTBI, in the absence of additional complicating factors (i.e., litigation, secondary gain, premorbid personality, and/or emotional disturbance) typically experience a full recovery.[43] These data are similar to more recent work noting that persistence of symptoms after mTBI is of relatively low incidence (e.g., 7 to 8 percent[44]; 10 to 20 percent[45]).

Most cases of mTBI do not result in PTA (or PTA of very short duration) and only temporary acute episodic memory disturbance (if any). However, there is a minority of individuals with mTBI who continue to suffer "postconcussive symptoms" (e.g., Ref. 46) for months or even years after the injury. These individuals report persisting complaints that may include episodic memory disturbance, slowed thinking, fatigue, irritability, or depression. That the magnitude and duration of these memory disturbances are disproportionate to the degree of injury has been a primary reason to attribute these postconcussive symptoms to a combination emotional and other premorbid risk factors. For example, emotional, personality, and other factors (e.g., litigation) have been shown to be related to persisting cognitive problems.[46–48]

More recently, positron emission tomography (PET) has corroborated the complaints of some individuals with postconcussion syndrome, suggesting differences in glucose metabolism between individuals exhibiting full recovery from TBI and individuals who experienced a prolonged or incomplete recovery curve.[49] Despite the difference in glucose metabolism between those who recover and those who do not, the cause for this difference remains unclear. Determining the causes of long-standing memory (and other cognitive) complaints in this "miserable minority"[47] has proven difficult. The reasons for their failure to achieve full recovery are likely linked to many factors including degree of neurologic injury, personality style, and premorbid emotional status.

It should also be recognized that suboptimal effort or motivation can have profound effects on test performance, particularly in mTBI. Recent studies have shown that 33 percent of mTBI patients who were seeking compensation had exaggerated their deficits on neuropsychological testing.[50] In addition, memory and other cognitive problems are often significantly worse in mTBI patients with suboptimal effort compared to moderately to severely injured persons with TBI.[51]

Learning and Memory in Moderate and Severe TBI Following moderate and severe TBI, the most rapid improvement in learning and memory function occurs during the first months of recovery,[52] although improvement in verbal memory has been noted up to 5 years postinjury.[8] Following the acute recovery process, individuals typically exhibit reduced information processing speed[53] and display significant impairment in working memory,[54] which can contribute to difficulties in episodic memory.[55]

Investigators have attempted to use markers of injury severity to predict memory functioning at 1 year postinjury. Levin and colleagues[56] determined that the GCS alone and measures of intracranial pressure did not predict memory dysfunction at 1 year following injury. However, these investigators did find that impaired consciousness and pupil reactivity at the time of the injury were predictive of later verbal memory performance.[56]

There is also evidence that learning and memory dysfunction following TBI may be characterized by a heterogeneous recovery curve irrespective of the nature or severity of TBI. For example, Ruff et al.[57] analyzed the memory performance of individuals recovering from severe TBI at three points in time (baseline, 6 months, and 12 months); their data revealed three separate subtypes within the sample. These recovery trajectories took the form of slow progressive recovery, dramatic linear recovery, and initial dramatic recovery followed by significant decline at around 1 year. Taken together, the results from these investigations do not indicate a clear relationship between markers of injury severity and long-term memory functioning months to years after TBI.

Nature of Learning and Memory Deficits following TBI

It is now well recognized that most individuals with moderate to severe TBI experience some level of learning memory disturbance.[5,58] In light of this, investigators have recently turned their attention away from documenting the presence of impaired memory after TBI and toward examining the precise mechanism underlying the memory disorder.[55,59]

One important question to be addressed concerns the nature of episodic memory deficits following TBI. That is, in terms of a processing theory approach, what stage in the learning and memory process (i.e., encoding-consolidation-retrieval) is primarily responsible for the observed deficit in learning and memory. While several studies support the hypothesis of impaired acquisition (or encoding)[60–62] or consolidation,[59] several others have concluded that individuals with TBI suffer from retrieval failure.[63–65] Still other studies have identified, within their samples, clusters of individuals with TBI who experienced primarily deficits in acquisition, some whose deficits were primarily in retrieval, and others with problems in both acquisition and retrieval.[66,67] These conflicting findings concerning the mechanism of impaired learning and memory were addressed by DeLuca et al.[55] They suggested that prior studies indicating retrieval failure did not adequately control for the amount of initial learning between TBI and control groups. Given that recall performance is dependent upon the amount of information initially learned, inferences drawn about retrieval performance are confounded[62] when acquisition is not controlled for.[62,68]

After controlling for initial acquisition (by training subjects with TBI and healthy groups to the same learning criteria), no significant differences in recall or recognition was observed between the moderate to severe TBI group versus healthy controls who were matched on initial learning.[55] These data clearly supported the hypothesis of impaired acquisition after TBI (see Fig. 40-4). However, approximately one-third of the sample in this study exhibited very severe learning deficits (i.e., they never met the learning criteria despite numerous trials). Figure 40-4 illustrates that those TBI subjects who did not meet the learning criteria showed recall and recognition performance significantly below that of the TBI subjects who met the learning criteria and as well as that of healthy controls. Rate of forgetting was also more rapid in these severely learning impaired TBI subjects,[55] which is consistent with the "deficient learners" examined by Millis and Ricker.[66] No differences were observed in injury

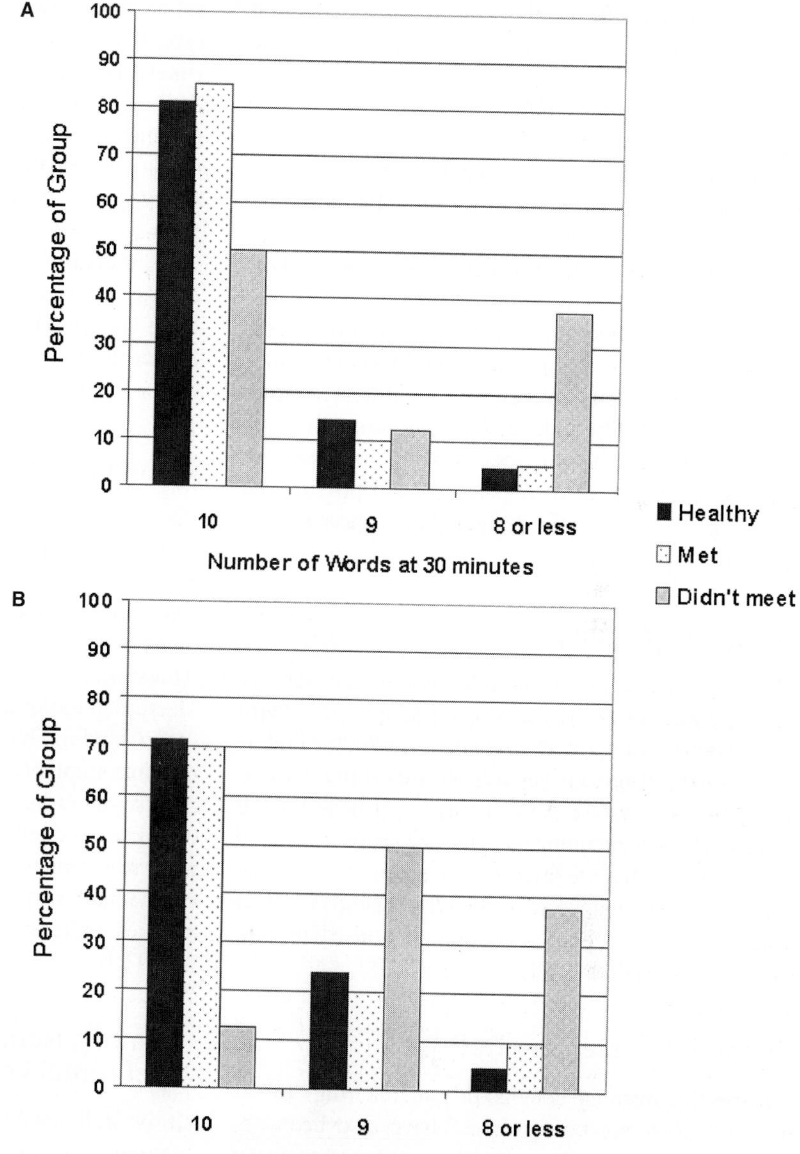

Figure 40-4
The performance of individuals with TBI who did not meet the verbal learning criteria compared to the performance of individuals with TBI who met the verbal learning criteria and healthy controls. A. 30-min recall condition. B. 90-min recall condition.

severity (e.g., initial GCS) or other demographic factors between the two TBI subgroups studied by DeLuca and colleagues.[55] However, this group of severely learning impaired individuals with TBI did show significantly greater executive impairment than the remainder of the TBI sample, which may explain the poor learning.

Overall, the study of DeLuca et al.[55] illustrates several important points: (1) patients with moderate to severe TBI suffer from significant difficulties in the acquisition of information; (2) given sufficient learning, recall and recognition performance is not impaired; (3) persons with TBI may not be suffering from "memory" problems (i.e., deficits in recall and recognition) but rather from cognitive factors that influence new learning (e.g., executive dysfunction, reduced processing efficiency); (4) a subgroup of TBI patients have such severe problems in acquiring information that, for them, learning becomes a primary cognitive problem affecting subsequent recall and recognition—a point that, as suggested by several others,[67] shows that the TBI population is a heterogeneous one; and (5) rehabilitation efforts must be tailored to the specific deficits of the individual. Interestingly, if the two TBI subgroups in the study of DeLuca et al.[55] were combined into one group (as is typically done in TBI research), the combined data would have shown a deficit in recall performance in the TBI group as a whole. This finding would have led to the erroneous conclusion that the primary deficit following TBI was in the retrieval of previously learned information. By recognizing the heterogeneity in memory impairment among individuals with TBI and the need to appropriately assess the nature of these deficits, investigators can profoundly alter theories of impairment and provide the theoretical foundation for designing appropriate interventions.

Semantic Memory

Deficits in semantic memory following TBI are relatively rare. However, the investigation of this form of memory impairment remains markedly under-researched.[69] There are suggestions that some individuals who have sustained a TBI may fail to benefit from deeper levels of encoding (semantically) during a word recall task.[70] There is greater evidence indicating that the ability to recognize semantic relationships is intact following TBI,[58,71] and these data are consistent with what is observed clinically.

Prospective Memory Deficits

Prospective memory deficits, or remembering "to" as opposed to remembering "that," have also been observed following TBI.[72–74] While there remains a paucity of prospective memory research following TBI, researchers have reported that the memory deficits actually reported by patients and family members are often prospective in nature.[75] Moreover, recent findings reveal that prospective memory deficits are predictive of day-to-day memory functioning and may be more sensitive to cognitive impairment following TBI than traditional psychometric tests of memory.[72]

Shum and colleagues[73] noted that the current prospective memory literature requires important refinement in two areas. First, prospective memory is typically tested with relatively few items and few trials (likely secondary to the time limitations in assessment). Second, these authors have pointed out that prospective memory has often been conceptualized as a unitary construct, even though separate subtypes of prospective memory (i.e., memory for a specific time and memory for a specified event) were noted over a decade ago.[76] Thus, there is a need for additional research in the area of prospective memory following TBI, with consideration given to prior methodologic limitations and what is known of the subtypes within prospective memory.

Procedural and Implicit Memory following TBI

As mentioned earlier, procedural memory is generally preserved following TBI. For instance, even during PTA, individuals show relatively normal procedural, or skill learning, memory across separate motor learning tasks (mirror reading, mazes, and a pursuit rotor task).[77] However, one recent study found some evidence of decreased motor learning in children with TBI.[78]

Findings have been more consistent, however, regarding implicit memory dysfunction following TBI. Investigators have noted intact implicit memory performance on stem-completion tasks in individuals with TBI who remain in PTA[79] and during priming tasks in individuals with chronic TBI.[80] Taken together, these studies indicate preserved implicit memory following TBI.

Memory, Neuroimaging, and the Frontal Lobes

It is well established from biomechanical investigations[81] and clinical research[82,83] that the prefrontal cortex (i.e., dorsolateral and ventrolateral) and the temporal poles are often damaged regardless of the mechanism of injury in moderate to severe TBI (i.e., impact, nonimpact). A schematic diagram of cortical regions commonly affected during TBI is presented in Fig. 40-5. Structural damage to frontal cortex leads directly to functional loss.[84,85] Subcortical shear injury can also affect frontal networks.

While the frontal lobes are commonly injured during TBI and such damage is observable using

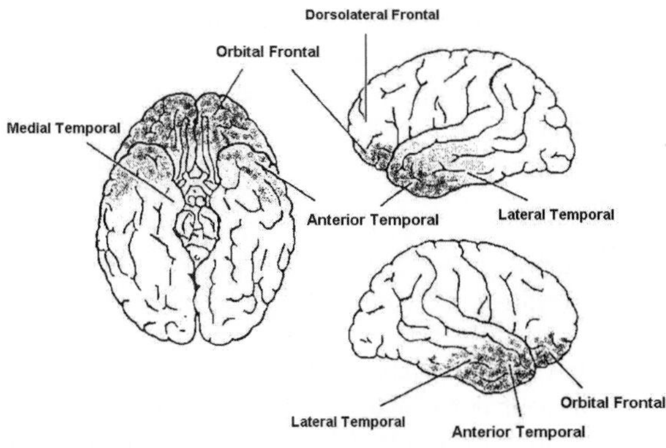

Figure 40-5
A schematic diagram of the areas predominantly affected by cortical contusions. Shading represents more frequently involved areas. Anterior temporal and orbitofrontal regions are commonly involved. Note the relative sparing of structures of the dorsolateral frontal and mediotemporal lobes. (Adapted from Courville,[101] with permission.)

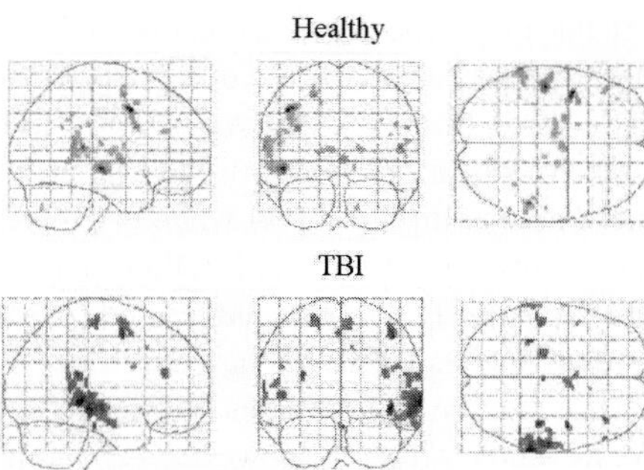

Figure 40-6
Statistical parametric maps of brain activation for healthy adults and individuals with TBI during a working memory study. (From Christodoulou et al.,[93] with permission.)

computed tomography (CT) or magnetic resonance imaging (MRI), studies examining the relationship between structural imaging and memory impairment have been disappointing.[86] For instance, localization of structural lesions as detected by CT or MRI has not been well correlated with neuropsychological functioning after TBI.[87] Others have noted that the physiologic and neurobehavioral consequences are often greater than that expected from focal contusions alone.[85–89]

Recent work with functional neuroimaging techniques [e.g., positron emission tomography (PET), functional magnetic resonance imaging (fMRI)] has led to a better understanding of the role of the frontal lobes in human learning and memory. PET and fMRI studies in healthy adults have determined that the frontal lobes play a critical role in several memory subsystems including working memory, encoding, maintenance of information for manipulation and richer encoding, and retrieval of information from long-term store (for review, see Refs. 90 and 91).

Given the predilection for frontal lobe damage in persons with TBI and the relationship between TBI and deficits in new learning and memory, it is not surprising that frontal lobe damage can significantly influence memory functions. For instance, the hemispheric encoding-retrieval asymmetry (HERA) model[92] postulates that the left frontal lobe has a preferential role during encoding, while the right frontal lobe plays a more important role during retrieval. Functional neuroimaging and the theoretical models of learning and memory that have emerged from these techniques now provide investigators with a new framework from which to study problems in learning and memory following TBI.

Recent studies using such techniques as fMRI and PET have shown that persons with TBI show altered functional cerebral representation during actual memory performance. In two working memory studies, subjects with moderate to severe TBI[93] and mTBI[94] have been found to show significantly increased cerebral activation in the contralateral hemisphere from that observed in healthy controls during the performance of a working memory task (see Fig. 40-6). Using PET, this same finding was observed in subjects with moderate to severe TBI during the performance of an episodic memory task.[95] In addition, these studies generally showed more widespread cerebral activation throughout the brain relative to controls.

While it is unclear at this time what these data suggest precisely, these functional neuroimaging findings may indicate that there are changes at the level of cerebral substrate that may include recruitment of additional brain regions in order to perform learning and memory tasks. Some have hypothesized that individuals with TBI require greater cerebral resources to perform learning and memory functions after TBI.[93,95] This latter interpretation appears to be consistent with subjective self-reports from individuals with TBI, who maintain that they expend greater mental energy to perform day-to-day tasks that were once "automatic."

The susceptibility of the frontal lobes following TBI may also result in errors in source memory (i.e., difficulty in the ability to report when or where information was initially encountered) rather than errors in actual item content (i.e., recall and/or recognition) during memory. Studies with other neurologic populations have shown that the frontal lobes are particularly susceptible to source errors.[96] However, very little work has been done in this area with TBI (e.g., Ref. 97), and it remains a fertile area of future work.

SUMMARY

Impairment of learning and memory is the most common cognitive symptom reported following TBI and is often associated with long-standing disability. While TBI comprises a heterogeneous clinical population, episodic memory decrement is clearly the primary source of learning and memory dysfunction. Recent research has indicated that these episodic deficits are typically problems in learning or acquiring new information, although deficits in retrieval and consolidation can be seen in those with the most severe learning problems. As such, what have been conceptualized as "memory" problems may more likely be problems in cognitive domains that affect learning (e.g., executive dysfunction) and not "memory" (i.e., recall and recognition) per se. Finally, functional imaging techniques are beginning to elucidate the functional changes observed at the level of the cerebral substrate associated with episodic and working memory impairment following TBI.

REFERENCES

1. National Institute of Health: Rehabilitation of Persons with Brain Injury. NIH Consensus Statement 16(1): 1–41, 1998.
2. Guerrero J, Thurman DJ, Sniezek JE: Emergency department visits association with traumatic brain injury: United States, 1995–1996. *Brain Inj* 14(2):181–186, 2000.
3. Thurman DJ, Guerrero J: Trends in hospitalization associated with traumatic brain injury. *JAMA* 282(10):954–957, 1999.
4. National Center for Health Statistics: Unpublished data from Multiple Cause of Death Public Use Data from the National Center for Health Statistics, 1996. Methods are described in Sosin DM, Sniezek JE, Waxweiler RJ: Trends in death associated with traumatic brain injury, 1979–1992. *JAMA* 273(22):1778–1780, 1995.
5. Rosenthal M, Ricker JH: Traumatic Brain Injury, in Frank R, Eliott T (eds): *Handbook of Rehabilitation Psychology*. Washington, DC: American Psychological Association, 2000, pp 49–74.
6. McKinlay W, Watkiss AJ: Cognitive and behavioral effect of brain injury, in Rosenthal M, Griffith ER, Kreutzer JS, Pentland B (eds): *Rehabilitation of the Adult and Child with Traumatic Brain Injury,* 3d ed. Philadelphia, Davis, 1999, pp 74–86.
7. Ryan TV, Sautter SW, Capps CF, et al: Utilizing neuropsychological measures to predict vocational outcome in a head trauma population. *Brain Inj* 6:175–182, 1992.
8. Millis SR, Rosenthal M, Novack TA, et al: Long-term neuropsychological outcome after traumatic brain injury. *J Head Trauma Rehabil* 16(4):343–355, 2001.
9. Zee RF, Zellers D, Belman J, et al: Long-term consequences of severe closed head injury on episodic memory. *J Clin Exp Neuropsychol* 23(5):671–691, 2001.
10. Schacter DL, Wagner AD, Buckner RL: Memory systems of 1999, in Tulving E, Craik FI (eds): *The Oxford Handbook of Memory*. New York: Oxford University Press, 2000, pp 627–643.
11. Tulving E: Concepts of memory, in Tulving E, Craik FI (eds): *The Oxford Handbook of Memory*. New York: Oxford University Press, 2000, p 37.
12. Baddeley A: Short-term and working memory, in Tulving E, Craik FI (eds): *The Oxford Handbook of Memory*. New York: Oxford University Press, 2000, pp 77–92.
13. Johnson MK: MEM: Mechanisms of recollection. *J Cogn Neurosci* 4(3):268–280, 1992.
14. Parkin AJ: The central executive does not exist. *J Int Neuropsychol Soc* 4(5):518–522, 1998.
15. Squire LR, Cohen NJ, Nadel L: The medial temporal region and memory consolidation: A new hypothesis, in Weingartner H, Parker E (eds): *Memory Consolidation*. Hillsdale, NJ: Erlbaum, 1983, pp 185–210.
16. Symonds CP: The differential diagnosis and treatment of cerebral states consequent upon head injuries. *Br Med J* 2:829–832, 1928.
17. Russell WR, Nathan PW: Traumatic amnesia. *Brain* 69:183–187, 1946.

18. Levin HS, High WM, Myers CA: Impairment of remote memory after closed head injury. *J Neurol Neurosurg Psychiatry* 48:556–563, 1985.
19. Wilson BA, Evans JJ, Emslie H, et al: Measuring recovery from post-traumatic amnesia. *Brain Inj* 13(7):505–520, 1999.
20. Corrigan JD, Mysiw WJ: Agitation following traumatic head injury: Equivocal evidence for a discrete stage of cognitive recovery. *Arch Phys Med Rehabil* 69(7):487–492, 1988.
21. Russell WR: Cerebral involvement in head injury: A study based on the examination of two hundred cases. *Brain* 55:549–603, 1932.
22. McMillan TM, Jongen EL, Greenwood RJ: Assessment of post-traumatic amnesia after severe closed head injury: Retrospective or prospective? *J Neurol Neurosurg Psychiatry* 60:422–427, 1996.
23. Zafonte RD, Mann NR, Millis SR, et al: Posttraumatic amnesia: its relation to functional outcome. *Arch Phys Med Rehabil* 78(10):1103–1106, 1999.
24. Haslam C, Batchelor J, Fearnside MR, et al: Post-coma disturbance and post-traumatic amnesia as nonlinear predictors of cognitive outcome following severe closed head injury: Findings from the Westmead Head Injury Project. *Brain Inj* 8(6):519–528, 1994.
25. Teasdale G, Jennett B: Assessment of coma and impaired consciousness: A practical scale. *Lancet* 2:81–83, 1974.
26. Ellenberg JH, Levin HS, Saydjari C: Posttraumatic amnesia as a predictor of outcome after severe closed head injury. Prospective assessment. *Arch Neurol* 53(8):782–791, 1996.
27. Levin HS, O'Donnell VM, Grossman RG: The Galveston Orientation and Amnesia Test: A practical scale to assess cognition after head injury. *J Nerv Ment Dis* 167:675–684, 1979.
28. Shores EA, Marosszeky JE, Sandman J, et al: Preliminary validation of a clinical scale for measuring duration of post-traumatic amnesia. *Med J Aust* 144:569–572, 1986.
29. Shiel A, Horn SA, Wilson BA, et al: The Wessex Head Injury Matrix (WHIM) main scale: A preliminary report on a scale to assess and monitor patient recovery after severe head injury. *Clin Rehabil* 14(4):408–416, 2000.
30. Levin HS, Benton AL, Grossman RG: *Neurobehavioral Consequences of Closed Head Injury*. New York: Oxford University Press, 1982.
31. Tate RL, Pfaff A, Jurjevic L: Resolution of disorientation and amnesia during post-traumatic amnesia. *J Neurol Neurosurg Psychiatry* 68(2):178–85 2000.
32. Wilson BA, Baddeley AD, Shiel A: How does post-traumatic amnesia differ from the amnesic syndrome and from chronic memory impairment? *Neuropsychol Rehabil* 2:231–243, 1992.
33. Gronwall D, Wrightson P: Duration of post-traumatic amnesia after mild head injury. *J Clin Neuropsychol* 2:51–60, 1980.
34. Stuss DT, Binns MA, Carruth FG, et al: The acute period of recovery from traumatic brain injury: Posttraumatic amnesia or posttraumatic confusional state? *J Neurosurg* 90(4):635–643, 1999.
35. McIntosh TK: Neurochemical sequelae of traumatic brain injury: Therapeutic implications. *Cerebrovasc Brain Metab* 6(2):109–162, 1994.
36. Hamm RJ, Temple MD, Buck DL, et al: Cognitive recovery from traumatic brain injury: Results of post-traumatic experimental interventions, in Levin HS, Grafman J (eds): *Cerebral Reorganization of Function After Brain Damage*. New York: Oxford University Press, 2000, pp 49–67.
37. Garnett MR, Blamire AM, Rajagopalan B, et al: Evidence for cellular damage in normal-appearing white matter correlates with injury severity in patients following TBI: A magnetic resonance spectroscopy study. *Brain* 123:1403–1409, 2000.
38. Friedman SD, Brooks WM, Jung RE, et al: Quantitative ^{1}H-MRS predicts outcome following traumatic brain injury. *Neurology* 52:1384–1391, 1999.
39. Brooks WM, Stidley CA, Petropoulos H, et al: Metabolic and cognitive response to human traumatic brain injury: A quantitative proton magnetic resonance study. *J Neurotrauma* 17(8):629–640, 2000.
40. American Congress of Rehabilitation Medicine: Definition of mild traumatic brain injury. References reprinted/adapted with permission from *J Head Trauma Rehabil* 8(3):86–87, 1993.
41. Gronwall D, Wrightson P: Delayed recovery of intellectual function after minor head injury. *Lancet* 2:604–609, 1974.
42. Rimel RW, Giordani B, Barth JT, et al: Disability caused by minor head injury. *Neurosurgery* 9:221–228, 1981.
43. Ruff RM, Levin HS, Mattis S, et al: Recovery of memory after mild head injury: A three-center study, in Levin HS, Eisenberg HM, Benton AL (eds): *Mild Head Injury*. New York: Oxford University Press, 1989, pp 176–188.
44. Binder LM: A review of mild head trauma: Part II. Clinical implications. *J Clin Exp Neuropsychol* 19:432–457, 1997.
45. Alexander MP: Mild traumatic brain injury: Pathophysiology, natural history, and clinical management. *Neurology* 45:1253–1260, 1995.

46. Putnam S, Millis S, Adams K: Mild traumatic brain injury: Beyond cognitive assessment, in Grant I, Adams KM (eds): *Neuropsychological Assessment of Neuropsychiatric Disorders*. New York: Oxford University Press, 1996, pp 531–532.
47. Ruff RM, Camenzuli L, Mueller J: Miserable minority: Emotional risk factors that influence the outcome of a mild traumatic brain injury. *Brain Inj* 10:551–565, 1996.
48. Ruff RM, Richardson AM: Mild traumatic brain injury, in Sweet J (ed): *Forensic Neuropsychology.* Lisse, Holland: Swets and Zeitlinger, 1999, pp 313–338.
49. Ruff RM, Couch JA, Troster AL, et al: Selected cases of poor outcome following minor brain trauma. Comparing neuropsychological and position emission tomography assessment. *Brain Inj* 8:297–308, 1994.
50. Binder LM: Assessment of malingering after mild head trauma with the Portland Digit Recognition Test. *J Clin Exp Neuropsychol* 15:170–182, 1993.
51. Green P, Rohling ML, Lees-Haley PR, et al: Effort has a greater effect on test scores than severe brain injury in compensation claimants. *Brain Inj* 15(12):1045–1060, 2001.
52. Novack TA, Alderson AL, Bush BA, et al: Cognitive and functional recovery at 6 and 12 months post-TBI. *Brain Inj* 14(11):987–996, 2000.
53. Madigan NK, DeLuca J, Diamond BJ, et al: Speed of information processing in traumatic brain injury: Modality-specific factors. *J Head Trauma Rehabil* 15(3):943–956, 2000.
54. McDowell S, Whyte J, D'Esposito M: Working memory impairments in traumatic brain injury: Evidence from a dual-task paradigm. *Neuropsychologia* 35(10):1341–1353, 1997.
55. DeLuca J, Schultheis MT, Madigan NK, et al: Acquisition versus retrieval deficits in traumatic brain injury: Implications for memory rehabilitation. *Arch Phys Med Rehabil* 81(10):1327–1333, 2000.
56. Levin HS, Gary HE Jr, Eisenberg HM, et al: Neurobehavioral outcome 1 year after severe head injury. Experience of the Traumatic Coma Data Bank. *J Neurosurg* 73(5):699–709, 1990.
57. Ruff RM, Barth J, Kreutzer J, et al: Verbal learning deficits following severe head injury: Heterogeneity in recovery over 1 year. *J Neurosurg* 75:S50–S58, 1991.
58. Goldstein FC, Levin HS, Boake C, et al: Facilitation of memory performance through induced semantic processing in survivors of severe closed head injury. *J Clin Exp Neuropsychol* 58:93–98, 1990.
59. Vanderploeg RD, Crowell TA, Curtiss G: Verbal learning and memory deficits in traumatic brain injury: Encoding, consolidation, and retrieval. *J Clin Exp Neuropsychol* 23(2):185–195, 2001.
60. Blachstein H, Vakil E, Hoofien D: Impaired learning in patients with closed-head injuries: An analysis of components in the acquisition process. *J Clin Psychol* 7:530–535, 1993.
61. Crosson B, Novack T, Trenerry MS, et al: California Verbal Learning Test (CVLT) performance in severely head-injured and neurologically normal adult males *J Clin Exp Neuropsychol* 10:754–768, 1988.
62. Hart RP: Forgetting in traumatic brain-injured patients with persistent memory impairment. *Neuropsychology* 8(3):325–332, 1994.
63. Brooks DN: Wechsler Memory Scale performance and its relationship to brain damage after severe closed head injury. *J Neurol Neurosurg Psychiatry* 39:593–601, 1976.
64. Levin HS, Grossman RG, Rose JE, et al: Long-term neuropsychological outcome of closed head injury. *J Neurosurg* 50:412–422, 1979.
65. Kear-Caldwell JJ, Heller M: The Wechsler Memory Scale and closed head injury. *J Clin Psychol* 36:782–787, 1980.
66. Millis SR, Ricker JH: Verbal learning patterns in moderate and severe traumatic brain injury. *J Clin Exp Neuropsychol* 16(4):498–507, 1994.
67. Deshpande SA, Millis SR, Reeder KP, et al: Verbal learning subtypes in traumatic brain injury: A replication. *J Clin Exp Neuropsychol* 18(6):836–842, 1996.
68. Carlesimo GA, Sabbadini M, Loasses A, et al: Forgetting long-term memory in severe closed head injury patients: Effects of retrieval conditions and semantic organization. *Cortex* 33:131–142, 1997.
69. Wilson BA: Semantic memory impairments following non-progressive brain injury: A study of four cases. *Brain Inj* 11(4):259–269, 1997.
70. Vakil E, Sigal J: The effect of level of processing on perceptual and conceptual priming: Control versus closed-head-injured patients. *J Int Neuropsychol Soc* 3(4):327–336, 1997.
71. Hough MS, Pierce RS, Difilippo M, et al: Access and organization of goal-derived categories after traumatic brain injury. *Brain Inj* 11(11):801–814, 1997.
72. Kinsela G, Murtagh A, Landry A, et al: Everyday memory following traumatic brain injury. *Brain Inj* 10(7):499–507, 1996.
73. Shum D, Valentine M, Cutmore T: Performance of individuals with severe long-term traumatic brain injury on time-, event-, and activity-based prospective memory tasks. *J Clin Exp Neuropsychol* 21(1):49–58, 1999.

74. Lynch WJ: You must remember this: Assistive devices for memory impairment. *J Head Trauma Rehabil* 10(1):94–97, 1995.
75. Mateer CA, Sohlberg MM, Crinean J: Perceptions of memory functioning in individuals with closed-head injury. *J Head Trauma Rehabil* 2:4–84, 1987.
76. Einstein GO, McDaniel MA: Normal aging and prospective memory. *J Exp Psychol Learn Mem Cogn* 16:717–726, 1990.
77. Ewert J, Levin HS, Watson MG, et al: Procedural memory during posttraumatic amnesia in survivors of severe closed head injury. Implications for rehabilitation. *Arch Neurol* 46(8):911–916, 1989.
78. Verger K, Serra-Grabulosa JM, Junque C, et al: Study of the long-term sequelae of traumatic brain injury: Evaluation of declarative and procedural memory, and its neuroanatomic substrate. *Rev Neurol* 33(1): 0–34, 2001.
79. Glisky EL, Delaney SM: Implicit memory and new semantic learning in posttraumatic amnesia. *J Head Trauma Rehabil* 11(2):31–42, 1996.
80. Watt S, Shores EA, Kinoshita S: Effects of reducing attentional resources on implicit and explicit memory after severe traumatic brain injury. *Neuropsychology* 13(3):338–349, 1999.
81. Gennarelli TA: Mechanisms of brain injury. *J Emerg Med* 11(suppl 1):5–11, 1993.
82. Whyte J, Hart T, Laborde A, et al: Rehabilitation of the patient with head injury, in DeLisa JA (ed): *Rehabilitation Medicine: Principles and Practice,* 3d ed. Philadelphia: Lippincott, 1998, pp 1191–1240.
83. Hillary FG, Moelter S, Schatz P, et al: Seatbelts contribute to location of lesion in moderate to severe head trauma. *Arch Clin Neuropsychol* 16(2):171–181, 2001.
84. Jansen HML, van der Naalt J, van Zomeren AH, et al: Cobalt-55 positron emission tomography in traumatic brain injury: A pilot study. *J Neurol Neurosurg Psychiatry* 60:221–224, 1996.
85. Langfitt TW, Obrist WD, Alavi A, et al: Computerized tomography, magnetic resonance imaging, and positron emission tomography in the study of brain trauma: Preliminary observations. *J Neurosurg* 64:760–767, 1986.
86. Ricker JH, Hillary FG, DeLuca J: Functionally activated brain imaging (O-15 PET and fMRI) in the study of memory after traumatic brain injury. *J Head Trauma Rehabil* 16(2):191–205, 2001.
87. Levin HS, Williams DH, Eisenberg HM, et al: Serial MRI and neurobehavioral findings after mild to moderate closed head injury. *J Neurol Neurosurg Psychiatry* 55(4):255–262, 1992.
88. Fontaine A, Azouvi P, Remy P, et al: Functional anatomy of neuropsychological deficits after severe traumatic brain injury. *Neurology* 53(9):1963–1968, 1999.
89. Bigler ED: Quantitative magnetic resonance imaging in traumatic brain injury. *J Head Trauma Rehabil* 16:117–134, 2001.
90. Cabeza R, Nyberg L: Neural bases of learning and memory: Functional neuroimaging evidence. *Curr Opin Neurol* 13(4):415–421, 2000.
91. Fletcher PC, Henson RN: Frontal lobes and human memory: Insights from functional neuroimaging. *Brain* 124(pt 5):849–881, 2001.
92. Tulving E, Kapur S, Craik FI, et al: Hemispheric encoding/retrieval asymmetry in episodic memory: Positron emission tomography findings. *Proc Natl Acad Sci USA* 91(6):2016–2020, 1994.
93. Christodoulou C, DeLuca J, Ricker JH, et al: Functional magnetic resonance imaging of working memory impairment after traumatic brain injury. *J Neurol Neurosurg Psychiatry* 71(2):161–168, 2001.
94. McAllister TW, Saykin AJ, Flashman LA, et al: Brain activation during working memory 1 month after mild traumatic brain injury: A functional MRI study. *Neurology* 53(6):1300–1308, 1999.
95. Ricker JH, Muller RA, Zafonte RD, et al: Verbal recall and recognition following traumatic brain injury: A [0–15]-water positron emission tomography study. *J Clin Exp Neuropsychol* 23(2):196–206, 2001.
96. Janowsky JS, Shimamura AP, Squire LR: Memory and metamemory: Comparisons between frontal lobe lesions and amnesic patients. *Psychobiology* 17:3–11, 1989.
97. Dywan J, Segalowitz SJ, Henderson D, et al: Memory for source after traumatic brain injury. *Brain Cogn* 21:20–43, 1993.
98. Squire LR: *Memory and Brain*. New York: Oxford University Press, 1987, p 170.
99. Jennet B: Assessment of the severity of head injury. *J Neurol Neurosurg Psychiatry* 39:647–655, 1976.
100. Friedman SD, Brooks WM, Jung RE, et al: Proton MR spectroscopic findings correspond to neuropsychological function in traumatic brain injury. *Am J Neuroradiol* 19:1879–1885, 1998.
101. Courville CB: *Mythology of the Central Nervous System.* Mountain View, CA: Pacific Press, 1937.

Chapter 41

MEMORY IMPAIRMENT FOLLOWING ANTERIOR COMMUNICATING ARTERY ANEURYSM*

John DeLuca
Deborah Bryant
Catherine E. Myers

The role of medial temporal and diencephalic structures in human memory and amnesia, reviewed in Chaps. 37 and 38, has been a focus of research for over 50 years. By contrast, our understanding of the role of the basal forebrain in human declarative memory began less than 20 years ago, with relatively few studies published to date. Much if not most of the work implicating the basal forebrain in human memory disorders comes from the examination of the amnestic syndrome often observed following anterior communicating artery (ACoA) aneurysms.[1,2] Survivors of ACoA aneurysms can present with a cluster of neurobehavioral impairments including amnesia, confabulation, and personality change—once collectively referred to as the "ACoA syndrome." However, the type and degree of cognitive and behavioral impairments (see Table 41-1) may range from no impairment to subtle cognitive (e.g., mild memory and attention problems) and emotional problems to profound amnesia, confabulation, and personality disturbances or abulic states.[3–5]

The purpose of this chapter is to outline and review disordered memory after ACoA aneurysm in humans. For an in-depth review of confabulation as well as other forms of cognitive and behavioral disturbances following ACoA aneurysm, the reader is referred to DeLuca and Chairavalloti (Ref. 6), DeLuca (Ref. 7), and DeLuca and Diamond (Ref. 2).

* **ACKNOWLEDGMENTS:** This work was supported in part by NIH grant HD07522. We would also like to thank Cassandra Racasi for preparing the manuscript for publication.

BACKGROUND ON ACoA

The ACoA lies at the anterior portion of the circle of Willis, connecting the two anterior cerebral arteries just rostral to the optic chiasm (see Fig. 41-1). Approximately 85 to 95 percent of all aneurysms develop at the anterior portion of the cerebral arterial supply, primarily at the circle of Willis.[8] Rupture of an ACoA aneurysm can markedly alter the hemodynamic circulation of the anterior portion of the circle of Willis, often resulting in cerebral infarction.[9] The ACoA is one of the most common sites of cerebral aneurysm in humans and is the most frequent site of cerebral infarct following aneurysmal rupture.[9,10] Infarcts are often observed along the distribution of the anterior cerebral arteries and the small perforating arteries that branch directly off the ACoA itself.[11,12] The vascular territory perfused by these small ACoA perforating branches includes the paraterminal gyrus (including the septal nuclei), the genu of the corpus callosum, the anterior cingulum, the optic chiasm, the columns of the fornix, the substantia inominata, the anterior hypothalamus, the medial anterior commissure, and the nucleus basalis of Meynert[13] (see Fig. 41-2). Lesions beyond the basal forebrain are frequent because of the proximity of the ACoA to other critical arterial vasculature. As such, ischemic lesions in the ventromedial portions of the frontal lobe can result from vasospasm of the anterior cerebral arteries. Also, lesions at the head of the caudate, anterior third of the putamen, outer portion of the globus pallidus, and anterior part of the internal capsule can result from involvement of the recurrent artery of Heubner because of its close proximity to the AcoA.[10,14]

Table 41-1
Frequently observed cognitive sequelae following aneurysm of the anterior communicating artery

"ACoA syndrome"	Severe memory deficit Confabulation Personality change
Other neuropsychological deficits	Decreased cognitive flexibility Decreased verbal fluency Poor problem solving Mild impairment in intelligence (decrease in PIQ*) Executive dysfunction Poor new learning Difficulty organizing stimuli
Other neurobehavioral dysfunction	Alien hand syndrome Akinesia Abulia

*Performance IQ.

Impaired Memory from a Historical Perspective

Impaired memory is clearly the most common and most studied symptom following ACoA aneurysm. It is well known from other populations that compromised declarative memory results from damage to the diencephalic and/or medial temporal structures in the brain.[15] But structural imaging techniques [computed tomography (CT) and magnetic resonance imaging (MRI)] reveal that patients with ACoA aneurysms do not have damage in these critical areas. So the question is: Why are these patients amnesic?

Prior to 1980, most published reports in the western literature were geared toward documenting the existence, nature, and severity of impaired memory after ACoA aneurysm (however, see the extensive work by Luria et al.[16]). It was believed that the amnesia resulted either from diencephalic damage (because of its similarity to Korsakoff's syndrome[17]) or frontal lobe impairment.[18] By the mid-1970s, it was discovered that the ACoA had significant perforating branches.[19,20] These small arterial branches were found to perfuse, among other structures, the basal forebrain.[14,19,20]

In 1982, Gade[12] was the first to suggest that the amnestic syndrome observed following ACoA aneurysm was due to reduced blood supply through the perforating branches of the ACoA, which supply the region of the basal forebrain. This hypothesis was suggested by several others during the 1980s (e.g., Refs. 11, 18, 21, and 22), but was not universally supported (e.g., Refs. 23 to 26). By the 1990s, the notion of behavioral heterogeneity following ACoA aneurysm was beginning to be incorporated into research, with

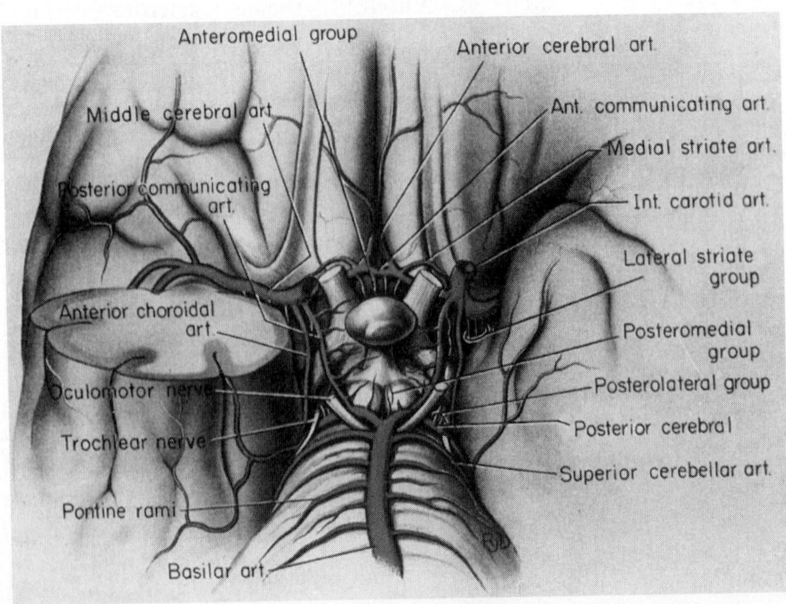

Figure 41-1
Cerebral arterial flow at the base of the brain. Note the perforating branches of the ACoA. (From Carpenter,[66] with permission.)

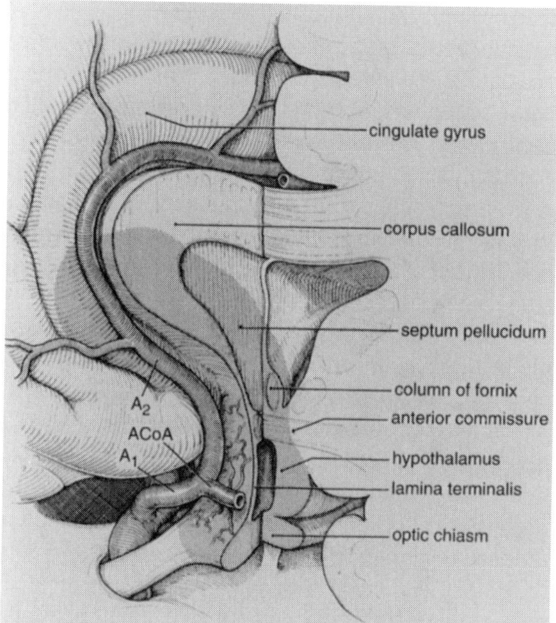

Figure 41-2
Cross section of mediobasal forebrain illustrating the vasculature and major structures. Tinted region represents area of perfusion from the perforating vessels off the ACoA (From Drumm et al.,[68] with permission.)

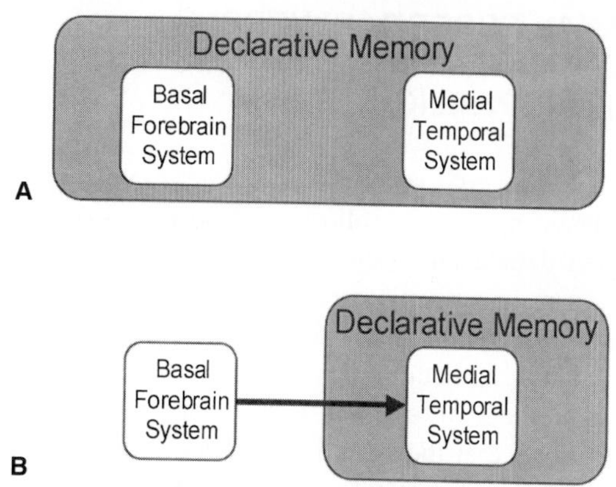

Figure 41-3
Two possible ways in which basal forebrain and mediotemporal lobes might contribute to declarative memory. A. *Both basal forebrain and mediotemporal structures could be directly involved in new declarative memory formation, either acting in concert or else each being primarily concerned with separate (as yet unspecified) aspects of declarative memory.* B. *The medial temporal system could be the primary site for new declarative memory formation, with the basal forebrain providing modulatory inputs that govern hippocampal function. In either model, disruption of new declarative memory formation would be observed following either basal forebrain or mediotemporal damage, and the two kinds of damage might lead to subtle differences in the amnesic syndrome.*

studies demonstrating differences in severity of amnesia ranging from severe to mild to none (e.g., Refs. 3 and 27 to 29). In addition, some researchers were reporting that the severity of amnesia was worse in patients who had damage extending beyond the basal forebrain into other proximal regions such as the basal ganglia and/or frontal lobes (e.g., Refs. 29 and 30). However, later research did not support the notion that the severity of amnesia was associated with lesions extending beyond the basal forebrain (e.g., Refs. 3 and 31). Instead, these newer studies suggested that damage to the diagonal band of Broca and/or septal region was key to the production of memory impairments (e.g., Refs. 3, 11, 22, and 31). Importantly, the nucleus basalis of Meynert, a region purported to be important in the memory disorder that accompanies Alzheimer's disease (e.g., Ref. 32), was not found to be damaged in patients with amnesia due to ACoA aneurysms.[22,31]

The studies mentioned so far suggest a direct role for the basal forebrain in human declarative memory; this idea is known as the basal forebrain hypothesis of ACoA amnesia. However, Damasio and colleagues[21] offered an alternative hypothesis—that ACoA amnesia may result from disruption of critical bidirectional connections between the basal forebrain and the hippocampus. According to this hypothesis (see Fig. 41-3), compromised declarative memory is a result of deficient hippocampal functioning secondary to faulty modulation from basal forebrain structures. Preliminary support for this latter hypothesis comes from functional neuroimaging studies, in which single photon emission computed tomography (SPECT) and positron emission tomography (PET) studies have revealed markedly reduced blood perfusion or metabolism in the hippocampus bilaterally.[31,33] However, with a total of three subjects with ACoA aneurysms between these two reports (and one more patient with a non-ACoA basal forebrain aneurysm[34]), such support remains speculative.

BASAL FOREBRAIN VERSUS MEDIAL TEMPORAL VERSUS DIENCEPHALIC AMNESIA

The controversy surrounding the ultimate origin of amnestic symptoms following ACoA aneurysm has fueled debate on whether or not amnesia following such an aneurysm represents a discrete amnestic syndrome, distinct from the amnestic syndromes associated with mediotemporal or diencephalic damage (e.g., Refs. 2, 21, and 35). Luria et al.[16] were the first to suggest that the nature of the amnestic syndrome in patients with ACoA aneurysms was qualitatively different from that seen in the typical mediotemporal amnesic. Demonstrations of differential learning in patients with ACoA aneurysm versus patients with mediotemporal damage support this view. For instance, Rajaram and Coslett[36] demonstrated verbal associative learning and transfer of this new learning in an individual with basal forebrain amnesia but not in an individual with medial temporal amnesia. Additionally, Kixmiller et al.[37] found that amnesic patients with ACoA aneurysms differed significantly from diencephalic (i.e., Korsakoff's syndrome) and mediotemporal amnesics in the encoding and/or recall of complex visuospatial memory task. These authors reported reduced encoding efficiency in those with ACoA aneurysms (due to reduced organizational and behavioral control inefficiencies) and Korsakoff's syndrome (due to perceptual impairment) relative to medial temporal subjects. Immediate and delayed recall performance was worst among the diencephalic amnesics, which was not attributed to differences in initial encoding. Palmer and McDonald[38] found that individuals who had undergone anterior temporal lobectomies exhibited retrospective and prospective memory deficits, while subjects with ACoA aneurysms exhibited only deficits in prospective memory.

Despite these apparently compelling findings, qualitative and quantitative differences in performance on tests of learning and memory among diencephalic, mediotemporal, and basal forebrain subjects are not always observed (see Corkin et al.[35]). In addition, the interpretation of differential patterns of performance between groups of amnesics with different primary sites of damage is clouded by several factors.[39] For instance, lesions outside the primary area of interest are not uncommon. ACoA lesions often extend into the basal ganglia and frontal lobes (see above), while patients with Korsakoff's syndrome also have frontal and basal forebrain lesions.[40] Such variability and overlap in lesion sites complicates an analysis of whether each of these primary sites results in lesion-specific contributions to impaired declarative memory.

Prior studies with animal models have suggested that the mediotemporal and basal forebrain regions make different contributions to memory and that qualitative differences can arise following damage to one or the other structure. For example, eyeblink conditioning is a canonical paradigm using a corneal air puff or paraorbital shock (the unconditioned stimulus, or US), which reliably evokes a protective eyeblink. If the US is repeatedly preceded by a neutral stimulus such as a tone or light (the conditioned stimulus, or CS), the CS itself comes to elicit an anticipatory eyeblink (the conditioned response, or CR), so that the eye is closed at the time of expected US arrival. Over 40 years of study with this paradigm have demonstrated that this simple form of classic conditioning is robust and reliable and that it depends on similar brain substrates in a variety of species including rabbits, rats, and humans.[41]

Delay eyeblink conditioning (where the CS and US overlap and coterminate) has repeatedly been shown to be spared following damage to the hippocampal region in animals (e.g., Ref. 42) or medial temporal amnesia in humans (e.g., Ref. 43). However, basal forebrain damage in the form of medioseptal lesions profoundly retards acquisition of an eyeblink CR in rabbits.[44] As such, animal models suggest that humans with basal forebrain damage should show impaired delayed eyeblink conditioning even though subjects with hippocampal damage do not. This finding was indeed observed in humans with basal forebrain amnesia resulting from rupture of an ACoA aneurysm [45] (see Fig. 41-4). These results suggest that a simple conditioning paradigm can be used to demonstrate qualitative differences between mediotemporal amnesia (spared delay eyeblink conditioning) and ACoA amnesia (impaired delay eyeblink conditioning).

One possible interpretation of the differences in conditioning between basal forebrain and mediotemporal subjects, suggested by animal and pharmacologic studies[46,47] and also by computational models,[48,49] is that the basal forebrain—specifically the medial septum/diagonal band complex—modulates hippocampal function (i.e., basal forebrain modulation hypothesis).

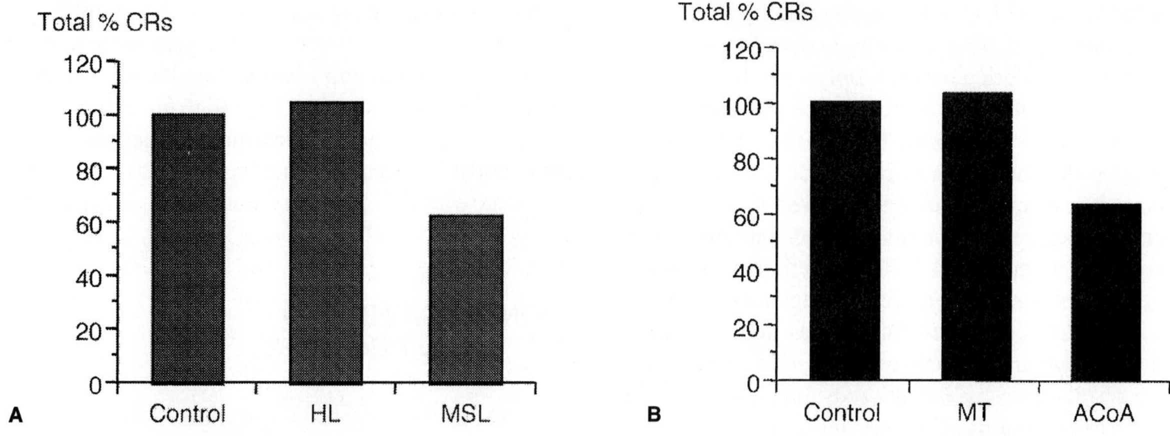

Figure 41-4
Delay eyeblink classic conditioning. A. *Animal data: hippocampal lesions (HL) but not medioseptal lesions (MSL) condition as strongly as controls. (Data for from Ref. 69.)* B. *Human data: MT amnesics but not ACoA amnesics condition as strongly as matched controls. (MT data from Ref. 43; ACoA data from Ref. 45.) Total percent CRs for patient groups shown as percentage of CRs given by control group in the corresponding study.*

Specifically, GABAergic projections from medial septum to hippocampus govern theta rhythm, an electroencephalographic (EEG) pattern associated with learning and exploration, whereas cholinergic projections from medial septum to hippocampus enhance synaptic plasticity while selectively suppressing inputs from other hippocampal region neurons more than inputs from outside the hippocampus. The net effect of these mechanisms may be to modulate hippocampal activity along a continuum from storage of new inputs to recall of previously-learned information.[48,49] Thus, basal forebrain disruption would in turn disrupt hippocampal processing—in the absence of direct hippocampal damage. As such, these data provide preliminary support for the basal forebrain modulation hypothesis in humans as described above. They also suggest that basal forebrain amnesics may perform differently than mediotemporal amnesics on those tasks where hippocampal disruption may be expected to have different behavioral effects than outright hippocampal destruction (see e.g., Ref. 46).

SPECIFIC MEMORY-RELATED SEQUELAE

Readers are referred elsewhere for a more detailed description of neuropsychological sequelae of ACoA aneurysm.[2,49] Neuropsychological consequences of ACoA aneurysm are dependent on several factors (e.g., chronicity, lesion location, medical complications). The information presented here represents the general case.

In general, verbal intellectual functions are largely preserved following ACoA aneurysm (e.g., Refs. 3, 27, and 50), although some select patients can show mild impairment (e.g., Ref. 29). In contrast, Performance IQ is often decreased compared to relatively intact verbal IQ,[50,51] although this is not always observed (e.g., Refs. 11 and 29). Simple attention (e.g., digit span) is often intact, while performance on more complex tasks (i.e., tests with increased challenge to the central executive of working memory) is often impaired. For instance, ACoA aneurysm results in impaired dual task performance[52] and increased susceptibility and/or release from proactive interference (e.g., Refs. 32, 53, and 54).

Deficits in executive control functions constitute a major difficulty among ACoA patients. Executive dysfunction plays a significant role in the memory abilities of ACoA patients for both anterograde[54,55] and retrograde[4] memory.

Declarative memory performance ranges from amnesic, to mild impairment, to normal performance. Immediate recall is generally far less impaired than delayed recall, particularly among patients with amnesia.[2] There is some suggestion that these patients show particular difficulty in discriminating temporal context during recall.[31] Only a handful of studies have been conducted on retrograde memory following ACoA aneurysm, with mixed results. Some studies suggest that the degree of retrograde memory impairment is less severe than that observed in diencephalic or mediotemporal amnesics, although one study found no group differences.[56] Still others find no retrograde impairment whatsoever, even among amnesic patients with ACoA aneurysms. D'Esposito and colleagues[4] showed that impairment of retrograde memory was the result of severe executive dysfunction secondary to bifrontal lesions. The very few studies examining implicit memory have consistently reported intact performance in patients with ACoA aneurysms.[57]

COURSE OF RECOVERY

While early studies reveal that up to 84 percent of ACoA survivors are able to return to work[26,58] or have a "good outcome,"[10] significant neuropsychological, psychological, and psychosocial consequences are often observed in ACoA and other aneurysm patients, even in the absence of obvious neurologic deficits (e.g., Ref. 59), with some evidence for particular difficulties in ACoA patients (e.g., Refs. 1 and 60). The pattern and degree of recovery from cognitive difficulties following ACoA aneurysm vary widely. A variety of factors influence recovery including surgical procedure (e.g., timing of surgery, duration of temporary clipping), medical factors (e.g., hydrocephalus, vasospasm, presence of lesions), premorbid functional status, premorbid employment status and the work environment to which the individual is returning, severity of postoperative cognitive abilities, personality changes, and emotional issues. [3,11,25,27,61–64] Preliminary evidence suggests that there is less structural brain damage and a better cognitive outcome in patients receiving an endovascular coiling procedure versus surgical clipping of a cerebral aneurysm.[65]

Studies of cognitive rehabilitation are extremely rare and have been primarily restricted to case studies. For instance, DeLuca and Locker[51] showed that an ACoA amnesic was able to return to his premorbid career as a college professor and to a lifestyle similar to premorbid levels after about 1 year of rehabilitation, despite remaining amnesic. Significant functional and employment gains were found to be related to significant improvements in executive functioning. Improvement in executive functions was also observed in subjects with ACoA aneurysms following systematic training.[67]

CONCLUSIONS AND FUTURE DIRECTIONS

It is now well established that the basal forebrain plays a critical role in human memory disorders. Whether structures within the basal forebrain (i.e., ventral nucleus of the diagonal band of Broca and septal nuclei) play a direct role in human declarative memory or act to modulate the activity of the hippocampal and mediotemporal system remains unclear (see Fig. 41-3). Nonetheless, future models outlining human declarative memory must incorporate the basal forebrain as a key contributor. Future research should be geared toward learning more about the specific contribution that the basal forebrain brings to human declarative memory. In addition, future work should also be geared toward evaluating rehabilitation techniques that may be effective in treating disordered memory after basal forebrain damage.

REFERENCES

1. Bornstein RA, Weir BK, Petruk KC, et al.: Neuropsychological function in patients after subarachnoid hemorrhage. *Neurosurgery* 21(5):651–654, 1987.
2. DeLuca J, Diamond BJ: Aneurysm of the anterior communicating artery: A review of neuroanatomical and neuropsychological sequelae. (review) (97 refs). *J Clin Exp Neuropsychol* 17(1):100–121, 1995.
3. Bottger S, Prosiegel M, Steiger HJ, et al: Neurobehavioural disturbances, rehabilitation outcome, and lesion site in patients after rupture and repair of anterior communicating artery aneurysm. *J Neurol Neurosurg Psychiatry* 65(1):93–102, 1998.
4. D'Esposito M, Alexander MP, Fischer R, et al: Recovery of memory and executive function following anterior communicating artery aneurysm rupture. *J Int Neuropsychol Soc* 2(6):565–570, 1996.

5. Ogden JA, Mee EW, Henning M: A prospective study of impairment of cognition and memory and recovery after subarachnoid hemorrhage. *Neurosurgery* 33(4):572–586; discussion 586–587, 1993.
6. DeLuca J, Chiaravalloti ND: Neuropsychological consequences of ruptured aneurysms of the anterior communicating artery, in Harrison JE, Owen AM (eds): *Cognitive Deficits in Brain Disorders.* London: Martin Duntz, 2002, pp 17–36.
7. DeLuca J: A cognitive neuroscience perspective on confabulation. *Neuropsychoanalysis* 2(2):119–132, 2000.
8. Adams HP, Biller J: Hemorrhagic intracranial vascular disease. *Clin Neurol* 2:1–64, 1992.
9. McCormick WF: Pathology and pathogenesis of intracranial saccular aneurysms. *Semin Neurol* 4(3):291–303, 1984.
10. Chalif DJ, Weinberg JS: Surgical treatment of aneurysms of the anterior cerebral artery. *Neurosurg Clin N Am* 9(4):797–821, 1998.
11. Alexander MP, Freedman M: Amnesia after anterior communicating artery aneurysm rupture. *Neurology* 34(6):752–757, 1984.
12. Gade A: Amnesia after operations on aneurysms of the anterior communicating artery. *Surg Neurol* 18(1):46–49, 1982.
13. Tatu L, Moulin T, Bogousslavsky J, et al: Arterial territories of the human brain: Cerebral hemispheres. *Neurology* 50(6):1699–1708, 1988.
14. Perlmutter D, Rhoton AL: Microsurgical anatomy of the anterior cerebral-anterior communicating-recurrent artery complex. *J Neurosurg* 45:259–272, 1976.
15. Squire LR, Shimamura AP, Graf P: Strength and duration of priming effects in normal subjects and amnesic patients. *Neuropsychologia* 25(1B):195–210, 1987.
16. Luria AR, Konovalov AN, Podgornaja AY: *Memory Disturbances in Anterior Communicating Artery Aneurysms.* Moscow: Moscow University Press, 1970.
17. Talland GA, Sweet WH, Ballantine HT Jr: Amnesic syndrome with anterior communicating artery aneurysm. *J Nerv Ment Dis* 145(3):179–192, 1967.
18. Vilkki J: Amnesic syndromes after surgery of anterior communicating artery aneurysms. *Cortex* 21(3):431–444, 1985.
19. Crowell RM, Morawetz RB: The anterior communicating artery has significant branches. *Stroke* 8(2):272–273, 1977.
20. Dunker RO, Harris AB: Surgical anatomy of the proximal anterior cerebral artery. *J Neurosurg* 44:359–367, 1976.
21. Damasio AR, Graff-Radford NR, Eslinger PJ, et al: Amnesia following basal forebrain lesions. *Arch Neurol* 42(3):263–271, 1985.
22. Phillips S, Sangalang V, Sterns G: Basal forebrain infarction. A clinicopathologic correlation. *Arch Neurol* 44(11):1134–1138, 1987.
23. Richardson JT: Cognitive performance following rupture and repair of intracranial aneurysm. *Acta Neurol Scand* 83(2):110–122, 1991.
24. Laiacona M, De Santis A, Barbarotto R, et al: Neuropsychological follow-up of patients operated for aneurysms of anterior communicating artery. *Cortex* 25(2):261–273, 1989.
25. Okawa M, Maeda S, Nukui H, et al.: Psychiatric symptoms in ruptured anterior communicating aneurysms: Social prognosis. *Acta Psychiatr Scand* 61(4):306–312, 1980.
26. Teissier du Cros J, Lhermitte F: Neuropsychological analysis of ruptured saccular aneurysms of the anterior communicating artery after radical therapy (32 cases). *Surg Neurol* 22(4):353–359, 1984.
27. Stenhouse LM, Knight RG, Longmore BE, et al: Long-term cognitive deficits in patients after surgery on aneurysms of the anterior communicating artery. *J Neurol Neurosurg Psychiatry* 54(10):909–914, 1991.
28. Tarel V, Pellat J, Naegele B, et al: Memory disorders following rupture of anterior communicating artery aneurysm: 22 cases. *Rev Neurol* 146(12): 746–751, 1990.
29. Irle E, Wowra B, Kunert HJ, et al: Memory disturbances following anterior communicating artery rupture. *Ann Neurol* 31(5):473–480, 1992.
30. Eslinger PJ, Grattan LM: Frontal lobe and frontal-striatal substrates for different forms of human cognitive flexibility. *Neuropsychologia* 31(1):17–28, 1993.
31. Abe K, Inokawa M, Kashiwagi A, et al: Amnesia after a discrete basal forebrain lesion. *J Neurol Neurosurg Psychiatry* 65:126–130, 1998.
32. Dringenberg HC: Alzheimer's disease: more than a "cholinergic disorder"—evidence that cholinergic-monoaminergic interactions contribute to EEG slowing and dementia. *Behav Brain Res* 115: 235–249, 2000.
33. Volpe BT, Hirst W: Amnesia following the rupture and repair of an anterior communicating artery aneurysm. *J Neurol Neurosurg Psychiatry* 46(8): 704–709, 1983.
34. Goldenberg G, Schuri U, Grömminger O, et al: Basal forebrain amnesia: Does the nucleus accumbens contribute to human memory? *J Neurol Neurosurg Psychiatry* 67:163–168, 1999.
35. Corkin S, Cohen NJ, Sullivan EV, et al: Analyses of global memory impairments of different etiologies. *Ann N Y Acad Sci* 444:10–40, 1985.
36. Rajaram S, Coslett HB: New verbal associative learning in annesia: A case study. *Neuropsychology* 14:427–455, 2000.

37. Kixmiller JS, Verfaellie M, Mather MM, et al: Role of perceptual and organizational factors in amnesics' recall of the Rey-Osterrieth complex figure: A comparison of three amnesic groups. *J Clin Exp Neuropsychol* 22(2):198–207, 2000.
38. Palmer HM, McDonald S: The role of frontal and temporal lobe processes in prospective remembering. *Brain Cogn* 44:103–107, 2000.
39. Parkin AJ: Amnesic syndrome: A lesion-specific disorder? *Cortex* 20:479–508, 1984.
40. Arendt T, Bigl V, Arendt A, et al: Loss of neurons in nucleus basalis of Meynert in Alzheimer' disease, paralysis agitans and Korsakoff's disease. *Acta Neuropathol* 61:101–108, 1983.
41. Gormezano I, Kehoe EJ, Marshall BS: Twenty years of classical conditioning research with the rabbit. *Prog Psychobiol Physiol Psychol* 10:197–275, 1983.
42. Solomon P, Moore J: Latent inhibition and stimulus generalization of the classically conditioned nictitating membrane response in rabbits (*Oryctolagus cuniculus*) following dorsal hippocampal ablation. *J Comp Physiol Psychol* 89:1192–1203, 1975.
43. Gabrieli J, McGlinchey-Berroth R, Carrillo M, et al: Intact delay-eyeblink classical conditioning in amnesia. *Behav Neurosci* 109(5):819–827, 1995.
44. Solomon P, Gottfried K: The septohippocampal cholinergic system and classical conditioning of the rabbit's nictitating membrane response. *J Comp Physiol Psychol* 95(2):322–330, 1981.
45. Myers C, DeLuca J, Schultheis M, et al: Impaired eyeblink classical conditioning in individuals with anterograde amnesia resulting from anterior communicating artery aneurysm rupture. *Behav Neurosci* 115:560–570, 2001.
46. Solomon P, Solomon S, Van der Schaaf E, et al: Altered activity in the hippocampus is more detrimental to classical conditioning than removing the structure. *Science* 220:329–331, 1983.
47. Solomon P, Groccia-Ellison M, Flynn D, et al: Disruption of human eyeblink conditioning after central cholinergic blockade with scopolamine. *Behav Neurosci* 107(2):271–279, 1993.
48. Hasselmo M, Schnell, E: Laminar selectivity of the cholinergic suppression of synaptic transmission in rat hippocampal region CA1: Computational modeling and brain slice physiology. *J Neurosci* 14(6):3898–3914, 1994.
49. Myers C, Ermita B, Hasselmo M, Gluck M: Further implications of a computational model of septohippocampal cholinergic modulation in eyeblink conditioning. *Psychobiology* 26(1):1–20, 1998.
50. DeLuca J: Cognitive dysfunction after aneurysm of the anterior communicating artery. *J Clin Exp Neuropsychol* 14(6):924–934, 1992.
51. DeLuca J, Locker R: Cognitive rehabilitation following anterior communicating artery aneurysm bleeding: A case report. *Disabil Rehabil* 18(5):265–272, 1996.
52. Leclercq M, Couillet J, Azouvi P, et al: Dual task performance after severe traumatic brain injury or vascular prefrontal damage. *J Clin Exp Neuropsychol* 22:339–350, 2000.
53. Parkin AJ, Leng NR, Stanhope N, et al: Memory impairment following ruptured aneurysm of the anterior communicating artery. *Brain Cogn* 7(2):231–243, 1988.
54. Luria AR: *The Neuropsychology of Memory*. Washington DC: Winston, 1976.
55. Diamond BJ, DeLuca J, Kelley SM: Memory and executive functions in amnesic and non-amnesic patients with aneurysms of the anterior communicating artery. *Brain* 120(6):1015–1025, 1997.
56. Gade A, Mortensen EL: Temporal gradient in the remote memory impairment of amnesic patients with lesions in the basal forebrain. *Neuropsychologia* 28(9):985–1001, 1990.
57. Bondi MW, Kaszniak AW, Rapcsak SZ, et al: Implicit and explicit memory following anterior communicating artery aneurysm rupture. *Brain Cogn* 22:213–229, 1993.
58. Hori S, Suzuki J: Early and late results of intracranial direct surgery of anterior communicating artery aneurysms. *J Neurosurg* 50(4):433–440, 1979.
59. Ljunggren B, Sonesson B, Saveland H, et al: Cognitive impairment and adjustment in patients without neurological deficits after aneurysmal SAH and early operation. *J Neurosurg* 62(5):673–679, 1985.
60. Sonesson B, Ljunggren B, Saveland H, et al: Cognition and adjustment after late and early operation for ruptured aneurysm. *Neurosurg* 21(3):279–287, 1987.
61. Tidswell P, Dias PS, Sagar HJ, et al.: Cognitive outcome after aneurysm rupture: Relationship to aneurysm site and perioperative complications. *Neurology* 45(5):875–882, 1995.
62. Storey PB: Psychiatric sequelae of subarachnoid haemorrhage. *BMJ* 3(560):261–266, 1967.
63. Storey PB: Brain damage and personality change after subarachnoid haemorrhage. *Br J Psychiatry* 117(537): 129–142, 1970.
64. Vilkki J, Holst P, Ohman J, et al: Social outcome related to cognitive performance and computed tomographic findings after surgery for a ruptured intracranial aneurysm. *Neurosurgery* 26(4):579–584, 1990.

65. Hadjivassiliou M, Tooth CL, Romanowski CAJ, et al: Aneurysmal SAH: Cognitive outcome and structural damage after clipping or coiling. *Neurology* 56:1672–1677, 2001.
66. Carpenter MB: Blood supply of the central nervous system, in Satterfield TS (ed): *Core Text of Neuroanatomy*. Baltimore: Lippincott, Williams, & Wilkins, 1988.
67. Stablum F, Umitla C, Mogentale C, et al: Rehabilitation of executive deficits in closed head injury and anterior communicating artery aneurysm patients. *Psychol Res* 63:265–278, 2000.
68. Drumm DA, Greene KA, Marciano FF, et al: Neurobehavioral deficits following rupture of ACoA aneurysms: The ACoA aneurysm syndrome. *BNI Quarterly* 9(2):7, 1993.
69. Berry S, Thompson R: Medial septal lesions retard classical conditioning of the nictitating membrane response in rabbits. *Science* 205:209–211, 1979.

Chapter 42

REHABILITATION OF MEMORY DYSFUNCTION*

Elizabeth L. Glisky

Rehabilitation of memory dysfunction has focused primarily on treating the kinds of memory problems that are most disruptive in everyday life—deficits of episodic or explicit memory that prevent the acquisition and retention of new information. The inability to acquire new long-term memories is associated with a variety of brain insults and neurologic conditions and may result from a deficit in encoding, storage, or retrieval processes or some combination of these (see Chaps. 37 and 38). At the same time, other kinds of memory may be unaffected—memory for the remote past, memory for world knowledge, or implicit memory, for example. For these reasons, no single treatment is likely to prove efficacious for all patients. Instead, it seems likely that treatments will have to take into account the particular pattern of impaired and spared cognitive functions in each case, the specific memory processes that are compromised, and the regions of the brain that are implicated.

Most attempts at rehabilitation have not considered all of these factors but instead have adopted more general approaches that have been applied broadly across a range of memory problems stemming from various etiologies and damage to different regions of the brain. This chapter provides an overview of these approaches, outlining their goals and assumptions, the treatment methodologies most commonly associated with each, the conditions under which they are most likely to be successful, and the extent to which they are based on well-established cognitive or neuropsychological principles.

* **ACKNOWLEDGMENT:** Preparation of this manuscript was supported by Grant No. AG 14792 from the National Institute on Aging.

APPROACHES TO MEMORY REHABILITATION

Approaches to memory rehabilitation have generally focused on one of two goals: (1) the repair or optimal use of damaged memory processes or (2) the alleviation of functional disabilities.[1] The first goal targets underlying impairment and assumes that if damaged processes can be repaired or trained to be used optimally, general improvements in memory *ability* will follow. The second goal targets disability rather than impairment and aims to improve memory *performance* or *function* on specific everyday tasks. The assumption here is that performance might be improved even though the underlying memory ability remains unchanged. Although both goals represent desirable outcomes for therapeutic intervention, the first has so far remained elusive, particularly when brain damage is severe. The bulk of the successful remedial work has been in the area of functional improvement. The four approaches outlined below focus on these goals to differing extents and are often combined in an attempt to achieve optimal outcomes.

Restoration of Damaged Function

This approach assumes that damaged memory processes can be restored through stimulation or activation and that premorbid memory ability can thereby be regained. Rehabilitation techniques developed within this framework have focused primarily on memory practice or on retraining of general memory skills with the expectation that such practice will lead to broad improvements in memory.[2] Such general improvements, however, have not yet been found. Also implicit in this view is the assumption that stimulation of damaged memory processes through exercise, practice, or retraining will result in neural as well as cognitive changes. Although recent evidence reveals some plasticity in the adult human brain (see Chap. 5) and the possibility of neurogenesis in areas important for memory,[3,4] the functional consequences of these changes are as yet unknown.[5,6]

Optimization of Residual Function

This approach to memory rehabilitation assumes that, in many cases, memory processes are not lost entirely but may be reduced in efficiency. Such may be the case in normal aging, for example, or in milder forms of head injury. Under these conditions, rehabilitation may focus on optimizing the use of residual function. The goal of this approach may be either a general improvement in memory ability or enhanced performance on specific functional tasks. It usually involves the training of mnemonic strategies or skills that were available premorbidly.[7]

Compensation for Lost Function

A more pragmatic approach to the treatment of memory problems assumes that, at least in some cases, cognitive and neural mechanisms cannot be restored; therefore interventions should focus on achieving behavioral outcomes that are important for an individual's functioning in everyday life. In this approach, the need to use internal memory processes is bypassed by the provision of external supports in the form of environmental restructurings and compensatory devices. Although a part of many treatment programs, the use of external aids is often thought to be the only intervention appropriate for patients with extensive brain damage and severe memory loss.

Substitution of Intact Function

This approach to memory remediation assumes that the cognitive and neural mechanisms normally involved in memory may no longer be available but that other *intact* processes may be recruited to serve as substitutes. Although the therapeutic goal of this approach is usually improved functional outcome, there is an underlying assumption that change may occur as a result of reorganization at both the cognitive and neural levels.[1,8] Neuroimaging studies suggesting that the brain may be able to use alternate regions to compensate for brain damage or decline[9,10] along with recent findings of plasticity in the human brain,[3,5] provide some support for this position. This approach may be most appropriate when the memory deficit is severe and memory function is minimal.

METHODS OF MEMORY REHABILITATION

Associated with each of the above approaches to rehabilitation are a number of different methodologies that have proved variously effective. Some of these are based on common sense, others on findings from the normal cognitive literature, and still others on consideration of neuropsychological factors. Their success has been primarily in the achievement of improved performance and specific functional goals; there is as yet little evidence that memory ability can be affected in any general sense.

Practice and Rehearsal Techniques

There is little doubt that, in order for memory-impaired individuals to acquire and retain new knowledge, they will have to spend considerable time practicing or rehearsing to-be-learned information. All rehearsal techniques, however, are not equally effective. A procedure frequently advocated for the restoration of memory ability is the presentation of computer-generated exercise and drill regimens that involve repeated practice of meaningless materials such as arbitrary lists of words, digits, pictures, locations, or shapes. Although this commonsense method may have face validity, there is no evidence that it leads to any general improvements in memory. Although people may learn the specific information that they practice (which in many cases is not very useful), benefits do not generalize beyond the training materials or context.[11,12]

Another rehearsal technique, borrowed from cognitive psychology and found to be effective for memory-impaired individuals, is *spaced retrieval.*[13] This method requires patients to retrieve information at gradually increasing time intervals. Using this technique, patients with memory disorders of varying severity and etiology, including Alzheimer's disease, have been able to learn specific information such as name-face associations,[14,15] the location of objects,[16] and items of orientation.[17] The method may rely on residual memory function or may tap into other preserved memory processes. Camp and McKitrick[16] have noted that acquisition of new information through spaced retrieval appears to occur effortlessly, and they have speculated that it may involve intact implicit memory systems.

Mnemonic Strategies

A variety of mnemonic strategies, including visual imagery and semantic elaboration, have been adapted from cognitive psychology, where they have proven effective in enhancing the memory performance of normal individuals. With neurologic patients, however, they have been useful only in limited circumstances (for reviews, see Refs. 18–20). For example, patients with unilateral lesions may benefit from a strategy that makes use of the preserved hemisphere.[7,21] Patients with bilateral lesions or severe memory impairments, however, tend not to be able to learn or use these strategies effectively,[7] consistent with the notion that mnemonic strategy training relies on the use of residual memory function. Even those patients who can learn the techniques tend not to use them spontaneously, so real-world benefits are minimal. Despite this lack of generalization, mnemonic strategies are often effective in helping those with mild to moderate impairments learn specific information that may be relevant in their everyday lives, such as people's names.[7,22,23]

Most mnemonic techniques are considered to be encoding strategies because they require meaningful organization of materials at input. Training of retrieval strategies has received much less attention. A recent attempt at training a retrieval skill[24] has shown some success in older adults. The technique involves a shaping procedure whereby the interval over which items have to be recollected is gradually increased, much like in the spaced retrieval method. Older adults were able to increase their span of retention to 28 intervening items and to demonstrate some maintenance of the skill over a 3- to 4-month period. This method likely depends on residual memory function and may be appropriate only for those with mild impairments.

External Aids

A way to compensate for the loss of memory is to use a variety of memory aids, such as notebooks, diaries, alarm watches, calendars, and so forth.[20] Many of these have been incorporated effectively into the everyday lives of memory-impaired individuals, although considerable training in their use is often required[25] (for review, see Ref. 26). Recently, micro- and pocket computers have begun to be used as cuing devices[27] and as external supports for a variety of everyday activities,[28,29] but as yet their potential as prosthetic devices has gone largely untapped (for reviews, see Refs. 30 and 31). The use of many of these devices, however, requires considerable training, and many memory-impaired individuals have great difficulty learning how to use them; they therefore may be appropriate only for mildly impaired patients. Simple electronic devices such as pagers and voice organizers, which deliver messages about daily activities to be performed, require little memory to operate, however, and have been found effective for even the most severely impaired individuals.[32–34]

Vanishing Cues

This method focuses on the acquisition of specific information and skills and has been used primarily for teaching large amounts of complex domain-specific knowledge such as that required to maintain a job or manage a home. The training technique involves the provision of partial information as a cue or prompt, which is then gradually withdrawn as learning progresses. The methodology has been used effectively with a range of memory-disordered patients who have learned vocational tasks such as computer data entry[35,36] and more general skills such as computer programming[37] and word processing.[29] The vanishing cues methodology has been hypothesized to tap into preserved implicit memory processes such as those involved in priming and procedural memory, which are often spared even in very severely impaired patients.

Errorless Learning

Baddeley and Wilson[38] suggested that the vanishing cues procedure may be successful because it prevents errors, and that for memory-impaired individuals, avoiding errors may be particularly important for learning. In a series of studies, Wilson and colleagues have demonstrated that individuals with memory deficits, including those with Alzheimer's disease,[39] benefited substantially from errorless learning and were able to acquire information such as names, the use of an electronic memory aid, and other items of general knowledge important for their daily functioning.[38,40] Recently it has been suggested that a combination of vanishing cues and errorless learning methods may provide optimal conditions for learning[41] and may be most beneficial for patients with the most severe disorders, who must rely on preserved implicit memory.[42]

FUTURE DIRECTIONS

Although several approaches to memory rehabilitation have been adopted and numerous individual treatments and therapies attempted, many of them have derived from practical concerns rather than from reliable empirical findings or strong theoretical formulations. In the past 20 years, however, with the growth of the fields of cognitive neuropsychology and cognitive neuroscience and the developing technologies in the field of neuroimaging, it has become possible to link rehabilitation methodologies to a firmer empiric and theoretical base and thus provide a clearer direction for clinicians to follow in the treatment of memory disorders. Much recent research in memory rehabilitation has suggested that memory-impaired patients may be learning new information through different processes and structures than normal individuals.[43,44] The multiple memory systems view[45] has provided a framework for interpreting these findings and a direction for rehabilitation. If there are several memory systems, each supporting different functions and relying on different underlying neural structures, then it might be possible to take advantage of preserved systems and structures to compensate for those that are damaged or lost. Similarly, as reviewed in Chapter 8, findings from neuroimaging studies suggest that the damaged brain may undergo reorganization following insult or may recruit intact regions to carry out functions previously handled by damaged areas.[46] These results seem consistent with a rehabilitation strategy that attempts to find new ways or alternate strategies to perform memory tasks. However, there will almost certainly not be a single therapy that works for everyone. Instead, different techniques will be appropriate for different patients depending on the nature of their memory deficit and the location of their brain damage. Neuropsychology now has the tools—neuropsychological, behavioral, and neuroanatomic—to construct detailed profiles of each individual patient, documenting his or her cognitive and neural strengths and weaknesses. Careful use of these assessments in the development of individualized treatment plans should increase the likelihood of successful rehabilitation outcomes in the future.

REFERENCES

1. Rothi LJ, Horner J: Restitution and substitution: Two theories of recovery with application to neurobehavioral treatment. *J Clin Neuropsychol* 5:73–81, 1983.
2. Sohlberg MM, Mateer CA: *Introduction to Cognitive Rehabilitation.* New York: Guilford Press, 1989.
3. Eriksson PS, Perfilieva E, Bjork-Eriksson T, et al: Neurogenesis in the adult human hippocampus. *Nat Med* 4:1313–1317, 1998.
4. Kolb B: *Brain Plasticity and Behavior.* Mahwah, NJ: Erlbaum, 1995.
5. Kolb B, Gibb R: Neuroplasticity and recovery of function after brain injury, in Stuss DT, Winocur W, Robertson IH (eds): *Cognitive Rehabilitation.* Cambridge, UK: Cambridge University Press, 1999, pp 9–25.
6. Stein DG: Brain injury and theories of recovery, in Christensen A-L, Uzzell BP (eds): *International Handbook of Neuropsychological Rehabilitation.* New York: Kluwer Academic/Plenum, 2000, pp 3–32.
7. Wilson B: *Rehabilitation of Memory.* New York: Guilford, 1987.
8. Luria AR: *Restoration of Function after Brain Injury.* New York: Macmillan, 1963.
9. Buckner RL, Corbetta M, Schatz J, et al: Preserved speech abilities and compensation following prefrontal damage. *Proc Nat Acad Sci U S A* 93:1249–1253, 1996.
10. Grady CL, Maisog JM, Horwitz B, et al: Age-related changes in cortical blood flow activation during visual processing of faces and location. *J Neurosci* 14:1450–1462, 1994.
11. Glisky EL, Schacter DL: Models and methods of memory rehabilitation, in Boller F, Grafman J (eds): *Handbook of Neuropsychology.* Amsterdam: Elsevier, 1989, vol 3, pp 233–246.

12. Berg IJ, Koning-Haanstra M, Deelman BG: Long-term effects of memory rehabilitation. *Neuropsychol Rehabil* 1:97–111, 1991.
13. Landauer TK, Bjork RA: Optimum rehearsal patterns and name learning, in Gruneberg MM, Morris PE, Sykes RN (eds): *Practical Aspects of Memory.* London: Academic Press, 1978, pp 625–632.
14. Camp CJ: Facilitation of new learning in Alzheimer's disease, in Gilmore GC, Whitehouse PJ, Wykle ML (eds): *Memory, Aging, and Dementia.* New York: Springer-Verlag, 1989, pp 212–225.
15. Schacter DL, Rich SA, Stampp MS: Remediation of memory disorders: Experimental evaluation of the spaced-retrieval technique. *J Clin Exp Neurolpsychol* 7:79–96, 1985.
16. Camp CJ, McKitrick LA: Memory interventions in Alzheimer's-type dementia populations: Methodological and theoretical issues, in West RL, Sinnott JD (eds): *Everyday Memory and Aging: Current Research and Methodology.* New York: Springer-Verlag, 1992, pp 155–172.
17. Moffat N: Strategies of memory therapy, in Wilson BA, Moffat N (eds): *Clinical Management of Memory Problems.* 2d ed. London: Chapman & Hall, 1992, pp 86–119.
18. Butters MA, Soety EM, Glisky EL: Memory rehabilitation, in Snyder PJ, Nussbaum PD (eds): *Clinical Neuropsychology.* Washington, DC: American Psychological Association, 1998, pp 450–466.
19. Glisky EL, Glisky ML: Learning and memory impairments, in Eslinger PJ (ed): *Neuropsychological Interventions.* New York: Guilford Press, 2002, pp 137–162.
20. Harris JE: Ways to help memory, in Wilson BA, Moffat N (eds): *Clinical Management of Memory Problems,* 2d ed. London: Chapman & Hall, 1992, pp 59–85.
21. Wilson B: Rehabilitation and memory disorders, in Squire LR (ed): *Neuropsychology of Memory,* 2d ed. New York: Guilford Press, 1992, pp 315–321.
22. Thoene AIT, Glisky EL: Learning of name-face associations in memory impaired patients: A comparison of different training procedures. *J Int Neuropsychol Soc* 1(1):29–38, 1995.
23. Wilson B: Success and failure in memory training following a cerebral vascular accident. *Cortex* 18:581–594, 1982.
24. Jacoby LL, Jennings JM, Hay JF: Dissociating automatic and consciously controlled processes: Implications for diagnosis and rehabilitation of memory deficits, in Herrmann DJ, McEvoy C, Hertzog C, et al (eds): *Basic and Applied Memory Research: Theory in Context.* Mahwah, NJ: Erlbaum, 1996, pp 161–193.
25. Sohlberg MM, Mateer CA: Training use of compensatory memory books: A three stage behavioral approach. *J Clin Exp Neuropsychol* 11:871–887, 1989.
26. Kapur N: Memory aids in the rehabilitation of memory disordered patients, in Baddeley AD, Wilson BA, Watts FN (eds): *Handbook of Memory Disorders.* Chichester, UK: Wiley, 1995, pp 534–556.
27. Kirsch NL, Levine SP, Lajiness-O'Neill R, Schnyder M: Computer-assisted interactive task guidance: Facilitating the performance of a simulated vocational task. *J Head Trauma Rehabil* 7(3):13–25, 1992.
28. Cole E, Dehdashti P, Petti L: Design and outcomes of computer-based cognitive prosthetics for brain injury: A field study of three subjects. *Neurorehabilitation* 4(3):174–186, 1994.
29. Glisky EL: Acquisition and transfer of word processing skill by an amnesic patient. *Neuropsychol Rehabil* 5(4):299–318, 1995.
30. Glisky EL: Computers in memory rehabilitation, in Baddeley AD, Wilson BA, Watts FN (eds): *Handbook of Memory Disorders.* New York: Wiley, 1995, pp 557–575.
31. Kapur N, Glisky EL, Wilson BA: External memory aids and computers in memory rehabilitation, in Baddeley AD, Wilson BA, Kopelman M (eds): *Handbook of Memory Disorders,* 2d ed. Chichester, UK: Wiley, 2002, pp 757–783.
32. Wilson BA, Evans JJ, Emslie H, Malinek V: Evaluation of NeuroPage: A new memory aid. *J Neurol Neurosurg Psychiatry* 63:113–115, 1997.
33. Wilson BA, Emslie H, Quirk K, Evans J: George: Learning to live independently with NeuroPage. *Rehabil Psychol* 44:284–296, 1999.
34. Van den Broek MD, Downes J, Johnson A, et al: Evaluation of an electronic memory aid in the neuropsychological rehabilitation of prospective memory deficits. *Brain Inj* 14:455–462, 2000.
35. Glisky EL, Schacter DL: Acquisition of domain-specific knowledge in organic amnesia: Training for computer-related work. *Neuropsychologia* 25:893–906, 1987.
36. Glisky EL: Acquisition and transfer of declarative and procedural knowledge by memory-impaired patients. *Neuropsychologia* 30:899–910, 1992.
37. Glisky EL, Schacter DL, Tulving E: Computer learning by memory-impaired patients: Acquisition and retention of complex knowledge. *Neuropsychologia* 24:313–328, 1986.
38. Baddeley AD, Wilson BA: When implicit learning fails: Amnesia and the problem of error elimination. *Neuropsychologia* 32:53–68, 1994.

39. Clare L, Wilson BA, Breen K, Hodges JR: Errorless learning of face-name associations in early Alzheimer's disease. *Neurocase* 5:37–46, 1999.
40. Wilson BA, Baddeley AD, Evans J, Shiel A: Errorless learning in the rehabilitation of memory impaired people. *Neuropsychol Rehabil* 4:307–326, 1994.
41. Komatsu S, Mimura M, Kato M, et al: Errorless and effortful processes involved in learning of face-name associations by patients with alcoholic Korsakoff's syndrome. *Neuropsychol Rehabil* 10:113–132, 2000.
42. Evans JJ, Wilson BA, Schuri U, et al: A comparison of "errorless" and "trial-and-error" learning methods for teaching individuals with acquired memory deficits. *Neuropsychol Rehabil* 10:67–101, 2000.
43. Glisky EL, Schacter DL, Butters MA: Domain-specific learning and remediation of memory disorders, in Riddoch MJ, Humphreys GW (eds): *Cognitive Neuropsychology and Cognitive Rehabilitation.* Hove, UK: Erlbaum, 1994, pp 527–548.
44. Verfaellie M: Semantic learning in amnesia, in Boller F, Grafman J (eds): *Handbook of Neuropsychology,* 2d ed. Amsterdam: Elsevier, 2000, vol 2, pp 335–354.
45. Schacter DL, Tulving E (eds): *Memory Systems 1994.* Cambridge, MA: MIT Press, 1994.
46. Grady CL, Kapur S: The use of neuroimaging in neurorehabilitative research, in Stuss DT, Winocur G, Robertson IH (eds): *Cognitive Neurorehabilitation.* Cambridge, UK: Cambridge University Press, 1999, pp 47–58.

Part 7

DELIRIUM, DEMENTIA, AND EPILEPSY

Chapter 43

DELIRIUM AND DEMENTIA: AN OVERVIEW*

Daniel I. Kaufer
Jeffrey L. Cummings

Delirium and dementia are distinctive clinical syndromes involving central nervous system dysfunction. Both have enormous social, economic, and epidemiologic ramifications, particularly in the elderly. Almost 4 million Americans are currently afflicted with Alzheimer's disease, and this number will rise severalfold in coming decades as longevity increases.[1,2] Beyond its toll on individuals and families, the overall cost of Alzheimer's disease to society approaches $100 billion annually.

In contrast to the typically insidious nature of dementia syndromes, delirium poses a more acute threat of morbidity and mortality. Although delirium in elderly general hospital patients is a common problem, studies suggest that up to two-thirds of cases go unrecognized.[3–6] The failure to detect delirium may have serious consequences, as it is associated with increased rates of medical complications, longer hospital stays, institutionalization, increased medical costs, and death.[5,7] Although dementia and delirium syndromes have many shared and independent risk factors, the strongest risk factor for both is advancing age.[1–3] Increased awareness and early recognition of these disorders in community, ambulatory, and inpatient settings may help minimize their devastating impact.

Delirium and dementia both involve acquired cognitive impairment frequently accompanied by behavioral disturbances. Each is a clinical syndrome with characteristic but variable patterns of expression. The multiplicity of clinical subtypes within each syndrome reflects the wide range of etiologies and pathophysiologic mechanisms underlying these disorders. Dementia and delirium are fundamentally distinguished by the clinical hallmarks of primary memory and attentional deficits, respectively.[8,9] Beyond these core deficits, considerable overlap in the clinical manifestations of these disorders can lead to diagnostic confusion. This highlights the need for valid and reliable definitional guidelines and a systematic approach to assessment. Accurate clinical characterization and distinction of dementia and delirium syndromes is essential to differential diagnosis. Knowledge of respective risk factors and etiologies, in turn, is crucial for guiding relevant laboratory diagnostic evaluation and therapeutic intervention.

As subsequent chapters focus on dementing disorders, delirium is reviewed in more detail here. The overview of dementia syndromes emphasizes general principles of classification, etiology, pathophysiology, and management. A principal aim is to elaborate a systematic and integrative approach to etiologic diagnosis based on recognizable constellations of brain-behavior relationships that are evident across a variety of conditions that impair cognition.

DELIRIUM

Definition

Historically, more than 30 different terms have been used to describe delirium.[10] The term *acute confusional state* (ACS) is commonly used by neurologists, and some authors reserve use of the term *delirium* for the syndrome of agitation, psychosis, and autonomic instability associated with alcohol withdrawal.[11] One of the major pitfalls in the assessment of delirium has been the absence of validated diagnostic criteria and rating instruments.[12] This problem has gradually been addressed by the increased availability of standardized definitions, operational criteria, and validated assessment

* **ACKNOWLEDGEMENTS:** This project was supported by National Institute on Aging Core Center Grants AG05133 and AG10123.

Table 43-1
DSM-IV criteria for delirium

Disturbance in consciousness impairing awareness of the environment
Reduced ability to focus, sustain, or shift attention
Cognitive or perceptual disturbance not attributable to dementia
Acute to subacute onset (hours to days)
Diurnal fluctuations
Clinical/laboratory evidence relating the disturbance to a general medical condition

Source: DSM-IV,[4] with permission.

tools.[8,13,14] The first widely used standardized criteria for delirium were presented in the *Diagnostic and Statistical Manual of Mental Disorders,* 3rd edition (DSM-III), published in 1980.[15] The nebulous term *clouding of consciousness* used as the anchoring criterion in DSM-III was replaced in subsequent editions by the term *disturbance of consciousness.*[8,16] The current definitional criteria for delirium presented in DSM-IV are outlined in Table 43-1. The core phenomenologic features of delirium are a disturbance in consciousness, attentional deficits, brief duration of symptoms, and fluctuation in symptoms over time.[8] The principal exclusionary criterion involves distinguishing delirium from a dementia syndrome, although the two disorders frequently coexist. Patients with dementia are often more susceptible to delirium-producing insults.[17] However, the initial diagnosis of a dementia cannot reliably be made in the presence of a delirium.

Clinical Features

Attentional Dysfunction Attentional impairment, the principal manifestation of delirium or ACS, is not a unitary phenomenon (see Chaps. 2 and 3).[9,18] The severity of attentional disturbance may vary from a marked decrease in level of consciousness (i.e., stupor or coma) to a seeming alertness in a subject exhibiting deficits only in the performance of attentionally demanding tasks. Determining level of alertness is a requisite first step of assessment. Simple bedside tests of attention and vigilance include digit span (the number of random, sequential spoken digits the subject is able to repeat) and a continuous performance test (e.g., the subject identifies a target stimulus, such as the letter "A," among a series of randomly presented target and nontarget stimuli).[18] Both tests have been shown to be as sensitive as formal instruments for detecting delirium.[19] More subtle deficits may be elicited by tests of divided attention such as reversing the sequence of spoken digits, spelling a word backward, or performing serial subtractions. Numerical scoring of these tests may be augmented informally by noting the degree of effort or length of time required to complete the task.

Nonattentional Cognitive Deficits Attentional deficits are associated with and contribute to other intellectual disturbances. Thought form may be rambling and incoherent, with bizarre content. When there is an associated language comprehension deficit, delirious speech may be confused with a Wernicke-type fluent aphasia. Delirium can usually be distinguished from the latter by the relative absence of paraphasic errors and a better-preserved ability to repeat.[20] Anomia is common and may be manifest as the syndrome of nonaphasic misnaming.[21–23] Nonaphasic misnaming entails a stilted or pedantic style, facetiousness, and a tendency for misidentifications along a particular theme. Anomic deficits associated with delirium also tend to be accompanied by more perseverative and visual perceptive errors compared to those seen in Alzheimer's disease.[24] Writing disturbances—such as poor legibility, spatial misalignment, agrammatism, and spelling errors (particularly at the ends of words)—are among the most sensitive indicators of delirium.[25] Similarly, mechanical, organizational, and spatial deficits may be apparent in figure copying and drawing. Learning and memory are virtually always affected, often reflecting the inability to encode or register new material. The inability to immediately recall newly presented information confounds formal testing of memory and may help distinguish delirium from a primary amnestic disorder. Confabulation is observed in about 15 percent of delirium patients[26,27]; other cognitive abnormalities may include concrete thinking, calculation errors, and perseverative tendencies in thinking, speech, and motor behavior. It is important to emphasize that disorientation to time and place are commonly present but are neither invariant nor pathognomonic features of delirium.

Neuropsychiatric Features Neuropsychiatric symptoms are frequent manifestations of delirium.

Hallucinations tend to be visual, although auditory and tactile hallucinations may also be present; the latter are particularly common in alcohol and drug withdrawal syndromes. Delusional beliefs, as discussed in Chap. 31, may be simple or complex and occasionally take on specific forms, such as the belief that significant others have been replaced by different, similar-appearing persons (Capgras's syndrome) or the belief that one is simultaneously in two locations (reduplicative paramnesia).[28,29] Psychotic symptoms may sometimes be florid, accompanied by persecutory fear and agitation. Emotional lability, hyperexcitability, and euphoria may produce a manic-like state, or the patient may appear depressed, apathetic, or perplexed. The polarity of these features has led to subtyping of delirium into "hyperactive-hyperalert" and "hypoactive-hypoalert," or "activated" and "somnolent" variants.[3,30] Ross et al.[30] observed paranoia, agitation, and psychosis much more frequently in patients with activated delirium, although admixtures of or alternations between these symptom complexes may occur in the same individual during the course of a delirious episode.[31]

Movement Disorders A variety of movement disorders may accompany delirium, particularly toxic-metabolic encephalopathies. A tremor may be present when the arms are held in extension or during movement.[32] Generalized tremulousness often accompanies withdrawal states. Asterixis is the brief, repetitive cessation of muscle activity best observed when the arms are held in a fixed posture extended at the elbow and wrist. Although colloquially referred to as the "liver flap" due to its association with hepatic encephalopathy, a wide variety of toxic and metabolic conditions may produce asterixis.[33,34] Myoclonus, like asterixis, is associated with drug toxicity and metabolic derangements, particularly uremia, but is otherwise a nonspecific finding. Generalized increased motor tone, hyperreflexia, and extensor plantar responses may also occur in delirium. *Catatonia* refers to a number of abnormal movements commonly including stereotyped mannerisms and bizarre posturing; it occurs in association with a wide variety of conditions including idiopathic psychiatric illnesses (schizophrenia and mood disorders), metabolic and toxic encephalopathies, and structural lesions of the limbic system and basal ganglia.[35]

Sleep-Wake Cycle Disturbances Disturbances of the sleep-wake cycle are a consistent feature of delirium. Sleep patterns may become fragmented, with an overall trend toward diminished physiologic sleep. The normal circadian cycle may be reversed, with daytime somnolence and nocturnal restlessness and agitation.[36]

Course and Prognosis

The estimated prevalence of delirium in elderly hospitalized patients varies between 11 and 16 percent, with incidence rates ranging between 3 and 31 percent.[37–40] Both rates are typically higher in surgical patient populations.[41] Advanced age, illness severity, fever, infection, and exposure to anticholinergic or sedative drugs are among the strongest risk factors for delirium. Dementia increases the risk of delirium two- to threefold, and up to half of all patients with delirium have preexisting or newly acquired dementia.

Short-term morbidity is increased in delirium patients, reflected by longer hospitalizations and an increased number of complications such as infections and decubitus ulcers.[42–45] Elderly patients with delirium are at higher risk for not being able to live independently, and, in more severe cases, may require nursing home placement. One-month mortality rates of 15 to 30 percent have been reported in patients admitted to hospital in a delirium.[44] Recovery from a delirium may be protracted and incomplete; intellectual and neuropsychiatric disturbances were noted to persist for more than 6 months in a majority of patients studied.[43] Delirium associated with comorbid medical illness often leads to further deterioration in functional or intellectual status over time.[45]

Laboratory Features

General Guidelines Laboratory evaluation of delirium is guided by available history, known factors, and clinical assessment. A toxicology panel and routine blood chemistries (electrolytes, blood glucose, blood urea nitrogen, creatinine, liver function tests) are appropriate screening tests. In certain situations, vitamin B_{12}, thyroid function tests, and collagen vascular disease screening tests may be useful. If respiratory status is compromised, an arterial blood gas is indicated. Focal or asymmetrical neurologic signs suggest an intracranial lesion and require radiographic evaluation.

If a hemorrhagic process is suspected by a history of apoplectic onset, severe and acute headache, or significant head trauma, a computed tomography (CT) scan is indicated. Pupillary or oculomotor dysfunction and other lesions implicating brainstem involvement are better assessed with magnetic resonance imaging (MRI). The presence of a fever dictates systemic evaluation for an infectious process including a lumbar puncture.

Electroencephalography The EEG is often useful in identifying the presence of a metabolic encephalopathy.[46] More recently, quantitative EEG methods have also been demonstrated to be useful in evaluating delirium.[47] Metabolic conditions are typically associated with diffuse slowing of background activity in the theta and delta range in proportion to the severity of cognitive impairment.[48] Triphasic waves are commonly seen in hepatic encephalopathy but are also variably present in uremic and anoxic encephalopathy.[49] Withdrawal states, particularly alcohol withdrawal, are associated with low-voltage, fast (beta) activity, but this pattern is also seen with barbiturate and benzodiazepine use. Focal structural or space-occupying lesions typically exhibit localized slowing or, less often, periodic lateralized epileptiform discharges (PLEDs).

Etiologies

Acute disruption of CNS function can result from a wide variety of etiologic factors, alone or in combination. The etiologic potential of a deliriogenic agent or condition is modified by a number of host and environmental factors. Advanced age, preexisting brain disease, constitutional compromise, absence of orienting stimuli in the environment, and sleep deprivation all may render an individual more susceptible. Within the CNS, lesions producing delirium may be broadly categorized into those with diffuse or multifocal involvement and those with more localized topography. Focal intracranial, multifocal to diffuse intracranial, and systemic etiologies of delrium are shown in Table 43-2.

Systemic The principal systemic etiologies of delirium include metabolic disturbances and the toxic

Table 43-2
Etiologies of delirium

Systemic	*Intracranial*
Metabolic conditions	*Multifocal/diffuse CNS*
Cardiac, pulmonary, renal, hepatic disease	Head trauma
Glucose and electrolyte disturbances	Encephalitis
Systemic inflammatory disorders	Epilepsy (ictal and postictal)
Hypoxia	Hypertensive encephalopathy
Anemia	Vasculitis
Porphyria	Migraine
Infection	Subdural hematoma
Systemic with fever	Neoplasm
Endocrine dysfunction	Cerebrovascular accident (acute phase)
Thyroid, parathyroid, adrenal, pituitary	*Focal CNS*
Nutritional deficiency	Right hemisphere:
Thiamine (Wernicke's encephalopathy)	Temporal (medial)
B_{12}, folate, biotin, niacin	Parietal (inferior)
Protein-calorie malnutrition	Frontal (inferior)
Intoxications	Occipitotemporal (bilateral or left)
Drugs (therapeutic and abused)	Caudate
Alcohol	Thalamus (paramedian)
Withdrawal syndromes	Midbrain (rostral)
Heavy metals, industrial solvents, pesticides	Internal capsule (genu)

effects of exogenous chemicals. Metabolic abnormalities arising from organ failure, endocrinopathies, nutritional deficiencies, infection, hypoxia, and withdrawal states may produce delirium. Dehydration and electrolyte abnormalities, particularly low sodium levels, are common precipitants of delirium in the elderly. Cardiac and respiratory compromise may have a generalized deleterious effect on neuronal aerobic metabolism secondary to hypoxemia. Renal and hepatic failure result in the accumulation of endogenous toxic metabolites. Therapeutic drugs are the most common cause of delirium in the elderly, whether iatrogenic, abused, or taken in standard doses by hypersensitive individuals. Although many drugs at excessive doses may produce a delirium, anticholinergic agents, sedative-hypnotics, and narcotic analgesics are among the most frequent offenders. The relatively high incidence of delirium postopertively is multifactorial and includes the routine use of drugs from one or more of these classes.[50,51]

Multifocal/Diffuse CNS A number of intracranial disorders may present as a delirium. Insults commonly resulting in diffuse or multifocal disturbances in CNS function include head trauma, encephalitides, epilepsy, hypertensive encephalopathy, vasculitis, migraine, subdural hematoma, neoplasms, and the acute phase of cerebrovascular accidents. Postictal confusion is common after partial or generalized tonic-clonic seizures and may persist after repeated seizures despite a normal EEG.[52] Basilar migraine may produce delirium in children and adolescents.[53] In many instances a delirium is present at the onset of a cerebrovascular accident, possibly due to the acute disruption of intrinsic neurovascular regulatory mechanisms.

Focal CNS In specific circumstances, focal cerebrovascular insults may result in a confusional state.[54,55] Delirium states with or without agitation have been observed with acute cerebrovascular lesions in the inferior division of the right middle cerebral artery and in the posterior circulation territories of the basilar and more distal posterior cerebral arteries.[56–64] Radiographic and pathologic studies have implicated lesions in right inferior parietal, right mediobasal temporal, right inferior frontal, unilateral or bilateral lingual, and fusiform gyri, rostral midbrain, and paramedian thalamic nuclei as areas most strongly associated with delirium. A confusional state with or without agitation has also been observed in some patients with infarcts principally involving the caudate nucleus.[65,66] Acute infarctions of the genu of the internal capsule may present with fluctuating attention and psychomotor slowing.[67] Mori and Yamadori have suggested that right hemispheric lesions involving frontostriatal regions are responsible for quiet delirum states, whereas confusional states marked by agitation are more intimately associated with right mediotemporal involvement.[62] These attributions are consistent with the dominant role of the right hemisphere in attentional processes (see Chaps. 25 and 26).

Management

Medical The first and most critical step in the management of delirium is to identify and address the underlying etiology. In many instances, a reversible toxic or metabolic disturbance will become apparent from the history, examination, and routine laboratory studies. A careful history may suggest the possibility of drug intoxication, alcoholism, or environmental toxin exposure. In the elderly, particular attention to alcohol and sedative-hypnotic withdrawal is necessary, as autonomic signs may be minimal or absent. Electrolyte disorders, hepatic and renal dysfunction, serum glucose abnormalities, endocrinopathies, and hypoxia can be identified by appropriate laboratory studies and treated accordingly. Febrile illnesses call for identifying the source of infection and empiric treatment. Although many elderly patients with delirium will have structural abnormalities evident on MRI, brain imaging has the highest yield in patients with focal neurologic signs or in whom trauma is suspected.[42,44] All prescribed medications known to cause delirium, including those taken on an "as needed" basis, should be scrutinized and adjusted if indicated.[68] Medication noncompliance or omission is a common cause of hospital admission in the elderly, warranting special attention to what medications are actually being taken.[69]

Pharmacologic Severe agitation impedes evaluation and treatment and increases the risk of self-harm. A general principle for the pharmacologic management of behavioral symptoms in the delirious patient is to use the lowest effective dose of a drug for the shortest possible time. Parenteral delivery is often necessary due to poor patient cooperation and has the advantage of rapid onset. High-potency neuroleptics such as haloperidol are generally favored due to their lack of cardiac, pulmonary, hypotensive, and anticholinergic side effects.[70] Droperidol can be administered intravenously and has a more rapid onset than haloperidol; it also has more sedative and hypotensive side effects. Both agents can cause extrapyramidal side effects and akathisia, which may be misinterpreted as worsening agitation. A parenteral form of the atypical antipsychotic olanzapine has recently been approved for use in acute agitation and may have advantages over standard neuroleptics.

Benzodiazepines are the drugs of choice for treating withdrawal from alcohol and sedative drugs, when sedation is desirable, or when extrapyramidal signs prohibit the use of neuroleptics.[71] Lorazepam is generally favored over diazepam due to its relatively shorter half-life and lack of active metabolites. Anticholinergic drugs may cause or exacerbate delirium symptoms; preliminary data suggest that treatment with the cholinesterase inhibitor, physostigmine is effective in controlling agitation and reducing complications from anticholinergic delirium.[72,73]

Nonpharmacologic Beyond identifying and correcting a specific etiology of delirium, the mainstay of care is supportive therapy. Careful attention to nutritional status, hydration, electrolyte balance, and sleep needs may ameliorate the risk or symptoms of delirium. Environmental manipulation to avoid sensory deprivation or overload is an important aspect of care, particularly in the intensive care unit setting. Orienting stimuli such as a nightlight or pictures of loved ones may also be helpful. Nursing staff have an important role in the serial assessment of the patient's status and providing reassurance and reorienting information. When such measures are put into effect, the need for sedating medications and restraints can be minimized or eliminated in many instances.

DEMENTIA

Definitions

As with delirium, the first widely used standardized guidelines for the diagnosis of dementia were contained in DSM-III.[15] The two essential diagnostic features of dementia as defined by DSM-III have been preserved in DSM-IV and include (1) an impairment in social and occupational functioning and (2) persistent memory and other cognitive deficits.[8] Specific domains of cognitive disturbance embraced by the definition include aphasia, apraxia, agnosia, and disturbances in executive functions such as planning, organizing, and abstract thinking. Additional requirements include the exclusion of a delirium or inability to better account for the symptoms by an axis I psychiatric disorder. Classification of dementia syndromes depends on evidence linking the clinical process to one or more medical etiologies (e.g., hypothyroidism), cerebrovascular disease (e.g., vascular dementia), or excluding other medical conditions (e.g., Alzheimer's disease).

Cummings and Benson[74] have proposed alternative criteria for dementia, highlighting the clinical and topographic heterogeneity of dementia syndromes. These are contrasted with DSM-IV criteria in Table 43-3. They define dementia as an acquired persistent impairment of intellectual function with compromise in at least three of the following spheres of mental activity: language, memory, visuospatial skills, emotion or personality, and cognition (abstraction, calculation, judgment, executive function, and so forth). In contrast to DSM-IV criteria, this definition allows for the possibility that memory disturbance may not be a presenting feature of a dementing illness, as is not infrequently the case with Pick's disease and other frontotemporal dementias (see Chap. 47). The DSM-IV stipulation of a decline in social or occupational functioning provides a measure of ecologic validity, but neurobiologic sensitivity is lost due to the variable social and functional demands an individual may face. Emphasis placed by DSM-IV on the "cortical" deficits of aphasia, apraxia, and agnosia may further diminish its sensitivity to other common manifestations of dementing illnesses, including apathy, psychosis, and other neuropsychiatric symptoms. Despite these differences, most patients meeting the criteria of Cummings and Benson for dementia would also be identified as demented using the DSM-IV approach.

Etiologic Classification

Degenerative and Nondegenerative The term *dementia* refers to a clinical *syndrome* of acquired

Table 43-3
Comparison of DSM-IV criteria for dementia and Cummings and Benson definition of dementia

DSM-IV	*Cummings and Benson*
Multiple cognitive deficits including: Memory impairment and one or more of the following: Aphasia Apraxia Agnosia Executive dysfunction	Acquired, persistent intellectual impairment involving at least three of the following domains: Language Memory Visuospatial skills Emotion or personality Executive functions
Impairment in social or occupational functioning	
Decline from a previous level of functioning	
Clinical/laboratory evidence relating the disturbance to a general medical condition	
Deficits do not occur exclusively in the course of a delirium	

Source: DSM-IV[4] and Cummings and Benson,[1] with permission.

intellectual disturbances encompassing a large number of *disease* processes. The key features distinguishing delirium and dementia syndromes are the primary attentional deficits associated with the former and the chronicity of the latter. However, these distinctions are more relative than absolute. Most etiologies of delirium may also result in a dementia. Reversibility of either syndrome is principally determined by the specific etiology.

Dementias may result from a wide variety of disorders including degenerative, vascular, traumatic, demyelinating, neoplastic, infectious, inflammatory, hydrocephalic, systemic, and toxic conditions. Etiologies of dementia may be classified into two broad categories, degenerative and nondegenerative. Collectively, degenerative brain diseases are the most common etiology of dementia, with Alzheimer's disease accounting for over one-half of all cases.

Degenerative dementias have a characteristic topography of involvement, although the underlying pathologic alterations are variable. Many degenerative brain diseases are associated with specific histopathologic markers composed of abnormal protein aggregates in affected regions. The pathologic hallmarks of Alzheimer's disease include beta amyloid–containing neuritic plaques and neurofibrillary tangles, which are formed by hyperphosphorylated tau protein cross-linking microtubules. Pathologic staging of Alzheimer's disease is based on the distribution of neurofibrillary tangles, which are typically most abundant in medial temporal, limbic, and neocortical association areas. Parkinson's disease is characterized by the presence of Lewy bodies, composed of alpha-synuclein, in pigmented nuclei of the brainstem. Dementia with Lewy bodies is a nosologically controversial degenerative condition that is distinguished by more widespread alpha synuclein–containing inclusions in limbic areas and cerebral cortex as well as the brainstem. Concomitant pathologic features of Alzheimer's disease (particularly neuritic plaques) are present in a majority of cases.[75–77] Progressive supranuclear palsy and corticobasal ganglionic degeneration are associated with abnormal tau-protein aggregates in cortical and subcortical regions. Frontotemporal dementia refers to a syndrome of selective frontal and anterior temporal lobe atrophy formerly known as "Pick's disease"; the presence of tau-staining Pick bodies is a variable feature.[78] A familial form of frontotemporal dementia is associated with a chromosome 17 mutation in the tau gene. Huntington's disease and spinocerebellar ataxias are autosomal dominant inherited conditions characterized by trinucleotide CAG repeats and regionally selective abnormal protein deposition (huntingtin and ataxins, respectively) in affected areas.

Hereditary forms or predisposing genetic factors have been identified in the majority of degenerative dementias; heritability is an uncommon feature of nondegenerative dementias. Wilson's disease, an autosomal recessive disorder of copper metabolism, and the most common forms of adult leukodystrophy, metachromatic (autosomal recessive) and adrenoleukodystrophy (X-linked), are metabolic-degenerative disorders usually expressed in youth or young adulthood. Similarly, autosomal dominant degenerative conditions, such as Huntington's disease and familial variants of Alzheimer's disease and frontotemporal dementia, tend to have earlier ages of onset. The apolipoprotein E type 4 allelle is a marker for earlier onset in sporadic forms and higher incidence in late-onset familial forms of Alzheimer's disease.[79,80]

Clinical Pathophysiology

Neuroimaging In contrast to the frequently "global" impact of attentional disturbances on intellectual functioning in delirium, dementing processes usually entail selective involvement of CNS areas. The differential nature and topography of involved neuronal systems results in distinctive patterns of intellectual and behavioral disturbances. The pathologic processes in dementia are diverse, ranging from intrinsic molecular ultrastructural or metabolic defects to exogenous neuronal toxins to gross alterations in brain structure. From a clinical perspective, structural imaging techniques such as computed tomography (CT) or magnetic resonance imaging (MRI) will often inform the evaluation and differential diagnosis of disorders with gross structural changes. Pertinent examples include mass lesions, cerebrovascular disease, demyelination, and focal or regional atrophy as seen in Huntington's disease (caudate), progressive supranuclear palsy (midbrain), and frontotemporal dementia (frontal and anterior temporal lobes). In the absence of radiographically demonstrable lesions, the underlying metabolic or cerebral perfusion derangements may be detectable by functional neuroimaging techniques such as single photon emission tomography (SPECT) and positron emission tomography (PET).[81] Such functional brain imaging techniques show promise for providing disease-specific patterns of altered cerebral perfusion (SPECT) or metabolism (PET).[82–84] Burgeoning research applications of PET imaging include preclinical detection of genetically determined dementias and in vivo neurotransmitter receptor ligand-binding techniques.[85–87]

Neurochemistry A broad range of neurochemical lesions may produce or contribute to dementia. Nutritional deficiencies of vitamin B_{12}, niacin, or, in the case of Wernicke's encephalopathy, thiamine typically have systemic and CNS manifestations due to their widespread roles as essential cofactors in intermediate metabolism (see Chap. 51). Disturbances in thyroid and pituitary function may also have pervasive deleterious effects on both peripheral and CNS metabolic pathways. Chronic exposure to alcohol, illicit substances such as cocaine, or heavy metals such as lead, mercury, or aluminum (chronic renal dialysis) may produce characteristic syndromes of dementia. Prolonged episodes of hypoxia and carbon monoxide poisoning may result in dementia syndromes that reflect the inherent vulnerabilities of the hippocampus and globus pallidus, respectively. The basal ganglia are particularly susceptible to injury due to abnormal metabolism or toxic levels of metallic substances. In Wilson's disease, selective deposition of unbound copper in the putamen occurs due to a deficiency in the copper transport protein, ceruloplasmin. Hallervorden-Spatz disease, idiopathic basal ganglia calcification (Fahr's disease), and manganese encephalopathy are associated with abnormal basal ganglia accumulations of iron, ferrocalcific aggregates, and manganese, respectively. Deficiency of the myelin synthetic enzyme arylsulfatase A underlies the dysmyelinating dementia of metachromatic leukodystrophy.[1] In many cases, etiologically based treatments of dementing disorders produced by specific neurochemical or biochemical alterations effect a reversal, or retard the progression of the dementia.

Neurochemical deficits typically have a less well defined etiologic role in most degenerative dementias. However, a variety of central neurotransmitter abnormalities may contribute to the clinical manifestations of many degenerative conditions. There are two general types of central neurotransmitter systems: (1) local or intrinsic neurotransmitters, such as gamma-aminobutyric acid (GABA) and glutamate, and (2) projection or extrinsic neurotransmitters, including acetylcholine, dopamine, serotonin, and norepinephrine.[88]

GABA and glutamate are the principal inhibitory and excitatory neurotransmitters of the CNS, respectively, and generally mediate the transfer of neuronal information along discrete channels in local cortical-cortical and cortical-subcortical circuits. The localized topography and channel specificity of these amino acid neurotransmitters reflect their integral role in neocortically based intellectual functions but render them less susceptible to pharmacologic manipulation.

Projection neurotransmitter systems arise from subcortical and brainstem nuclei and primarily exert a modulatory influence on widely distributed neuronal networks.[88,89] Cholinergic projections from the brainstem reticular system (lateral dorsal tegmentum and pedunculopontine nucleus) terminate in nonspecific thalamic nuclei and basal forebrain regions, activating cortical arousal and attentional mechanisms. Basal forebrain cholinergic nuclei have diffuse projections to neocortical and limbic areas such as the amygdala and hippocampus; disruption of these cholinergic pathways is implicated in the pathogenesis of memory and other intellectual disturbances seen in Alzheimer's disease.

Dopaminergic projections from the substantia nigra to the putamen are disrupted in Parkinson's disease, producing the characteristic motor disturbances of tremor, rigidity, and bradykinesia. Dopaminergic efferents from the ventral tegmental area to the nucleus accumbens, septal area, amygdala (mesolimbic pathway), and anterior cingulate, medial temporal, and frontal lobe regions (mesocortical pathway) are affiliated with cognitive functioning and neuropsychiatric disturbances such as depression, mania, and psychosis.[90,91]

Locus ceruleus is the origin of two primary ascending noradrenergic projections—a dorsal pathway arising from midbrain nuclei and terminating in neocortical, thalamic, basal forebrain, and medial temporal regions and a ventral pathway arising from lower brainstem areas that project to the hypothalamus and midbrain reticular nuclei. These noradrenergic projections are thought to influence arousal, selective attention, and anxiety states.[89,92]

Serotoninergic projections arise from median and paramedian raphe nuclei in the brainstem and are widely distributed throughout the cerebral hemispheres. Serotonin principally acts as an inhibitor of diffuse neuronal systems; anxiety, disinhibition, and aggression are associated with altered serotonergic function.[92,93]

Together, these diffusely projecting neurotransmitter systems regulate the excitatory and inhibitory tone of multiple, discrete neural circuits underlying specific domains of intellectual function. Regional variations in receptor density and receptor subtypes superimpose a response topography on these "diffuse" systems. Their generally indirect influence on cognition is paralleled by their integrated role in the modulation of behavioral states. Selective disturbances in this regulatory mosaic may produce characteristic patterns of neuropsychological and neuropsychiatric symptoms.

Clinical Features

Cortical and Subcortical Syndromes Dementia has many different etiologies, each with its own range of symptoms. In addition, a multitude of individual-specific factors— including genetic predisposition, education, gender differences, age-related changes, preexisting brain disease, environmental exposures, and medical and psychiatric comorbidity— may impinge on the expression of a dementing illness. Despite the etiologic and individual heterogeneity of dementing illnesses, two basic patterns of neurobehavioral features have been observed and named according to the predominant neuroanatomic regions involved.[1]

One syndromic constellation includes *cortical* dementias such as Alzheimer's disease. Cerebral cortical regions are the primary locus of involvement in Alzheimer's disease, although restricted pathologic alterations in subcortical regions are also present. *Subcortical* dementias—including extrapyramidal disorders such as Parkinson's disease, Huntington's disease, progressive supranuclear palsy, subcortical vascular disease, white matter diseases, and hydrocephalus— are distinguished by clinical symptoms principally referable to involvement of basal ganglia, limbic-related thalamic nuclei, and portions of the brainstem. From a functional anatomic perspective, striatum, globus pallidus, anterior and medial thalamus, and substantia nigral portion of the midbrain are interconnected with prefrontal cortical regions in a series of circuits with unique neurobehavioral affiliations.[94,95] Similar clinical deficits may result from lesions anywhere in these circuits or reflect circuit dysfunction at both cortical and subcortical levels, as in frontotemporal dementia. A third category, *mixed,* includes conditions such as dementia with Lewy bodies, corticobasal ganglionic degeneration, some vascular dementias, and slow virus infections, which typically produce symptoms attributable to dysfunction of both cortical and subcortical structures.

From a clinical viewpoint, distinguishing cortical and subcortical patterns of signs and symptoms facilitates a systematic approach to differential diagnosis. A classification of dementia based on degenerative versus nondegenerative etiology and cortical-subcortical typography is presented in Table 43-4.

The clinical features of cortical and subcortical dementias arise from differential involvement of neural components underlying specific cognitive and behavioral functions. The neuropsychological and neurobehavioral concomitants of cortical dementias generally reflect the functional specificity of pathologically disturbed neocortical regions. Cerebral cortex can be viewed as consisting of functionally specialized domains that are linked together in serial and parallel modular networks for information processing.[89] Structural or functional disturbances in these cortical networks may produce deficits in instrumental intellectual skills such as language, visuospatial functions, and mathematical abilities. Elementary sensory and motor functioning is typically preserved. Subcortical dementias, in contrast, are characterized by slowing

Table 43-4
Etiologic classification of dementias based on cortical and subcortical features

Degenerative	*Nondegenerative*
Cortical Dementias	
Alzheimer's disease	Multiple cortical infarcts
	Angular gyrus syndrome
Subcortical Dementias	
Extrapyramidal syndromes:	Vascular dementias:
Parkinson's disease	Binswanger's disease
Progressive supranuclear palsy	Lacunar state
Striatonigral degeneration	Infectious dementia:
Shy-Drager syndrome	HIV dementia
Spinocerebellar degeneration	Whipples disease
Huntington's disease	Neurosyphilis
Wilson's disease	Demyelinating dementia:
Neuroacanthocytosis	Multiple sclerosis
Hallervorden-Spatz	Miscellaneous:
Progressive subcortical gliosis	Symptomatic hydrocephalus
Idiopathic basal ganglia calcification	Dementia syndrome of depression
Mixed Cortical/Subcortical Dementias	
Frontotemporal dementia (includes motor neuron disease with dementia)	Multiple cerebral infarctions
	Toxic/metabolic disorders:
Dementia with Lewy bodies	Deficiencies (B_{12}, niacin, etc.)
Corticobasal ganglionic degeneration	Endocrinopathies (thyroid, etc.)
Leukodystrophies:	Chronic alcohol/drug abuse
Metachromatic leukodystrophy	Industrial/environmental toxins
Adrenoleukodystrophy	Posttraumatic encephalopathy
	Vasculitides (systemic and CNS)
Prion (slow virus) diseases	
Schizophrenia (developmental)	

Table 43-5
Clinical features of cortical and subcortial dementias and delirium

Feature	*Cortical dementia*	*Subcortical dementia*	*Delirium*
Onset	Insidious	Insidious	Sudden
Duration	Months to years	Months to years	Hours to days
Course	Progressive	Progressive or constant	Fluctuating
Attention	Normal	Normal (slow response time)	Fluctuating
Speech	Normal	Hypophonic, dysarthric, mute	Slurred, incoherent
Language	Aphasic	Normal or anomic	Anomia, dysgraphia
Memory	Learning deficit (AD)	Retrieval deficit	Encoding deficit
Cognition	Acalculia, concrete (AD)	Slow, dilapidated	Disorganized
Awareness	Impaired	Usually preserved	Impaired
Demeanor	Unconcerned, disinhibited	Apathetic, abulic	Apathetic, agitated
Psychosis	May be present	May be present	Often florid
Motor signs	None	Tremor, chorea, rigidity, dystonia	Tremor, asterixis
EEG	Mild diffuse slowing	Normal or mild slowing (diffuse or focal)	Moderate to severe diffuse slowing

and dilapidation of executive functions, affective and personality disturbances, forgetfulness, and movement disorders.[96,97] These features are attributable to disruption of one or more of the structures participating in the frontal-subcortical circuits, the nodes of which are less functionally specialized than neocortical neural regions. Some features of subcortical dementias are reminiscent of delirium. A comparison between the features of cortical and subcortical dementias and their relationship to delirium are presented in Table 43-5.

Differential Diagnosis

Detailed information pertaining to the major classes of dementing illnesses is provided in subsequent chapters. As a prelude, salient examples of differential diagnosis related to cortical, subcortical, and mixed dementias are highlighted here. Table 43-6 presents a summary of clinicopathoanatomic profiles for the major causes of degenerative and other dementias. Attention to concomitant features such as extrapyramidal and focal or lateralizing neurologic signs complements a systematic approach to the differential diagnosis of dementia syndromes based on the cortical-subcortical organizing principle. Identifying reversible or treatable etiologies of dementia is of paramount concern.

The Quality Standards Committee of the American Academy of Neurology recently published an evidence-based review of guidelines for diagnosing dementia.[98] Research diagnostic criteria for Alzheimer's disease and Creutzfeldt-Jakob disease were endorsed as being acceptably valid and reliable, whereas criteria for diagnosing dementia with Lewy bodies, vascular dementia, and frontotemporal dementia, although potentially useful in clinical practice, were found to be lacking. Other recommendations included structural brain imaging in the initial evaluation of dementia and routine screening for depression, hypothyroidism, and vitamin B_{12} deficiency. Functional brain imaging and genetic testing were not endorsed for routine use due to insufficient data.

Cortical Dementia Alzheimer's disease is the prototype cortical dementia syndrome. Deficits in short-term memory, visuospatial functions, naming, and verbal fluency are the common initial manifestations of Alzheimer's disease. Apathetic indifference, diminished insight or lack of awareness of these deficits, and poor abstract thinking frequently accompany the core neuropsychological deficits. Insidious onset is the rule, although the initial clinical symptoms may be precipitated by a surgical procedure, infection, or minor head injury. Focal neurologic signs are conspicuously absent early in the course; later, motor dysfunction, myoclonus, and seizures may develop.

The principal distinguishing features of Alzheimer's disease are the nature of the memory

Table 43-6
Differential diagnostic profiles of clinicopathoanatomic features of dementia

Etiology	*Clinical features*	*Pathoanatomic correlates*
Cortical dementias:		
Alzheimer's disease	Memory deficit (learning)	Hippocampus, nucleus basalis (cholinergic)
	Aphasia, apraxia, agnosia	Temporal and parietal neocortex
	Apathy/indifference	Anterior cingulate, parietal neocortex
Mixed dementias:		
Frontotemporal dementia	Memory deficit (retrieval)	Dorsolateral prefrontal cortex
	Speech/language stereotypies	Frontal/temporal neocortex
	Disinhibition	Orbitofrontal cortex
	Hyperorality (Kluver-Bucy)	Amygdala/anterior temporal cortex
Dementia with Lewy bodies	Memory deficit (mixed)	Nucleus basalis, hippocampal formation
	Extrapyramidal signs	Substantia nigra (dopamine)
	Fluctuating attentional deficits	Pedunculopontine nucleus (cholinergic)?
	Visual hallucinations, delusions	Neocortex (serotonin/cholinergic imbalance)?
Corticobasal ganglionic degeneration	Unilateral limb signs (dystonia, clumsiness, myoclonus)	Subthalamic nucleus, thalamus, globus pallidus
	Cortical sensory loss, apraxia, alien hand phenomena	Parietal and frontal neocortex (asymmetrical)
	Rigidity	Substantia nigra (dopamine)
	Supranuclear gaze palsy (late)	Midbrain
Subcortical dementias:		
Progressive supranuclear palsy	Supranuclear gaze palsy	Midbrain
	Dysarthria/dysphagia	Bulbar cranial nerves
	Gait/balance disturbances, axial rigidity	Globus pallidus, subthalamic nucleus, substantia nigra
	Pseudobulbar palsy	Brainstem, prefrontal cortex
Parkinson's disease	Memory deficit (retrieval)	Caudate; nucleus basalis (cholinergic)
	Executive dysfunction	Caudate nucleus
	Tremor, rigidity, bradykinesia	Substantia nigra, putamen (dopamine)
Huntington's disease	Memory deficit (retrieval)	Caudate nucleus
	Executive dysfunction	Caudate nucleus
	Choreiform movements	Putamen, subthalamic nucleus, globus pallidum
Symptomatic hydrocephalus	Gait disturbance	Midline subcortical structures and connections
	Memory deficit (retrieval)	
	Executive dysfunction	
	Incontinence	
Dementia syndrome of depression	Memory deficit (retrieval)	Subcortical white or gray matter
	Impaired concentration/attention	
	Executive dysfunction	
	Parkinsonian features (except tremor)	
Vascular dementia (multiple lacunar strokes or Binswanger's disease)	Memory deficit (retrieval)	Thalamic or basal ganglia—frontal disconnection
	Executive dysfunction	
	Focal or asymmetrical elementary neurologic signs	Location-dependent

deficits, the presence of other intellectual disturbances, and the relative absence of elementary neurologic signs. Primary attentional functions are preserved in Alzheimer's disease, distinguishing it from toxic and other systemic etiologies of delirium. More isolated disturbances in language or visuospatial functions may reflect cerebrovascular insults or focal cortical degenerative syndromes. The angular gyrus syndrome is a symptom complex of fluent aphasia, constructional disturbances, and elements of the Gerstmann syndrome (acalculia, finger agnosia, dysgraphia, and right-left disorientation).[99] It may result from left hemispheric cerebrovascular lesions in the distribution of the posterior branches of the middle cerebral artery and is distinguished from Alzheimer's disease by its abrupt onset and the relative absence of nonverbal memory deficits. Focal degenerative conditions such as primary progressive aphasia (a form of frontotemporal dementia) and corticobasal ganglionic degeneration are also characterized by asymmetrical hemispheric involvement and relatively preserved memory— but, as with Alzheimer's disease, these have a more insidious onset and progressive course.[100–102] In corticobasal ganglionic degeneration, unilateral sensory and motor disturbances including apraxia, astereognosis, dystonia, myoclonus, and the alien hand syndrome are often present.

Subcortical Dementias Extrapyramidal system involvement is a common feature of subcortical dementias. Parkinsonian features concurrent with a dementia syndrome characterized by retrieval memory deficits, cognitive slowing, and executive dysfunction have a wide differential diagnosis (see Chap. 48). Parkinson's disease, progressive supranuclear palsy, multiple system atrophies, the rigid form of Huntington's disease, and many secondary basal ganglia disorders produce parkinsonism with dementia. Most patients with idiopathic Parkinson's disease exhibit some degree of intellectual impairment; 30 to 40 percent will have deficits severe enough to meet criteria for dementia.[103] The subcortical dementia of Parkinson's disease and progressive supranuclear palsy exhibit overlapping executive deficits[104,105] and are both associated with reductions in frontal lobe metabolism or blood flow.[106,107] Progressive supranuclear palsy is principally distinguished by the early features of gait imbalance and bulbar symptoms (dysarthria and pseudobulbar affect), axial rigidity, and a supranuclear vertical gaze palsy.[108]

Communicating or normal-pressure hydrocephalus is an uncommon but potentially reversible syndrome produced by impaired egress of cerebrospinal fluid via arachnoid granulations from the intracranial compartment (see Chap. 53). A subcortical dementia syndrome of apathy, psychomotor slowing, retrieval memory deficits, and executive dysfunction may develop over a period of months and is typically preceded by a characteristic "magnetic" or "apraxic" gait.[109] Incontinence generally appears later if at all. The rapidity of decline and prominent gait and balance disturbances help distinguish normal-pressure hydrocephalus from Parkinson's disease and other extrapyramidal syndromes. CT or MRI often shows panventricular enlargement, particularly in the anterior ventricular regions, out of proportion to the degree of cortical gyral atrophy. However, these radiographic findings lack absolute specificity, emphasizing the diagnostic primacy of clinical features. Radionuclide cisternography may lend support to the diagnosis.

Depression may influence the symptomatic expression of dementia or may induce cognitive impairment on its own (dementia syndrome of depression). About 40 percent of Parkinson's disease patients exhibit significant depressive symptoms, which are often associated with memory impairment relative to Parkinson's disease patients without depression.[110,111] Depression is also common in Huntington's disease, vascular dementia, and other subcortical syndromes. The dementia syndrome of depression is a reversible dementia most commonly seen in elderly patients with a history of severe or psychotic depression. Impaired attention and concentration, forgetfulness, psychomotor slowing, decreased motivation, and impaired ability to grasp the meaning of situations are characteristic features.[112,113]

Vascular dementia is a heterogenous syndrome with multiple clinical presentations depending on lesion type and location (see Chap. 49).[114,115] Whereas infarctions in the territory of large cerebral vessels produce characteristic syndromes of cortically based higher intellectual functions, diffuse or multifocal small vessel ischemic disease affecting periventricular white matter or basal ganglia and thalamic nuclei results in a classic subcortical dementia syndrome. Dementia arising from multiple lacunar infarcts is associated with a preponderance of lesion sites in the frontal lobe white matter, implicating disruption of frontal-subcortical circuit pathways as the relevant pathologic mechanism.[116] More diffuse involvement of subcortical white matter secondary to small vessel ischemia (Binswanger's disease) also functionally disconnects cortical and subcortical regions. Hypertension and other risk factors for vascular disease are commonly present. Correlation of radiographically evident lesions with relevant historical and clinical data is essential to diagnosing vascular dementia, which occurs more commonly in conjunction with Alzheimer's disease than in isolation.

Huntington's disease is a hyperkinetic extrapyramidal syndrome with choreiform movements and a subcortical dementia. The genetic defect in Huntington's disease is an autosomal dominant trinucleotide repeat mutation on chromosome four.[117] Severe atrophy of the caudate nuclei is the pathologic feature accompanying the frequently prominent behavioral and mood disturbances, including depression, irritability, and impulsivity.

Human immunodeficiency virus (HIV) infection is the most common cause of infectious dementia (see Chap. 50). Typical manifestations reflect subcortical dysfunction—psychomotor slowing, memory and concentration impairment, and apathy—due to direct CNS invasion of the virus.[118] Gait, motor, and sensory disturbances may be present due to a vacuolizing myelopathy. Opportunistic infections such as toxoplasmosis and progressive multifocal leukoencephalopathy may produce superimposed deficits.

Mixed Cortical and Subcortical Dementias

Dementia with Lewy bodies comprises one or more clinical syndromes with overlapping features of Alzheimer's disease and Parkinson's disease.[75–77] A characteristic clinical profile including fluctuating cognitive impairments, prominent psychiatric features (hallucinations, delusions, and depression), gait and balance difficulties, and unexplained loss of consciousness has been suggested, although these criteria appear to lack diagnostic sensitivity. Cognitive disturbances may reflect more severe deficits in attention, verbal fluency, and visuospatial processing compared to "pure" Alzheimer's disease.[77] Extrapyramidal motor signs are frequently but not invariably present, and the clinical picture may be dominated by neuropsychiatric symptoms, particularly florid visual hallucinations. Whereas Parkinson's disease is characterized by Lewy bodies primarily affecting the midbrain substantia nigra and other brainstem nuclei (e.g., locus ceruleus and raphe nuclei), the additional presence of Lewy bodies in limbic (hippocampus and amygdala), paralimbic (anterior cingulate), and neocortical regions is the pathologic hallmark of dementia with Lewy bodies. Pathologic features of Alzheimer's disease, most notably amyloid plaques, are present in a majority of individuals with dementia with Lewy bodies, although neurofibrillary tangles are typically sparse or absent.[75] Abundant clinical and pathologic overlap among dementia with Lewy bodies, Alzheimer's disease, and Parkinson's disease underlies their controversial nosologic relationship.[119]

Frontotemporal dementia encompasses a dementia syndrome with variable clinical and pathologic features involving selective frontal and anterior temporal degeneration (see Chap. 47). The core features of frontotemporal dementia are typically neuropsychiatric and may include behavioral disinhibition, apathy, inappropriate behavior, lack of social awareness, distractibility, impulsivity, and stereotyped or perseverative behaviors.[78,101] Behavior and personality changes often appear many years before the appearance of frank neuropsychological deficits.[82] Memory function, calculations, and visuospatial skills are preserved early in the course, contrasting with the initial manifestations of Alzheimer's disease. Two subtypes of frontotemporal dementia that primarily affect language functions have been identified.[101] Primary progressive aphasia involves primary expressive language disturbances akin to a transcortical motor aphasia, with relatively preserved general cognitive functions.[100] Semantic dementia comprises a syndrome of fluent speech, word-finding difficulty, impaired word comprehension, and visual associative agnosia. Pathologic involvement in frontotemporal dementia syndromes is concentrated in frontal and anterior temporal lobes and is typically bilateral, although asymmetrical involvement of the left hemisphere is seen in primary progressive aphasia. Lobar or "knife edge" atrophy may be demonstrable on MRI imaging, particularly in the midsagittal plane.[120] Gliosis and regional atrophy are characteristic pathologic features; the presence of Pick bodies and swollen neurons is variable. Clinical and pathologic features of frontotemporal dementia may occur in the setting of motor neuron disease, with additional degenerative changes in lower brainstem and spinal cord motor neurons.

Treatment and Management of Dementia

Pharmacologic Therapy The growing prevalence of Alzheimer's disease has motivated intensive efforts to develop rational therapies to ameliorate clinical symptoms, slow disease progression, and ultimately prevent clinical expression of the disease. To date, two types of symptomatic treatments based on modulating CNS transmitter function have been shown to be beneficial in treating Alzheimer's disease. Several acetylcholinesterase-inhibitor agents—including tacrine, donepezil, rivastigmine, and galantamine—have been shown in large-scale, placebo-controlled trials to slow the progression of the decline in cognitive and behavioral function.[121] Although all of these agents are approved for treating mild to moderate Alzheimer's disease, their use for other indications is being investigated.[122] One large-scale controlled study of rivastigmine in dementia with Lewy bodies showed a beneficial impact on psychotic and other neuropsychiatric symptoms as well as a computer-based measure of attention.[123] Psychotic and agitated behaviors in Alzheimer's disease patients have also been shown to benefit from atypical antipsychotic drugs risperidone and olanzapine.[124–126] Vitamin E at a dose of 1000 international units twice a day and the monoamine oxidase-inhibitor selegilene at a dose of 5 mg twice in the morning were both shown in one large, multicenter controlled trial to slow disease progression in moderate Alzheimer's disease.[127] Vitamin E was more beneficial than selegilene and has a more favorable cost and side-effect profile, which supports its widespread use in treating Alzheimer's disease patients.[122] Interestingly, the combination of vitamin E and selegilene produced less benefit than either agent alone. Large-scale placebo-controlled studies of estrogen in women with Alzheimer's disease have not shown benefit in altering disease course, but epidemiologic studies suggest that estrogen replacement therapy in postmenopausal women may reduce the risk of developing Alzheimer's disease by up to 50 percent.[128–130] Anti-inflammatory agents also have not been demonstrated to alter the progression of Alzheimer's disease, but may reduce disease risk in asymptomatic individuals.[131–133] Preliminary studies with disease-modifying agents, such as an antiamyloid vaccine and gamma secretase-inhibitors, are currently underway.

Therapeutic strategies in cerebrovascular disease are aimed at both limiting the acute damage of cerebral ischemia and secondary prevention. Excitotoxic mechanisms have been widely implicated in neuronal damage produced by acute ischemia and other neurologic conditions and may prove amenable to intervention.[134] The progression of vascular dementia may be impeded by aggressive control of risk factors such as hypertension and by the use of platelet antiaggregating agents such as aspirin and antiplatelet agents. Preliminary data suggest that cholinesterase-inhibitor agents may be beneficial in mixed Alzheimer's disease and vascular dementia.

Transient improvement in the symptoms of hydrocephalic dementia (particularly gait) following lumbar puncture helps to confirm the diagnosis and may have prognostic significance. The response to shunting in normal-pressure hydrocephalus is highly variable, but this measure is usually beneficial if there is an identifiable cause and symptom duration has been brief.[135,136]

Toxic and metabolic dementias often respond to removal of the offending agent or reversal of the metabolic abnormality. Cognitive symptoms in depression may respond at least partially to antidepressant therapy, with selective serotonin reuptake inhibitors (SSRIs) being the class of drugs most commonly used. Residual cognitive symptoms may indicate the presence of an underlying dementia syndrome. Steroid and other immunosuppressive agents may ameliorate the cognitive and neuropsychiatric disturbances associated with vasculitis and other CNS inflammatory disorders. The dementia and movement disorders of Wilson's disease may be prevented or reversed with penicillamine treatment. Evacuation of subdural hematomas and surgical resection of CNS neoplasms produce variable improvement, depending on the size, location, and nature of the mass lesion.

Nonpharmacologic Therapy The overarching goal of all therapeutic interventions for dementia is to optimize adaptive functioning and preserve quality of life. Although these therapeutic aims need to be individualized, there are several general aspects of care that should be addressed proactively and revisited on an ongoing basis. These include recommendations for a structured, secure, and safe environment; routinizing tasks such as medication tracking and dispensation; encouraging participation in constructive activities and social interaction; and informing caregivers of educational and supportive resources. Other aspects of comprehensive management include addressing concurrent medical conditions and remediable physical limitations (e.g., sensory impairment), promoting adequate nutrition and sleep, and improving or maintaining mobility through prescriptions for regular exercise and physical therapy. Whether employed as preventative measures, a first-line approach to overt symptoms, or in conjunction with symptomatic pharmacologic treatments, nonpharmacologic behavioral and environmental manipulations play an integral role in the comprehensive management of dementia syndromes.

Conclusions and Future Directions

Delirium and dementia respectively denote acute and chronic disorders of brain function producing cognitive impairment. They are common nemeses of aging but differ in their temporal course and the nature of the core neuropsychological deficit—attention in the case of delirium and memory disturbance in dementia. The clinical distinction between attentional and memory dysfunction has important neuroanatomic and etiologic implications. Attention forms the substrate of memory and is subserved by a hierarchical network linking brainstem, thalamic, basal forebrain, and neocortical areas. The broadly distributed nature of pathways subserving attentional function renders it susceptible to a wide variety of toxic and metabolic insults as well as strategically located lesions, particularly those involving the right cerebral hemisphere. Dementia syndromes may also be produced by a large number of brain diseases. Degenerative dementing illnesses have selective and characteristic topographies of pathologic involvement and associated lesions that reflect abnormal protein accumulation. Memory processes that are compromised in dementia are mediated by distributed cortical and subcortical networks, and two general clinical patterns of dementia can be distinguished on the basis of a cortical or subcortical locus of primary involvement. Cortical dementias such as Alzheimer's disease produce impaired learning of new information and other deficits in intellectual domains associated with dysfunction of cortically based neural networks. Retrieval memory deficits characterize the subcortical dementia syndrome, which is associated with less discretely localized executive and neuropsychiatric disturbances. The subcortical dementia syndrome results from lesions that disrupt the integrity of functional circuits linking prefrontal, basal ganglia, and thalamic areas. Distinguishing subcortical and cortical syndromes of dementia facilitates the etiologic differential diagnosis of dementing disorders and provides insight into functional clinicopathologic relationships. Improved accuracy in the diagnosis of degenerative and other dementias will derive from a more precise understanding of how genetic determinants influence the appearance of pathologic disturbances in brain function and lead to the associated clinical manifestations. Integrated knowledge of these relationships provides a basis for unraveling the mechanisms of dementing brain diseases and may help identify therapeutic targets to reverse or prevent these disorders.

REFERENCES

1. Cummings JL, Benson DF: *Dementia: A Clinical Approach,* 2d ed. Boston: Heinemann-Butterworths, 1992.
2. Max W: The economic impact of Alzheimer's disease. *Neurology* 43(Suppl 4):S6–S10, 1993.
3. Lipowski ZJ: *Delirium: Acute Confusional States.* New York: Oxford Univerity Press, 1990.
4. Francis J: Delirium in older patients. *J Am Geriatr Soc* 40:829–838, 1992.
5. Inouye SK: The dilemma of delirium: Clinical and research controversies regarding diagnosis and evaluation of delirium in hospitalized elderly medical patients. *Am J Med* 97:278–288, 1994.
6. Rockwood K, Cosway S, Stolee P, et al: Increasing the recognition of delirium in elderly patients. *J Am Geriatr Soc* 42:252–256, 1994.
7. Francis J, Hilko E, Kapoor W: Delirium and prospective payment: The economic impact of acute confusion. *J Am Geriatr Soc* 41:SA9, 1993.
8. *Diagnostic and Statistical Manual of Mental Disorders,* 4th ed. Washington, DC: American Psychiatric Association, 1994.

9. Geschwind N: Disorders of attention: A new frontier in neuropsychology. *Philos Trans R Soc Lond [Biol]* 298:173–185, 1982.
10. Liston EH: Delirium in the aged. *Psychiatr Clin North Am* 5:49–66, 1982.
11. Adams RD, Victor M: *Principles of Neurology,* 4th ed. New York: McGraw-Hill, 1989.
12. Liptzin B, Levkoff SE, Cleary PD, et al: An empiric study of diagnostic criteria for delirium. *Am J Psychiatry* 148:454–457, 1991.
13. Trzepacz P, Baker RW, Greenhouse J: A simple rating scale for delirium. *Psychiatry Res* 23:89–97, 1988.
14. Inouye SK, van Dyck CH, Alessi CA, et al: Clarifying confusion: The confusion assessment method: A new method for detection of delirium. *Ann Intern Med* 113:941–948, 1990.
15. *Diagnostic and Statistical Manual of Mental Disorders,* 3d ed. Washington, DC: American Psychiatric Association, 1980.
16. *Diagnostic and Statistical Manual of Mental Disorders,* 3d ed rev. Washington, DC: American Psychiatric Association, 1987.
17. Sunderland T, Tariot P, Cohen RM, et al: Anticholinergic sensitivity in patients with dementia of the Alzheimer type and age-matched controls. *Arch Gen Psychiatry* 44:418–426, 1987.
18. Mesulam M-M: Attention, confusional states, and neglect, in Mesulam M-M (ed): *Principles of Behavioral Neurology.* Philadelphia: Davis, 1985, pp 125–168.
19. Strub RL, Black FW: *The Mental Status Examination in Neurology,* 3d ed. Philadelphia: Davis, 1993.
20. Pompei P, Foreman M, Cassel CK, et al: Detecting delirium among hospitalized older patients. *Arch Intern Med* 155:301–307, 1995.
21. Cummings JL: *Clinical Neuropsychiatry.* Orlando, FL: Grune & Stratton, 1985.
22. Weinstein EA, Kahn RL: Nonaphasic misnaming (paraphasia) in organic brain disease. *Arch Neurol Psychiatry* 67:72–79, 1952.
23. Cummings J, Hebben NA, Obler L, Leonard P: Nonaphasic misnaming and other neurobehavioral features of an unusual toxic encephalopathy. *Cortex* 16:316–323, 1980.
24. Wallesch CW, Hundsalz A: Language function in delirium: A comparison of single word processing in acute confusional states and probable Alzheimer's disease. *Brain Lang* 46:592–606, 1994.
25. Chedru F, Geschwind N: Writing disturbances in acute confusional states. *Neuropsychologia* 10:343–353, 1972.
26. Mercer B, Wagner W, Gardner H, et al: A study of confabulation. *Arch Neurol* 34:429–433, 1977.
27. Stuss DT, Alexander MP, Lieberman A, Levine H: An extraordinary form of confabulation. *Neurology* 28:1166–1172, 1978.
28. Cummings JL: Organic delusions: phenomenology, anatomic correlations, and review. *Br J Psychiatry* 46:184–197, 1985.
29. Alexander MP, Stuss DT, Benson DF: Capgras syndrome: A reduplicative phenomenon. *Neurology* 29:334–339, 1979.
30. Ross CA, Peyser CE, Shapiro I, et al: Phenomenologic and etiologic subtypes. *Int Psychogeriatr* 3:135–147, 1991.
31. Liptzin B, Levkoff SE: An empirical study of delirium subtypes. *Br J Psychiatry* 161:843–845, 1992.
32. Jankovic J, Fahn S: Physiologic and pathologic tremors. *Ann Intern Med* 93:460–465, 1980.
33. Adams RD, Foley JM: The neurological changes in the more common types of liver disease. *Trans Am Neurol Assoc* 74:217–219, 1949.
34. Young RR, Shahani BT: Asterixis: One type of negative myoclonus, in Fahn S, Marsden CD, Van Woert M (eds): *Advances in Neurology: Myoclonus.* New York: Raven Press, 1986, vol 43, pp 137–156.
35. Taylor MA: Catatonia: A review of a behavioral neurologic syndrome. *Neuropsychiatry Neuropsychol Behav Neurol* 3:48–72, 1990.
36. Henry WD, Mann AM: Diagnosis and treatment of delirium. *Can Med Assoc J* 93:1156–1166, 1965.
37. Erkinjuntti T, Wikstrom J, Palo J, et al: Dementia among medical inpatients: Evaluation of 2000 consecutive admissions. *Arch Intern Med* 146:1923–1926, 1986.
38. Rockwood K: Acute confusion in elderly medical patients. *J Am Geriatr Soc* 37:150–154, 1989.
39. Francis J, Martin D, Kapoor WN: A prospective study of delirium in the elderly. *JAMA* 263:1097–1101, 1990.
40. Schor JD, Levkoff SE, Lipsitz LA, et al: Risk factors for delirium in hospitalized elderly. *JAMA* 267:827–831, 1992.
41. Gustafson Y, Berggren D, Brannstrom B, et al: Acute confusional states in elderly patients treated for femoral neck fractures. *J Am Geriatr Soc* 36:525–530, 1988.
42. Francis J, Kapoor W. Prognosis after hospital discharge of older medical patients with delirium. *J Am Geriatr Soc* 40:601–606, 1992.
43. Levkoff SE, Evans DA, Liptzin B, et al: Delirium: The occurrence and persistence of symptoms among elderly hospitalized patients. *Arch Intern Med* 152:334–340, 1992.

44. Beresin EV: Delirium in the elderly. *J Geriatr Psychiatr Neurol* 1:127–143, 1988.
45. Katz IR, Curyto KJ, TenHave T, et al: Validating the diagnosis of delirium and evaluating its association with deterioration over a one-year period. *Am J Geriatr Psychiatry* 9:148–159, 2001.
46. Brenner RP: Utility of EEG in delirium: Past views and current practice. *Int Psychogeriatr* 3:211–229, 1991.
47. Leuchter AF, Jacobsen SA: Quantitative measurement of brain electrical activity in delirium. *Int Psychogeriatr* 3:231–247, 1991.
48. Engel GL, Romano J: Delirium, a syndrome of cerebral insufficiency. *J Chronic Dis* 9:260–277, 1959.
49. Brenner RP: The electroencephalogram in altered states of consciousness. *Neurol Clin* 3:615–631, 1985.
50. Tune L, Carr S, Cooper TC, et al: Association of anticholinergic activity of prescribed medications with postoperative delirium. *J Neuropsychiatry Clin Neurosci* 5:208–210, 1993.
51. Marcantonio ER, Juarez G, Goldman L, et al: The relationship of postoperative delirium with psychoactive medications. *JAMA* 272:1518–1522, 1994.
52. Engel J Jr: *Seizures and Epilepsy.* Philadelphia: Davis, 1989.
53. Bickerstaff ER: Impairment of consciousness in migraine. *Lancet* 2:1057–1059, 1961.
54. Krasuki JS, Gaviria M: Neuropsychiatric sequelae of ischemic cerebrovascular disease: Clinical and neuroanatomic correlates and implications for the concept of dementia. *Neurol Res* 16:241–250, 1994.
55. Trzepacz PT: The neuropathogenesis of delirium: a need to focus our research. *Psychosomatics* 35:374–391, 1994.
56. Horenstein S, Chamberlain W, Conomy J: Infarction of the fusiform and calcarine regions: Agitated delirium and hemianopia. *Trans Am Neurol Assoc* 92:85–88, 1967.
57. Medina JL, Rubino FA, Ross E: Agitated delirium caused by infarctions of the hippocampal formation and fusiform and lingual gyri: A case report. *Neurology* 24:1181–1183, 1974.
58. Mesulam M-M, Waxman SG, Geschwind N, Sabin TD: Acute confusional states with right middle cerebral artery infarctions. *J Neurol Neurosurg Psychiatry* 39:84–89, 1976.
59. Caplan LR: "Top of the basilar" syndrome. *Neurology* 30:72–79, 1980.
60. Caplan LR, Kelly M, Kase CS, et al: Infarcts of the inferior division of the right middle cerebral artery: mirror image of Wernicke's aphasia. *Neurology* 36:1015–1020, 1986.
61. Katz DI, Alexander MP, Mandell AM: Dementia following strokes in the mesencephalon and diencephalon. *Arch Neurol* 44:1127–1133, 1987.
62. Mori E, Yamadori A: Acute confusional state and agitated delirium: Occurrence after infarction in the right middle cerebral artery territory. *Arch Neurol* 44:1139–1143, 1987.
63. Devinsky O, Bear D, Volpe BT: Confusional states following posterior cerebral artery infarction. *Arch Neurol* 45:160–163, 1988.
64. Mehler MF: The rostral basilar artery syndrome. *Neurology* 39:9–16, 1989.
65. Mendez MF, Adams NL, Lewandowski S: Neurobehavioral changes associated with caudate lesions. *Neurology* 39:349–354, 1989.
66. Caplan LR, Schahmann JD, Kase CS, et al: Caudate infarcts. *Neurology* 47:133–143, 1990.
67. Tatemichi TK, Desmond DW, Prohovnik I, et al: Confusion and memory loss from capsular genu infarction: A thalamocortical disconnection syndrome. *Neurology* 42:1966–1979, 1992.
68. Drugs that cause psychiatric symptoms. *Med Lett* 31:113–118, 1989.
69. Chan M, Nicklason F, Vial JH: Adverse drug events as a cause of hospital admission in the Elderly. *Int Med J* 31:199–205, 2001.
70. Fish DN: Treatment of delirium in the critically ill patient. *Clin Pharm* 10:456–466, 1991.
71. Menza MA, Murray GB, Holmes VF, Rafuls WA: Controlled study of extrapyramidal reactions in the management of delirious, medically ill patients: intravenous haloperidol vs haloperidol plus benzodiazepines. *Heart Lung* 17:238–241, 1988.
72. Han L, McCusker J, Cole M, et al: Use of medications with anticholinergic effect predicts clinical severity of of delirium symptoms in older medical in-patients. *Arch Intern Med* 161:1099–1105, 2001.
73. Burns MJ, Linden CH, Graudins A, et al: A comparison of physostigmine and benzodiazepines for the treatment of anticholinergic poisoning. *Ann Emerg Med* 35:374–381, 2000.
74. Cummings JL, Benson DF, LoVerme S Jr: Reversible dementia. *JAMA* 243:2434–2439, 1980.
75. McKeith IG, Galasko D, Kosaka K, et al: Consensus guidelines for the clinical and pathological diagnosis of dementia with Lewy bodies (DLB): report on the consortium on DLB international workshop. *Neurology* 47:1113–1124, 1996.
76. Perry R, Irving D, Blessed G, et al: Senile dementia of the Lewy body type: A clinically and neuropathologically distinct form of dementia in the elderly. *J Neurol Sci* 95:119–139, 1990.

77. Hansen L, Salmon D, Galasko D, et al: The Lewy body variant of Alzheimer's disease: A clinical and pathological entity. *Neurology* 40:1–8, 1990.
78. Lund and Manchester Groups: Clinical and neuropathological criteria for frontotemporal dementia. *J Neurol Neurosurg Psychiatry* 57:416–418, 1994.
79. van Duijn CM, de Knijff P, Cruts A, et al: Apolipoprotein E4 allele in a population-based study of early-onset Alzheimer's disease. *Nat Genet* 7:74–78, 1994.
80. Strittmatter WJ, Saunders AM, Schmechel D, et al: Apolipoprotein E: High-avidity binding to beta-amyloid and increased frequency of type 4 allele in late-onset familial Alzheimer's disease. *Proc Natl Acad Sci U S A* 90:1977–1981, 1993.
81. Prichard JW, Brass LM: New anatomical and functional imaging methods. *Ann Neurol* 32:395–400, 1992.
82. Miller BL, Cummings JL, Vilanueva-Meyer J, et al: Frontal lobe degeneration: Clinical, neuropsychological, and SPECT characteristics. *Neurology* 41:1374–1382, 1991.
83. Minoshima S, Giordani B, Berent S, et al: Metabolic reduction in the posterior cingulate cortex in very early Alzheimer's disease. *Ann Neurol* 42:85–94, 1997.
84. Silverman DHS, Small GW, Chang CY, et al: Positron emission tomography in evaluation of dementia: Regional brain metabolism and long-term outcome. *JAMA* 286:2120–2127, 2001.
85. Grafton ST, Mazziota JC, Pahl JJ, et al: A comparison of neurological, metabolic, structural, and genetic evaluations in persons at risk for Huntington's disease. *Ann Neurol* 28:614–621, 1990.
86. Small GW, Mazziota JC, Collins MT, et al: Apolipoprotein E type 4 allele and cerebral glucose metabolism in relatives at risk for familial Alzheimer's disease. *JAMA* 273:942–947, 1995.
87. Kuhl DE, Koeppe RA, Minoshima S, et al: In vivo mapping of cerebral acetylcholinesterase activity in aging and Alzheimer's disease. *Neurology* 52:691–699, 1999.
88. Cummings JL, Coffey CE: Neurobiological basis of behavior, in Coffey CE, Cummings JL (eds): *Textbook of Geriatric Neuropsychiatry.* Washington DC: American Psychiatric Association Press, 1994, pp 72–96.
89. Mesulam M-M. Large scale neurocognitive networks and distributed processing for attention, language, and memory. *Ann Neurol* 28:597–613, 1990.
90. Wolfe N, Katz DI, Albert ML, et al: Neuropsychological profile linked to low dopamine: in Alzheimer's disease, major depression, and Parkinson's disease. *J Neurol Neurosurg Psychiatry* 53:915–917, 1990.
91. Cummings JL: Behavioral complications of drug treatment of Parkinson's disease. *J Am Geriatr Soc* 39:708–716, 1991.
92. Hoehn-Saric R: Neurotransmitters in anxiety. *Arch Gen Psychiatry* 39:735–742, 1982.
93. Palmer AM, Stratmann GC, Procter AW, Bowen DM: Possible neurotransmitter basis of behavioral changes in Alzheimer's disease. *Ann Neurol* 23:616–620, 1988.
94. Alexander GE, Delong MR, Strick PL: Parallel organization of functional circuits linking basal ganglia and cortex. *Annu Rev Neurosci* 9:357–381, 1986.
95. Cummings JL: Frontal-subcortical circuits and human behavior. *Arch Neurol* 50:873–880, 1993.
96. Albert ML, Feldman RG, Willis AL: The "subcortical dementia" of progressive supranuclear palsy. *J Neurol Neurosurg Psychiatry* 37:121–130, 1974.
97. Cummings JL, Benson DF: Subcortical dementia. *Arch Neurol* 41:874–879, 1984.
98. Knopman DS, DeKosky ST, Cummings JL, et al: Practice parameter: Diagnosis of dementia (an evidence-based review). *Neurology* 56:1143–1153, 2001.
99. Benson DF, Cummings Jl, Tsai SY: Angular gyrus syndrome simulating Alzheimer's disease. *Arch Neurol* 39:616–620, 1982.
100. Mesulam M-M: Slowly progressive aphasia without generalized dementia. *Ann Neurol* 11:592–598, 1982.
101. Neary D, Snowden JS, Gustafson L, et al: Frontotemporal lobar degeneration: A consensus on clinical diagnostic criteria. *Neurology* 51:1546–1554, 1998.
102. Wenning GK, Litvan I, Jankovic J, et al: Natural history and survival of 14 patients with corticobasal degenration. *J Neurol Neurosurg Psychiatry* 64:184–189, 1998.
103. Cummings JL: Intellectual impairment in Parkinson's disease: Clinical, pathological, and biochemical correlates. *J Geriatr Psychiatry Neurol* 1:24–36, 1988.
104. Robbins TW, James M, Owen AM, et al: Cognitive deficits in progressive supranuclear palsy, Parkinson's disease, and multiple system atrophy in tests sensitive to frontal lobe dysfunction. *J Neurol Neurosurg Psychiatry* 57:79–88, 1994.
105. Pillon B, Gouider-Khouja N, Deweer B, et al: Neuropsychological pattern of striatonigral degeneration: comparison with Parkinson's disease and progressive supranuclear palsy. *J Neurol Neurosurg Psychiatry* 58:174–179, 1995.
106. Foster NL, Gilman S, Berent S, et al: Cerebral hypometabolism in progressive supranuclear palsy studied with positron emission tomography. *Ann Neurol* 24:399–406, 1988.
107. Sawada H, Udaka F, Kameyama M, et al: SPECT findings in Parkinson's disease associated with dementia. *J Neurol Neurosurg Psychiatry* 55:960–963, 1992.
108. Collins SJ, Ahlskog JE, Parisi JE, Maraganore DM: Progressive supranuclear palsy: neuropathologically based

diagnostic clinical criteria. *J Neurol Neurosurg Psychiatry* 58:167–173: 1995.

109. Benson DF: Hydrocephalic dementia, in Fredericks JAM (ed): *Handbook of Clinical Neurology: Neurobehavioral Disorders.* New York: Elsevier, 1985, vol 2, pp 323–333.
110. Cummings JL: Depression and Parkinson's disease: A review. *Am J Psychiatry* 149:443–445, 1992.
111. Tröster AI, Paolo AM, Lyons KE, et al: The influence of depression on cognition in Parkinson's disease: A pattern of impairment distinguishable from Alzheimer's disease. *Neurology* 45:672–676, 1995.
112. Folstein MF, McHugh PR: Dementia syndrome of depression, in Katzman R, Terry RD, Bick Kl (eds): *Alzheimer's Diease, Senile Dementia and Related Disorders.* New York: Raven Press, 1978, pp 87–93.
113. Caine ED: Pseudodementia. Current concepts and future directions. *Arch Gen Psychiatry* 38:1359–1364, 1981.
114. Roman GC, Tatemichi TK, Erkinjutti T, et al: Vascular dementia: Diagnostic criteria for research studies. Report of the NINDS-AIREN International Workshop. *Neurology* 43:250–260, 1993.
115. Chui HC, Vicoroff JI, Margolin D, et al: Criteria for the diagnosis of vascular dementia proposed by the state of California Alzheimer's Disease Diagnostic and Treatment Centers. *Neurology* 42:473–480, 1992.
116. Ishii N, Nishihara Y, Imamura T: Why do frontal lobe symptoms predominate in vascular dementia with lacunes? *Neurology* 36:340–345, 1986.
117. Huntington's Disease Research Collaborative Group: A novel gene containing a trinucleotide repeat that is expanded and unstable on Huntington's disease chromosomes. *Cell* 72:971–983, 1993.
118. Navia B, Jordan BJ, Price RW: The AIDS dementia complex: I. Clinical features. *Ann Neurol* 19:514–517, 1986.
119. Perl DP, Olanow CW, Calne D: Alzheimer's disease and Parkinson's disease: Distinct entities or extremes of a spectrum of neurodegeneration? *Ann Neurol* 44(Suppl 3):S19–S31, 1998.
120. Kaufer DI, Miller BL, Itti L, et al: Midline cerebral morphometry distinguishes frontotemporal dementia and Alzheimer's disease. *Neurology* 48:978–984, 1997.
121. Doody RS, Stevens JC, Beck C, et al: Practice parameter: Management of dementia (an evidence-based review). *Neurology* 56:1154–1166, 2001.
122. Cummings JL: Cholinesterase-inhibitors: A new class of psychotropic compounds. *Am J Psychiatry* 157:4–15, 2000.
123. McKeith IG, Del Ser T, Spano P, et al: Efficacy of rivastigmine in dementia with Lewy bodies: A randomised, double-blind, placebo-controlled international study. *Lancet* 356:2031–2036, 2000.
124. Katz IR, Jeste DV, Mintzer JE, et al: Comparison of risperidone and placebo for psychosis and behavioral disturbances associated with dementia: A randomized, double-blind trial. *J Clin Psychiatry* 60:107–115, 1999.
125. De Duyn PP, Rabheru K, Rasmussen A, et al: A randomized trial of risperidone, placebo, and haloperidol for behavioral symptoms of dementia. *Neurology* 53:946–955, 1999.
126. Street JS, Clark WS, Gannon KS, et al: Olanzapine treatment of psychotic and behavioral symptoms in patients with Alzheimer disease in nursing care facilities: a double-blind, randomized, placebo-controlled trial. *Am J Psychiatry* 57:968–976, 2000.
127. Sano M, Ernesto C, Thomas RG, et al: A controlled trial of selegiline, alpha-tocopherol, or both as treatment for Alzheimer's disease. *N Engl J Med* 336:1216–1222, 1997.
128. Mulnard R, Cotman C, Kawas C, et al: Estrogen replacement therapy for treatment of mild to moderate Alzheimer's disease in women: A randomized, double-blind placebo-controlled trial. *JAMA* 283:1007–1015, 2000.
129. Henderson V, Paginini-Hill A, Miller V, et al: Estrogen for Alzheimer's disease in women: Randomized, double-blind placebo-controlled trial. *Neurology* 54:295–301, 2000.
130. Kawas C, Resnick S, Morrison A, et al: A prospective study of estrogen replacement therapy and the risk of developing Alzheimer's disease: The Baltimore Longitudinal Study of Aging. *Neurology* 48:1517–1521, 1997.
131. Aisen PS, Davis KL, Berg JD, et al: A randomized controlled trial of prednisone in Alzheimer's disease. *Neurology* 54:588–593, 2000.
132. Stewart WF, Kawas C, Corrada M, Metter EJ: Risk of Alzheimer's disease and duration of NSAID risk. *Neurology* 48:626–632, 1997.
133. Veld B, Ruitenberg A, Hofman A, et al: Nonsteroidal antiinflammatory drugs and the risk of Alzheimer's disease. *N Engl J Med* 345:1515–1521, 2001.
134. Lipton SA, Rosenberg PA: Excitatory amino acids as a final common pathway for neurological disorders. *N Eng J Med* 330:613–622, 1994.
135. Graff-Radford NR, Godersky JC, Jones MP: Variables predicting surgical outcome in symptomatic hydrocephalus in the elderly. *Neurology* 39:1601–1604, 1989.
136. Clarfield AM. Normal-pressure hydrocephalus: Saga or swamp? *JAMA* 262:2592–2593, 1989.

Chapter 44

ALZHEIMER'S DISEASE: CLINICAL AND ANATOMIC ISSUES

François Boller
Charles Duyckaerts

Alzheimer's disease (AD) is a degenerative disease of the central nervous system (CNS), characterized clinically by progressive dementia and histologically by senile plaques (SPs) and neurofibrillary tangles (NFTs). The disease usually starts after the age of 40, and its incidence increases with age. In recent years, there has been a marked sharpening of diagnostic criteria and some new ancillary tests. However, in clinical practice, the diagnosis is still based on the exclusion of other conditions and on probability.

Strange as it may seem today, AD was long considered a rare disorder, and its recognition by the medical communiy has been slow. Until about 20 to 30 years ago, classic textbooks either failed to mention it[1] or dismissed it in a few lines.[2] According to Medline, only 42 papers including AD as a keyword were published in 1975. This long oblivion was followed by a major upsurge and, since the 1980s, a very large number of articles on AD have been appearing in medical journals (over 3500 entries in Medline in 2001, a total of 1421 as "major topic") as well as in the lay press. In the near future, however, the pendulum may swing back, since there are at present several questions about the homogeneity of AD and even about its usefulness as a single nosologic entity.[3]

It has taken even more time for AD to be "accepted" as a meaningful area of research and clinical investigation by behavioral neurologists and neuropsychologists. In the "classic" age, there had been very important clinical observations. Pick's 1892 paper is an outstanding early example of a single case description.[4] Alzheimer's patient[5] had probably been well studied. Seglas's careful study of the language disorders of the "insane"[6] also goes back to 1892. In later years, however, particularly after World War II, when neuropsychology arrived or rather returned to the scientific scene, mention of AD was strangely absent. It was as if diseases that produce dementia were not considered worthy of investigation, perhaps because the lesions were considered too "diffuse."* Of course, the disease is not diffuse, clinically or neuropathologically, and important dissociations and "focal signs" can be observed in behavior and cognition. Our knowledge concerning the neuropsychology of memory and attention, among others things, has expanded greatly thanks to the study of patients with AD and other degenerative disorders.

In this chapter, AD is first defined and placed in its historical context, past and present, and the diagnostic criteria currently in use are reviewed. After a description of the clinical picture, the known and supposed risk factors of AD are outlined, as well as current laboratory tests including positron emission tomography (PET) and single photon emission tomography (SPECT) imaging. The neuropathology of AD is then presented in detail. The chapter concludes with a review of the "borderland" of AD, particularly diffuse Lewy body disease (DLBD). In recent years, the so-called non-Alzheimer degenerative dementias (NADD), including progressive aphasia, have been isolated from AD and are also briefly discussed.

* There were a few noticeable exceptions. Sjögren et al. included results of neuropsychological tests in their masterful description of AD and Pick's disease.[293] Language disorders in dementia were studied by Pichot, by Critchley, and in a more complete and systematic fashion by DeRenzi and Vignolo as well as by Irigaray,[294–297] Other aspects of behavior and dementia had also been studied sporadically.[298,299] In North America, Frank Benson was probably one of the first to make patients with dementia "acceptable" for systematic neuropsychological studies. A survey shows that 80 percent of behavioral neurology fellowship programs in the United States include dementia as a major part of their teaching.[300]

HISTORICAL BACKGROUND OF AD

Until recently, the term *Alzheimer's disease* applied only to progressive dementias starting in the presenile years.[7] The distinction is still thought to be valid by some researchers,[8] but in the past 25 years or so it has become customary, following Katzman and coworkers[9] to deemphasize the distinction, "since the two conditions, except for their age of onset, are clinically and pathologically indistinguishable."[10]

The diseases that may produce dementia obviously existed long before Alois Alzheimer's short description of the condition. On the other hand, many prominent people were actively involved in that area of research, not only in Munich (Fig. 44-1) but also in other centers. The Prague group, led by Arnold Pick, came very close to getting the credit for first describing the disease, mainly thanks to the work of Pick's assistant Oskar Fischer. Following Perusini's work,[11] which confirmed that senile plaques (SPs) represented "a specific finding in senile dementia cases," the name *Fisher's plaques* began to appear in the literature. As for Nissl, he began to work with Alzheimer in 1889 and their professional relationship was so close that it was impossible to decide which owed more to the other.[12] While the work of Nissl and Perusini[13] was important, one gets a feeling that Alzheimer was the driving force of the group and therefore deserves credit for the eponym given to this most common form of dementia. The historical development of studies related to dementia and AD is discussed elsewhere.[14]

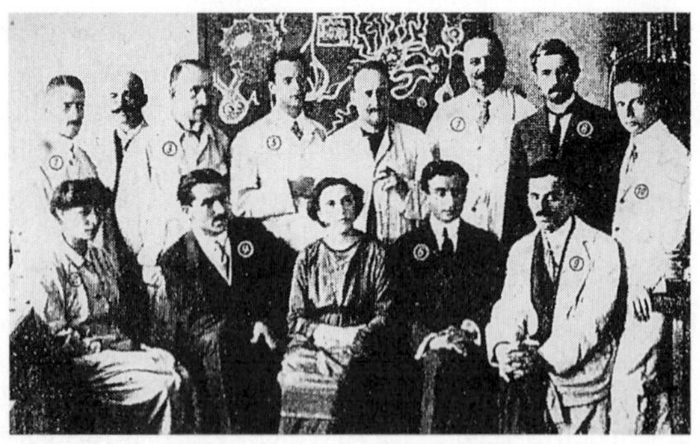

Figure 44-1
Picture of Alois Alzheimer (7) and his coworkers taken around 1907 at what is today the Max Planck Institute of Munich. The head of the group, Kraepelin, is in the center, smoking a cigar. The picture also includes Cerletti (4) who was to become responsible for the introduction of electroshock, Bonfiglio (6) and Perusini (9),both responsible for the publication of cases of presenile dementia, and Lewy (10), after whom the Lewy bodies are named.

NEUROPSYCHOLOGICAL TESTS IN ALZHEIMER'S DISEASE

Neuropsychological tests, formal or informal, have always been the keystone of the clinical diagnosis of AD. A recent article[15] has reviewed the application to AD of standard batteries and of short screening tests. In particular the article discusses "global tests" [such as the Wechsler Adult Intelligence Scale (WAIS)] and batteries specifically designed to test dementia, including the Cambridge Examination for Mental Disorders in the Elderly (CAMDEX),[16,17] the Alzheimer's Disease Assessment Scale (ADAS),[18,19] and the battery of the Consortium to Establish a Registry for AD (CERAD) (see below). In addition to these tests, it is useful for the neuropsychologist to have at his or her disposal tests that assess the specific deficits of the disease, including attention, short-term memory and executive functions, language, memory and apraxia. In developing new tests to assess these cognitive changes, researchers have shown that they realize the need to develop and use tests developed in a rational manner, with high sensitivity and specificity, not only in the moderate stages of the disease but also in the very early and even "preclinical" stages as well as during the late stages (severe dementia).[20]

DIAGNOSTIC CLINICAL CRITERIA

The diagnostic criteria for dementia proposed by the *Diagnostic and Statistical Manual of Mental Disorders*[21] are presented in detail in Chap. 43. In 1984, a consensus conference met in Bethesda, Maryland, under the auspices of the Neurology Institute of the National Institutes of Health (then called NINCDS) and the Alzheimer's Disease and Related Disorders Association (ADRDA). The so-called NINCDS/ADRDA criteria defined at that conference[22] remain valid today and are now in use in many countries around the world. One of their merits is to have introduced the notion of probable and possible AD, the certainty of the diagnosis being provided only in cases where neuropathology (i.e., an autopsy or a biopsy) confirms the clinical findings. The validity of the NINCDS/ADRDA criteria has been demonstrated by clinical studies and by clinicopathologic correlations.[23,24]

Criteria of the Consortium to Establish a Registry for AD (CERAD)

Soon after the creation in the United States of the first 10 Alzheimer's Disease Research Centers (ADRCs) by the National Institute on Aging in 1985, it was felt that there was a need and an opportunity to establish standardized diagnostic criteria that could be used not only in North America but in other countries as well. The CERAD criteria were therefore proposed in the late 1980s under the leadership of different centers, particularly those of Duke University in Durham, North Carolina, and Washington University in St. Louis, Missouri.[25]

The CERAD criteria are for the most part an operational adaptation of those proposed by NINCDS-ADRDA[22] and include the foundations for three diagnoses: no dementia, possible AD, and probable AD. The clinical evaluation battery includes a semistructured interview with the patient and with another person who knows the patient well (if possible a close family member). The CERAD examination includes general physical and neurologic examinations, laboratory tests aimed especially at ruling out other conditions such as thyroid disease or B_{12} deficiency, and a depression scale. As originally proposed, the neuropsychological battery consisted of 7 tests, J1 to J7, which are listed in Table 44-1. This short battery was shown[25] to have high interrater and retest reliability. The study of Morris et al.[25] also found that the battery discriminated all of 350 AD patients from 275 controls. Another study[26] found that the test can distinguish even the patients with the mildest cases of AD from nondemented controls. Nevertheless, the battery has been augmented by the addition of further measures (L1 to L7), including delayed verbal recall, Trails A and B, and a simple test of verbal intelligence aimed at estimating the subject's premorbid IQ. In addition, finger tapping and clock drawing (which were already part of the neurologic examination) are now considered part of the battery.

Table 44-1
Neuropsychological tests of CERAD

J 1: Word fluency (category-animal)*
J 2: Boston Naming Test*
J 3: MMSE*
J 4: Word list memory*
J 5: Constructional praxis*
J 6: Word list–delayed recall*
J 7: Word list–recognition*
L 1: Shipley-Hartford Vocabulary
L 2: Verbal Paired Associate Learning test (from WMS-R)
L 3: Recall of constructional praxis items
L 4: Verbal Paired Associate recall
L 5: Trails A and B
L 6: Nelson Adult reading Test (NART)
L 7: Word fluency (letter: "F" and "P")
Finger tapping
Clock drawing

*The "J" tests are those included in the earliest version of the battery.

An estimate of the overall degree of deterioration is provided by the Mini-Mental State (MMS) examination,[27] the Blessed test,[28] and the Clinical Dementia Rating Scale (CDR),[29] which relies on subjective assessment by the clinician. Administration of the CDR requires training, for which video cassettes have been developed in the United States; these are also available in other countries. it's the scoring of the CDR has been simplified by using the "sum of boxes." Recent studies have shown an 83 percent rate of agreement among users of the CDR.

The introduction of the criteria listed above may be responsible for a marked improvement in diagnostic accuracy witnessed in recent years. If the "gold standard" is an autopsy with positive findings for AD, the percentage of accurate diagnoses during the 1970s may have been as low as 50 percent.[30] According to a later (1989) study,[31] this figure had reached around 80 percent. Two studies based on small series[32,33] reported 100 percent accuracy—a rather unlikely result. The latest CERAD data concerning neuropathology[34] indicate a reliability of the order of 85 percent.

CLINICAL PICTURE

Thanks to personal experience or readings of the literature, most people are aware of the "typical" appearance of AD and how it evolves. Very schematically, one can distinguish three stages. The first *(amnestic)* is dominated by disorders of memory, particularly episodic memory, but also semantic memory, with therefore a fairly frequent impairment in language even in the initial stages. In the second stage (*dementia*), the loss of intellectual abilities reflects itself in everyday life and it becomes more and more difficult for the patient to live independently. Each of these two stages lasts an average of 2 years, but there is, of course, considerable variation from patient to patient. Even within the same patient, the course may fluctuate a great deal, with relatively long stable periods alternating with precipitous declines.[35] The third stage (known as the *vegetative stage*) is characterized by the patients' inability to take care of themselves, to feed, and to communicate. One of the tragic aspects of AD is that with proper care, this stage can go on for many years. AD patients do not die *of* the disease, they die *with* it from some other cause. It has been shown that survival is affected more by loss of autonomy than by the severity of the dementia.[36]

This brief outline of the clinical picture belies the fact that no two patients are alike, as there is an almost infinite number of combination of clinical symptoms of varying severity, particularly in the early stages. Among the most atypical forms are those where a specific symptom—for instance, language impairment or apraxia— dominates the picture for a long time. Some of these forms are discussed below. The early phases of AD may also be dominated by noncognitive disorders such as agitation, hallucinations, sleep disturbances, or, on the contrary, apathy and depression. This extremely important aspect of AD has been reviewed by Absher and Cummings.[37] Details concerning cognitive changes of AD are found in Chap. 45.

RISK FACTORS

Age is of course the main "risk factor" for AD, even though we hesitate to qualify as such a process that can hardly be dissociated from life itself. AD can start at age 45 or even younger, but it is mainly after the age of 60 to 65 that the proportion of AD patients becomes sizable. The proportion increases up to 80 to 90 years of age and then seems to become stable.

Chromosomal Abnormalities and Family History

Even though it had been known for years that patients with trisomy 21 (Down's syndrome) develop AD-like neuropathologic changes after the age of 40, it was only in the mid to late 1980s that the first reports of chromosomal abnormality associated with AD were published.[38] These reports indicated an association with the gene of the APP precursor. It became apparent shortly thereafter that chromosome 21 is not the only chromosome where abnormalities can be found in AD. A tie between early-onset forms and chromosome 14 (S182) was established by the Seattle group.[39] Implication of chromosome 19 has also been shown, particularly in familial forms with late onset.[40] The latest episode in the chromosomal "saga" comes again from the Seattle group. Studies of a special form of familial Alzheimer's disease (FAD) in a group known as the Volga Germans reveals the presence of an AD locus on chromosome 1 (STM2).[41]

An association has been found between AD and the locus of the gene coding apolipoprotein E (ApoE), located on chromosome 19. A particular allele of the gene, the Apoε4, responsible for the synthesis of the ApoE4 phenotype, is genetically associated not only with familial[42] but also with sporadic forms of the disease.[43] It has been shown that as the number of Apoε4 alleles (which code for the ApoE4 protein) increases (from 0 to 2), so does the risk of developing the disease. According to one group, octogenarians with AD carry the genotype 4/4 three times more often than healthy octogenarians.[44]

After age, ApoE4 is the most significant risk factor for AD. It is not yet clear to what extent these genetic associations are reflected in the course, severity, and other clinical aspects of the disease.[45,46] They might increase Aβ deposition even in intellectually normal subjects.[47] The specificity of ApoE is also the subject of an ongoing debate. ApoE ε4 alleles are reported to be associated not only with AD but also with other conditions, particularly PSP, Pick's disease, corticobasal degeneration,[48] amyloid angiopathy,[49] Down's syndrome,[50] and possibly Creutzfeldt- Jakob disease.[51] However, one report indicates no association with Parkinson's disease (PD) without or with dementia.[52] The significance of ApoE as a biological marker is discussed below.

Cases of FAD have been known for many years (see Ref. 53 for a review); in some families, several dozens of members have been studied, with unequivocal demonstration of autosomal dominant pattern of transmission, which has also been found in apparently sporadic cases.[54] A study based on two pairs of twins aged 62 to 73 years shows high concordance for subjects who are $\varepsilon4$ homozygous, but it also shows that there is little genetic influence in early-onset AD patients without the $\varepsilon4$ allele.[55]

Families where genetic transmission is apparent are, however, exceptional, and in clinical practice, it is quite rare to obtain a positive family history. The discrepancy between research and clinical data is probably related to the fact that AD is almost unique in having such a late clinical expression. Meanwhile, there is no question that having a case in a family considerably increases the chances of other family members developing it. Epidemiologic studies have also shown associations of AD with Parkinson's disease[56] and Down's syndrome,[57] even though the latter finding has been contradicted.[58]

Geographic Distribution

Available epidemiologic data suggest that AD has a similar incidence everywhere in the world. There may be two exceptions to this rule. In Japan, numerous cases of dementia appear to be caused not by AD but by cerebrovascular diseases. Recent findings suggest that in some African countries, AD is less frequent than in industrialized areas.[59]

Gender

In clinical practice, one is struck by a marked gender difference: many more women than men seem to be affected. In their review, Fratiglioni and Rocca[60] show that many but not all studies confirm these data. In addition, survival to AD is shorter for male patients than for females.[36]

Level of Instruction

Several studies have shown that the prevalence of dementia is related to the level of instruction and is much greater among illiterate subjects (see Ref. 60, page 205). This finding has yet to receive a clear explanation. The possibility of a bias related to the difficult administration and interpretation of cognitive tests in patients with no or little instruction has not been entirely ruled out. On the other hand, one can also hypothesize that education actually increases the density of neocortical synapses, allowing the accumulation of "reserves" and therefore delaying the appearance of dementia.[61] Paradoxically, there is an increased risk of mortality in AD patients with more advanced educational and occupational attainment.[62] It is felt that this is because lower education is accompanied by an earlier expression and therefore a longer survival.

Other factors—including parental age at birth, some thyroid diseases, depression, and head injuries—are thought by many to be associated with an increased incidence of AD, but these effects cannot be said to have been demonstrated with certainty. The possible protective role of tobacco and alcohol consumption[63,64] could be due to a side effect of the ApoE4 genotype, which is also a significant risk factor for vascular diseases. The proportion of old smokers and drinkers with ApoE4 genotype could be abnormally low due to attrition by death from vascular causes.

LABORATORY TESTS

Until fairly recently, no laboratory test could be used to diagnose AD. In routine clinical use, neurophysiologic tests can help corroborate a diagnosis of dementia and rule out some other conditions. The use of more sophisticated techniques such as the study of P300 has been advocated in the detection of early cases.[65] The new imaging techniques provided by computed tomography (CT) and magnetic resonance imaging (MRI) have been found to be invaluable not only in ruling out other conditions but also in pointing out some specific features such as atrophy of the temporal lobe,[66] of the hippocampal formation,[67] and of the amygdala.[68] MRI spectroscopy has shown anomalies that may reflect lesions of the neuronal membrane.[69]

Metabolic abnormalities associated with AD are reflected in PET and SPECT studies.[70] While PET studies remain limited to few patients by practical considerations, SPECT has reached a level of practical interest because it is relatively cheap and, with the use of technetium-99m hexa methylpropyleneamine oxime (HMPAO), is said to have demonstrated between 90 and 100 percent ability to detect AD.[71] In most cases (around 80 percent), one can demonstrate a "characteristic" pattern of bilateral parietotemporal perfusion deficit. The SPECT and PET changes have been shown to correlate with different cognitive profiles[72–75] and even to possibly precede the clinical changes.[76]

The neurochemical changes that accompany AD are described in detail in Chap. 46.

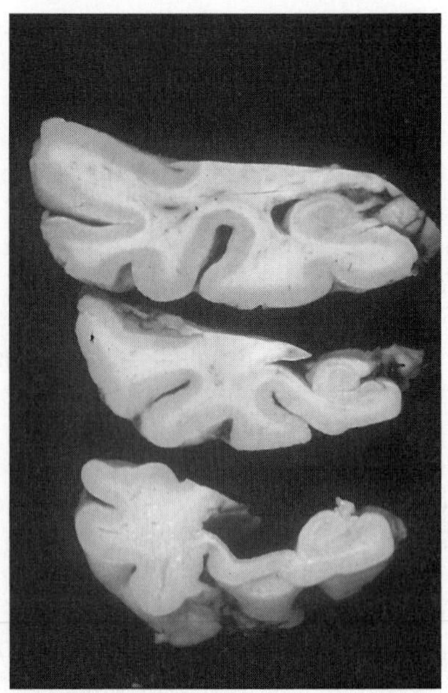

Figure 44-2 (Plate 10)
Atrophy of the hippocampus. The upper section comes from a control without neurologic symptoms. The hippocampus has a normal volume. The two other sections come from patients with Alzheimer's disease at various stages. Maximal atrophy is seen on the lowest section.

NEUROPATHOLOGY OF AD

Anatomy

AD affects the very structure of the brain; unlike tumors, it does not invade the parenchyma nor does it destroy it, as infarcts do. The disease, however, affects cerebral organization without causing much destruction or inflammation. In order to comprehend AD pathology and its progression, it may therefore be useful to discuss some points concerning the anatomic organization of the brain. In the following section, we distinguish schematically the cortex and the subcortex; in the cortex, we recognize three main divisions: the *hippocampus* (including the dentate gyrus and the subiculum) necessary to normal memory acquisitions (Fig. 44-2, Plate 10); the *isocortex* (sometimes also called neocortex), which covers most of the brain surface; and finally the interface region between hippocampus and isocortex—i.e., the *entorhinal area*—limited by the rhinal sulcus (*ento-* is the Greek word for "inside" or "limited by"). The neocortex may be subdivided into broad categories depending on their functions.[77] The sensory inputs (somesthetic, auditory, visual) reach areas known as primary. At this stage, the signal is still raw, close to its physical origin. Its main characteristics are manifest in specialized cortical areas. In the visual mode, for example, color, movement, and three-dimensional perception are selectively analyzed[78] in so-called association cortices, which are said to be unimodal, since only one type of signal—visual, somesthetic, or auditory—is treated in each one. The unimodal association cortical areas are connected with large multimodal areas, located mainly in the prefrontal and in the parietotemporal regions. The information is funneled from these areas onto the entorhinal area, which receives signals that have been processed through the various association cortices. This set of corticocortical connections from the primary to the entorhinal areas ("feed forward") is paralleled by connections that go back from the multimodal areas to the primary cortex ("feed backward") (see Ref. 79 for review). These corticocortical connections are thought to play a major role in memory processes by providing the necessary relays between the hippocampus and the isocortex.

The laminar organization of the cortex may give some insight into the preferential topography of the microscopic lesions (SPs and NFTs).[80] The isocortex is made up of six layers. Layer IV comprises small neurons known as *granules,* which receive sensory inputs coming, for example, from the thalamus. The output of the cortex stems from pyramidal neurons. Those located in layer II and, to a greater extent, layer III project to other cortical areas, some through the corpus callosum. This is the layer where most SPs are found, as elaborated further on. The large pyramidal neurons of layer V send the majority of their axons to subcortical targets such as the lenticular nucleus, the brainstem nuclei, or the spinal motor neuron. The spindle-shaped cells of layer VI contribute to transcortical connections. Layer I contains mainly dendritic expansions from the undelying layers. This brief outline is highly schematic but emphasizes the hierarchical organization of the cortex, through corticocortical connections, for which layer III plays a major role.

Main Lesions and Diagnosis

We should now consider how the two major lesions seen in AD—the SPs and the NFTs—are integrated within this complex circuitry. SPs and NFTs (Fig. 44-3, Plate 11) differ in shape, topography, and biochemical/immunohistochemical markers. This has led some authors to consider that only one type of alteration has a diagnostic or pathogenetic meaning. Several diagnostic criteria take only SPs into account,[81,82] the tangles being considered poorly specific, but it has also been said that the clinical symptoms were more tightly linked to the NFTs than to the SPs.[83] The most recent diagnostic criteria take both the SPs and the NFTs into account.[84]

It is probably artificial to consider the plaques and the tangles separately: no patient with Alzheimer's disease has ever been reported *without* NFTs in the entorhinal and hippocampal regions, although they may be absent in the isocortex.[85] Cases with a large predominance of NFTs and a scarcity of plaques have also been identified.[86]

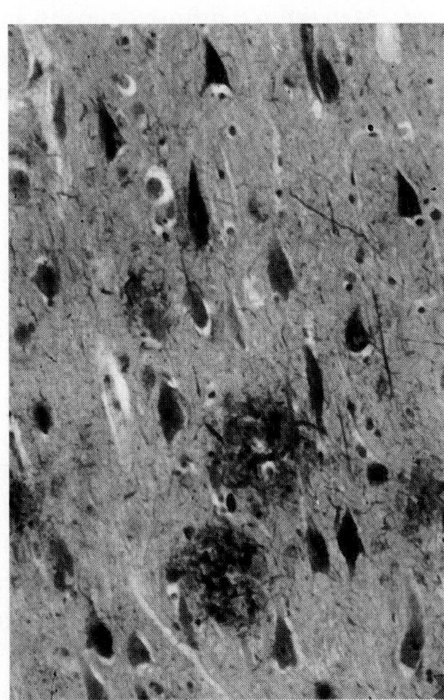

Figure 44-3 (Plate 11)
The two main lesions of Alzheimer's disease: (1) neurofibrillary tangles (NFT) are located in the neuronal cell body and appear in black; (2) SPs are seen as spheres made of entangled neurites. Bielschowsky silver impregnation counterstained by cresyl violet. Staining performed by Dr. Joachim Kauss. Initial magnification: x750.

Senile Plaques SPs are composite and complex lesions. That complexity makes them difficult to analyze: their density as evaluated on microscopic sections is highly dependent on the staining technique, which may reveal more specifically one of the three main components of the plaque[87] (Fig. 44-4, Plate 12): the extracellular deposit, the neurites, or the cells (macrophages and astrocytes). This deposit makes up the core of the plaque and the neurites draw a crown around it. They

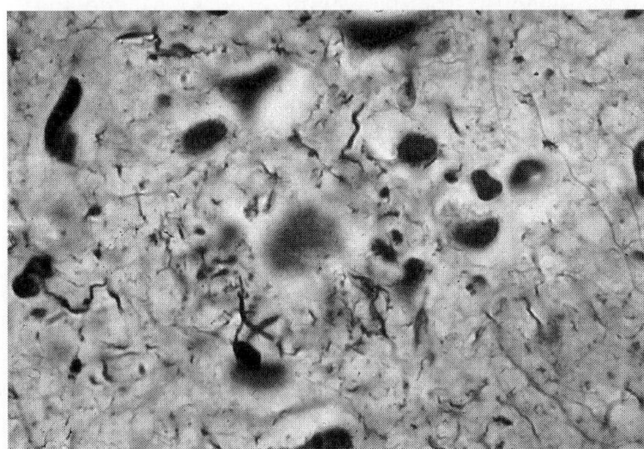

Figure 44-4 (Plate 12)
Senile plaques. The SP, in the center of the picture, is a composite lesion. Its center, stained gray, is made of amorphous extracellular material, mainly composed of Aβ peptide. Other stains, such as Congo red, would show its "amyloid" nature. Around the amyloid center a crown of degenerating neurites is clearly seen. The nuclei that are in contact with the plaque belong for the most part to microglial cells. Initial magnification: x1200.

are principally made up of axons.[88] The astrocytes surround the plaques with their processes, whereas the macrophages are usually located in the core or close to it.[89,90] Other constituents, belonging to the extracellular matrix, have also been identified.

The Extracellular Deposit A number of proteins have been recognized in the core of the plaque, the most significant probably being Aβ and apolipoprotein E.

Aβ Properties of Congo red staining, known as "birefringence" (light reflection in two directions) and "dichroism" (change of color due to a change in light wavelength) have been used to define the amyloid substance. They are thought to be related to the highly repetitive three-dimensional structure of the proteins when they exhibit the β-pleated sheet arrangement. Many proteins or peptides may take on this three-dimensional structure and become "amyloid." Proteins with the β-pleated sheet structure become highly insoluble and therefore difficult to isolate and analyze. It remained unknown until 1984, when Glenner and Wong (Glenner and Wong 1984) described a hitherto unknown peptide they named A4 peptide (A for amyloid and 4 for its weight of 4 kDa) and that is also known as Aβ peptide (β stands for β-pleated sheet). It was rapidly found that the peptide came from a large and ubiquitous protein, the APP (amyloid precursor protein),[303] which is probably located across cellular membranes. It has a hydrophobic moiety located between two hydrophilic extremities. The neuron itself contains high amounts of mRNA coding for APP. The Aβ peptide is cleaved from APP through two enzymatic activities: the β secretase cuts APP at the N-terminal part of the protein, outside the membrane, while the γ secretase cleaves it within the membrane. The enzyme responsible for β-secretase activity has been isolated and called beta-secretase cleavage (BACE).[91] Enzymes responsible for the γ cleavage have been elusive. Some authors believe that presenilin (a protein mutated in some familial cases of Alzheimer's disease) could be γ secretase itself (Selkoe and Wolfe, 2000). For others, presenilin regulates γ-secretase activity but is different from it (Armogida, Petit, et al., 2001; Checler, 2001). Immunohistochemistry labels some Aβ deposits that are not stained by Congo red—i.e., are not amyloid. They are not surrounded by a crown of abnormal neurites and appear less dense than the core of the senile plaques. These so-called diffuse deposits can be observed in AD patients as well as in old and apparently normal individuals (Delaère et al., 1990, 1993), in young patients with trisomy 21 (Mann and Esiri, 1989) and possibly after severe head trauma (Roberts et al., 1991), although this has been contradicted (Adle-Biassette et al., 1996). Diffuse deposits should be distinguished from SPs, since they may be seen in intellectually normal (or nearly normal) old patients. They could indicate "pathologic aging" according to Dickson (Dickson et al., 1992). It is established that at least some of these diffuse deposits will never mature into true SPs since they are located in regions that are always devoid of true neuritic plaques.

Apolipoprotein E ApoE, a cholesterol transporter, is present in the Aβ diffuse deposits, in the core of neuritic plaques, and in the microglial cells.[92–95] It has been suggested that it could accumulate in the early stage of plaque formation and even precede Aβ deposition as punctate deposits.[96] The role of ApoE has been emphasized in a mouse model of Alzheimer's disease, a transgenic line bearing a human APP mutation found in familial cases. In these mice, the packing density of Aβ deposits is dramatically decreased when ApoE is absent because its gene gene has been knocked out.[97–99] Apolipoprotein E could play a role in the abnormal folding of Aβ into a β-pleated, insoluble, protein—a role described by the term *chaperone protein*.[95] The presence of ApoE in the senile plaque is probably related to the accumulation of cholesterol, which has recently been detected within the core of the plaque.[100] The cell responsible for the presence of ApoE in the plaque core has not yet been determined convincingly: it could be the astrocyte, the microglial cell, or the neuron itself.[94]

Components of the Extracellular Matrix Various components of the extracellular matrix—such as ICAM1,[101] thrombospondin,[102] and heparan sulfate proteoglycan[103]— have been shown to accumulate in the senile plaque.

Other Constituents of Senile Plaques Alpha$_1$-antichymotrypsin, a serine protease inhibitor synthesized in the liver, has been thoroughly studied. It consistently colocalizes with Aβ amyloid deposits[104,105] and is associated with activated astrocytes.[106] Cathepsin D, a lysosomal enzyme, is also abundant in the processes around the plaque and in the plaques themselves; it could be related to an activation of the endosomal-lysosomal pathway.[107]

Inflammation in the Senile Plaque Inflammation is a general process that involves both cells, such as macrophages (microglial cell in the brains) or lymphocytes, and various molecules, among which cytokines, which are produced by inflammatory cells and circulating proteins such as components of the complement cascade. Several elements suggest that an inflammation of a special type is taking place in the senile plaque. Unlike inflammation elsewhere, it does not recruit lymphocytes but only macrophages (microglial cells).[108,109] Only the first components of the complement cascade[110,111] are present as well as a few cytokines (interleukins- 1[112] and -6[113]).

The activated microglia seem to be better correlated with the neurofibrillary alterations than with the density of Aβ peptide[114] in the hippocampus; but in the isocortex, they are closely linked to the amyloid deposits.[89] Microglia may play an important role in the production of the amyloid fibrils themselves.[115,116] The density of activated microglia correlates better with the density of amyloid (i.e., Congo red–positive) deposits than with any other type of Aβ deposits,[89] suggesting that the amyloid itself may be responsible for the macrophage activation.

The Neurites of the Senile Plaque The neurites are major constituents of the plaque. They are revealed by silver-staining methods, which show a crown of dark, sometimes dilated fibers coming into contact with the deposit. Some of them contain APP or ubiquitin epitopes ("dystrophic neurites").[117] In mature plaques, most are immunolabeled by anti-tau antibodies. At electron microscopy, they appear to be filled with "paired helical filaments" (PHF),[118,119] a structure characteristic of the NFTs to be described further on. The great majority of neurites is made of axons, as shown by the presence of presynaptic vesicles at electron microscopy[120] and of neurofilament epitopes[88]; dendrites are rare[121] or absent.[88] Most clinicopathologic studies have demonstrated that the density of SPs with neurites ("true SPs") is correlated with dementia.[83,122–125] The correlation may be low when diffuse deposits of Aß peptide without the crown of abnormal neurites are taken into account. Detailed morphologic analysis of the plaque suggests that it should not be considered as a "scar" of some unusual type but rather as a living set of abnormal nervous connections. There must be some relationship between NFTs and plaques. The presence of PHF in the plaque demonstrates the intricacy of the relationship between these two lesions, but it is not yet known whether SPs are physically connected to tangle-bearing neurons.

The Cells In looking at sections stained with the usual hematoxylin-eosin (H&E) stain, one finds good evidence of the presence of SPs is the microglial cell: it is usually found close to the amyloid core deposit.[89] Microglial cells can be considered the histiocytes of the brain: under some circumstances, they become activated and exhibit phagocytic activity. They belong to the macrophage system, although their origin remains debated. Microglial cells have attracted much attention because the macrophages play a major role in amyloid formation outside the brain during chronic inflammation.[126] It has been suggested that the microglial cell could be responsible for the formation of amyloid.[116] Amyloid has indeed been seen in the microglial cell, but its presence could be related either to its production or to phagocytosis of the deposit.[89]

Astrocytes are found in the vicinity of SPs. Immunohistochemistry of the GFAp (glial fibrillary acid protein), specific for astrocytes, reveals a meshwork of astrocytic processes surrounding the SP. The role played by astrocytes is still debated. It could produce significant components of the plaque (it has been said that it could synthesize ApoE[127]) or circumscribe the lesion and limit its extent. It has been shown in culture that astrocytes prevent the phagocytosis of amyloid deposit by microglia.[128]

Plaques are often in close contact with capillaries. Some authors have suggested in the past that a capillary was always present in the plaque.[129] Other studies have shown that capillaries and amyloid deposits are topographically unrelated.[130]

NFTs and Neuropile Threads

The term *neurofibrillary tangle* (NFT) denotes fibrillary material in the neuronal cell body or perikaryon (Fig. 44-5, Plate 13). These tangles were first described by Alzheimer himself,[131] using a (then new) silver technique (Bielschowsky method). When ionic silver, soluble and invisible, is "reduced" to metallic silver by chemical agents used in photography, the metal precipitates on fibrillary material present in the tissue section. The fibrillary material is either normal (as normal axons) or abnormal (as neurofibrillary tangles). Since the time of Bielschowsky, the silver impregnations have improved in specificity: one of the techniques described by Gallyas stains only the abnormal neurofibrillary structures. Nowadays, however, labeling by antibodies (immunohistochemistry) allows identifying more specifically the proteins present in the lesions and immunohistochemistry tends, therefore, to replace silver methods. NFTs have been frequently examined with electron microscopy. The first observations revealed their filamentous and helical (or twisted) structure,[119,120] beautifully illustrated with scanning electron microscopy.[132] It was initially thought that they were made of two filaments (hence the term *paired helical filaments,* or PHFs). New data suggest that they are actually twisted ribbons.[133,134]

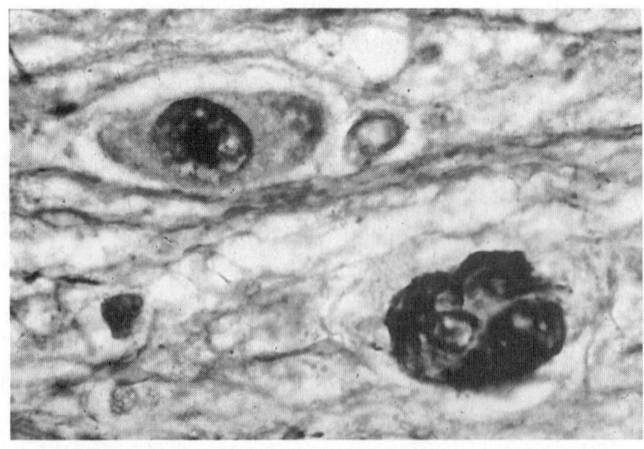

Figure 44-5 (Plate 13)
Neurofibrillary tangle. This high-power view of the nucleus basalis of Meynert shows two neurons; the cytoplasm of the normal neuron appears light brown. The second neuron contains a NFT made of deep black fibrils surrounding and partly overlapping the nucleus. Bodian silver impregnation. Initial magnification: x2500.

It has been possible to isolate PHFs and inject them in animals in order to obtain antibodies. Various anti-NFTs have been produced in this way, but a major step was taken when it was shown that NFTs were specifically labeled by an antibody directed against tau proteins, a group of proteins associated with neurotubules and resistant to heat.[135] Tau has several phosphorylation sites and in NFTs appears to be "abnormally phosphorylated," meaning that tau has bound too many phosphate radicals.[136–140] The very existence of this hyperphosphorylation in vivo has been challenged; it could be an artifact due to the relative inefficiency of phosphatases, postmortem or after sampling, in patients with Alzheimer's disease.[141] Tau antibodies have provided a very useful tool for the study of all types of neurofibrillary pathology. Tau is actually present in normal brain parenchyma. After the usual histology techniques (formalin fixation, alcoholic dehydration, toluene or xylene, paraffin), it becomes undetectable except in various inclusions such as NFTs. It should be mentioned here that NFTs are seen not only in AD but also in progressive supranuclear palsy (PSP), corticobasal ganglionic degeneration (CBD or CGD),[142] and various tauopathies due to tau gene mutations.

Tau immunocytochemistry has clearly demonstrated that neurofibrillary pathology is not limited to the cell body but also involves neuronal processes, which indeed contain PHFs. Tau antibodies (as well as Gallyas stain) show in AD brains a great number of small, fragmented, tortuous processes weaving between the cell bodies (i.e., in the "neuropil"—that part of the brain tissue which is not the cell bodies or the white matter tracts). These "tortuous fibers"[143] contain PHFs and are mainly dendrites.[144] They are called *neuropil threads*[145] and, at least in Alzheimer's disease, invariably accompany tangles and plaques when they are numerous.

SPs and NFTs do not have the same distribution. Both lesions are exclusively found in the gray matter (although a few Aβ deposits without neurites have been found in the white matter.[94] The great majority of plaques is found in the isocortex; the hippocampus is relatively spared, and true neuritic plaques are exceptional in the subcortex except for the amygdala. Neuritic plaques are never seen in the cerebellum, where only diffuse deposits may occasionally occur.

Plaques are rare in the brainstem and found there only in specific locations.[146] In the isocortex, the plaques are diffusely distributed: they are present in primary areas as well as in unimodal and multimodal cortical areas.[147] However, they do not involve all the layers of the cortex evenly, being much more numerous in layer III,[80] implicated, as we have seen, in the corticocortical connection. The density of neuritic SPs in the isocortex is linked with the cognitive status.[28]

NFTs involve specifically some areas, and in those, only some neurons.[148] The medium-sized pyramidal neurons are selectively affected.[147,149] They are located in layers III and V. The granule cells—e.g., of the dentate gyrus or of layer IV—are largely spared. So are the giant pyramidal cells of Betz, in area 4. The islands of pyramidal cells in layer II of the entorhinal cortex are thought to be the first involved. They contain NFTs in all the cases of Alzheimer's disease.[149] The pyramidal layers of the hippocampus and adjoining subiculum are the next most sensitive areas. It has been noticed that when tangles were present in those areas, they were also present in the previously mentioned entorhinal region. Finally, in advanced cases, one can find numerous tangles in layers III and V of the isocortical associative areas. In those cases, as could be expected, the tangles are also numerous in the entorhinal area, hippocampus, and subiculum. The primary isocortical areas contain NFTs only in the most advanced cases.[147,150]

The distribution of SPs and of NFTs can thus be contrasted: SPs involve all the isocortical areas and their density increases with the severity of the disease. NFTs involve an increasing number of areas in a stereotyped order: entorhinal area, hippocampus-subiculum, isocortex. Figure 44-6, Plates 14 and 15, compares two maps: the distribution of NFTs[147] on the one hand and the functional organization of the cortical areas (as illustrated by Mesulam[77]) on the other. It shows that the distribution of NFTs is precisely constrained by cytoarchitectonic borders. NFTs are rarely found in primary cortices. Their density is low in unimodal association cortices, increases in multimodal association cortices, and reaches a peak in the paralimbic areas.

This explains why the *mapping* of the areas involved by the neurofibrillary pathology (Braak stages[149]) may help to evaluate the severity of the disease. The distinct distribution of the lesions may also explain some of the apparent paradoxes of the clinicopathologic correlations: severe memory disorders may be observed in the absence of isocortical SPs. At this stage, described as "limbic,"[149] NFTs may be numerous in the entorhinal-hippocampal region.[151] Isocortical plaques may be seen in the isocortex at a stage where tangles involve only the entorhinal-hippocampal region

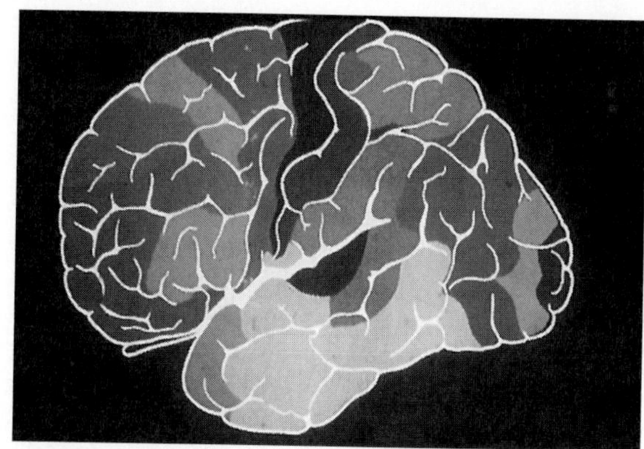

A

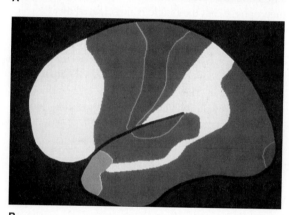

B

Figure 44-5 (Plates 14 and 15)
Comparison of the distribution of neurofibrillary tangles with the functional organization of the cortical areas. Upper panel: *Distribution of the cortical NFTs. (From Arnold et al.,[147] with permission.) The density of the lesions is indicated by the following color scale: dark blue (no lesion); light blue, green, yellow, and orange (maximal density of lesions).* Lower panel: *Classification of functional cortical zones in relation with Brodmann's map according to Mesulam.[77] Blue: primary sensory areas. Yellow:unimodal association cortex. Purple: multimodal association areas. Green: paralimbic areas.*

("plaque-only AD"). In addition, were the plaques the main cause of the deficit, all cortical functions would have to be affected simultaneously, since SPs tend to be diffusely spread over the neocortex. The progression of NFTs, from limbic to isocortical areas, beginning in multimodal association cortices to later involve unimodal and finally primary cortices, clearly follows the usual course of the symptoms, which involve first memory and secondarily language, gnosis, and praxis. NFTs may also be located outside of a neuron, the shape of which they retain. These "ghost tangles" are direct evidence of neuronal death, leaving the tangle in the extracellular space.[152] The cell is phagocytosed by the macrophage, but the tangle is not cleared away.

The atrophy of the cortex also seems better correlated with the presence of tangles than with plaques. As gross atrophy is the direct consequence of neuronal loss, one may conclude that the tangle is the main cause of cell death in AD. It should, however, be added that some cell populations devoid of tangles, most noticeably in the retina, can also be reduced.[153] This could imply other mechanisms of neuronal death.

Neuronal Loss and Neuronal Atrophy

Much has been written about neuronal loss in aging and AD and extreme values have been suggested: for some authors, neuronal loss is the main determinant of dementia[154]; for others, neuronal loss does not even exist.[155] Such discrepancies reflect the methodologic difficulties involved in evaluating the number of neurons in the cortex. This number is much too high for direct assessment. Results are extrapolated from samples on which the density of neurons (i.e., their number by unit volume) has been measured. The mean neuronal density evaluated in the samples is then multiplied by the volume of the cortex. The procedure implies two different quantitative evaluations, both of which are subject to errors: one of neuronal density and one of cortical volume. Both measures are necessary. One may indeed imagine extreme and ideal situations in which the volume of the cortex does not change but the neuronal density declines or, on the contrary, the volume of the cortex shrinks and the neuronal density does not change.[156] Atrophy seen in AD shows that the latter mechanism indeed is in play. The reader may imagine that the death of a neuron leaves a hole in the cortex. It would then suffice to count the number of the neurons in the sample to detect the presence of "holes," responsible for a decline in neuronal density. In fact, the death of a neuron is immediately followed by shrinkage of the neuropile, which, so to speak, fills the holes. Shrinkage has two consequences: the number of neurons per unit volume (i.e., neuronal density) remains the same but the volume of a small part of the cortex decreases—a process which, when repeated, leads to what is known as cortical atrophy.[157] Cortical atrophy explains why neuronal density is only slightly affected in Alzheimer's disease: the shrinkage of the cortex masks the neuronal loss on the microscopical sections.

On the other hand, counting neurons in a microscopic sample does not provide a correct evaluation of neuronal density because it is not only influenced by the density of the neurons in the sample volume but also by their size. To understand this last point, one may consider that the microscopic section is a haphazard hit by the blade of the microtome: the large neurons are more likely to be hit. They are thus oversampled and their density is overestimated. If a population of neurons changes size, its probability of being hit by the microtome blade also changes. For example, if some neurons have become smaller (have shrunk), they are less often cut by the microtome and appear less numerous: however, their number is in fact not reduced and there is no loss. This process, described as "pseudoloss,"[158] should throw some doubts on the idea that neuronal loss involves the large neurons selectively. It may, in fact, be explained by the neuronal atrophy occurring in aging without actual loss. Various methods have been devised to avoid the interference of pseudoloss in the assessment of neuronal density. The most famous is the technique of cell counting known as the "disector"[159]: it consists in using two real or virtual ("optical") sections (hence *di-* for two sections). Only the cells visible in the first section and absent from the second are counted. In so doing, one actually counts one of the poles of the cell, a structure whose presence on the section is said to be independent of the cell size. Using this technique, Regeur et al.[155] were unable to detect neuronal loss in Alzheimer disease's. This result does not indicate that neuronal loss does not take place: it shows that it, in that study, it was below the sensitivity of the count. In other words, neuronal loss was of a lower magnitude than interindividual variation in the number of neurons. That neuronal loss is difficult to ascertain is clearly reflected in the various diagnostic criteria: none mention it.

The use of the disector method in restricted areas of the cortex has, on the contrary, shown that a severe neuronal loss can be measured when the counts are focused on specific regions, such as the entorhinal cortex[160] or associative isocortical areas.[161] In another study, where the neurons of a sample from the supramarginal gyrus (an associative area) were fully mapped, the neuronal loss could be shown only in the most affected cases, but then appeared severe.[162]

Synaptic Loss

The loss of synapses may be revealed by antibodies labeling their constituents. Synaptophysin has been the most widely used marker of synapses. Immunohistochemistry or immunoblots have shown a dramatic decrease in the concentration of synaptophysin in the cerebral cortex of AD patients. On the other hand, observations with electron microscopy have resulted in the conclusion that the decrease in the number of synapses was associated with an increase in apposition length: the synapses are less abundant but bigger in AD.[163,164] This could explain why markers of the synaptic membrane (such as SNAP25) are relatively less affected[165] than those of the synaptic vesicles.[166] It has been said that synaptic loss was the best correlate of dementia in AD[167]—an opinion that has been challenged.[168]

CLINICOPATHOLOGIC FRONTIERS OF AD

Dementia with Lewy Bodies

A large number of Lewy bodies has been found in the isocortex of patients with dementia and parkinsonism. First described in two American patients,[169] the disease was later named "diffuse Lewy body disease"[170–172] or "diffuse cortical Lewy body disease."[173–175]

Lewy bodies are spherical inclusions found in the cytoplasm of neurons. Their shape is somewhat different in the brainstem and in the cortex. With standard H&E stain, they appear bright red and surrounded by a clear halo when they involve brainstem neurons. In the cortex, the halo is lacking. Lewy bodies are ubiquitinated. Ubiquitin is a normal constituent of the cell that recognizes misfolded proteins and targets them toward the proteasome, a multicatalytic system that destroys them. Antiubiquitin antibodies label Lewy bodies with a high sensitivity.[176,*] Rare familial cases of PD appear to be due to mutations of the alpha-synuclein gene. This finding has helped to show that Lewy bodies contain alpha synuclein or perhaps are principally made of it. Synucleins are synaptic proteins whose functions remain unknown. Anti–alpha synuclein and ubiquitin antibodies label not only the Lewy bodies but also processes ("Lewy processes"), probably mostly axons that are enlarged and are filled by ubiquitinated alpha synuclein.

In Parkinson's disease, Lewy bodies involve pigmented neurons of the *substantia nigra,* locus ceruleus, and dorsal vagal nucleus. They are also abundant in the nucleus basalis of Meynert[177,178] and in the amygdala.[179] A small number of Lewy bodies is almost constantly found in the cortex of PD patients who were not demented during life.[180] Lewy processes, located in a small sector of the hippocampus called CA2-3, are also quite frequently observed.[181–183]

Cortical Lewy bodies are also found in cases presenting with severe dementia that is evolving rapidly. In the latter situation, Lewy bodies tend to be associated with Alzheimer pathology of a sufficient severity to warrant the diagnosis of AD according to current criteria. The abundance of senile plaques and the scarcity of NFTs could be characteristic.[184]

Various terms have been used to describe those cases: *Lewy body dementia,*[185] *senile dementia of the Lewy body type,*[186] and *Lewy body variant of AD.*[175] Consensus conferences[187,188] have proposed the term *dementia with Lewy bodies,* which has gained general acceptance. The term indicates that the diagnosis is clinicopathologic. The clinician makes the diagnosis of dementia. The most frequently observed characteristics include fluctuation of symptoms, visual hallucinations, and parkinsonism. The pathologist may then classify the case according to the abundance and topography

* This antibody is not specific for Lewy bodies and stains also the tangles which can be recognized on account of their shape.

of the Lewy bodies (brainstem type = usual PD; diffuse type = a large number of Lewy bodies in the cortex; transitional type = intermediate between brainstem type and diffuse type[189]). The "common type" is associated with Alzheimer pathology, while the "pure type" is devoid of it.[189] The diagnosis of "dementia with Lewy bodies" applies to cases with numerous cortical Lewy bodies in which the cognitive alterations were the first symptoms or followed parkinsonism by less than a year.

There is some controversy concerning the significance of the Lewy bodies. It has recently been stressed that Lewy bodies can be found in patients with familial AD due to mutations of APP or presenilin or with trisomy 21.[190–192] It has also been noticed that in dementia with Lewy bodies and Alzheimer pathology the ApoE4 allele, a risk factor for AD, was overrepresented.[193] The prevalence of dementia with Lewy bodies varies considerably from one geographic area to another and can reach one-third of the cases in some centers, whereas it amounts only to a small percentage in others. A report by Hansen[175] has stated that of 36 patients with dementia, fulfilling AD criteria (which exclude patients presenting with parkinsonism), 13 (36 percent) had Lewy bodies. A report based on 150 unselected cases[194] and a review by Lennox[195] have presented data suggesting that close to 20 percent of patients with dementia may have cortical Lewy bodies. This would make dementia with Lewy bodies (DLB) the most frequent cause of primary dementia after AD. Some data indicate that the disease is more frequent among males, thus following the pattern of PD rather than AD. The average duration of the disease, about 6 years, tends to be shorter than that of the duration of either AD or PD. It parallels, however, the duration found in PD patients with dementia and AD-like neuropathologic changes.[196] Several recent studies suggest that patients with DLB have a better response to anticholinesterase drugs than AD patients.[303]

Argyrophilic Grains Disease

While systematically screening patients with dementia, H. and E. Braak observed lesions that had previously escaped the attention of the neuropathologists.[197] Entorhinal cortex and hippocampus contained spindle-shaped grains a few micrometers in diameter. They were visible after Gallyas silver stain. In 8 of the 56 cases examined, grains were the only lesions. In 8 other cases, they were associated with AD. Further studies revealed accumulation of argyrophilic material in oligodendrocytes, an alteration that was called a *coiled body*[198] and was found mainly in the white matter. Grains and coiled bodies are also found in the amygdala (basolateral nuclei) and in the lateral tuberal nucleus of the hypothalamus.[198] In the areas that contain grains, antibodies against tau protein reveal accumulation of the protein within the cell body without tangle formation, an aspect known as a *pretangle*.. Grains are also tau-positive and appear to be located in the dendrites of the tau-positive neurons.[199,200] Ballooned neurons are commonly found in the amygdala.[201] Grains, pretangles, and coiled bodies define a disease that is frequently but not necessarily associated with AD. The ApoE4 allele is not associated with an increased risk of argyrophilic grains disease. The prevalence of the grains is very high in autopsy series and may be compared to the prevalence of AD lesions.[202] The clinical symptoms associated with grains are still little known. It seems to be clearly established that dementia is not constantly associated with the presence of grains. The extent of the lesions could be an important factor.[203] A clinicopathologic study concerning four cases mentioned memory difficulties and "emotional disorder with aggression or ill temper."[204] Argyrophilic grains disease is presently a purely neuropathologic diagnosis. To our knowledge, it has never been identified in a living individual. Much remains to be done to elucidate the clinical correlates of these lesions and their mechanisms.

Focal Cortical Atrophies

DLB was first defined on the basis of autopsy findings. Other types of dementia have been defined not by their pathology but by their clinical peculiarities. The features of these clinical syndromes are determined mainly by the topography of the lesions and not by their nature. They do not fully correspond to the pathologic classification of the dementias. It may be useful at the present time to keep separate the clinical and the pathologic classifications in order to correctly apprehend the complexity of these diseases. Clinical data have led to separate cases of "typical" AD, where the symptoms suggest a limbic and parieto-temporo-occipital location of the lesions, from cases with a predominant sign, such as apraxia, semantic disorder, frontal syndrome, or visual disturbances.[205–207] On the other hand, pathologic classifications rely on the presence of morphologic markers: NFTs and SPs for AD, Pick bodies in Pick's disease, chromatolytic neurons and cytoskeletal pathology in CBD, Lewy bodies in the just discussed DLD, and tau accumulation in dementia due to mutations on the tau gene. In other instances, no specific pathologic markers can be found; the dementia "lacks distinctive pathology."[208,209] Our current ignorance of the causes of these focal degenerations of the cortex has led to two contrasting approaches: The first, covering all the circumscribed atrophy, would group them together in one large category called *Pick complex.*[210–212] This was really the point of view of Pick himself, who used only gross examination to describe the first cases of focal cortical degenerations. The second approach would employ an analytical point of view, attempting to distinguish by clinical and pathologic means phenomena appearing similar at first sight. We would favor this second approach, which, historically, was followed by Alzheimer himself, who was the first to describe the inclusion bodies found in the condition that ironically now bears the name of Pick.[213,214] In the following sections, we will use the clinical syndromes as the main thread and try to correlate them with the pathologic data.

Primary progressive aphasia (PPA) In 1982, Mesulam[215] described six patients with a slowly progressive aphasia without obvious dementia. No pathology was available (except for a biopsy in one case, which had yielded no specific findings). Mesulam pointed out the differences with other known pathologic entities and thought that, together with a few cases described previously,[216,217] this could represent a new entity.* Since that time, many more cases have been described (see summary of 63 cases in Ref. 218).

The diagnostic criteria proposed by the group of Mesulam[218] emphasize three points:

1. Language disturbances may or may not be accompanied by a disorder of speech; their onset is insidious and their progression gradual.
2. This deficit must remain isolated or nearly so for at least 2 years.
3. It may, however, coexist with disorders such as constructional apraxia and acalculia.

In the majority of the clinicopathologic cases that have been published up to now, no pathologic markers have been found: neuronal loss and gliosis, poorly specific laminar spongiosis (different from the status spongiosis of Creutzfeldt-Jakob disease), and some chromatolytic neurons were present in large cortical regions, encompassing the language areas. In a high proportion of cases, AD pathology was the main finding; this suggests that it may be localized for a long period of time, although no neuropathologic evidence of focal AD pathology has been published. Finally, Pick bodies have been found in some cases,[219–221] justifying the diagnosis of Pick's disease. In view of the focal nature of Pick's pathology, the latter findings are less surprising than those of AD-like pathology. These findings do not contradict the existence of PPA as a real clinical entity, since Mesulam has insisted on the clinical nature of this diagnosis, stating that it may be associated with different neuropathologic substrates. Familial incidence of the condition is known to occur.[222]

Frontal Lobe Degeneration (FLD), Dementia of Frontal Lobe Type (DFT), Frontotemporal Lobar Degeneration, Other Lobar Atrophies Dementias with predominant frontal syndrome have been identified for a long time.[223,224] Pathology showed Pick bodies, chromatolytic neurons and neuronal loss (Pick disease of "type A" according to Constantinidis[225,226]), chromatolytic neurons and neuronal loss (type B), or isolated neuronal loss (type C). A new interest in those dementias came from Sweden, where "frontal lobe dementia" or FLD was described anew as a pathologic entity[227] with matching neuropsychiatric and cerebral blood flow changes. Neary and colleagues in Manchester[228] had previously pointed out that cerebral atrophy and cognitive changes need not

* To these, one should add the carefully documented case of Wechsler[301]; it has been argued that the composer Maurice Ravel, who suffered from a neurodegenerative disease in the last years of his life, may also represented an early case of progressive aphasia.[302]

be synonymous with AD or Pick's disease. Since that time, both groups have written extensively on these topics, pointing out that the cortex was not the only region of the nervous system to be involved. A consensus conference tried to unify the terminology and proposed the term *frontotemporal lobar degeneration* (FTLD). FTLD includes three "prototypic" syndromes: frontotemporal dementia, progressive nonfluent aphasia, and semantic dementia.[229] FTLD occurs more often in males below the age of 65, and about half of these patients have a positive family history. Initial symptoms include mainly personality changes, social misconduct, and language or speech disorders often evolving toward mutism. Later, neurologic signs such as primitive reflexes and extrapyramidal signs (mainly akinesia and rigidity) emerge. Electroencephalography (EEG) and SPECT tend to show changes in the frontal regions. FLD and other lobar atrophies are discussed in detail in an issue of the journal *Neurocase* (the issue of July 2001). As is the case with practically all neurologic syndromes, the clinical picture found in patients with this pathology reflects the topographic distribution of the lesions rather than the specific histologic features. Bilateral frontal lobe lesions are related to the syndrome of DFT. When the left cerebral hemisphere is predominantly affected, the clinical picture is characterized mainly by nonfluent aphasia. Fluent aphasia and visual agnosia are associated with bilateral involvement of the temporal lobes.

Progressive Apraxia (Corticobasal Degeneration) Isolated, sometimes unilateral apraxia, usually accompanied by parkinsonism, may develop over years. Neuropathologic examination often discloses neuronal loss in the substantia nigra. Some remaining neurons contain a fibrillary, tau-positive inclusion. Neuronal loss and gliosis are marked in the parietal lobe, and large "achromatic" neurons are seen: this condition, first described by Rebeiz et al.[230] under the name of *corticodentatonigral degeneration,* is now more often identified as corticobasal degeneration[231] (*basal* stands for the lesions of the substantia nigra located at the base of the brain). Tau immunohistochemistry has shown extensive cytoskeletal pathology both in subcortical nuclei and in the affected areas (mainly the parietal and premotor cortex). Tau accumulates in neurons as neurofibrillary tangles and in glia as astrocytic plaques and coiled bodies.[232] Astrocytic plaques are considered the marker of the disease[233]; tau accumulates at the end of the astrocytic processes and spares the proximal part, which appears empty on immunohistochemistry (see diagram in Ref. 234). Coiled bodies are less specific: they synthesize the accumulation of tau in the cytoplasm of the oligodendrocytes and between the myelin lamellae.[235] The markers of corticobasal degeneration were found in several cases of frontal lobe dementia, clinically resembling Pick's disease,[236] and of primary progressive aphasia.[237] On the other hand, typical pathology of progressive supranuclear palsy (PSP, or Steele-Richardson-Olzewski disease) has also been seen in patients with progressive apraxia.[238] In PSP, accumulation of tau in the astrocytes fills the entire cellular processes—a neuropathologic lesion called a *tufted astrocyte.* In addition, the predominant sign of AD at onset may also be apraxia.[239–241]

NORMAL AGING

Not all the persons who develop AD are old, yet AD is a typical example of age-associated disease. The symptoms of AD are so closely tied to age that it has been hard to separate AD from "senility." It was long thought normal for elderly persons to lose their memory. The finding of lesions typical of Alzheimer's disease (previously thought to be a "presenile" disease in those cases) explains the rather awkward term *senile dementia of the Alzheimer type*[242] that was used for several years. AD is now being considered a disease, whatever its age of onset. Is that fully justified? Is it necessary to include descriptions of AD changes in the context of the changes that accompany normal aging?

Several factors complicate the study of normal aging. Clinicians and researchers alike are aware that the variability in intellectual functioning found in normal adults increases greatly with age.[243] This is probably because age is often accompanied by other events (arterial hypertension, diabetes, traumas, etc.) that may affect the brain to a greater or lesser extent. The methods used in selecting subjects included in studies of aging are a major factor of bias in research, and it is necessary to stress that all studies on "normal" aging must be interpreted in the light of the selection of the subjects involved. *Longitudinal* studies use a group of individuals who are studied for as long as the study lasts. Limitations on these kinds of studies include, obviously, their cost as well as logistic difficulties. In addition, the sample is bound to dwindle more or less rapidly because of death, loss of motivation, etc. Examples of large and fruitful longitudinal studies include the Seattle Longitudinal Study[244,245] and the Framingham Study.[246,247]

On the other hand, *cross-sectional* studies are performed at a given time (sometimes, when the question concerns the prevalence of a given disorder, on a single day) and often use several groups of different ages. Obviously these cross-sectional studies do not suffer from a loss of sampled subjects. They are faced, however, with another drawback, the so-called *cohort effect.* In neuropsychology, this term refers to the changes in performance related to the different socioeconomic and educational characteristics of people of different ages (presumably more important for younger people) and differences in number of relevant medical events (usually greater for older persons). It is not surprising that longitudinal studies tend to show a lesser decline of performance with age than cross-sectional studies do. Cohort effects also apply to other aspects of the study of aging, such as the study of brain weight in relation to aging.[248]

Neuropathology and Normal Aging

To include within one title the words normal and pathology may look like an oxymoron. However, even when the methodologic problems mentioned above are taken into account, the great majority of research confirms the intuitive notion that intellectual abilities deteriorate with age, at least to some extent (see Ref. 249 for a review). It is therefore necessary to attempt to establish the morphologic basis of these changes. Two categories of changes have been identified: AD-like changes and cerebral atrophy with neuronal loss. The latter have been extensively studied, with contrasting results.

Atrophy and Neuronal Loss

Macroscopically, the most "obvious" changes concern loss of volume and weight. An age-related decrease in *normal* adult brain weight[250] was overestimated because of a cohort effect in cross-sectional studies: young brains came from patients born much later in the century.[248] Once the secular increase in adult body length and brain weight are taken into account, the volume of the cerebral hemispheres does not change significantly until age 50; from then on, it decreases by 2 percent per decade.[251,252] In a series of 51 normal brains, the decline appeared to occur mostly after age 55.[253] Atrophy is best assessed by comparing the volume of a given brain to that of its own cranial capacity.[254] The brain fills about 92 percent of the cavity in the sixth decade, 83 percent in the ninth, and 81 percent in the tenth. Tomlinson et al.[255] found no case with marked or generalized cortical atrophy in elderly normal individuals at neuropathologic examination. A slight atrophy in the parasagittal gyri of the frontal and parietal lobes or generalized isolated frontal atrophy was sometimes observed, contrasting with the normal shape of the cerebellum. With CT, gyral atrophy is first seen at about age 40 and increases thereafter.[256] Studies have attempted to follow longitudinally the decrease in brain volume with age[257,258]: using MRI, the mean annual rate of decrease in hippocampal volume was found to be 1.55 +/− 1.38 percent per year in intellectually normal individuals aged 70 to 89. It reached 4 percent in those with Alzheimer's disease. However, atrophy is lacking in some aged individuals. Some people with atrophy have normal brain function and, finally, brains at autopsy sometimes fail to exhibit the atrophy that had been seen with CT. The volume of the brain in vivo is indeed highly dependent on the individual's hydration status and can thus fluctuate.

The microscopic changes that accompany aging vary and are controversial. Neuronal loss, when it occurs, is not uniform. Authors were probably not as aware of the stereologic bias before 1984,[159] when Gundersen, under the pseudonym of Sterio, published the disector method (see above), showing that when profiles of sectioned neurons are counted, large neurons, which will be often cut, are overrepresented compared to small ones. The disector method (using two sections) avoids the bias. We do not believe that this bias was of a sufficient magnitude[158] to justify dismissing previous literature. Our discussion is therefore not confined to the results obtained with the disector method.

A neuronal loss (amounting to 12 percent of the neuronal profiles) has been documented in the hippocampus during aging.[259,260] This loss involves mainly the hilar region and the subiculum. In Alzheimer's disease, CA1 is mainly affected, as shown by studies using the disector method.[261,262] The loss of isocortical neurons with aging has been discussed. Brody[263] found a high correlation between age and the number of neuronal profiles included in five strips of cortex taken perpendicular to the pial surface. The greatest changes were found in the superotemporal and precentral gyri, while the postcentral gyrus and the area striata (visual cortex) were the least affected.[263] By contrast, Haug[264] and Terry[253] did not find any significant change in the density of the neuronal profiles but observed a negative correlation between the size of the perikaryon and age. The ratio large/small neurons was also found to decrease with age in the studies by Henderson et al.[265] This atrophy of the cell body of the neurons reduces their apparent number on sections (pseudoloss).[158]

The total number of neurons in the neocortex in relation to aging has been studied more recently with the disector[266]: the loss of neocortical neurons during a life period extending from 20 to 90 years of age was considered to reach 10 percent. Such a decrease in neuronal number would cause "an 'average' loss of about 85000 neurons per day." It is interesting to note that this figure was reached previously by other means.[267] In summary, the density of neuronal profiles in sections does not change much with age, but the volume of the brain decreases slightly. The net effect is a relatively mild loss of neurons in view of the individual variations (which can reach 200 percent).

In the brainstem, neuronal loss during aging has been documented, but it appears heterogeneous. Some nuclei—such as the ventral cochlear, trochlear, and abducens, or the inferior olive—show no cell loss with age.[268–271] On the contrary, the number of neurons decreases in the locus ceruleus[268,272]—a finding that has been discussed[273,274]—and the Purkinje cell layer.[275] In the substantia nigra, the neuronal loss was thought to involve mainly the medial and dorsal tiers of the pars compacta, while the brunt of the pathology is located in the lateral tier in Parkinson's disease.[276–278] Recent results, however, show large individual variations. Centenarians may exhibit a high density of neurons.[279]

Neuronal loss has been documented in the thalamus[280]; putamen[281]; mediocentral, medial, and cortical nuclei of the amygdala[282]; and nucleus basalis of Meynert.[283,284]

AD-Like Changes AD-like microscopic changes—Aβ diffuse deposits, neuritic SPs, and NFTs—are often found in the cortex of old individuals considered to be intellectually normal.[285,286] NFTs tend to increase with age and can be observed in most individuals past the seventh decade; they are localized mainly in the hippocampus and the entorhinal cortex.[287–289] Half the population in a large cohort of cases studied by Braak[289] had at least a few tangles in the entorhinal region at the age of 47. All the 12 centenarians studied by Delaère et al. and Hauw et al.[290,291] had at least a few tangles and some Aβ deposits.

These lesions have been interpreted as being part of normal aging or as evidence of presymptomatic AD. It is presently impossible to determine whether the presence of a few lesions in the entorhinal cortex is evidence of AD at onset[286] or will remain anatomically limited and clinically silent. Are they, like cataracts, an

Table 44-2
Location of neurofibrillary tangles (NFT) and senile plaques (SPs) in normal aging and in Alzheimer's disease (AD)

Structure	*NFT aging*	*NFT AD*	*SP aging*	*SP AD*
Hippocampus and entorhinal cortex	++	+++	++	+++
Parahippocampal gyrus	+	+++	±	++
Amygdala	+	+++	++	+++
Neocortex	±	++	+	+++
Subcortical gray nuclei	±	++	±	++

Key: ± = minimal or borderline lesions; + = moderate lesions; ++ = clearcut lesions; + + + = severe lesions.
Source: Based on data of Hauw and Delaère,[292] with permission.

inescapable consequence of time? Are they evidence of a disease against which most individuals have efficient barriers (as in the case of rubella in young children)? Are they the stigmata of the early phases of a disease, which would have been full-blown if the patient had survived long enough? These three possibilities remain open at the present time. It is, however, important to stress that while these lesions can be found in both intellectually normal persons and AD patients, their location tends to be different, as shown in Table 44-2, adapted from data of Hauw and Delaère.[292]

CONCLUSIONS

What is the position of AD in current nosology? It has been thought by some to be inevitable, as if it were part of the history of the human race—an unavoidable scourge of phylogeny. However, recent studies have shown that AD may well represent a stereotyped mode of reaction of the brain to different types of aggression—a syndrome rather than a disease. Such a stereotyped reaction of the nervous system is probably due to the fact that it is deeply linked to normal functioning of the brain. In AD, the pathologic process dissects, within the nerves' parenchyma, networks of neurons and fibers connected to the hippocampal-entorhinal complex. According to our present knowledge, these connections are mainly involved in the "making of memories" at all levels, including the neocortex, where they are stored. AD pathology may then not be adequately covered by our usual neurologic reasoning in terms of "areas" of the cortex, since it rapidly implicates a great number of them and does not fully abolish their functions, as for instance, infarcts would do. AD can therefore be said to be "transareal"—i.e., it probably implicates the same network within different cortical regions. This naturally leads us to consider that the functions of the brain are distributed within two different systems of organization: one being areal and corresponding to the old concept of "cerebral localization" and the other transareal or laminar and involving the linkage of different cortices within a given domain, such as memory. These questions concerning the mechanisms of AD relate to the functioning of the brain itself. The solution of the problems they raise may unveil some of the mysteries of the most complex object of the known universe: the human brain.

REFERENCES

1. Walshe F: *Diseases of the Nervous System.* London: Livingstone, 1958.
2. Merritt H: *A Textbook of Neurology.* Philadelphia: Lea & Febiger, 1967.
3. Boller F, Muggia S: Non-Alzheimer dementias, in Denes G, Pizzamiglio G (eds): *Handbook of Clinical and Experimental Neuropsychology.* Hove, England: Psychology Press, 1999.
4. Pick A: Über die Beziehungen der senilen Hirnatrophie zur Aphasie. *Prager Med Wochenschr* 17:165, 1892.
5. Alzheimer A: Uber Eine eigenartige Erkrankung der Hirnrinde. *Allge Zeitschr Psychiatrie Psych Gericht Med* 64:146, 1907.
6. Seglas J: *Les troubles du langage chez les aliénés.* Paris: Rueff, 1892.
7. Amaducci L, Rocca W, Schoenberg B: Origin of the distinction between Alzheimer's disease and senile dementia. How history can clarify nosology. *Neurology* 36:1497, 1986.
8. Roth M: Aging of the brain and dementia: An overview, in Amaducci L, Davison A, Antuono P (eds): *Aging of the Brain and Dementia.* New York: Raven Press, 1980.
9. Katzman R, Terry R, Bick K: Alzheimer's disease: Senile dementia and related disorders, in *Aging.* New York: Raven Press, 1978, vol 5, p 595.
10. Adams RD, Victor M: *Principles of Neurology.* New York: McGraw-Hill, 1993.
11. Perusini G: Sul valore nosografico di alcuni reperti istopatologici caratteristici per la senilità. *Riv Ital Neuropatolo Psichiatria Elettroter* 4:145, 1911.
12. Lewey F: Alois Alzheimer, in Haymaker W, Schiller F (eds): *The Founders of Neurology.* Springfield IL: Charles C Thomas, 1970 pp. 315–319.
13. Pomponi M, Marta M: "On the suggestion of Dr. Alzheimer I examined the following four cases." Dedicated to Gaetano Perusini. *Aging* 5:135, 1993.
14. Boller F, Forbes MA: History of dementia and dementia in history: An overview. *J Neurol Sci* 158:125, 1998.
15. Boller F, Dalla Barba G: Neuropsychological tests in Alzheimer's disease. *Aging (Milan)* 13:210, 2001.
16. van Hout H, Teunisse S, Derix M, et al: CAMDEX, can it be more efficient? Observational study on the contribution of four screening measures to the diagnosis of dementia by a memory clinic team. *Int J Geriatr Psychiatry* 16:64, 2001.

17. Roth M, Tym E, Mountjoy C, et al: CAMDEX: A standardized instrument for the diagnosis of mental disorder in the elderly with special reference to the early detection of dementia. *Br J Psychiatry* 149:698, 1986.
18. Rosen W, Mohs R, Davis K: A new rating scale for Alzheimer's disease. *Am J Psychiatry* 141:1356, 1984.
19. Pena-Casanova J: Alzheimer's Disease Assessment Scale–Cognitive in clinical practice. *Int Psychogeriatr* 9(suppl 1):105, 1997.
20. Boller F, Verny M, Hugonot L, et al: Clinical features of severe dementia. A review. *Eur J Neurol.* In press.
21. American Psychiatric Association: *Diagnostic and Statistical Manual of Mental Disorders.* Washington, DC: American Psychiatric Association, 1994.
22. McKhann G, Drachman D, Folstein M, et al: Clinical diagnosis of Alzheimer's disease: Report of the NINCDS-ADRDA Work Group under the auspices of the Department of Health and Human Services Task Force on Alzheimer's Disease. *Neurology* 34:939, 1984.
23. Huff FJ, Becker JT, Belle SH, et al: Cognitive deficits and diagnosis of Alzheimer's Disease. *Neurology* 36:1198, 1987.
24. Tierney MC, Fisher RH, Lewis AJ, et al: The NINCDS-ADRDA Work Group criteria for the clinical diagnosis of probable Alzheimer's disease: A clinicopathological study of 57 cases. *Neurology* 38:359, 1988.
25. Morris JC, Heyman A, Mohs RC, et al: The Consortium to Establish a Registry for Alzheimer's Disease (CERAD). Part I. Clinical and neuropsychological assessment of Alzheimer's disease. *Neurology* 39:1159, 1989.
26. Welsh KA, Butters N, Hughes JP, et al: Detection of abnormal memory decline in mild cases of Alzheimer's disease using CERAD neuropsychological measures. *Arch Neurol* 48:278, 1991.
27. Folstein MF, Folstein SE, McHugh PR: "Mini Mental State": A practical method for grading the cognitive state of patients for the clinician. *J Psychiatr Res* 12:189, 1975.
28. Blessed G, Tomlinson BE, Roth M: The association between quantitative measures of dementia and senile change in the cerebral grey matter of elderly subjects. *Br J Psychiatry* 114:797, 1968.
29. Hughes CP, Berg L, Danziger WL, et al: A new clinical scale for the staging of dementia. *Br J Psychiatry* 140:566, 1982.
30. Todorov A, Go R, Constantinidis J, et al: Specificity of the clinical diagnosis of dementia. *J Neurol Sci* 26:81, 1975.
31. Boller F, Lopez OL, Moossy J: Diagnosis of dementia: Clinicopathologic correlations. *Neurology* 39:76, 1989.
32. Martin EM, Wilson RS, Penn RD, et al: Cortical biopsy results in Alzheimer's disease: Correlation with cognitive deficits. *Neurology* 37:1201, 1987.
33. Morris JC, Berg L, Fulling K, et al: Validation of clinical diagnostic criteria in senile dementia of the Alzheimer type. *Ann Neurol* 22:122, 1987.
34. Mirra S, Gearing M, Mckeel D, et al: Interlaboratory comparison of neuropathology assessments in Alzheimer's disease: A study of the consortium to establish a registry for Alzheimer's disease (CERAD). *J Neuropathol Exp Neurol* 53:303, 1994.
35. Bracco L, Gallato R, Lippi A, et al: Factors affecting course and survival in Alzheimer's disease. A nine-year longitudinal study. *Arch Neurol* 51:1213, 1994.
36. Hébert M, Parlato V, Lese GB, et al: Survival in institutionalized patients: Influence of dementia and loss of functional capacities. *Arch Neurol* 52:469, 1995.
37. Absher JR, Cummings J: Noncognitive behavioral alterations in dementia syndromes, in Boller F, Grafman J (eds): *Handbook of Neuropsychology.* Amsterdam: Elsevier, 1993.
38. St George-Hyslop PH, et al: The genetic defect causing familial Alzheimer's disease maps on chromosome 21. *Science* 235:885, 1987.
39. Schellenberg GD, Bird TD, Wijsman EM, et al: Genetic linkage evidence for a familial Alzheimer's disease locus on chromosome-14. *Science* 258:668, 1992.
40. Pericak-Vance MA, Bebout JL, Gaskell PC, et al: Linkage studies in familial Alzheimer disease—evidence for chromosome-19 linkage. *Am J Hum Genet* 48:1034, 1991.
41. Levy-Lahad E, Wijsman E, Nemens E, et al.: A familial Alzheimer's disease locus on chromosome 1. *Science* 269:970, 1995.
42. Corder EH, Saunders AM, Strittmatter WJ, et al: Gene dose of apolipoprotein E type 4 allele and the risk of Alzheimer's disease in late onset families. *Science,* 261:921, 1993.
43. Saunders AM, Schmader K, Breither JC, et al: Apolipoprotein E e4 allele distribution in late-onset Alzheimer's disease and other amyloid-forming diseases. *Lancet* 342:710, 1993.
44. Poirier J, Davignon J, Bouthillier D, et al: Apolipoprotein E polymorphism and Alzheimer's disease. *Lancet* 342:697, 1993.
45. West H, Rebeck G, Growdon J, et al: Apolipoprotein E4 affects neuropathology but not clinical progression in Alzheimer's disease (abstr). *Neurobiol Aging* 15(suppl 1): S28, 1994.

46. Bird T: Apolipoprotein E genotyping in the diagnosis of Alzheimer's disease: A cautionary view. *Ann Neurol* 38:2, 1995.
47. Berr C, Hauw JJ, Delaere P, et al: Apoliprotein E allele epsilon 4 is linked to increased deposition of the amyloid beta-peptide (A-beta) in cases with or without Alzheimer's disease. *Neurosci Lett* 178:221, 1994.
48. Schneider J, Gearing M, Robbins R, et al: Apolipoprotein E genotype in diverse neurodegenerative disorders. *Ann Neurol* 38:131, 1995.
49. Greenberg S, Rebeck G, Vonsattel J, et al: Apolipoprotein E e4 and cerebral hemorrhage associated with amyloid angiopathy. *Ann Neurol* 38:254, 1995.
50. vanGool W, Evenhuis H, vanDuijn C: A case-control study of apolipoprotein E genotypes in Alzheimer's disease associated with Down's syndrome. *Ann Neurol* 38:225, 1995.
51. Amouyel P, Vidal O, Launay J, et al: The apolipoprotein E alleles as major susceptibility factors for Creutzfeldt-Jakob disease. *Lancet* 344:1315, 1994.
52. Marder K, Maestre G, Cote L, et al: The apolipoprotein e 4 allele in Parkinson's disease with and without dementia. *Neurology* 44:1330, 1994.
53. Rossor M, Kennedy A, Newman S: Heterogeneity in familial Alzheimer's disease, in Boller F, Forette F, Khatchaturian Z, et al (eds): *Heterogeneity of Alzheimer's Disease.* Berlin: Springer-Verlag, 1992.
54. Huff F, Auerbach J, Chakravarti A, et al: Risk of dementia in relatives of patients with Alzheimer's disease. *Neurology* 38:786, 1988.
55. Breitner J, Welsh K, Gau B, et al: Alzheimer's disease in the National Academy of Sciences–National Research Council Registry of Aging Twin Veterans. *Arch Neurol* 52:763, 1995.
56. Hofman A, Schulte W, Tanja T, et al: History of dementia and Parkinson's disease in 1st-degree relatives of patients with Alzheimer's disease. *Neurology* 39:1589, 1989.
57. Heyman A, Wilkinson W, Hurwitz B, et al: Alzheimer's disease: Genetic aspects and associated clinical disorders. *Ann Neurol* 14:507, 1983.
58. Berr C, Borghi E, Rethoré M, et al: Absence of familial association between dementia and Down syndrome. *Am J Med Genet* 33:545, 1989.
59. Ogunniyi A, Baiyewu O, Gureje O, et al: Epidemiology of dementia in Nigeria: Results from the Indianapolis-Ibadan study. *Eur J Neurol* 7:485, 2000.
60. Fratiglioni L, Rocca W: Epidemiology of dementia, in Boller F, Cappa S (eds): *Handbook of Neuropsychology.* Amsterdam: Elsevier, 2001.
61. Katzman R: Education and the prevalence of dementia and Alzheimer's disease. *Neurology* 43:13, 1993.
62. Stern Y, Tang M, Denaro J, et al: Increased risk of mortality in Alzheimer's disease patients with more advanced educational and occupational attainment. *Ann Neurol* 37:590, 1995.
63. Letenneur L, Dartigues J, Commenges D, et al: Tobacco consumption and cognitive impairment in elderly people. A population-based study. *Ann Epidemiol* 4:449, 1994.
64. Letenneur L, Dartigues J, Orgogozo J: Wine consumption in the elderly. *Ann Intern Med* 118:317, 1993.
65. Polich J, Laish C, Bloom F: P300 assessment of early Alzheimer's disease. *Electroencephalogr Clin Neurophysiol* 77:179, 1990.
66. George AE, De Leon MJ, Stylopoulous LA, et al: CT diagnostic features of Alzheimer disease. Importance of the choroidal/hippocampal fissure complex. *AJNR* 11:101, 1990.
67. Jack CR Jr, Petersen RC, O'Brien PC, et al: MR-based hippocampal volumetry in the diagnosis of Alzheimer's disease. *Neurology* 42:183, 1992.
68. Cuénod CA, Denys A, Michot JL, et al: Amygdala atrophy in Alzheimer's disease: An in vivo Magnetic resonance imaging study. *Arch Neurol* 50:941, 1993.
69. Cuénod C, Kaplan D, Michot J, et al: Phospholipid abnormalities in early Alzheimer's disease: In vivo 31P NMR spectroscopy. *Arch Neurol* 52:89, 1995.
70. Perani D, Cappa S: Brain imaging in normal aging and dementia, in Boller F, Cappa S (eds): *Handbook of Neuropsychology.* Amsterdam: Elsevier, 2001.
71. O'Brien J, Eagger S, Syed G, et al: A study of regional cerebral blood flow and cognitive performance in Alzheimer's disease. *J Neurol Neurosurg Psychiatry* 55:1182, 1992.
72. Foster NL, Chase TH, Fedio P, et al: Alzheimer's disease: Focal cortical changes shown by positron emission tomography. *Neurology* 33:961, 1983.
73. Haxby J: Cognitive deficits and local metabolic changes in dementia of the Alzheimer type, in Rapoport S, Petit H, Leys D, Christen Y (eds): *Imaging, Cerebral Topography and Alzheimer's Disease.* Berlin: Springer-Verlag, 1990.
74. Steinling M, Leys D: Patterns of dementia in Alzheimer's disease. *J Nucl Med* 33:1431, 1992.
75. Keilp J, Prohovnik I: Intellectual decline predicts the parietal perfusion deficit in Alzheimer's disease. *J Nucl Med* 36:1347, 1995.
76. Scheltens PH: Structural neuroimaging of Alzheimer's disease and other dementias. *Aging (Milan)* 13:203, 2001.

77. Mesulam M-M: *Principles of behavioral Neurology.* Philadelphia: Davis, 1985
78. Zeki S: *A Vision of the Brain.* Oxford: Blackwell, 1993.
79. Delacoste MC, White CL: The role of cortical connectivity in Alzheimer's disease pathogenesis—a review and model system. *Neurobiol Aging* 14:1, 1993.
80. Duyckaerts C, Hauw J-J, Bastenaire F, et al: Laminar ditribution of neocortical plaques in senile dementia of the Alzheimer type. *Acta Neuropathol (Berl)* 70:249, 1986.
81. Khachaturian ZS: Diagnosis of Alzheimer's disease. *Arch Neurol* 42:1097, 1985.
82. Mirra SS, Heyman A, McKeel D, et al: The consortium to establish a registry in Alzheimer's disease (CERAD). Part II: Standardization of the neuropathologic assessment of Alzheimer's disease. *Neurology* 41:479, 1991.
83. Wilcock GK, Esiri MM: Plaques, tangles and dementia. A quantitative study. *J Neurol Sci* 57:407, 1982.
84. WorkingGroup: Consensus recommendations for the postmortem diagnosis of Alzheimer's disease. The National Institute on Aging and Reagan Institute Working Group on Diagnostic Criteria for the Neuropathological Assessment of Alzheimer's Disease. *Neurobiol Aging* 18(4 suppl):S1, 1997.
85. Terry RD, Hansen LA, DeTeresa R, et al: Senile dementia of the Alzheimer type without neocortical neurofibrillary tangles. *J Neuropathol Exp Neurol* 46:262, 1987.
86. Bancher C, Jellinger KA: Neurofibrillary tangle predominant form of senile dementia of Alzheimer type: A rare subtype in very old subjects. *Acta Neuropathol (Berl)* 88:565, 1994.
87. Lamy C, Duyckaerts C, Delaère P, et al: Comparison of seven staining methods for senile plaques and neurofibrillary tangles in a prospective study of 15 elderly patients. *Neuropathol Appl Neurobiol* 15:563, 1989.
88. Schmidt M, Lee V, Trojanowski J: Comparative epitope analysis of neuronal cytoskeletal proteins in Alzheimer's disease senile plaque, neurites and neuropil threads. *Lab Invest* 64:352, 1991.
89. Arends YM, Duyckaerts C, Rozemuller JM, et al: Microglia, amyloid and dementia in Alzheimer disease. A correlative study. *Neurobiol Aging* 21:39, 2000.
90. Uchihara T, Kondo H, Akiyama H, et al: White matter amyloid in Alzheimer's disease brain. *Acta Neuropathol (Berl)* 90:51, 1995.
91. Vassar R, Bennett BD, Babu-Khan S, et al: Beta-secretase cleavage of Alzheimer's amyloid precursor protein by the transmembrane aspartic protease BACE. *Science* 286:735, 1999.
92. Dickson TC, Saunders HL, Vickers JC: Relationship between apolipoprotein E and the amyloid deposits and dystrophic neurites of Alzheimer's disease. *Neuropathol Appl Neurobiol* 23:483, 1997.
93. Namba Y, Tomonaga M, Kawasaki H, et al: Apolipoprotein E immunoreactivity in cerebral amyloid deposits and neurofibrillary tangles in Alzheimer's disease and kuru plaque amyloid in Creutzfeldt-Jakob disease. *Brain Res* 541:163, 1991.
94. Uchihara T, Duyckaerts C, He Y, et al: ApoE immunoreactivity and microglial cells in Alzheimer's disease brain. *Neurosci Lett* 195:5, 1995.
95. Wisniewski T, Frangione B: Apolipoprotein E. A pathological chaperone protein in patients with cerebral and systemic amyloid. *Neurosci Lett* 135:235, 1992.
96. Yamaguchi H, Ishiguro K, Sugihara S, et al: Presence of apolipoprotein E on extracellular neurofibrillary tangles and on meningeal blood vessels precedes the Alzheimer ß-amyloid deposition. *Acta Neuropathol (Berl)* 88:413, 1994.
97. Irizarry MC, Cheung BS, Rebeck GW, et al: Apolipoprotein E affects the amount, form, and anatomical distribution of amyloid beta-peptide deposition in homozygous APP(V717F) transgenic mice. *Acta Neuropathol (Berl)* 100:451, 2000.
98. Bales KR, Verina T, Cummins DJ, et al: Apolipoprotein E is essential for amyloid deposition in the APP(V717F) transgenic mouse model of Alzheimer's disease. *Proc Natl Acad Sci U S A* 96:15233, 1999.
99. Bales KR, Verina T, Dodel RC, et al: Lack of apolipoprotein E dramatically reduces amyloid beta-peptide deposition. *Nat Gene* 17:263, 1997.
100. Mori T, Paris D, Town T, et al: Cholesterol accumulates in senile plaques of Alzheimer disease patients and in transgenic APP(SW) mice. *J Neuropathol Exp Neurol* 60:778, 2001.
101. Verbeek MM, Otte-Höller I, Westphal JR, et al: Accumulation of intercellular adhesion molecule-1 in senile plaques in brain tissue of patients with Alzheimer's disease. *Am J Pathol* 144:104, 1994.
102. Buée L, Hof PR, Roberts DD, et al: Immunohistochemical identification of thrombospondin in normal human brain and in Alzheimer's disease. *Am J Pathol* 141:783, 1992.
103. Snow AD, Sekiguchi R, Nochlin D, et al: An important role of heparan sulfate proteoglycan (Perlecan) in a model system for the deposition and persistence of fibrillar A beta-amyloid in rat brain. *Neuron* 12:219, 1994.
104. Abraham CR, Selkoe DJ, Potter H: Immunochemical identification of the serine protease inhibitor a-1

antichymotrypsin in the brain amyloid deposits of Alzheimer's disease. *Cell* 52:487, 1988.

105. Abraham CR, Shirama T, Potter H: a-1 Antichymotrypsin is associated solely with amyloid deposits containing the ß-protein: Amyloid and cell localization of a-1 antichymotrypsin. *Neurobiol Aging* 11:123, 1990.
106. Licastro F, Mallory M, Lawrence AH, et al: Increased levels of alpha-1-antichymotrypsin in brains of patients with Alzheimer's disease correlate with activated astrocytes and are affected by ApoE 4 genotype. *J Neuroimmunol* 88:105, 1998.
107. Nixon RA, Cataldo AM, Mathews PM: The endosomal-lysosomal system of neurons in Alzheimer's disease pathogenesis: A review. *Neurochem Res* 25:1161, 2000.
108. McGeer PL, Kawamata T, Walker DG, et al: Microglia in degenerative neurological diseases. *Glia* 7:84, 1993.
109. McGeer EG, McGeer PL: The importance of inflammatory mechanisms in Alzheimer disease. *Exp Gerontol* 371, 1998.
110. Veerhuis R, Janssen I, Hack CE, et al: Early complement components in Alzheimer's disease brains. *Acta Neuropathol* 91:53, 1996.
111. McGeer PL, Akiyama H, Itagaki S, et al: Complement activation in amyloid plaques in Alzheimer's dementia. *Neurosci Lett* 107:341, 1989.
112. Mrak RE, Griffin WS: Interleukin-1, neuroinflammation, and Alzheimer's disease. *Neurobiol Aging* 22:903, 2001.
113. Huell M, Strauss S, Volk B, et al: Interleukin-6 is present in early stages of plaque formation and is restricted to the brains of Alzheimer's disease patients. *Acta Neuropathol* 89:544, 1995.
114. DiPatre PL, Gelman BB: Microglial cell activation in aging and Alzheimer disease: Partial linkage with neurofibrillary tangle burden in the hippocampus. *J Neuropathol Exp Neurol* 56:143, 1997.
115. Wegiel J, Wisniewski HM: The complex of microglial cells and amyloid star in three-dimensional reconstruction. *Acta Neuropathol* 81:116, 1990.
116. Wegiel J, Wang KC, Tarnawski M, et al: Microglia cells are the driving force in fibrillar plaque formation, whereas astrocytes are a leading factor in plaque degradation. *Acta Neuropathol (Berl)* 100:356, 2000.
117. Dickson DW: The pathogenesis of senile plaques. *J Neuropathol Exp Neurol* 56:321, 1997.
118. Gonatas NK, Anderson W, Evangelista I: The contribution of altered synapses in the senile plaque: An electron microscopic study in Alzheimer's dementia. *J Neuropathol Exp Neurol* 26:25, 1967.
119. Kidd M: Alzheimer's disease. An electron microscopic study. *Brain* 87:307, 1964.
120. Terry RD, Gonatas JK, Weiss M: Ultrastructural studies in Alzheimer presenile dementia. *Am J Pathol* 44:269, 1964.
121. Probst A, Basler V, Bron B, et al: Neuritic plaques in senile dementia of the Alzheimer type : A Golgi analysis in the hippocampal region. *Brain Res* 268:249, 1983.
122. Dickson D: Qualitative differences between senile plaques (SP) in pathological aging (PA) and Alzheimer's disease. *Brain Pathol* 7:1054, 1997.
123. Delaère P, Duyckaerts C, He Y, et al: Subtypes and differential laminar distributions of ßA4 deposits in Alzheimer's disease: Relationship with the intellectual status of 26 cases. *Acta Neuropathol (Berl)* 81:328, 1991.
124. Berg L, McKeel DWJ, Miller JP, et al: Clinicopathologic studies in cognitively healthy aging and Alzheimer's disease: Relation of histologic markers to dementia severity, age, sex, and apolipoprotein E genotype. *Arch Neurol* 55:326, 1998.
125. Bancher C, Jellinger K, Lassmann H, et al: Correlations between mental state and quantitative neuropathology in the Vienna Longitudinal Study on Dementia. *Eur Arch Psychiatr Clin Neurosci* 246:137, 1996.
126. Glenner GG: Amyloid deposits and amyloidosis. The ß-fibrilloses. *N Engl J Med* 302:1283, 1980.
127. Pitas RE, Boyles JK, Lee SH, et al: Astrocytes synthetise apolipoprotein E and metabolize apolipoprotein E–containing lipoproteins. *Biochem Biophys Acta* 917:148, 1987.
128. DeWitt DA, Perry G, Cohen M, et al: Astrocytes regulate microglial phagocytosis of senile plaque cores of Alzheimer's disease. *Exp Neurol* 149:329, 1998.
129. Miyakawa T, Shimoji A, Kuramoto R, et al: The relationship between senile plaques and cerebral blood vessels in Alzheimer's disease and senile dementia. *Virchows Arch* 40:121, 1982.
130. Kawai M, Cras P, Perry G: Serial reconstruction of ß-protein amyloid plaques: Relationship to microvessels and size distribution. *Brain Res* 592:278, 1992.
131. Alzheimer A: Uber eigenartige Krankheitsfälle des späteren Alters. *Zentralbl Gesamte Neurol Psychiatry* 4:356, 1911.
132. Itoh Y, Amano N, Inoue M, et al: Scanning electron microscopical study of the neurofibrillary tangles of Alzheimer's disease. *Acta Neuropathol (Berl)* 94:78, 1997.
133. Pollanen P, Markiewicz P, Bergeron C, et al: Twisted ribbon structure of paired helical filaments revealed by atomic force microscopy. *Am J Pathol* 144:869, 1994.

134. Ruben GC, Iqbal K, Grundke-Iqbal I: Helical ribbon morphology in neurofibrillary tangles of paired helical filaments, in Iqbal K, Mortimer JA, Winblad B, Wisniewski HM (eds): *Research Advances in Alzheimer's Disease and Related Disorders.* Chichester, England: Wiley, 1995.
135. Brion JP, Passareiro H, Nunez J, et al: Mise en évidence immunologique de la protéine tau au niveau des lésions de dégénérescence neurofibrillaire de la maladie d'Alzheimer. *Arch Biol (Brux)* 95:229, 1985.
136. Grundke-Iqbal I, Iqbal K, Tung YC, et al: Abnormal phosphorylation of the microtubule associated protein (tau) in Alzheimer cytoskeletal pathology. *Proc Natl Acad Sci USA* 83:4913, 1986.
137. Delacourte A, Defossez A: Alzheimer's disease: Tau proteins, the promoting factors of microtubule assembly are major components of paired helical filaments. *J Neurol Sci* 76:173, 1986.
138. Flament S, Delacourte A, Hemon B, et al: Démonstration directe d'une phosphorylation anormale des protéines microtubulaires tau au cours de la maladie d'Alzheimer. *CR Acad Sci (Paris)* 208:77, 1989.
139. Flament S, Delacourte A: Abnormal tau species are produced during Alzheimer's disease neurodegenerating process. *FEBS Lett* 247:213, 1989.
140. Delacourte A: Pathological tau proteins of Alzheimer's disease as a biochemical marker of neurofibrillary degeneration. *Biomed Pharmacother* 48:287, 1994.
141. Matsuo ES, Shin RW, Billingsley ML, et al: Biopsy-derived adult human tau is phosphorylated at many of the same sites as Alzheimer's disease paired helical filament tau. *Neuron* 13:989, 1994.
142. Feany M, Ksiezak-Reding H, Liu W, et al: Epitope expression and hyperphosphorylation of tau protein in corticobasal degeneration: Differentiation from progressive supranuclear palsy. *Acta Neuropathol (Berl)* 90:37, 1995.
143. Duyckaerts C, Kawasaki H, Delaère P, et al: Fiber disorganization in the neocortex of patients with senile dementia of the Alzheimer type. *Neuropathol Appl Neurobiol* 15:233, 1989.
144. Braak H, Braak E: Neuropil threads occur in dendrites of tangle-bearing nerve cells. *Neuropathol Appl Neurobiol* 14:39, 1988.
145. Braak H, Braak E, Grundke-Iqbal I, et al: Occurrence of neuropil threads in the senile human brain and in Alzheimer's disease. A third location of paired helical filaments outside of neurofilament tangles and neuritic plaques. *Neurosci Lett* 65:351, 1986.
146. Parvizi J, Van Hoesen GW, Damasio A: The selective vulnerability of brainstem nuclei to Alzheimer's disease. *Ann Neurol* 49:53, 2001.
147. Arnold SE, Hyman BT, Flory J, et al: The topographical and neuroanatomical distribution of neurofibrillary tangles and neuritic plaques in the cerebral cortex of patients with Alzheimer's disease. *Cereb Cortex* 1:103, 1991.
148. Delaère P, Duyckaerts C, Brion JP, et al: Tau, paired helical filaments and amyloid in the neocortex : A morphometric study of 15 cases with graded intellectual status in aging and senile dementia of Alzheimer type. *Acta Neuropathol* 77:645, 1989.
149. Braak H, Braak E: Neuropathological staging of Alzheimer-related changes. *Acta Neuropathol (Berl)* 82:239, 1991.
150. Duyckaerts C, Bennecib M, Grignon Y, et al: Modeling the relation between neurofibrillary tangles and intellectual status. *Neurobiol Aging* 18:267, 1997.
151. Bancher C, Jellinger KA: Neurofibrillary tangle predominant form of senile dementia of Alzheimer's disease: A rare subtype in very old subjects. *Acta Neuropathol (Berl)* 88:565, 1994.
152. Cras P, Smith MA, Richey PL, et al: Extracellular neurofibrillary tangles reflect neuronal loss and provide further evidence of extensive protein cross-linking in Alzheimer disease. *Acta Neuropathol (Berl)* 89:291, 1995.
153. Blanks J, Hinton D, Sadun A, et al: Retinal ganglion cell degeneration in Alzheimer's disease. *Brain Res* 501:364, 1989.
154. Mann DMA: Pathological correlates of dementia in Alzheimer's disease. *Neurobiol Aging* 15:357, 1994.
155. Regeur L, Badsberg Jensen G, Pakkenberg H, et al: No global neocortical nerve cell loss in brains from patients with senile dementia of Alzheimer's type. *Neurobiol Aging* 15:347, 1994.
156. Hauw J-J, Duyckaerts C, Partridge M: Neuropathological aspects of brain aging and SDAT, in *Modern Trends in Aging Research: Colloque Inserm-Eurage.* London: John Libbey Eurotext, 1986.
157. Duyckaerts C, Hauw J-J, Piette F, et al: Cortical atrophy in senile dementia of the Alzheimer type is mainly due to a decrease in cortical length. *Acta Neuropathol (Berl)* 66:72, 1985.
158. Duyckaerts C, Llamas E, Delaère P, et al: Neuronal loss and neuronal atrophy. Computer simulation in connection with Alzheimer's disease. *Brain Res* 504:94, 1989.
159. Sterio DC: The unbiased estimation of number and sizes of arbitrary particles using the disector. *J Microsc* 134:127, 1984.

160. Gomez-Isla T, Price JL, McKeel DW, et al: Profound loss of layer II entorhinal cortex neurons occurs in very mild Alzheimer's disease. *J Neurosci* 16:4491, 1996.
161. Gomez-Isla T, Hollister R, West H, et al: Neuronal loss correlates with but exceeds neurofibrillary tangles in Alzheimer's disease. *Ann Neurol* 41:17, 1997.
162. Grignon Y, Duyckaerts C, Bennecib M, et al: Cytoarchitectonic alterations in the supramarginal gyrus of late onset Alzheimer's disease. *Acta Neuropathol (Berl)* 95:395, 1998.
163. Scheff SW, Price DA: Synapse loss in the temporal lobe in Alzheimer's disease. *Ann Neurol* 33:190, 1993.
164. Scheff SW, Sparks DL, Price DA: Quantitative assessment of synaptic density in the outer molecular layer of the hippocampal dentate gyrus in Alzheimer's disease. *Dementia* 7:226, 1996.
165. Dessi F, Colle MA, et al: Accumulation of SNAP-25 immunoreactive material in axons of Alzheimer's disease. *Neuroreport* 8:3685, 1997.
166. Shimohama S, Kamiya S, Taniguchi T, et al: Differential involvement of synaptic vesicle and presynaptic plasma membrane proteins in Alzheimer's disease. *Biochem Biophys Res Commun* 236:239, 1997.
167. Terry RD, Masliah E, Salmon DP, et al: Physical basis of cognitive alterations in Alzheimer's disease—synapse loss is the major correlate of cognitive impairment. *Ann Neurol* 30:572, 1991.
168. Dickson DW, Crystal HA, Bevona C, et al: Correlations of synaptic and pathological markers with cognition of the elderly. *Neurobiol Aging* 16:285, 1995.
169. Okasaki H, Lipkin LE, Aronson SM: Diffuse intracytoplasmatic ganglionic inclusions (Lewy type) associated with progressive dementia and quadriparesis in flexion. *J Neuropathol Exp Neurol* 20:237, 1961.
170. Kosaka K: Diffuse Lewy body disease in Japan. *J Neurol* 237:197, 1990.
171. Kosaka K, Matsushita M, Oyanagi S, et al: A clinicopathological study of the "Lewy body disease." *Psychiatr Neurol Jpn* 82:292, 1980.
172. Byrne EJ, Lennox G, Lowe J, et al: Diffuse Lewy body disease: Clinical features in 15 cases. *J Neurol Neurosurg Psychiatry* 52:709, 1989.
173. Gibb WRG, Esiri MM, Lees AJ: Clinical and pathological features of diffuse cortical Lewy body disease (Lewy body dementia). *Brain* 110:1131, 1985.
174. Dickson DW, Wu E, Crystal HA, et al: Alzheimer's disease and age-related pathology in diffuse Lewy body disease, in Boller F, Forette F, Khatchaturian Z, et al (eds): *Heterogeneity of Alzheimer's Disease.* Berlin: Springer-Verlag, 1992.
175. Hansen L, Salmon D, Galasko D, et al: Lewy body variant of Alzheimer's disease: A clinical and pathological entity. *Neurology* 40:1, 1990.
176. Lennox G, Lowe B, Morrell K, et al: Antiubiquitin immunocytochemistry is more sensitive than conventional techniques in the detection of difuse Lewy body disease. *J Neurol Neurosurg Psychiatry* 52:67, 1989.
177. Jellinge KA: Post mortem studies in Parkinson's disease—Is it possible to detect brain areas for specific symptoms? *J Neural Transm Suppl* 56:1, 1999.
178. Tagliavini F, Pilleri G, Bouras C, et al: The basal nucleus of Meynert in idiopathic Parkinson's disease. *Acta Neurol Scand* 70:20, 1984.
179. Braak H, Braak E, Yilmazer D, et al: Amygdala pathology in Parkinson's disease. *Acta Neuropathol* 88:493, 1994.
180. Hughes AJ, Daniel SE, Blankson S, et al: A clinicopathologic study of 100 cases of Parkinson's disease. *Arch Neurol* 50:140, 1993.
181. Dickson DW, Ruan D, Crystal H, et al: Hippocampal degeneration differentiates diffuse Lewy body disease (DLBD) from Alzheimer's disease: Light and electron microscopic immunocytochemistry of CA2-3 neurites specific to DLBD. *Neurology* 41:1402, 1991.
182. Dickson DW, Schmidt ML, Lee VMY, et al: Immunoreactive profile of hippocampal Ca2/3 neurites in diffuse Lewy body disease. *Acta Neuropathol (Berl)* 87:269, 1994.
183. Mattila PM, Rinne JO, Helenius H, et al: Neuritic degeneration in the hippocampus and amygdala in Parkinson's disease in relation to Alzheimer pathology. *Acta Neuropathol (Berl)* 98:157, 1999.
184. Hansen LA, Masliah E, Galasko D, et al: Plaque only Alzheimer disease is usually the Lewy body variant and vice versa. *J Neuropathol Exp Neurol* 52:648, 1993.
185. Gibb WRG, Luthert PJ, Janota I, et al: Diffuse Lewy body dementia: Clinical features and classification. *J Neurol Neurosurg Psychiatry* 52:185, 1989.
186. Perry EK, Marshall E, Perry RH, et al: Cholinergic and dopaminergic activities in senile dementia of Lewy body type. *Alzheimer Dis Assoc Disord* 4:87, 1990.
187. McKeith IG, Galasko D, Kosaka K, et al: Consensus guidelines for the clinical and pathological diagnosis of dementia with Lewy bodies (DLB): Report of the consortium on DLB international workshop. *Neurology* 47:1113, 1996.
188. McKeith IG, Perry EK, Perry RH: Report of the second dementia with Lewy body international workshop: Diagnosis and treatment. Consortium on Dementia with Lewy Bodies. *Neurology* 53:902, 1999.

189. Kosaka K: Dementia and neuropathology in Lewy Body disease, in Narabayashi H, Nagatsu T, Yanagisawa N, Misuno Y (eds): *Parkinson's Disease: From Basic Research to Treatment.* New York: Raven Press, 1993.
190. Lantos PL, Ovenstone IMK, Johnson J, et al: Lewy bodies in the brain of two members of a family with the 717 (Val to Ile) mutation of the amyloid precursor protein gene. *Neurosci Lett* 172:77, 1994.
191. Lippa CF, Fujiwara H, Mann DMA, et al: Lewy bodies contain altered alpha-synuclein in brains of many familiar Alzheimer's disease patients with mutations in presenilin and amyloid precursor protein genes. *Am J Pathol* 153:1365, 1998.
192. Lippa CF, Schmidt ML, Lee VM, et al: Antibodies to alpha-synuclein detect Lewy bodies in many Down's syndrome brains with Alzheimer's disease. *Ann Neurol* 45:353, 1999.
193. Galasko D, Saitoh T, Xia Y, et al: The apolipoprotein E allele e4 is overrepresented in patients with the Lewy body variant of Alzheimer's disease. *Neurology* 44:1950, 1994.
194. Joachim CL, Morris JH, Selkoe DJ: Cinically diagnosed Alzheimer's disease: Autopsy results in 150 cases. *Ann Neurol* 24:50, 1988.
195. Lennox G: Lewy body dementia, in Rossor MN (ed): *Baillière's Clinical Neurology.* London: Baillière Tindall, 1992.
196. Boller F, Mizutani T, Roessmann U, et al: Parkinson disease, dementia and Alzheimer disease: Clinicopathological correlations. *Ann Neurol* 7:329, 1980.
197. Braak H, Braak E: Argyrophilic grains: Characteristic pathology of cerebral cortex in cases of adult onset dementia without Alzheimer changes. *Neurosci Lett* 76:124, 1987.
198. Braak H, Braak E: Cortical and subcortical argyrophilic grains characterize a disease associated with adult onset dementia. *J Neuropathol Appl Neurobiol* 15:13, 1989.
199. Tolnay M, Spillantini MG, Goedert M, et al: Argyrophilic grain disease: Widespread hyperphosphorylation of tau protein in limbic neurons. *Acta Neuropathol (Berl)* 93:477, 1997.
200. Tolnay M, Mistl C, Ipsen S, et al: Argyrophilic grains of Braak: Occurrence in dendrites of neurons containing hyperphosphorylated tau protein. *Neuropathol Appl Neurobiol* 24:53, 1998.
201. Tolnay M, Probst A: Ballooned neurons expressing alphaB-crystallin as a constant feature of the amygdala in argyrophilic grain disease. *Neurosci Lett* 246:165, 1998.
202. Braak H, Braak E: Argyrophilic grain disease: Frequency of occurrence in different age categories and neuropathological diagnostic criteria. *J Neural Transm* 105:801, 1998.
203. Tolnay M, Schwietert M, Monsch AU, et al: Argyrophilic grain disease: Distribution of grains in patients with and without dementia. *Acta Neuropathol (Berl)* 94:353, 1997.
204. Ikeda K, Akiyama H, Arai T, et al: Clinical aspects of argyrophilic grain disease. *Clin Neuropathol* 19:278, 2000.
205. Benson DF: Posterior cortical atrophy: A new entity or Alzheimer's disease? *Arch Neurol* 46:843, 1989.
206. Benson D: Progressive frontal dysfunction. *Dementia* 4:149, 1993.
207. Jacquet MF, Boucquey D, Theaux R, et al: L'atrophie corticale postérieure: Variante anatomo-clinique de la maladie d'Alzheimer. *Acta Neurol Belg* 20:265, 1990.
208. Knopman D, Mastri A, Frey W, et al: Dementia lacking distinctive histologic features: A common non-Alzheimer degenerative dementia. *Neurology* 40:251, 1990.
209. Knopman DS: Overview of dementia lacking distinctive histology—pathological designation of a progressive dementia. *Dementia* 4:132, 1993.
210. Kertesz A: Pick complex and Pick's disease, the nosology of frontal lobe dementia, primary progressive aphasia, and corticobasal ganglionic degeneration. *Eur J Neurol* 3:280, 1996.
211. Kertesz A, Munoz D: Clinical and pathological overlap between frontal dementia, progressive aphasia and corticobasal degeneration. The Pick complex. *Neurology* 48:293, 1997.
212. Kertesz A, Munoz D: Pick's disease, frontotemporal dementia, and Pick complex: Emerging concepts. *Arch Neurol* 55:302, 1998.
213. Duyckaerts C, Dürr A, Uchihara T, et al: Pick complex: Too simple? *Eur J Neurol* 3:283, 1996.
214. Duyckaerts C, Hauw J-J: Diagnostic controversies: Another view. *Adv Neurol* 82:233, 2000.
215. Mesulam M-M: Slowly progressive aphasia without generalized dementia. *Ann Neurol* 11:592, 1982.
216. Dejerine J, Sérieux P: Un cas de surdité verbale pure terminée par aphasie sensorielle suivie d'autopsie. *Comptes Rendus Soc Biol* 49:1074, 1897.
217. Cole M, Wright D, Banker BQ: Familial aphasia due to Pick's disease. *Ann Neurol* 6:158, 1979.
218. Weintraub S, Mesulam MM: Four neuropsychological profiles in dementia, in Boller F, Grafman J (eds): *Handbook of Neuropsychology.* Amsterdam: Elsevier, 1993.
219. Holland AL, McBurney DH, Moossy J, et al: The dissolution of language in Pick's disease with neurofibrillary tangles: A case study. *Brain Lang* 24:36, 1985.

220. Fustinoni O, Mangone CA, Abiusi GRP, et al: Primary progressive aphasia: Clinical subtypes, with one postmortem study (abstr). *Neurology* 44:A387, 1994.
221. Kertesz A, Munoz DG: The pathology and nosology of primary progressive aphasia. *Neurology* 44:2065, 1994.
222. Morris JC, Cole M, Banker BQ, et al: Hereditary dysphasic dementia and the Pick-Alzheimer spectrum. *Ann Neurol* 16:455, 1984.
223. Delay J, Brion S: Les démences tardives. 1962.
224. Escourolle R: *La maladie de Pick. Etude critique d'ensemble et synthèse anatomo-clinique*. Paris: Foulon, 1958.
225. Constantinidis J, Richard J, Tissot R: Pick's disease. Histological and clinical correlations. *Eur Neurol* 11:208, 1974.
226. Tissot R, Constantinidis J, Richard J: *La Maladie de Pick*. Paris: Masson, 1975.
227. Brun A: Frontal lobe degeneration of non-Alzheimer type. I Neuropathology. *Arch Gerontol Geriatr* 6:193, 1987.
228. Neary D, Snowden JS, Bowen DM, et al: Neuropsychological syndromes in presenile dementia due to cerebral atrophy. *J Neurol Neurosurg Psychiatry* 49:163, 1986.
229. Neary D, Snowden JS, Gustafson L, et al: Frontotemporal lobar degeneration: A consensus on clinical diagnostic criteria. *Neurology* 51:1546, 1998.
230. Rebeiz J, Kolodney E, Richardson E: Corticodentatonigral degeneration with neuronal achromatasia. *Arch Neurol*, 18:20, 1968.
231. Gibb W, Luthert P: Corticobasal degeneration. *Brain* 112:1171, 1989.
232. Feany MB, Dickson DW: Widespread cytoskeletal pathology characterizes corticobasal degeneration. *Am J Pathol* 146:1388, 1995.
233. Komori T, Arai N, Oda M, et al: Astrocytic plaques and tufts of abnormal fibers do not coexist in corticobasal degeneration and progressive supranuclear palsy. *Acta Neuropathol (Berl)* 96:401, 1998.
234. Tolnay M, Probst A: Tau protein pathology in Alzheimer's disease and related disorders. *Neuropathol Appl Neurobiol* 25:171, 1999.
235. Ikeda K, Akiyama H, Aral T, et al: Glial tau pathology in neurodegenerative diseases: Their nature and comparison with neuronal tangles. *Neurobio Aging* 19:S85, 1998.
236. Tsuchiya K, Ikeda K, Uchihara T, et al: Distribution of cerebral cortical lesions in corticobasal degeneration: A clinicopathological study of five autopsy cases in Japan. *Acta Neuropathol (Berl)* 94:416, 1997.
237. Ikeda K, Akiyama H, Iritani S, et al: Corticobasal degeneration with primary progressive aphasia and accentuated cortical lesion in superior temporal gyrus: Case report and review. *Acta Neuropathol (Berl)* 92:534, 1996.
238. Cordato NJ, Halliday GM, McCann H, et al: Corticobasal syndrome with tau pathology. *Mov Disord* 16:656, 2001.
239. Crystal HA, Horoupian DS, Katzman R, et al: Biopsy-proved Alzheimer disease presenting as right parietal lobe syndrome. *Ann Neurol* 12:186, 1981.
240. Jagust W, Davies P, Tiller-Borcich J, et al: Focal Alzheimer's disease. *Neurology* 14, 1990.
241. Léger J-M, Levasseur M, Benoit M, et al: Apraxie d'aggravation lentement progressive: Etude par IRM et tomographie à positons dans 4 cas. *Rev Neurol (Paris)* 147:183, 1991.
242. Terry RD: Aging, senile dementia and Alzheimer disease, in Katzman R, Terry RD, Bick KL (eds): *Alzheimer's Disease: Senile Dementia and Related Disorders.* New York: Raven Press, 1978.
243. Thuillard F, Assal G: Données neuropsychologiques chez le sujet agé normal, in Habib M, Joanette Y, Puel M (eds): *Démences et syndromes démentiels.* Paris: Masson, 1991.
244. Schaie K: The Seattle Longitudinal Study: A 35-year inquiry of adult intellectual development. *Zeitschr Gerontol* 26:129, 1993.
245. Willis S, Schaie W: Cognitive training in the normal elderly, in Forette F, Christen Y, Boller F (eds): *Plasticité cérébrale et stimulation cognitive.* Paris: Fondation Nationale de Gérontologie, 1993.
246. Bachman DL, Wolf PA, Linn R, et al: Prevalence of dementia and probable senile dementia of the Alzheimer's type in the Framingham Study. *Neurology* 42:115, 1992.
247. Linn R, Wolf PA, Bachman DL, et al: The "preclinical phase" of probable Alzheimer's disease. *Neurology* 52:485, 1995.
248. Miller A, Corsellis J: Evidence for a secular increase in human brain weight during the past century. *Ann Hum Biol* 4:253, 1977.
249. Corkin S: Aging, age-related disorders and dementia, in Boller F, Grafman J (eds): *Handbook of Neuropsychology.* Amsterdam: Elsevier, 1991.
250. Pakkenberg H, Voigt J: Brain weight of the Danes. A forensic material. *Acta Anat* 56:297, 1964.
251. Dekaban AS, Sadowsky D: Changes in brain weight during the span of human life: Relation of brain weight to body height and body weight. *Ann Neurol* 4:345, 1978.
252. Miller AKH, Alston RL, Corsellis JAN: Variations with age in the volumes of gray and white matter in the

cerebral hemispheres of man: Measurements with an image analyser. *Neuropathol Appl Neurobiol* 6:119, 1980.

253. Terry RD, DeTeresa R, Hansen LA: Neocortical cell counts in normal human adult aging. *Ann Neurol* 21:530, 1987.
254. Davis PJM, Wright EA: A new method for measuring cranial capacity volume and its application to the assessment of cerebral atrophy at autopsy. *Neuropathol Appl Neurobiol* 3:341, 1977.
255. Tomlinson BE, Blessed G, Roth M: Observation on the brains of non-demented old people. *J Neurol Sci* 7:331, 1968.
256. Jacoby RJ, Levy R: Computed tomography in the elderly II: Senile dementia: Diagnosis and functional impairment. *Br J Psychiatry* 136:256, 1980.
257. Jack CJ, Petersen R, Xu Y, et al: Rate of medial temporal lobe atrophy in typical aging and Alzheimer's disease. *Neurology* 51:993, 1998.
258. Jack CJ, Petersen R, Xu Y, et al: Prediction of AD with MRI-based hippocampal volume in mild cognitive impairment. *Neurology* 52:1397, 1999.
259. Ball MJ: Neuronal loss, neurofibrillary tangles and granulovacuolar degeneration in the hippocampus with ageing and dementia. *Acta Neuropathol (Berl)* 37:111, 1977.
260. Dam AM: The density of neurons in the human hippocampus. *Neuropathol Appl Neurobiol* 5:249, 1979.
261. West MJ: Regionally specific loss of neurons in the aging human hippocampus. *Neurobiol Aging* 14:287, 1993.
262. West MJ, Coleman PD, Flood DG, et al: Differences in the pattern of hippocampal neuronal loss in normal aging and Alzheimer disease. *Lancet* 344:769, 1994.
263. Brody H: Organization of cerebral cortex. III. A study of aging in the human cerebral cortex. *J Comp Neurol* 102:511, 1955.
264. Haug H, Barmwater U, Eggers R, et al: Anatomical changes in aging brain: Morphometric analysis of the human prosencephalon, in Cervos Navarro J, Sarkander H-I (eds): Brain *Aging: Neuropathology And Neuropharmacology.* New York, Raven Press, 1983, vol 21.
265. Henderson G, Tomlinson BE, Gibson PH: Cell counts in human cerebral cortex in normal adults throughout life using an image analysing machine. *J Neurol Sci* 46:113, 1980.
266. Pakkenberg B, Gundersen HJG: Neocortical neuron number in humans: Effect of sex and age. *J Comp Neurol* 384:312, 1997.
267. Brody H: Cell counts in cerebral cortex and brainstem in Alzheimer's disease, in Katzman R, Terry RD, Bick KL (eds): *Senile Dementia and Related Disorders.* New York: Raven Press, 1978.
268. Vijayashankar N, Brody H: The neuronal population of the nuclei of the trochlear nerve and the locus coeruleus in the human. *Anat Rec* 172:421, 1973.
269. Vijayashankar N, Brody H: A study of aging in the human abducens nucleus. *J Comp Neurol* 173:433, 1977.
270. Konigsmark BW, Murphy EA: Volume of ventral cochlear nucleus in man: Its relationship to neuronal population and age. *J Neuropathol Exp Neurol* 31:304, 1972.
271. Monagle RD, Brody H: The effects of age upon the main nucleus of the inferior olive in the human. *J Comp Neurol* 155:61, 1974.
272. Vijayashankar N, Brody H: A quantitative study of the pigmented neurons in the nuclei coeruleus and subcoeruleus in man as related to aging. *J Neuropathol Exp Neurol* 38:490, 1979.
273. Mouton PR, Pakkenberg B, Gundersen HJ, et al: Absolute number and size of pigmented locus coeruleus neurons in young and aged individuals. *J Chem Neuroanat* 7:185, 1994.
274. Ohm TG, Busch C, Bohl J: Unbiased estimation of neuronal numbers in the human nucleus coeruleus during aging. *Neurobiol Aging* 18:393, 1997.
275. Hall TC, Miller AKH, Corsellis JAN: Variation in human Purkinje cell population according to age and sex. *Neuropathol Appl Neurobiol* 1:267, 1975.
276. Fearnley JM, Lees AJ: Ageing and Parkinson's disease: Substantia nigra regional selectivity. *Brain* 114:2283, 1991.
277. Mann DMA, Yates PO: The effects of ageing on the pigmented nerve cells of the human locus coeruleus and substantia nigra. *Acta Neuropathol (Berl)* 47:93, 1979.
278. McGeer PL, McGeer EG, Suzuki PS: Aging and extrapyramidal function. *Arch Neurol* 34:33, 1977.
279. Kubis N, Faucheux BA, Ransmayr G, et al: Preservation of midbrain catecholaminergic neurons in very old human subjects. *Brain* 123:366, 2000.
280. Brody H, Vijayashankar N: Anatomical changes in the nervous system, in Finch DE, Hayflick L (eds): *Handbook of the Biology of Aging.* New York: Van Nostrand, 1977.
281. Bugiani O, Salvarani S, Perdelli F, et al: Nerve cell loss with aging in the putamen. *Eur Neurol* 17:286, 1978.
282. Herzog AG, Kemper TL: Amygdaloid changes in aging and dementia. *Arch Neurol* 37:625, 1980.
283. de Lacalle S, Iraizoz I, Ma Gonzalo L: Differential changes in cell size and number in topographic subdivisions of human basal nucleus in normal aging. *Neuroscience* 43:445, 1991.

284. Szenborn M: Neuropathological study on the nucleus basalis of Meynert in mature and old age. *Patol Pol* 44:211, 1993.
285. Berg L, McKeel DW, Miller P, et al: Neuropathological indexes of Alzheimer's disease in demented and non-demented persons aged 80 years and older. *Arch Neurol* 50:349, 1993.
286. Morris JC, Storandt M, McKeel DW Jr, et al: Cerebral amyloid deposition and diffuse plaques in "normal" aging: Evidence for presymptomatic and very mild Alzheimer's disease. *Neurology* 46:707, 1996.
287. Arriagada PV, Marzloff K, Hyman BT: Distribution of Alzheimer-type pathologic changes in nondemented elderly individuals matches the pattern in Alzheimer's Disease. *Neurology* 42:1681, 1992.
288. Frigard B, Vermersch P, David JP, et al: Le processus neurodegeneratif au cours du vieillissement cerebral et de la maladie d'Alzheimer, in Albarède JL, Vellas P, Garry PJ (eds): *L'année gérontologique. Facts and Research in Gerontology.* New York: Springer-Verlag, 1994.
289. Braak H, Braak E: Frequency of stages of Alzheimer-related lesions in different age categories. *Neurobiol Aging* 18:351, 1997.
290. Delaère P, He Y, Fayet G, et al: ßA4 deposits are constant in the brain of the oldest old: An immunocytochemical study of 20 French centenarians. *Neurobiol Aging* 14:191, 1993.
291. Hauw J-J, Delaère P, He Y, et al: The centenarian's brain. *Adv Biosci* 87:127, 1993.
292. Hauw J-J, Delaère P: Topographie des lésions, in Signoret J, Huw J-J (eds): *Maladie d'Alzheimer et autres démences.* Paris: Flammarion, 1991.
293. Sjögren T, Sjögren H, Lindgren A: Morbus Alzheimer and morbus Pick. A genetic, clinical and pathoanatomical study. *Acta Psychiatr Neurol Scand Suppl* 82:1, 1952.
294. Pichot P: Language disturbances in cerebral disease. *Arch Neurol Psychiatry* 74:92, 1955.
295. Critchley M: The neurology of psychotic speech. *Br J Psychiatry* 110:353, 1964.
296. De Renzi E, Vignolo L: I disturbi del linguaggio nei dementi. *Lavoro Neuropsichiatr* 12:1, 1966.
297. Irigaray L: Approche psycholinguistique du langage des déments. *Neuropsychologia* 5:25, 1967.
298. Ajuriaguerra JD, Strejilevitch M, Tissot R: A propos de quelques conduites devant le miroir de sujets atteints de syndrome démentiels du grand âge. *Neuropsychologia* 1:59, 1963.
299. Pollock M, Hornabrook RW: The prevalence, natural history and dementia of Parkinson's disease. *Brain* 89:429, 1966.
300. Green R, Benjamin S, Cummings J: Fellowship programs in behavioral neurology. *Neurology* 45:412, 1995.
301. Wechsler AF: Presenile dementia presenting as aphasia. *J Neurol Neurosurg Psychiatry* 40:303, 1977.
302. Amaducci L, Grassi E, Boller F: Maurice Ravel and right-hemisphere musical creativity: Influence of disease on his last musical works? *Eur J Neurol* 9:75, 2002.
303. Kang J, Lemaire H-G, Unterbeck A, et al: The precursor of Alzheimer's disease amyloid A4 protein resembles a cell-surface receptor. *Nature* 325:733, 1987.
304. Grace J, Daniel S, Stevens J, et al: Long-term use of rivastigmine in patients with dementia with Lewy bodies: An open label trial. *Int Psychogeriatr* 13:199, 2001.

Chapter 45

ALZHEIMER'S DISEASE: BIOCHEMICAL AND PHARMACOLOGIC ISSUES*

Gang Tong
Leon J. Thal

Nearly a century ago, Alzheimer described abnormal extracellular and intracellular deposits in the cerebral cortex of a 51-year-old woman who suffered from severe presenile dementia.[1] It was assumed that such neuropathology was only rarely associated with senility in the general population, but we now know that senile plaques (SPs) and neurofibrillary tangles (NFTs) he observed are in fact commonly found in the brains of elderly persons with impaired cognitive functions or sometimes even in elderly persons with normal cognitive functions. When seen in the context of a slowly progressive dementia, these lesions are diagnostic of Alzheimer's disease (AD).[2,3] There have been considerable advances in neuropathology which—coupled with clinicopathologic correlation, molecular genetics, cellular and molecular techniques, elucidation of neurotransmitters and their receptors, and well-designed clinical trials—have made major contributions to our understanding of AD. Our increased understanding of AD has suggested various pharmacologic treatment strategies, some of which have already found practical clinical applications.

STRUCTURAL LESIONS CHARACTERISTIC OF ALZHEIMER'S DISEASE

Grossly, the volume of brain parenchyma typically shrinks in AD, while the volume of the fluid spaces expands. These volumetric changes are paralleled on the microscopic level by neuronal loss, intraneuronal NFTs and extracellular SPs, a reduced density of synaptic contacts between neurons in both cortical and subcortical regions, and synaptic alteration. A subset of patients meeting clinical and pathologic criteria for AD also have neuronal inclusions called Lewy bodies, which were traditionally thought to be exclusively associated with idiopathic Parkinson's disease. This chapter discusses the role these lesions play in AD and the biochemical changes associated with them, emphasizing their implications for treating AD.

The Senile Plaque

Structure of SPs The major component of the SPs is the β-amyloid protein (Aβ), whose fibrils aggregate themselves into pleated sheets that bind with high avidity to Congo red stain and which, due to their amyloid conformation, have the property of birefringence when viewed under polarized light.[4] All pathologically confirmed AD patients by definition have SPs, and nearly all will have deposits of Aβ in the walls of cerebral blood vessels.[5] There are two main types of SPs: (1) diffuse plaques, which consist mainly of minute wisps of formed filamentous amyloid and nonstructured Aβ, containing no abnormal neurites; and (2) neuritic plaques, which include dense bundles of amyloid fibrils and dystrophic neuronal processes called neurites. Diffuse plaques are found in some nondemented elderly persons as well as in AD. Many investigators presume that there is a progression from the first to the second type that roughly parallels the increasing severity of AD and that the most "mature" plaque is neuritic, with a dense core of Aβ. The dystrophic neurites may contain paired helical filaments (PHFs) characteristic of NFTs and may show signs of regenerative as well as degenerative axons and dendrites.[6]

* **ACKNOWLEDGMENT:** This work was supported by a VA fellowship and by grants from the National Institutes of Health: AG 05131, AG 10483. We thank Mrs. Barbara Reader and Dr. Hiroto Takahashi for expert assistance.

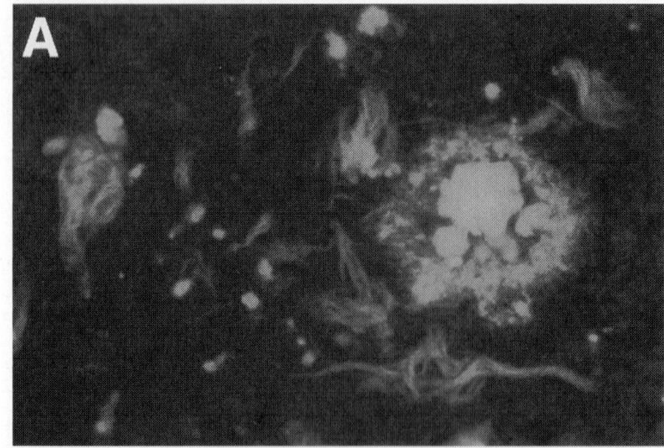

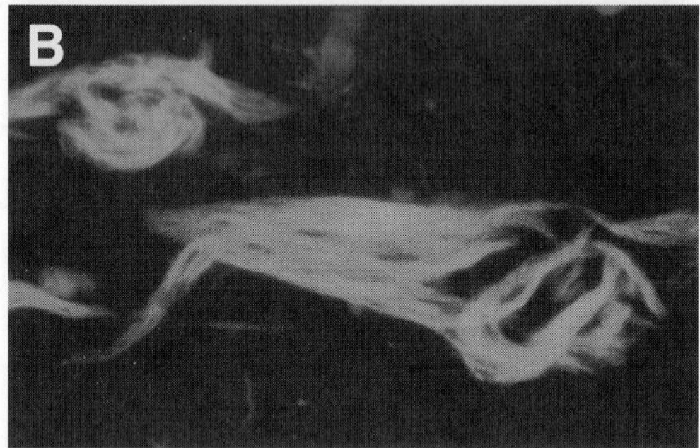

Figure 45-1 (Plate 16)
The classic lesions of AD, as seen using thioflavin S staining and fluorescent microscopy. A. *Mature plaque with dense amyloid core.* B. *NFTs in the entorhinal cortex. (Photographs provided by Dr. Robert D. Terry.)*

An example of the microscopic appearance of SPs is shown in Fig. 45-1*A*, Plate 16.

Biochemistry of SPs

The Aβ protein is 39 to 43 amino acids long[7] and is derived from a much larger amyloid precursor protein (APP)[8,9] (Fig. 45-2, Plate 17) that functions as a kinesin-I membrane receptor, mediating the axonal transport of β-secretase and presenilin (PS).[10] The dense cores of neuritic plaques contain mixtures of Aβ_{42} and Aβ_{40} peptides. Even though Aβ_{40} is the more abundant form (about 90 percent) of total Aβ in the brain, Aβ_{42} is much more likely to aggregate into a fibrillar structure than Aβ_{40}. The Aβ fragment is generated by a cleavage at amino acid 671 and a more variable cleavage of the molecule at about amino acid 713. The enzymes required to make these cleavages are called secretases. There are three major forms of secretases. The principal cleavage is carried out by α-secretase. The cleavage creates a large, soluble ectodomain fragment (APPs-α). Alpha-secretase is probably membrane-anchored proteases that are capable of cleaving single transmembrane proteins. Some of APP can be cut by β-secretase.[11–13] This cleavage releases a truncated form of APPs (APPs-β) from the cell and leaves a 99-residue C-terminal fragment (C99) embedded within the membrane. C99 can then be cleaved by γ-secretase to create Aβ. Increases in Aβ production are associated with decreased α-secretase or increased β- or γ-secretase activities.

Only a minority of cases of AD result from increased Aβ production. Recent evidence suggests that decreasing clearance of Aβ plays an important role in AD pathogenesis.[14] Several proteases have been implicated in the degradation of Aβ. Neprilysin, one of these proteases, has been shown to be a major Aβ_{42}-degrading protease in rat brain.[15,16] Insulin-degrading enzyme (IDE) has also been implicated in the degradation of more soluble monomeric Aβ; of note, it has less ability to degrade Aβ once it becomes insoluble and/or oligomeric.[17]

Controversy remains as to whether the deposition of Aβ in SPs is merely a marker for AD or a causative agent. However, much indirect evidence supports Aβ as a causative substance in AD, since Aβ_{40} has been shown to cause neuronal loss and gliosis when applied to neuronal cells grown in culture and when injected in solubilized form into rat or monkey cortex. Even a fragment of the Aβ peptide from the 25th to 35th amino acid has a neurotoxic effect.[18] Evidence suggests that Aβ in soluble form or deposited as amorphous aggregates does not significantly damage neurons but that Aβ in fibrillar form may be neurotoxic.[19] Aβ_{42} is much more likely to aggregate into a fibrillar structure than Aβ_{39} or Aβ_{40}. Prior deposition of Aβ_{42} can seed subsequent fibrillar aggregation and enhance deposition of the more soluble shorter forms.[20–22]

The mechanism by which fibrillar Aβ might inflict neuronal damage is unknown. The aggregated peptide could directly damage cell membranes and cause cell death. More subtly, fibrillar Aβ may interfere with ion channels that regulate calcium influx,

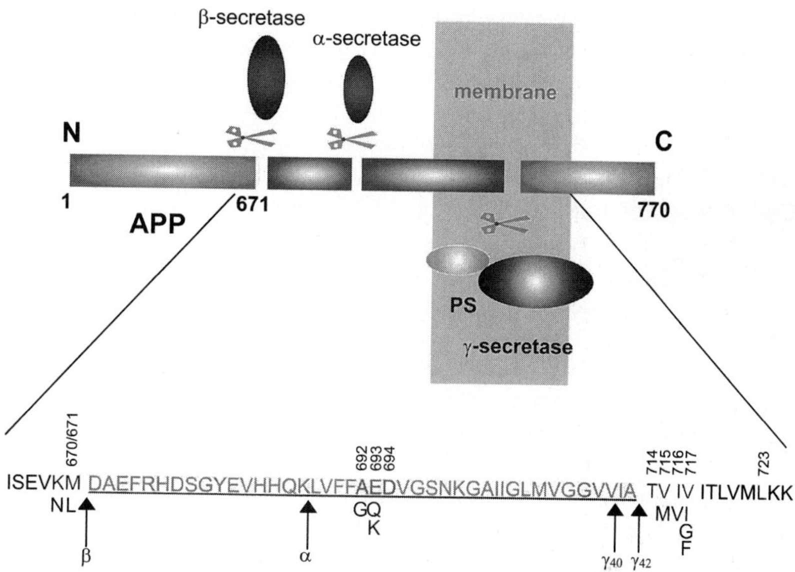

Figure 45-2 (Plate 17) *Schematic diagram of APP and its mutations genetically linked to familial AD. The sequence in APP that contains the Aβ and the transmembrane region is expanded. The underlined residues represent $A\beta_{1-42}$. The letters below the line indicate the currently known missense mutations linked to familial AD.*

leading to excess intracellular calcium, vulnerability to excitotoxicity, and cell death.[23,24] Aside from excitatory amino acids, other chemical mechanisms have been proposed for the neurotoxicity of fibrillar $A\beta$, including the production of free radicals and damage to mitochondria. Many proteins are found to be associated with $A\beta$ deposits or with SPs, and these may play roles in $A\beta$ solubility, inflammation, or neuronal sprouting. Examples of plaque-associated proteins are α_1-antichymotrypsin and proteoglycans, which, along with complement proteins, are suggestive of an inflammatory reaction.[25–28] Fibroblast growth factor[29] and apolipoprotein E[30] are also found in the SP. Neuritic plaques are typically surrounded by reactive astrocytes and microglial cells, which, like complements, are suggestive of an inflammatory process. Plaque neurites contain APP,[31,32] epidermal growth factor receptor,[33] the GAP 43, growth-associated protein,[34] ubiquitin,[35] neurofilaments,[36] and neurotransmitters.[37]

$A\beta$ in Familial AD

Some of the most impressive evidence for a causative role of $A\beta$ in AD pathogenesis is provided by a small number of families who suffer from familial AD due to specific mutations in APP (see Fig. 45-2, Plate 17). Affected members of these families typically develop the disease early, often before the age of 50. All mutations are located adjacent to the three secretase sites. No other mutations have been found in the other sites of APP. Although identification of these mutations has not had any clinical impact on diagnosis and treatment of AD, it has promoted research into AD animal models. Transgenic mice have been produced by overexpressing the human APP gene with a mutant codon 717. The brains of these animals show extensive SPs, synapse loss, and inflammatory changes, but no NFTs have been found.[38] Transgenic models are very useful tools in searching for effective therapeutic interventions such as selective secretase inhibitors and inhibitors of amyloid aggregations and for developing methods for immunization.

Another genetically related observation that points to the central role of $A\beta$ in AD pathogenesis is the striking similarity between $A\beta$ deposits seen in AD and Down's syndrome.[39,40] Down's syndrome is most often caused by trisomy of chromosome 21 and is associated with mental retardation and the formation of SPs (and of NFTs) in the same brain regions commonly affected in AD. Many Down's syndrome patients undergo cognitive decline in their sixth or seventh decade. The SPs seen in Down's syndrome are composed of $A\beta_{42}$, particularly in the earlier stages of plaque formation, though $A\beta_{40}$ may also be seen in older plaques, perhaps because its deposition has been promoted by the prior accumulation of $A\beta_{42}$.[41] Since the gene coding for APP is located on chromosome 21, it is likely that an extra copy of this gene in Down's syndrome leads to overproduction of $A\beta$, including $A\beta_{42}$.

Cell Biology of the PSs PS1 and PS2 are highly homologous proteins containing eight putative transmembrane domains that localize primarily to the endoplasmic reticulum and Golgi apparatus in mammals.[42] The PS holoproteins are found to undergo constitutive endoproteolysis, which occurs within a hydrophobic portion of the cytoplasmic loop.[43] Therefore the PS exists in part as stable heterodimers composed of the N- and C-terminal fragments. The fragments are the principal biologically functional form of PSs. Once formed, PS fragments can also associate into higher-molecular-mass complexes (~100 to 200 kDa) with other proteins.[44]

Human PS1 and PS2 mutations have been linked to early-onset familial AD. More than 80 missense mutations in PS1 and PS2 have been found in families with early-onset AD. Even though it is unclear whether PS serves either as the "γ-secretase" or as a necessary cofactor, accumulating data suggest that PSs are physically inseparable from γ-secretase activities. Knockout mice with no PS1 activity have reduced γ-cleavage of APP.[45,46] Mutation of either of two conserved aspartate residues in PS1 also interferes with γ-cleavage.[47,48] In addition, transition-state analogue inhibitors of γ-secretase bind directly and specifically to PS1 and PS2.[49–52]

Since the discovery of the PSs in 1995, it has become apparent that these proteins are important for Notch signaling, APP processing, and perhaps other cellular processes. The Notch pathway controls cell-fate specifications in all multicellular animals.[53,54] When the Notch receptor binds to one of its ligands, it results in expression of target genes via downstream transcription factors. A large number of studies have shown that the PSs are important in the intramembranous cleavage of the Notch receptor for Notch signaling in *Drosophila,* mice, and human cells.[55–57] Since the Notch pathway plays a critical role in the mammalian immune system, digestive tract, and other tissues, the development of nontoxic γ-secretase inhibitors will be very difficult.

The Neurofibrillary Tangle

Structure of NFTs Neurons depend on three types of cytoskeletal filament systems to maintain their shape and assist with the internal transport of nutrients and the constituents of cell products such as neurotransmitters: (1) microfilaments, (2) intermediate filaments oriented longitudinally within axons and dendrites, and (3) microtubules with side-arm projections to which microtubule-associated proteins can bind. In AD brains, NFTs and neuropil thread pathology are found intracellularlly in conjunction with the deposition of $A\beta$ in the extracellular space (Fig. 45-1*B*). By light microcopy, NFTs of AD are stained with anti-tau antibodies. Tau protein deposits occur as fine neuropil threads in dystrophic neurites or as massive NFTs in neuronal perikarya, which become extracellular ghost tangles after the death of the cell. Ultrastructurally, the dominant components of NFTs are PHFs and straight filaments.[58] PHFs are composed of two strands of filament twisted around each other with a periodicity, whereas straight filaments lack this periodicity.[59]

Biochemistry of NFTs Both PHFs and straight filaments are composed predominantly of abnormally hyperphosphorylated tau protein.[60] Tau is one of the microtubule-associated proteins (MAPs) that bind and stabilize neuronal microtubules for their roles in the development of cell processes, establishment of cell polarity, and intracellular transport.[61] In natural conditions, tau is very hydrophilic and soluble; it displays a natively unfolded structure and can be phosphorylated at multiple sites, some of which regulate its microtubule-binding properties.

The phosphorylation state of tau depends on a balance between kinases and phosphatases. Studies using antibodies specific for various phospho-tau epitopes have established residues that are phosphorylated in PHF tau.[62] Tau detaches from microtubules when phosphorylated at Ser262 or at Ser214, two sites that are also phosphorylated in AD. Although a variety of kinases have been shown to be capable of phosphorylating tau in vitro at various sites in AD brain,[63] it is unclear whether one or more kinases are involved for initiating the hyperphosphorylation of tau in vivo. The phosphorylating sites include targets for proline-directed kinases such as glycogen synthase kinase 3, cyclin-dependent kinase (Cdk5), MAP kinase, protein kinase A, microtubule-affinity-regulating kinase (MARK), or Ca^{2+}/calmodulin-dependent protein kinase. Recent evidence suggests that unregulated Cdk5 may serve as one of the major kinases in hyperphosphorylating tau.[64] Other kinases (e.g., Fyn) and phosphatases (e.g., protein phosphatase 2A) may also play a role in the formation of NFTs. The mechanisms underlying tau aggregation and PHF formation are still unclear. When highly phosphorylated at specific sites, tau becomes incapable of binding to microtubules, at least in vitro, resulting in an accumulation of unbound tau in dendrites, which is followed by self-aggregation into paired helical filaments.[19] The loss of tau's normal functions is likely to be severely disruptive to the microtubule and transport system, ultimately leading to cell death.

Atrophy and Neuron Loss

Gross atrophy of the brain is a hallmark of AD, although such changes are seen among the cognitively normal elderly as well (Fig. 45-3). Terry and coworkers[65] reported the average brain weight of 14 AD patients as 1055 g and that of 10 age-matched controls as 1152 g; the difference between these groups was statistically significant, but in both the weight was lower than the 1450 g expected for a normal 30-year-old. Cerebral atrophy can be visualized on computed tomography (CT) or magnetic resonance imaging (MRI) of the living patient.[66–69] Paralleling this decline in brain weight and size is a loss of large neocortical neurons[70,71] and thinning of the cortical ribbon, which also occurs in normal aging but is accelerated in AD.[72] In the hippocampal formation and the entorhinal region, focal neuronal death seems closely related to the presence of NFTs.[73,74] Whitehouse et al. were first to report the loss of neurons in the cholinergic nucleus basalis of Meynert.[75,76] This affects cholinergic activity in the hippocampus and neocortex. The locus ceruleus[77] and the dorsal raphe nuclei[78] also sustain major neuronal loss, resulting in widespread loss of noradrenergic and 5-HT activity. Along with the loss of neurons, there are an increased number of astrocytes scattered throughout the neocortex, especially in association with plaques.[79]

Synapse Alterations

Given the prominent changes in brain structure and physiology of AD, it would be expected that even the smallest structural component of brain function, the synapse, would also be impaired. Quantitative electron microscopic (EM) studies of AD biopsy and autopsy tissue have shown a 27 to 42 percent reduction

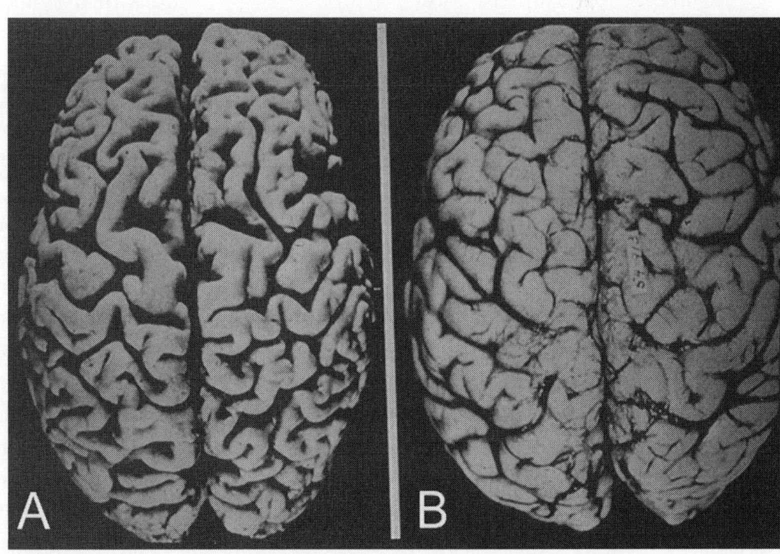

Figure 45-3
Gross brain atrophy in AD. Gross appearance of the brain of an AD patient (A) *and that of a normal elderly person* (B). *(Photographs provided by Dr. Robert D. Terry.)*

in synapses of layers 2, 3, and 5 of the frontal and temporal cortices, which are often accompanied by extensive pathologic changes in the synapses.[80–83] Immunochemical and immunocytochemical studies of synaptic density in AD neocortex using antibodies against the presynaptic vesicle proteins synaptophysin and spectrin have shown an average 45 percent decrease in the population density of presynaptic terminals.[84–89] Synaptophysin immunoreactivity is also altered in certain regions of the hippocampus,[90,91] although to a lesser degree. The nucleus basalis and locus ceruleus also show significant synaptic loss. It is not known whether synaptic pathology in AD precedes cytoskeletal changes or is related to Aβ deposition. However, this loss of synapses is relevant to neurotransmitter-based therapies in AD; for example, loss of neurons in a subcortical center with widespread neocortical projections such as the nucleus basalis could cause a loss of synapses throughout its projection zone. Alternatively, synapse loss might precede neuron loss, since cortical synaptic loss is greater than the decline of neuronal cell bodies. In transgenic animal models, decline of the density of presynaptic terminals and neurons occurs well before these mice develop amyloid plaques, which supports the view that plaque-independent Aβ toxicity plays an important role in the development of synaptic deficits in AD.[92,93]

Lewy Bodies

A subgroup comprising 15 to 30 percent of AD patients is afflicted with extensive neocortical SPs sufficient to meet pathologic criteria for AD but few if any NFTs.[94] Subcortical and neocortical Lewy bodies are present in at least 75 percent of this "plaque predominant" form of AD.[95] Though AD-type dementia is the presenting complaint of patients with the Lewy body variant of AD, these patients typically develop some parkinsonian features, including bradykinesia, rigidity, gait instability, and masked facies.[96] In addition, visual hallucination and fluctuations in attention are common.[97,98] Neocortical Lewy bodies had previously been overlooked because they are not well visualized using routine hematoxylin and eosin stains. However, antibodies to ubiquitin protein immunostain Lewy bodies very well. Lewy bodies are found in subcortical nuclei (nucleus basalis, locus ceruleus, substantia nigra) as well as in the hippocampus, cingulate gyrus, and neocortex. The frequency of neocortical Lewy bodies has been found to correlate with the severity of neuropsychological impairment among Lewy body–variant patients.[99,100] Lewy bodies are found in 20 to 40 percent of cases of AD when using α-synuclein immunostaining, which are mainly located in the amygdala.[101,102]

Biochemistry of Lewy Bodies

Lewy bodies are rounded intracytoplasmic inclusions, usually circular in outline, with a brightly eosinophilic, hyaline core surrounded by a pale halo. Their precise chemical composition is unknown, but they are composed of filamentous structures and give a positive reaction for neurofilament protein, ubiquitin, and α-synuclein. Alpha-synuclein is a major component of Lewy bodies. Immunohistochemistry for α-synuclein shows predominantly a presynaptic pattern of localization in AD and in control brains.

Alpha-synuclein is a 140–amino acid protein that is encoded by *SNCA,* a gene on chromosone 4.[103] Alpha-synuclein is a natively unfolded protein with several structural motifs, including a hydrophobic central region that contains the non-Aβ component (NAC) sequence. Even though the principal biochemical component of neuritic plaques in AD is the Aβ, NAC comprises about 10 percent of the total protein that remains insoluble after SDS detergent extraction.[104] The functions of α-synuclein and the NAC fragment are unknown.

Risk and Protective Factors

Age Age is the number one risk factor for AD. The prevalence and incidence rise exponentially as a function of age in the 65- to 85-year-old range, and AD doubles approximately every 5 years in persons between the ages of 65 and 95 years of age.[105,106] The most important consequence of this relationship is that delaying the onset of AD by 5 years would decrease the prevalence by half.

Education It is generally believed that lack of education is a risk factor for AD.[107–110] When uneducated persons are compared with those who have more than 6 years of education, the relative risk (RR) is about 2. In addition, several studies have found a dose-response curve, with the prevalence and incidence of dementia, especially AD, being lower among persons with higher education.[111,112]

Family History One of the most predominant risk factors for AD is a family history of AD.[113] The RR is 3.5 if a first-degree relative has AD. The RR is highest in those with relatively early onset (at 60 to 69 years of age) (RR, 5.3), but it is still significant in those with late onset (at greater than 70 years of age). The RR increases to 7.5 in persons who have two or more first-degree relatives with AD.

Gender Even though there are inconsistencies, the prevalence rates for AD in several studies are significantly higher in women than in men of same age.[105,108] AD occurs in about twice as many women as men. The factors that are responsible for this are unknown. Factors that may account for this finding include an abrupt decline in estrogen production in postmenopausal women. Other factors include differential longevity of demented women and differences in education between men and women.

Apolipoprotein E Apolipoprotein E (ApoE) is a protein found both in the peripheral tissues and in the brain; it functions as a cholesterol transporter.[114,115] Its synthesis occurs mainly in the liver. In the brain, ApoE is primarily produced by glial cells, whereas its receptors are expressed in neurons.[116] There are three major isoforms of ApoE ($\varepsilon 2$, $\varepsilon 3$, and $\varepsilon 4$), each of which is coded by a slightly different allele of the ApoE gene on chromosome 19. Since one allele is inherited from each parent, six combinations are possible in a given individual. Among Caucasians in the general population, the $\varepsilon 3/\varepsilon 3$ and $\varepsilon 3/\varepsilon 2$ combinations are most prevalent (72 percent); about 24 percent of people have one $\varepsilon 4$ allele ($\varepsilon 4/\varepsilon 3$ or $\varepsilon 4/\varepsilon 2$), and only 3 percent are $\varepsilon 4/\varepsilon 4$ homozygotes; $\varepsilon 2/\varepsilon 2$ homozygotes are very rare.[117] An association between the $\varepsilon 4$ allele and late-onset AD was discovered.[118,119] In Caucasian populations, individuals who carry the $\varepsilon 4$ allele are three (heterozygotes) to eight (homozygotes) times more likely to develop AD than individuals who do not have the $\varepsilon 4$ allele. The frequency of the $\varepsilon 4$ allele is increased to 40 to 65 percent in AD patients. There is a similarly increased frequency of the $\varepsilon 4$ allele among those with the Lewy body variant of AD.[120] One of the effects of the $\varepsilon 4$ allele is to decrease the age of onset of AD. In the original study of families with late-onset AD, the mean age at onset was 68 for $\varepsilon 4/\varepsilon 4$ homozygotes, 76 for $\varepsilon 4$ heterozygotes, and 86 for patients lacking an $\varepsilon 4$ allele.[118] The mechanisms by which the ApoE $\varepsilon 4$ allele promotes the pathogenesis of AD are unclear; however, there are several ways in which ApoE may be involved in the pathogenesis of AD, including interactions with APP, modulation of Aβ clearance from the extracellular space, modulation of tau phosphorylation, and transmission of signals to neurons.

THERAPEUTIC IMPLICATIONS OF ALZHEIMER'S DISEASE

Dementia involves acquired cognitive impairment and behavioral alterations of multiple domains. Adult-onset dementing disorders are among the major medical problems of modern society. Until the last decade, neurodegenerative diseases, including AD, were considered to be among the most obscure and intractable disorders in medicine. Major advances in neuropathology, molecular genetics, and cellular and molecular biology have resulted in contributions to our understanding of AD. Our increasing level of understanding of AD pathogenesis is reflected in both current and prospective therapeutic interventions. One approach toward treatment of AD aims at symptomatic relief of its primary manifestations (e.g., memory impairment) or secondary ones (neurobehavioral change—e.g., depression or agitation) without influencing the basic neurodegenerative process. A second approach aims at slowing disease progression or delaying disease onset. The third approach aims at the primary prevention in people at risk for developing AD.

Therapies Aimed at Symptomatic Relief

Table 45-1 lists several neurotransmitter systems that are dysfunctional in AD and indicates presently available or prospective therapies for these deficits.

Treatment with Cholinergic Agents The basal forebrain provides the major source of cholinergic innervation for the cerebral cortex and hippocampal formation.[121] AD is associated with a significant decline of cortical acetylcholinesterase (AChE) and

Table 45-1
Major neurotransmitters and neuropeptides involved in AD

Neurotransmitter or neuropeptide	*Main sites of production*	*Main axonal projections relevant to AD*	*Current or potential therapies*
Acetylcholine (ACh)	Nucleus basalis of Meynert, septal nuclei	Neocortex, thalamus, striatum, hippocampus	1. AChE inhibitors 2. Selective muscarinic receptor agonists 3. Nicotinic receptor agonists 4. Trophic factors
Glutamate	Throughout CNS	Throughout CNS	1. NMDA receptor antagonists 2. AMPAkine
Gamma-aminobutyric acid (GABA)	Inhibitory neurons, widely distributed	Neocortex, hippocampus	1. GABA receptor agonists
Norepinephrine (NE)	Locus ceruleus	Neocortex, thalamus	1. Tricyclics and some SSRIs
Dopamine (DA)	Substantia nigra, ventral tegmental nuclei	Striatum, neocortex, limbic system	1. Levodopa 2. Dopamine agonists 3. MAO-B inhibitors
Serotonin (5-HT)	Midbrain raphe nuclei	Neocortex, thalamus, reticular formation	1. Reuptake inhibitors
Somatostatin	Inhibitory neurons, widely distributed	Neocortex hippocampus	1. Somatostatin analogues

Key: AMPAkine = alpha-amino-3-hydroxy-5-methyl-4-isoxazolepropionate; CNS = central nervous system; AChE = acetylcholinesterase; NMDA = *N*-methyl-D-aspartate; SSRIs = selective serotonin reuptake inhibitors; MAO = monoamine oxidase.

choline acetyltransferase (ChAT),[122] both of which are markers for cholinergic activity. In addition, the nucleus basalis is commonly afflicted by NFT and SP depositions, by neuron and synapse loss, and (in the Lewy body variant) by Lewy body formation. Patients with the Lewy body variant have even lower levels of neocortical ChAT than those with pure AD.[123] The degree of decline in cholinergic markers has been found to correlate significantly with the severity of dementia in AD.[124] Animals in whom the nucleus basalis is selectively lesioned show impairments in attention, learning, and memory that appear analogous to the deficits seen in AD patients.[125–127]

Based on the above findings, the cholinergic deficit in AD is a logical target for treatments aimed at improving memory and cognition, and this has been achieved through inhibition of AChE, the enzyme that breaks down acetylcholine (ACh). So far, AChE inhibitors are the only drugs that have been approved by the U.S. Food and Drug Administration (FDA) for the treatment of AD. In addition to AChE inhibitors, several other approaches directed at the cholinergic system have been pursued. These include (1) precursor loading with choline and lecithin (a source of choline) or (2) using muscarinic and nicotinic ACh receptor agonists.

AChE Inhibitors AChE inhibitors prolong the action of ACh at postsynaptic receptors by preventing its hydrolysis. Numerous AChE inhibitors have undergone development during the past decade; so far, four of them received FDA approval for the treatment of AD (Table 45-2).

<u>Tacrine</u> Tacrine (Cognex) was approved for use in AD patients in 1993, after three double-blind placebo-controlled multicenter trials showed small but statistically significant benefits for the tacrine-treated as compared to the placebo-treated group in terms of the Alzheimer Disease Assessment Scale-Cognitive Component (ADAS-COG) scores and global ratings of functional ability.[128–130] About 15 to 20 percent of the AD patients treated with this drug improve by 4 or more

Table 45-2
Characteristics of AChE inhibitors

	Tacrine	*Donepezil*	*Rivastigmine*	*Galantamine*
Trade name	Cognex	Aricept	Exelon	Reminyl
Type of molecule	Aminoacridine	Piperidine	Carbamate	Tertiary alkaloid
Type of AChE inhibition	Noncompetitive, reversible	Noncompetitive, reversible	Pseudoirreversible	Competitive, reversible
ADAS-COG (treatment-placebo difference*)	1.4–2.2	2.5–2.9	2.3–3.8	3.1–3.9
Dosage	80–160 mg	5–10 mg	3–12 mg	8–32 mg
Frequency	qid	qd	bid	bid
Titration period	Every 6 weeks	After 4–6 weeks	Every 4 weeks	Every 4–8 weeks
Half-life (hours)	~3	~70	~1.5	~7
Route of elimination	Hepatic (cytochrome P450 1A2)	Hepatic (cytochrome P450 2D6 and 3A4)	Hepatic	Hepatic (cytochrome P450 2D6 and 3A4)
Typical side effects	Nausea, vomiting, diarrhea, hepatotoxicity	Nausea, vomiting, anorexia, muscle cramps	Nausea, vomiting	Nausea, vomiting, anorexia, diarrhea

*Treatment differences from placebo based on intention to treat, last observation carried forward method of analyses in clinical trials lasting 12 to 28 weeks.

points on the ADAS-COG, which is felt to be clinically significant. Unfortunately, nearly 50 percent of those receiving tacrine developed liver toxicity. The effects of tacrine are dose-dependent and are more noticeable at the higher dose of 160 mg daily. Tacrine did not achieve widespread use because of hepatotoxicity and the need for frequent monitoring for hepatotoxicity.

Donepezil Donepezil (Aricept) was the second AChE inhibitor approved by the FDA for the treatment of mild to moderate AD. Like tacrine, donepezil is a reversible AChE inhibitor. However, it has several advantages over tacrine. It is administered once daily due to a long plasma half-life of approximately 70 h and appears to be well tolerated, with gastrointestinal side effects occurring in fewer than 20 percent of subjects who take a 10-mg dose. It is not associated with liver toxicity.

The efficacy of donepezil has been demonstrated in several clinical trials.[131–135] Efficacy from a 24-week study revealed that donepezil was associated with a 1.5- to 2.5-point improvement compared with placebo on the ADAS-COG at a dose of 5 mg daily and with a 2.9-point improvement at a dose of 10 mg daily. Results on the Clinician Interview-Based Impression of Change (CIBIC) Plus indicate that approximately 25 percent of subjects treated with donepezil at doses of 5 or 10 mg demonstrate noticeable clinical improvement, compared with 11 to 14 percent for placebo groups. The long-term (>1 year) efficacy and safety of donepezil have been evaluated in two clinical trials.[136,137] The donepezil-treated group was associated with a 38 percent reduction in the risk of functional decline compared with placebo group[137] and with benefits on global assessment, cognition, and activities of daily living (ADL) over placebo.[136]

Rivastigmine Rivastigmine (Exelon) was the third AChE inhibitor approved by the FDA for the treatment of mild-to-moderate AD. Rivastigmine is a pseudoirreversible AChE inhibitor and a butyrylcholinesterase inhibitor.[138] Since rivastigmine is metabolized principally by AChE itself and has a low plasma protein binding, it has few interactions with other drugs. Rivastigmine is dosed twice daily.

Rivastigmine has been evaluated in three large, 26-week clinical trials. Over 2100 patients with mild-to-moderate AD have been enrolled in one of three randomized, placebo-controlled, double-blind studies.[139–141] The 26-week U.S. trial revealed an ADAS-COG treatment-placebo difference of 3.8

points for high-dose and 2.1 points for low-dose rivastigmine.[139] The long-term efficacy and safety of rivastigmine have been evaluated in a 6-month U.S. study with a 6-month open-label extension.[141] At 12 months, a mean decline of 3.8 points on ADAS-COG scores for patients treated with rivastigmine was noted, which was less than the 8 points that would have been predicted based on historical data.

Galantamine Galantamine (Reminyl), a tertiary alkaloid, is the fourth AChE inhibitor approved by the FDA. It is a selective, reversible, competitive inhibitor of AChE that enhances central nervous system (CNS) cholinergic functions through two mechanisms: inhibition of AChE and potentiation of nicotinic ACh receptors.[142] The drug is administered twice daily, preferably with breakfast and dinner. Galantamine is generally well tolerated by patients with AD.

Galantamine has been evaluated in large clinical trials of 3 to 24 months' duration.[143–145] Over 3000 patients with mild-to-moderate AD have been enrolled in one of three randomized, placebo-controlled, double-blind studies. Results from these studies suggest a statistically significant treatment effect for galantamine versus placebo on cognitive performance, global function, and ADL. In the 6-month U.S. study,[145] mean change from baseline on the ADAS-COG for the treatment group was 3.9 points better than that of the placebo group at the end of the study. A similar result was observed in a 5-month U.S. study, where more galantamine-treated patients (~35 percent) achieved a clinically meaningful improvement in ADAS-COG score (≥4 points) than placebo. In addition, galantamine-treated patients had significantly better outcomes with regard to behavioral disturbances and psychiatric symptoms as measured by the Neuropsychiatric Inventory (NPI) total score. Galantamine reduced both the distress associated with patients' behavioral symptoms and caregiver burden as well as the daily time required by caregivers to supervise patients.

The long-term efficacy of galantamine has been evaluated in the 6-month U.S. study with a 6-month open-label extension.[145] An 18-month open-label extension has been reported.[146] The ADAS-COG scores of patients treated with galantamine did not decline from baseline for the first 12 months of the study. At 24 months, a mean decline of 5.4 points on ADAS-COG scores for patients treated with galantamine was noted, which was less than that which would have been predicted based on historical data.

AChE inhibitors are the only therapy approved by the FDA for the treatment of AD. Even though the size of the treatment effect is only modest on ADAS-COG, the cognitive gains are detectable on clinical ratings by both clinician and caregivers and on functional ratings, independent of the cognitive measures. These agents also have benefits on behavioral symptoms of AD patients. In some trials, small differences in ADLs can be detected. In addition, several studies have revealed long-term benefits (>1 year) of AChE inhibitors in treating mild to moderate AD.

Selective Muscarinic Receptor Agonists and Nicotinic Acetylcholine Receptor Agonists Cholinergic agonists act directly on the pre- or postsynaptic cholinergic receptors. In the CNS, cholinergic receptors can be divided into two subtypes, nicotinic and muscarinic receptors. Both muscarinic and nicotinic receptors are reduced in AD brains.[147] Muscarinic receptors can be further divided into M_1, M_2, and M_3. It is known that the cortex and hippocampus contain abundant M_1 receptors, consistent with its role as a major postsynaptic muscarinic receptor.[148] M_2 receptors are present centrally and peripherally in brainstem and heart, while M_1, M_2, and M_3 receptors are present in gut. Several nonselective muscarinic agonists have been tried in AD, but the use of these agonists has been hindered by peripheral side effects. Several selective M_1 agonists underwent clinical trials, but none have shown sufficient efficacy and tolerability for clinical use.

The effects of nicotine and its analogues have also been examined in AD patients. Nicotine appears to increase anxiety as well as to improve attention and short-term memory.[149–151] However, nicotine never achieved clinical use in AD due to adverse effects. Several other nicotinic receptor agonists are currently in development, but it is too early to foresee their clinical use.

Other Cholinergic Strategies Precursor loading using choline and lecithin has been tried in many studies in combination or alone. This approach has been ineffective.

Excitatory Amino Acids Glutamate is a major excitatory neurotransmitter in the CNS, which activates at least two types of glutamate receptors, *N*-methyl-D-aspartate (NMDA) receptors and alpha-amino-3-hydroxy-5-methyl-4-isoxazolepropionate (AMPA) receptors. AMPA receptors are the principal mediators of fast excitatory transmission, whereas NMDA receptors are involved in synaptic plasticity and neuroexcitotoxicity, which has been implicated in the pathogenesis of a variety of neurodegenerative disorders, including AD. In several clinical trials, the NMDA receptor modulators milacemide and D-cycloserine have failed to improve cognition in AD patients.[152,153]

Memantine Memantine, a noncompetitive NMDA antagonist, has been approved for use in the treatment of dementia in Germany for over 10 years. It exhibits none of the undesirable side effects associated with competitive NMDA antagonists such as dizocilpine or high-affinity noncompetitive antagonists such as MK-801. In a 12-week double-blind placebo-controlled trial, 166 severely demented [Mini-Mental State Examination (MMSE) score <10] patients with either AD (49 percent) or vascular dementia (51 percent) were randomized to receive either 10 mg memantine daily or placebo.[154] A positive response in the Clinical Global Impression of Change (CGIC) was seen in 73 percent of the memantine group versus 45 percent of the placebo group. In a 28-week, double-blind, placebo-controlled U.S. phase III trial of severely demented AD patients (MMSE score 3 to14), memantine-treated group also showed better scores on CIBIC plus.[155] Another multicenter phase III trial is in progress to assess the efficacy of memantine in treating severely demented AD patients.

AMPAkine AMPAkines are a family of approximately 300 small synthetic compounds. A number of AMPAkine compounds show positive modulatory effects on AMPA receptor function in animal studies.[156,157] Three double-blind placebo-controlled phase II studies are in progress to determine the tolerability and primary efficacy of one of the AMPAkine compounds in patients with AD.

Somatostatin and Other Neuropeptides Somatostatin is a neuropeptide that is concentrated in large neurons of the cortex and hippocampus and, among other roles, modulates the activity of neurons whose primary neurotransmitter is the inhibitory gamma-aminobutyric acid (GABA), which is widely distributed in the brain.[158] Immunocytochemistry has demonstrated reactivity to somatostatin and other neuropeptides (neuropeptide Y, cholecystokinin, vasoactive intestinal peptide, corticotrophin-releasing factor) in neuritic plaques. Levels of somatostatin and many neuropeptides are diminished overall in AD brains.[159] The neuropathologic and clinical implications of these changes are not well understood, and treatments aimed at correcting these deficiencies are still in development.

Treatment of the Behavioral Manifestations of AD

Although the primary symptoms of AD are memory impairment and loss of cognitive abilities, AD patients also display characteristic neuropsychiatric symptoms at some stage of the illness. These symptoms include depression, anxiety, agitation, delusions, hallucinations, psychosis, wandering, and sleep disturbance, which have significant impacts on the quality of life of the patients and the caregiver. In addition, noncognitive symptoms are also associated with an increased risk for institutionalization. While psychotropic drugs are frequently used to control these symptoms, they have the potential for significant side effects, which include sedation, disinhibition, falls, incontinence, parkinsonism, tardive dyskinesia, and akathisias.

In general, there have been few double-blind, placebo-controlled trials for behavioral treatment in AD. Most clinicians, therefore, make decisions regarding therapy based on personal experience and the side-effect profile of each medication (Table 45-3).

Depression Up to 25 percent of patients with AD have depressed mood at the time of onset of memory loss.[160] In addition, major depression occurs in 5 to 8 percent of patients.[161] Depression is more prominent early in AD, when patients still have some awareness of their cognitive impairments. Depression can itself mimic dementia. It should be treated, since depression can contribute to cognitive impairment.[162]

If the depression requires therapy, one of the selective serotonin reuptake inhibitors (SSRIs:

Table 45-3
Psychotropic treatments in AD

Psychotropic treatments in AD
Cholinergic agents
Tacrine (Cognex)
Donepezil (Aricept)
Rivastigmine (Exelon)
Galantamine (Reminyl)
Disease-modifying agents
Vitamine E
Selegiline
Psychotropic agents
Depression
Tricyclics
Nortriptyline (Pamelor)
Selective serotonin reuptake inhibitors
Fluoxetine (Prozac)
Paroxetine (Paxil)
Sertraline (Zoloft)
Fluvoxamine (Luvox)
Citalopram (Celexa)
Venlafaxine (Effexor)
Anxiety
Lorazepam (Ativan)
Alprazolam (Xanax)
Buspirone (Buspar)
Agitation
Trazodone (Desyrel)
Haloperidol (Haldol)
Thioridazine (Mellaril)
Risperidone (Risperdal)
Olanzapine (Zyprexa)
Quetiapine (Seroquel)
Delusions
Risperidone (Risperdal)
Olanzapine (Zyprexa)
Quetiapine (Seroquel)
Haloperidol (Haldol)
Insomnia
Warm milk
Trazodone (Desyrel)
Diphenhydramine (Benadryl)
Zolpidem (Ambien)
Short-acting benzodiazepine
Anticonvulsants
Valproic acid
Carbamazepine
Gabapentin (Neurontin)

fluoxetine, sertraline, fluvoxamine, paroxetine, or citalopram) is commonly used. Venlafaxine is an inhibitor of both serotonin and norepinephrine reuptake that may be useful in some refractory cases. Trazodone is an antidepressant with serotonin reuptake inhibition properties, α-adrenergic antagonism, and antihistaminergic properties. In addition to depression, serotoninergic agents such as the SSRIs are useful for a variety of behavioral symptoms in AD. Tricyclic antidepressants such as nortriptyline, amitriptyline, and imipramine may also be effective in treating AD patients with depression. However, the SSRIs and some other newer antidepressants are preferred to tricyclics, not only because of their greater efficacy but also because they produce fewer side effects, such as confusion, orthostatic hypotension, dry mouth, and cardiac problems. SSRIs are better tolerated but cause insomnia, anorexia, and ejaculatory dysfunctions.

Anxiety Anxiety may accompany AD, especially in its early stages. It can be treated with small doses of benzodiazepines, such as lorazepam and alprazolam, or buspirone, as needed.

Agitation and Psychosis Agitation, a common neuropsychiatric symptom complex in AD, includes three behavioral symptoms: aggressive behaviors, inappropriate physically nonaggressive behaviors, and inappropriate verbal agitated behaviors.[163] Psychotic behaviors, such as hallucinations and delusions, may coexist, especially at the later stages of the disease. Agitation can have serious emotional, medical, and health care system consequences. It results in decreased quality of life for both the patient and caregiver and is often cited as an important factor for institutionalization.

Since the causes of agitation are multifactorial, its management must be multidisciplinary. Precipitating factors, such as medical illnesses, should be sought for and corrected. Neuroleptics, which block dopamine receptors, are often used to treat these symptoms,[164–166] but they can produce disabling side effects, such as akathisia, tardive dyskinesia, and parkinsonism. The deficits in aminergic neurotransmitters make AD patients more sensitive to the therapeutic effects and extrapyramidal side effects of neuroleptics. Newer "atypical" neuroleptics—such as risperidone (Risperdal), olanzapine (Zyprexa), and quetiapine

(Seroquel)—which have more selective receptor specificity than older agents, may be useful for controlling agitation in AD with a lesser risk of side effects. Several placebo-controlled trials of risperidone in agitated AD patients have demonstrated a significant reduction in some behavioral symptoms.[165,167] Low doses of olanzapine (5 to 10 mg daily) may be also useful in reducing agitation while producing few extrapyramidal symptoms.[168] All such medications should be given in the lowest effective doses, and alternatives, such as behavioral management, should be considered before neuropsychiatric drugs are prescribed.

Anticonvulsants such as carbamazepine and divalproex sodium have been used in treating behavioral disturbances in AD patients. Carbamazepine[169] and divalproex sodium[170] have been reported to reduce agitation in demented nursing home patients in two small studies. A multicenter, double-blind, placebo-controlled trial is in progress to assess the efficacy and safety of valproic acid in treating the behavioral symptoms of AD patients.

Sleep Disturbance Disturbances of sleep and the sleep-wake cycle are a common clinical observation in AD, as is "sundowning," or the onset or exacerbation of delirium during the evening or night and that disappears or improves during the daytime.[171] About 10 percent of AD outpatient and 30 percent of institutionalized AD patients have sleep disturbances.[172] These are best managed by environmental manipulation. Keeping the patient awake during the day, reducing daytime naps, restriction of time in bed, reducing nighttime fluids, and adequate exposure to daytime bright light may be helpful, but these measures have not been rigorously investigated.[171,173] Pharmacologic treatments range from neuroleptics to sedative drugs, all of which have adverse effects. A nighttime dose of trazodone 25 to 100 mg or diphenhydramine 25 to 50 mg might suffice. Alternatively, short-acting benzodiazepines such as zolpidem can be used intermittently to prevent the development of tolerance.

Wandering Wandering, one of the most disturbing symptoms, includes behaviors such as aimless walking, purposeful attempts to leave the home or health care facility, and nighttime walking and pacing. Altering the physical environment by concealing doorways and encouraging movement under supervision may limit wandering.[174,175] Behavioral therapy involving structured programs to help instill a sense of stability and security has also been shown to be helpful. Other treatments include use of SSRI antidepressants[176] and AChE inhibitors, but again, no controlled trials have been conducted.

Therapies Aimed at Slowing Disease Progression or Delaying Disease Onset

Although there are no fully effective therapies for AD currently, there are several potential mechanisms specifically related to the pathogenesis of AD that may modify the appearance or progression of this disease. Since the prevalence of AD rises rapidly with aging, a treatment that delays the onset of the disease would have enormous medical, social, and economic consequences.

Antiamyloid Treatment The Aβ protein, which is widely believed to be the leading candidate for a causative agent in AD, is cleaved from the much larger APP. α-Secretase involves the nonamyloidogenic pathway, whereas β- and γ-secretases are involved in Aβ production. Thus, inhibition of the β- or γ-secretase activity would reduce the Aβ production. Alternatively, increasing clearance of Aβ would also reduce Aβ deposits in the brain.

γ- and β-Secretase Inhibitors A major therapeutic advance in the treatment of AD has been the development of β- and γ-secretase inhibitors. Several pharmaceutical companies have developed γ-secretase inhibitors and at least one agent was in a phase I clinical trial in the years 2000 and 2001. Furthermore, the identifications of β-secretase may pave the way for developing specific β-secretase inhibitors.

Immunotherapy An exciting approach to the reduction of Aβ deposits comes from recent studies in APP transgenic mice.[177–180] The PDAPP mouse, which is transgenic for a human APP gene containing a mutation at codon 717, exhibits age- and region-specific neuritic plaques, astrogliosis, synaptic loss, and behavioral abnormalities.[38] In older transgenic mice with fully developed neuritic plaques, parental immunization with synthetic human Aβ peptide led to a reduction of the total plaque burden. Immunization of young mice before the development of AD-type pathology is associated with a significant decline of subsequent plaque formation.[177,178] In addition, immunization also prevents cognitive decline in a different APP transgenic mouse model.[179,180]

Data from single- and multiple-dose phase I safety studies in approximately 80 patients with mild to moderate AD has shown that immunization with Aβ plus adjuvant is well tolerated, and no significant side effects have been noted. A double-blind, placebo-controlled, multicenter international phase II trial to evaluate the safety and efficacy of immunization in mild to moderate AD patients was initiated but stopped due to the development of encephalitis in a minority of the immunized subjects.

Metal Chelator to Decrease Aβ Plaques Recent studies suggest that metals such as Cu^{2+} and Zn^{2+} may play an important role in the pathogenesis of AD. Cu^{2+} and Zn^{2+} are elevated in the neocortex in AD, particularly in neuritic plaques.[181,182] In the APP2576 transgenic mouse brain, both Zn^{2+} and Fe are enriched in amyloid deposits.[183,184] When clioquinol, a Cu/Zn chelator, is given to 12-month-old APP2576 mice for 12 weeks, there is a 65 percent reduction in sedimentable Aβ in the clioquinol-treated mice, and some of the mice treated with clioquinol show no detectable Aβ deposits.[185] Similar results were obtained with older 21-month-old mice. A phase I trial of clioquinol with B_{12} supplementation in AD patients revealed no adverse side effects. A phase II clinical trial is currently in progress.[185,186]

Anti-Inflammatory Approaches Although AD has classically been considered to be a neurodegenerative disease, large amounts of data suggest that inflammatory processes play important roles in the pathogenesis of AD. Activated microglia and at least 40 proteins associated with immune responses are present in the AD brain.[187]

Nonsteroidal Anti-Inflammatory Drugs (NSAIDs) and COX-2 Inhibitors Many epidemiologic studies have shown that anti-inflammatory drugs including both steroids and NSAIDs delay the onset and progression of AD.[188,189] In a twin study, the twin with prior exposure to either glucocorticoids or NSAIDs is less likely to become demented.[190] In a recent prospective, population-based cohort study of 6989 subjects who were followed for a period of 6.8 years, long-term use (>24 months) of NSAIDs is associated with a significantly lower risk of developing AD.[191] In an early study, AD patients treated with indomethacin for 6 months appeared to have a slower rate of progression than those given placebo, despite a high dropout rate in the indomethacin-treated group.[192] In a 25-week pilot study, 41 patients with mild to moderate AD were randomized to receive either placebo or diclofenac (50 mg daily); only nonsignificant trends in favor of diclofenac are noted.[193]

Traditional NSAIDs act by nonselective inhibition of cyclooxygenase (COX). There are two types of COX, a constitutive form, COX-1, and a mitogen-inducible form, COX-2. The major advantage of selective COX-2 inhibitors is their reduced gastrointestinal side effects. Recent studies suggest that COX-2 may contribute to the pathogenesis of AD, and inhibition of COX-2 may be a useful theaputic target.[194] However, in a 52-week double-blind, placebo-controlled trial of 425 subjects with mild to moderate AD, celecoxib at 200 mg twice daily failed to demonstrate efficacy in slowing cognitive decline.[195] In light of the recent discovery that some NSAIDs can reduce Aβ_{42} independent of inhibition of COX activity,[196] several additional NSAIDs are in clinical development.

Prednisone Among the classes of anti-inflammatory drugs, glucocorticoids are the most potent and the broadest anti-inflammatory/immunosuppressive drugs in clinical use. In a randomized, double-blind, placebo-controlled, multicenter trial,[197] prednisone or placebo were given to 138 patients with AD. The active treatment regimen consisted of prednisone 20 mg daily for 4 weeks, tapered to 10 mg for the duration of 1 year, followed by gradual withdrawal over an additional 16 weeks. The primary outcome measure was the 1-year change on the ADAS-COG. Unfortunately, the study was negative: there was no difference in cognitive decline between the prednisone and placebo treatment groups. Furthermore, subjects treated with prednisone displayed a greater behavioral decline.

Hydroxychloroquine Since the 1950s, because of its broad scope of anti-inflammatory activity, the antimalarial drug hydroxychloroquine has been used to treat inflammatory diseases such as rheumatoid arthritis. It is well tolerated and readily passes across the blood-brain barrier. However, in an 18-month double-blind, placebo-controlled multicenter trial, hydroxychloroquine at 200 or 400 mg daily failed to show any benefit in cognition, behavior, or ADL for patients with mild AD.[198]

Estrogens Estrogens may play an important role in cognitive functions. Estrogen-sensitive neurons are found in both male and female brains. Estrogen receptors colocalize with low-affinity nerve growth factor (NGF) receptors on basal forebrain ACh-producing neurons, including those in the nucleus basalis.[199] Estrogen has been reported to regulate NMDA receptors in the hippocampus.[200] Estrogen is a free radical scavenger, thus protecting against oxidation and oxidative stress,[201–203] and it has neurotrophic activity.[204,205] AD occurs in approximately twice as many women as men.[105] An abrupt decline in estrogen production among postmenopausal women is thought to be one of the major factors. A number of epidemiologic, preclinical, and clinical studies support the concept of using supplemental estrogen to improve cognition in women with AD.

Epidemiologic studies examining the relationship between estrogen replacement therapy (ERT) and AD have been mixed. Early studies failed to demonstrate a protective effect of estrogen.[206–210] However, more recent epidemiologic studies suggest that estrogen is associated with a reduced risk of developing dementia.[211–216] Three very small open-label clinical trials[217–219] reported improvement in some areas of cognitive function in women with dementia who were receiving ERT.

The results of four double-blind, placebo-controlled clinical trials have been reported.[220–223] Only one small pilot study reported slight improvement in attention and verbal memory in postmenopausal women with mild to moderate AD treated with 17 β-estradiol patches for 8 weeks. The other three trials revealed no improvement in cognition in AD women treated with conjugated equine estrogens (Premarin) for 3 to 12 months.[221–223] In the large multicenter study,[223] hysterectomized women with AD were randomized to placebo, Premarin 0.625 mg per day, or Premarin 1.25 mg per day for 12 months. No differences were observed between the treatment and placebo groups in cognitive, global, or functional decline.

Neurotrophic Factors

NGF Neurotrophic factors are polypeptides that promote the growth and differentiation of neurons in the developing nervous system and support survival of neurons in the adult. NGF, the best-characterized neurotrophic factor, has a profound effect on central cholinergic neurons.

Since NGF is a protein, it is inactive with oral administration and cannot cross the blood-brain barrier when administrated systemically. In animal studies, intraventricular administration of NGF can partially reverse lesions and age-related behavioral, biochemical, and histologic deficits. Treatment with NGF ameliorates memory and learning deficits in the Morris water maze task,[224,225] increases the activity of ChAT,[225] and increases cortical ACh synthesis.[226] Histologic reversal of cellular atrophy due to lesioning[227] or aging[224] of cholinergic basal forebrain neurons has also been demonstrated after intraventricular NGF administration. However, intraventricular administration of NGF is associated with significant adverse effects, including an increase in APP expression,[228] an increase in sympathetic innervation of cerebral blood vessels,[229] the stimulation of sympathetic and sensory neurite sprouting,[230] Schwann cell hyperplasia,[231] and stimulation of other CNS NGF-responsive neurons.[232] NGF has been infused intraventricularly in three patients with AD.[233] Even though the treatment was associated with cognitive improvement on some neuropsychological tests, it was also associated with severe back pain and weight loss.

The gene therapy approach has been used as an alternative route for administering NGF to reverse the atrophy of cholinergic neurons in the basal forebrain of aged monkeys.[234] A phase I study is in progress using similar techniques. In this study, eight patients will receive autologous transplants of skin fibroblasts modified to secrete NGF. These cells will be transplanted to the basal forebrain in the region of the nucleus basalis of Meynert.

Propentofylline Because of the difficulty of delivering NGF to the brain, orally bioavailable agents capable of stimulating or upregulating brain NGF have been studied. Propentofylline, a xanthine derivative, stimulates the synthesis and release of NGF in the basal forebrain.[235,236] In a 12-month double-blind, placebo-controlled clinical trial of AD and vascular dementia, the patients with AD show a very small degree of efficacy.[237] In a total of 901 patients with AD given propentofylline in other clinical trials, the scores on the MMSE improved slightly, but the ADAS-COG was not used in these trials.[237,238]

AIT-082 AIT-082 (Neotrofin) is a neurotrophic agent under development as a potential treatment for AD. AIT-082 is a paraaminobenzoic acid derivative of hypoxanthine that mimics the action of NGF in cell culture, enhancing the effect of NGF on neuritogenesis.[239] AIT-082 has been shown to enhance cognition, improve both long- and short-term memory in young mice, and restore memory in mice with mild to moderate age-related memory deficits.[240] This agent is orally bioavailable, well tolerated, and currently undergoing phase II clinical trials in patients with AD.[241,242]

In addition to NGF, numerous additional neurotrophic factors have recently been identified and proposed for use in a wide variety of neurodegenerative diseases.[243] A potential therapeutic approach is suggested by the recent discovery of humanin,[244,245] a short polypeptide, which prevented neuronal death caused by multiple different types of familial AD genes and Aβ peptides.

Antioxidants

Vitamin E and Selegiline Free radicals, such as peroxide and superoxide, are reactive species derived mainly from oxygen and lipids that are produced by oxidative metabolism. In general, cells with high levels of oxidative metabolism and high lipid content (e.g., neurons) are at particularly high risk for free radical–induced damage.[246] These substances, particularly in combination with iron and ferritin, which are frequently deposited in the course of AD, may overwhelm neuronal antioxidant defenses.[247] The defenses consist primarily of enzymes such as superoxide dismutase and glutathione peroxidase, reductase, and transferase along with free radical acceptors (i.e., reducing agents) such as vitamins E and C, β-carotene, and membrane lipids. There are several lines of evidence implicating free radical mechanisms in AD, including promotion of free radical formation by Aβ toxicity or neurotransmitter catabolism, impairment of mitochondrial function, and lipid peroxidation. There is also a significant increase in monoamine oxidase (MAO-B) activity in AD brain.[248]

Population-based and epidemiologic studies suggest that antioxidant vitamin intake is associated with a lower incidence of AD.[249] A number of small clinical trials using MAO inhibitors in AD have demonstrated modest improvement in behavior; some studies have shown small effects on a variety of verbal learning tasks or rate of decline (see review, Ref. 250). In a 2-year pivotal trial[251] of moderately demented AD patients with mean MMSE scores between 11 and 13, vitamin E (1000 IU twice daily) and selegiline (10 mg daily) were effective at delaying progression to a more advanced disease stage and subsequent institutionalization. There was no difference in the rate of decline on the MMSE or the ADAS-COG during the 2 years of the trial. In addition, there was no added benefit from the combination of vitamin E and selegiline.

Vitamin C Vitamin C has been shown to be effective in preventing the development of AD in a prospective study of 633 individuals over 65 years of age. Over an average 4.3 year follow-up, none of 23 subjects who took a high dose of vitamin C developed AD, while 11 of 68 multivitamin users and 80 of 542 nonvitamin users developed probable AD.[249]

Idebenone Idebenone is a benzoquinone compound structurally related to coenzyme Q. It has antioxidant properties and is a free radical scavenger. It protects cell membranes from lipid peroxidation, and against glutamate and Aβ-induced neurotoxicity in neuronal cell cultures.[252–255] In an earlier double-blind, placebo-controlled clinical trial, idebenone was found to be effective in enhancing memory, attention, and orientation in AD patients.[256] However, in a more recent 1-year trial, idebenone was found not to be effective, and subsequent trials were suspended because of lack of sufficient efficacy.

Ginkgo Biloba The extract of ginkgo biloba, derived from the leaves of a subtropical tree, is believed to act as an antioxidant. Ginkgo biloba extract is approved in Germany for the treatment of dementia, including AD and vascular dementia. It is widely used in the United States as an alternative therapy for AD. Only one U.S. trial studied the efficacy and safety of EGb761, an extract of ginkgo biloba,[257] in which, EGb-761 showed a small effect on cognition (1.7 points improvement on the ADAS-COG over 52 weeks when compared to placebo). However, less than half of the subjects completed the trial, which raises questions about the validity of the result.

Decreasing Tau Hyperphosphorylation NFTs are composed of hyperphosphorylated tau. The phosphorylation state of tau depends on a balance between kinases and phosphatase; inhibition of the former or enhancement of the latter could potentially diminish PHF formation. Recent evidence suggests that unregulated Cdk5 may function as one of the major kinases in hyperphosphorylation of tau.[64] In theory, specific Cdk5 inhibitors may significantly decrease tau hyperphosphorylation and thus slow the progression of AD. Several agents have been shown to reduce the degree of tau phosphorylation in vitro.[258–261] However, it is too early to predict whether these agents will translate into effective treatments of AD.

Statins Increasing evidence suggests that cholesterol plays an important role in the pathogenesis of AD. The normal cellular function of ApoE is the uptake and delivery of lipids.[116] ApoE $\varepsilon 4$, the major genetic risk factor for AD, correlates with increasing atherosclerosis and plaque formation.[262,263] An elevated cholesterol level increases plaque formation and Aβ deposition in animal models.[264,265] The formation of Aβ was completely blocked by reducing the cellular cholesterol level of living hippocampal neurons with statins.[266,267] Two recent epidemiologic studies revealed a significant decrease in the prevalence of AD and other dementias for patients treated with statins.[268,269] Several double-blind, placebo-controlled trials are currently under way to determine the efficacy of statins in preventing cognitive decline.[270] The SUN Health Study is a double-blind, placebo-controlled trial comparing atorvastatin to placebo in AD patients. The Prospective Study of Pravastatin in Elderly at Risk (PROSPER) trial[270] is a double-blind, placebo-controlled trial to investigate the effect of pravastatin in an elderly nondemented population; 5804 persons with cardiovascular disease or at increased risk have been randomized. Even though the major endpoints of this study are stroke, myocardial infarction, and mortality, the data from annual neuropsychological tests should provide information on the effect of pravastatin on cognitive decline in the elderly nondemented population.

MCI Trials Mild cognitive impairment (MCI) has been used to identify subjects as having a memory complaint and objective memory loss on psychometric testing but with little or no loss of other cognitive functions and no or minimal impairment in ADL.[271] The rate of progression to AD in MCI is much higher than that of the general population, reaching 12 to 15 percent per year.[272,273] Due to the high conversion rate, it is more efficient to study MCI patients than normal controls, who develop AD at rates of 1 to 2 percent per year, especially for medications that are expensive or have significant side effects.

Currently, there are at least four secondary prevention MCI trials and one treatment trial using MCI subjects. One secondary prevention trial is examining the efficacy of vitamin E and donepezil to prevent the progression of MCI to AD. This is a double-blind, placebo-controlled trial with approximately 760 participants diagnosed with MCI. Subjects will be followed for 3 years and the primary outcome is the conversion rate to AD. There are two additional trials examining the efficacy of the AChE inhibitors rivastigmine and galantamine in the prevention of MCI conversion to AD. In a fourth trial, the efficacy of the selective COX-2 inhibitor rofecoxib (Vioxx) is being compared to placebo in delaying the onset of AD. Finally, a fifth treatment trial of donepezil in patients with MCI has been completed, although the results of this study are not yet available.

Primary Prevention Trials Due to our increased understanding of pathogenesis of AD, it is now possible to develop strategies to prevent AD. Currently, several clinical trials are in progress for primary AD prevention.

Estrogens Two important estrogen primary prevention trials are currently under way. In the first study, the Women's Health Initiative Memory Study (WHIMS),[274] 8300 women aged 65 and older with normal cognition have been randomized to placebo or hormone replacement therapy. The progesterone/estrogen arm was recently discontinued because of an increase in the risk of myocardial infarction, stroke, and breast cancer; the unopposed estrogen arm is continuing.[275] The second is the PREPARE study, in which approximately 900 women over the age of 75 with a positive family history of AD are being enrolled.

Ginkgo Biloba A study is currently under way to evaluate the efficacy of ginkgo biloba in the prevention of primary dementia. This is a randomized, double-blind, placebo-controlled trial of approximately 3000 elderly individuals with normal cognition. The subjects are receiving either placebo or ginkgo biloba at a dose of 240 mg daily and are being examined every 6 months for 5 years. The incidence of dementia is the primary outcome.

Nonsteroidal Anti-Inflammatory Drugs A large three-arm prevention trial in elderly normal individuals is in progress (ADAPT) that will compare naproxen, a traditional NSAID; celecoxib (Celebrex), a selective COX-2 inhibitor; and placebo for the incidence of dementia.

CONCLUSION

Major advances in our understanding of AD pathogenesis allow us to develop different therapeutic strategies for symptomatic treatments, disease modification, and primary and secondary prevention of AD. Four AChE are already approved by the FDA for the treatment of AD. Vitamin E is widely used in clinical practice for slowing the progression of AD. Progress in delineating the AD pathogenesis cascade has provided several potential targets for the treatment of AD. Inhibition of Aβ production by γ- or β-secretase inhibitors could be a therapeutic target in the early clinical stages of the disease. Increasing clearance of Aβ deposits by either immunization or other small compounds may also provide a useful approach. In addition, an alternate approach would be to administrator anti-inflammatory drugs that could interfere with aspects of the microglial, astrocytic, and cytokine responses that occur in AD brains. The rate of scientific advance and progress in clinical trials indicates that some level of practical success in treating and preventing AD is on the horizon.

REFERENCES

1. Alzheimer A: Uber eine eigenartige Erkrangkung der Hirnrinde. *All Z Psychiatr* 64:146–148, 1907.
2. Mirra SS, Hart MN, Terry RD: Making the diagnosis of Alzheimer's disease. A primer for practicing pathologists. *Arch Pathol Lab Med* 117:132–144, 1993.
3. Khachaturian ZS: Diagnosis of Alzheimer's disease. *Arch Neurol* 42:1097–1105, 1985.
4. Robbins SL, Cotran RS, Kumar V: *Pathologic Basis of Disease*, 3d ed. Philadelphia: Saunders, 1984.
5. Glenner GG: Congophilic microangiopathy in the pathogenesis of Alzheimer's syndrome (presenile dementia). *Med Hypoth* 5:1231–1236, 1979.
6. McKee AC, Kowall NW, Kosik KS: Microtubular reorganization and dendritic growth response in Alzheimer's disease. *Ann Neurol* 26:652–659, 1989.
7. Masters CL, Simms G, Weinman NA, et al: Amyloid plaque core protein in Alzheimer disease and Down syndrome. *Proc Natl Acad Sci U S A* 82:4245–4249, 1985.
8. Selkoe DJ: Translating cell biology into therapeutic advances in Alzheimer's disease. *Nature* 399:A23–A31, 1999.
9. Selkoe DJ: Alzheimer's disease: genes, proteins, and therapy. *Physiol Rev* 81:741–766, 2001.
10. Kamal A, Almenar-Queralt A, LeBlanc JF, et al: Kinesin-mediated axonal transport of a membrane compartment containing beta-secretase and presenilin-1 requires APP. *Nature* 414:643–648, 2001.
11. Yan R, Bienkowski MJ, Shuck ME, et al: Membrane-anchored aspartyl protease with Alzheimer's disease beta-secretase activity. *Nature* 402:533–537, 1999.
12. Vassar R, Bennett BD, Babu-Khan S, et al: Beta-secretase cleavage of Alzheimer's amyloid precursor protein by the transmembrane aspartic protease BACE. *Science* 286:735–741, 1999.
13. Sinha S, Anderson JP, Barbour R, et al: Purification and cloning of amyloid precursor protein beta-secretase from human brain. *Nature* 402:537–540, 1999.
14. Selkoe DJ: Clearing the brain's amyloid cobwebs. *Neuron* 32:177–180, 2001.
15. Iwata N, Tsubuki S, Takaki Y, et al: Metabolic regulation of brain Aβ by neprilysin. *Science* 292:1550–1552, 2001.

16. Iwata N, Tsubuki S, Takaki Y, et al: Identification of the major $A\beta_{42}$-degrading catabolic pathway in brain parenchyma: Suppression leads to biochemical and pathological deposition. *Nat Med* 6:143–150, 2000.
17. Qiu WQ, Walsh DM, Ye Z, et al: Insulin-degrading enzyme regulates extracellular levels of amyloid beta-protein by degradation. *J Biol Chem.* 273:32730–32738, 1998.
18. Kowall NW, McKee AC, Yankner BA, Beal MF: In vivo neurotoxicity of beta-amyloid (β_{1-40}) and the β_{25-35} fragment. *Neurobiol Aging* 13:537–542, 1992.
19. Busciglio J, Lorenzo A, Yeh J, Yankner BA: Beta-amyloid fibrils induce tau phosphorylation and loss of microtubule binding. *Neuron* 14:879–888, 1995.
20. Jarrett JT, Berger EP, Lansbury PT Jr: The C-terminus of the beta protein is critical in amyloidogenesis. *Ann NY Acad Sci* 695:144–148, 1993.
21. Jarrett JT, Berger EP, Lansbury PT Jr: The carboxy terminus of the beta amyloid protein is critical for the seeding of amyloid formation: implications for the pathogenesis of Alzheimer's disease. *Biochemistry* 32:4693–4697, 1993.
22. Jarrett JT, Lansbury PT Jr: Seeding "one-dimensional crystallization" of amyloid: A pathogenic mechanism in Alzheimer's disease and scrapie? *Cell* 73:1055–1058, 1993.
23. Mattson MP, Cheng B, Davis D, et al: Beta-amyloid peptides destabilize calcium homeostasis and render human cortical neurons vulnerable to excitotoxicity. *J Neurosci* 12:376–389, 1992.
24. Cotman CW, Pike CJ, Copani A: Beta-amyloid neurotoxicity: A discussion of in vitro findings. *Neurobiol Aging* 13:587–590, 1992.
25. Mattson MP, Rydel RE: Beta-amyloid precursor protein and Alzheimer's disease: The peptide plot thickens. *Neurobiol Aging* 13:617–621, 1992.
26. Abraham CR, Selkoe DJ, Potter H: Immunochemical identification of the serine protease inhibitor alpha 1-antichymotrypsin in the brain amyloid deposits of Alzheimer's disease. *Cell* 52:487–501, 1988.
27. Snow AD, Mar H, Nochlin D, et al: The presence of heparan sulfate proteoglycans in the neuritic plaques and congophilic angiopathy in Alzheimer's disease. *Am J Pathol* 133:456–463, 1988.
28. Eikelenboom P, Hack CE, Rozemuller JM, Stam FC: Complement activation in amyloid plaques in Alzheimer's dementia. *Virchows Arch B Cell Pathol Mol Pathol* 56:259–262, 1989.
29. Gomez-Pinilla F, Cummings BJ, Cotman CW: Induction of basic fibroblast growth factor in Alzheimer's disease pathology. *Neuroreport* 1:211–214, 1990.
30. Namba Y, Tomonaga M, Kawasaki H, et al: Apolipoprotein E immunoreactivity in cerebral amyloid deposits and neurofibrillary tangles in Alzheimer's disease and kuru plaque amyloid in Creutzfeldt-Jakob disease. *Brain Res* 541:163–166, 1991.
31. Cole GM, Masliah E, Shelton ER, et al: Accumulation of amyloid precursor fragment in Alzheimer plaques. *Neurobiol Aging* 12:85–91, 1991.
32. Joachim C, Games D, Morris J, et al: Antibodies to non-beta regions of the beta-amyloid precursor protein detect a subset of senile plaques. *Am J Pathol* 138:373–384, 1991.
33. Birecree E, Whetsell WO Jr, Stoscheck C, et al: Immunoreactive epidermal growth factor receptors in neuritic plaques from patients with Alzheimer's disease. *J Neuropathol Exp Neurol* 47:549–560, 1988.
34. Masliah E, Mallory M, Hansen L, et al: Localization of amyloid precursor protein in GAP43-immunoreactive aberrant sprouting neurites in Alzheimer's disease. *Brain Res* 574:312–316, 1992.
35. Perry G, Friedman R, Shaw G, Chau V: Ubiquitin is detected in neurofibrillary tangles and senile plaque neurites of Alzheimer disease brains. *Proc Natl Acad Sci U S A* 84:3033–3036, 1987.
36. Arai H, Lee VM, Otvos L Jr, et al: Defined neurofilament, tau, and beta-amyloid precursor protein epitopes distinguish Alzheimer from non-Alzheimer senile plaques. *Proc Natl Acad Sci USA* 87:2249–2253, 1990.
37. Armstrong DM, Benzing WC, Evans J, et al: Substance P and somatostatin coexist within neuritic plaques: Implications for the pathogenesis of Alzheimer's disease. *Neuroscience* 31:663–671, 1989.
38. Games D, Adams D, Alessandrini R et al: Alzheimer-type neuropathology in transgenic mice overexpressing V717F beta-amyloid precursor protein. *Nature* 373:523–527, 1995.
39. Glenner GG, Wong CW: Alzheimer's disease and Down's syndrome: Sharing of a unique cerebrovascular amyloid fibril protein. *Biochem Biophys Res Commun* 122:1131–1135, 1984.
40. Hof PR, Bouras C, Perl DP, et al: Age-related distribution of neuropathologic changes in the cerebral cortex of patients with Down's syndrome. Quantitative regional analysis and comparison with Alzheimer's disease. *Arch Neurol* 52:379–391, 1995.
41. Iwatsubo T, Mann DM, Odaka A, et al: Amyloid beta protein (A beta) deposition: A beta 42(43) precedes A beta 40 in Down syndrome. *Annu Neurol* 37:294–299, 1995.
42. Steiner H, Haass C: Intramembrane proteolysis by presenilins. *Nat Rev Mol Cell Biol* 1:217–224, 2000.

43. Li X, Greenwald I: Additional evidence for an eight-transmembrane-domain topology for *Caenorhabditis elegans* and human presenilins. *Proc Natl Acad Sci U S A* 95:7109–7114, 1998.
44. Yu G, Chen F, Levesque G, et al: The presenilin 1 protein is a component of a high molecular weight intracellular complex that contains beta-catenin. *J Biol Chem* 273:16470–16475, 1998.
45. De Strooper B, Saftig P, Craessaerts K, et al: Deficiency of presenilin-1 inhibits the normal cleavage of amyloid precursor protein. *Nature* 391:387–390, 1998.
46. Naruse S, Thinakaran G, Luo JJ, et al: Effects of PS1 deficiency on membrane protein trafficking in neurons. *Neuron* 21:1213–1221, 1998.
47. Wolfe MS, Xia W, Ostaszewski BL, et al: Two transmembrane aspartates in presenilin-1 required for presenilin endoproteolysis and gamma-secretase activity. *Nature* 398:513–517, 1999.
48. Steiner H, Duff K, Capell A, et al: A loss of function mutation of presenilin-2 interferes with amyloid beta-peptide production and Notch signaling. *J Biol Chem* 274:28669–28673, 1999.
49. Li YM, Xu M, Lai MT, et al: Photoactivated gamma-secretase inhibitors directed to the active site covalently label presenilin 1. *Nature* 405:689–694, 2000.
50. Esler WP, Kimberly WT, Ostaszewski BL, et al: Transition-state analogue inhibitors of gamma-secretase bind directly to presenilin-1. *Nat Cell Biol* 2:428–434, 2000.
51. Seiffert D, Bradley JD, Rominger CM, et al: Presenilin-1 and -2 are molecular targets for gamma-secretase inhibitors. *J Biol Chem* 275:34086–34091, 2000.
52. Li YM, Lai MT, Xu M, et al: Presenilin 1 is linked with gamma-secretase activity in the detergent solubilized state. *Proc Natl Acad Sci U S A* 97:6138–6143, 2000.
53. Artavanis-Tsakonas S, Rand MD, Lake RJ: Notch signaling: cell fate control and signal integration in development. *Science* 284:770–776, 1999.
54. Weinmaster G: The ins and outs of Notch signaling. *Mol Cell Neurosci* 1997;9:91-102, 1999.
55. Ray WJ, Yao M, Mumm J, et al: Cell surface presenilin-1 participates in the gamma-secretase-like proteolysis of Notch. *J Biol Chem* 274:36801–37807, 1999.
56. Song W, Nadeau P, Yuan M, et al: Proteolytic release and nuclear translocation of Notch-1 are induced by presenilin-1 and impaired by pathogenic presenilin-1 mutations. *Proc Natl Acad Sci U S A* 96:6959–6963, 1999.
57. Zhang Z, Nadeau P, Song W, et al: Presenilins are required for gamma-secretase cleavage of beta-APP and transmembrane cleavage of Notch-1. *Nat Cell Biol* 2:463–465, 2000.
58. Kidd M: Paired helical filaments in electron microscopy of Alzheimer's disease. *Nature* 197:192–194, 1963.
59. Lee VM, Balin BJ, Otvos L Jr, Trojanowski JQ: A68: A major subunit of paired helical filaments and derivatized forms of normal Tau. *Science* 251:675–678, 1991.
60. Lee VM, Trojanowski JQ: The disordered neuronal cytoskeleton in Alzheimer's disease. *Curr Opin Neurobiol* 2:653–656, 1992.
61. Drewes G, Ebneth A, Mandelkow EM: MAPs, MARKs and microtubule dynamics. *Trends Biochem Sci* 23:307–311, 1998.
62. Goedert M, Trojanowski JQ, Lee VM: The neurofibrillary pathology of Alzheimer's disease, in Rosenberg RN, Prusiner SB, DiMauro S, Barchi RL (eds): *The Molecular and Genetic Basis of Neurological Disease*. Boston, MA: Butterworth-Heinemann, 1996, pp 613–627.
63. Illenberger S, Zheng-Fischhofer Q, Preuss U, et al: The endogenous and cell cycle-dependent phosphorylation of tau protein in living cells: Implications for Alzheimer's disease. *Mol Biol Cell* 9:1495–1512, 1998.
64. Patrick GN, Zukerberg L, Nikolic M, et al: Conversion of p35 to p25 deregulates Cdk5 activity and promotes neurodegeneration. *Nature* 402:615–622, 1999.
65. Terry RD, Peck A, DeTeresa R, et al: Some morphometric aspects of the brain in senile dementia of the Alzheimer type. *Ann Neurol* 10:184–192, 1981.
66. Jobst KA, Smith AD, Szatmari M, et al: Detection in life of confirmed Alzheimer's disease using a simple measurement of medial temporal lobe atrophy by computed tomography. *Lancet* 340:1179–1183, 1992.
67. Luxenberg JS, Haxby JV, Creasey H, et al: Rate of ventricular enlargement in dementia of the Alzheimer type correlates with rate of neuropsychological deterioration. *Neurology* 37:1135–1140, 1987.
68. Kesslak JP, Nalcioglu O, Cotman CW: Quantification of magnetic resonance scans for hippocampal and parahippocampal atrophy in Alzheimer's disease. *Neurology* 41:51–54, 1991.
69. Jack CR Jr, Petersen RC, O'Brien PC, Tangalos EG: MR-based hippocampal volumetry in the diagnosis of Alzheimer's disease. *Neurology* 42:183–188, 1992.
70. Mann DM, Marcyniuk B, Yates PO, et al: The progression of the pathological changes of Alzheimer's disease in frontal and temporal neocortex examined both at biopsy and at autopsy. *Neuropathol Appl Neurobiol* 14:177–195, 1988.

71. Gomez-Isla T, Hollister R, West H, et al: Neuronal loss correlates with but exceeds neurofibrillary tangles in Alzheimer's disease. *Ann Neurol* 41:17–24, 1997.
72. Terry RD: Neuronal populations in normal and abnormal aging, in Goldstein AL (ed): *Biomedical Advances in Aging*. New York: Plenum Press, 1990, pp 435–440.
73. Ball MJ: Neuronal loss, neurofibrillary tangles and granulovacuolar degeneration in the hippocampus with ageing and dementia. A quantitative study. *Acta Neuropathol (Berl)* 37:111–118, 1977.
74. Hyman BT, Van Horsen GW, Damasio AR, Barnes CL: Alzheimer's disease: cell-specific pathology isolates the hippocampal formation. *Science* 225:1168–1170, 1984.
75. Whitehouse PJ, Price DL, Struble RG, et al: Alzheimer's disease and senile dementia: loss of neurons in the basal forebrain. *Science* 215:1237–1239, 1982.
76. Vogels OJ, Broere CA, ter Laak HJ, et al: Cell loss and shrinkage in the nucleus basalis Meynert complex in Alzheimer's disease. *Neurobiol Aging* 11:3–13, 1990.
77. Bondareff W, Mountjoy CQ, Roth M: Loss of neurons of origin of the adrenergic projection to cerebral cortex (nucleus locus ceruleus) in senile dementia. *Neurology* 32:164–168, 1982.
78. Aletrino MA, Vogels OJ, Van Domburg PH, Ten Donkelaar HJ: Cell loss in the nucleus raphes dorsalis in Alzheimer's disease. *Neurobiol Aging* 13:461–468, 1992.
79. Schechter R, Yen SH, Terry RD: Fibrous astrocytes in senile dementia of the Alzheimer type. *J Neuropathol Exp Neurol* 40:95–101, 1981.
80. DeKosky ST, Scheff SW: Synapse loss in frontal cortex biopsies in Alzheimer's disease: correlation with cognitive severity. *Ann Neurol* 27:457–464, 1990.
81. Scheff SW, DeKosky ST, Price DA: Quantitative assessment of cortical synaptic density in Alzheimer's disease. *Neurobiol Aging* 11:29–37, 1990.
82. Masliah E, Hansen L, Albright T, et al: Immunoelectron microscopic study of synaptic pathology in Alzheimer's disease. *Acta Neuropathol (Berl)* 81:428–433, 1991.
83. Scheff SW, Price DA: Synapse loss in the temporal lobe in Alzheimer's disease. *Ann Neurol* 33:190–199, 1993.
84. Masliah E, Terry RD, Alford M, et al: Cortical and subcortical patterns of synaptophysinlike immunoreactivity in Alzheimer's disease. *Am J Pathol* 138:235–246, 1991.
85. Brion JP, Couck AM, Bruce M, et al: Synaptophysin and chromogranin A immunoreactivities in senile plaques of Alzheimer's disease. *Brain Res* 539:143–150, 1991.
86. Davies CA, Mann DM, Sumpter PQ, Yates PO: A quantitative morphometric analysis of the neuronal and synaptic content of the frontal and temporal cortex in patients with Alzheimer's disease. *J Neurol Sci* 78:151–164, 1987.
87. Terry RD, Masliah E, Salmon DP, et al: Physical basis of cognitive alterations in Alzheimer's disease: Synapse loss is the major correlate of cognitive impairment. *Ann Neurol* 30:572–580, 1991.
88. Honer WG, Dickson DW, Gleeson J, Davies P: Regional synaptic pathology in Alzheimer's disease. *Neurobiol Aging* 13:375–382, 1992.
89. Masliah E, Iimoto DS, Saitoh T, et al: Increased immunoreactivity of brain spectrin in Alzheimer disease: A marker for synapse loss? *Brain Res* 531:36–44, 1990.
90. Samuel W, Masliah E, Hill LR, et al: Hippocampal connectivity and Alzheimer's dementia: Effects of synapse loss and tangle frequency in a two-component model. *Neurology* 44:2081–2088, 1994.
91. Scheff SW, Sparks DL, Price DA: Quantitative assessment of synaptic density in the outer molecular layer of the hippocampal dentate gyrus in Alzheimer's disease. *Dementia* 7:226–232, 1996.
92. Hsia AY, Masliah E, McConlogue L, et al: Plaque-independent disruption of neural circuits in Alzheimer's disease mouse models. *Proc Natl Acad Sci U S A* 96:3228–3233, 1999.
93. Mucke L, Masliah E, Yu GQ, et al: High-level neuronal expression of $A\beta_{1-42}$ in wild-type human amyloid protein precursor transgenic mice: Synaptotoxicity without plaque formation. *J Neurosci* 20:4050–4058, 2000.
94. Terry RD, Hansen LA, DeTeresa R, et al: Senile dementia of the Alzheimer type without neocortical neurofibrillary tangles. *J Neuropathol Exp Neurol* 46:262–268, 1987.
95. Hansen LA, Masliah E, Galasko D, Terry RD: Plaque-only Alzheimer disease is usually the Lewy body variant, and vice versa. *J Neuropathol Exp Neurol* 52:648–654, 1993.
96. Hansen L, Salmon D, Galasko D, et al: The Lewy body variant of Alzheimer's disease: a clinical and pathologic entity. *Neurology* 40:1–8, 1990.
97. McKeith IG, Perry EK, Perry RH: Report of the second dementia with Lewy body international workshop: Diagnosis and treatment. Consortium on Dementia with Lewy Bodies. *Neurology* 53:902–905, 1999.
98. McKeith IG, Galasko D, Kosaka K, et al: Consensus guidelines for the clinical and pathologic diagnosis of dementia with Lewy bodies (DLB): Report of the consortium on DLB international workshop. *Neurology* 47:1113–1124, 1996.

99. Lennox G, Lowe J, Landon M, et al: Diffuse Lewy body disease: correlative neuropathology using anti-ubiquitin immunocytochemistry. *J Neurol Neurosurg Psychiatry* 52:1236–1247, 1989.
100. Samuel W, Galasko D, Masliah E, Hansen LA: Neocortical Lewy body counts correlate with dementia in the Lewy body variant of Alzheimer's disease. *J Neuropathol Exp Neurol* 55:44–52, 1996.
101. Hamilton RL: Lewy bodies in Alzheimer's disease: A neuropathological review of 145 cases using alpha-synuclein immunohistochemistry. *Brain Pathol* 10:378–384, 2000.
102. Arai Y, Yamazaki M, Mori O, et al: Alpha-synuclein-positive structures in cases with sporadic Alzheimer's disease: Morphology and its relationship to tau aggregation. *Brain Res* 888:287–296, 2001.
103. Touchman JW, Dehejia A, Chiba-Falek O, et al: Human and mouse alpha-synuclein genes: Comparative genomic sequence analysis and identification of a novel gene regulatory element. *Genome Res* 11:78–86, 2001.
104. Ueda K, Fukushima H, Masliah E, et al: Molecular cloning of cDNA encoding an unrecognized component of amyloid in Alzheimer disease. *Proc Natl Acad Sci U S A* 90:11282–11286, 1993.
105. Jorm AF, Korten AE, Henderson AS: The prevalence of dementia: A quantitative integration of the literature. *Acta Psychiatr Scand* 76:465–479, 1987.
106. Hofman A, Rocca WA, Amaducci LA: A collaborative study of the prevalence of dementia in Europe: The EURODEM findings, in Gottfries CG, Levy SR, Clinche G, Tritsmans L (eds): *Diagnostic and Therapeutic Assessments in Alzheimer's Disease*. Wrightson Biomedical, 1991, pp 100–106.
107. Kawas C, Katzman R: Epidemiology of dementia and Alzheimer disease, in Terry R, Katzman R, Bick KL, Sisodia SS (eds): *Alzheimer Disease,* 2d ed. Philadelphia: Lippincott Williams & Wilkins, 1999, pp 95-116.
108. Zhang MY, Katzman R, Salmon D, et al: The prevalence of dementia and Alzheimer's disease in Shanghai, China: Impact of age, gender, and education. *Ann Neurol* 27:428–437, 1990.
109. Butler SM, Ashford JW, Snowdon DA: Age, education, and changes in the Mini-Mental State Exam scores of older women: Findings from the nun Study. *J Am Geriatr Soc* 44:675–681, 1996.
110. Snowdon DA, Ostwald S K, Kane RL: Education, survival, and independence in elderly Catholic sisters, 1936–1988. *Am J Epidemiol* 130:999–1012, 1989.
111. Ott A, Breteler MMB, van Harskamp F, et al: Prevalence of Alzheimer's disease and vascular dementia: Association with education. The Rotterdam study. *BMJ* 310:970–973, 1995.
112. Schmand B, Smit JH, Geerlings MI, Lindeboom J: The effects of intelligence and education on the development of dementia. A test of the brain reserve hypothesis. *Psychol Med* 27:1337–1344, 1997.
113. Van Duijn CM, Clayton DG, Chandra V, et al: Interaction between genetic and environmental risk factors for Alzheimer's disease: a reanalysis of case-control studies. EURODEM Risk Factors Research Group. *Genet Epidemiol* 11:539–551, 1994.
114. Swertfeger DK, Hui DY: Apolipoprotein E: a cholesterol transport protein with lipid transport-independent cell signaling properties. *Front Biosci* 6:D526–D535, 2001.
115. Herz J, Beffert U: Apolipoprotein E receptors: Linking brain development and Alzheimer's disease. *Nat Rev Neurosci* 1:51–58, 2000.
116. Mahley RW: Apolipoprotein E: Cholesterol transport protein with expanding role in cell biology. *Science* 240:622–630, 1988.
117. Menzel HJ, Kladetzky RG, Assmann G: Apolipoprotein E polymorphism and coronary artery disease. *Arteriosclerosis* 3:310–315, 1983.
118. Corder EH, Saunders AM, Strittmatter WJ, et al: Gene dose of apolipoprotein E type 4 allele and the risk of Alzheimer's disease in late onset families. *Science* 261:921–923, 1993.
119. Saunders AM, Strittmatter WJ, Schmechel D, et al: Association of apolipoprotein E allele epsilon 4 with late-onset familial and sporadic Alzheimer's disease. *Neurology* 43:1467–1472, 1993.
120. Galasko D, Saitoh T, Xia Y, et al: The apolipoprotein E allele epsilon 4 is overrepresented in patients with the Lewy body variant of Alzheimer's disease. *Neurology* 44:1950–1951, 1994.
121. Mesulam MM, Geula C: Nucleus basalis (Ch4) and cortical cholinergic innervation in the human brain: Observations based on the distribution of acetylcholinesterase and choline acetyltransferase. *J Comp Neurol* 275:216–240, 1988.
122. Hansen LA, DeTeresa R, Davies P, Terry RD: Neocortical morphometry, lesion counts, and choline acetyltransferase levels in the age spectrum of Alzheimer's disease. *Neurology* 38:48–54, 1988.
123. Perry EK, Haroutunian V, Davis KL, et al: Neocortical cholinergic activities differentiate Lewy body dementia from classical Alzheimer's disease. *Neuroreport* 5:747–749, 1994.

124. Mountjoy CQ: Correlations between neuropathological and neurochemical changes. *Br Med Bull* 42:81–85, 1986.
125. Dekker AJ, Connor DJ, Thal LJ: The role of cholinergic projections from the nucleus basalis in memory. *Neurosci Biobehav Rev* 15:299–317, 1991.
126. Saper CB, German DC, White CL III: Neuronal pathology in the nucleus basalis and associated cell groups in senile dementia of the Alzheimer's type: Possible role in cell loss. *Neurology* 35:1089–1095, 1985.
127. Muir JL, Page KJ, Sirinathsinghji DJ, et al: Excitotoxic lesions of basal forebrain cholinergic neurons: Effects on learning, memory and attention. *Behav Brain Res* 57:123–131, 1993.
128. Davis KL, Thal LJ, Gamzu ER, et al: A double-blind, placebo-controlled multicenter study of tacrine for Alzheimer's disease. The Tacrine Collaborative Study Group. *N Engl J Med* 327:1253–1259, 1992.
129. Farlow M, Gracon SI, Hershey LA, et al: A controlled trial of tacrine in Alzheimer's disease. The Tacrine Study Group. *JAMA* 268:2523–2529, 1992.
130. Knapp MJ, Knopman DS, Solomon PR, et al: A 30-week randomized controlled trial of high-dose tacrine in patients with Alzheimer's disease. The Tacrine Study Group. *JAMA* 271:985–991, 1994.
131. Burns A, Rossor M, Hecker J, et al: The effects of donepezil in Alzheimer's disease—results from a multinational trial. *Dement Geriatr Cogn Disord* 10:237–444, 1999.
132. Rogers SL, Doody RS, Mohs RC, Friedhoff LT: Donepezil improves cognition and global function in Alzheimer disease: A 15-week, double-blind, placebo-controlled study. Donepezil Study Group. *Arch Intern Med* 158:1021–1031, 1998.
133. Rogers SL, Friedhoff LT: Long-term efficacy and safety of donepezil in the treatment of Alzheimer's disease: An interim analysis of the results of a US multicentre open label extension study. *Eur Neuropsychopharmacol* 8:67–75, 1998.
134. Rogers SL, Farlow MR, Doody RS, et al: A 24-week, double-blind, placebo-controlled trial of donepezil in patients with Alzheimer's disease. Donepezil Study Group. *Neurology* 50:136–145, 1998.
135. Rogers SL, Friedhoff LT: The efficacy and safety of donepezil in patients with Alzheimer's disease: Results of a US Multicentre, Randomized, Double-Blind, Placebo-Controlled Trial. The Donepezil Study Group. *Dementia* 7:293–303, 1996.
136. Winblad B, Engedal K, Soininen H, et al: A 1-year, randomized, placebo-controlled study of donepezil in patients with mild to moderate AD. *Neurology* 57:489–495, 2001.
137. Mohs RC, Doody RS, Morris JC, et al: A 1-year, placebo-controlled preservation of function survival study of donepezil in AD patients. *Neurology* 57:481–488, 2001.
138. Cutler NR, Polinsky RJ, Sramek JJ, et al: Dose-dependent CSF acetylcholinesterase inhibition by SDZ ENA 713 in Alzheimer's disease. *Acta Neurol Scand* 97:244–250, 1998.
139. Corey-Bloom J, Anand R, Veach J: A randomized trial evaluating the efficacy and safety of ENA713 (rivastigmine tartrate), a new acetylcholinesterase inhibitor, in patients with mild to moderately severe Alzheimer's disease. *Int J Geriatr Psychopharmacol* 1:55–65, 1998.
140. Rosler M, Anand R, Cicin-Sain A, et al: Efficacy and safety of rivastigmine in patients with Alzheimer's disease: International randomised controlled trial. *BMJ* 318:633–638, 1999.
141. Farlow M, Anand R, Messina J Jr, et al: A 52-week study of the efficacy of rivastigmine in patients with mild to moderately severe Alzheimer's disease. *Eur Neurol* 44:236–241, 2000.
142. Scott LJ, Goa KL: Galantamine: A review of its use in Alzheimer's disease. *Drugs* 60:1095–1122, 2000.
143. Tariot PN, Solomon PR, Morris JC, et al: A 5-month, randomized, placebo-controlled trial of galantamine in AD. The Galantamine USA-10 Study Group. *Neurology* 54:2269–2276, 2000.
144. Wilcock GK, Lilienfeld S, Gaens E: Efficacy and safety of galantamine in patients with mild to moderate Alzheimer's disease: Multicentre randomised controlled trial. *Br Med J* 321:1445–1449, 2000.
145. Raskind MA, Peskind ER, Wessel T, Yuan W: Galantamine in AD: A 6-month randomized, placebo-controlled trial with a 6-month extension. The Galantamine USA-1 Study Group. *Neurology* 54:2261–2268, 2000.
146. Doody R, Kershaw P: The cognitive benefits of galantamine are sustained for at least 24 months: Results of a long-term extension trial in Alzheimer's disease. *Neurology* 56:A456, 2001.
147. Whitehouse PJ, Martino AM, Marcus KA, et al: Reductions in acetylcholine and nicotine binding in several degenerative diseases. *Arch Neurol* 45:722–724, 1988.
148. Levey AI, Kitt CA, Simonds WF, et al: Identification and localization of muscarinic acetylcholine receptor proteins in brain with subtype-specific antibodies. *J Neurosci* 11:3218–3226, 1991.
149. Newhouse PA, Sunderland T, Narang PK, et al: Neuroendocrine, physiologic, and behavioral responses

following intravenous nicotine in nonsmoking healthy volunteers and in patients with Alzheimer's disease. *Psychoneuroendocrinology* 15:471–484, 1990.

150. Jones GM, Sahakian BJ, Levy R, et al: Effects of acute subcutaneous nicotine on attention, information processing and short-term memory in Alzheimer's disease. *Psychopharmacology (Berl)* 108:485–494, 1992.
151. Parks RW, Becker RE, Rippey RF, et al: Increased regional cerebral glucose metabolism and semantic memory performance in Alzheimer's disease: A pilot double blind transdermal nicotine positron emission tomography study. *Neuropsychol Rev* 6:61–79, 1996.
152. Dysken MW, Mendels J, LeWitt P, et al: Milacemide: A placebo-controlled study in senile dementia of the Alzheimer type. *J Am Geriatr Soc* 40:503–506, 1992.
153. Randolph C, Roberts JW, Tierney MC, et al: D-Cycloserine treatment of Alzheimer disease. *Alzheimer Dis Assoc Disord* 8:198–205, 1994.
154. Winblad B, Poritis N: Memantine in severe dementia: Results of the 9M-Best Study (benefit and efficacy in severely demented patients during treatment with memantine). *Int J Geriatr Psychiatry* 14:135–146, 1999.
155. Reisberg B, Windscheif U, Ferris SH et al: Memantine in moderately severe to severe Alzheimer's disease (AD): Results of a placebo-controlled 6-month trial. *Neurobiol Aging* 21:S275, 2000.
156. Hampson RE, Rogers G, Lynch G, Deadwyler SA: Facilitative effects of the ampakine CX516 on short-term memory in rats: Correlations with hippocampal neuronal activity. *J Neurosci* 18:2748–2763, 1998.
157. Hampson RE, Rogers G, Lynch G, Deadwyler SA: Facilitative effects of the ampakine CX516 on short-term memory in rats: Enhancement of delayed-nonmatch-to-sample performance. *J Neurosci* 18:2740–2747, 1998.
158. Chan-Palay V: Somatostatin immunoreactive neurons in the human hippocampus and cortex shown by immunogold/silver intensification on vibratome sections: Coexistence with neuropeptide Y neurons, and effects in Alzheimer-type dementia. *J Comp Neurol* 260:201–223, 1987.
159. Kowall NW, Beal MF: Cortical somatostatin, neuropeptide Y, and NADPH diaphorase neurons: Normal anatomy and alterations in Alzheimer's disease. *Ann Neurol* 23:105–114, 1988.
160. Devanand DP, Sano M, Tang MX, et al: Depressed mood and the incidence of Alzheimer's disease in the elderly living in the community. *Arch Gen Psychiatry* 1996;53:175–182, 1988.
161. Greenwald BS, Kramer-Ginsberg E, Marin DB, et al: Dementia with coexistent major depression. *Am J Psychiatry* 146:1472–1478, 1989.
162. McDonald WM, Krishnan KR: Pharmacologic management of the symptoms of dementia. *Am Fam Physician* 42:123–132, 1990.
163. Cohen-Mansfield J, Marx MS, Werner P: Agitation in elderly persons: An integrative report of findings in a nursing home. *Int Psychogeriatr* 4:221–240, 1992.
164. Devanand DP, Marder K, Michaels KS, et al: A randomized, placebo-controlled dose-comparison trial of haloperidol for psychosis and disruptive behaviors in Alzheimer's disease. *Am J Psychiatry* 155:1512–1520, 1998.
165. De Deyn PP, Rabheru K, Rasmussen A, et al: A randomized trial of risperidone, placebo, and haloperidol for behavioral symptoms of dementia. *Neurology* 53:946–955, 1999.
166. Teri L, Logsdon RG, Peskind E, et al: Treatment of agitation in AD: A randomized, placebo-controlled clinical trial. *Neurology* 55:1271–1278, 2000.
167. Katz IR, Jeste DV, Mintzer JE, et al: Comparison of risperidone and placebo for psychosis and behavioral disturbances associated with dementia: A randomized, double-blind trial. Risperidone Study Group. *J Clin Psychiatry* 60:107–115, 1999.
168. Street JS, Clark WS, Gannon KS, et al: Olanzapine treatment of psychotic and behavioral symptoms in patients with Alzheimer disease in nursing care facilities: A double-blind, randomized, placebo-controlled trial. The HGEU Study Group. *Arch Gen Psychiatry* 57:968–976, 2000.
169. Tariot PN, Erb R, Podgorski CA, et al: Efficacy and tolerability of carbamazepine for agitation and aggression in dementia. *Am J Psychiatry* 155:54–61, 1998.
170. Porsteinsson AP, Tariot PN, Erb R, et al: Placebo-controlled study of divalproex sodium for agitation in dementia. *Am J Geriatr Psychiatry* 9:58–66, 2001.
171. Vitiello MV, Bliwise DL, Prinz PN: Sleep in Alzheimer's disease and the sundown syndrome. *Neurology* 42:83–93, 1992; discussion 93–94.
172. Cohen-Mansfield J, Waldhorn R, Werner P, Billig N: Validation of sleep observations in a nursing home. *Sleep* 13:512–525, 1990.
173. Cohen-Mansfield J, Garfinkel D, Lipson S: Melatonin for treatment of sundowning in elderly persons with dementia—a preliminary study. *Arch Gerontol Geriatr* 31:65–76, 2000.
174. Logsdon RG, Teri L, McCurry SM, et al: Wandering: A significant problem among community-residing individuals with Alzheimer's disease. *J Gerontol B Psychol Sci Soc Sci* 53:P294–P299, 1998.
175. Namazi KH, Rosner TT, Calkins MP: Visual barriers to prevent ambulatory Alzheimer's patients from exiting

through an emergency door. *Gerontologist* 29:699–702, 1989.

176. Luxenberg JS: Clinical issues in the behavioural and psychological symptoms of dementia. *Int J Geriatr Psychiatry* 15:S5–S8, 2000.
177. Schenk D, Barbour R, Dunn W, et al: Immunization with amyloid-beta attenuates Alzheimer-disease-like pathology in the PDAPP mouse. *Nature* 400:173–177, 1999.
178. Bard F, Cannon C, Barbour R, et al: Peripherally administered antibodies against amyloid beta-peptide enter the central nervous system and reduce pathology in a mouse model of Alzheimer disease. *Nat Med* 6:916–919, 2000.
179. Janus C, Pearson J, McLaurin J, et al: A beta peptide immunization reduces behavioural impairment and plaques in a model of Alzheimer's disease. *Nature* 408:979–982, 2000.
180. Morgan D, Diamond DM, Gottschall PE, et al: A beta peptide vaccination prevents memory loss in an animal model of Alzheimer's disease. *Nature* 408:982–985, 2000.
181. Lovell MA, Robertson JD, Teesdale WJ, et al: Copper, iron and zinc in Alzheimer's disease senile plaques. *J Neurol Sci* 158:47–52, 1998.
182. Suh SW, Jensen KB, Jensen MS, et al: Histochemically-reactive zinc in amyloid plaques, angiopathy, and degenerating neurons of Alzheimer's diseased brains. *Brain Res* 852:274–278, 2000.
183. Lee JY, Mook-Jung I, Koh JY: Histochemically reactive zinc in plaques of the Swedish mutant beta-amyloid precursor protein transgenic mice. *J Neurosci* 19:RC10, 1999.
184. Smith MA, Harris PL, Sayre LM, Perry G: Iron accumulation in Alzheimer disease is a source of redox-generated free radicals. *Proc Natl Acad Sci U S A* 94:9866–9868, 1997.
185. Cherny RA, Atwood CS, Xilinas ME, et al: Treatment with a copper-zinc chelator markedly and rapidly inhibits beta-amyloid accumulation in Alzheimer's disease transgenic mice. *Neuron* 30:665–676, 2001.
186. Gouras GK, Beal MF: Metal chelator decreases Alzheimer beta-amyloid plaques. *Neuron* 30:641–642, 2001.
187. McGeer PL, McGeer EG: The inflammatory response system of brain: implications for therapy of Alzheimer and other neurodegenerative diseases. *Brain Res Brain Res Rev* 21:195–218, 1995.
188. Andersen K, Launer LJ, Ott A, et al: Do nonsteroidal anti-inflammatory drugs decrease the risk for Alzheimer's disease? The Rotterdam Study. *Neurology* 45:1441–1445, 1995.
189. Breitner JC, Welsh KA, Helms MJ, et al: Delayed onset of Alzheimer's disease with nonsteroidal anti-inflammatory and histamine H2 blocking drugs. *Neurobiol Aging* 16:523–530, 1995.
190. Breitner JC, Gau BA, Welsh KA, et al: Inverse association of anti-inflammatory treatments and Alzheimer's disease: Initial results of a co-twin control study. *Neurology* 44:227–232, 1994.
191. Veld BA, Ruitenberg A, Hofman A, et al: Nonsteroidal antiinflammatory drugs and the risk of Alzheimer's disease. *N Engl J Med* 345:1515–1521, 2001.
192. Rogers J, Kirby LC, Hempelman SR, et al: Clinical trial of indomethacin in Alzheimer's disease. *Neurology* 43:1609–1611, 1993.
193. Scharf S, Mander A, Ugoni A, et al: A double-blind, placebo-controlled trial of diclofenac/misoprostol in Alzheimer's disease. *Neurology* 53:197–201, 1999.
194. Ho L, Pieroni C, Winger D, et al: Regional distribution of cyclooxygenase-2 in the hippocampal formation in Alzheimer's disease. *J Neurosci Res* 57:295–303, 1999.
195. Saninati SM, Ingram DM, Talwalker S, Geis GS: Results of a double-blind, randomized, placebo-controlled study of celecoxib in the treatment of progression of Alzheimer's disease. Sixth International Stockholm/Springfield Symposium on Advances in Alzheimer Therapy. Stockholm, Sweden; 2000.
196. Weggen S, Eriksen JL, Das P, et al: A subset of NSAIDs lower amyloidogenic $A\beta_{42}$ independently of cyclooxygenase activity. *Nature* 414:212–216, 2001.
197. Aisen PS, Davis KL, Berg JD, et al: A randomized controlled trial of prednisone in Alzheimer's disease. *Neurology* 54:588–593, 2000.
198. Van Gool WA, Weinstein HC, Scheltens PK, Walstra GJ: Effect of hydroxychloroquine on progression of dementia in early Alzheimer's disease: An 18-month randomised, double-blind, placebo-controlled study. *Lancet* 358:455–460, 2001.
199. Toran-Allerand CD, Miranda RC, Bentham WD, et al: Estrogen receptors colocalize with low-affinity nerve growth factor receptors in cholinergic neurons of the basal forebrain. *Proc Natl Acad Sci U S A* 89:4668–46672, 1992.
200. Woolley CS: Effects of oestradiol on hippocampal circuitry. *Novartis Found Symp* 230:173–180, 2000; discussion 181–187.
201. Regan RF, Guo Y: Estrogens attenuate neuronal injury due to hemoglobin, chemical hypoxia, and excitatory amino acids in murine cortical cultures. *Brain Res* 764:133–140, 1997.

202. Romer W, Oettel M, Menzenbach B, et al: Novel estrogens and their radical scavenging effects, iron-chelating, and total antioxidative activities: 17 alpha-substituted analogs of delta 9(11)-dehydro-17 beta-estradiol. *Steroids* 62:688–694, 1997.
203. Romer W, Oettel M, Droescher P, Schwarz S: Novel "scavestrogens" and their radical scavenging effects, iron-chelating, and total antioxidative activities: delta 8,9-dehydro derivatives of 17 alpha-estradiol and 17 beta-estradiol. *Steroids* 62:304–310, 1997.
204. Brinton RD, Tran J, Proffitt P, Montoya M: 17 beta-Estradiol enhances the outgrowth and survival of neocortical neurons in culture. *Neurochem Res* 22:1339–1351, 1997.
205. Brinton RD, Proffitt P, Tran J, Luu R: Equilin, a principal component of the estrogen replacement therapy Premarin, increases the growth of cortical neurons via an NMDA receptor-dependent mechanism. *Exp Neurol* 147:211–220, 1997.
206. Heyman A, Wilkinson WE, Stafford JA, et al: Alzheimer's disease: A study of epidemiological aspects. *Ann Neurol* 15:335–341, 1984.
207. Amaducci LA, Fratiglioni L, Rocca WA, et al: Risk factors for clinically diagnosed Alzheimer's disease: A case-control study of an Italian population. *Neurology* 36:922–931, 1986.
208. Broe GA, Henderson AS, Creasey H, et al: A case-control study of Alzheimer's disease in Australia. *Neurology* 40:1698–1707, 1990.
209. Graves AB, White E, Koepsell TD, et al: A case-control study of Alzheimer's disease. *Ann Neurol* 28:766–774, 1990.
210. Barrett-Connor E, Kritz-Silverstein D: Estrogen replacement therapy and cognitive function in older women. *JAMA* 269:2637–2641, 1993.
211. Paganini-Hill A, Henderson VW: Estrogen deficiency and risk of Alzheimer's disease in women. *Am J Epidemiol* 140:256–261, 1994.
212. Paganini-Hill A, Henderson VW: Estrogen replacement therapy and risk of Alzheimer disease. *Arch Intern Med* 156:2213–2217, 1996.
213. Henderson VW, Paganini-Hill A, Emanuel CK, et al: Estrogen replacement therapy in older women. Comparisons between Alzheimer's disease cases and nondemented control subjects. *Arch Neurol* 51:896–900, 1994.
214. Tang MX, Jacobs D, Stern Y, et al: Effect of oestrogen during menopause on risk and age at onset of Alzheimer's disease. *Lancet* 348:429–432, 1996.
215. Kawas C, Resnick S, Morrison A et al: A prospective study of estrogen replacement therapy and the risk of developing Alzheimer's disease: The Baltimore Longitudinal Study of Aging. *Neurology* 48:1517–1521, 1997.
216. Carlson MC, Zandi PP, Plassman BL, et al: Hormone replacement therapy and reduced cognitive decline in older women: The Cache County Study. *Neurology* 57:2210–2216, 2001.
217. Fillit H, Weinreb H, Cholst I, et al: Observations in a preliminary open trial of estradiol therapy for senile dementia-Alzheimer's type. *Psychoneuroendocrinology* 11:337–345, 1986.
218. Honjo H, Ogino Y, Naitoh K, et al: In vivo effects by estrone sulfate on the central nervous system-senile dementia (Alzheimer's type). *J Steroid Biochem* 34:521–525, 1989.
219. Ohkura T, Isse K, Akazawa K, et al: Evaluation of estrogen treatment in female patients with dementia of the Alzheimer type. *Endocr J* 41:361–371, 1994.
220. Asthana S, Craft S, Baker LD, et al: Cognitive and neuroendocrine response to transdermal estrogen in postmenopausal women with Alzheimer's disease: Results of a placebo-controlled, double-blind, pilot study. *Psychoneuroendocrinology* 24:657–677, 1999.
221. Henderson VW, Paganini-Hill A, Miller BL, et al: Estrogen for Alzheimer's disease in women: Randomized, double-blind, placebo-controlled trial. *Neurology* 54:295–301, 2000.
222. Wang PN, Liao SQ, Liu RS, et al: Effects of estrogen on cognition, mood, and cerebral blood flow in AD: A controlled study. *Neurology* 54:2061–2066, 2000.
223. Mulnard RA, Cotman CW, Kawas C, et al: Estrogen replacement therapy for treatment of mild to moderate Alzheimer disease: A randomized controlled trial. Alzheimer's Disease Cooperative Study. *JAMA* 283:1007–1015, 2000.
224. Fischer W, Wictorin K, Bjorklund A, et al: Amelioration of cholinergic neuron atrophy and spatial memory impairment in aged rats by nerve growth factor. *Nature* 329:65–68, 1987.
225. Dekker AJ, Gage FH, Thal LJ: Delayed treatment with nerve growth factor improves acquisition of a spatial task in rats with lesions of the nucleus basalis magnocellularis: Evaluation of the involvement of different neurotransmitter systems. *Neuroscience* 48:111–119, 1992.
226. Dekker AJ, Langdon DJ, Gage FH, Thal LJ: NGF increases cortical acetylcholine release in rats with lesions of the nucleus basalis. *Neuroreport* 2:577–580, 1991.
227. Gage FH, Armstrong DM, Williams LR, Varon S: Morphological response of axotomized septal neurons to nerve growth factor. *J Comp Neurol* 269:147–155, 1988.

228. Mobley WC, Neve RL, Prusiner SB, McKinley MP: Nerve growth factor increases mRNA levels for the prion protein and the beta-amyloid protein precursor in developing hamster brain. *Proc Natl Acad Sci U S A* 85:9811–9815, 1988.
229. Isaacson LG, Saffran BN, Crutcher KA: Intracerebral NGF infusion induces hyperinnervation of cerebral blood vessels. *Neurobiol Aging* 11:51–55, 1990.
230. Lewin GR, Ritter AM, Mendell LM: Nerve growth factor-induced hyperalgesia in the neonatal and adult rat. *J Neurosci* 13:2136–2148, 1993.
231. Winkler J, Ramirez GA, Kuhn HG, et al: Reversible Schwann cell hyperplasia and sprouting of sensory and sympathetic neurites after intraventricular administration of nerve growth factor. *Ann Neurol* 41:82–93, 1997.
232. Williams LR: Hypophagia is induced by intracerebroventricular administration of nerve growth factor. *Exp Neurol* 113:31–37, 1991.
233. Eriksdotter Jonhagen M, Nordberg A, Amberla K, et al: Intracerebroventricular infusion of nerve growth factor in three patients with Alzheimer's disease. *Dement Geriatr Cogn Disord* 9:246–257, 1998.
234. Smith DE, Roberts J, Gage FH, Tuszynski MH: Age-associated neuronal atrophy occurs in the primate brain and is reversible by growth factor gene therapy. *Proc Natl Acad Sci U S A* 96:10893–10898, 1999.
235. Meskini N, Nemoz G, Okyayuz-Baklouti I, et al: Phosphodiesterase inhibitory profile of some related xanthine derivatives pharmacologically active on the peripheral microcirculation. *Biochem Pharmacol* 47:781–788, 1994.
236. Grome JJ, Hofmann W, Gojowczyk G, Stefanovich V: Effects of a xanthine derivative, propentofylline, on local cerebral blood flow and glucose utilization in the rat. *Brain Res* 740:41–46, 1996.
237. Marcusson J, Rother M, Kittner B, et al: A 12-month, randomized, placebo-controlled trial of propentofylline (HWA 285) in patients with dementia according to DSM III-R. The European Propentofylline Study Group. *Dement Geriatr Cogn Disord* 8:320–328, 1997.
238. Rother M, Erkinjuntti T, Roessner M, et al: Propentofylline in the treatment of Alzheimer's disease and vascular dementia: A review of phase III trials. *Dement Geriatr Cogn Disord* 9:36–43, 1998.
239. Middlemiss PJ, Glasky AJ, Rathbone MP, et al: AIT-082, a unique purine derivative, enhances nerve growth factor mediated neurite outgrowth from PC12 cells. *Neurosci Lett* 199:131–134, 1995.
240. Glasky AJ, Melchior CL, Pirzadeh B, et al: Effect of AIT-082, a purine analog, on working memory in normal and aged mice. *Pharmacol Biochem Behav* 47:325–329, 1994.
241. Grundman M, Farlow M, Peavy G: A phase I study of AIT-082 in healthy elderly volunteers. *Soc Neurosci Abst* 24:1217, 1998.
242. Wieland S, Molloy W, Targum S, et al: Neotrofin: Novel approach for Alzheimer's disease treatment. *Neurobiol Aging* 21:S274, 2000.
243. Winkler J, Thal LJ: Clinical potential of growth factors in neurological disorders. *CNS Drugs* 2:465–478, 1994.
244. Hashimoto Y, Niikura T, Tajima H, et al: A rescue factor abolishing neuronal cell death by a wide spectrum of familial Alzheimer's disease genes and Aβ. *Proc Natl Acad Sci USA* 98:6336–6341, 2001.
245. Hashimoto Y, Ito Y, Niikura T, et al: Mechanisms of neuroprotection by a novel rescue factor humanin from Swedish mutant amyloid precursor protein. *Biochem Biophys Res Commun* 283:460–468, 2001.
246. Jenner P: Oxidative damage in neurodegenerative disease. *Lancet* 344:796–798, 1994.
247. Connor JR, Snyder BS, Beard JL, et al: Regional distribution of iron and iron-regulatory proteins in the brain in aging and Alzheimer's disease. *J Neurosci Res* 31:327–335, 1992.
248. Oreland L, Gottfries CG: Brain and brain monoamine oxidase in aging and in dementia of Alzheimer's type. *Prog Neuropsychopharmacol Biol Psychiatry* 10:533–540, 1986.
249. Morris MC, Beckett LA, Scherr PA, et al: Vitamin E and vitamin C supplement use and risk of incident Alzheimer disease. *Alzheimer Dis Assoc Disord* 12:121–126, 1998.
250. Corey-Bloom J, Thal L: Monoamine oxidase inhibitors in Alzheimer's disease, in Lieberman A, Olanow CW, Youdim MBH, Tipton K (eds): *Monoamine Oxidase Inhibitors in Neurological Disease*. New York: Chapman and Hall, 1994, pp 279–294.
251. Sano M, Ernesto C, Thomas RG, et al: A controlled trial of selegiline, alpha-tocopherol, or both as treatment for Alzheimer's disease. The Alzheimer's Disease Cooperative Study. *N Engl J Med* 336:1216–1222, 1997.
252. Gillis JC, Benefield P, McTavish D: Idebenone. A review of its pharmacodynamic and pharmacokinetic properties, and therapeutic use in age-related cognitive disorders. *Drugs Aging* 5:233–252, 1994.
253. Bruno V, Battaglia G, Copani A, et al: Protective action of idebenone against excitotoxic degeneration in cultured cortical neurons. *Neurosci Lett* 178:186–193, 1994.
254. Wieland E, Schutz E, Armstrong VW, et al: Idebenone protects hepatic microsomes against oxygen

radical-mediated damage in organ preservation solutions. *Transplantation* 60:444–451, 1995.

255. Hirai K, Hayako H, Kato K, Miyamoto M: Idebenone protects hippocampal neurons against amyloid beta-peptide-induced neurotoxicity in rat primary cultures. *Naunyn Schmiedebergs Arch Pharmacol* 358:582–585, 1998.
256. Bergamasco B, Scarzella L, La Commare P: Idebenone, a new drug in the treatment of cognitive impairment in patients with dementia of the Alzheimer type. *Funct Neurol* 9:161–168, 1994.
257. Le Bars PL, Katz MM, Berman N, et al: A placebo-controlled, double-blind, randomized trial of an extract of Ginkgo biloba for dementia. North American EGb Study Group. *JAMA* 278:1327–1332, 1997.
258. Bi X, Haque TS, Zhou J, et al: Novel cathepsin D inhibitors block the formation of hyperphosphorylated tau fragments in hippocampus. *J Neurochem* 74:1469–1477, 2000.
259. Alvarez G, Munoz-Montano JR, Satrustegui J, et al: Lithium protects cultured neurons against beta-amyloid-induced neurodegeneration. *FEBS Lett* 453:260–264, 1999.
260. Rapoport M, Ferreira A: PD98059 prevents neurite degeneration induced by fibrillar beta-amyloid in mature hippocampal neurons. *J Neurochem* 74:125–133, 2000.
261. Gong CX, Lidsky T, Wegiel J, et al: Phosphorylation of microtubule-associated protein tau is regulated by protein phosphatase 2A in mammalian brain. Implications for neurofibrillary degeneration in Alzheimer's disease. *J Biol Chem* 275:5535–5544, 2000.
262. Hofman A, Ott A, Breteler MM, et al: Atherosclerosis, apolipoprotein E, and prevalence of dementia and Alzheimer's disease in the Rotterdam Study. *Lancet* 349:151–154, 1997.
263. Bales KR, Verina T, Dodel RC, et al: Lack of apolipoprotein E dramatically reduces amyloid beta-peptide deposition. *Nat Genet* 17:263–264, 1997.
264. Sparks DL, Scheff SW, Hunsaker JC III, et al: Induction of Alzheimer-like beta-amyloid immunoreactivity in the brains of rabbits with dietary cholesterol. *Exp Neurol* 126:88–94, 1994.
265. Refolo LM, Pappolla MA, Malester B, et al: Hypercholesterolemia accelerates the Alzheimer's amyloid pathology in a transgenic mouse model. *Neurobiol Dis* 7:321–331, 2000.
266. Simons M, Keller P, De Strooper B, et al: Cholesterol depletion inhibits the generation of beta-amyloid in hippocampal neurons. *Proc Natl Acad Sci U S A* 95:6460–6464, 1998.
267. Fassbender K, Simons M, Bergmann C, et al: Simvastatin strongly reduces levels of Alzheimer's disease beta-amyloid peptides $A\beta_{42}$ and $A\beta_{40}$ in vitro and in vivo. *Proc Natl Acad Sci USA* 98:5856–5861, 2001.
268. Wolozin B, Kellman W, Ruosseau P, et al: Decreased prevalence of Alzheimer disease associated with 3-hydroxy-3-methyglutaryl coenzyme A reductase inhibitors. *Arch Neurol* 57:1439–1443, 2000.
269. Jick H, Zornberg GL, Jick SS, et al: Statins and the risk of dementia. 356:1627–1631, 2000.
270. Shepherd J, Blauw GJ, Murphy MB, et al: The design of a prospective study of Pravastatin in the Elderly at Risk (PROSPER). PROSPER Study Group. PROspective Study of Pravastatin in the Elderly at Risk. *Am J Cardiol* 84:1192–1197, 1999.
271. Petersen RC: Aging, mild cognitive impairment, and Alzheimer's disease. *Neurol Clin* 18:789–806, 2000.
272. Tierney MC, Szalai JP, Snow WG, et al: Prediction of probable Alzheimer's disease in memory-impaired patients: A prospective longitudinal study. *Neurology* 46:661–665, 1996.
273. Grundman M, Petersen RC, Morris JC, et al: Rate of dementia of the Alzheimer type (DAT) in subjects with mild cognitive impairment. *Neurology* 46:A403, 1996.
274. Shumaker SA, Reboussin BA, Espeland MA, et al: The Women's Health Initiative Memory Study (WHIMS): a trial of the effect of estrogen therapy in preventing and slowing the progression of dementia. *Control Clin Trials* 19:604–621, 1998.
275. Writing Group for the Women's Health Initiative Investigators: Risks and benefits of estrogen plus progestin in healthy postmenopausal women. *JAMA* 288:321–333, 2002.

Chapter 46

ALZHEIMER'S DISEASE: COGNITIVE NEUROPSYCHOLOGICAL ISSUES*

William Milberg
Regina McGlinchey-Berroth

Alzheimer's disease (AD) is the most common dementing illness affecting older adults. It was the first to be identified and clearly defined clinically, and more is known about the pathology, genetics, and molecular biology of AD than about any other degenerative dementia. It has also received a great deal of attention from investigators interested in defining its clinical neuropsychological character and trying to relate these observations to normal models of cognition. Yet progress in this latter enterprise has been slow and marked in some cases by a surprising amount of disagreement about even fundamental theoretical issues. There are several good reasons for the lack of consensus. First, the experimental paradigms and theoretical constructs of experimental and cognitive psychology rest on the assumption that neural functions are represented focally and are for the most part independent or modular. The field of cognitive neuropsychology was founded on this assumption and has indeed provided powerful tools for the description and analysis of syndromes that are based on single focal lesions or lesions of a single neural syndrome. For example, deficits in language, memory, and vision following stroke or other focal lesions have been very effectively studied using the paradigms of cognitive neuropsychology. Patients with AD may suffer from deficits in all of these domains simultaneously, making it more difficult to conclude that deficits on an experimental task are solely attributable to a single domain.

Second, cognitive neuropsychology rests on the assumption that the underlying lesion itself is ablative. That is, the entire function residing in a circumscribed area of brain tissue has been removed via an ablative lesion. The "lesion" of AD is likely not to be ablative, at least in the stages that allow patients to be sufficiently intact to perform psychological tasks.

While it is true that AD patients do suffer from neural atrophy, this does not appear to be a factor that distinguishes AD from many other disorders. Neural atrophy appears in such diseases as Huntington's chorea, Parkinson's disease, schizophrenia, and alcoholism as well as others.[1] Neural atrophy can also be present to the same extent in older normal adults without AD. None of these other populations have been associated with the extensive semantic memory disorder described in patients with AD.

Furthermore, for most patients, neural atrophy appears to be more important later in the course of the disorder, appearing as a consequence of pathophysiologic factors specific to AD that occur early in the disease. In a longitudinal study, Fox et al.[2] measured cerebral atrophy in clinically normal individuals who were at high risk for developing AD. Blinded assessment of the scans revealed "the appearance of diffuse cerebral and medial temporal lobe atrophy in subjects *only once they were clinically affected*" (our italics) by the clinical signs of dementia. These patients, however, did show preclinical cognitive decline on neuropsychological measures well before the appearance of detectable atrophy or clinically significant dementia. This finding suggests that incipient pathologic changes were occurring in these patients before atrophy itself could be observed.

In fact, the critical early marker for the disorder is the effect on synaptic connectivity caused by neuritic plaques and neurofibrillary tangles (see Chap. 44).[3–6] There is now considerable evidence that affected neurons sprout new dystrophic neural connections.[7] Last, there is increasing evidence that the reduction of such

* **ACKNOWLEDGMENT**: This research was supported by Department of VA Medical Research Service VA Merit Review Awards to Regina McGlinchey-Berroth and William Milberg.

neurotransmitters as acetylcholine has the effect of demodulating existing neural connections by increasing the likelihood of activation (for a review see Ref. 8; see also Chap. 45).

A more realistic model of the pathology of AD should at least make some reference to the changes and disregulation of connectivity that characterize the disease during its early stages. In fact, very recently there have been some attempts to develop models of the pathology of AD that are more closely derived from the notion that connectivity is disrupted.[8,9] In these models, the pathologic mechanism is an interruption of the modulation of activation rather than a loss of activation per se. For example, Hasselmo[8] has suggested that the mechanism underlying the advancement of AD within the nervous system is what he terms "runaway synaptic modification," a cascade of synaptic overactivation that gradually induces pathology in ever increasing areas of a neural network. Models such as Hasselmo's have not been applied to the problem of providing an account for the neuropsychological deficits of AD, but they at least represent a biologically plausible pathologic mechanism that does not rely on the notion of degraded knowledge to account for functional deficits.

A third reason for the lack of theoretical consensus, and perhaps the one causing the most difficulty, is that the clinical syndrome of AD is in itself an evolving phenomenon, potentially changing its fundamental nature as the disease progresses. While the early stages of the disease may be accompanied by extensive neural disconnection affecting strategic focal regions, the later stages of the disease may indeed be more ablative in nature, though more neural regions and systems may be affected.

With these issues in mind we review below two areas of cognitive function that have been most intensively investigated: semantic memory and attention.

SEMANTIC MEMORY IN ALZHEIMER'S DISEASE

Semantic memory encompasses our general knowledge of word meanings and categories (see Chap. 39). Martin and Fedio made what was probably the first strong theoretical statement regarding semantic memory in AD.[10] Based on logic first outlined by Warrington and others,[11,12] they argued that AD patients' consistent pattern of deficits on a number of language tasks could be attributed to a "disruption in the organization of semantic knowledge" or a "loss of semantic knowledge." Subsequently, the view favored by Martin and Fedio was widely echoed by other laboratories,[13–15] who continued to document AD patients' poor performance on a variety of tasks designed to directly assess the integrity of their semantic knowledge base (i.e., facts, word meanings, etc.).

Nebes and colleagues[16] were the first to challenge the semantic loss or degradation view by using a semantic priming paradigm that had previously uncovered evidence of preserved semantic processing in aphasic patients.[17] This paradigm differed in an important way from those used in most of the previous studies examining the semantic memory of patients with AD. Specifically, the priming paradigm assessed semantic knowledge indirectly or implicitly by observing changes in the time and accuracy with which individuals performed simple word-nonword decisions (lexical decisions) or in overlearned language tasks such as word reading. This was in contrast to prior studies that asked patients to directly access and retrieve semantic information or make explicit judgments upon that information. Having set out to support further the already overwhelming case for degraded representations (R.D. Nebes, personal communication, July 14, 1998), the investigators were surprised to find that AD patients showed normal sensitivity to semantic relationships (i.e., semantic priming).[16,18] Since the initial reports by Nebes and colleagues, these findings have also been extended and replicated in a number of laboratories.[19–24] It was the assumption of these investigators that the presence of preserved semantic priming constituted a prima facie case that AD patients suffered not from a degradation or loss of semantic knowledge but from a loss of retrieval or other attentionally mediated access processes.[21]

There is no question that these two theoretical positions have had considerable heuristic value, galvanizing a great deal of research focused on an important clinical issue. There is also little question that this work provided a foundation for the emergence of semantic memory as a topic central to the field of experimental clinical neuropsychology. It is therefore disconcerting that the theoretical dividing lines drawn by these views have changed little since Nebes reviewed what was already a fully formed debate a decade ago.[25] The lack of evolution toward a theoretical common ground suggests that there must be something singularly unconvincing about the constituent positions of an explanatory dichotomy that has allowed for more steadfast and unrelenting partisanship than a congressional debate on taxes. With only a little reflection, it becomes evident that each position has both empiric and logical disadvantages that have prevented the development of a consensus on how to describe the pathology of semantic memory of AD.

The primary empiric disadvantage of each of these theoretical positions is that neither knowledge degradation nor retrieval-based models can account for the wide range of experimental phenomenon characterizing the semantic memory deficit of AD. This probably derives from the fact that each position has primarily drawn support from a specific and limited set of experimental paradigms. For example, most studies that provide evidence for degraded knowledge or degraded representations have used tasks that require explicit access or direct judgments to be made upon semantic information (e.g., word reading, picture identification, providing definitions, category attribute ranking or judgment, matching category members or features to objects, etc.). On the other hand, most of the studies that have concluded that semantic knowledge is preserved in AD have relied almost entirely on implicit measures like the semantic priming paradigm. The alliance of paradigm with theory has been so nearly complete in this literature as if to establish a virtual operational identity between the two.

One important exception was a study by Chertkow and coworkers,[26] who assessed implicit priming performance relative to explicit performance on a variety of semantic knowledge tasks. Using this multimeasure approach, they documented a critical observation regarding a possible priming abnormality in patients with AD. They found larger-than-normal priming or "hyperpriming" in patients with AD. This effect was most pronounced for exemplars from categories found to be "degraded" in the tasks requiring more explicit access to semantic knowledge. They thereby operationalized degraded knowledge as a failure to perform normally on explicit semantic tasks. Because of this association, they concluded that "hyperpriming" was a reflection of degraded knowledge.

The study by Chertkow et al.[26] represents one of the only attempts to reconcile direct/explicit and indirect/implicit semantic memory measures and to document potential abnormalities in both kinds of tasks. Though hyperpriming has been offered as a possible example of an implicit phenomenon that could be associated with knowledge degradation, the arguments of Chertkow and colleagues depends on the acceptance of the assumption that failure of a semantic judgment task can be caused only by degradation of knowledge. As we discuss below, failure to perform on tasks requiring the use of semantic knowledge does *not* necessarily implicate the unavailability of that information, since the performance of these tasks requires the participation of retrieval operations and other attentionally mediated functions.

Furthermore, "knowledge degradation" theories predict a reduction of priming for all semantic relationships. For example, computational models of semantic memory in AD simulate the differential loss of weak compared to strong semantic relationships by the addition of "noise" or to a random loss of nodes or internodal connectivity (see Chap. 10).[27,28] In these models, all relationships are degraded, but weaker associates may drop below threshold before stronger associates. There is indeed evidence that weak semantic associates may produce less reliable priming effects in patients with AD than normal adults.[29,30]

Hyperpriming is but one of several patterns of results obtained with implicit measures of semantic knowledge that presents an empiric challenge to both degradation and retrieval accounts. Recall that the data of Chertkow et al.[26] contrast to the initial findings of Nebes et al.,[16] who found normal semantic priming effects. Indeed, some studies showed priming effects of a normal magnitude,[16,18] still others showed diminished priming,[21,30] and some have even shown negative priming.[19,31]

Ober and Shenaut[24] have suggested that variations in the magnitude of semantic priming effects may be due to the degree to which automatic and controlled processing contribute to performance in a particular semantic priming experiment. In a metanalysis of approximately 21 priming studies conducted between 1984 and 1991, Ober and Shenaut concluded that hyperpriming was observed only in those experiments that employed "a pairwise, long stimulus onset asynchrony (SOA) priming paradigm, with relatedness proportions from 0.33 to 0.67." They speculated that such conditions allowed for controlled processing to contribute to performance. In contrast, normal priming was observed in experimental paradigms using "short-SOA, pairwise paradigms, or continuous paradigms" that only allowed automatic processing to contribute to performance. They interpreted these results as an indication that automatic processes are intact in AD, leading to normal magnitude priming effects during these conditions. They hypothesized that controlled processing is the central impairment of semantic memory in AD, leading to abnormal hyperpriming. Though in principle Ober and Shenaut's claim may be true, the automatic-controlled dichotomy does not account for the fact that some studies show reduced priming for prime-target relationships that do not have a strong associative relationship.[29,30] It also does not account for that fact that AD patients may also show "negative priming."[19,31]

In addition to their ties to limited sets of empiric phenomena, the degradation and retrieval-based theoretical positions require the acceptance of either vague or questionable assumptions and logic. First consider the retrieval-based account of the semantic memory deficits in AD. Though retrieval processes or other attentionally mediated processes may be involved in both explicit and implicit semantic tasks, these constructs are at best vague and do not provide a blueprint to account for the wide variety of deficits that have been consistently documented in AD patients. The phenomenon of hyperpriming is an important example. To posit a retrieval-based account of hyperpriming as due to impaired controlled processes is at best descriptive because, in the context of a semantic priming paradigm, there are at least two candidate processes that could be responsible for variations in priming effects at long SOAs: prime-target expectancies[32] and postlexical checking.[33] Both involve the retrieval or recognition of the semantic relationship between prime and target to help reduce response time in making target-based responses to related word targets. We know from the explicit studies that AD patients have an impaired ability to retrieve semantic information. The inability to retrieve or recognize prime-target relations should *reduce, not increase,* attentionally mediated or controlled-based priming. A controlled-based account of hyperpriming must posit a deficit based on a greater-than-normal tendency or ability to retrieve and/or predict semantically based relationships between prime and target. Such an explanation is at best counterintuitive, though it is possible, as we argue, that under some circumstances highly overlearned semantic associations may attain abnormally salient status for patients with AD. As such, it may be possible to describe a controlled processing mechanism to account for hyperpriming, but such a description has not been forthcoming.

Another empiric difficulty with controlled processing–based accounts is that, at least in the context of semantic priming tasks, these processes are never directly measured or observed. The operation of controlled processes is only indirectly observed by varying experimental conditions (such as SOA or relatedness proportion) that would merely allow such processes to occur. There has yet to be a direct demonstration of controlled processing abnormalities in a semantic priming task in AD patients. The difficulty in operationalizing such constructs (as retrieval and controlled processing) probably accounts for the fact that they have failed to find their way into formal models of the pathology of semantic memory.

Although the construct of knowledge degradation may be more easily operationalized than that of retrieval or controlled processes, acceptance of this position is based on the assumption that performance on semantic memory tasks is solely dependent on the availability of knowledge structures. This leads to the related premise that performance deficits on semantic tasks are functionally equivalent to "degraded representations." This logic was first advanced by Warrington and Shallice,[12] who suggested that certain criteria could be used to infer the presence of deficits in stored information by comparing performance to criterial patients (e.g., agnosics or aphasics), for whom such deficits could be assumed to be true.

More recently, several laboratories have explored specific processes intrinsic to the retrieval of semantic information without implicating retrieval per se. The most intriguing example of this type of approach is in the work of Balota and his colleagues,[20,34,35] who have suggested that dysfunction in inhibitory control systems contributes to the impairments seen in attention, semantic memory, and language comprehension in AD. This position is appealing because it is quite specific as an account of deficits on tasks requiring explicit retrieval of semantic information without the inherent difficulties of knowledge degradation–based accounts. However, this model also asserts that facilitatory processes are preserved (e.g., Ref. 34). As described, the phenomena of hyperpriming and negative priming suggest that semantic facilitation is not always normal in AD. Although inhibitory control may still work as an account for a variety of judgment-based deficits, it remains to be seen whether the data from implicit tasks may ultimately be incorporated into this type of model.

Milberg et al.[36] recently proposed that small disruptions in the rate and peak levels of activation (caused by alterations in the time constant of the function relating activation to time) can be used to account for a wide variety of implicit and explicit data as well as some of the critical phenomena that are considered clinical benchmarks of the semantic memory disorder of AD (see Ref. 31). The gain/decay hypothesis suggests that variations in the strength of association will lead to empirically different consequences than variations in the time constant. This simple change has many specific empiric implications, accounting for both implicit and explicit semantic memory findings.

ATTENTION IN AD

Most studies investigating attentional processing in AD (and in normal individuals) have adopted the paradigm and basic premises of Posner's attentional orienting task.[37,38] Posner and colleagues proposed a model of attentional orienting consisting of three component processes: (1) disengagement of attention from the current focus, (2) moving or shifting of attention to a new focus, and (3) engagement of attention at the new focus. These shifts of attention can occur overtly, meaning that eye movements accompany them, or they can occur covertly, without eye movements. Posner and his colleagues proposed that facilitation of response times (RTs) at the validly cued location reflects the RT savings in having already oriented to the target location based on the cue, whereas the lengthened RTs to invalidly cued targets are due to the time required to disengage and reorient attention from an incorrect to a correct spatial location.[39,40]

Using this logic, investigators have examined the phenomenon of inhibition of return (IOR) in patients with AD. *IOR* refers to a tendency to inhibit the orienting of attention to a previously attended location; a very early visual attentional biasing mechanism thought to automatically orient the visual system to novel stimuli in the environment. A number of studies investigating IOR using cuing paradigms have indicated that this function is intact in patients with AD (e.g., Ref. 34), but that it can break down in the context of more complex processing requirements.[41]

In a classic demonstration, Parasuraman and colleagues[42] investigated AD patients' ability to orient their attention spatially. It was found that AD patients were not impaired in their ability to focus attention to a validly cued target location (indicated by RT benefits that did not differ between AD patients and controls) but were markedly impaired in their ability to shift attention from an invalidly cued location to a new location (greater costs), particularly with centrally located cues (that initiate more effortful shifts) and at longer SOAs. This "disengage deficit" has been replicated in numerous, more complex visual search tasks and may be most pronounced for AD patients in conjunction searches in which the precue does not precisely indicate the correct location of the target, suggesting a restriction in the dynamic range of spatial attention in AD.[43–45]

Taken together, these studies suggest that AD patients can use the advanced information provided by a cue to select stimuli, but also that their ability to shift the focus of attention from a cued location to an unexpected location is greatly compromised. This story is complicated, however, by the findings of Duncan et al.[46] This target detection experiment was similar to the study of Parasuraman et al.[42] in that targets were lateralized and preceded by valid, invalid, and neutral cues with varying SOAs. Consistent with the earlier study, the data indicated that control participants showed significant benefits for valid cues and significant costs for invalid cues. The AD patients, however, showed significant benefits for valid cues but no significant costs from invalid cues. In fact, AD patients were actually *faster* to respond to invalid cues than normal (see also Freed et al.,[47] who found a subgroup of AD patients who responded "anomalously" to targets following an invalid cue in that they were faster to respond in the invalid compared to valid condition). A possible reconciling factor between the study of Duncan and colleagues and that of Parasuraman et al. is that in the latter study patients had a mean score on the Folstein Mini-Mental State Exam (MMSE) of 21.3. The sample of patients in the study of Duncan et al. had a mean MMSE score of 18.6, and there was a significant positive correlation between MMSE and costs. Thus it is possible that our patients were functionally more impaired and manifesting a greater inhibitory deficit (see below).

The "Posner paradigm" has also been used extensively to investigate selective attention. Selective attention refers to a set of mechanisms that function to limit or focus the stream of incoming information from the environment that subsequently receives more elaborative processing. In this way, stimuli in the environment are either "selected" for more elaborative processing,[37,48–50] or they can passively decay over time, [51,52] or they are actively suppressed.[53–55]

The concepts of selection and inhibition in attentional functioning have been examined across a broad range of tasks, from simple target detection to semantic activation. Overall, this research has indicated that the selection component of attention remains relatively intact in patients with AD, but there is a selective impairment in the inhibitory component that, while present to some degree in "normal aging," is more severe in patients with AD.

For example, in an early study, Nebes and Brady[56] asked subjects to detect a target letter in an array of six letters. The target letter was always black, but on half of the trials, four of the distractors were red (reducing the relevant distractors to only two). The difference between search times for targets in mixed distractor arrays compared to all-black arrays was similar in their patients and their control subjects, indicating intact selection.

Sullivan and coworkers[35] investigated selective attention in a group of AD patients, age-matched normal controls, and young controls using a priming paradigm similar to that developed by Tipper and colleagues.[53,54] Sullivan et al. found that AD patients could successfully discriminate a target from a distractor (indicating intact selection) but were disproportionately impaired relative to the young and age-matched normal controls in their ability to inhibit distracting information.

In a similar study, Grande et al.[57] used a semantic priming task in which two vertically aligned drawings of objects (one orange, one blue) served as the priming stimuli and object names served as target stimuli. Subjects attended to the drawing of only one color and read aloud a centrally presented word target that was the name of either the attended object, the unattended object, or an object unrelated to either in the prime display. Normal control participants showed semantic facilitation only for target items that were the name of the attended prime object, while AD patients demonstrated facilitation for both the attended and unattended prime objects. Grande et al. suggested that these findings were due to an impairment in AD patients that resulted in semantic activation of information that is normally inhibited.

Duncan et al.[46] also examined semantic facilitation and inhibition in a priming task. In this experiment, precues indicated the probable location of a critical priming stimulus (left or right visual field) that always appeared with a nonsense priming stimulus in the opposing visual field. The target stimuli were centrally presented words that could be either semantically related, unrelated, or neutral with regard to the priming stimulus. Findings indicated that for normal control participants, the cue was sufficient to orient attention only to the validly cued primes; semantic facilitation was observed only following validly cued primes. AD patients, however, showed significant semantic facilitation regardless of the validity of the cue. This finding was interpreted to indicate a deficit in the ability of AD patients to inhibit semantic information appearing at an invalidly cued location.

Further support for an inhibitory breakdown in AD comes from studies utilizing the Stroop task. In general, a number of studies have reported that older control subjects are slowed in the incongruent condition (greater interference effect) to a greater extent than are younger subjects,[58–60] but that AD patients are disproportionately slowed compared to age-matched normal control participants.[61,62] These studies support the notion of an inhibitory dysfunction in normal aging and an accelerated breakdown in inhibition in patients with AD.

REFERENCES

1. Hopkins A: *Clinical Neurology: A Modern Approach.* London: Oxford University Press, 1993.
2. Fox NC, Warrington EK, Seiffer AL, et al: Presymptomatic cognitive deficits in individuals at risk of familial Alzheimer's disease—a longitudinal prospective study. *Brain* 121:1631-1639, 1998.
3. Callahan LM, Coleman PD: Neurons bearing neurofibrillary tangles are responsible for selected synaptic deficits in Alzheimer's disease. *Neurobiol Aging* 16(3):311–314, 1995.
4. Cook IA, Leuchter AF: Synaptic dysfunction in Alzheimer's disease: clinical assessment using quantitative EEG. *Behav Brain Res* 78:15–23, 1996.
5. Dickson DW, Crystal HA, Bevona C, et al: Correlations of synaptic and pathological markers with cognition of the elderly. *Neurobiol Aging* 16(3):285–304, 1995.
6. Nielson KA, Cummings BJ, Cotman CW: Constructional apraxia in Alzheimer's disease correlates with neuritic neuropathology in occipital cortex. *Brain Res* 741(1–2): 284–293, 1996.
7. Clinton J, Blackman SE-A, Royston MC, et al: Differential synaptic loss in the cortex in Alzheimer's disease: A study using archival material. *Neuroreport* 5: 497–500, 1994.
8. Hasselmo ME: Runaway synaptic modification in models of cortex: Implications for Alzheimer's disease. *Neur Netw* 7(1):13–40, 1994.
9. Ruppin E, Horn D, Levy N, et al: Computational studies of synaptic alterations in Alzheimer's disease, in Reggia JA, Ruppin E, Berndt RS (eds): *Neural Modeling of Brain and Cognitive Disorders.* Singapore: World Scientific, 1996, pp 63–87.
10. Martin A, Fedio P: Word production and comprehension in Alzheimer's disease: The breakdown of semantic knowledge. *Brain Lang* 19:124–141, 1983.
11. Warrington EK: The selective impairment of semantic memory. *Q J Exp Psychol* 27:635–657, 1975.
12. Warrington EK, Shallice T: Semantic access dyslexia. *Brain* 102:43–63, 1979.
13. Bayles KA, Tomoeda CK, Trosset MW: Naming and categorical knowledge in Alzheimer's disease: The process of semantic memory deterioration. *Brain Lang* 39:498–510, 1990.
14. Grober E, Buschke H, Kawas C, et al: Impaired ranking of semantic attributes in dementia. *Brain Lang* 26(2):276–286, 1985.
15. Hodges JR, Salmon DP, Butters N: Semantic memory impairment in Alzheimer's disease: Failure of access or degraded knowledge. *Neuropsychologia* 30(4):301–314, 1992.
16. Nebes RD, Martin DC, Horn LC: Sparing of semantic memory in Alzheimer's disease. *J Abnorm Psychol* 93(3):321–330, 1984.
17. Milberg W, Blumstein S: Lexical decision and aphasia: Evidence for semantic processing. *Brain Lang* 14:371–385, 1981.
18. Nebes RD, Boller F, Holland A: Use of semantic context by patients with Alzheimer's disease. *Psychol Aging* 1(3):261–269, 1986.
19. Albert M, Milberg W: Semantic processing in patients with Alzheimer's disease. *Brain Lang* 37:163–171, 1989.
20. Balota DA, Duchek JM: Semantic priming effects, lexical repetition effects, and contextual disambiguation effects in healthy aged individuals and individuals with senile dementia of the Alzheimer's type. *Brain Lang* 40:181–201, 1991.
21. Ober BA, Shenaut GK: Lexical decision and priming in Alzheimer's disease. *Neuropsychologia* 26(2):273–286, 1988.
22. Ober BA, Shenaut GK, Jagust WJ, et al: Automatic semantic priming with various category relations in Alzheimer's disease and normal aging. *Psychol Aging* 6(4):647–660, 1991.
23. Ober BA, Shenaut GK, Reed BR: Assessment of associative relations in Alzheimer's disease: evidence for preservation of semantic memory. *Aging Cogn* 2(4):254–267, 1995.
24. Ober BA, Shenaut GK: Semantic priming in Alzheimer's disease: Meta-analysis and theoretical evaluation, in Allen PA, Bashore TR (eds): *Age Differences in Word and Language Processing.* Amsterdam: North Holland, 1995.
25. Nebes RD: Semantic memory in Alzheimer's disease. *Psychol Bull* 106(3):377–394, 1989.
26. Chertkow J, Bub D, Seidenberg M: Priming and semantic memory loss in Alzheimer's Disease. *Brain Lang* 36:420–446, 1989.
27. Devlin JT, Andersen ES, Seidenberg MS: Category coordinate errors in a dynamic system: Simulating the naming errors in Alzheimer's disease. *Brain Lang* 65(1):81–83, 1998.
28. Tippett LJ, McAuliffe S, Farah MJ: Preservation of categorical knowledge in Alzheimer disease: A computational account. *Memory* 3:519–533, 1995.
29. Glosser G, Friedman RB: Lexical but not semantic priming in Alzheimer's disease. *Psychol Aging* 6:522–527, 1991.

30. Glosser G, Friedman RB, Grugan PK, et al: Lexical semantic and associative priming in Alzheimer's disease. *Neuropsychology* 12(2):218–224, 1998.
31. McGlinchey-Berroth R, Milberg WP: Preserved semantic memory structure in Alzheimer's disease, in Cerella J et al (eds): *Adult Information Processing: Limits on Loss*. San Diego: Academic Press, 1993, pp 407–422.
32. Neely JH: Semantic priming effects in visual word recognition: a selection review of current findings and theories, in Besner D, Humphreys GW (eds): *Basic Processes in Reading: Visual Word Recognition*. Hillsdale, NJ: Erlbaum, 1991.
33. de Groot AMB: Primed lexical decision: Combined effects of proportion of related prime-target pairs and the stimulus-onset asynchrony of prime and target. *Q J Exp Psychol* 96:29–44, 1984.
34. Faust ME, Balota DA, Duchek JM, et al: Inhibitory control during sentence comprehension in individuals with dementia of the Alzheimer's type. *Brain Lang* 57:225–253, 1997.
35. Sullivan MP, Faust ME, Balota DA: Identity negative priming in older adults and individuals with dementia of the Alzheimer's type. *Neuropsychology* 9(4):1–19, 1995.
36. Milberg WP, McGlinchey-Berroth R, Duncan K, et al: Evidence for alterations in the dynamics of semantic activation in Alzheimer's disease: The gain/decay hypothesis of a disorder of semantic memory. *J Int Neuropsychol Soc* 5:641–658, 1999.
37. Posner MI, Cohen Y: Components of visual orienting, in Bouma H, Bouwhuis D (eds): *Attention and Performance X*. Hillsdale, NJ: Erlbaum, 1984, pp 531–556.
38. Posner MI, Inhoff AW, Friedrich FJ, et al: Isolating attentional systems: A cognitive-anatomical analysis. *Psychobiology* 15(2):107–121, 1987.
39. Posner MI: Structures and functions of selective attention, in Boll T, Bryant B (eds): *Master Lectures in Clinical Neuropsychology*. Washington DC: American Psychological Association, 1988.
40. Posner MI, Peterson S: The attentional system of the human brain. *Annu Rev Neurosci* 13:25–42, 1990.
41. Langley LK, Fuentes LJ, Hochhalter AK, et al: Inhibition of return in aging and Alzheimer's disease: Performance as a function of task demands and stimulus timing. *J Clin Exp Neuropsychol* 23(4):431–446, 2001.
42. Parasuraman R, Greenwood PM, Haxby JV, et al: Visuospatial attention in dementia of the Alzheimer type. *Brain* 115:711–733, 1992.
43. Greenwood PM, Parasuraman R, Alexander GE: Controlling the focus of spatial attention during visual search: Effects of advanced aging and Alzheimer's disease. *Neuropsychologia* 11(3):3–12, 1997.
44. Parasuraman R, Greenwood PM, Alexander GE: Selective impairment of spatial attention during visual search in Alzheimer's disease. *Neuroreport* 6(14):1861–1864, 1995.
45. Parasuraman R, Greenwood PM, Alexander GE: Alzheimer's disease constricts the dynamic range of spatial attention in visual search. *Neuropsychologia* 38(8):1126–1135, 2000.
46. Duncan K, Tunick R, McGlinchey-Berroth R, et al: Covert attention and semantic priming in Alzheimer's disease. Presented at the 27th Annual Meeting of the International Neuropsychological Society, Boston, 1999.
47. Freed DM, Corkin S, Growden JH, et al: Selective attention in Alzheimer's disease: Characterizing cognitive subgroups of patients. *Neuropsychologia* 27(3):325–339, 1989.
48. Houghton G, Tipper P: A model of inhibitory mechanisms in selective attention, in Dagenbach D, Carr TH (eds): *Inhibitory Processes in Attention, Memory, and Language*. San Diego, CA: Academic Press, 1994, pp 53–112.
49. Kahneman D: *Attention and Effort*. Englewood Cliffs, NJ: Prentice-Hall, 1973.
50. Shiffrin RM, Schneider W: Controlled and automatic human information processing: II. Perceptual learning, automatic attending, and a general theory. *Psychol Rev* 84(2):127–190, 1977.
51. Broadbent DE: *Decision and Stress*. London: Academic Press, 1971.
52. Kahneman D, Treisman A: Changing views. of attention and automaticity, in Parasuraman R, Davies R, Beatty J (eds): *Varieties of Attention*. New York: Academic Press, 1984.
53. Tipper SP, Cranston M: Selective attention and priming: Inhibitory and facilitory effects of ignored primes. *Q J Exp Psychol* 37A:591–611, 1985.
54. Tipper SP: The negative priming effect: Inhibitory priming by ignored objects. *Q J Exp Psychol* 37A:571–590, 1985.
55. Tipper SP, Driver J: Negative priming between pictures and words in a selective attention task: Evidence for semantic processing of ignored stimuli. *Mem Cogn* 16(1):64–70, 1988.
56. Nebes RD, Brady CB: Focused and divided attention in Alzheimer's disease. *Cortex* 25(2):305–315, 1989.
57. Grande LJ, McGlinchey-Berroth R, Milberg W, et al: Facilitation of unattended semantic information in Alzheimer's disease: Evidence from a selective attention task. *Neuropsychology* 10(4):475–484, 1996.

58. Cohn NB, Dustman RE, Bradford DC: Age-related decrements in Stroop color test performance. *J Clin Psychol* 40:1244–1250, 1984.
59. Comalli PE, Wapner S, Werner H: Interference effects of Stroop Color-Word Test in childhood, adulthood, and aging. *J Genet Psychol* 100:47–53, 1962.
60. Panek P, Rush M, Slade L: Locus of age-Stroop interference relationships. *J Genet Psychol* 25:201–216, 1984.
61. Fisher LM, Freed DM, Corkin S: Stroop color-word test performance in patients with Alzheimer's disease. *J Clin Exp Neuropsychol* 12(5):745–758, 1990.
62. Speiler DH, Balota DA, Faust ME: Stroop performance in younger adults, healthy older adults and individuals with senile dementia of the Alzheimer's type. *J Exp Psychol Hum Percept Perform* 22(2):461–479, 1996.

Chapter 47

FRONTOTEMPORAL DEMENTIA AND VARIANTS

Mario F. Mendez

Frontotemporal lobar degeneration (FTLD) is a broad category of degenerative disease that emcompasses frontotemporal dementia (FTD) and variants including primary progressive aphasia and semantic dementia. Beginning in 1892, Arnold Pick described a series of patients with dementia and circumscribed lobar atrophy, particularly of the left temporal lobe.[1] Alzheimer and Altman went on to describe prominent lobar atrophy of gray and white matter and argentophilic intraneuronal inclusions known as Pick's bodies. On neuropathologic examination, however, most patients with FTD lack these pathognomonic Pick bodies necessary for the clinicopathologic diagnosis of "Pick's disease." In fact, FTD is not a single entity but part of a spectrum of disorders that have in common circumscribed and progressive atrophy of the frontotemporal lobes (Table 47-1).[2–4] Converging evidence now suggests that these FTLDs are "taupathies," stemming from tau protein abnormalities in the brain.[2]

EPIDEMIOLOGY

The FTLDs are the second most common degenerative dementia[5] after Alzheimer's disease (AD). FTD is especially common when the age of onset is less than 65 years.[4] The age of onset of FTD averages about 56 to 58 years, with a range beginning as young as 22; the average duration of the disease is 8 to 11 years, with motor variants having a shorter, more malignant course.[4,5] Males and females are equally affected, and the main risk factor is familial; 42 to 50 percent of patients with FTD have a first-degree relative with a FTD.[6,7]

FTD CLINICAL FEATURES

In most patients with FTD, personality changes are dramatic symptoms, and these usually precede or overshadow the cognitive disabilities.[5] Clinical Consensus Criteria for diagnosing FTD include a progressive course, qualitative impairments in social interactions, quantitative changes in personal regulation, impaired emotional ability or blunting, and loss of insight (Table 47-2).[4] Patients lose social tact and become socially intrusive and inappropriate. They are often disinhibited, with impulsive behavior; apathetic, with decreased initiative; or both. FTD patients lack empathy and appear emotionally shallow and indifferent. Other emotional changes include depression, mania, lability, anger, and irritability.[5] As the disease progresses, FTD patients neglect their hygiene and may wander unclothed or urinate or defecate in public. In addition, FTD patients tend toward decreased verbal output, later progressing to complete mutism.

Prominent compulsive-like behaviors are other manifestations of this disease.[8] Perseverative and stereotyped behaviors encompass simple repetitive acts, and verbal or motor stereotypies such as lip smacking, hand rubbing or clapping, counting aloud, and humming. They also encompass complex repetitive motor routines such as wandering a fixed route, collecting and hoarding objects, counting money, and rituals involving unusual toileting behavior, oral behaviors, singing the same songs, touching, grabbing, or superstitious acts.

In midstages of FTD, bilateral temporal lobe involvement with damage to the amygdalar nuclei predisposes to the Klüver-Bucy syndrome.[4,5] This syndrome

Table 47-1
Frontotemporal dementia (FTD) and its variants

FTD, bilateral frontotemporal involvement
- FTD, lacking distinctive histology on neuropathology
- FTD, with Pick bodies and Pick cells on neuropathology

Primary progressive aphasia from asymmetrical left hemisphere frontotemporal lobar degeneration (FTLD)

Semantic dementia from asymmetrical temporal lobe FTLD

FTD with motor neuron disease or amyotrophic lateral sclerosis

FTD with parkinsonism linked to chromosome 17 (FTDP-17)

Corticobasal ganglionic degeneration (CBGD)

Table 47-2
Consensus clinical diagnostic features of FTD[4]

I. Core diagnostic features (all must be present)
   A. Insidious onset and gradual progression
   B. Early decline in social interpersonal conduct
   C. Early impairment in regulation of personal conduct
   D. Early emotional blunting
   E. Early loss of insight

II. Supportive diagnostic features
   A. Behavioral disorder
      1. Decline in personal hygiene and grooming
      2. Mental rigidity and inflexibility
      3. Distractibility and impersistence
      4. Hyperorality and dietary changes
      5. Perseverative and stereotyped behavior
      6. Utilization behavior
   B. Speech and language: Altered speech output (aspontaneity and economy of speech, press of speech), stereotypy of speech, echolalia, perseveration, mutism
   C. Physical signs: Primitive reflexes, incontinence, akinesia, rigidity, tremor, low and labile blood pressure
   D. Investigations
      1. Neuropsychology: impaired frontal tests without amnesia or perceptual deficits
      2. EEG: normal on conventional EEG despite clinically evident dementia
      3. Brain imaging: predominant frontal and/or anterior temporal abnormality

Source: From Neary et al.,[4] with permission.

includes hypermetamorphosis or the compulsion to attend and touch every visual stimulus, hyperorality and altered dietary changes, altered sexual behavior, visual agnosia, and placidity. Hypermetamorphosis is the compulsion to attend to any visual stimulus. Patients are driven to explore and manipulate objects, particularly with their mouths. Hyperorality results in overeating and the eating of inedible items; it may require restraints to prevent suffocation.[9]

On neuropsychologic testing, frontal-executive functions are compromised early, memory is less impaired, and occipitoparietal functions are relatively preserved.[10] Frontal-executive functions such as planning and follow-through, set shifting and sequencing, and judgment are abnormal. Memory is eventually compromised, but there is relative preservation of recognition memory compared to free recall. Visuospatial functions, however, remain intact in most patients. As the disease advances, patients develop global cognitive impairments and compromised activities of daily living.

On neurologic examination, abnormalities are usually confined to the presence of primitive reflexes such as grasp, snout, and sucking reflexes. In subsets of FTD patients, however, the neurologic examination discloses dysarthria, dysphagia, fasciculations, muscle wasting, parkinsonism, ideomotor apraxia, or dystonia.

FTLD Variants: Primary Progressive Aphasia, Semantic Dementia, and Motor Variants

Investigators have identified several variants of FTLD.[11,12] The left hemisphere–predominant patients have early speech and language difficulty or a primary progressive aphasia syndrome (see below) but otherwise normal behavioral status. In contrast, the right hemisphere–predominant patients have preserved speech and language but prominent personality changes. In addition to the usual frontotemporal combination, there are patients with predominant frontal or predominant temporal involvement.[12] The predominant frontal patients have more dysexecutive cognitive changes and the predominant temporal patients may have elements of the Klüver-Bucy syndrome or of semantic dementia (see below).

Table 47-3
Consensus clinical criteria for progressive nonfluent aphasia

I. Core diagnostic features
  A. Insidious onset and gradual progression
  B. Nonfluent spontaneous speech with at least one of the following: agrammatism, phonemic paraphasias, anomia
II. Supportive diagnostic features
  A. Speech and language
    1. Stuttering or oral apraxia
    2. Impaired repetition
    3. Alexia, agraphia
    4. Early preservation of word meaning
    5. Late mutism
  B. Behavior
    1. Early preservation of social skills
    2. Late behavioral changes similar to FTD
  C. Physical signs: late contralateral primitive reflexes, akinesia, rigidity, and tremor
  D. Investigations
    1. Neuropsychology: nonfluent aphasia without amnesia or perceptual disorder
    2. EEG: normal or minor asymmetrical slowing
    3. Brain imaging (structural and/or functional): asymmetric abnormality predominantly affecting dominant (usually left) hemisphere

Source: From Neary et al.,[4] with permission.

Some patients with FTLD lateralized to the left hemisphere present with an isolated primary progressive aphasia (PPA) for at least 2 years before other clinical manifestations appear.[13] PPA is characterized by difficulty in verbal expression, anomia, and shortened phrase length in the presence of relative preservation of comprehension (Table 47-3).[4] Speech is hesitant, broken, telegraphic (agrammatism), dysarthric, and effortful. There may be phonologic (phonemic paraphasic) errors, particularly in repetition, a decreased repetition span, and comparably impaired reading and writing. PPA that progresses anteriorly to affect frontal functions is usually associated with FTD, but the syndrome is etiologically heterogeneous, with some patients found at postmortem to have had AD.[13]

Another asymmetrical FTLD variant is semantic dementia (Table 47-4).[4] In this syndrome, which some consider to be a semantic form of PPA, speech production is fluent, but there are deficiencies in single-word comprehension. There may be semantic paraphasias characterized by the replacement of correct words with semantically related ones. Reading is consistent with surface dyslexia; there is preserved ability to read phonologically, with regular spelling-to-sound correspondence, but difficulty reading orthographically irregular words. The rest of the cognitive profile in semantic dementia reflects early profound semantic loss in other domains with preservation of other cognitive abilities. There may be impairments of object meaning

Table 47-4
Consensus clinical criteria for semantic dementia

I. Core diagnostic features
  A. Insidious onset and gradual progression
  B. Language disorder characterized by
    1. Progressive, fluent, empty spontaneous speech
    2. Loss of word meaning, manifest by impaired naming and comprehension
    3. Semantic paraphasias *and/or*
  C. Perceptual disorder characterized by
    1. Prosopagnosia: impaired recognition of identity of familiar faces *and/or*
    2. Object agnosia: impaired recognition of object identity
  D. Preserved perceptual matching and drawing reproduction
  E. Preserved single-word repetition
  F. Preserved ability to read aloud and write to dictation orthographically regular words
II. Supportive diagnostic features
  A. Speech and language: Press of speech, idiosyncratic word usage, absence of phonemic paraphasias, surface dyslexia and dysgraphia, preserved calculation
  B. Behavior: Loss of sympathy and empathy, narrowed preoccupations, parsimony
  C. Physical signs: Absent or late primitive reflexes, akinesia, rigidity, and tremor
  D. Investigations: Neuropsychology: Profound semantic loss, manifest in failure of word comprehension and naming and/or face and object recognition; preserved phonology, syntax, perceptual/spatial skills, memorizing. EEG: normal; Brain imaging: predominant anterior temporal abnormality-symmetrical or asymmetrical

Source: From Neary et al.,[4] with permission.

or identity (object agnosia) or of the recognition of familiar faces (prosopagnosia). These are not perceptual disturbances, because patients can match objects and demonstrate normal performance on perceptual matching for identity. These patients usually have a temporal variant of FTLD affecting the inferior and middle temporal gyri,[14] and they can have other FTLD-spectrum findings such as motor neuron disease.[15]

Motor variants of FTLD include FTD with motor neuron disease or amyotrophic lateral sclerosis (ALS-FTD), FTD with parkinsonism linked to chromosome 17 (FTDP-17), and corticobasal ganglion degeneration (CBGD). Approximately 10 percent of FTD patients have accompanying ALS with prominent bulbar involvement and a rapid disease course.[16] In some cases, FTD with parkinsonism occurs as a hereditary autosomal dominant disorder linked to chromosome 17q21-22.[17] These FTDP-17 patients make up about 13 to 14 percent of those with a positive family history of FTD, and, in addition to early parkinsonism, manifest a more rapidly progressive course and an earlier age of onset than most FTD patients.[18] Finally, the combination of FTD with asymmetrical involvement of the parietal lobe and basal ganglia plus brainstem basophilic (corticobasal) inclusions may be identical with the syndrome of CBGD. These patients have asymmetrical parkinsonism, myoclonus, ideomotor apraxia, and an "alien limb" that feels foreign with involuntary, semipurposeful movements.[19]

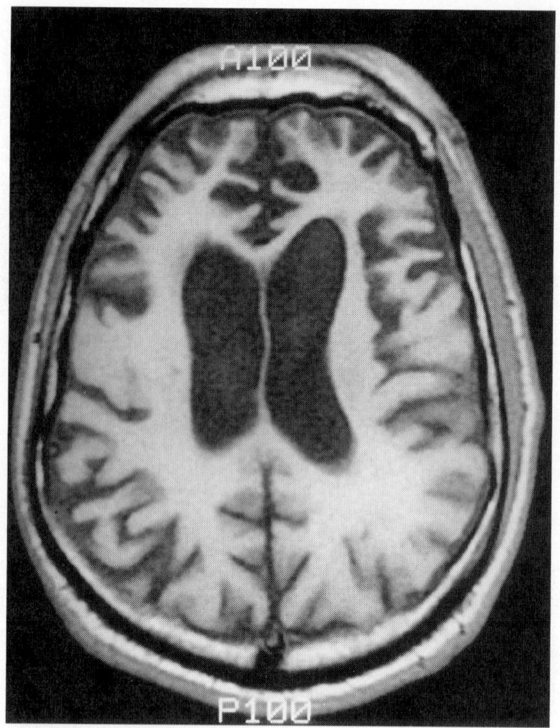

Figure 47-1
Magnetic resonance imaging scans of patient with frontotemporal dementia proven to be Pick's disease on autopsy. T1-weighted horizontal (A) and sagittal (B) images demonstrating frontotemporal atrophy.

DIFFERENTIAL DIAGNOSIS

Clinicians diagnose FTD after excluding other conditions that can present with similar behavioral changes, such as primary psychiatric disease and other frontally predominant dementias. Other diseases involving the frontal or frontal and temporal lobes include AD with frontal features, vascular dementia, normal-pressure hydrocephalus, neurosyphilis, AIDS dementia, Huntington's disease, Creutzfeldt-Jakob disease, adult-onset neuronal intranuclear hyaline inclusion disease, adult polyglucason body disease, and frontotemporal mass lesions.

During life, FTD is most commonly confused with AD.[5] In early AD, there is amnesia with preserved social skills and personal propriety; in early FTD,

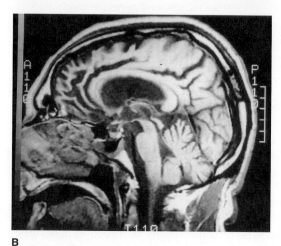

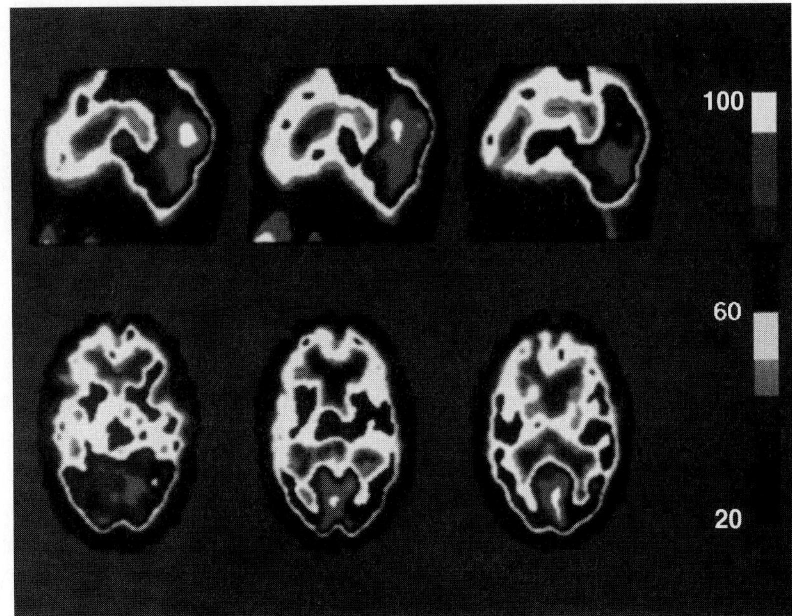

Figure 47-2 (Plate 18) *Single photon emission computed tomography (SPECT) scans of patient with Pick's disease demonstrating frontal hypometabolism.*

there are interpersonal and other personality changes with the relative preservation of memory.[5] In these early stages, FTD patients also perform significantly better than the AD patients on elementary drawings and calculations.[20] Loss of personal awareness, eating changes or hyperorality, stereotyped and perseverative behavior, progressive reduction of speech rather than fluent logorrhea, and preserved spatial orientation differentiated 100 percent of patients with FTD from those with AD.[21]

NEUROIMAGING

There are no definitive laboratory tests for FTD, but neuroimaging can help confirm the presence of this syndrome. Although absent early, most FTD patients eventually show frontotemporal atrophy, which is often asymmetrical, on computed tomography (CT) or magnetic resonance imaging (MRI) (Fig. 47-1). In contrast, AD patients have more generalized atrophy with smaller hippocampal formations.[22,23] Functional imaging is more sensitive than structural imaging for the diagnosis of FTD. Single photon emission computed tomography (SPECT) and positron emission tomography (PET) show decreased regional cerebral blood flow and hypometabolism in the frontal cortex and anterior temporal lobes (Fig. 47-2, Plate 18).[24] In contrast, SPECT and PET scans show predominant posterior temporoparietal changes in AD.[24] Patients with the PPA and semantic dementia show asymmetrical changes in the left hemisphere or temporal lobes, respectively (Fig. 47-3).

NEUROPATHOLOGIC FEATURES

At autopsy, the brains of patients with FTD show a lobar distribution of atrophy involving the frontal lobes, temporal lobes, or both. Coronal sections reveal deep sulci and knife-edged gyri in the atrophic areas (Fig. 47-4). An abrupt transition may be evident between involved and uninvolved cortical regions, and there is a tendency for sparing of the precentral gyrus and the posterior one-third of the superior temporal gyrus. The cortical degeneration mainly involves the gray matter. Further studies of FTD patients disclose Pick bodies in about 20 to 25 percent, motor neuron changes in 10 percent, early parkinsonian changes in 3 to 4 percent, and CBGD in a small percentage.[2,16,17,19,25]

There are several major histopathologic variants of FTLD.[25] First, the most common is a nonspecific

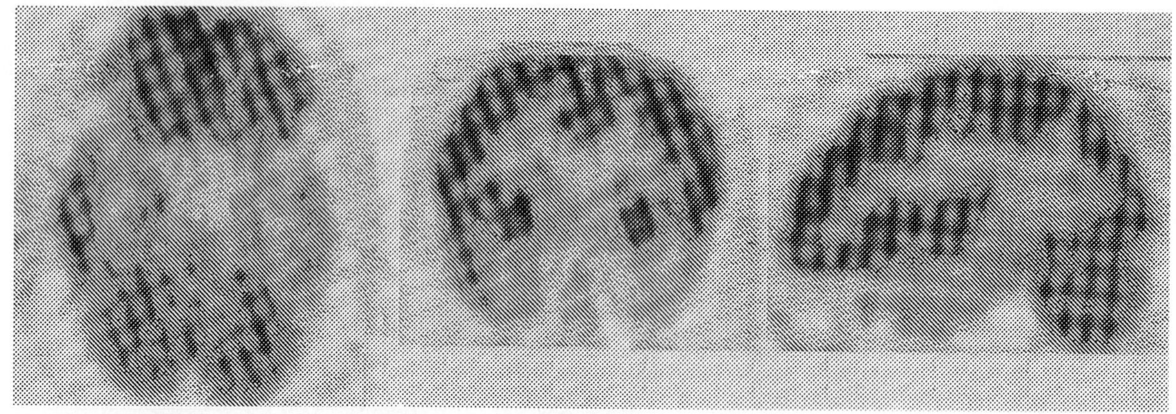

Figure 47-3
Fluorodeoxyglucose positron emission tomography (PET) of patient with semantic dementia demonstrating bilateral anterior temporal hypoperfusion, greater on the left. This image was greatly magnified.

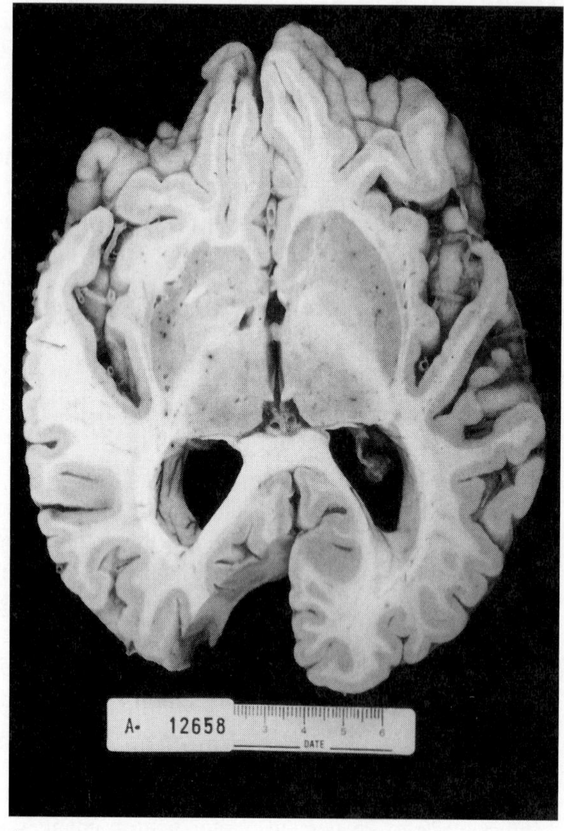

A

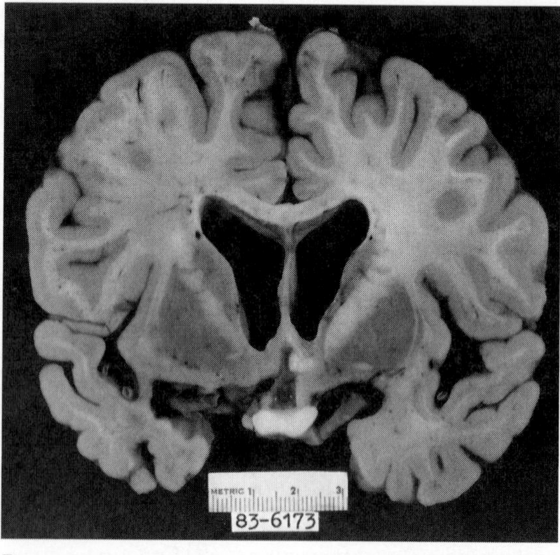

B

Figure 47-4
Gross neuropathologic features of Pick's disease demonstrating disproportionate atrophy of the frontal (A) *and temporal* (B) *lobes (Courtesy of Drs. Linda Chang and Bruce L. Miller.)*

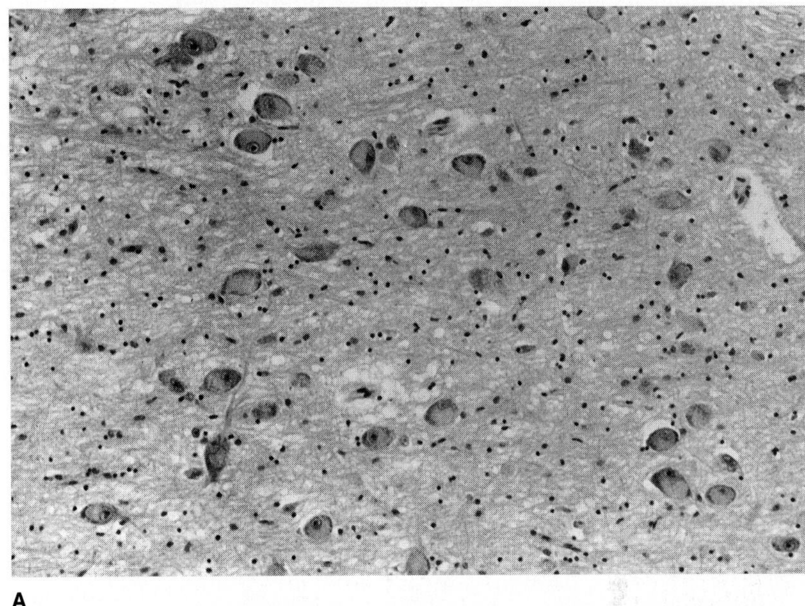

A

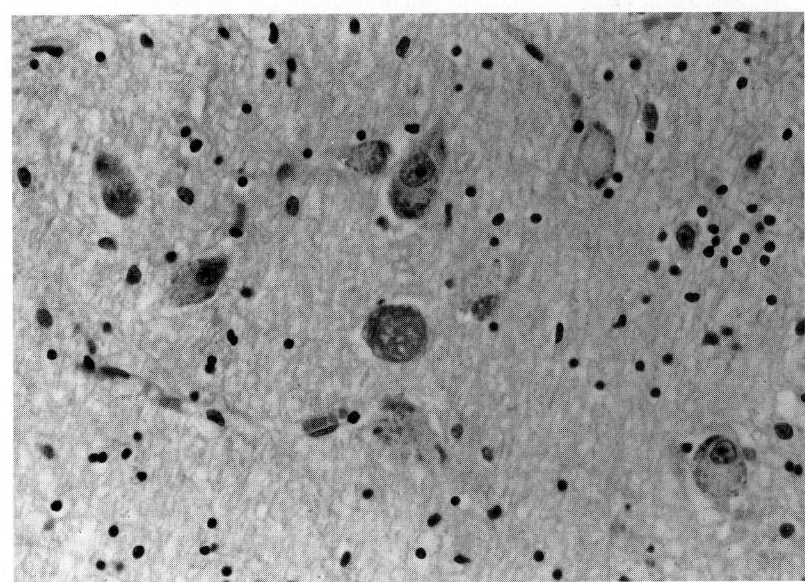

B

Figure 47-5
Microscopic neuropathologic features of Pick's disease demonstrating neocortical Pick bodies. These intracytoplasmic inclusions have a dark rim and displace the nuclei laterally.

frontotemporal atrophy "lacking distinctive histology." There is neuronal loss and astrogliosis with spongiosis (minute cavities or microvacuolation) of the outer, supragranular layers (II to III) of the frontotemporal cortex, with variable involvement of subcortical and limbic structures. Second, in addition to these changes, there may be pathognomonic changes of Pick's disease. These include severe frontotemporal atrophy often with "knife-like" gyri, ballooned neurons or Pick cells, and tau-positive, ubiquitin-positive Pick bodies (Fig. 47-5). Pick bodies are spherical, argentophilic intraneuronal inclusions consisting of straight 10- to 20-nm neurofilaments and constricted 160-nm fibrils, particularly concentrated in neocortical layers II to III and V to VI and in the granular layer of the dentate gyrus and CA1 sector of the hippocampus.[26] Third, there may be evidence of additional involvement of anterior horn cells with or without ubiquitin-positive inclusions. Finally, smaller numbers of FTLD patients have involvement of the substantia nigra, striatopallidum, parietal cortex, thalamus, and other structures.

The neurotransmitter's changes primarily involve serotonin. There are decreases in serotonin receptors and in postsynaptic serotonin.[27] On the other hand, choline acetyltransferase activity is comparable with that of normal controls, and scopolamine infusion may not improve memory in FTD. Cerebrospinal fluid and brain tissue studies suggest that dopamine is relatively spared but somatostatin is decreased.

PATHOPHYSIOLOGY

The underlying cause of FTLD is unknown, but genetic factors are strongly implicated. A positive family history of a similar dementia in a first-degree relative is present in as many as 38 to 50 percent of patients with FTD.[6,7] Analysis of the frequency of apolipoprotein alleles in patients with FTD indicates an increased frequency of the $\varepsilon 4$ allele, but this is not as strong as for AD.[7,28] Most molecular studies have shown autosomal dominant mutations on chromosome 17[17]; however, there is an FTD pedigree with trinucleotide repeat expansions linked to chromosome 3.[29]

The chromosome 17 mutations involve primarily the gene for tau protein. The most common known tau mutations are located in the microtubular binding domain of tau and are either missplicing mutations in the intronic "stem-loop" site following exon 10 or missense mutations in or outside the exon 10 coding region.[30] These mutations may result in neuronal damage from hyperphosphorylation of tau and disruption of its microtubular binding and stabilization properties.[31] Hyperphosphorylated tau impairs microtubule function and axonal transport, leading to inability to bind to microtubules and allowing the abnormal tau to aggregate into wide, twisted, ribbon-like filaments. In patients with FTDP-17, one common mechanism leading to this abnormal tau function and aggregation is an increase in the ratio of the tau protein isoform with four microtubular binding repeats over the three repeat isoforms. Another mechanism for abnormal tau expression in some FTDP-17 patients results from mutations located outside the exon 10 region, which lead to neuronal inclusions with both 4R and 3R tau isoforms, similar to the paired helical and straight filaments seen in AD.

TREATMENT

Currently, there is no specific treatment for FTD. In addition to managing the general aspects of dementia, the management of these patients focuses on behavioral interventions. Given the decreased serotonin receptor binding in FTD, many of the behavioral symptoms of FTD may respond to selective serotonin reuptake inhibitors (SSRIs).[32] Marked disinhibition, aggressive behavior, or verbal outbursts may respond to small doses of risperidone or quetiapine, trazodone, or to anticonvulsants such as carbamazepine and valproate. There is no evidence of benefit, however, from the acetylcholinesterase inhibitors used for AD. Patients with PPA and semantic dementia may respond to speech therapy techniques. Methods for the effective treatment of FTLD patients require much more research and investigation. In the future, drugs directed at altering the pathophysiology, such as the abnormally phosphorylated tau residues, may be the key to treating the FTLD disorders.

REFERENCES

1. Kertesz A, Kalvach P: Arnold Pick and German neuropsychiatry in Prague. *Arch Neurol* 53:935, 1996.
2. Kertesz A, Davidson W, Munoz DG: Clinical and pathological overlap between frontotemporal dementia, primary progressive aphasia and corticobasal degeneration: The Pick complex. *Dement Geriatr Cogn Disord* 10:46, 1999.
3. Pasquier F, Lebert F, Lavenu I, et al: The clinical picture of frontotemporal dementia: Diagnosis and follow-up. *Dement Geriatr Cogn Disord* 10:10, 1999.
4. Neary D, Snowden JS, Gustafson L, et al: Frontotemporal lobar degeneration: A consensus on clinical diagnostic criteria. *Neurology* 51:1546, 1998.
5. Mendez MF, Selwood A, Mastri AR, et al: Pick's disease versus Alzheimer's disease: A comparison of clinical characteristics. *Neurology* 43:289, 1993.

6. Chow TW, Miller BL, Hayashi VN, et al: Inheritance of frontotemporal dementia. *Arch Neurol* 56:817, 1999.
7. Stevens M, van Duijn CM, Kamphorst W, et al: Familial aggregation in frontotemporal dementia. *Neurology* 50:1541, 1998.
8. Mendez MF, Perryman KM, Miller BL, et al: Compulsive behaviors as presenting symptoms of frontotemporal dementia. *J Geriatr Psychiatry Neurol* 10:154, 1997.
9. Mendez MF, Foti DJ: Lethal hyperoral behavior from the Klüver-Bucy syndrome. *J Neurol Neurosurg Psychiatry* 62:293, 1997.
10. Hodges JR, Gurd JM: Remote memory and lexical retrieval in a case of frontal Pick's disease. *Arch Neurol* 51:821, 1994.
11. Miller BL, Chang L, Mena I, et al: Progressive right frontotemporal degeneration: Clinical, neuropsychological, and SPECT characteristics. *Dementia* 4:204, 1993.
12. Edwards-Lee T, Miller BL, Benson DF, et al: The temporal variant of frontotemporal dementia. *Brain* 120:1027, 1997.
13. Mesulam MM: Primary progressive aphasia. *Ann Neurol* 49:425, 2001.
14. Mummery CJ, Patterson K, Price CJ, et al: A voxel-based morphometry study of semantic dementia: Relationship between temporal lobe atrophy and semantic memory. *Ann Neurol* 47:36, 2000.
15. Rossor MN, Revesz T, Lantos PL, et al: Semantic dementia with ubiquitin-positive tau-negative inclusion bodies. *Brain* 123:267, 2000.
16. Neary D, Snowden JS, Mann DM: Cognitive change in motor neurone disease/amyotrophic lateral sclerosis (MND/ALS). *J Neurol Sci* 180:15, 2000.
17. Wilhelmsen KC: Chromosome 17-linked dementias. *Cell Mol Life Sci* 54:920, 1998.
18. Basun H, Almkvist O, Axelman K, et al: Clinical characteristics of a chromosome 17-linked rapidly progressive familial frontotemporal dementia. *Arch Neurol* 54:539, 1997.
19. Jendroska K, Rossor MN, Mathias CJ, et al: Morphological overlap between corticobasal degeneration and Pick's disease: A clinicopathological report. *Mov Disord* 10:111, 1995.
20. Mendez MF, Cherrier M, Perryman KM, et al: Frontotemporal dementia versus Alzheimer's disease: Differential cognitive features. *Neurology* 47:1189, 1996.
21. Miller BL, Ikonte C, Ponton M, et al: A study of the Lund-Manchester research criteria for frontotemporal dementia: Clinical and single-photon emission CT correlations. *Neurology* 48:937, 1997.
22. Frisoni GB, Beltramello A, Geroldi C, et al: Brain atrophy in frontotemporal dementia. *J Neurol Neurosurg Psychiatry* 61:157, 1996.
23. Kitagaki H, Mori E, Yamaji S, et al: Frontotemporal dementia and Alzheimer disease: Evaluation of cortical atrophy with automated hemispheric surface display generated with MR images. *Radiology* 208:431, 1998.
24. Duara R, Barker W, Luis CA: Frontotemporal dementia and Alzheimer's disease: Differential diagnosis. *Dement Geriatr Cogn Disord* 10:37, 1999.
25. Jackson M, Lowe J: The new neuropathology of degenerative frontotemporal dementias. *Acta Neuropathol* 91:127, 1996.
26. Hof PR, Bouras C, Perl DP, et al: Quantitative neuropathologic analysis of Pick's disease cases: Cortical distribution of Pick bodies and coexistence with Alzheimer's disease. *Acta Neuropathol* 87:115, 1994.
27. Francis PT, Holmes C, Webster MT, et al: Preliminary neurochemical findings in non-Alzheimer dementia due to lobar atrophy. *Dementia* 4:172, 1993.
28. Geschwind D, Karrim J, Nelson SF, et al: The apolipoprotein E epsilon 4 allele is not a significant risk factor for frontotemporal dementia. *Ann Neurol* 44:134, 1998.
29. Brown J: Chromosome 3-linked frontotemporal dementia. *Cell Mol Life Sci* 54:925, 1998.
30. Goedert M, Crowther RA, Spillantini MG: Tau mutations cause frontotemporal dementias. *Neuron* 21:955, 1998.
31. Arawaka S, Usami M, Sahara N, et al: The tau mutation (val337met) disrupts cytoskeletal networks of microtubules. *Neuroreport* 10:993, 1999.
32. Swartz JR, Miller BL, Lesser IM, et al: Frontotemporal dementia: Treatment response to serotonin selective reuptake inhibitors. *J Clin Psychiatry* 58:212, 1997.

Chapter 48

DEMENTIA IN PARKINSON'S DISEASE, HUNTINGTON'S DISEASE, AND RELATED DISORDERS*

Diane M. Jacobs
Gilberto Levy
Karen Marder

OVERVIEW

This chapter describes the epidemiology, clinical characteristics, and pathology of dementia in Parkinson's disease, Huntington's disease, progressive supranuclear palsy, corticobasal ganglionic degeneration, multiple system atrophy, and spinocerebellar ataxia. Each of these conditions is associated with degeneration of subcortical nuclei and is characterized by prominent motor symptomatology; the presence of cognitive change or dementia varies somewhat depending upon the specific condition. Although some cognitive characteristics are associated more with one of these disorders than another, in general they share a common neuropsychological profile often referred to as subcortical dementia or subcorticofrontal dysfunction.

Examples of cognitive symptoms associated with these disorders include slowed information processing, impaired attention and executive functioning, and poor memory retrieval in the context of relatively preserved encoding and consolidation. Primary language abilities are also typically preserved. A summary of cognitive characteristics is provided in Table 48-1. This pattern of performance is distinct from that associated with "cortical dementias" (e.g., Alzheimer disease), which are characterized by amnesia, aphasia, and agnosia. The subcorticofrontal dysfunction associated with these disorders can be explained by damage to connections between subcortical structures (in the basal ganglia, basal forebrain, brainstem, and cerebellum) and neocortical association areas.

* **ACKNOWLEDGMENTS:** This work was supported by federal grant NS36630 and the Parkinson's Disease Foundation.

PARKINSON'S DISEASE

Epidemiology

Idiopathic Parkinson's disease (PD) is characterized clinically by tremor at rest, rigidity, bradykinesia, and postural instability. Accuracy of clinical diagnosis is improved by additional characteristics, such as asymmetrical onset and the absence of atypical features suggestive of a parkinsonian disorder other than PD.[1] PD affects approximately 1 per 1000 persons.[2] The prevalence of PD increases with advancing age, affecting 1.6 percent of those over 65 years of age.[3] The average incidence rate of PD is about 10 per 100,000 person-years of observation.[2,4]

Estimates of the prevalence of dementia among PD patients vary widely, from under 10 percent to over 80 percent.[5–8] The type of assessment of cognitive impairment (nonstandardized clinical examination versus screening cognitive tests or neuropsychological battery) and the diagnostic criteria for dementia partly account for this variation. In community-based studies, which provide less biased estimates than hospital-based studies, dementia as defined by the *Diagnostic and Statistical Manual of Mental Disorders,* revised third edition (DSM-III-R)[9] criteria is present in about 20 to 40 percent of PD patients assessed with either the Mini-Mental State Examination or a neuropsychological battery.[10–15]

The risk of incident dementia among patients with PD is increased compared to that of individuals of the same age without PD, ranging from 1.7- to 5.9-fold.[13,16–18] Estimates of the incidence rate of dementia in PD range from 42.6 to 112.5 per 1000 person-years of observation.[13,18–22] The identification of dementia

Table 48-1
*Neuropsychological characteristics of dementia in degenerative disease**

	Alzheimer's disease	*Parkinson's disease*	*Huntington's disease*	*Progressive supranuclear palsy*	*Corticobasal ganglionic degeneration*
Orientation	Impaired	Normal	Normal	Normal	Normal
Memory					
Immediate recall	Impaired	Impaired	Impaired	Normal–mildly impaired	Normal–mildly impaired
Delayed recall	Severely impaired	Impaired	Impaired	Normal–mildly impaired	Normal–mildly impaired
Delayed recognition	Severely impaired	Normal	Normal	Normal	Normal
Percent retained†	0–50	50–80‡	50–80‡	50–80‡	50–80‡
Executive functions/ problem solving	Severely impaired	Severely impaired‡	Severely impaired	Severely impaired‡	Severely impaired
Language					
Naming	Severely impaired; anomia, paraphasia	Normal–mildly impaired; anomia	Normal; visual misperceptions	Normal; visual misperceptions	Normal–mildly impaired
Verbal fluency	Impaired	Severely impaired	Severely impaired	Severely impaired	Severely impaired
Visuospatial skills	Impaired	Impaired	Severely impaired	Impaired	Impaired
Praxis	Normal	Normal	Normal	Normal	Severely impaired; asymmetrical

*Distinct neuropsychological characteristics are most commonly observed when overall severity of dementia is mild.
†Percent retained = (delayed recall/immediate recall) × 100.
‡Executive functions often are disproportionately impaired relative to other cognitive abilities.

in patients with PD is of clinical significance for several reasons. First, dementia is the single most important factor limiting standard pharmacotherapy of PD.[23] Second, cognitive impairment in PD affects quality of life,[24] contributes to caregiver distress,[25] and has been associated with nursing home placement.[26] Last, the development of dementia has been associated with reduced survival in patients with PD.[27–30]

Among PD patients, risk factors for developing dementia include advancing age, severity of extrapyramidal motor signs, depressive symptoms, and levodopa-induced psychosis or confusional states.[11,13,18,20,22,31–37] Low education was significantly associated with dementia in PD in one study.[38] This may suggest a nonspecific effect of education in the expression of cognitive impairment, given the association of lower education with Alzheimer's disease.[39] Some studies have shown a higher frequency of dementia in males with PD[17,22,38,40,41]; in females, an inverse association between estrogen replacement therapy and dementia in PD has been reported.[42] An association of a family history of dementia[41] and Alzheimer's disease[43] with dementia in PD has been found. However, with the exception of one study,[44] no increased frequency of the ApoE-ε4 allele was found in demented PD patients.[45–48] While an inverse association between smoking and PD has been consistently demonstrated, a positive association was observed between smoking and dementia in the setting of PD.[31,49]

Cognitive Characteristics

Cognitive impairment occurs frequently in patients with PD, even in the absence of overt dementia. Estimates of the prevalence of neuropsychological abnormalities among nondemented patients with PD indicate that as many as 93 percent[50] experience some difficulty on tests requiring speeded mental processing, attention, and executive functioning, abstract reasoning, visuospatial skills, recall memory, and verbal fluency. Often these impairments are subtle and do not interfere with daily functioning. This mild or relatively circumscribed cognitive dysfunction, which is evident in many patients with PD, does not progress to frank dementia in all affected individuals. As described above, cognitive impairment sufficient to warrant a diagnosis of dementia occurs in 20 to 40 percent of PD patients.[10–15]

Whether dementia in PD represents a worsening of the cognitive symptoms present in nondemented PD patients or the introduction of additional cognitive deficits is a matter of some controversy and has implications regarding the pathophysiology of dementia in PD. Girotti et al.,[51] for example, observed that demented PD patients had more severe and widespread cognitive deficits than nondemented patients, but mostly on those measures that already discriminated nondemented PD patients from control subjects. In contrast, Stern et al.[52] concluded that although cognitive problems preceding dementia in PD patients continue to worsen with the onset of dementia, there is also a qualitative shift in the pattern of cognitive deficits, with substantial broadening and worsening of memory dysfunction as dementia emerges.

The dementia associated with PD is generally characterized by predominant impairment on tests of executive functioning (e.g., planning, initiating, sequencing, monitoring, and shifting between responses; adapting to novel situations; abstract reasoning), visuospatial and visuomotor skills, free recall memory, and verbal fluency. Language functions other than verbal fluency typically are relatively preserved, as are orientation, cued recall, and recognition memory. Impairment of executive functions—particularly on measures requiring response initiation, planning, set-shifting, and ability to benefit from feedback—may be disproportionately severe relative to deficits in other cognitive domains.

Performance on neuropsychological tests of memory yields important clues as to the nature of the memory deficit in PD. Specifically, memory in Parkinson dementia is associated with impaired ability to retrieve information from memory stores.[53,54] The ability to register, store, and consolidate new memories, however, is relatively preserved. As a result, performance on tests requiring free recall is impaired, while cued recall or recognition memory may be relatively intact. Another way of examining this phenomenon is by examining retention of recently learned material over time, often referred to as "savings" scores. Although initial level of recall may be low for PD patients, retention of material after a delay interval typically is commensurate with the level of initial recall; that is, there is little forgetting over time (i.e., good "savings"). In contrast, patients with Alzheimer's disease rapidly forget recently learned material, often retaining less than half of initially recalled material after an interval of only a few minutes. While the memory impairment associated with PD is considered primarily a retrieval deficit, Alzheimer's disease is characterized by deficient encoding or consolidation of new information. The encoding deficit of Alzheimer's disease reflects the prominent pathology of the hippocampus and entorhinal cortex associated with this disorder,[55–57] while the poor retrieval of new information by PD patients may be secondary to executive dysfunction (i.e., inability to plan and initiate systematic searches of memory stores) and reflects dysfunction of subcorticofrontal circuits.[58]

There is mounting evidence that many of the cognitive impairments observed in Parkinson patients, including poor memory and visuospatial functioning, are associated with limited or slowed processing resources that characterize cognition in PD.[59–61] For example, Stebbins et al.[61] found significant group differences between PD patients and normal control subjects on tests of explicit memory (i.e., free recall, cued recall, and delayed recognition) and working memory (i.e., listening span and digit ordering); however, once the effects of psychomotor processing speed were removed from the analysis, group differences were no longer significant. Similarly, Pillon et al.[60] concluded that impaired memory for spatial locations observed in PD results mainly from a disturbance of strategic processes and from decreased attentional resources.

Pathology

The pathologic hallmark of PD is loss of pigmented cells in the substantia nigra and other pigmented brainstem nuclei. Lewy bodies are found within remaining neurons in the affected areas.[62,63] Small numbers of cortical Lewy bodies have also been described as a constant finding in PD cases in neuropathologic series.[64,65] The pattern of neuropsychological deficit typical of dementia in PD, including prominent impairment on "frontal-lobe" or executive tasks, has been attributed to subcortical degeneration of dopaminergic (medial substantia nigra and ventral tegmental area),[66–68] noradrenergic (locus ceruleus),[68–70] and cholinergic (nucleus basalis of Meynert)[71–75] structures. Other pathologic entities that have been proposed as the neuropathologic basis for dementia in PD include concomitant Alzheimer's disease[76–78] and dementia with Lewy bodies.[79,80] Recently, α-synuclein was found to be a major component of Lewy bodies, leading to the description of PD as a "synucleinopathy."[81] Two studies using α-synuclein immunostaining found a stronger association of cortical Lewy bodies than Alzheimer cortical changes with dementia in PD.[82,83]

HUNTINGTON'S DISEASE

Epidemiology

Huntington's disease (HD) is characterized by an extrapyramidal movement disorder, cognitive, and psychiatric impairment. The movement disorder includes impairment in both involuntary movements (chorea, dystonia, tremor, and rigidity) and voluntary movements (saccadic and smooth pursuit, gait, and speech). Impairment in memory, executive function, and visuomotor skills may be seen. Psychiatric impairment may include irritability, depression, mania, psychosis, and obsessive-compulsive disorder.[84–86]

There are currently 30,000 individuals in the United States who have HD and an additional 150,000 who are at risk by virtue of having a parent with HD. In North America and western Europe, the prevalence of HD is 4 to 7 per 100,000,[87] while among African blacks, Japanese, Chinese, and Finnish, the prevalence is tenfold lower due to a lower CAG repeat length.[88] The mean age of onset is from 36 to 45 years, but it has been reported as early as age 2 and as late as age 90.[84] Death occurs on average 15 to 20 years after onset (usually dated from the onset of the extrapyramidal movement disorder). Approximately 6 percent of HD presents before the age of 20. This form of the disease is known as juvenile HD or the Westphal variant.[84]

HD is an autosomal dominant disorder and the disease gene was localized to chromosome 4p16.3 in 1983.[89] In 1993, when the mutation was identified,[90] direct testing became a possibility for any at-risk individual. HD alleles range from 36 to 121 repeats, with the vast majority exhibiting repeat lengths $\geq$40 (mean 42 to 46).[91] A highly significant negative correlation between age of onset of HD and length of the repeat has been demonstrated, such that higher polyglutamine repeat length is associated with earlier age of onset.[92,93]

This negative correlation is strongest for those with a high number of repeats, who generally have juvenile HD (>60 repeats). The correlation is weaker for alleles within the range of 40 to 50 repeats, which constitutes the majority of HD alleles. Because repeat length accounts for approximately 50 percent of the variance in age of onset,[92,94] there may be other genes[92,95,96] or environmental modifiers[97] that affect the age of onset.

Cognitive dysfunction is a common feature of HD; however, the severity of impairment does vary from patient to patient. The juvenile onset form is associated with severe and rapidly progressive dementia, while cognitive dysfunction is relatively mild and slowly progressive in patients with onset of motor symptoms after age 50.[98] The dementia associated with midlife onset of HD, the most frequent presentation, is intermediate between the juvenile and late onset in terms of severity and rapidity of course. Degree of dementia is closely associated with severity of motor involvement.[99]

Cognitive Characteristics

A metanalysis of 36 studies published between 1980 and 1997 confirmed the characterization of HD as a prototypical subcortical dementia.[100] Specifically, dementia in HD is characterized by impaired performance on tests of learning and memory, attention and executive functions, and visuospatial skills. Patients typically are very slow to initiate responses. As in PD, language functions are relatively preserved in patients with HD with the exception of verbal fluency, which can be markedly impaired.

The memory impairment of HD, like that of PD, is characterized by poor performance on tests of recall memory. Nevertheless, rates of retention from immediate to delayed testing are relatively preserved[101]; that is, once something is learned, it is retained in long-term memory. This is further demonstrated by the fact that performance of HD patients on memory tests using a recognition format improves dramatically. These findings suggest that the memory impairment of HD, as in PD, is characterized by impaired retrieval of stored information. Specifically, patients have difficulty initiating and organizing spontaneous retrieval strategies.

Since the discovery of the genetic mutation for HD in 1993, there have been several studies comparing cognitive functioning of presymptomatic gene carriers who have no motor or psychiatric symptoms to non–gene carriers. These studies have yielded mixed results, with some finding significant differences on measures of memory[102] as well as attention and problem solving[103] while others found no differences on neuropsychological testing between these two groups.[104] Differences in test selection, small sample sizes, and the cross-sectional methodology of many of these studies undoubtedly contribute to these disparate findings. Variation in gene repeat length may be associated with cognitive symptomatology, although there have been conflicting findings in this regard.[102,105] Longitudinal analyses of gene carriers suggest that abnormalities on neuropsychological testing are more evident as conversion to clinical disease nears.[105,106] Nevertheless, impairments on tests of executive function (i.e., Symbol-Digit and Stroop Tests) may be observed as long as 2 years before the onset of clinically significant motor signs.[106] These findings suggest that, at least in some individuals, cognitive change may be the earliest manifestation of disease onset.

Pathology

The core pathologic feature of HD is atrophy of the caudate, putamen, and deep layers of the cortex. Striatal degeneration begins dorsomedially and extends ventrolaterally, such that neuronal loss in the caudate precedes neuronal loss in the putamen and ventral striatum.[107] Striatal medium spiny neurons are selectively impaired. These GABAergic projection neurons, which also express D1 and D2 receptors, make up 90 percent of all striatal neurons.[108] In contrast, large aspiny cholinergic interneurons that are adjacent to the medium spiny neurons are preserved until late in the illness.[109]

HD is one of nine triplet repeat disorders caused by expansion of a trinucleotide repeat (CAG) that codes for glutamine.[110,111] All share certain features: (1) they are neurodegenerative—in all, there is neuronal cell death in an overlapping set of brain regions including basal ganglia, cortex, brainstem, and cerebellum; (2) with the exception of spinobulbar muscular atrophy, which is x-linked recessive, they are autosomal dominant; (3) despite widespread tissue distribution of the protein both centrally and peripherally, the affected region is primarily in the brain; (4) they show genetic anticipation (the earlier onset of disease in succeeding generations, which has long been observed in HD, particularly when disease is inherited from the father); and (5) neuronal intranuclear inclusions have been found in most (HD, dentatorubropallidoluysian atrophy, spinobulbar muscular atrophy, and spinocerebellar ataxias 1, 3, and 7).

PROGRESSIVE SUPRANUCLEAR PALSY

Epidemiology

Clinical characteristics of progressive supranuclear palsy (PSP) include early gait impairment and postural instability with falls, supranuclear ophthalmoplegia primarily affecting vertical gaze, dysarthria, dysphagia, and axial and nuchal rigidity.[112–115] Litvan et al.[114] found that supranuclear downward gaze abnormalities and postural instability with unexplained falls were the best predictors of the diagnosis of PSP pathologically proven. Conversely, the absence of supranuclear gaze palsy is a common reason for the misdiagnosis of PSP as PD.[116] In two studies, the prevalence of PSP has been estimated as 1.4 and 6.4 per 100,000.[117,118] Incidence rates of PSP have ranged from 0.3 to 1.1 per 100,000 person-years.[119–122] Age and male gender may be risk factors for PSP.[117,119,121–124] Mean age at onset in most series is between 60 and 70 years,[113,115,117,124,125] and median duration of disease from onset to death ranges from 5 to 10 years.[113,117,121,124]

Dementia commonly occurs in individuals with PSP. Cognitive or behavioral symptoms were reported in 7 of the 9 cases described by Steele and colleagues.[112] Subsequent estimates of the prevalence of dementia in PSP range from 50 to 80 percent.[113,116,121,126,127] Diagnostic criteria for dementia are likely to influence prevalence estimates of dementia in PSP. Daniel et al.[116] found that only 10 out of 17 autopsy cases of PSP were demented using DSM-III-R criteria, which requires memory impairment. In a study by Pillon et al.,[126] dementia was defined as performance on a global cognitive score at least two standard deviations lower than that of a control group. If the global cognitive score included tests of attention, orientation, memory, and reasoning, the prevalence of dementia in PSP was 58 percent; if the global cognitive score additionally included frontal lobe tests, the prevalence of dementia increased to 71 percent.

Cognitive Characteristics

Comparisons of cognitive functioning in PSP, PD, and multiple system atrophy (MSA) generally have found that cognitive decline is more frequent and severe in PSP than either PD or MSA.[126,128–130] For example, Pillon et al.[126] reported that dementia, defined by a global intellectual performance two standard deviations lower than mean control values, was diagnosed in 58 percent of patients with PSP but only 18 percent of those with PD. Despite differences in the frequency and severity of cognitive dysfunction, however, the neuropsychological pattern of cognitive compromise in PSP, PD, and MSA is similar.

PSP is considered a prototypical subcortical dementia. In fact, the seminal paper on cognition in PSP by Albert et al.[131] was among the first to introduce the term *subcortical dementia*. Albert et al.[131] described forgetfulness, slowed thought processes, emotional or personality changes, and impaired ability to manipulate acquired knowledge as typical cognitive changes in PSP. Executive dysfunction is a prominent feature at all stages of the disease course.[126,132] Although performance on relatively simple attentional tasks may be normal, performance on more complex tasks—such as those requiring sequencing, mental flexibility, abstraction, and reasoning—is severely impaired. PSP patients score lower on tests of executive and frontal lobe functions than PD patients matched for overall level of intellectual deterioration.[126] Slowness of information processing in PSP is pervasive and marked. Dubois et al.[133] found processing time in patients with PSP to be increased, even relative to patients with PD. Albert et al.[131] reported that when patients were allowed additional time to respond (sometimes as long as 4 to 5 min for a single question), their performance improved by as much as 50 percent. Verbal fluency is generally very severely impaired; however, other language functions remain preserved, and paraphasic errors are uncommon. Although language is relatively preserved, severe dysarthria often impairs communicative ability.[134] The memory disorder of PSP is generally mild.[135] Although PSP patients may be impaired on memory tasks requiring free recall, they are able to benefit from retrieval cues and perform normally on tests of cued recall.[136]

Pathology

Cell loss and neurofibrillary changes occur in various regions of the basal ganglia, brainstem, and cerebellum in PSP, including the pallidum, striatum, subthalamic nucleus, substantia nigra, red nucleus, superior colliculi, nuclei cuneiformis and subcuneiformis, periaqueductal gray matter, pontine tegmentum, and the dentate nucleus.[112,137–139] Involvement of the cholinergic pedunculopontine nucleus[140,141] and nucleus basalis of Meynert[142] as well as neurofibrillary degeneration in the cerebral cortex[143,144] have also been reported in PSP. Together with corticobasal ganglionic degeneration and Pick's disease, PSP is now classified as a "tauopathy."[145] The neurofibrillary tangle in PSP differs from that in Alzheimer's disease and consists of straight filaments composed almost entirely of four-repeat tau protein.[145] Both the A0 allele, a dinucleotide repeat polymorphism of the gene coding for tau, and the A0/A0 genotype are significantly overrepresented in PSP patients versus controls.[146,147] Higgins et al.[148] have also identified an extended 5′-tau haplotype consisting of four single nucleotide polymorphisms (SNP) that are associated with the disease phenotype in sporadic PSP.

CORTICOBASAL GANGLIONIC DEGENERATION

Epidemiology

Corticobasal ganglionic degeneration (CBGD) is an uncommon disorder characterized by asymmetrical akinetic-rigid syndrome, limb ideomotor apraxia, focal dystonia or myoclonus, alien limb sign, cortical sensory loss, tremor, supranuclear gaze palsy, postural instability, and gait impairment.[149–152] Signs and symptoms are often strikingly asymmetrical. Asymmetrical signs and symptoms and late postural instability and falls help distinguish CBGD from PSP, while marked apraxia, alien limb sign, and poor response to levodopa distinguish CBGD from PD.[153] The alien limb sign is defined as a feeling that one limb is foreign or "has a will of its own," together with involuntary motor activity; spontaneous levitation and posturing may be more common in CBGD than in alien limb sign due to cerebrovascular disease.[154]

The low sensitivity (<50 percent) of the clinical diagnosis of CBGD suggests that this disorder is underdiagnosed.[153] Mean age at onset in clinical and pathologic series is between 60 and 65 years, and median duration of disease from onset to death is 6 to 8 years.[152,153,155] Cases of CBGD reported in the literature have been sporadic, but two families presenting with dementia and with a neuropathologic diagnosis of CBGD have been described.[156] Although dementia or behavioral manifestations were not a prominent feature in the initial report of this disorder,[149,150] subsequent studies have reported pathologically proven CBGD manifesting as dementia, frontal lobe symptomatology, or progressive aphasia.[157–159] In a pathologic series of 13 patients with CBGD followed in movement disorders or memory clinics, 9 presented with dementia, suggesting that dementia may be a common initial manifestation of CBGD.[160]

Cognitive Characteristics

The neuropsychological profile of dementia associated with CBGD is characterized by a prominent dysexecutive syndrome; deficient dynamic motor control (e.g., bimanual coordination, temporal organization); asymmetrical praxis disorders; and poor free recall but intact cued recall and recognition memory.[136] Massman et al.[161] found a dissociation in neuropsychological functioning between CBGD and Alzheimer's disease patients matched for dementia severity, such that CBGD patients performed significantly better than Alzheimer's disease patients on tests of immediate and delayed verbal recall memory, whereas Alzheimer's disease patients (with or without extrapyramidal symptoms) performed better on tests of praxis, finger-tapping speed, and motor programming. Both groups were severely impaired on tests of sustained attention/mental control and verbal fluency, and mildly impaired on tests of confrontation naming. Similarly, Pillon et al.[136] found that CBGD patients, like patients with PSP, had more severe executive dysfunction than Alzheimer's disease patients, while Alzheimer disease patients were more impaired on tests of learning and memory than either CBGD or PSP.

The presence of apraxia is among the most frequent and distinguishing behavioral features of CBGD. Leiguarda et al.[162] assessed praxis in the least affected limb of 10 patients with CBGD and found that 70 percent of patients were impaired on tests of ideomotor apraxia (e.g., waving goodbye, using a hammer), 30 percent had both ideomotor apraxia and ideational apraxia (i.e., inability to complete multistep purposeful tasks), and none showed buccofacial apraxia. Ideomotor praxis correlated significantly with scores on the Mini-Mental State Examination and Picture Arrangement subtest of the Wechsler Adult Intelligence Scale, which requires planning and abstract reasoning. It is not uncommon that patients can accurately describe an action (e.g., using a key to open a door) that they are completely unable to perform.

Pathology

CBGD is characterized pathologically by atrophy of frontal and parietal cortex, often greater contralateral to the side of the body, with pronounced motor involvement, cortical cell loss, gliosis, swollen and achromatic neurons, neuropil threads, and sometimes neurofibrillary tangles. Basophilic inclusions, cell loss, and gliosis are observed in the substantia nigra and other subcortical structures, including the thalamus, striatum, pallidum, subthalamic nucleus, red nucleus, and dentate nucleus.[138,149,150,157] As in the case of PSP, CBGD brains contain tau-immunoreactive neuronal and glial inclusions composed predominantly of four-repeat tau protein.[145,163] Despite a significant neuropathologic overlap, there are morphological and regional differences between CBGD and PSP.[163] Glial inclusions have been reported to be relatively specific; astrocytic plaques and tufted astrocytes are seen in CBGD and PSP, respectively.[144,164] A tau haplotype overrepresented in PSP has also been associated with CBGD, suggesting a similar genetic background for these disorders.[165,166]

MULTIPLE SYSTEM ATROPHY

Epidemiology

The term *multiple system atrophy* (MSA) encompasses striatonigral degeneration, Shy-Drager syndrome, and sporadic olivopontocerebellar atrophy but excludes familial autosomal dominant olivopontocerebellar atrophy. The clinical features of MSA include parkinsonism and cerebellar, pyramidal, and autonomic dysfunction in different combinations.[167] Some clinical features are useful in distinguishing MSA from PD, including poor response to levodopa, absence of levodopa-induced confusion, speech or bulbar dysfunction, falls, and absence of dementia up to death.[168] The prevalence of MSA has been estimated as 4.4 per 100,000 in one study.[118] Mean age of onset ranges from 50 to 55 years old, and median survival estimates range from 5 to 10 years.[167,169,170] Dementia seems to be a most unusual manifestation of MSA. In a review of 203 pathologically proven cases of MSA, severe intellectual impairment was described in only 1 case and moderate intellectual impairment in 4 cases during the course of the disease.[169]

Cognitive Characteristics

Although clinically significant dementia is not a common symptom associated with MSA, a number of studies have reported neuropsychological abnormalities in patients with these disorders.[128,129,171–173] Most of these investigations have examined patients with probable striatonigral degeneration–type illness. While there have been reports of global impairment on neuropsychological testing in MSA patients compared to control subjects,[129] the majority of studies have found a relatively circumscribed dysexecutive syndrome, as evidenced by poor performance on tests of attentional set shifting, spatial working memory, speeded mental processing, visuospatial organization, abstract reasoning, constructional skill, and verbal fluency.[128,171–173] These deficits have been observed in the context of relatively preserved memory, language, visual perception, and general intellectual functioning.[171,173] The pattern of cognitive dysfunction in MSA is similar to that observed in patients with PD and not as severe as that seen in patient with PSP.[129,173] Studies comparing PD and

MSA patients suggest that patients with MSA are more impaired on tests of verbal fluency[129] and motor movement time,[172] while PD patients are more impaired on the Wisconsin Card Sorting Test.[173]

Pathology

Pathologically, MSA is characterized by cell loss and gliosis in the striatum, pallidum, substantia nigra, locus ceruleus, inferior olives, pontine nuclei, cerebellar Purkinje cells, and intermediolateral cell columns of the spinal cord.[169] The description of oligodendroglial cytoplasmic and other inclusions, which contain α-synuclein, has linked MSA to PD as a synucleinopathy.[81,174]

SPINOCEREBELLAR ATAXIA

Spinocerebellar ataxia (SCA) is an autosomal dominant disorder characterized clinically by progressive gait and limb ataxia and dysarthria. Additional clinical features are characteristic of specific genotypes, as several different mutations, mostly CAG repeat expansions (see "Huntington's Disease," above), have been identified in SCA.[111] Cognition in SCA is characterized by poor performance on tests of attention and executive functioning, despite normal learning, memory, and general intellectual functioning.[175–177] These findings suggest that cognitive deficits in patients with SCA reflect disruption of subcorticofrontal pathways.

REFERENCES

1. Hughes AJ, Ben Shlomo Y, Daniel SE, Lees AJ: What features improve the accuracy of clinical diagnosis in Parkinson's disease: A clinicopathologic study. *Neurology* 42:1142–1146, 1992.
2. Mayeux R, Marder K, Cote LJ, et al: The frequency of idiopathic Parkinson's disease by age, ethnic group, and sex in northern Manhattan, 1988–1993 [published erratum appears in *Am J Epidemiol* 143:528, 1996]. *Am J Epidemiol* 142:820–827, 1995.
3. de Rijk MC, Tzourio C, Breteler MM, et al: Prevalence of parkinsonism and Parkinson's disease in Europe: The EUROPARKINSON Collaborative Study. European Community Concerted Action on the Epidemiology of Parkinson's disease. *J Neurol Neurosurg Psychiatry* 62:10–15, 1997.
4. Bower JH, Maraganore DM, McDonnell SK, Rocca WA: Incidence and distribution of parkinsonism in Olmsted County, Minnesota, 1976–1990. *Neurology* 52:1214–1220, 1999.
5. Brown RG, Marsden CD: How common is dementia in Parkinson's disease? *Lancet* 2:1262–1265, 1984.
6. Cummings JL: Intellectual impairment in Parkinson's disease: Clinical, pathologic, and biochemical correlates. *J Geriatr Psychiatry Neurol* 1:24–36, 1988.
7. Dubois B, Boller F, Pillon B, Agid Y: Cognitive deficits in Parkinson's disease, in Boller F, Grafman J (eds): *Handbook of Neuropsychology.* Amsterdam: Elsevier, 1991, pp 195–240.
8. Marder K, Mayeux R: The epidemiology of dementia in patients with Parkinson's disease. *Adv Exp Med Biol* 295:439–445, 1991.
9. American Psychiatric Association: *Diagnostic and Statistical Manual of Mental Disorders,* 3d rev ed (DSM-III-R). Washington, DC: American Psychiatric Press, 1987.
10. Ebmeier KP, Calder SA, Crawford JR, et al: Dementia in idiopathic Parkinson's disease: Prevalence and relationship with symptoms and signs of parkinsonism. *Psychol Med* 21:69–76, 1991.
11. Mayeux R, Denaro J, Hemenegildo N, et al: A population-based investigation of Parkinson's disease with and without dementia. Relationship to age and gender. *Arch Neurol* 49:492–497, 1992.
12. Tison F, Dartigues JF, Auriacombe S, et al: Dementia in Parkinson's disease: A population-based study in ambulatory and institutionalized individuals. *Neurology* 45:705–708, 1995.
13. Marder K, Tang MX, Cote L, et al: The frequency and associated risk factors for dementia in patients with Parkinson's disease. *Arch Neurol* 52:695–701, 1995.
14. Aarsland D, Tandberg E, Larsen JP, Cummings JL: Frequency of dementia in Parkinson disease. *Arch Neurol* 53:538–542, 1996.
15. Giladi N, Treves TA, Paleacu D, et al: Risk factors for dementia, depression and psychosis in long-standing Parkinson's disease. *J Neural Transm (Budapest)* 107:59–71, 2000.
16. Rajput AH, Offord KP, Beard CM, Kurland LT: A case-control study of smoking habits, dementia, and other illnesses in idiopathic Parkinson's disease. *Neurology* 37:226–232, 1987.

17. Breteler MM, de Groot RR, van Romunde LK, Hofman A: Risk of dementia in patients with Parkinson's disease, epilepsy, and severe head trauma: A register-based follow-up study. *Am J Epidemiol* 142:1300–1305, 1995.
18. Aarsland D, Andersen K, Larsen JP, et al: Risk of dementia in Parkinson's disease: A community-based, prospective study. *Neurology* 56:730–736, 2001.
19. Mayeux R, Chen J, Mirabello E, et al: An estimate of the incidence of dementia in idiopathic Parkinson's disease. *Neurology* 40:1513–1517, 1990.
20. Biggins CA, Boyd JL, Harrop FM, et al: A controlled, longitudinal study of dementia in Parkinson's disease. *J Neurol Neurosurg Psychiatry* 55:566–571, 1992.
21. Mahieux F, Fenelon G, Flahault A, et al: Neuropsychological prediction of dementia in Parkinson's disease. *J Neurol Neurosurg Psychiatry* 64:178–183, 1998.
22. Hughes TA, Ross HF, Musa S, et al: A 10–year study of the incidence of and factors predicting dementia in Parkinson's disease. *Neurology* 54:1596–1602, 2000.
23. Mayeux R: A current analysis of behavioral problems in patients with idiopathic Parkinson's disease. *Mov Disord* 4 (Suppl 1):S48–S56, 1989.
24. Schrag A, Jahanshahi M, Quinn N: What contributes to quality of life in patients with Parkinson's disease? *J Neurol Neurosurg Psychiatry* 69:308–312, 2000.
25. Aarsland D, Larsen JP, Karlsen K, et al: Mental symptoms in Parkinson's disease are important contributors to caregiver distress. *Int J Geriatr Psychiatry* 14:866–874, 1999.
26. Aarsland D, Larsen JP, Tandberg E, Laake K: Predictors of nursing home placement in Parkinson's disease: A population-based, prospective study. *J Am Geriatr Soc* 48:938–942, 2000.
27. Mindham RH, Ahmed SW, Clough CG: A controlled study of dementia in Parkinson's disease. *J Neurol Neurosurg Psychiatry* 45:969–974, 1982.
28. Marder K, Leung D, Tang M, et al: Are demented patients with Parkinson's disease accurately reflected in prevalence surveys? A survival analysis. *Neurology* 41:1240–1243, 1991.
29. Piccirilli M, D'Alessandro P, Finali G, Piccinin GL: Neuropsychological follow-up of parkinsonian patients with and without cognitive impairment. *Dementia* 5: 17–22, 1994.
30. Roos RA, Jongen JC, van der Velde EA: Clinical course of patients with idiopathic Parkinson's disease. *Mov Disord* 11:236–242, 1996.
31. Ebmeier KP, Calder SA, Crawford JR, et al: Clinical features predicting dementia in idiopathic Parkinson's disease: A follow-up study. *Neurology* 40:1222–1224, 1990.
32. Stern Y, Marder K, Tang MX, Mayeux R: Antecedent clinical features associated with dementia in Parkinson's disease. *Neurology* 43:1690–1692, 1993.
33. Piccirilli M, Piccinin GL, Agostini L: Characteristic clinical aspects of Parkinson patients with intellectual impairment. *Eur Neurol* 23:44–50, 1984.
34. Elizan TS, Sroka H, Maker H, et al: Dementia in idiopathic Parkinson's disease. Variables associated with its occurrence in 203 patients. *J Neural Transm* 65:285–302, 1986.
35. Starkstein SE, Mayberg HS, Leiguarda R, et al: A prospective longitudinal study of depression, cognitive decline, and physical impairments in patients with Parkinson's disease. *J Neurol Neurosurg Psychiatry* 55:377–382, 1992.
36. Starkstein SE, Bolduc PL, Mayberg HS, et al: Cognitive impairments and depression in Parkinson's disease: A follow-up study. *J Neurol Neurosurg Psychiatry* 53:597–602, 1990.
37. Guillard A, Chastang C, Fenelon G: Etude a long terme de 416 cas de maladie de Parkinson. Facteurs de pronostic et implications therapeutiques. *Rev Neurol* 142:207–214, 1986.
38. Glatt SL, Hubble JP, Lyons K, et al: Risk factors for dementia in Parkinson's disease: effect of education. *Neuroepidemiology* 15:20–25, 1996.
39. Katzman R: Education and the prevalence of dementia and Alzheimer's disease. *Neurology* 43:13–20, 1993.
40. Guillard A, Chastang C: Maladie de Parkinson. Les facteurs de pronostic a long terme. *Rev Neurol* 134:341–354, 1978.
41. Marder K, Flood P, Cote L, Mayeux R: A pilot study of risk factors for dementia in Parkinson's disease. *Mov Disord* 5:156–161, 1990.
42. Marder K, Tang MX, Alfaro B, et al: Postmenopausal estrogen use and Parkinson's disease with and without dementia. *Neurology* 50:1141–1143, 1998.
43. Marder K, Tang MX, Alfaro B, et al: Risk of Alzheimer's disease in relatives of Parkinson's disease patients with and without dementia. *Neurology* 52:719–724, 1999.
44. Arai H, Muramatsu T, Higuchi S, et al: Apolipoprotein E gene in Parkinson's disease with or without dementia. *Lancet* 344:889, 1994.
45. Marder K, Maestre G, Cote L, et al: The apolipoprotein epsilon 4 allele in Parkinson's disease with and without dementia. *Neurology* 44:1330–1331, 1994.
46. Koller WC, Glatt SL, Hubble JP, et al: Apolipoprotein E genotypes in Parkinson's disease with and without dementia. *Ann Neurol* 37:242–245, 1995.

47. Inzelberg R, Chapman J, Treves TA, et al: Apolipoprotein E4 in Parkinson disease and dementia: new data and meta-analysis of published studies. *Alzheimer Dis Assoc Disord* 12:45–48, 1998.
48. Whitehead AS, Bertrandy S, Finnan F, et al: Frequency of the apolipoprotein E epsilon 4 allele in a case-control study of early onset Parkinson's disease. *J Neurol Neurosurg Psychiatry* 61:347–351, 1996.
49. Levy G, Tang MX, Cote LJ, et al: Do risk factors for Alzheimer's disease predict dementia in Parkinson's disease? An exploratory study. *Mov Disord.* 17:250–257, 2002.
50. Pirozzolo FJ, Hansch EC, Mortimer JA, et al: Dementia in Parkinson disease: A neuropsychological analysis. *Brain Cogn* 1:71–83, 1982.
51. Girotti F, Soliveri P, Carella F, et al: Dementia and cognitive impairment in Parkinson's disease. *J Neurol Neurosurg Psychiatry* 51:1498–1502, 1988.
52. Stern Y, Richards M, Sano M, Mayeux R: Comparison of cognitive changes in patients with Alzheimer's and Parkinson's disease. *Arch Neurol* 50:1040–1045, 1993.
53. Helkala EL, Laulumaa V, Soininen H, Riekkinen PJ: Recall and recognition memory in patients with Alzheimer's and Parkinson's diseases. *Ann Neurol* 24:214–217, 1988.
54. Taylor AE, Saint-Cyr JA, Lang AE: Memory and learning in early Parkinson's disease: Evidence for a "frontal lobe syndrome." *Brain Cogn* 13:211–232, 1990.
55. Hyman BT, Van Horsen GW, Damasio AR, Barnes CL: Alzheimer's disease: Cell-specific pathology isolates the hippocampal formation. *Science* 225:1168–1170, 1984.
56. Van Hoesen GW, Hyman BT, Damasio AR: Entorhinal cortex pathology in Alzheimer's disease. *Hippocampus* 1:1–8, 1991.
57. Braak H, Braak E: Evolution of the neuropathology of Alzheimer's disease. *Acta Neurol Scand Suppl* 165: 3–12, 1996.
58. Taylor AE, Saint-Cyr JA, Lang AE: Frontal lobe dysfunction in Parkinson's disease. The cortical focus of neostriatal outflow. *Brain* 109:845–883, 1986.
59. Bondi MW, Kaszniak AW, Bayles KA, Vance KT: Contributions of frontal system dysfunction to memory and perceptual abilities in Parkinson's disease. *Neuropsychology* 7:89–102, 1993.
60. Pillon B, Deweer B, Vidailhet M, et al: Is impaired memory for spatial location in Parkinson's disease domain specific or dependent on "strategic" processes? *Neuropsychologia* 36:1–9, 1998.
61. Stebbins GT, Gabrieli JD, Masciari F, et al: Delayed recognition memory in Parkinson's disease: A role for working memory? *Neuropsychologia* 37:503–510, 1999.
62. Gibb WR, Scott T, Lees AJ: Neuronal inclusions of Parkinson's disease. *Mov Disord* 6:2–11, 1991.
63. Jellinger K: New developments in the pathology of Parkinson's disease. *Adv Neurol* 53:1–16, 1990.
64. Hughes AJ, Daniel SE, Blankson S, Lees AJ: A clinicopathologic study of 100 cases of Parkinson's disease. *Arch Neurol* 50:140–148, 1993.
65. Duyckaerts C, Gaspar P, Costa C, et al: Dementia in Parkinson's disease. Morphometric data. *Adv Neurol* 60:447–455, 1993.
66. Rinne JO, Rummukainen J, Paljarvi L, Rinne UK: Dementia in Parkinson's disease is related to neuronal loss in the medial substantia nigra. *Ann Neurol* 26:47–50, 1989.
67. Paulus W, Jellinger K: The neuropathologic basis of different clinical subgroups of Parkinson's disease. *J Neuropathol Exp Neurol* 50:743–755, 1991.
68. Zweig RM, Cardillo JE, Cohen M, et al: The locus ceruleus and dementia in Parkinson's disease. *Neurology* 43:986–991, 1993.
69. Mann DM, Yates PO: Pathological basis for neurotransmitter changes in Parkinson's disease. *Neuropathol Appl Neurobiol* 9:3–19, 1983.
70. Cash R, Dennis T, L'Heureux R, et al: Parkinson's disease and dementia: Norepinephrine and dopamine in locus ceruleus. *Neurology* 37:42–46, 1987.
71. Gaspar P, Gray F: Dementia in idiopathic Parkinson's disease. A neuropathological study of 32 cases. *Acta Neuropathol* 64:43–52, 1984.
72. Nakano I, Hirano A: Parkinson's disease: Neuron loss in the nucleus basalis without concomitant Alzheimer's disease. *Ann Neurol* 15:415–418, 1984.
73. Tagliavini F, Pilleri G, Bouras C, Constantinidis J: The basal nucleus of Meynert in idiopathic Parkinson's disease. *Acta Neurol Scand* 70:20–28, 1984.
74. Whitehouse PJ, Hedreen JC, White CL III, Price DL: Basal forebrain neurons in the dementia of Parkinson disease. *Ann Neurol* 13:243–248, 1983.
75. Dubois B, Pillon B, Lhermitte F, Agid Y: Cholinergic deficiency and frontal dysfunction in Parkinson's disease. *Ann Neurol* 28:117–121, 1990.
76. Hakim AM, Mathieson G: Dementia in Parkinson disease: A neuropathologic study. *Neurology* 29:1209–1214, 1979.
77. Boller F, Mizutani T, Roessmann U, Gambetti P: Parkinson disease, dementia, and Alzheimer disease: Clinicopathological correlations. *Ann Neurol* 7:329–335, 1980.

78. Bancher C, Braak H, Fischer P, Jellinger KA: Neuropathological staging of Alzheimer lesions and intellectual status in Alzheimer's and Parkinson's disease patients. *Neurosci Lett* 162:179–182, 1993.
79. Kosaka K, Tsuchiya K, Yoshimura M: Lewy body disease with and without dementia: A clinicopathological study of 35 cases. *Clin Neuropathol* 7:299–305, 1988.
80. McKeith IG, Galasko D, Kosaka K, et al: Consensus guidelines for the clinical and pathologic diagnosis of dementia with Lewy bodies (DLB): Report of the consortium on DLB international workshop. *Neurology* 47:1113–1124, 1996.
81. Galvin JE, Lee VM, Trojanowski JQ: Synucleinopathies: Clinical and pathological implications. *Arch Neurol* 58:186–190, 2001.
82. Hurtig HI, Trojanowski JQ, Galvin J, et al: Alpha-synuclein cortical Lewy bodies correlate with dementia in Parkinson's disease. *Neurology* 54:1916–1921, 2000.
83. Mattila PM, Rinne JO, Helenius H, et al: Alpha-synuclein-immunoreactive cortical Lewy bodies are associated with cognitive impairment in Parkinson's disease. *Acta Neuropathol* 100:285–290, 2000.
84. Folstein SE: *Huntington's Disease. A Disorder of Families*. Baltimore: The Johns Hopkins University Press, 1989.
85. Rosenblatt A, Leroi I: Neuropsychiatry of Huntington's disease and other basal ganglia disorders. *Psychosomatics* 41:24–30, 2000.
86. De Marchi N, Mennella R: Huntington's disease and its association with psychopathology. *Harvard Rev Psychiatry* 7:278–289, 2000.
87. Harper PS: The epidemiology of Huntington's disease. *Hum Genet* 89:365–376, 1992.
88. Squitieri F, Andrew SE, Goldberg YP, et al: DNA haplotype analysis of Huntington disease reveals clues to the origins and mechanisms of CAG expansion and reasons for geographic variations of prevalence. *Hum Mol Genet* 3:2103–2114, 1994.
89. Gusella JF, Wexler NS, Conneally PM, et al: A polymorphic DNA marker genetically linked to Huntington's disease. *Nature* 306:234–238, 1983.
90. The Huntington's Disease Collaborative Research Group: A novel gene containing a trinucleotide repeat that is expanded and unstable on Huntington's disease chromosomes. *Cell* 72:971–983, 1993.
91. Albin RL, Tagle DA: Genetics and molecular biology of Huntington's disease. *Trends Neurosci* 18:11–14, 1995.
92. Brinkman RR, Mezei MM, Theilmann J, et al: The likelihood of being affected with Huntington disease by a particular age, for a specific CAG size. *Am J Hum Genet* 60:1202–1210, 1997.
93. The American College of Medical Genetics/American Society of Human Genetics Huntington Disease Genetic Testing Working Group: ACMG/ASHG statement. Laboratory guidelines for Huntington disease genetic testing. *Am J Hum Genet* 62:1243–1247, 1998.
94. Andrew SE, Goldberg YP, Kremer B, et al: The relationship between trinucleotide (CAG) repeat length and clinical features of Huntington's disease. *Nat Genet* 4:398–403, 1993.
95. Kremer B, Almqvist E, Theilmann J, et al: Sex-dependent mechanisms for expansions and contractions of the CAG repeat on affected Huntington disease chromosomes. *Am J Hum Genet* 57:343–350, 1995.
96. Rubinsztein DC, Leggo J, Chiano M, et al: Genotypes at the GluR6 kainate receptor locus are associated with variation in the age of onset of Huntington disease. *Proc Natl Acad Sci U S A* 94:3872–3876, 1997.
97. Sudarsky L, Myers RH, Walshe TM: Huntington's disease in monozygotic twins reared apart. *J Med Genet* 20:408–411, 1983.
98. Bird ED: The brain in Huntington's chorea. *Psychol Med* 8:357–360, 1978.
99. Brandt J, Strauss ME, Larus J, et al: Clinical correlates of dementia and disability in Huntington's disease. *J Clin Neuropsychol* 6:401–412, 1984.
100. Zakzanis KK: The subcortical dementia of Huntington's disease. *J Clin Exp Neuropsychol* 20:565–578, 1998.
101. Troster AI, Butters N, Salmon DP, et al: The diagnostic utility of savings scores: Differentiating Alzheimer's and Huntington's diseases with the logical memory and visual reproduction tests. *J Clin Exp Neuropsychol* 15:773–788, 1993.
102. Hahn-Barma V, Deweer B, Durr A, et al: Are cognitive changes the first symptoms of Huntington's disease? A study of gene carriers. *J Neurol Neurosurg Psychiatry* 64:172–177, 1998.
103. Kirkwood SC, Siemers E, Hodes ME, et al: Subtle changes among presymptomatic carriers of the Huntington's disease gene. *J Neurol Neurosurg Psychiatry* 69:773–779, 2000.
104. de Boo GM, Tibben AA, Hermans JA, et al: Memory and learning are not impaired in presymptomatic individuals with an increased risk of Huntington's disease. *J Clin Exp Neuropsychol* 21:831–836, 1999.
105. Campodonico JR, Codori AM, Brandt J: Neuropsychological stability over two years in asymptomatic carriers of the Huntington's disease mutation. *J Neurol Neurosurg Psychiatry* 61:621–624, 1996.

106. Paulsen JS, Zhao H, Stout JC, et al: Clinical markers of early disease in persons near onset of Huntington's disease. *Neurology* 57:658–662, 2001.
107. Vonsattel JP, Myers RH, Stevens TJ, et al: Neuropathological classification of Huntington's disease. *J Neuropathol Exp Neurol* 44:559–577, 1985.
108. Graveland GA, Williams RS, DiFiglia M: Evidence for degenerative and regenerative changes in neostriatal spiny neurons in Huntington's disease. *Science* 227:770–773, 1985.
109. Ferrante RJ, Kowall NW, Richardson EP Jr: Proliferative and degenerative changes in striatal spiny neurons in Huntington's disease: A combined study using the section-Golgi method and calbindin D28k immunocytochemistry. *J Neurosci* 11:3877–3887, 1991.
110. Ross CA: Intranuclear neuronal inclusions: A common pathogenic mechanism for glutamine-repeat neurodegenerative diseases? *Neuron* 19:1147–1150, 1997.
111. Subramony SH, Filla A: Autosomal dominant spinocerebellar ataxias ad infinitum? (letter; comment). *Neurology* 56:287–289, 2001.
112. Steele JC, Richardson JC, Olszweski J: Progressive supranuclear palsy. *Arch Neurol* 10:333–358, 1964.
113. Maher ER, Lees AJ: The clinical features and natural history of the Steele-Richardson-Olszewski syndrome (progressive supranuclear palsy). *Neurology* 36:1005–1008, 1986.
114. Litvan I, Agid Y, Jankovic J, et al: Accuracy of clinical criteria for the diagnosis of progressive supranuclear palsy (Steele-Richardson-Olszewski syndrome). *Neurology* 46:922–930, 1996.
115. Litvan I, Agid Y, Calne D, et al: Clinical research criteria for the diagnosis of progressive supranuclear palsy (Steele-Richardson-Olszewski syndrome): Report of the NINDS-SPSP international workshop. *Neurology* 47:1–9, 1996.
116. Daniel SE, de Bruin VM, Lees AJ: The clinical and pathological spectrum of Steele-Richardson-Olszewski syndrome (progressive supranuclear palsy): A reappraisal. *Brain* 118:759–770, 1995.
117. Golbe LI, Davis PH, Schoenberg BS, Duvoisin RC: Prevalence and natural history of progressive supranuclear palsy. *Neurology* 38:1031–1034, 1988.
118. Schrag A, Ben Shlomo Y, Quinn NP: Prevalence of progressive supranuclear palsy and multiple system atrophy: A cross-sectional study. *Lancet* 354:1771–1775, 1999.
119. Radhakrishnan K, Thacker AK, Maloo JC, et al: Descriptive epidemiology of some rare neurological diseases in Benghazi, Libya. *Neuroepidemiology* 7:159–164, 1988.
120. Rajput AH, Offord KP, Beard CM, Kurland LT: Epidemiology of parkinsonism: Incidence, classification, and mortality. *Ann Neurol* 16:278–282, 1984.
121. Bower JH, Maraganore DM, McDonnell SK, Rocca WA: Incidence of progressive supranuclear palsy and multiple system atrophy in Olmsted County, Minnesota, 1976 to 1990. *Neurology* 49:1284–1288, 1997.
122. Golbe LI: The epidemiology of progressive supranuclear palsy. *Adv Neurol* 69:25–31, 1996.
123. Kristensen MO: Progressive supranuclear palsy—20 years later. *Acta Neurol Scand* 71:177–189, 1985.
124. Litvan I, Mangone CA, Mckee A, et al: Natural history of progressive supranuclear palsy (Steele-Richardson-Olszewski syndrome) and clinical predictors of survival: A clinicopathological study. *J Neurol Neurosurg Psychiatry* 60:615–620, 1996.
125. Santacruz P, Uttl B, Litvan I, Grafman J: Progressive supranuclear palsy: A survey of the disease course. *Neurology* 50:1637–1647, 1998.
126. Pillon B, Dubois B, Ploska A, Agid Y: Severity and specificity of cognitive impairment in Alzheimer's, Huntington's, and Parkinson's diseases and progressive supranuclear palsy. *Neurology* 41:634–643, 1991.
127. Collins SJ, Ahlskog JE, Parisi JE, Maraganore DM: Progressive supranuclear palsy: Neuropathologically based diagnostic clinical criteria. *J Neurol Neurosurg Psychiatry* 58:167–173, 1995.
128. Robbins TW, James M, Owen AM, et al: Cognitive deficits in progressive supranuclear palsy, Parkinson's disease, and multiple system atrophy in tests sensitive to frontal lobe dysfunction. *J Neurol Neurosurg Psychiatry* 57:79–88, 1994.
129. Monza D, Soliveri P, Radice D, et al: Cognitive dysfunction and impaired organization of complex motility in degenerative parkinsonian syndromes. *Arch Neurol* 55:372–378, 1998.
130. Soliveri P, Monza D, Paridi D, et al: Neuropsychological follow-up in patients with Parkinson's disease, striatonigral degeneration-type multisystem atrophy, and progressive supranuclear palsy. *J Neurol Neurosurg Psychiatry* 69:313–318, 2000.
131. Albert ML, Feldman RG, Willis AL: The "subcortical dementia" of progressive supranuclear palsy. *J Neurol Neurosurg Psychiatry* 37:121–130, 1974.
132. Litvan I: Cognitive disturbances in progressive supranuclear palsy. *J Neural Transm Suppl* 42:69–78, 1994.
133. Dubois B, Pillon B, Legault F, et al: Slowing of cognitive processing in progressive supranuclear palsy. A comparison with Parkinson's disease. *Arch Neurol* 45:1194–1199, 1988.

134. Podoll K, Schwarz M, Noth J: Language functions in progressive supranuclear palsy. *Brain* 114:1457–1472, 1991.
135. Milberg W, Albert M: Cognitive differences between patients with progressive supranuclear palsy and Alzheimer's disease. *J Clin Exp Neuropsychol* 11:605–614, 1989.
136. Pillon B, Blin J, Vidailhet M, et al: The neuropsychological pattern of corticobasal degeneration: Comparison with progressive supranuclear palsy and Alzheimer's disease. *Neurology* 45:1477–1483, 1995.
137. Jellinger K, Riederer P, Tomonaga M: Progressive supranuclear palsy: Clinicopathological and biochemical studies. *J Neural Transm Suppl* 111–128, 1980.
138. Hauw JJ, Daniel SE, Dickson D, et al: Preliminary NINDS neuropathologic criteria for Steele-Richardson-Olszewski syndrome (progressive supranuclear palsy). *Neurology* 44:2015–2019, 1994.
139. Litvan I, Hauw JJ, Bartko JJ, et al: Validity and reliability of the preliminary NINDS neuropathologic criteria for progressive supranuclear palsy and related disorders. *J Neuropathol Exp Neurol* 55:97–105, 1996.
140. Hirsch EC, Graybiel AM, Duyckaerts C, Javoy-Agid F: Neuronal loss in the pedunculopontine tegmental nucleus in Parkinson disease and in progressive supranuclear palsy. *Proc Natl Acad Sci U S A* 84:5976–5980, 1987.
141. Zweig RM, Whitehouse PJ, Casanova MF, et al: Loss of pedunculopontine neurons in progressive supranuclear palsy. *Ann Neurol* 22:18–25, 1987.
142. Tagliavini F, Pilleri G, Gemignani F, Lechi A: Neuronal loss in the basal nucleus of Meynert in progressive supranuclear palsy. *Acta Neuropathol* 61:157–160, 1983.
143. Vermersch P, Robitaille Y, Bernier L, et al: Biochemical mapping of neurofibrillary degeneration in a case of progressive supranuclear palsy: Evidence for general cortical involvement. *Acta Neuropathol* 87:572–577, 1994.
144. Bergeron C, Pollanen MS, Weyer L, Lang AE: Cortical degeneration in progressive supranuclear palsy. A comparison with cortical-basal ganglionic degeneration. *J Neuropathol Exp Neurol* 56:726–734, 1997.
145. Morris HR, Lees AJ, Wood NW: Neurofibrillary tangle parkinsonian disorders—tau pathology and tau genetics. *Mov Disord* 14:731–736, 1999.
146. Conrad C, Andreadis A, Trojanowski JQ, et al: Genetic evidence for the involvement of tau in progressive supranuclear palsy. *Ann Neurol* 41:277–281, 1997.
147. Higgins JJ, Litvan I, Pho LT, et al: Progressive supranuclear gaze palsy is in linkage disequilibrium with the tau and not the alpha-synuclein gene. *Neurology* 50:270–273, 1998.
148. Higgins JJ, Golbe LI, De Biase A, et al: An extended 5′-tau susceptibility haplotype in progressive supranuclear palsy. *Neurology* 55:1364–1367, 2000.
149. Rebeiz JJ, Kolodny EH, Richardson EP Jr: Corticodentatonigral degeneration with neuronal achromasia: A progressive disorder of late adult life. *Trans Am Neurol Assoc* 92:23–26, 1967.
150. Rebeiz JJ, Kolodny EH, Richardson EP Jr: Corticodentatonigral degeneration with neuronal achromasia. *Arch Neurol* 18:20–33, 1968.
151. Kompoliti K, Goetz CG, Boeve BF, et al: Clinical presentation and pharmacological therapy in corticobasal degeneration. *Arch Neurol* 55:957–961, 1998.
152. Rinne JO, Lee MS, Thompson PD, Marsden CD: Corticobasal degeneration. A clinical study of 36 cases. *Brain* 117:1183–1196, 1994.
153. Litvan I, Agid Y, Goetz C, et al: Accuracy of the clinical diagnosis of corticobasal degeneration: a clinicopathologic study. *Neurology* 48:119–125, 1997.
154. Doody RS, Jankovic J: The alien hand and related signs. *J Neurol Neurosurg Psychiatry* 55:806–810, 1992.
155. Wenning GK, Litvan I, Jankovic J, et al: Natural history and survival of 14 patients with corticobasal degeneration confirmed at postmortem examination. *J Neurol Neurosurg Psychiatry* 64:184–189, 1998.
156. Brown J, Lantos PL, Roques P, et al: Familial dementia with swollen achromatic neurons and corticobasal inclusion bodies: a clinical and pathological study. *J Neurol Sci* 135:21–30, 1996.
157. Bergeron C, Pollanen MS, Weyer L, et al: Unusual clinical presentations of cortical-basal ganglionic degeneration. *Ann Neurol* 40:893–900, 1996.
158. Lang AE: Cortical basal ganglionic degeneration presenting with "progressive loss of speech output and orofacial dyspraxia." (letter; comment). *J Neurol Neurosurg Psychiatry* 55:1101, 1992.
159. Lippa CF, Cohen R, Smith TW, Drachman DA: Primary progressive aphasia with focal neuronal achromasia. *Neurology* 41:882–886, 1991.
160. Grimes DA, Lang AE, Bergeron CB: Dementia as the most common presentation of cortical-basal ganglionic degeneration. *Neurology* 53:1969–1974, 1999.
161. Massman PJ, Kreiter KT, Jankovic J, Doody RS: Neuropsychological functioning in cortical-basal ganglionic degeneration: Differentiation from Alzheimer's disease. *Neurology* 46:720–726, 1996.
162. Leiguarda R, Lees AJ, Merello M, et al: The nature of apraxia in corticobasal degeneration. *J Neurol Neurosurg Psychiatry* 57:455–459, 1994.

163. Feany MB, Mattiace LA, Dickson DW: Neuropathologic overlap of progressive supranuclear palsy, Pick's disease and corticobasal degeneration. *J Neuropathol Exp Neurol* 55:53–67, 1996.
164. Komori T, Arai N, Oda M, et al: Astrocytic plaques and tufts of abnormal fibers do not coexist in corticobasal degeneration and progressive supranuclear palsy. *Acta Neuropathol* 96:401–408, 1998.
165. Di Maria E, Tabaton M, Vigo T, et al: Corticobasal degeneration shares a common genetic background with progressive supranuclear palsy. *Ann Neurol* 47:374–377, 2000.
166. Houlden H, Baker M, Morris HR, et al: Corticobasal degeneration and progressive supranuclear palsy share a common tau haplotype. *Neurology* 56:1702–1706, 2001.
167. Wenning GK, Ben Shlomo Y, Magalhaes M, et al: Clinical features and natural history of multiple system atrophy. An analysis of 100 cases. *Brain* 117:835–845, 1994.
168. Wenning GK, Ben Shlomo Y, Hughes A, et al: What clinical features are most useful to distinguish definite multiple system atrophy from Parkinson's disease? *J Neurol Neurosurg Psychiatry* 68:434–440, 2000.
169. Wenning GK, Tison F, Ben Shlomo Y, et al: Multiple system atrophy: A review of 203 pathologically proven cases. *Mov Disord* 12:133–147, 1997.
170. Ben Shlomo Y, Wenning GK, Tison F, Quinn NP: Survival of patients with pathologically proven multiple system atrophy: a meta-analysis. *Neurology* 48:384–393, 1997.
171. Robbins TW, James M, Lange KW, et al: Cognitive performance in multiple system atrophy. *Brain* 115 Pt 1:271–291, 1992.
172. Testa D, Fetoni V, Soliveri P, et al: Cognitive and motor performance in multiple system atrophy and Parkinson's disease compared. *Neuropsychologia* 31:207–210, 1993.
173. Pillon B, Gouider-Khouja N, Deweer B, et al: Neuropsychological pattern of striatonigral degeneration: comparison with Parkinson's disease and progressive supranuclear palsy. *J Neurol Neurosurg Psychiatry* 58:174–179, 1995.
174. Jaros E, Burn DJ: The pathogenesis of multiple system atrophy: past, present, and future. *Mov Disord* 15:784–788, 2000.
175. Storey E, Forrest SM, Shaw JH, et al: Spinocerebellar ataxia type 2: Clinical features of a pedigree displaying prominent frontal-executive dysfunction. *Arch Neurol* 56:43–50, 1999.
176. Maruff P, Tyler P, Burt T, et al: Cognitive deficits in Machado-Joseph disease. *Ann Neurol* 40:421–427, 1996.
177. Gambardella A, Annesi G, Bono F, et al: CAG repeat length and clinical features in three Italian families with spinocerebellar ataxia type 2 (SCA2): Early impairment of Wisconsin Card Sorting Test and saccade velocity. *J Neurol* 245:647–652, 1998.

Chapter 49

VASCULAR DEMENTIA

John V. Bowler
Vladimir Hachinski

Over the past century, our concept of vascular dementia has evolved remarkably. It has developed from a poorly described condition, confused first with neurosyphilis and more recently with Alzheimer's disease, to the position of being recognized as the second commonest cause of dementia. However, it has not yet reached clinical maturity, as there are several fundamental problems regarding its diagnosis and classification. These include but are not limited to problems relating to the following:

1. Vascular dementia is not a single condition but has several etiologies, the clinical features and treatments of which may differ.
2. The current definition is based on Alzheimer's disease, requiring prominent memory loss, and may be inappropriate.
3. The level of cognitive impairment required for dementia is too severe and will prevent identification of early cases.
4. Major stroke is included.
5. Intracerebral and subarachnoid hemorrhage are included.
6. The role of leukoaraiosis is problematic.
7. The volumes and sites of infarction that are consistent with dementia require definition.

The current uncertainty profoundly limits the observations that can be made regarding the behavioural and psychological aspects of vascular dementia; interpretation of the data that do exist must be done in the context of these uncertainties, which are reviewed below.

CRITERIA FOR VASCULAR DEMENTIA

Because Alzheimer's disease (AD) was recognized as the commonest cause of dementia in western society, the criteria used to define dementia[1,2] were based on AD. Thus the prominent features of dementia have come to include early and prominent memory loss, progression, irreversibility, and a level of cognitive impairment sufficient to affect normal daily activities. Rather than using specific criteria for vascular dementia, it has been traditional to identify dementia according to AD-based criteria and then to separate AD from vascular dementia using clinical features thought to reflect vascular risk factors, vascular events, and the manifestations of systemic and cerebral vascular disease. These elements are often operationalized using the ischemic score.[3–6] Thus, for historical reasons, the criteria for vascular dementia have come to emphasize memory loss and the progression and irreversibility of cognitive decline. None of these necessarily apply in cognitive decline due to cerebrovascular disease.[7,8] Furthermore, patients cannot be diagnosed as demented until they have developed impairment in normal day-to-day activities—a degree of severity that will prevent treatment until it is too late.

The available criteria for the diagnosis of vascular dementia fall into two groups. The first of these are the criteria contained in general diagnostic tools—i.e., the fourth edition of the *Diagnostic and Statistical Manual of Mental Disorders* (DSM-IV)[2] and the tenth revision of the *International Classification of Diseases* (ICD-10).[1] Both are very general in nature and do not operationalize their criteria. The second group, the criteria, those of the State of California Alzheimer Disease Diagnostic and Treatment Centers[9] and the criteria of the National Institute of Neurological Disorders and Stroke and the Association Internationale pour la Recherche at L'Enseignement en Neurosciences (NINDS-AIREN)[6] are developments of the first two and attempt to operationalize the criteria.

The Criteria of the State of California Alzheimer Disease Diagnostic and Treatment Centers

These criteria are given in Table 49-1.[9] Hemorrhagic and anoxic lesions are not included. The number and type of cognitive defects are deliberately not specified but are not confined to a single narrow category, and memory loss is not emphasized. The severity should be sufficient to interfere with the conduct of the patient's customary affairs of life, and this judgment is to be made on clinical criteria—not by neuropsychological testing. Two or more ischemic strokes, by history and examination or imaging, are required, though rarely one stroke with a clear temporal relationship to the onset of dementia may be allowed. Unlike most of the other criteria, these criteria do not require a clear temporal relationship between infarcts and dementia except where a single infarct is the alleged cause of the dementia. The reason for this is that vascular dementia may progress gradually, without a clear-cut association between events and cognitive decline, such that establishing a temporal relationship can be difficult. These points are valid, but the criteria risk is in diagnosing all cases of dementia with two or more infarcts as vascular dementia.

NINDS-AIREN Criteria

The NINDS-AIREN criteria[6] define dementia according to the ICD-10, requiring impaired functioning in daily living and a decline in memory and at least two other domains. The memory deficits may be less severe than in Alzheimer disease and a diagnosis of vascular dementia is made uncertain or unlikely by the presence of early-onset memory deficit and progressive worsening of memory without corresponding focal lesions. A temporal association between stroke and onset of dementia is required and is arbitrarily set at 3 months. An abrupt deterioration in cognition or a stepwise progression of dementia is acceptable if the 3-month criterion is not met. Neuroimaging is required as the absence of a vascular lesion on magnetic resonance imaging (MRI) or computed tomography (CT) excludes the possibility of vascular dementia, but there are no criteria regarding lesion volume. A single lesion is acceptable. Specific recommendations regarding the sites of lesions and the minimum amount of white matter disease are given in Table 49-2. The recommendations regarding white matter changes should be treated with caution, as the correlation between white matter changes on MRI and cognition is extremely weak.[10] Correlation of the MRI or CT changes with the clinical picture is required on the grounds that there are no pathognomonic CT or MRI correlates of vascular dementia. Hemorrhagic lesions are permitted.

These elements are synthesized by requiring evidence of (1) dementia, (2) vascular disease, and (3) an association between the two, without evidence of any other cause, for a diagnosis of probable vascular dementia to be made. A diagnosis of possible vascular dementia is made if (1) there are no neuroimaging data but there is clinical evidence of cerebrovascular disease, (2) in the absence of a clear temporal relationship between dementia and stroke, or (3) in those patients with a subtle onset and variable course. Definite vascular dementia is diagnosed if probable dementia exists, it is accompanied by histopathologic evidence of cerebrovascular disease, and there is no histopathologic evidence of other possible causes of the cognitive loss. Mixed dementia is not recognized, but the coexistence of vascular dementia with AD is termed AD with cerebrovascular disease.

Limitations

While these criteria are the only operational criteria available, it is important to realize that they are based on supposition and not on fact. The NINDS-AIREN criteria were also developed with a view to epidemiologic convenience rather than clinical accuracy. They are at fault in several fundamental respects; the reader is therefore encouraged to review them critically and use them cautiously.

Pattern of Cognitive Deficit in Vascular Dementia The adoption of criteria from AD, in which the mesial temporal lobes are affected early and prominently, is erroneous, as the mesial temporal lobes are not especially involved in cerebrovascular disease. The available data show that executive, subcortical, and frontal lobe functions are affected at least as prominently as memory.[11–27] Thus a diagnostic paradigm based on early memory loss is

Table 49-1

Criteria for Alzheimer's disease from the State of California Alzheimer Disease Diagnostic and Treatment Centers

I. Dementia

Dementia is a deterioration from a known or estimated prior level of intellectual function sufficient to interfere broadly with the conduct of the patient's customary affairs of life, which is not isolated to a single narrow category of intellectual performance, and which is independent of level of consciousness.

This deterioration should be supported by historical evidence and documented by either bedside mental status testing or ideally by more detailed neuropsychological examination, using tests that are quantifiable, reproducible, and for which normative data are available.

II. Probable IVD

A. The criteria for the clinical diagnosis of "probable ischemic vascular dementia (IVD)" include *all* of the following:

1. Dementia
2. Evidence of two or more ischemic strokes by history, neurologic signs, and/or neuroimaging studies (CT or T1-weighted MRI) or occurrence of a single stroke with a clearly documented temporal relationship to the onset of dementia
3. Evidence of at least one infarct outside the cerebellum by CT or T1-weighted MRI

B. The diagnosis of "probable IVD" is supported by

1. Evidence of multiple infarcts in brain regions known to affect cognition
2. A history of multiple transient ischemic attacks
3. History of vascular risk factors (e.g., hypertension, heart disease, diabetes mellitus)
4. Elevated score on the Hachinski Ischemic Scale (original or modified version)

C. Clinical features that are thought to be associated with IVD but await further research include

1. Relatively early appearance of gait disturbance and urinary incontinence
2. Periventricular and deep white matter changes on T2-weighted MRI that are excessive for age
3. Focal changes in electrophysiologic studies (e.g., EEG, evoked potentials) or physiologic neuroimaging studies (e.g., SPECT, PET, NMR, spectroscopy)

D. Other clinical features that do not constitute strong evidence either for or against a diagnosis of "probable IVD" include

1. Periods of slowly progressive symptoms
2. Illusions, psychosis, hallucinations, delusions
3. Seizures

E. Clinical features that cast doubt on a diagnosis of "probable IVD" include

1. Transcortical sensory aphasia in the absence of corresponding focal lesions on neuroimaging studies
2. Absence of central neurologic symptoms/signs, other than cognitive disturbance
3. Possible IVD

A clinical diagnosis of "possible IVD" may be made when there is

a. Dementia

and one or more of the following:

b. A history or evidence of a single stroke (but not multiple strokes) without a clearly documented temporal relationship to the onset of dementia

or

c. Binswanger's syndrome (without multiple strokes) that includes all of the following:

1. Early onset urinary incontinence not explained by urologic disease, or gait disturbance (e.g., parkinsonian, magnetic, apraxic, or "senile" gait) not explained by peripheral cause
2. Vascular risk factors
3. Extensive white matter changes on neuroimaging
4. Definite IVD

A diagnosis of "definite IVD" requires histopathologic examination of the brain as well as

A. Clinical evidence of dementia*

B. Pathologic confirmation of multiple infarcts, some outside the cerebellum

5. Mixed dementia

A diagnosis of "mixed dementia" should be made in the presence of one or more other systemic or brain disorders that are thought to be causally related to the dementia.

The degree of confidence in the diagnosis of IVD should be specified as possible, probable, or definite, and the other disorder(s) contributing to the dementia should be listed. For example: "Mixed dementia due to probable IVD and possible Alzheimer's disease or mixed dementia due to definite IVD and hypothyroidism."

6. Research classification

Classification of IVD for research purposes should specify features of the infarcts that may differentiate subtypes of the disorder, such as

Location: cortical, white matter, periventricular, basal ganglia, thalamus

Size: volume

Distribution: large, small, or microvessel

Severity: chronic ischemia versus infarction

Etiology: embolism, atherosclerosis, arteriosclerosis, cerebral amyloid angiopathy, hypoperfusion.

Source: From Chui et al.,[9] with permission.

Note: If there is evidence of Alzheimer's disease or some other pathologic disorder that is thought to have contributed to the dementia, a diagnosis of *mixed* dementia should be made.

Table 49-2
Radiologic Features Considered Compatible with Vascular Dementia by the NINDS-AIREN Criteria

1. Site
   A. Large-vessel strokes in the following territories:
      a. Bilateral anterior cerebral artery
      b. Posterior cerebral artery
      c. Parietotemporal and temporooccipital association areas
      d. Superior frontal and parietal watershed territories
   B. Small vessel disease:
      a. Basal ganglia and frontal white matter lacunes
      b. Extensive periventricular white matter lesions
      c. Bilateral thalamic lesions
2. Severity
   a. Large vessel lesions of the dominant hemisphere
   b. Bilateral large vessel hemispheric strokes
   c. Leukoencephalopathy involving at least 25% of the total white matter

Source: From Roman et al.,[6] with permission.

inappropriate and will fail to identify many cases of vascular dementia. New paradigms are required that give greater emphasis to more appropriate domains and that remove emphasis from memory. Such tests as the EXIT25, CLOX,[28,29] and a modification of the ADAS-Cog termed VaDAS-Cog may all represent appropriate steps in this direction.[30,31]

Severity of Dementia Current criteria define dementia on the basis of a clear loss of cognitive function. This will deny early cases the most appropriate opportunity for secondary preventive measures by failing to be detected.[8,32–35] Early cases need to be identified. There is now some evidence to suggest that the very first manifestation of leukoaraiosis—vascular cognitive impairment—may be symptoms[36] rather than signs or measureable cognitive deficits.

Infarct Volume That an infarct volume of 50 to 100 cm^3 distinguished between vascular dementia and "senile dementia" was suggested in early work.[37] However, these data were based on highly selected cases. Dementia can exist with much smaller infarct volumes[7,38–41] and cognitive impairment short of dementia can be seen with very small infarct volumes.[24,42] Correlation between infarct volume and neuropsychological deficit is poor when all etiologies of vascular dementia are studied together.[23,41,43,44] This is not surprising, as site is at least as important as size. It is therefore unlikely that there is a precise volume of infarction other than at meaninglessly large volumes that can reliably predict vascular dementia. The current criteria are not, in any case, concerned with infarct volumes but concentrate on numbers of infarcts. This might, fortuitously, be more appropriate as in subcortical regions, where a count of the number of infarcts correlates more closely with cognitive loss than infarct volume.[24] However, infarcts by themselves are found in less than 50 percent of cases of established vascular dementia[45,46] and the presence of infarcts is therefore not essential for that diagnosis to be made. Indeed, there is good evidence that microvascular disease is crucial in the development of dementia in many cases.[47] If this is the case, there will be a further weakening of the correlation between infarct volume and cognitive status.

Infarct Site Infarct site is crucial,[48] but such data as exist are inconsistent because of variability in the study populations and protocols. The following sites are putatively important in the production of cognitive loss: bilateral,[38,40,49] left-sided,[22,40,41,50] thalamic,[49] anterior cerebral,[22] and frontal lesions.[27] Some work favors a special role for "lacunar" and other deep lesions over cortical lesions,[7,50–53] but other work does not.[22,39–41] Fisher felt that dementia in association with lacunes was rare[54] but cognitive impairment in association with small numbers and volumes of subcortical infarcts was readily detectable.[24,55]

Multiple Types of Vascular Dementia The term *vascular dementia* describes dementia due to cerebrovascular disease in general[56] and has replaced *multi-infarct dementia,* as multiple infarcts are not the only etiology. All of the current criteria largely treat vascular dementia as a single condition. This is an important error, since vascular lesions capable of causing cognitive loss arise from many different etiologies, and differing causes require different treatments. In addition, events falling short of stroke may be relevant. Episodes of hypotension, leukoaraiosis, and incomplete infarction are all associated with cognitive impairment and all have some vascular basis but do not necessarily cause or consist of infarcts.[19,25,26,57–66] The movement away from multi-infarct dementia has now reached the point where subcortical vascular dementia is now increasingly recognized as the most common single variety of vascular dementia, and this is based on leukoaraiosis and lacunar infarcts with no requirement for cortical lesions. Criteria have been proposed for this entity,[67] although they have not yet been validated.

The most important aspect of vascular dementia must always be the treatment and prevention of disease. Prevention, in particular, will depend on etiology, and it is important that this be specified routinely in each case. Current practice does not emphasize this.[8,32–35]

Leukoaraiosis Leukoaraiosis seen on CT impairs cognition.[55,59,63,66,68,69] Leukoaraiosis demonstrated on MRI has a weaker association with cognitive loss. Some studies have found a correlation between neuropsychological deficits and the extent of leukoaraiosis,[19,25,26,58,61,62,64,65] but in others the correlation becomes insignificant after correction for age.[70,71] Other studies have been negative[72–75] but may have been negative for methodologic reasons, including the use of insensitive tests of cognition,[74] the summarizing of data from several neuropsychological tests together in a way that may mask changes in a few positive tests,[70] too little disease,[73] too few cases,[74] and the use of a simple dichotomy between demented and nondemented.[72,75] In early vascular dementia there is a weak association between leukoaraiosis and cognitive loss[42]; a large population study has produced clear evidence of an association between leukoaraiosis and impaired cognition.[76] Overall, it seems the evidence shows that leukoaraiosis of relatively minor degree can affect cognition but that the effects can be very subtle.

Subcortical Vascular Dementia (Binswanger's Disease) Interest in Binswanger's disease was stimulated during the 1980s by numerous reports of Binswanger disease diagnosed by MRI. However, Binswanger's disease is a clinical syndrome and cannot be diagnosed by MRI alone; extensive leukoaraiosis on MRI without clinical correlates is not Binswanger's disease. Furthermore, there have always been doubts as to the nosology of Binswanger's disease.[77–79] With the increasing recognition that subcortical vascular dementia may be the most common and most homogeneous of the vascular dementias, *Binswanger's disease* is becoming a redundant term and is now to be considered as no more than an well-advanced form of subcortical vascular dementia. Diagnostic criteria for Binswanger's disease have been published.[80]

The clinical picture is typically that of a patient slightly more often male than female in the sixth or seventh decade. A history of hypertension is present in 80 percent or more, and it is often poorly controlled. Other risk factors for vascular disease, especially diabetes, are often present.[78,81] Dementia is variable and not necessarily the presenting symptom. It evolves over 3 to 10 years and is intermittently progressive but may become gradually progressive without further clear-cut vascular events. Aphasia, amnestic intervals, and neglect are seen in some cases. Memory loss is not prominent.[82] Dysarthria, focal motor signs, and a gait disturbance—with features of spasticity, parkinsonism, and ataxia[83]—evolve during the illness and may appear relatively early. Incontinence develops later but may occur while cognition is still at least grossly intact.[82,84] The dysarthria is part of a pseudobulbar palsy, and while both are variable in degree, they are nearly universally present.[82] Dizziness, faints, and, less commonly, epilepsy also occur.[77] A history of stroke at some stage is almost universal, but exceptions occur and rarely focal signs may be absent even late in the disease.[85] Behavioral changes are early and prominent and may be the presenting feature. Some patients exhibit an early manic phase, but in most progressively increasing abulia develops later in the illness.[82] Depression is common[80] and mood disturbances are seen.[84] Diagnostic criteria for clinical trials in subcortical vascular dementia have also been proposed[67] but not yet validated.

Atrophy Atrophy is largely ignored in the current criteria but is often assumed to be due to degenerative dementia and its presence is sometimes used as an argument against a patient having vascular dementia.[86] However, increasing evidence suggests that atrophy is a common feature in cerebrovascular disease even where this is limited to leukoaraiosis. The process may begin with risk factors alone, without definite vascular events, which are associated with both a relative increase in lateral ventricle volume, suggesting central atrophy,[87] and cognitive decline.[88–90] In other words, cognitive impairment may correlate more closely with ventricular enlargement than it does with infarct volume, and this trend is continued in more fully established cerebrovascular disease.[24,42,91] Similar findings have been reported in multiple sclerosis, a condition that can be regarded as closely analogous to subcortical vascular dementia.[92] Atrophy may progress at the same rate in vascular dementia, Alzheimer's disease, and Lewy body dementia.[93] Atrophy may therefore be associated with both vascular disease and degenerative dementia rather than just being a hallmark of degenerative dementia, as previously supposed.

Inclusion of Major Stroke Whether major stroke should be included within vascular dementia largely depends on the purpose of the study in question. Major stroke—identified by the production of substantial motor, sensory, visual, or language deficits—comprises a group of conditions for which the epidemiology, risk factors, primary and secondary preventative therapy, and prognoses are relatively well established. If the purpose of defining vascular dementia is to identify a group of conditions for which there may be special risk factors, perhaps different from stroke in general, for which patients may benefit from appropriate preventative therapy, then the inclusion of patients with major stroke is inappropriate. Alternatively, if, for example, the purpose is to describe the economic burden of cognitive decline due to stroke, a more inclusive approach is necessary. All of the current criteria implicitly or explicitly include major stroke. We would recommend that studies should explicitly state whether or not major stroke is included and present, or make their data available in such a way that they can be analyzed with or without the contribution from major stroke.

Inclusion of Subarachnoid and Intracerebral Hemorrhage The inclusion or exclusion of intracerebral and subarachnoid haemorrhage within VCI is a matter of opinion and, like the inclusion of major stroke, will vary in appropriateness according to the purpose of the study in question. Once again, the solution is to state clearly whether such cases have been included or excluded and to tabulate, or to make available to others, the data with and without these cases so that others may interpret the data as necessary.

Inclusion of Poststroke Dementia Over one-quarter of patients admitted with stroke become demented,[20,50] but much of this is due to coexistent degenerative dementia, either preexistent or developed subsequently.[94–97] Most of these cases therefore fall outside of pure vascular dementia and might best be considered as mixed dementia unless there is a high level of confidence that only cerebrovascular disease is present.

Mixed Dementia The recognition of the coexistence of vascular dementia with degenerative dementia, particularly Alzheimer's disease, is a new development. Mixed dementia may account for between 18 and almost 50 percent of all dementia and may be more common than any other single group.[44,98–102] In one autopsy-based series based on a dementia clinic, none of 87 patients had pure vascular dementia, while 32 had mixed disease.[103] Furthermore, the interaction between the vascular component and other components more than doubles the rate of progression when compared to pure Alzheimer's disease alone.[99,104] Thus mixed dementia is far more important than was realized when the current criteria were prepared and poses a major problem in that no good method yet exists for identifying mixed dementia in life. Criteria that first select Alzheimer-like cases and then subselect those with vascular features might form an excellent basis for doing so; unfortunately this is precisely what the current criteria for vascular dementia do, and it is very likely that much of the reported data about vascular dementia are in fact about mixed disease, albeit not yet recognized as such.

A Solution—Vascular Cognitive Impairment

Given the limitations of the current criteria, progress in this field would best be served by moving away from vascular dementia toward a new concept. This concept should be broader, including not only those now described as vascular dementia, but also those with early cognitive changes, regardless of whether memory was primarily affected or not. To encompass this concept, vascular cognitive impairment (VCI)[34] has been proposed. It is imperative that VCI be characterized prospectively and on the basis of fact, not preconception, to avoid the misconceptions contained within the current criteria for vascular dementia. This will require wholesale revision of the current criteria; indeed, it would probably be best to start again rather than to attempt to revise fatally flawed criteria.[105–107]

The identification of patients with VCI will lead to the identification of risk factors for VCI. These will differ between different etiologies but would allow the identification of presymptomatic subjects, a stage termed *brain at risk*.[34] VCI and brain-at-risk are the most appropriate stages for early secondary and primary preventative therapy respectively.

Formal criteria have not yet been proposed for VCI because insufficient data exist as yet. More data are needed about the functional, neuropsychological, and imaging changes in each of the etiologic subgroups of VCI before this can be done. At present it is essential to gather cognitive, imaging, and risk-factor data on patients with cerebrovascular disease, beginning from those with known risk factors but without MRI, functional or cognitive changes, through to those with several minor strokes and clear cognitive and functional deficits who might meet current criteria for vascular dementia. Data from such populations can then be analysed to produce objective criteria, rather than the dogmatic criteria currently on offer. One of the most important steps in the development of the concept of VCI is the determination to acknowledge our own ignorance and not to create criteria not supported by data. Successful development of this concept offers the prospect of prevention or significant amelioration of the second commonest cause of dementia, something that the current criteria cannot. For this reason VCI offers the best way forward in this important field.

THE MECHANISM OF COGNITIVE IMPAIRMENT IN CEREBROVASCULAR DISEASE

Lesions interact synergistically in impairing cognition.[108,109] Neural nets may explain this as they provide scope for recovery after lesions, but as lesions' numbers increase the scope for recovery decreases; the net sequelae of each successive lesion thus increasing. Neural nets also give clues to the likely order of cognitive decline produced by multiple lesions, suggesting that frontal involvement may be the most prominent.[16,110] Evidence of prominent frontal system involvement following multiple lacunar infarction supports this.[16] Memory, which also depends on an extensive neural net,[110] may also be affected relatively early but not most prominently. The predicted recovery is also evident in that subcortical processes are commonly affected by stroke, and these processes can show considerable improvement,[23] an observation consistent with disturbance of an underlying, complex, and flexible network[110] capable of rerouting to bypass damaged signal pathways. Where the basis of vascular dementia was a single lesion or a few large ones, this would not hold and the pattern of cognitive loss would be closely linked to the site of the lesion. Even so, patients with right-sided lesions exhibit impairment in verbal IQ and patients with left-sided lesions exhibit impairment in performance IQ,[18] clearly showing the importance of generalized cognitive processing, presumably based on neural nets, as opposed to the more traditional localization of function. Support for a role for neural nets in global cognitive decline after stroke also comes from factorial analyses of neuropsychological deficits after stroke. These show that a relatively small number of factors,[43,111,112] distinct from the traditionally recognized cognitive domains, may form a mechanism by which dementia could occur based on multiple infarcts. These factors may reflect neural nets. Further support comes from emission tomography that shows extensive diaschisis, extending to the contralateral hemisphere, after a variety of lesions.[51,113–116] While there is doubt about whether these changes are causative or simply consequences,[117–119] they do reflect functional disconnection and so might indicate the more important projections of the affected neural nets.

NEUROPSYCHOLOGICAL ASPECTS OF VASCULAR DEMENTIA AND ALZHEIMER DISEASE CONTRASTED

In comparing these two conditions, selection bias almost certainly affects the published data. Many studies report data from patients seen in memory clinics. Between 1992 and 1995, only 1 of 136 new cases seen by us in a memory clinic had vascular dementia while 43 percent had AD (Bowler and Hachinski, unpublished observations). Historically, in the same clinic, cases of vascular dementia were equally rare, amounting to only 4.6 percent. Conversely, the Canadian Study of Health and Aging,[120] which is a population-based study, established that vascular dementia was responsible for 29 percent of all dementia. Furthermore, in 100 consecutive referrals to the vascular clinic, we found that 25 percent were cognitively impaired and 10 percent demented (Bowler and Hachinski, unpublished observations) according to Folstein Mini-Mental State Examination[121] using cutoffs of 26 and 24 respectively. These discrepancies suggest that cases of vascular dementia detected in memory clinics, as opposed to those detected in population surveys or vascular clinics, represent a subset of all cases of vascular dementia. We speculate that this is a subgroup in which the presentation mimics AD unusually closely, or which have mixed disease.

Methodologic differences also make comparisons of the two conditions difficult. Many studies identifying differences between AD and vascular dementia have not matched their cases for severity. In one series language and orientation were worse in vascular dementia,[122] but the patients with vascular dementia were globally worse than those with AD. Other series[11–13] reported extensive neuropsychological differences between AD and vascular dementia, but in this work the AD patients were globally much more impaired than those with vascular disease, which could explain all the differences. Greater difficulty in accessing the lexicon in AD compared to greater difficulty with syntax in vascular dementia has been reported,[123] but in this series the patients with vascular dementia were 10 years younger than those with AD and there is no mention of, or correction for, education, occupation, or overall level of cognition.

In studies in which the cases are matched for severity, differences between AD and vascular dementia are typically sparse or nonexistent except that aspects of memory are often more severely impaired in AD,[21,124–128] although others have found no difference.[129–134] Shuttleworth and Huber[130] found that only picture absurdities, which were worse in AD,[130] distinguished early AD and early vascular dementia, while visual memory, Raven matrices, geographic orientation, and copying of figures were not different. Patients with vascular dementia have better recognition memory for faces and famous faces than those with AD but are not better at block design and line orientation.[135] Erkinjuntti also found little neuropsychological difference between AD and vascular dementia.[131,132] In his series, motor functions, reading, and writing were worse in the vascular cases while most cognitive functions, including memory, did not differ between the two groups. Fischer et al. also found no differences in semantic memory.[133] Several aspects of language may be relatively more impaired in AD,[127,136] including understanding temporal relationships and complex grammatical structures, repetition of sentences and stories, and word span,[127,136,137] while mechanical problems may be greater in vascular dementia.[137] Functions thought to have frontal or subcortical components—including motor performance, picture arrangement, writing, object assembly, and block design—are more severely affected in vascular dementia,[127] findings largely supported in other work in which patients with AD were better on measures of attention, executive function, self-regulation, and fine motor control while those with vascular dementia were better oriented and had better recall and language.[21]

BEHAVIORAL CHANGES IN VASCULAR DEMENTIA

The study of behavioral changes in vascular dementia has been impaired by the use of behavioral changes in some criteria used for vascular dementia. The International Classification of Diseases[1] specifically suggests that personality is relatively well preserved but allows that personality changes may occur in some cases with features of apathy, disinhibition, or accentuation of previous traits such as egocentricity, paranoid attitudes, or irritability. The ischemic score,[4] which is often used to help identify vascular dementia, includes several behavioral items. The NINDS-AIREN criteria for vascular dementia[6] attaches significance to incontinence, mood (particularly depression), and personality changes. Data obtained using any of these criteria cannot properly be used to determine the behavioral changes seen in vascular dementia because of the selection of cases for the very features under investigation and the consequent inevitable tautology.

Only incontinence, among various behavioral changes, distinguished demented from nondemented stroke patients,[7] while in lacunar infarcts, behavioral changes may be more prominent than intellectual differences,[39] suggesting that behavioral changes may be important in identifying vascular dementia. Comparison of patients with lacunar infarcts with controls without infarcts suggests that depression, apathy, and perseveration[16] are associated with lacunar infarcts.

In a comparison of AD and vascular dementia, delusions were not more common in AD than in vascular dementia,[138] occurring in about half of all cases in each condition. Hallucinations occur only rarely in both conditions. Severe depression occurs in up to 25 percent of patients with vascular dementia, while depression of any severity occurs in about 60 percent of such individuals. The comparative incidence of depression in vascular dementia as compared to AD lies between $2^1/_2$ and 8,[138–140] and anxiety is twice as common.[140] A further comparative study of AD and vascular dementia, which used patients with dementia of moderate severity, found that distractibility, perplexity, disorientation, speech defects, and long-term memory[141] were worse in the AD group, while there were no differences between the two groups on 10 other measures of behavioral disturbance.

A comparative study of AD and vascular dementia confirmed the differences outlined above but also rated leukoaraiosis on a four-point scale and included this as a covariant in the analysis. The differences between the two groups appeared to be accounted for by the leukoaraiosis with respect to decreased affect and withdrawal, but leukoaraiosis did not account for psychomotor slowing.[142] It should be noted, however, that there were only 36 patients with vascular dementia, and 21 of these were thought to have mixed disease, which will have reduced differences between the groups. Furthermore, the patients came from an Alzheimer center and were identified using NINCDS/ADRDA and ADDTC criteria. These factors are likely to have biased the study population in favor of AD and mixed disease. Depression is also associated with frontal leukoaraiosis in particular as opposed to periventricular or basal ganglia disease.[143]

THE EPIDEMIOLOGY OF VASCULAR DEMENTIA

Dementia from all causes affects about 8 percent of the population over the age of 65; between 9 and 43 percent are of vascular origin and many additional cases are of mixed origin, such that mixed dementia may be the single commonest form.[44,98–102,144,145] The prevalence of vascular dementia varies considerably, from 0 to 2 percent in the 60-to-69 age group to up to 16 percent for males aged 80 to 89, though more typical figures are between 3 and 6 percent.[146–148] As a proportion of cases of dementia, one study in men and women aged 60 to 79 suggested figures of 13.6 and 12 percent respectively, falling to 4.8 and 7 percent at age 80 to 89.[146] More recent work generally produces higher figures.[148] One study suggested that vascular dementia accounted for 47 percent of dementia cases in 85-year-olds and that the overall prevalence of vascular dementia was 14 percent at that age.[149] Males are more commonly affected than females in most but not all studies.[51,145,146,150] Vascular dementia accounts for half of dementia in Japan.[147,151] After stroke, the incidence of dementia may be as high as 26 percent,[20,50] though exclusion of possible preexisting cases of AD reduces this to 16.3 percent,[20,22] and blacks may be at greater risk than whites.[20] The risk increases with age, from 14.8 percent in those aged 60 to 69 to 52.3 percent for those over 80, but 36.4 percent of these individuals were felt to have both AD and the sequelae of stroke.[20]

RISK FACTORS FOR VASCULAR DEMENTIA

The risk of developing vascular dementia begins in midlife. The Honolulu-Asia aging study has now shown that midlife systolic hypertension is associated with impairment of cognition in later life independent of stroke.[89]

Other data on risk factors is, to some extent, contradictory because of differences in the populations studied and the definitions used. There is increasing evidence that the risk factors that affect cognition do so even after correction for prevalent stroke, suggesting an additional effect. As vascular dementia may be more often due to small vessel disease than stroke in general, hypertension may be a disproportionate risk factor for vascular dementia, but this remains an unproven hypothesis. Nevertheless, hypertension is consistently identified in all studies investigating risk factors in this field. Identified risk factors include hypertension, age, male sex, education, race, prior stroke, diabetes, impaired glucose tolerance, elevated low-density-lipoprotein (LDL) cholesterol, cardiac disease, electrocardiographic (ECG) changes, elevated hematocrit, smoking, history of myocardial infarction, alcohol, and proteinuria.[39,40,49–51,150–155,155–157] The same studies have often yielded negative results for many other common stroke risk factors[50,150] including cardiac disease, increased viscosity, and fibrinogen in one[49] and obesity, cholesterol, alcohol, cigarettes, and glucose intolerance in a Japanese study,[151] both diabetes and smoking in the first report from the Canadian Study of Heath and Aging,[152] the lack of effect of smoking being confirmed in the second report[156] and cholesterol, smoking, and alcohol among others in the Honolulu-Asia Aging Study.[155] The Eurodem study did not confirm male sex as a risk factor, although the figures were higher for men.[158] Interestingly, in elderly blacks with and without multi-infarct dementia who had been hospitalized for cerebral infarction, elevated systolic blood pressure and obesity were protective.[150] The authors suggest that protection by elevated systolic blood pressure may be a true finding because the suggestion that a window of systolic blood pressure exists below which cognition declines.[159] However, the finding has not been replicated, is unexpected, and contradicts such other evidence as is available.

DIFFERENTIAL DIAGNOSIS OF VASCULAR DEMENTIA

The principal differential diagnosis is from AD. In 90 percent of cases where multiple infarcts are responsible, there is also a history of stroke or of transient ischemic attacks. The ischemic scale score,[4] classifying those with a score of 4 or less as having AD and 7 or more as having vascular dementia, has a sensitivity and specificity of 89 percent, although distinguishing between vascular and mixed cases remains problematic.[160] The use of computed tomography (CT) to identify infarcts increases diagnostic accuracy. Of at least equal importance to the identification of vascular dementia itself is identification of the cause of the vascular events, as it is upon these that the treatment and prognosis depend. The remainder of the differential diagnosis is that of dementia.

THE INVESTIGATION OF VASCULAR DEMENTIA

The clinical history and examination alone can identify dementia. The examination should include an assessment for depression, as this is both a common cause of pseudodementia and treatable. Imaging is required to confirm the occurrence of infarction and to exclude structural causes. In the past we have suggested that CT is sufficient in routine clinical practice and that magnetic resonance imaging (MRI) was necessary only if certain conditions, such as cerebral autosomal-dominant anteriopathy with subcortical infarcts and leukoencephalopathy (CADASIL),[161–163] were suspected. Certainly, the presence of white matter lesions on CT (but not on MRI) may help to distinguish vascular dementia from AD.[164,165] However, the increasing recognition of the effect of small amounts of cerebrovascular disease couple with the increasing recognition of mixed dementia makes our original recommendation untenable. MRI is required if imaging evidence of small amounts of vascular disease sufficient to convert a diagnosis of AD into one of mixed dementia is not to be missed. Cortical sulcal atrophy and left ventricular enlargement are more severe in patients with multiple infarcts and dementia than in those with multiple infarcts without dementia,[40] but there is no evidence to suggest that this is sufficiently discriminating to be a useful part of the evaluation. Atrophy has previously been associated with degenerative dementias.[86] However, in one study based on subcortical infarcts, it was ventricular enlargement and not infarct volume that correlated best with cognitive impairment,[24] and similar findings have been reported in cerebral microangiopathy[91] and multiple sclerosis.[92] Another study comparing progressive atrophy in vascular dementia, Alzheimer's disease, and Lewy body dementia found the rate of progression to be the same in all three groups,[93] and we have recently identified a powerful association between atrophy and VCI.[42] This evidence suggests that the assumption that atrophy means degenerative dementia is wrong and that atrophy is a common feature in cerebrovascular disease even where this is limited to leukoaraiosis. Syphilis and HIV serology are necessary and thyroid function, vitamin B_{12}, and red cell folic acid are needed to exclude abnormalities in these as possible causes of cognitive decline.

The vascular component of the investigations should be directed by clinical suspicion. Not all investigations are routinely required. However, a complete blood count, erythrocyte sedimentation rate, glucose, and electrocardiogram should be done. Where appropriate, carotid duplex Doppler, chest x-ray, echocardiography, Holter monitoring, coagulation screen, lipid profile, lupus anticoagulant, anticardiolipin antibodies,[166] and autoantibody screen are justifiable. A glycosylated hemoglobin may detect unsuspected diabetes.[167] Cerebral angiography is indicated if carotid surgery is considered or to demonstrate beading of the smaller cerebral vessels if a cerebral vasculitis is suspected, but this is not a routine investigation. Examination of the cerebrospinal fluid may be required if an infectious or inflammatory etiology is suspected as, rarely, may be dural or brain biopsy.

A number of investigations have been proposed as being useful in the diagnosis of multi-infarct dementia. Focal abnormalities on electroencephalography favor multi-infarct dementia[168,169] but are a poor discriminator. Intracranial hemodynamics may help distinguish multi-infarct dementia from AD and normal subjects,[170] but this has not been confirmed. Single photon emission computed tomography demonstrates more perfusion defects in AD than in multi-infarct dementia[171–173] but has not been assessed as a discriminatory test. These investigations are not recommended.

THE PREVENTION AND TREATMENT OF VASCULAR DEMENTIA

Data are now becoming available for both the prevention of vascular dementia, by which is meant disease-modifying drugs, and symptomatic treatment, by which is meant drugs that improve the cognitive or behavioral aspects of the disease without affecting the underlying rate of progression. However, there are still very few trials in pure vascular dementia. Aspirin has been proposed on the basis of a pilot study done without placebo.[174] Interestingly, nonaspirin NSAIDs do not seem to protect against vascular dementia, while the use of aspirin is associated with a higher incidence of vascular dementia, presumably because of the treatment of patients with vascular disease with aspirin.[175] In a small uncontrolled, unblinded study, cessation of cigarette smoking was suggested, along with lowering blood pressure to a window of 135 to 150 mmHG systolic. Reductions below a systolic of 135 mmHg were detrimental.[159] Cessation of smoking[176] and control of blood pressure[177] increase cerebral blood flow, but the implications of these observations for therapy are unclear. A large study of lowering blood pressure with beta blockers or diuretics produced showed no benefit for cognition after more than 4 years of follow-up.[178] However, the Syst-Eur study suggested that treatment of those aged over 60 with a systolic blood pressure of 160 to 219 mmHg and a diastolic of less than 95 mmHg with nitrendipine, enalapril, or hydrochlorothiazide to produce a systolic below 150 mmHg might prevent 19 cases for each 1000 subjects treated for 5 years.[179] The PROGRESS study[180] supports the notion that the lowering of blood pressure helps cognition, but the cognitive data from this study have yet to be formally published. Vitamins E and C may have a protective effect, as may an Occidental as opposed to an Oriental diet.[155,181] There is some evidence for a weak effect, mostly from single studies for pentoxifylline,[182,183] vincamine,[184] posatirelin,[185] and propentofylline,[186–188] but these findings have not yet been confirmed and the drugs have not entered into clinical practice. Memantine may also have a role in this field,[189] although major studies have yet to be published. Donepezil and rivastigmine[190] may have a role, but once again data for pure vascular dementia remain to be published. The status of nimodipine remains uncertain; it has not yet been shown to be helpful.[191,192]

At present, therefore, the medical management of vascular dementia remains largely the management of stroke and risk factors for stroke with some symptomatic therapeutic interventions available that overlap with those of AD. The social, economic, and legal management is similar to that for AD.

THE PROGNOSIS OF VASCULAR DEMENTIA

Multi-infarct dementia shortens life expectancy[193] to about 50 percent of normal at 4 years from initial evaluation.[194,195] Vascular cognitive impairment short of dementia is still associated with a 52 percent 5-year mortality and 46 percent progression to dementia.[196] Those with higher education and those who perform well on some neuropsychological tests do better, but the data for the effect of female sex are contradictory.[194,196] In the very elderly, 3-year mortality may reach two-thirds, almost three times that of controls[149]; in one study, the 6-year survival was only 11.9 percent, about one-quarter of that expected,[197] though many of these patients were elderly and severely demented at entry. About one-third die from complications of the dementia itself, one-third from cerebrovascular disease, 8 percent from other cardiovascular disease, and the rest from miscellaneous causes, including malignancy.[197]

CONCLUSIONS

Vascular disease is a common cause of dementia, but, despite this, relatively little is known about it. Knowledge is increasing as a result of the recognition of the importance of vascular dementia, particularly when it coexists with AD as mixed dementia. It is still necessary to be very cautious in interpreting published data because of the use of inappropriate criteria for the diagnosis of vascular dementia. This has almost certainly resulted in the selection and study of a subset of all the vascular dementias, selecting only more advanced cases and those in which memory loss is a prominent feature. It is now clear that frontal dysfunction and a subcortical pattern of dementia are the most prominent cognitive deficits seen when vascular dementia is studied as a single entity. Memory is affected, but this is not a preeminent feature. Depression, apathy, perseveration, and incontinence have been identified as common behavioral changes in vascular dementia, but it must be borne in mind that the criteria used to diagnose vascular dementia specify similar deficits, and some part of the findings may ultimately prove to be tautologic. There is also the very considerable risk that much of the data reported in fact refers to cases with mixed disease. The current criteria require an AD-like cognitive deficit with vascular risk factors and events, and this paradigm would seem perfect for the detection of mixed disease. Clarification of the diagnostic criteria and subsequent study of well-defined cases is a major challenge to be addressed over the next decade.

REFERENCES

1. World Health Organization: *The ICD-10 Classification of Mental and Behavioural Disorders. Diagnostic Criteria for Research.* Geneva: World Health Organization, 1993.
2. American Psychiatric Association: *Diagnostic and Statistical Manual of Mental Disorders*, 4th ed. (DSM-IV). Washington, DC: American Psychiatric Association, 1994.
3. Hachinski VC, Lassen NA, Marshall J: Multi-infarct dementia: A cause of mental deterioration in the elderly. *Lancet* 2:207–209, 1974.
4. Hachinski VC, Iliff LD, Zilkha E, et al: Cerebral blood flow in dementia. *Arch Neurol* 32:632–637, 1975.
5. Wade JPH, Mirsen T, Hachinski VC, et al: The clinical diagnosis of Alzheimer's disease. *Arch Neurol* 44: 24–29, 1987.
6. Roman GC, Tatemichi TK, Erkinjuntti T, et al: Vascular dementia: Diagnostic criteria for research studies. Report of the NINDS-AIREN international workshop. *Neurology* 43:250–260, 1993.
7. del Ser T, Bermejo F, Portera A, et al: Vascular dementia. A clinicopathological study. *J Neurol Sci* 96:1–17, 1990.
8. Hachinski VC: Preventable senility: A call for action against the vascular dementias. *Lancet* 340:645–647, 1992.
9. Chui HC, Victoroff JI, Margolin D, et al: Criteria for the diagnosis of ischemic vascular dementia proposed by the State of California Alzheimer's Disease Diagnostic and Treatment Centers. *Neurology* 42:473–480, 1992.
10. Kinkel WR, Jacobs L, Polachini I, et al: Subcortical arteriosclerotic encephalopathy (Binswanger's disease). Computed tomographic, nuclear magnetic resonance, and clinical correlations. *Arch Neurol* 42:951–959, 1985.
11. Perez FI, Gay JR, Taylor RL: WAIS performance of neurologically impaired aged. *Psychol Rep* 37:1043–1047, 1975.

12. Perez FI, Gay JR, Taylor RL, Rivera VM: Patterns of memory performance in the neurologically impaired aged. *Can J Neurol Sci* 2:347–355, 1975.
13. Perez FI, Rivera VM, Meyer JS, et al: Analysis of intellectual and cognitive performance in patients with multi-infarct dementia, vertebrobasilar insufficiency with dementia, and Alzheimer's disease. *J Neurol Neurosurg Psychiatry* 38:533–540, 1975.
14. Wade DT, Parker V, Langton Hewer R: Memory disturbance after stroke: Frequency and associated losses. *Int Rehabil Med* 8:60–64, 1986.
15. Wade DT, Wood VA, Hewer RI: Recovery of cognitive function soon after stroke: A study of visual neglect, attention span and verbal recall. *J Neurol Neurosurg Psychiatry* 51:10–13, 1988.
16. Wolfe N, Linn R, Babikian VL, et al: Frontal systems impairment following multiple lacunar infarcts. *Arch Neurol* 47:129–132, 1990.
17. Babikian VL, Wolfe N, Linn R, et al: Cognitive changes in patients with multiple cerebral infarcts. *Stroke* 21:1013–1018, 1990.
18. Hom J, Reitan RM: Generalized cognitive function after stroke. *J Clin Exp Neuropsychol* 12:644–654, 1990.
19. Pujol J, Junque C, Vendrell P, et al: Cognitive correlates of ventricular enlargement in vascular patients with leukoaraiosis. *Acta Neurol Scand* 84:237–242, 1991.
20. Tatemichi TK, Desmond DW, Mayeux R, et al: Dementia after stroke: Baseline frequency, risks, and clinical features in a hospitalized cohort. *Neurology* 42:1185–1193, 1992.
21. Villardita C: Alzheimer's disease compared with cerebrovascular dementia. Neuropsychological similarities and differences. *Acta Neurol Scand* 87:299–308, 1993.
22. Tatemichi TK, Desmond DW, Stern Y, et al: Cognitive impairment after stroke: Frequency, patterns, and relationship to functional abilities. *J Neurol Neurosurg Psychiatry* 57:202–207, 1994.
23. Bowler JV, Hadar U, Wade JPH: Cognition in stroke. *Acta Neurol Scand* 90:424–429, 1994.
24. Corbett A, Bennett H, Kos S: Cognitive dysfunction following subcortical infarction. *Arch Neurol* 51:999–1007, 1994.
25. Breteler MM, van Amerongen NM, van Swieten JC, et al: Cognitive correlates of ventricular enlargement and cerebral white matter lesions on magnetic resonance imaging. The Rotterdam Study. *Stroke* 25:1109–1115, 1994.
26. Breteler MMB, van Swieten JC, Bots ML, et al: Cerebral white matter lesions, vascular risk factors, and cognitive function in a population-based study: The Rotterdam Study. *Neurology* 44:1246–1252, 1994.
27. Fukuda H, Kobayashi S, Okada K, Tsunematsu T: Frontal white matter lesions and dementia in lacunar infarction. *Stroke* 21:1143–1149, 1990.
28. Royall DR, Cordes JA, Polk M: CLOX: An executive clock drawing task. *J Neurol Neurosurg Psychiatry* 64:588–594, 1998.
29. Roman GC, Royall DR: Executive control function: A rational basis for the diagnosis of vascular dementia. *Alzheimer Dis Assoc Disord* 13(suppl 3):S69–S80, 1999.
30. Ferris SH: Cognitive outcome measures. *Alzheimer Dis Assoc Disord* 13(Suppl 3):S140–S142, 1999.
31. Gauthier S, Ferris S: Outcome measures for probable vascular dementia and Alzheimer's disease with cerebrovascular disease. *Int J Clin Pract Suppl* 29–39, 2001.
32. Hachinski VC: The decline and resurgence of vascular dementia. *Can Med Assoc J* 142:107–111, 1990.
33. Hachinski VC: Multi-infarct dementia: A reappraisal. *Alzheimer Dis Assoc Disord* 5:64–68, 1991.
34. Hachinski VC, Bowler JV: Vascular dementia. *Neurology* 43:2159–2160, 1993.
35. Erkinjuntti T, Hachinski VC: Rethinking vascular dementia. *Cerebrovasc Dis* 3:3–23, 1993.
36. de Groot JC, de Leeuw FE, Oudkerk M, et al: Cerebral white matter lesions and subjective cognitive dysfunction: The Rotterdam Scan Study. *Neurology* 56:1539–1545, 2001.
37. Tomlinson BE, Blessed G, Roth M: Observations on the brains of demented old people. *J Neurol Sci* 11:205–242, 1970.
38. Erkinjuntti T, Haltia M, Palo J, et al: Accuracy of the clinical diagnosis of vascular dementia: A prospective clinical and post-mortem neuropathological study. *J Neurol Neurosurg Psychiatry* 51:1037–1044, 1988.
39. Loeb C, Gandolfo C, Bino G: Intellectual impairment and cerebral lesions in multiple cerebral infarcts. A clinical-computed tomography study. *Stroke* 19:560–565, 1988.
40. Gorelick PB, Chatterjee A, Patel D, et al: Cranial computed tomographic observations in multi-infarct dementia. A controlled study. *Stroke* 23:804–811, 1992.
41. Liu CK, Miller BL, Cummings JL, et al: A quantitative MRI study of vascular dementia. *Neurology* 42:138–143, 1992.
42. Bowler JV, Hachinski V, Steenhuis R, Lee D: Vascular cognitive impairment: Clinical, neuropsychological and imaging findings in early vascular dementia. *Lancet* 352(supple 4):63, 1998.
43. Bowler JV: Cerebral infarction and $^{99}Tc^{m}$ HMPAO SPECT. MD Thesis. University of London, 1993.

44. Anonymous: Pathological correlates of late-onset dementia in a multicentre, community-based population in England and Wales. Neuropathology Group of the Medical Research Council Cognitive Function and Ageing Study (MRC CFAS). *Lancet* 357:169–175, 2001.
45. Wetterling T, Kanitz RD, Borgis KJ: Comparison of different diagnostic criteria for vascular dementia (ADDTC, DSM-IV, ICD-10, NINDS-AIREN). *Stroke* 27:30–36, 1996.
46. Pohjasvaara T, Mantyla R, Ylikoski R, et al: Comparison of different clinical criteria (DSM-III, ADDTC, ICD-10, NINDS-AIREN, DSM-IV) for the diagnosis of vascular dementia. National Institute of Neurological Disorders and Stroke-Association Internationale pour la Recherche et l'Enseignement en Neurosciences. *Stroke* 31:2952–2957, 2000.
47. Esiri MM, Wilcock GK, Morris JH: Neuropathological assessment of the lesions of significance in vascular dementia. *J Neurol Neurosurg Psychiatry* 63:749–753, 1997.
48. Hijdra A: Vascular dementia, in Bradley WG et al (eds): *Neurology in Clinical Practice*. Boston: Butterworth-Heinemann, 1991, pp 1425–1435.
49. Ladurner G, Iliff LD, Lechner H: Clinical factors associated with dementia in ischaemic stroke. *J Neurol Neurosurg Psychiatry* 45:97–101, 1982.
50. Tatemichi TK, Desmond DW, Paik M, et al: Clinical determinants of dementia related to stroke. *Ann Neurol* 33:568–575, 1993.
51. Meyer JS, McClintic KL, Rogers RL, et al: Aetiological considerations and risk factors for multi-infarct dementia. *J Neurol Neurosurg Psychiatry* 51:1489–1497, 1988.
52. Meyer JS, Rogers RL, Mortel KF: Multi-infarct dementia: demography, risk factors and therapy, in Ginsberg MD et al (eds): *Cerebrovascular Diseases. Sixteenth Research (Princeton) Conference*. New York: Raven Press, 1989, pp 199–206.
53. Parnetti L, Mecocci P, Santucci C, et al: Is multi-infarct dementia representative of vascular dementias? A retrospective study. *Acta Neurol Scand* 81:484–487, 1990.
54. Fisher CM: Lacunes: small, deep cerebral infarcts. *Neurology* 15:774–784, 1965.
55. Miyao S, Takano A, Teramoto J, Takahashi A: Leukoaraiosis in relation to prognosis for patients with lacunar infarction. *Stroke* 23:1434–1438, 1992.
56. Loeb C: Vascular dementia. *Dementia* 1:175–184, 1990.
57. Lassen NA: Incomplete cerebral infarction—focal incomplete ischaemic tissue necrosis not leading to emollision. *Stroke* 13:522–523, 1982.
58. Cummings JL, Benson DF: Subcortical dementia. Review of an emerging concept. *Arch Neurol* 41:874–879, 1984.
59. Steingart A, Hachinski VC, Lau C, et al: Cognitive and neurologic findings in subjects with diffuse white matter lucencies on computed tomographic scan (leukoaraiosis). *Arch Neurol* 44:32–35, 1987.
60. Goto K, Ishii N, Fukasawa H: Diffuse white matter disease in the geriatric population. A clinical, neuropathological and CT study. *Radiology* 141:687–695, 1989.
61. Kertesz A, Polk M, Carr T: Cognition and white matter changes on magnetic resonance imaging in dementia. *Arch Neurol* 47:387–391, 1990.
62. Bowen BC, Barker WW, Loewenstein DA, et al: MR signal abnormalities in memory disorder and dementia. *AJNR* 11:283–290, 1990.
63. Diaz JF, Merskey H, Hachinski VC, et al: Improved recognition of leukoaraiosis and cognitive impairment in Alzheimer's disease. *Arch Neurol* 48:1022–1025, 1991.
64. Wahlund LO, Andersson-Lundman G, Julin P, et al: Quantitative estimation of brain white matter abnormalities in elderly subjects using magnetic resonance imaging. *Magn Reson Imaging* 10:859–865, 1992.
65. Almkvist O, Wahlund L, Andersson-Lundman G, et al: White-matter hyperintensity and neuropsychological functions in dementia and healthy aging. *Arch Neurol* 49:626–632, 1992.
66. Skoog I, Berg S, Johansson B, et al: The influence of white matter lesions on neuropsychological functioning in demented and non-demented 85 year olds, in Skoog I (ed): *Mental Disorders in the Elderly. A Population Study in 85-Year-Olds*. Göteborg: University of Göteborg, 1993.
67. Erkinjuntti T, Inzitari D, Pantoni L, et al: Research criteria for subcortical vascular dementia in clinical trials. *J Neural Transm Suppl* 59:23–30, 2000.
68. Steingart A, Hachinski VC, Lau C, et al: Cognitive and neurologic findings in demented patients with diffuse white matter lucencies on computed tomographic scan (leukoaraiosis). *Arch Neurol* 44:36–39, 1987.
69. Skoog I, Palmertz B, Andreasson L-A: The prevalence of white matter lesions on computed tomography of the brain in demented and non-demented 85 year olds. *J Geriatr Psychiatry Neurol* 7:169–175, 1994.
70. Hunt AL, Orrison WW, Yeo RA, et al: Clinical significance of MRI white matter lesions in the elderly. *Neurology* 39:1470–1474, 1989.
71. Tupler LA, Coffey CE, Logue PE, et al: Neuropsychological importance of subcortical white matter hyperintensity. *Arch Neurol* 49:1248–1252, 1992.

72. Hershey LA, Modic MT, Greenough PG, Jaffe DF: Magnetic resonance imaging in vascular dementia. *Neurology* 37:29–36, 1987.
73. Rao SM, Mittenberg W, Bernardin L, et al: Neuropsychological test findings in subjects with leukoaraiosis. *Arch Neurol* 46:40–44, 1989.
74. Mirsen TR, Lee DH, Wong CJ, et al: Clinical correlates of white-matter changes on magnetic resonance imaging scans of the brain. *Arch Neurol* 48:1015–1021, 1991.
75. Erkinjuntti T, Gao F, Lee DH, et al: Lack of difference in brain hyperintensities between patients with early Alzheimer's disease and control subjects. *Arch Neurol* 51:260–268, 1994.
76. Longstreth WT, Manolio TA, Arnold A, et al: Clinical correlates of white matter findings on cranial magnetic resonance imaging of 3301 elderly people. The Cardiovascular Health Study. *Stroke* 27:1274–1282, 1996.
77. Olszewski J: Subcortical arteriosclerotic encephalopathy: Review of the literature on the so-called Binswanger's disease and presentation of two cases. *World Neurol* 3:359–375, 1962.
78. Babikian V, Ropper AH: Binswanger's disease: A review. *Stroke* 18:2–12, 1987.
79. Hachinski VC, Potter P, Merskey H: Leukoaraiosis. *Arch Neurol* 44:21–23, 1987.
80. Bennett DA, Wilson RS, Gilley DW, Fox JH: Clinical diagnosis of Binswanger's disease. *J Neurol Neurosurg Psychiatry* 53:961–965, 1990.
81. Loizou LA, Kendall BE, Marshall J: Subcortical arteriosclerotic encephalopathy: A clinical and radiological investigation. *J Neurol Neurosurg Psychiatry* 44:294–304, 1981.
82. Caplan LR, Schoene WC: Clinical features of subcortical arteriosclerotic encephalopathy (Binswanger disease). *Neurology* 28:1206–1215, 1978.
83. Thompson PD, Marsden CD: Gait disorder of subcortical arteriosclerotic encephalopathy: Binswanger's disease. *Mov Disord* 2:1–8, 1987.
84. Delong GR, Kemper TL, Pogacar S, Lee HY: Clinical neuropathological conference. *Dis Nerv Syst* 35:286–291, 1974.
85. Burger PC, Burch JG, Kunze U: Subcortical arteriosclerotic encephalopathy (Binswanger's disease). A vascular etiology of dementia. *Stroke* 7:626–631, 1976.
86. Pohjasvaara T, Mantyla R, Aronen HJ, et al: Clinical and radiological determinants of prestroke cognitive decline in a stroke cohort. *J Neurol Neurosurg Psychiatry* 67:742–748, 1999.
87. Salerno JA, Murphy DGM, Horwitz B, et al: Brain atrophy in hypertension. A volumetric magnetic resonance imaging study. *Hypertension* 20:340–348, 1992.
88. Wilkie F, Eisdorfer C: Intelligence and blood pressure in the aged. *Science* 172:959–962, 1971.
89. Launer LJ, Masaki K, Petrovitch H, et al: The association between midlife blood pressure levels and late-life cognitive function. The Honolulu-Asia Aging Study. *JAMA* 274:1846–1851, 1995.
90. Launer LJ, Ross GW, Petrovitch H, et al: Midlife blood pressure and dementia: The Honolulu-Asia Aging Study. *Neurobiol Aging* 21:49–55, 2000.
91. Sabri O, Ringelstein EB, Hellwig D, et al: Neuropsychological impairment correlates with hypoperfusion and hypometabolism but not with severity of white matter lesions on MRI in patients with cerebral microangiopathy. *Stroke* 30:556–566, 1999.
92. Zivadinov R, Sepcic J, Nasuelli D, et al: A longitudinal study of brain atrophy and cognitive disturbances in the early phase of relapsing-remitting multiple sclerosis. *J Neurol Neurosurg Psychiatry* 70:773–780, 2001.
93. O'Brien JT, Paling S, Barber R, et al: Progressive brain atrophy on serial MRI in dementia with Lewy bodies, AD, and vascular dementia. *Neurology* 56:1386–1388, 2001.
94. Desmond DW, Moroney JT, Paik MC, et al: Frequency and clinical determinants of dementia after ischemic stroke. *Neurology* 54:1124–1131, 2000.
95. Barba R, Martínez-Espinosa S, Rodríguez-Garcia E, et al: Poststroke dementia: Clinical features and risk factors. *Stroke* 31:1494–1501, 2000.
96. Pohjasvaara T, Erkinjuntti T, Vataja R, Kaste M: Comparison of stroke features and disability in daily life in patients with ischemic stroke aged 55 to 70 and 71 to 85 years. *Stroke* 28:729–735, 1997.
97. Pohjasvaara T, Erkinjuntti T, Ylikoski R, et al: Clinical determinants of poststroke dementia. *Stroke* 29:75–81, 1998.
98. Bowler JV, Munoz DG, Merskey H, Hachinski VC: Fallacies in the pathological confirmation of the diagnosis of Alzheimer's disease. *J Neurol Neurosurg Psychiatry* 64:18–24, 1998.
99. Snowdon DA, Greiner LH, Mortimer JA, et al: Brain infarction and the clinical expression of Alzheimer disease. The nun study. *JAMA* 227:813–817, 1997.
100. Lim A, Tsuang D, Kukull W, et al: Clinico-neuropathological correlation of Alzheimer's disease in a community-based case series. *J Am Geriatr Soc* 47: 564–569, 1999.
101. Holmes C, Cairns N, Lantos P, Mann A: Validity of current clinical criteria for Alzheimer's disease, vascular

dementia and dementia with Lewy bodies. *Br J Psychiatry* 174:45–50, 1999.

102. Gold G, Giannakopoulos P, Montes-Paixao JC, et al: Sensitivity and specificity of newly proposed clinical criteria for possible vascular dementia. *Neurology* 49:690–694, 1997.
103. Nolan KA, Lino MM, Seligmann AW, Blass JP: Absence of vascular dementia in an autopsy series from a dementia clinic. *J Am Geriatr Soc* 46:597–604, 1998.
104. Heyman A, Fillenbaum GG, Welsh-Bohmer KA, et al: Cerebral infarcts in patients with autopsy-proven Alzheimer's disease: CERAD, part XVIII. Consortium to Establish a Registry for Alzheimer's Disease. *Neurology* 51:159–162, 1998.
105. Bowler JV, Hachinski V: Criteria for vascular dementia: Replacing dogma with data. *Arch Neurol.* 57:170–171, 2000.
106. Bowler JV: Vascular dementia: Changing concepts and criteria. *Stroke Rev* 4:1–4, 2000.
107. Chui HC, Mack W, Jackson JE, et al: Clinical criteria for the diagnosis of vascular dementia: A multi-center study of comparability and inter-rater reliability. *Arch Neurol* 57:191–196, 2000.
108. Hachinski VC: Multi-infarct dementia. *Neurol Clin* 1:27–36, 1983.
109. Wolfe N, Babikian VL, Linn RT, et al: Are multiple cerebral infarcts synergistic? *Arch Neurol* 51:211–215, 1994.
110. Mesulam M-M: Large-scale neurocognitive networks and distributed processing for attention, language and memory. *Ann Neurol* 28:597–613, 1990.
111. Fillenbaum GG, Heyman A, Wilkinson WE, Haynes CS: Comparison of two screening tests in Alzheimer's disease. The correlation and reliability of the mini-mental state examination and modified Blessed test. *Arch Neurol* 44:924–927, 1987.
112. Brandt J, Welsh KA, Breitner JCS, et al: Hereditary influences on cognitive functioning in older men. A study of 4000 twin pairs. *Arch Neurol* 50:599–603, 1993.
113. D'Antona R, Baron JC, Pantano P, et al: Effects of thalamic lesions on cerebral cortex metabolism in humans (abstr). *J Cereb Blood Flow Metab* 5(suppl 1):S457–S458, 1985.
114. Dobkin JA, Levine RL, Lagreze HL, et al: Evidence for transhemispheric diaschisis in unilateral stroke. *Arch Neurol* 46:1333–1336, 1989.
115. Szelies B, Herholz K, Pawlik G, et al: Widespread functional effects of discrete thalamic infarction. *Arch Neurol* 48:178–182, 1991.
116. Baron JC, Levasseur M, Mazoyer B, et al: Thalamocortical diaschisis: Positron emission tomography in humans. *J Neurol Neurosurg Psychiatry* 55:935–942, 1992.
117. Bowler JV, Wade JPH: Ipsilateral cerebellar diaschisis following pontine infarction. *Cerebrovasc Dis* 1:58–60, 1991.
118. Bowler JV, Costa DC, Jones BE, et al: High resolution SPECT, small deep infarcts and diaschisis. *J R Soc Med* 85:142–146, 1992.
119. Bowler JV, Wade JPH, Jones BE, et al: The contribution of diaschisis to the clinical deficit in human cerebral infarction. *Stroke* 26:1000–1006, 1995.
120. Canadian Study of Health and Aging Working Group: The Canadian study of health and aging: Study methods and prevalence of dementia. *Can Med Assoc J.* 150:899–913, 1994.
121. Folstein MF, Folstein SE, McHugh PR: "Mini-mental state": A practical method for grading the cognitive state of patients for the clinician. *J Psychiatr Res* 12:189–198, 1975.
122. Baldy-Moulinier M, Valmier J, Touchon J, et al: Clinical and neuropsychological rating scales for differential diagnosis of dementias. *Gerontology* 32(suppl 1):89–97, 1986.
123. Hier DB, Hagenlocker K, Shindler AG: Language disintegration in dementia: Effects of etiology and severity. *Brain Lang* 25:117–133, 1985.
124. Carlesimo GA, Fadda L, Bonci A, Caltagirone C: Differential rates of forgetting from long-term memory in Alzheimer's and multi-infarct dementia. *Int J Neurosci* 73:1–11, 1993.
125. Gainotti G, Parlato V, Monteleone D, Carlomagno S: Neuropsychological markers of dementia on visual-spatial tasks: A comparison between Alzheimer's type and vascular forms of dementia. *J Clin Exp Neuropsychol* 14:239–252, 1992.
126. Muramoto O: Selective reminding in normal and demented aged people: Auditory verbal versus visual spatial task. *Cortex* 20:461–478, 1984.
127. Kertesz A, Clydesdale S: Neuropsychological deficits in vascular dementia vs Alzheimer's disease. Frontal lobe deficits prominent in vascular dementia. *Arch Neurol* 51:1226–1231, 1994.
128. Looi JC, Sachdev PS: Differentiation of vascular dementia from AD on neuropsychological tests. *Neurology* 53:670–678, 1999.
129. Almkvist O, Backman L, Basun H, Wahlund LO: Patterns of neuropsychological performance in Alzheimer's disease and vascular dementia. *Cortex* 29:661–673, 1993.

130. Shuttleworth EC, Huber SJ: The picture absurdities test in the evaluation of dementia. *Brain Cogn* 11:50–59, 1989.
131. Erkinjuntti T: Differential diagnosis between Alzheimer's disease and vascular dementia: Evaluation of common clinical methods. *Acta Neurol Scand* 76:433–442, 1987.
132. Erkinjuntti T, Laaksonen R, Sulkava R, et al: Neuropsychological differentiation between normal aging, Alzheimer's disease and vascular dementia. *Acta Neurol Scand* 74:393–403, 1986.
133. Fischer P, Gatterer G, Marterer A, Danielczyk W: Nonspecificity of semantic impairment in dementia of Alzheimer's type. *Arch Neurol* 45:1341–1343, 1988.
134. Bowler JV, Eliasziw M, Steenhuis R, et al: Comparative evolution of Alzheimer disease, vascular dementia and mixed dementia. *Arch Neurol* 54:697–703, 1997.
135. Ricker JH, Keenan PA, Jacobson MW: Visuoperceptual-spatial ability and visual memory in vascular dementia and dementia of the Alzheimer type. *Neuropsychologia* 32:1287–1296, 1994.
136. Kontiola P, Laaksonen R, Sulkava R, Erkinjuntti T: Pattern of language impairment is different in Alzheimer's disease and multi-infarct dementia. *Brain Lang* 38:364–383, 1990.
137. Powell AL, Cummings JL, Hill MA, Benson DF: Speech and language alterations in multi-infarct dementia. *Neurology* 38:717–719, 1988.
138. Cummings JL, Miller B, Hill MA, Neshkes R: Neuropsychiatric aspects of multi-infarct dementia and dementia of the Alzheimer type. *Arch Neurol* 44:389–393, 1987.
139. Newman SC: The prevalence of depression in Alzheimer's disease and vascular dementia in a population sample. *J Affect Disord* 52:169–176, 1999.
140. Ballard C, Neill D, O'Brien J, et al: Anxiety, depression and psychosis in vascular dementia: Prevalence and associations. *J Affect Disord* 59:97–106, 2000.
141. Bucht G, Adolfsson R: The Comprehensive Psychopathological Rating Scale in patients with dementia of Alzheimer type and multiinfarct dementia. *Acta Psychiatr Scand* 68:263–270, 1983.
142. Hargrave R, Geck LC, Reed B, Mungas D: Affective behavioural disturbances in Alzheimer's disease and ischaemic vascular disease. *J Neurol Neurosurg Psychiatry* 68:41–46, 2000.
143. O'Brien J, Perry R, Barber R, et al: The association between white matter lesions on magnetic resonance imaging and noncognitive symptoms. *Ann NY Acad Sci* 903:482–489, 2000.
144. Kase CS, Wolf PA, Bachman DL, et al: Dementia and stroke: The Framingham study, in Ginsberg MD et al (eds): *Cerebrovascular Diseases. Sixteenth Research (Princeton) Conference*. New York: Raven Press, 1989, pp. 193–197.
145. Kase CS: Epidemiology of multi-infarct dementia. *Alzheimer Dis Assoc Disord* 5:71–76, 1991.
146. Rocca WA, Hofman A, Brayne C, et al: The prevalence of vascular dementia in Europe: Facts and fragments from 1980–1990 studies. EURODEM-Prevalence Research Group. *Ann Neurol* 30:817–824, 1991.
147. Ikeda M, Hokoishi K, Maki N, et al: Increased prevalence of vascular dementia in Japan: A community-based epidemiological study. *Neurology* 57:839–844, 2001.
148. Rockwood K, Wentzel C, Hachinski V, et al: Prevalence and outcomes of vascular cognitive impairment. *Neurology* 54:447–451, 2000.
149. Skoog I, Nilsson L, Palmertz B, et al: A population-based study of dementia in 85-year-olds. *N Engl J Med* 328:153–158, 1993.
150. Gorelick PB, Brody J, Cohen D, et al: Risk factors for dementia associated with multiple cerebral infarcts. A case-control analysis in predominantly African-American hospital-based patients. *Arch Neurol* 50:714–720, 1993.
151. Ueda K, Kawano H, Hasuo Y, Fujishima M: Prevalence and etiology of dementia in a Japanese community. *Stroke* 23:798–803, 1992.
152. Lindsay J, Hebert R, Rockwood K: The Canadian Study of Health and Aging: Risk factors for vascular dementia. *Stroke* 28:526–530, 1997.
153. Curb JD, Rodriguez BL, Abbott RD, et al: Longitudinal association of vascular and Alzheimer's dementias, diabetes, and glucose tolerance. *Neurology* 52:971–975, 1999.
154. Moroney JT, Tang MX, Berglund L, et al: Low-density lipoprotein cholesterol and the risk of dementia with stroke. *JAMA* 282:254–260, 1999.
155. Ross GW, Petrovitch H, White LR, et al: Characterization of risk factors for vascular dementia: The Honolulu-Asia Aging Study. *Neurology* 1999;53:337–343.
156. Hebert R, Lindsay J, Verreault R, et al: Vascular dementia: Incidence and risk factors in the Canadian study of health and aging. *Stroke* 31:1487–1493, 2000.
157. Guo Z, Viitanen M, Fratiglioni L, Winblad B: Low blood pressure and dementia in elderly people: The Kungsholmen project. *Br Med J* 312:805–808, 1996.
158. Andersen K, Launer LJ, Dewey ME, et al: Gender differences in the incidence of AD and vascular dementia:

The EURODEM Studies. EURODEM Incidence Research Group. *Neurology* 53:1992–1997, 1999.

159. Meyer JS, Judd BW, Tawaklna T, et al: Improved cognition after control of risk factors for multi-infarct dementia. *JAMA* 256:2203–2209, 1986.
160. Moroney JT, Bagiella E, Desmond DW, et al: Meta-analysis of the Hachinski Ischemic Score in pathologically verified dementias. *Neurology* 49:1096–1105, 1997.
161. Bousser MG, Lasserve ET: Summary of the proceedings of the first international workshop on CADASIL. *Stroke* 25:704–707, 1994.
162. Bowler JV, Hachinski VC. Progress in the genetics of cerebrovascular disease: Inherited subcortical arteriopathies. *Stroke* 25:1696–1698, 1994.
163. Tournier Lasserve E, Joutel A, Melki J, et al: Cerebral autosomal dominant arteriopathy with subcortical infarcts and leukoencephalopathy maps to chromosome 19q12. *Nat Genet* 3:256–259, 1993.
164. Erkinjuntti T, Ketonen L, Sulkava R, et al: Do white matter changes on MRI and CT differentiate vascular dementia from Alzheimer's disease? *J Neurol Neurosurg Psychiatry* 50:37–42, 1987.
165. Erkinjuntti T, Ketonen L, Sulkava R, et al: CT in the differential diagnosis between Alzheimer's disease and vascular dementia. *Acta Neurol Scand* 75:262–270, 1987.
166. Coull BM, Bourdette DN, Goodnight SH Jr, et al: Multiple cerebral infarctions and dementia associated with anticardiolipin antibodies. *Stroke* 18:1107–1112, 1987.
167. Riddle MC, Hart J: Hyperglycemia, recognized and unrecognized, as a risk factor for stroke and transient ischemic attacks. *Stroke* 13:356–359, 1982.
168. Erkinjuntti T, Larsen T, Sulkava R, et al: EEG in the differential diagnosis between Alzheimer's disease and vascular dementia. *Acta Neurol Scand* 77:36–43, 1988.
169. Leuchter AF, Newton TF, Cook IA, et al: Changes in brain functional connectivity in Alzheimer-type and multi-infarct dementia. *Brain* 115:1543–1561, 1992.
170. Ries F, Horn R, Hillekamp J, et al: Differentiation of multi-infarct and Alzheimer dementia by intracranial hemodynamic parameters. *Stroke* 24:228–235, 1993.
171. Smith FW, Besson JA, Gemmell HG, Sharp PF: The use of technetium-99m-HM-PAO in the assessment of patients with dementia and other neuropsychiatric conditions. *J Cereb Blood Flow Metab* 8:S116–S122, 1988.
172. Neary D, Snowden JS, Shields RA, et al: Single photon emission tomography using 99mTc-HM-PAO in the investigation of dementia. *J Neurol Neurosurg Psychiatry* 50:1101–1109, 1987.
173. Launes J, Sulkava R, Erkinjuntti T, et al: 99Tcm-HMPAO SPECT in suspected dementia. *Nucl Med Commun* 12:757–765, 1991.
174. Meyer JS, Rogers RL, McClintic K, et al: Randomized clinical trial of daily aspirin therapy in multi-infarct dementia. A pilot study. *J Am Geriatr Soc* 37:549–555, 1989.
175. in 't Veld BA, Ruitenberg A, Hofman A, et al: Nonsteroidal anti-inflammatory drugs and the risk of Alzheimer's disease. *N Engl J Med* 345:1515–1521, 2001.
176. Rogers RL, Meyer JS, Judd BW, Mortel KF: Abstention from cigarette smoking improves cerebral perfusion among elderly chronic smokers. *JAMA* 253:2970–2974, 1985.
177. Meyer JS, Rogers RL, Mortel KF: Prospective analysis of long term control of mild hypertension on cerebral blood flow. *Stroke* 16:985–990, 1985.
178. Prince M, Bird AS, Blizard RA, Mann AH: Is the cognitive function of older patients affected by antihypertensive treatment? Results from 54 months of the Medical Research Council's treatment trial of hypertension in older adults. *Br Med J* 312:801–805, 1996.
179. Forette F, Seux M-L, Staessen JA, et al: Prevention of dementia in randomised double-blind placebo-controlled Systolic Hypertension in Europe (Syst-Eur) trial. *Lancet* 352:1347–1351, 1998.
180. PROGRESS Collaborative Group: Randomised trial of a perindopril-based blood-pressure-lowering regimen among 6,105 individuals with previous stroke or transient ischaemic attack. *Lancet* 358:1033–1041, 2001.
181. Masaki KH, Losonczy KG, Izmirlian G, et al: Association of vitamin E and C supplement use with cognitive function and dementia in elderly men. *Neurology* 54:1265–1272, 2000.
182. Black RS, Barclay LL, Nolan KA, et al: Pentoxifylline in cerebrovascular dementia. *J Am Geriatr Soc* 40:237–244, 1992.
183. European Pentoxifylline Multi-Infarct Dementia Study Group: European Pentoxifylline Multi-Infarct Dementia Study. *Eur Neurol* 36:315–321, 1996.
184. Fischhof PK, Moslinger GR, Herrmann WM, et al: Therapeutic efficacy of vincamine in dementia. *Neuropsychobiology* 34:29–35, 1996.
185. Parnetti L, Ambrosoli L, Agliati G, et al: Posatirelin in the treatment of vascular dementia: A double-blind multicentre study vs placebo. *Acta Neurol Scand* 93:456–463, 1996.
186. Mielke R, Moller HJ, Erkinjuntti T, et al: Propentofylline in the treatment of vascular dementia and Alzheimer-type dementia: Overview of phase I and

phase II clinical trials. *Alzheimer Dis Assoc Disord* 12 (suppl 2):S29–S35, 1998.
187. Rother M, Erkinjuntti T, Roessner M, et al: Propentofylline in the treatment of Alzheimer's disease and vascular dementia: A review of phase III trials. *Dement Geriatr Cogn Disord* 9(suppl 1):36–43, 1998.
188. Kittner B: Clinical trials of propentofylline in vascular dementia. European/Canadian Propentofylline Study Group. *Alzheimer Dis Assoc Disord* 13(suppl 3):S166–S171, 1999.
189. Winblad B, Poritis N: Memantine in severe dementia: Results of the 9M-Best Study (Benefit and efficacy in severely demented patients during treatment with memantine). *Int J Geriatr Psychiatry* 14:135–146, 1999.
190. Anand R, Messina J, Hartman R, Veach J: An efficacy and safety analysis of Exelon in Alzheimer's disease patients with concurrent vascular risk factors. *Eur J Neurol* 7:159–169, 2000.
191. Pantoni L, Bianchi C, Beneke M, et al: The Scandinavian Multi-Infarct Dementia Trial: A double-blind, placebo-controlled trial on nimodipine in multi-infarct dementia. *J Neurol Sci* 175:116–123, 2000.
192. Pantoni L, Rossi R, Inzitari D, et al: Efficacy and safety of nimodipine in subcortical vascular dementia: A subgroup analysis of the Scandinavian Multi-Infarct Dementia Trial. *J Neurol Sci* 175:124–134, 2000.
193. Martin DC, Miller JK, Kapoor W, et al: A controlled study of survival with dementia. *Arch Neurol* 44:1122–1126, 1987.
194. Hier DB, Warach JD, Gorelick PB, Thomas J: Predictors of survival in clinically diagnosed Alzheimer's disease and multi-infarct dementia. *Arch Neurol* 46:1213–1216, 1989.
195. Barclay LL, Zemcov A, Blass JP, Sansone J: Survival in Alzheimer's disease and vascular dementias. *Neurology* 35:834–840, 1985.
196. Wentzel C, Rockwood K, MacKnight C, et al: Progression of impairment in patients with vascular cognitive impairment without dementia. *Neurology* 57:714–716, 2001.
197. Molsa PK, Marttila RJ, Rinne UK: Survival and cause of death in Alzheimer's disease and multi-infarct dementia. *Acta Neurol Scand* 74:103–107, 1986.

Chapter 50

INFECTIVE CAUSES OF DEMENTIA INCLUDING HUMAN IMMUNODEFICIENCY VIRUS

Clement T. Loy
Bruce J. Brew

Infective causes of dementia are uncommon but important because of the potential for efficacious therapy in most. In a systematic review including 16 case series and 1551 patients, Weytingh et al. found that 15.2 percent of dementia patients had a potentially reversible cause, and about 2 percent of these patients had an infective cause.[1] Moreover, increasing global importance of both AIDS dementia complex (ADC) and variant Creutzfeldt-Jakob disease make the consideration of an infective cause for dementia crucial, especially in the presenile dementia patient group. In this chapter, we review dementias caused primarily by an infective agent itself and dementias that occur as a sequela of initial infection. Roughly in the order of disease frequency, we review ADC, progressive multifocal leukoencephalopathy, prion diseases, neurosyphilis, Lyme disease, Whipple's disease, subacute sclerosing panencephalitis, progressive rubella panencephalitis, and postmeningitic syndromes.

AIDS DEMENTIA COMPLEX

Direct involvement of the human immunodeficiency virus (HIV) in the brain leads to a subcortical dementia. This syndrome of subcortical dementia has been named variously as HIV encephalitis, AIDS-related dementia, AIDS dementia complex (ADC), as well as HIV-1-associated minor cognitive/motor deficit and HIV-1-associated dementia. The term *ADC* is used here as it is inclusive and highlights the distinctive complex of symptoms and signs associated with this syndrome.

ADC is characterized by cognitive, motor, and behavioral features, often in the absence of substantial memory disturbance. It occurred in 20 to 30 percent of patients[2] with advanced HIV disease (median CD4 cell count ~$50/\mu L$)[3] in the past. However, with the advent of highly active antiretroviral therapy (HAART), the incidence has been halved,[4] and the median CD4 cell count has risen to $160/\mu L$.[5] As patients are now living longer because of HAART, it is expected that the prevalence of ADC will increase.

The cognitive, motor, and behavioral symptoms of ADC have been studied in a prospective series by Brew with 549 patients, of whom 111 had ADC.[6] In terms of cognition, approximately 80 percent of patients complained of decreased concentration and forgetfulness that is *constant* and independent of the usual precipitating factors such as fatigue. In terms of motor deficits, three-quarters complained of gait unsteadiness; 50 percent noted clumsiness including poor handwriting and typing, while one-third complained of tremor. In regard to behavior, approximately half noted that they had lost interest in keeping up with their friends, appearing to some extent to be depressed but without the inner feeling of dysphoria. Other clinical features associated with ADC include urinary urgency/hesitancy, nonspecific headaches, and unexplained generalized seizures. These symptoms usually develop subacutely over weeks to months, though rarely presentation can be fulminant, over days to weeks.

Neurologic examination may show few abnormalities in the early stage of ADC except for subtle signs, such as slowing and inaccuracy of saccadic and pursuit eye movements. Importantly, the Mini-Mental State Examination (MMSE) is normal, although responses may be delayed. As the disease progresses, slowing of fine finger movements and hyperreflexia (especially of the legs) occur in almost every patient,

Table 50-1
Modified staging scheme for AIDS dementia complex

Stage 0 (normal)	Normal mental and motor function.
Stage 0.5 (subclinical)	Minimal or equivocal symptoms without impairment of work or activities of daily living (ADL). "Background" neurologic signs, such as slowed fine finger movements or primitive reflexes, may be present.
Stage 1 (mild)	Cognitive deficit that compromises the performance of the more demanding aspects of work or ADL.
Stage 2 (moderate)	Cognitive deficit makes the patient unable to perform work or the more demanding aspects of ADL. The patient may require assistance with walking.
Stage 3 (severe)	Cognitive deficit makes it possible for the patient to perform only the most rudimentary tasks; for example, the patient cannot follow news or sustain a conversation of any complexity. The patient often requires some support for walking.
Stage 4 (end stage)	Cognitive deficit has reached the point where the patient has virtually no understanding of his or her surroundings and is virtually mute. The patient is paraparetic or paraplegic, often with double incontinence.

and half or more of the patients will manifest facial hypomotility, failure of tandem gait, and an action tremor. Less common findings include mild leg weakness (just under 50 percent), a positive glabellar tap/snout response (one-quarter), and peripheral neuropathy characterized by depressed or absent ankle jerks (one-third). Myoclonus and chorea are found in only a very small percentage of patients. As the disorder progresses, patients become globally demented, mute, paraparetic, and incontinent of urine and feces. The modified staging scheme for ADC is listed in Table 50-1, with median survival of 10, 4.6, and 1.4 months for stages 1, 2, 3, and 4 (combined) respectively in patients not treated with HAART.[7]

At present, there are no investigations diagnostic of ADC; such studies are done predominantly to exclude other causes of cognitive impairment. However, reduced *N*-acetylaspartate and increased choline levels on magnetic resonance spectroscopy[8,9] and increased cerebrospinal fluid (CSF) HIV viral load[10,11] are supportive of a diagnosis of ADC. Neuropsychological testing showing impaired attention and slowing of motor-based processes, with sparing of recognition memory, is also characteristic of ADC.[12]

The pathogenesis of ADC is complicated and only partly understood. HIV is thought to enter the brain either directly through infected lymphocytes/monocytes or via the meningeal macrophage/CSF compartment.[13] Once in the brain, HIV productively infects microglial cells, leading to the formation of whole intact virions. Other neural elements, such as astrocytes, support restricted infection, where components of the virus, usually the regulatory proteins, are released rather than whole virions. A variety of toxins is then elaborated by both HIV (env, tat, nef, and vpr) and the host, including quinolinic acid, tumor necrosis factor-alpha, and platelet-activating factor, among many others.[14] Neuronal death and dysfunction are subsequently mediated via activation of the *N*-methyl-D-aspartate receptor,[15] with myelin damage secondary to alterations in the blood-brain barrier[16] and cytokines. These changes affect predominantly the deeper structures of the brain, in particular the basal ganglia, perhaps paralleling the dominant distribution of microglia.

Combination antiretroviral treatment of patients with ADC should ideally include at least two drugs that are able to enter the brain (zidovudine, stavudine, abacavir, lamivudine, nevirapine, efavirenz, and indinavir), although definite proof of the superior efficacy of such a strategy is lacking at present. Genotypic resistance testing to antiretroviral drugs in the CSF and blood should also be employed to assist in the selection of an appropriate drug regimen. Clinical effect of treatment may be expected by week 6,[17] though sustained improvement may continue up to 6 months.[18] Symptomatic treatment of mood disturbance is also important, and drugs with minimal extrapyramidal side effects (such as olanzapine) should be used if a neuroleptic is needed.

PROGRESSIVE MULTIFOCAL LEUKOENCEPHALOPATHY

Progressive multifocal leukoencephalopathy (PML) is a demyelinating disease of the central nervous system caused by infection of B cells and oligodendrocytes by the polyoma JC virus.[19] Prior to the HIV epidemic, PML was a rare disease associated predominantly with hematologic malignancies such as lymphoproliferative disorders.[20] PML is now relatively common, occurring in up to 4 percent of patients with advanced HIV disease (mean CD4 cells 30 to 104/μL) in the pre-HAART era.[21,22]

PML presents characteristically with a neurologic deficit (hemiparesis, altered mental status, headache, and ataxia) over several weeks with no fever or raised intracranial pressure. In 60 percent of HIV-related PML, there is a single localization, as opposed to non-HIV-related PML.[21] About 36 percent of HIV-related cases of PML present with cognitive abnormalities as the initial neurologic problem.[21,22]

Diagnosis is aided by magnetic resonance imaging (MRI) demonstrating predominantly white matter nonenhancing, high signal intensities on T2-weighted images, though the MRI can rarely be normal.[23] CSF polymerase chain reaction (PCR) for JC virus has a sensitivity and specificity of 65 and 92 percent[24] respectively in HIV-related PML, and brain biopsy may be needed for definitive diagnosis.

Treatment with HAART in HIV-related PML has been demonstrated to improve most but not all patients, reducing the risk of death by up to 63 percent, but the improvement in neurologic deficit is variable.[25] Anecdotal reports have suggested that cidofovir is efficacious, but a larger controlled study has not confirmed this.[26] There are also some case reports on the usefulness of interferon alpha.[27] Cytosine arabinoside probably has only a very limited role.[28] There are no randomized controlled trials for the treatment of non-HIV-related PML. The only data that exist relate to a case series where some efficacy for cytosine arabinoside was found.[29]

PRION DISEASES

Prions are disease-causing isoforms of cellular prion proteins (cellular PrP). Cellular PrPs are membrane proteins of uncertain physiologic function normally present in cells. The pathogenic isoform of PrP produces a protease-resistant residue that polymerizes into amyloid, forming plaques that are pathognomonic of prion diseases. Prions are devoid of nucleic acids and reproduce by converting normal PrP into the pathogenic isoform instead.[30] Other histologic findings include spongiform changes, atrophy, and gliosis, all without inflammatory cell infiltrates.

Clinically, prion diseases may present as Gerstmann-Straussler-Scheinker (GSS) syndrome, fatal familial insomnia (FFI), kuru, classic Creutzfeldt-Jakob disease (CJD), or variant Creutzfeldt-Jakob disease (vCJD). GSS is caused by mutations of the human prion protein (PRNP) gene, leading to large multicentric PrP-containing amyloid plaques. It presents predominantly as an ataxic disorder with an autosomal dominant mode of inheritance and can be distinguished from CJD with its milder degrees of subcortical dementia and myoclonus.[31] FFI is caused by a D178N mutation of the PRNP gene, leading to neuronal loss predominantly in the thalami. It presents with nocturnal insomnia, episodic stupor, dementia, and dysautonomia and can be distinguished from CJD by the absence of 14-3-3 protein in the CSF.[32] Kuru, a progressive ataxic disease with tremor, emotional lability, and dementia, has all but disappeared upon the banning of cannibalism in Papua New Guinea in the 1960s.[32]

Creutzfeldt-Jakob Disease

The incidence rate of CJD is 0.5 to 1 per million per year,[33–35] with 8 percent of the cases being familial and 5 percent iatrogenic; but the majority are sporadic with no clear etiology.[34] Sixteen point mutations and 15 insertions have been described in exon 2 of the human prion protein gene on chromosome 20, accounting for many of the familial CJD cases.[31] Contaminated cadaveric growth hormone and dura grafts account for 94 percent of the 268 reported cases of iatrogenic CJD,[36] the rest being linked to neurosurgery/stereotactic electroencephalography (EEG), corneal implants, and gonadotropin administration. Etiologic agents are rarely found for cases of sporadic CJD.[37]

Clinically, CJD patients most commonly present with a progressive subcortical dementia with myoclonus (>80 percent) or cerebellar (>50 percent), pyramidal (>50 percent), or extrapyramidal (>50 percent) dysfunction.[38] The sporadic or familial forms of CJD more commonly present with cognitive deficits, while iatrogenic cases tend to present with cerebellar dysfunction.[39] Periodic sharp wave complexes on EEG have been regarded as characteristic for CJD in the appropriate clinical context, though they are not an early finding. They have a sensitivity of 66 to 67 percent and specificity of 74 to 86 percent.[40,41] Protein 14-3-3 is a cellular signal transduction protein released into the CSF upon neuronal damage and has been demonstrated to be highly sensitive and specific for patients with clinical features of CJD (sensitivity 94 to 97 percent, specificity 84 to 87 percent[40,42]). However, the release of CSF 14-3-3 is not an exclusively CJD-related pathologic process, and its positive predictive value can be as low as 14 percent among unselected dementia patients.[43] Several clinical diagnostic criteria have been established for probable CJD, including the Masters criteria[44] and the European study criteria[45] (which requires EEG changes or CSF 14-3-3 detection). When compared against autopsy as the reference standard, the Masters criteria are sensitive (95.9 percent) but not specific (17.5 percent), while the European study criteria are specific (95 percent) but less sensitive (65.3 percent).[46] To date there is no proven therapy for CJD, though a trial has been announced using the antimalarial quinacrine,[47] which has been demonstrated to inhibit the pathogenic conversion of prion protein in vitro.[48] Recombinant antibodies have also been developed that inhibit prion propagation in vitro.[49]

Variant Creutzfeldt-Jakob Disease

In 1996, as part of a national CJD surveillance program set up in response to the 1986 bovine spongiform encephalopathy (BSE) epidemic in the United Kingdom, a new variant of CJD (vCJD) was identified. vCJD affects a younger population than classic CJD (mean age 29 versus 60) and presents with early psychiatric and sensory features—both atypical for classic CJD.[50] These psychiatric features characteristically include depression and apathy, while the sensory features include foot pain and paresthesia in the lower limbs. Although periodic sharp waves are absent on EEG examination, a bilateral increased pulvinar signal on MRI is highly specific.[51] The neuropathology of vCJD is also characteristic, with florid PrP plaques surrounded by vacuoles. The clinical diagnostic criteria incorporating the EEG and MRI features have been established with a sensitivity of 77 percent and specificity of 64 percent.[52] There has been some controversy over the origin of vCJD, but there is a growing consensus that vCJD has emerged from BSE-contaminated mechanically recovered beef, which in turn entered the cattle population via contaminated feeds (meat and bone meals, or MBM) manufactured from sheep carcasses with scrapies.[53] The BSE epidemic is hypothesized to have started in Britain due to its unusual practice of feeding MBM not only to older cattle but also younger calves, which may be more susceptible to BSE.[54] The first case of BSE in a cow born outside Europe was found in Japan in September 2001[55]—though no vCJD has been reported from Japan to date.

NEUROSYPHILIS

Treponema pallidum infection may present as a cognitive deficit associated with syphilitic vasculitis or dementia paralytica. The former may present in different ways depending on the vessels involved, though the middle cerebral and basilar arterial territories are most commonly affected.[56] Dementia paralytica has a peak incidence of 10 to 20 years after primary infection and presents initially with a memory and cognitive deficit similar to that of Alzheimer's disease. Psychiatric symptoms (including mania, psychosis, or depression), dysarthria, optic atrophy, and seizures may follow in the ensuing 3 to 4 years. None of the antibody assays is perfect for the diagnosis of neurosyphilis,[57] but the serum *T. pallidum* hemagglutination assay (TPHA) is regarded as the best screening test, with a specificity of over 98 percent[58] and a sensitivity of 98 percent in late syphilis.[59] CSF examination may demonstrate elevated protein and a lymphocytosis (in about 63 percent of cases[58]). Both the CSF-TPHA and the CSF fluorescent treponemal antibody absorption tests (FTA-ABS IgG) are subject to false positives due to passive immunoglobulin transfer across the meninges; therefore a positive result is of little diagnostic value. With a near 100 percent specificity, the CSF Venereal Disease Research Laboratory (VDRL) test is therefore used to 'rule in' neurosyphilis despite its low sensitivity (27 to 79 percent).[58,60] An additional problem with serum syphilis screening is a high false-positive rate (for neurosyphilis) in the elderly, as demonstrated by a 10.9 percent FTA-ABS positivity rate among a cohort of demented patients with no clinical evidence of neurosyphilis.[61] Neurosyphilis occurs in up to 9 percent of neurologically symptomatic HIV-infected individuals,[62] and these patients are more likely to lose reactivity to syphilis serologic tests[63]; thus the index of suspicion should be high in this patient group. Recommended treatment for neurosyphilis has been 3 weeks of intramuscular procaine penicillin with oral probenecid or 3 weeks of IV benzylpenicillin,[64] though there are early data raising the possibility of using ceftriaxone.[65] Poor prognosis has been associated with persistent CSF-VDRL serology[66] and medial temporal atrophy on MRI.[67]

LYME DISEASE

Lyme disease is a tick-borne disorder caused by the spirochete *Borrelia burgdorferi.* It typically presents with erythema migrans, myalgia, and arthritis and may be associated with atrioventricular heart block.[57] Neurologic manifestations occur in up to 40 percent of the patients[68] and can be protean—ranging from myopathy, peripheral neuropathy, and meningitis to demyelinating encephalopathy.[69,70] Cognitive deficit following Lyme disease predominantly involves deficits in memory and verbal skills.[71] Antibody testing for *B. burgdorferi* is prone to false positives, though the sensitivity and specificity can be improved to 83 and 95 percent using a strict criterion on Western blotting after the first weeks of infection.[72] CSF antibody testing is thought to be specific, but prospective data evaluating this are scarce[73] and a positive result may persist after successful treatment.[57] PCR for *B. burgdorferi* in CSF is positive in only about 40 percent of patients with Lyme meningitis.[74] The treatment of choice for neurologic complications of Lyme disease is intravenous penicillin[75] or cephalosporin,[76] though the role of antibiotics in Lyme disease–associated cognitive deficits is unclear.[71]

WHIPPLE'S DISEASE

Whipple's disease is a multisystem chronic granulomatous disease caused by *Tropheryma whippelii,* primarily involving the small bowel. Neurologic complications occur in up to 50 percent of patients[77] and may occur without involvement of other systems in 5 percent.[78] Psychiatric manifestations accompany cognitive deficit in up to half the patients. Oculomasticatory myorhythmia (pendular nystagmus with synchronous jaw contraction), while pathognomonic, is present in only 20 percent.[78] Vertical gaze palsy can be helpful in the appropriate clinical context. Diagnosis of Whipple's disease is usually established by small bowel biopsy, which may be aided by PCR amplification of the bacteria's 16S ribosomal RNA.[77] CSF can also be tested with cytology or PCR. However, around 70 percent of patients with Whipple's disease may test positive by cytology or PCR regardless of the presence of any clinical neurologic involvement.[79] Trimethoprim-sulfamethoxazole (TMP-SMX) is one standard treatment regimen with good central nervous system penetration, but treatment failure has been reported in a number of cases.[80] This has led Schnider et al.[80] to suggest a treatment regimen of 2 weeks of IV ceftriaxone plus streptomycin or intravenous TMP-SMX followed by 1 year of oral TMP-SMX.

SUBACUTE SCLEROSING PANENCEPHALITIS

The measles virus was first isolated from a patient with subacute sclerosing panencephalitis (SSPE) in 1969.[81] SSPE is caused by persistent infection of genetically mutated forms of the measles virus that escape immune clearance due to defective envelope proteins (especially the matrix or "M"-protein).[82] Its incidence is 4 per 100,000 postmeasles, and 0.14 postvaccination[83]; it has therefore become a rare disease in countries with mass measles vaccination programs. SSPE typically presents 6 to 15 years after the initial infection, with behavioral symptoms such as poor school performance, irritability, and attention problems.[84] Periodic myoclonic spasms typically occur next, with spasticity, extrapyramidal symptoms, and optic atrophy progressing over the ensuing 1 to 2 years. SSPE also occurs in an adult form (age 20 to 35), where visual symptoms may be more prominent.[85] Findings on investigation may include elevated serum and CSF measles-specific antibody titers[84] and a nonspecific EEG with bilateral high-amplitude symmetrical periodic complexes.[86] MRI typically shows asymmetrical gray matter and subcortical white matter lesions in the early stages, progressing to high signal changes in deep white matter and severe cerebral atrophy.[87] Data on treatment efficacy are based on small patient numbers, but insoprinosine (with or without intraventricular interferon) seems most effective, while amantadine and cimetidine have also been used in this setting.[88]

PROGRESSIVE RUBELLA PANENCEPHALITIS

Progressive rubella panencephalitis is rare and was first described in 1975. It is characterized by a cognitive deficit accompanied by ataxia and myoclonic seizures.[89] It forms a differential for SSPE, though the age of presentation is later and signs of congenital rubella syndrome are present in most.[90] MRI may show diffuse atrophy and antirubella IgG may be detected in the CSF. There is no specific therapy.

POSTMENINGITIC SYNDROMES

Dementia-like syndromes have been reported following anthropod-borne encephalitides[91] and chronic meningitides caused by tuberculosis,[92] histoplasmosis, and candidiasis.[93] Cognitive and memory disturbances have also been observed up to 12 years after acute bacterial meningitis.[94,95] However, it is not clear whether these cognitive deficits are truly progressive.

SUMMARY

Generally speaking, dementias with infective causes tend to present as subcortical dementias, with cognitive deficits, behavioral disturbances, and motor/movement disorders. In the past, these conditions had been difficult to diagnose with certainty antemortem, and treatment options had been limited. However, with increasingly well validated molecular techniques and magnetic resonance imaging/spectroscopy, diagnostic accuracy has improved. Treatment options of varying efficacy have also emerged, rendering infective causes an essential consideration in the workup for dementing patients.

REFERENCES

1. Weytingh MD, Bossuyt PM, Van Crevel H: Reversible dementia: more than 10% or less than 1%? A quantitative review. *J Neurol* 242:466–71, 1995.
2. McArthur JC, Hoover DR, Bacellar H, et al: Dementia in AIDS patients: Incidence and risk factors. Multicenter AIDS Cohort Study. *Neurology* 43:2245–2252, 1993.
3. Portegies P, Enting RH, de Gans J, et al: Presentation and course of AIDS dementia complex: 10 years of follow-up in Amsterdam, the Netherlands. *AIDS* 7:669–675, 1993.
4. Dore G, Correll P, Kaldor J, et al: Changes to the natural history of AIDS dementia complex in the era of HAART. *AIDS* 13:1249–1253, 1999.
5. Dore GJ, Hoy J, Mallal SA, et al: Trends in incidence of AIDS illnesses in Australia from 1983 to 1994: the Australian AIDS Cohort. *JAIDS* 16(1):39–43: 1997.
6. Brew BJ: *HIV Neurology*. New York, Oxford University Press, 2001; pp 53–90.
7. Pan Y, Dore C, van der Bij A, et al: Prognosis of AIDS dementia complex (ADC) and predictors of post ADC survival. Australian Society for HIV Medicine Annual Meeting. Melbourne, October 12–14, 2000.
8. Navia BA, Lee PL, Chang L, et al: Metabolite changes in the basal ganglia provide a signature for the AIDS dementia complex: a multicenter proton magnetic resonance study. *Neurology* 52(S2):A253, 1999.
9. Chang L, Ernst T, Leonido-Yee M, et al: Cerebral metabolites correlate with clinical severity of HIV-cognitive motor complex. *Neurology* 52:100–108, 1999.
10. Brew BJ, Pemberton L, Cunningham P, et al: Levels of HIV-1 RNA correlate with AIDS dementia. *J Infect Dis* 175:963–966, 1997.
11. McArthur JC, McClernon DR, Cronin MF, et al: Relationship between human immunodeficiency virus–associated dementia and viral load in cerebrospinal fluid and brain. *Ann Neurol* 42:689–698: 1997.

12. Dunbar N, Brew BJ: Neuropsychological dysfunction in HIV infection: a review. *J NeuroAIDS* 1(3):73–102, 1996.
13. Brew BJ, Wesselingh SL, Gonzales M, et al: How HIV leads to neurological disease. *Med J Aust* 164:233–234, 1996.
14. Price RW: The cellular basis of central nervous system HIV-1 infection and the AIDS dementia complex: introduction. *J NeuroAIDS* 1:1–30, 1996.
15. Lipton SA, Gendelman HE: Dementia associated with the acquired immunodeficiency syndrome. *N Engl J Med* 332(14):934–940, 1995.
16. Power C, Kong PA, Crawford TO, et al: Cerebral white matter changes in acquired immunodeficiency syndrome dementia: alterations of the blood brain barrier. *Ann Neurol* 34:339–359, 1993.
17. Brew BJ, Brown SJ, Catalan J, et al: Safety and efficacy of Abacavir (ABC, 1592) in AIDS dementia complex (Study CNAB 3001). 12th World AIDS Conference. Geneva, June 28–July 3, 1998.
18. Tozzi V, Balestra P, Galgani S, et al: Positive and sustained effects of highly active antiretroviral therapy on HIV-1 associated neurocognitive impairment. *AIDS* 13:1889–1897, 1999.
19. Berger JR, Major EO: Progressive multifocal leukoencephalopathy. *Semin Neurol* 19(2):193–200, 1999.
20. Brooks BR, Walker DL: Progressive multifocal leukoencephalopathy. *Neurol Clin* 2:299–313, 1984.
21. Adcock J, Davies M, Turner J, et al: Progressive multifocal leukoencephalopathy: a retrospective series of 30 patients. *J Clin Neurosci* 4: 463–468, 1997.
22. Berger JR, Pall L, Lanska D, et al: Progressive multifocal leukoencephalopathy in patients with HIV infection. *J Neurovirol* 59–68, 1998.
23. Sweeney NJ, Manji H, Miller RF, et al: Cortical and subcortical JC virus infection: two unusual cases of AIDS associated progressive multifocal leukoencephalopathy. *J Neurol Neurosurg Psych* 57:994–997, 1994.
24. Cinque P, Scarpellinin P, Vago L, et al: Diagnosis of central nervous system complications in HIV infected patients: cerebrospinal fluid analysis by polymerase chain reaction. *AIDS* 11:1–17, 1997.
25. Gasnault J, Taoufik Y, Kousignian P, et al: Effects of protease inhibitors on neurological course in AIDS-PML. *J Neurvirol* 4:351, 1998.
26. Gasnault J, Toufik Y, Abbed K, et al: Experience of cidofovir in HIV-associated progressive multifocal leukoencephalopathy: clinical and virological monitoring. Sixth Conference on Retroviruses and Opportunistic Infections. Chicago, January 31–February 4, 1999.
27. Huang SS, Skolansky RL, Dal Pan GJ, et al: Survival prolongation in HIV-associated progressive multifocal leukoencephalopathy treated with alpha-interferon: an observational study. *J Neurovirol* 4: 324–332, 1998.
28. Hall C, Dafni I, Simpson D, et al: Failure of cytarabine in progressive multifocal leukoencephalopathy associated with human immunodeficiency virus infection. *N Eng J Med* 338: 1345–1351, 1998.
29. Aksamit AJ: Treatment of non-AIDS progressive multifocal leukoencephalopathy with cytosine arabinoside. *J Neurovirol* 7:386–390, 2001.
30. Prusiner SB: Shattuck lecture—neurodegenerative diseases and prions. *N Engl J Med* 344(20):1516–1526, 2001.
31. Windl O, Kretzschmar HA: Prion diseases, in: Pulst S (ed): *Neurogenetics*. New York: Oxford University Press, 2000, pp 191–218.
32. Collins S, McLean CA, Masters CL: Gerstmann-Straussler-Scheinker syndrome, fatal familial insomnia, and kuru: a review of these less common human transmissible spongiform encephalopathies. *J Clin Neurosci* 8(5):387–397, 2001.
33. Gibbons RV, Holman RC, Belay ED, et al: Creutzfeldt-Jakob disease in the United States: 1979–1998. *JAMA* 284(18):2322–2323, 2000.
34. Will RG, Alperovitch A, Poser S, et al: Descriptive epidemiology of Creutzfeldt-Jakob disease in six European countries, 1993–1995. EU Collaborative Study Group for CJD. *Ann Neurol* 43(6):763–767, 1998.
35. Nakamura Y, Yanagawa H, Hoshi K, et al: Incidence rate of Creutzfeldt-Jakob disease in Japan. *Int J Epilepsy* 28(1):130–134, 1999.
36. Brown P, Preece M, Brandel JP, et al: Iatrogenic Creutzfeldt-Jakob disease at the millennium. *Neurology* 55(8):1075–1081, 2000.
37. Wientjens DP, Davanipour Z, Hofman A, et al: Risk factors for Creutzfeldt-Jakob disease: a reanalysis of case-control studies. *Neurology* 46(5):1287–1291, 1996.
38. Johnson RT, Gibbs CJ: Creutzfeldt-Jakob disease and related transmissible spongiform encephalopathies. *N Engl J Med* 339(27):1994–2004, 1998.
39. Weihl CC, Roos RP: Creutzfeldt-Jakob disease, new variant Creutzfeldt-Jakob disease, and bovine spongiform encephalopathy. *Neurol Clin* 17(4):835–859, 1999.
40. Zerr I, Pocchiari M, Collins S, et al: Analysis of EEG and CSF 14-3-3 proteins as aids to the diagnosis of Creutzfeldt-Jakob disease. *Neurology* 55(6):811–815, 2000.
41. Steinhoff BJ, Racker S, Herrendorf G, et al: Accuracy and reliability of periodic sharp wave complexes

in Creutzfeldt-Jakob disease. *Arch Neurol* 53(2):162–166,1996.

42. Lemstra AW, van Meegen MT, Vreyling JP, et al: 14-3-3 testing in diagnosing Creutzfeldt-Jakob disease: a prospective study in 112 patients. *Neurology* 55(4): 514–516: 2000.
43. Burkhard PR, Sanchez JC, Landis T, et al: CSF detection of the 14-3-3 protein in unselected patients with dementia. *Neurology* 56(11):1528–1533, 2001.
44. Masters CL, Harris JO, Gajdusek DC, et al: Creutzfeldt-Jakob disease: patterns of worldwide occurrence and the significance of familial and sporadic clustering. *Ann Neurol* 5(2):177–188, 1979.
45. Concerted action of the EU: Surveillance of Creutzfeldt-Jakob disease in the European Community. Minutes of the meeting in Amsterdam, June 12–13; 1998.
46. Brandel JP, Delasnerie-Laupretre N, Laplanche JL, et al: Diagnosis of Creutzfeldt-Jakob disease: effect of clinical criteria on incidence estimates. *Neurology* 54(5):1095–1099, 2000.
47. Anonymous: News in brief. *Nature* 413(6854): 340–341, 2001.
48. Korth C, May BCH, Cohen FE, et al: Acridine and phenothiazine derivatives as pharmacotherapeutics for prion disease. *PNAS* 98(17):9836–9841, 2001.
49. Peretz D, Williason RA, Kaneko K, et al: Antibodies inhibit prion propagation and clear cell cultures of prion infectivity. *Nature* 412 (6848):739–743, 2001.
50. Zeidler M, Stewart GE, Barraclough CR, et al: New variant Creutzfeldt-Jakob disease: neurological features and diagnostic tests. *Lancet* 350:903–907, 1997.
51. Zeidler M, Sellar RJ, Collie DA, et al: The pulvinar sign on magnetic resonance imaging in variant Creutzfeldt-Jakob disease. *Lancet* 355:1412–1418, 2000.
52. Will RG, Zeidler M, Stewart GE, et al: Diagnosis of new variant Creutzfeldt-Jakob disease. *Ann Neurol* 47(5):575–582, 2000.
53. Brown P: Bovine spongiform encephalopathy and variant Creutzfeldt-Jakob disease. *Br Med J* 322(7290):841–844, 2001.
54. Adam D: Review blames BSE outbreak on calf feed. *Nature* 412(6846):467, 2001.
55. Giles J: Mad cow disease comes to Japan. *Nature* 413(6853):240, 2001.
56. Scheck DN, Hook EW: Neurosyphilis. *Inf Dis Clin North Am* 8(4):769–795, 1994.
57. Estanislao LB, Pachner AR: Spirochetal infection of the nervous system. *Neurol Clin* 17(4):783–800, 1999.
58. Black ER, Bordley DR, Tape TG, et al (eds): *Diagnostic Strategies for Common Medical Problems,* 2d ed. Philadelphia: American College of Physicians, 1999, pp 315–319.
59. Roos KL: Neurosyphilis. *Sem Neurol* 12(3):209–212, 1992.
60. Al-Semari AM, Bohlega SI, Cupler EJ, et al: Pitfalls in cerebrospinal fluid test for the diagnosis of neurosyphilis. *Saudi Med J* 22(1):26–29, 2001.
61. Powell AL, Coyne AC, Jen L: A retrospective study of syphilis seropositivity in a cohort of demented patients. *Alzheimer Dis Assoc Disord* 7(1):33–38, 1993.
62. Holtom PD, Larsen RA, Leal ME, et al: Prevalence of neurosyphilis in human immunodeficiency virus–infected patients with latent syphilis. *Am J Med* 93:9–12, 1992.
63. Johnson PD, Graves SR, Stewart L, et al: Specific syphilis serological tests may become negative in HIV infection. *AIDS* 5:419–423, 1991.
64. Clinical Effectiveness Group (Association of Genitourinary Medicine and the Medical Society for the Study of Venereal Diseases): National guideline for the management of late syphilis. *Sex Transm Infect* 75(S1):S34–S37, 1999.
65. Marra CM, Boutin P, McArthur JC, et al: A pilot study evaluating ceftriaxone and penicillin G as treatment agents for neurosyphilis in human immunodeficiency virus–infected individuals. *Clin Infect Dis* 30(3):540–544, 2000.
66. Roberts MC, Emsley RA: Cognitive change after treatment for neurosyphilis: correlation with CSF laboratory measures. *Gen Hosp Psychiatry* 17(4):305–309, 1995.
67. Kodama K, Okada S, Komatsu N, et al: Relationship between MRI findings and prognosis for patients with general paresis. *J Neuropsychiatr Clin Neurosci* 12(2):246–250, 2000.
68. Fallon BA, Nields JA: Lyme disease: a neuropsychiatric illness. *Am J Psychiatry* 151(11):1571–1583, 1994.
69. Haass A: Lyme neuroborreliosis. *Curr Opin Neurol* 11(3):253–258, 1998.
70. Reik L, Smith L, Khan A, et al: Demyelinating encephalopathy in Lyme disease. *Neurology* 35: 267–269, 1985.
71. Benke T, Gasse T, Hittmair-Delazer M, et al: Lyme encephalopathy: long-term neuropsychological deficits years after acute neuroborreliosis. *Acta Neurol Scand* 91:353–357, 1995.
72. Dressler F, Whalen JA, Reinhardt BN, et al: Western blotting in the serodiagnosis of Lyme disease. *J Infect Dis* 167:392–400, 1993.
73. Tugwell P, Dennis DT, Weintstein A, et al: Laboratory evaluation in the diagnosis of Lyme disease. *Ann Intern Med* 127(12):1109–1123, 1997.

74. Lebech AM, Hansen K: Detection of *Borrelia burgdorferi* DNA by polymerase chain reaction in urine and cerebrospinal fluid of patients with early and late Lyme neuroborreliosis. *J Clin Microbiol* 30:1646–1653, 1992.
75. Steere AC, Pachner AR, Malawista SE: Successful treatment of neurologic abnormalities of Lyme disease with high dose intravenous penicillin. *Ann Intern Med* 99: 767–772, 1983.
76. Logigian EL, Kaplan RF, Steere AC: Chronic neurologic manifestations of Lyme disease. *N Engl J Med* 323: 1438–1444, 1990.
77. Ratnaike RN: Whipple's disease. *Postgrad Med J* 76: 760–766, 2000.
78. Louis ED, Lynch T, Kaufmann P, et al: Diagnostic guidelines in central nervous system Whipple's disease. *Ann Neurol* 40(4):561–568, 1996.
79. Von Herbay A, Ditton HJ, Schuhmacher F, et al: Whipple's disease: staging and monitoring by cytology and polymerase chain reaction analysis of cerebrospinal fluid. *Gastroenterology* 113:434–441, 1997.
80. Schnider PJ, Reisinger EC, Berger T, et al: Treatment guidelines in central nervous system Whipple's disease. *Ann Neurol* 41(4):561–562, 1997.
81. Payne FE, Baublis JV, Itabashi HH: Isolation of measles virus from cell cultures of brain from a patient with subacute sclerosing panencephalitis. *N Engl J Med* 281:585–589, 1969.
82. Norrby E, Kristensson K: Measles virus in the brain. *Brain Res Bull* 44(3):213–220, 1997.
83. Miller C, Farrington CP, Harbert K: The epidemiology of subacute sclerosing panencephalitis in England and Wales 1970–1989. *Int J Epidemiol* 21(5):998–1006, 1992.
84. Gascon GG: Subacute sclerosing panencephalitis. *Semin Pediatr Neurol* 3(4):260–269, 1996.
85. Singer C, Lang AE, Suchowersky O: Adult-onset subacute sclerosing panencephalitis: case reports and review of the literature. *Mov Disord* 12(3):342–353, 1997.
86. Gurses C, Ozturk A, Baykan B, et al: Correlation between clinical stages and EEG findings of subacute sclerosing panencephalitis. *Clin Electroencephalogr* 31(4):201–206, 2000.
87. Tuncay R, Akman-Demir G, Gokyigit A, et al: MRI in subacute sclerosing panencephalitis. *Neuroradiol* 38(7):636–640, 1996.
88. Panagariya A, Sureka RK, Aurora A: Current developments in the management of subacute sclerosing panencephalitis. *JAPI* 46(2):218–220, 1998.
89. Weil ML, Itabashi H, Cremer NE, et al: Chronic progressive panencephalitis due to rubella virus simulating subacute sclerosing panencephalitis. *N Engl J Med* 292(19):994–998, 1975.
90. Kuroda Y, Matsui M: Progressive rubella panencephalitis. *Jpn J Clin Med* 55:922–925, 1997.
91. Bailey P, Baker AB (eds): Sequelae of the arthropod-borne encephalitides. *Neurology* 8:878–896, 1958.
92. Williams M, Smith HV: Mental disturbances in tuberculous meningitis. *J Neurol Neurosurg Psychiatry* 17:173–182, 1954.
93. Cummings JL, Benson DF: *Dementia: A Clinical Approach,* 2d ed. Boston: Butterworth-Heinemann, 1992, p 208.
94. Merkelbach S, Sittinger H, Schweizer I, et al: Cognitive outcome after bacterial meningitis. *Acta Neurol Scand* 102:118–123, 2000.
95. Grimwood K, Anderson P, Anderson V, et al: Twelve-year outcomes following bacterial meningitis: further evidence for persisting effects. *Arch Dis Child* 83:111–116, 2000.

Chapter 51

WERNICKE-KORSAKOFF AND RELATED NUTRITIONAL DISORDERS OF THE NERVOUS SYSTEM*

Mieke Verfaellie

CLINICAL PRESENTATION

In 1881, Wernicke described a neurologic syndrome of acute onset characterized by ataxia, ophthalmoplegia, nystagmus, polyneuropathy in the arms and legs, and a global confusional state. Shortly thereafter, Korsakoff[1,2] described the chronic changes in mental status and memory he observed in patients with disorders involving polyneuropathy. Not until several years later[3] was it realized that the symptoms described by Wernicke and Korsakoff often occur sequentially in the same patients and represent a functional syndrome now generally referred to as Wernicke-Korsakoff syndrome (WKS). Although most commonly associated with chronic alcoholism, the syndrome is also seen in a number of other disorders leading to nutritional insufficiency, including prolonged vomiting, gastrointestinal carcinoma, dialysis, and AIDS.

The onset of WKS is usually marked by an acute phase in which the patient is disoriented, confused and apathetic, and unable to maintain a coherent conversation. This confusional state is often accompanied by ataxia and oculomotor problems. Traditionally, this triad of neurologic signs was a prerequisite for a diagnosis of Wernicke's encephalopathy, but it is now clear that these problems do not necessarily co-occur in a single patient.[4] More recently, it has been suggested that a diagnosis of Wernicke's encephalopathy be based on at least two of the following criteria: (1) dietary deficiencies; (2) oculomotor abnormalities; (3) cerebellar dysfunction; and (4) altered mental status.[5]

* **ACKNOWLEDGMENTS:** Preparation of this chapter was supported by grants NS26985 and MH57681 to Boston University School of Medicine and by the Medical Research Service of the U.S. Department of Veterans Affairs.

Unless treated with thiamine (vitamin B_1), the patient is in danger of having fatal midbrain hemorrhages. Given appropriate treatment, however, the neurologic signs improve rapidly and markedly. Once the acute confusion clears, the patient is frequently left with an enduring dense amnesia characteristic of the Korsakoff stage of the disorder. Although some patients have been described to recover to a premorbid level of functioning, this is a rare occurrence.[4] Because of considerable variability in its presentation, Wernicke's encephalopathy may at times go unrecognized until autopsy.[6] Indeed, some patients may evolve to the Korsakoff stage of the disorder without clinical evidence of an antecedent Wernicke's encephalopathy.[7,8]

The hallmark of the chronic stage of WKS is the inability to retrieve recent memories and learn new information in the context of otherwise relatively preserved cognitive functioning. The selective and acute nature of the memory disorder sets it apart from alcoholic dementia, a syndrome characterized by more global impairments in intellectual functioning that evolve gradually over time.[9,10] Despite differences in clinical presentation between these two syndromes, controversy remains as to whether a nosologic distinction is justified on neuropathologic grounds.[11–13]

The incidence of WKS is rare, having been estimated in one study at approximately 10 per million of first psychiatric admissions.[14] Other statistics, based on hospital admissions as well as general population studies, estimate its occurrence at approximately 50 per million.[7,15] Notwithstanding its rare occurrence, the neuropsychological sequelae of WKS have been studied in extensive detail because patients with WKS provided one of the first opportunities to systematically examine the information processing deficits underlying selective amnesia.[16,17]

NEUROPSYCHOLOGICAL PROFILE

General Cognitive Status

Despite severe amnesia, general intelligence is commonly well preserved in WKS.[16,17] Accordingly, many group studies of WKS patients have reported mean IQ scores as measured by the revised Wechsler Adult Intelligence Scale (WAIS-R) in the average range (see e.g., Ref. 18). Our experience to date suggests that patients also perform in the normal range on the WAIS-III.[19] Table 51-1 illustrates the WAIS-III performance of a representative group of 7 patients followed at the Memory Disorders Research Center. As can be seen, these patients perform in the average range on all subtests of the WAIS-III with the exception of the Digit Symbol subtest, a measure of visuomotor performance. The same table also illustrates the severity of these patients' memory deficit as indicated by performance on the Wechsler Memory Scale-III.[20] A discrepancy of more than two standard deviations between IQ and both Immediate and Delayed Memory is commonly observed. Of note is the average Working Memory Quotient, a finding indicative of patients' simple attentional functions as well as their ability to maintain and manipulate information over brief periods of time. The difference between Working Memory and General Memory therefore provides a good indication of the severity of amnesia in this patient group.

Table 51-1
*Mean WAIS-III (selected subtests) and WMS-III scores in a representative group of Korsakoff patients**

WAIS-III	
Full-Scale IQ	96.6
Working Memory	102.9
Processing Speed	95.0
Verbal IQ	97.0
Vocabulary	8.7
Similarities	8.0
Arithmetic	11.1
Digit Span	10.6
Information	9.1
Performance IQ	96.0
Matrix Reasoning	10.7
Symbol Search	10.7
Picture Completion	9.0
Digit Symbol	7.7
Block Design	9.7
WMS-III	
Immediate Memory	63.6
Auditory Immediate	76.1
Visual Immediate	63.0
General Memory	64.4
Auditory Delay	66.6
Visual Delay	65.3
Auditory Recognition	81.4
Working Memory	99.6

*WAIS-III subtest scores are age-scaled.

Despite their relatively well-preserved intellectual abilities, WKS patients do demonstrate deficits in a number of domains other than memory. Impairments in visuospatial and visuoperceptual functioning have been observed in a number of tasks. These include Digit Symbol and Symbol Digit Substitution,[21–23] embedded figures tests,[17,21,23] and tests of figure-ground reversal.[17] Since early processing of visual information is intact,[24] these deficits have often been attributed to impaired analysis of contour or configural information (see also Ref. 25).

Deficits in olfactory and gustatory functioning have also consistently been observed. WKS patients have difficulty in making qualitative discriminations between smells and tastes,[26,27] but it is still unclear whether these deficits are related to heightened sensory thresholds.[27,28] Regardless of the exact level at which these processing deficits occur, they can be linked directly to atrophy of diencephalic structures associated with these sensory systems.

Gross motor deficits (gait ataxia and postural sway) are well recognized in WKS, but perhaps less recognized is the fact WKS patients also show deficits in fine motor control.[29] Dysfunction of frontal and cerebellar systems may contribute to impairments in fine motor movements, although their relative role remains unknown.

The extramemorial deficits most commonly noted in WKS are deficits in problem solving and concept formation,[30,31] deficits linked to impaired frontal executive control. Indeed, WKS patients typically perform poorly on clinical tests of frontal lobe functioning, such as the Wisconsin Card Sorting Test,[17,32] Verbal Fluency,[22,32,33] and Trails B.[22] Although perseveration and poor planning are frequently cited as underlying causes, executive deficits are likely to be multidetermined.[34]

An often-cited clinical characteristic of WKS that may be linked to impaired executive control is patients' tendency to confabulate when faced with questions they cannot answer. This is by no means a central feature of the disorder, however, and occurs almost exclusively during the acute phase of the disorder. Even then, confabulations are mostly provoked by the examiner's questioning and rarely occur spontaneously.

Anterograde Amnesia

The cardinal symptom of WKS is a profound inability to acquire new verbal and nonverbal information. Patients typically are unable to learn new names, faces, or facts, even in the face of multiple repetitions, and they forget events that occurred just minutes before. These deficits are not due to impairments in the immediate registration of information, as patients are able to repeat information in the absence of any delay.[35–38] However, given distracting activity for as little as 9 s, performance can be markedly impaired.[16,37,39,40] Some information may be learned on an initial learning trial, but on subsequent trials, marked deficits occur because of interference from information that was presented earlier. This increased sensitivity to interference is generally considered to be the most prominent feature of the anterograde amnesia. Some theorists [41,42] have suggested that interference occurs because the patient is unable to inhibit competition from irrelevant material at the time of *retrieval,* a hypothesis supported by the fact that retrieval cues that eliminate response competition improve performance.[41,43] Other investigators[16,39] have suggested that the learning deficits are due primarily to a failure to *encode* all the attributes of a stimulus. When left to their own devices, patients analyze the phonemic and associative features of stimuli, but they fail to analyze the semantic features.[44–46] In the past, the relative contribution of encoding and retrieval deficits has been vigorously debated (for reviews, see Refs. 47 and 48); but there is now general agreement that a true understanding of the anterograde amnesia of WKS lies in the interaction between these factors.[49]

Although the anterograde amnesia of WKS is in many respects quite similar to that seen in patients with amnesias from other etiologies, the question arises as to whether frontal executive deficits influence the character of the memory disorder in this patient group. One feature that distinguishes WKS patients from patients with amnesia of other etiologies is their increased propensity to commit prior-item intrusions—a finding that has been attributed to superimposed frontal pathology.[50] Another feature of the memory disturbance in WKS that has been linked to frontal dysfunction is patients' failure to demonstrate release from proactive interference (PI).[32] However, more recent studies have suggested that frontal dysfunction by itself is neither sufficient[51,52] nor necessary[53] to cause impaired release from PI. In comparison to other amnesic subgroups, WKS patients also show disproportionate impairment on tasks that tap memory for temporal information.[32,54–57] Since similar contextual deficits occur in patients with focal frontal lesions,[58] it has been suggested that these deficits in WKS may be secondary to superimposed frontal deficits.[32] The absence of reliable correlations between contextual memory performance and both structural and behavioral indices of frontal dysfunction, however, casts doubt on this view.[54] It appears that contextual memory deficits are an inseparable feature of WKS amnesia.

In addition to primary cognitive disturbances, motivational and arousal deficits may also contribute to patients' severe learning and memory problems. WKS patients generally display a profound apathy, passivity, and lack of initiative, features that are indicative of defective arousal and activation mechanisms. Several investigators have suggested that these deficits may interfere with the encoding and retrieval of information.[17,59] Partial support for this view comes from studies demonstrating that WKS patients show better learning when the information is emotionally salient or otherwise arousing.[60–62] These arousal effects appear to be transient, however, as no benefits are observed in the long-term retention of this information.[63,64] Motivational and arousal deficits may also contribute to WKS patients' lack of insight into their memory problems. Kopelman and colleagues[65] recently demonstrated that subjective evaluations of memory are severely impaired in WKS patients—more so than in patients with equally severe amnesia resulting from mediotemporal lesions.

Notwithstanding the severe impairments in new learning, several areas of preserved memory capacity should be mentioned briefly. These include the ability to acquire new motor[66,67] and perceptual skills[68,69] as well as preserved performance on a range of implicit memory tasks in which memory is indicated by changes in speed, accuracy, or bias of processing a stimulus as a consequence of prior experience with that stimulus (for a review, see Ref. 70).

Retrograde Amnesia

WKS patients have significant difficulty retrieving public as well as personal autobiographical events that occurred prior to the onset of their illness. This retrograde impairment is usually very extensive, but memories from childhood and early adulthood are typically remembered better than memories from the recent past. Such a temporal gradient has been observed in tests of autobiographical knowledge[71–73] as well as tests of public events and famous faces.[73–76] Even when events from recent and remote time periods are carefully equated in terms of task difficulty,[77–79] this pattern remains, suggesting that it is not just an artifact of differential exposure and overlearning.

A popular explanation[77,78] for this temporal gradient posits that two factors may jointly contribute to the observed remote memory impairment in WKS: a gradually developing anterograde memory deficit that is related to patients' alcohol abuse, and a general retrieval deficit that appears acutely during the Wernicke's phase of the illness and affects all time periods equally. The gradually building new learning deficit is thought to account for the presence of a temporal gradient, while the general retrieval deficit explains the fact that across all decades, remote memory is worse in WKS patients than in chronic alcoholics.

The contribution of new learning deficits to retrograde amnesia, however, was called into question by the report of patient P.Z.,[80] a college professor who had written his autobiography 2 years prior to developing WKS. This patient demonstrated a temporally graded remote memory loss for material mentioned in his autobiography. Clearly, this could not be due to an inability to learn this material originally. Instead, Cermak and colleagues[80,81] explained the existence of a gradient in P.Z. by suggesting that information from different time periods may tap qualitatively different forms of memory. Information from the recent past seems anchored in a temporal and spatial context, but information from the distant past often loses its contextual qualities through continued rehearsing and retelling. As a consequence, recent items may tap primarily episodic memory, whereas remote items may tap primarily semantic memory. According to this view, P.Z.'s performance may reflect the fact that episodic memories are more vulnerable to disruption than are semantic memories. Recent evidence, however, challenges this view. Memory for semantic information acquired prior to the onset of amnesia is also impaired in WKS and is characterized by a similar temporal gradient.[82] Thus, it appears that more recent memories, whether episodic or semantic, are more vulnerable to disruption than are remote memories. Even though P.Z. was able to describe recent events in his autobiography, these memories may have been less well established and less frequently rehearsed, hence their higher vulnerability.

Of note, several studies[71,82] have demonstrated that the extent of retrograde amnesia in WKS is correlated with performance on tests of frontal lobe functioning. A number of investigators[83,84] have suggested that the frontal lobes play an important role in the planning and initiation of systematic memory search. Such deficits in strategic control may underlie the inability to retrieve premorbidly acquired information regardless of its recency of occurrence.

ETIOLOGY OF WKS

It is now generally accepted that Wernicke's encephalopathy is directly linked to severe avitaminosis and especially deficiency of thiamine. Autopsied brain samples of patients with WKS have been found to be severely and selectively deficient in thiamine-dependent enzymes.[85] Furthermore, in animals with induced thiamine deficiency, neurologic symptoms of Wernicke's encephalopathy have been observed[86,87] as well as significant memory disorders.[88–90] This thiamine deficiency is due primarily to inadequate dietary intake of the vitamin, but impaired metabolism, possibly because of a genetic predisposition, is also thought to play a role.[91,92] Severe reductions in thiamine may trigger a series of metabolic events[90,93] leading to compromised energy metabolism and ultimately cell death.

In addition to thiamine deficiency, direct toxic effects of alcohol may also contribute to the neuropathology seen in patients with alcoholic WKS. There is now impressive evidence to suggest that patients with chronic alcohol abuse but without signs of WKS have signs of cognitive impairment and brain damage.[94–96] The similarity between the visuoperceptual and problem-solving deficits of WKS patients and chronic alcoholics has led to the suggestion that direct toxic effects of alcohol on association cortex may underlie these nonmnemonic deficits.[97] The link between frontal deficits and alcohol abuse per se remains controversial, however,[36] in part because frontal deficits have also been documented in patients with WKS of nonalcoholic origin.[98] It is likely, therefore, that multiple neuropathologic mechanisms contribute to the observed frontal deficits. Whether these deficits reflect direct structural damage to frontal cortex or a functional disconnection resulting from disruption of subcortical-frontal pathways also remains unclear.

NEUROPATHOLOGIC FINDINGS

The main pathology of WKS, described in detail by Victor and colleagues,[4] consists of symmetrically placed punctate lesions in the area of the third ventricle, fourth ventricle, and aqueduct, areas known to be very sensitive to thiamine deficiency. For many years, it was thought that lesions in the midbrain and cerebellum were responsible for the neurologic symptoms of the Wernicke's stage,[99] while diencephalic lesions were responsible for the amnesic syndrome. Later studies, however, indicated that all alcoholics with Wernicke's encephalopathy, regardless of level of memory functioning, have characteristic diencephalic lesions.[5,100]

The location of the lesion responsible for the amnesia that accompanies the WKS syndrome remains controversial. Victor and coworkers[4] reported that of 43 brains in which the thalamus was systematically examined, 38 had widespread atrophy of the dorsomedial nucleus (DMN). The 5 patients without DMN damage were not amnesic, even though they showed severe atrophy of the mammillary bodies. Based on these findings, the authors concluded that involvement of the DMN was responsible for the memory deficit, but it should be noted that these findings are also consistent with the notion that combined damage to the DMN and mammillary bodies is critical.[101] Casting doubt on either conclusion, however, is a recent study by Harding and colleagues[102] comparing Korsakoff patients, patients with Wernicke's encephalopathy, and nonamnesic alcoholics without Wernicke's encephalopathy. This study revealed shared pathology in the DMN as well as the mammillary bodies in all three groups. In contrast, neuronal loss in anterior thalamic nuclei was found only in the Korsakoff group. The anterior nucleus receives hippocampal input via the mammillary bodies as well as directly via the fornix and therefore forms an intrinsic part of the hippocampal memory system. It is clear that damage to the hippocampal-anterior thalamic system can lead to memory dysfunction. However, the pervasive memory deficits in recall and recognition that characterize dense amnesia require lesions not only in the hippocampal-anterior thalamic system but also in the perirhinal-dorsomedial thalamic system.[103] Although some exceptions have been described,[101,104] Korsakoff patients typically have damage to both systems. In contrast, patients with Wernicke's encephalopathy and nonamnesic alcoholics have damage to the latter system only (Fig. 51-1).[102]

Other neuropathologic studies have questioned whether diencephalic damage is sufficient to account for the amnesia seen in WKS, raising the possibility that damage to the basal forebrain and hippocampus may also play a role.[5,104,105] Lesions in these latter areas, however, are not always present. Although they may contribute to the observed behavioral deficits, they do not appear to be mandatory.

Structural neuroimaging studies have confirmed the presence of diencephalic lesions in WKS,[106–109] and studies examining structure-function correlations have found that long-term memory correlates significantly with volume of the third ventricle, thought to reflect atrophy of the midline thalamic nuclei, but not with volume of the mammillary bodies.[110,111] In addition to examining structures of the limbic system, neuroimaging studies have also focused attention on the presence of neocortical involvement, especially in the parietal and frontal lobes. Evidence for cortical atrophy comes from findings of enlargement of the lateral ventricles and widening of the sylvian and interhemispheric fissure, particularly between the frontal lobes. It should be noted, however, that the presence of frontal

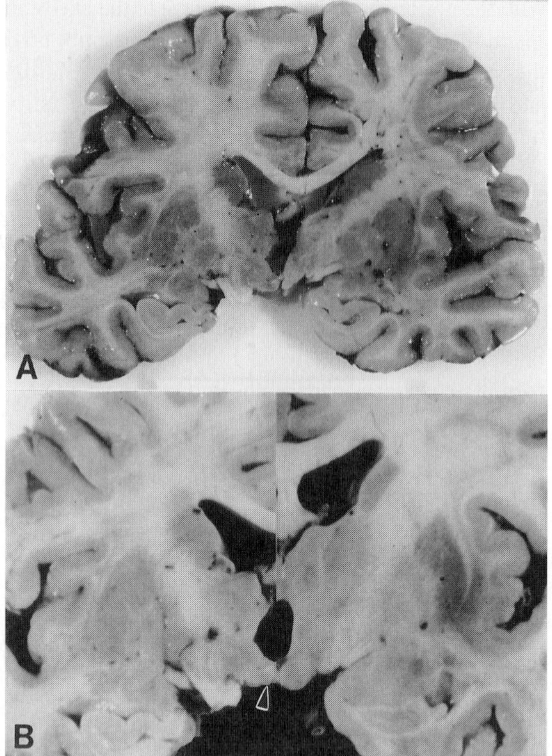

Figure 51-1
Coronal section of a Korsakoff brain (A) *illustrating sulcal widening, loss of white matter, and enlarged ventricles. Significant atrophy of the mammillary bodies is highlighted by comparing the left hemisphere of the Korsakoff brain with the right hemisphere of an age-matched control* (B).

atrophy is characteristic of alcoholics both with and without WKS.[112]

To date, few studies have focused on quantitative measurements of cerebral blood flow and metabolism in WKS. In the acute phase, widespread depression of metabolism has been observed in both cortical and subcortical areas, but significant recovery has been noted following thiamine treatment.[113,114] In the chronic phase, decreased metabolism in diencephalic areas is the most noticeable feature.[114–116] Frontal metabolic deficits have also been observed,[116–118] although not consistently[115]—a finding that again points to the variability in the neuropathology of WKS.

In comparison to a wealth of structural neuroanatomic studies, relatively little research has addressed the biochemical deficiencies that may underlie the amnesia in WKS. One exception, however, is the work of McEntee and colleagues.[119,120] They have drawn attention to the fact that the areas in the midbrain and diencephalon that are typically compromised in WKS are the very areas in which the monoaminergic pathways are located. Consistent with a monoaminergic disruption, they found significant reductions in the concentration of MHPG, the primary metabolite of norepinephrine, in the CSF of WKS patients. Moreover, the magnitude of this reduction was correlated with the severity of the patients' memory impairment,[121] and administration of the norepinephrine agonist clonidine had a beneficial effect on patients' anterograde memory capabilities.[122] This latter effect, however, has been difficult to replicate.[123] Serotoninergic mechanisms have also been implicated in a study demonstrating a selective improvement in memory following administration of the serotonin uptake inhibitor fluvoxamine.[124] Finally, another neurotransmitter that deserves further scrutiny is acetylcholine. As a consequence of thiamine depletion, cholinergic deficiencies are present in the acute phase of WKS.[90] It is less clear to what extent cholinergic systems are involved in the chronic stage of the disorder, but a recent report of significant improvement in cognition and comportment in two Korsakoff patients treated with anticholinesterase drugs suggests that cholinergic depletion must be considered in later stages of the disorder as well.[125]

REFERENCES

1. Korsakoff SS: Medico-psychological study of a memory disorder. Banks WP, Karam SJ, trans. *Conscious Cogn* 5:2–21, 1996.
2. Victor M, Yakovlev PI: SS Korsakoff's psychic disorder in conjunction with peripheral neuritis. A translation of Korsakoff's original article with brief comments on the author and his contribution to clinical medicine. *Neurology* 5:394–406, 1955.
3. Gudden H: Klinische und anatomische Beitraege zur Kenntniss der multiplen Alkoholneuritis nebst Bemerkungen ueber die Regenerationsvorgaenge im perihperen Nervensystem. *Arch Psychiatrie Nervenkrankh* 28:643–741, 1896.
4. Victor M, Adams RA, Collins GH: *The Wernicke-Korsakoff Syndrome and Related Neurologic Disorders*

Due to Alcoholism and Malnutrition. Philadelphia: Davis, 1989.

5. Caine D, Halliday G, Kril J, et al: Operational criteria for the classification of chronic alcoholics: Identification of Wernicke's encephalopathy. *J Neurol Neurosurg Psychiatry* 62:51–60, 1997.
6. Harper CG, Giles M, Finlay-Jones R: Clinical signs in the Wernicke-Korsakoff complex: A retrospective analysis of 131 cases diagnosed at necropsy. *J Neurol Neurosurg Psychiatry* 49:341–345, 1986.
7. Blansjaar BA, Van Dijk JG: Korsakoff minus Wernicke syndrome. *Alcohol* 27:435–437, 1992.
8. Jauhar P, Montaldi D: Wernicke-Korsakoff syndrome and the use of brain imaging. *Alcohol* 35 (suppl 1):21–23, 2000.
9. Cutting J: The relationship between Korsakov's syndrome and alcoholic dementia. *Br J Psychiatry* 132: 240–251, 1978.
10. Jacobson RR, Lishman WA: Selective memory loss and global intellectual deficits in alcoholic Korsakoff syndrome. *Psychol Med* 17:649–655, 1987.
11. Bowden SC: Separating cognitive impairment in neurologically asymptomatic alcoholism from Wernicke-Korsakoff syndrome: Is the neuropsychological distinction justified? *Psychol Bull* 107:355–366, 1990.
12. Joyce EM: Aetiology of alcoholic brain damage: Alcoholic neurotoxicity or thiamine malnutrition? *Br Med Bull* 50:90–114, 1994.
13. Victor M, Adams RA: The alcoholic dementias, in Frederiks J (ed): *Handbook of Clinical Neurology*. Amsterdam: Elsevier, 1985, pp 335–352.
14. Centerwall BS, Criqui MH: Prevention of the Wernicke-Korsakoff syndrome. A cost-benefit analysis. *N Engl J Med* 299:285–289, 1978.
15. Victor M, Laureno R: Neurologic complications of alcohol abuse: Epidemiologic aspects, in Schoenberg B (ed): *Advances in Neurology: Neuroepidemiology*. New York: Raven Press, 1978, vol 19.
16. Butters N, Cermak LS: *Alcoholic Korsakoff's Syndrome: An Information Processing Approach to Amnesia*. London: Academic Press, 1980.
17. Talland G: *Deranged Memory: A Psychonomic Study of the Amnesic Syndrome*. New York: Academic Press, 1965.
18. Parkin AJ, Leng NR: *Neuropsychology of the Amnesic Syndrome*. London: Erlbaum, 1993.
19. Wechsler D: *Wechsler Adult Intelligence Scale—III*. San Antonio, TX: Psychological Corporation, 1997.
20. Wechsler D: *Wechsler Memory Scale—III*. San Antonio, TX: Psychological Corporation, 1997.
21. Glosser G, Butters N, Kaplan E: Visuoperceptual processes in brain-damaged patients on the digit-symbol substitution test. *Int J Neurosci* 7:59–66, 1977.
22. Jacobson RR, Acker CF, Lishman WA: Patterns of neuropsychological deficit in alcoholic Korsakoff's syndrome. *Psychol Med* 20:321–334, 1990.
23. Kapur N, Butters N: Visuoperceptive deficits in long-term alcoholics with Korsakoff's psychosis. *J Stud Alcohol* 38:2025–2035, 1977.
24. Deary IJ, Hunter R, Langan SJ, et al: Inspection time, psychometric intelligence and clinical estimates of cognitive ability in pre-senile Alzheimer's disease and Korsakoff's psychosis. *Brain* 114:2543–2554, 1991.
25. Dricker J, Butters N, Berman G, et al: Recognition and encoding of faces by alcoholic Korsakoff and right hemisphere patients. *Neuropsychologia* 16:683–695, 1978.
26. Jones BP, Moskowitz HR, Butters N: Olfactory discrimination in alcoholic Korsakoff patients. *Neuropsychologia* 13:173–179, 1975.
27. Jones BP, Butters N, Moskowitz HR, et al: Olfactory and gustatory capacities of alcoholic Korsakoff patients. *Neuropsychologia* 16:323–337, 1978.
28. Mair RG, Capra C, McEntee WL, et al: Odor discrimination and memory in Korsakoff's psychosis. *J Exp Psychol Hum Percept Perform* 6:445–448, 1980.
29. Welch LW, Cunningham AT, Eckardt MJ, et al: Fine motor speed deficits in alcoholic Korsakoff's syndrome. *Alcohol Clin Exp Res* 21:134–139, 1997.
30. Becker JT, Butters N, Rivoira P, et al: Asking the right questions: Problem solving in male alcoholics and male alcoholics with Korsakoff's syndrome. *Alcohol Clin Exp Res* 10:641–646, 1986.
31. Oscar-Berman M: Hypothesis testing and focusing behavior during concept formation by amnesic Korsakoff patients. *Neuropsychologia* 11:191–198, 1973.
32. Squire LR: Comparisons between forms of amnesia: Some deficits are unique to Korsakoff's syndrome. *J Exp Psychol Learni Mem Cogn* 8:560–571, 1982.
33. Butters N, Granholm E, Salmon DP, et al: Episodic and semantic memory: A comparison of amnesic and demented patients. *J Clin Exp Neuropsychol* 9:479–497, 1987.
34. Delis DC, Squire LR, Bihrle A, et al: Componential analysis of problem-solving ability: Performance of patients with frontal lobe damage and amnesic patients on a new sorting test. *Neuropsychologia* 30:683–697, 1992.
35. Haxby JV, Lundgren SL, Morley GK: Short-term retention of verbal, visual shape and visuospatial location

information in normal and amnesic subjects. *Neuropsychologia* 21:25–33, 1983.
36. Joyce EM, Robbins TW: Frontal lobe function in Korsakoff and non-Korsakoff alcoholics: Planning and spatial working memory. *Neuropsychologia* 29:709–723, 1991.
37. Kopelman MD: Rates of forgetting in Alzheimer-type dementia and Korsakoff's syndrome. *Neuropsychologia* 23:623–638, 1985.
38. Wiegersma S, De Jong E, Dieren MV: Subjective ordering and working memory in alcoholic Korsakoff patients. *J Clin Exp Neuropsychol* 13:847–853, 1991.
39. Kinsbourne M, Wood F: Short-term memory processes and the amnesic syndrome, in Deutsch DD, Deutsch JA (eds): *Short-Term Memory*. New York: Academic Press, 1975.
40. Meudell PR, Butters N, Montgomery K: Role of rehearsal in the short-term memory performance of patients with Korsakoff's and Huntington's disease. *Neuropsychologia* 16:507–510, 1978.
41. Warrington EK, Weiskrantz L: Amnesic syndrome: Consolidation or retrieval? *Nature* 228:628–630, 1970.
42. Warrington EK, Weiskrantz L: An analysis of short-term and long-term memory defects in man, in Deutsch J (ed): *The Physiological Basis of Memory*. New York: Academic Press, 1973, pp 365–395.
43. Warrington EK, Weiskrantz L: The effect of prior learning on subsequent retention in amnesic patients. *Neuropsychologia* 12:419–428, 1974.
44. Biber C, Butters N, Rosen J, et al: Encoding strategies and recognition of faces by alcoholic Korsakoff and other brain-damaged patients. *J Clin Neuropsychol* 3:315–330, 1981.
45. Cermak LS, Reale L: Depth of processing and retention of words by alcoholic Korsakoff patients. *J Exp Psychol Hum Learn Mem* 4:165–174, 1978.
46. McDowall J: Effects of encoding instructions and retrieval cuing on recall in Korsakoff patients. *Mem Cogn* 7:232–239, 1979.
47. Butters N, Stuss DT: Diencephalic amnesia, in Squire LR (ed): *Handbook of Neuropsychology*. Amsterdam: Elsevier, 1991, vol 3, pp 107–148.
48. Cermak LS: Models of memory loss in Korsakoff and alcoholic patients, in Parsons O, Butters N, Nathan P (eds): *Neuropsychology of Alcoholism*. New York: Guilford Press, 1987, pp 207–226.
49. Verfaellie M, Cermak LS: Neuropsychological issues in amnesia, in Martinez J, Kesner R (eds): *Learning and Memory: A Biological View*. San Diego, CA: Academic Press, 1992, pp 467–497.
50. Kixmiller JS, Verfaellie M, Chase KA, et al: Comparison of figural intrusion errors in three amnesic subgroups. *J Int Neuropsychol Soc* 1:561–567, 1995.
51. Freedman M, Cermak LS: Semantic encoding deficits in frontal lobe disease and amnesia. *Brain Cogn* 5:108–114, 1986.
52. Kopelman MD: Frontal dysfunction and memory deficits in the alcoholic Korsakoff syndrome and Alzheimer-type dementia. *Brain* 114:117–137, 1991.
53. Becker JT, Furman JM Panisset M, et al: Characteristics of the memory loss of a patient with Wernicke-Korsakoff's syndrome without alcoholism. *Neuropsychologia* 28:171–179, 1990.
54. Hunkin NM, Parkin AJ: Recency judgements in Wernicke-Korsakoff and post-encephalitic amnesia: Influences of proactive interference and retention interval. *Cortex* 29:485–499, 1993.
55. Parkin AJ, Leng NRC, Hunkin NM: Differential sensitivity to context in diencephalic and temporal lobe amnesia. *Cortex* 26:373–380, 1990.
56. Shimamura AP, Janowski JS, Squire LR: Memory for the temporal order of events in patients with frontal lobe lesions and amnesic patients. *Neuropsychologia* 28:803–813, 1990.
57. Kopelman MD, Stanhope N, Kingsley D: Temporal and spatial context memory in patients with focal frontal, temporal lobe, and diencephalic lesions. *Neuropsychologia* 35:1533–1545, 1997.
58. Milner B, Petrides M, Smith ML: Frontal lobes and the temporal organisation of memory. *Hum Neurobiol* 4:137–142, 1985.
59. Oscar-Berman M: Neuropsychological consequences of long-term alcoholism. *Am Sci* 68:410–419, 1980.
60. Kopelman MD: Recall of anomalous sentences in dementia and amnesia. *Brain Lang* 29:154–170, 1986.
61. Kovner R, Mattis S, Goldmeier E: A technique for promoting robust free recall in chronic organic amnesia. *J Clin Exp Neuropsychol* 5:65–71, 1983.
62. Markowitsch HJ, Kessler J, Denzler P: Recognition memory and psychophysiological responses to stimuli with neutral or emotional content: A study of Korsakoff patients and recently detoxified and long-term abstinent alcoholics. *Int J Neurosci* 29:1–35, 1986.
63. Davidoff D, Butters N, Gerstman L, et al: Affective-motivational factors in the recall of prose passages by alcoholic Korsakoff patients. *Alcohol* 1:63–69, 1984.
64. Granholm E, Wolfe J, Butters N: Affective-arousal factors in the recall of thematic stories by amnesic and demented patients. *Dev Neuropsychol* 4:317–333, 1985.
65. Kopelman MD, Stanhope N, Guinan E: Subjective memory evaluations in patients with focal frontal,

diencephalic, and temporal lobe lesion. *Cortex* 34:191–207, 1998.
66. Brooks DN, Baddeley AD: What can amnesic patients learn? *Neuropsychologia* 14:111–122, 1976.
67. Cermak LS, Lewis R, Butters N, et al: Role of verbal mediation in performance of motor tasks by Korsakoff patients. *Percept Motor Skills* 37:259–262, 1973.
68. Cohen NJ, Squire LR: Preserved learning and retention of pattern-analyzing skill in amnesia: Dissociation of knowing how and knowing that. *Science* 210:207–210, 1980.
69. Martone M, Butters N, Payne M, et al: Dissociations between skill learning and verbal recognition in amnesia and dementia. *Arch Neurol* 41:965–970, 1984.
70. Moscovitch M, Vriezen E, Gottstein J: Implicit tests of memory in patients with focal lesions or degenerative brain disorders, in Spinnler H, Boller F (eds): *Handbook of Neuropsychology*. Amsterdam: Elsevier, 1993, vol 8, pp 133–173.
71. Kopelman MD: Remote and autobiographical memory, temporal context memory and frontal atrophy in Korsakoff and Alzheimer patients. *Neuropsychologia* 27:437–460, 1989.
72. Zola-Morgan S, Cohen NJ, Squire LR: Recall of remote episodic memory in amnesia. *Neuropsychologia* 21:487–500, 1983.
73. Kopelman MD, Stanhope N, Kingsley D: Retrograde amnesia in patients with diencephalic, temporal lobe or frontal lesions. *Neuropsychologia* 37:939–958, 1999.
74. Albert MS, Butters N, Levin J: Temporal gradients in the retrograde amnesia of patients with alcoholic Korsakoff's disease. *Arch Neurol* 36:211–216, 1979.
75. Marslen-Wilson ND, Teuber H-L: Memory for remote events in anterograde amnesia: Recognition of public figures from news photographs. *Neuropsychologia* 13:347–352, 1975.
76. Seltzer B, Benson DF: The temporal pattern of retrograde amnesia in Korsakoff's disease. *Neurology* 24:527–530, 1974.
77. Butters N, Albert MS: Processes underlying failures to recall remote events, in Cermak LS (ed): *Human Memory and Amnesia*. Hillsdale, NJ: Erlbaum, 1982, pp 257–274.
78. Cohen NJ, Squire LR: Retrograde amnesia and remote memory impairment. *Neuropsychologia* 19:337–356, 1981.
79. Squire LR, Cohen NJ: Remote memory, retrograde amnesia and the neuropsychology of memory, in Cermak LS (ed): *Human Memory and Amnesia*. Hillsdale, NJ: Erlbaum, 1982, pp 275–303.
80. Butters N, Cermak LS: A case study of the forgetting of autobiographical knowledge: Implications for the study of retrograde amnesia, in Rubin D (ed): *Autobiographical Memory*. New York: Cambridge University Press, 1986, pp 253–272.
81. Cermak LS: The episodic/semantic distinction in amnesia, in Squire LR, Butters N (eds): *The Neuropsychology of Memory*. New York: Guilford Press, 1984, pp 55–62.
82. Verfaellie M, Reiss L, Roth HL: Knowledge of new English vocabulary in amnesia: An examination of premorbidly acquired semantic memory. *J Int Neuropsychol Soc* 1:443–453, 1995.
83. Dall'Ora P, Della Sala S, Spinnler H: Autobiographical memory. Its impairment in amnesic syndromes. *Cortex* 25:197–217, 1989.
84. Stuss DT, Benson DF: *The Frontal Lobes*. New York: Raven Press, 1986.
85. Butterworth RF, Krill JK, Harper CG: Thiamine-dependent enzyme changes in the brains of alcoholics: Relationship to the Wernicke-Korsakoff syndrome. *Alcohol Clin Exp Res* 17:1084–1088, 1993.
86. Dreyfus PM: Diseases of the nervous system in chronic alcoholics, in Kissin B, Begleiter H (eds): *The Biology of Alcoholism: Clinical Pathology*. New York: Plenum Press, 1974, vol 3, pp 265–291.
87. Mesulam M-M, Van Hoesen G, Butters N: Clinical manifestations of chronic thiamine deficiency in the rhesus monkey. *Neurology* 27:239–245, 1977.
88. Mair RG, Knoth RL, Rabchenuk SA, et al: Impairment of olfactory, auditory, and spatial serial reversal learning in rats recovered from pyrithiamine-induced thiamine deficiency. *Behav Neurosci* 105:360–374, 1991.
89. Markowitsch HJ, Pritzel M: The neuropathology of amnesia. *Prog Neurobiol* 25:189–287, 1985.
90. Witt ED: Neuroanatomical consequences of thiamine deficiency: A comparative analysis. *Alcohol Alcohol* 20:202–221, 1985.
91. Blass JP, Gibson GE: Abnormality of a thiamine-requiring enzyme in Wernicke-Korsakoff syndrome. *N Engl J Med* 297:1367–1370, 1977.
92. Martin PR, McCool BA, Singleton CK: Genetic sensitivity to thiamine deficiency and development of alcoholic organic brain disease. *Alcohol Clin Exp Res* 17:31–37, 1993.
93. Todd KG, Butterworth RF: Mechanisms of selective neuronal cell death due to thiamine deficiency. *Ann NY Acad Sci* 893:404–411, 1999.
94. Butters N, Brandt J: The continuity hypothesis: The relationship of long-term alcoholism to the Wernicke-

Korsakoff syndrome, in Galanter M (ed): *Recent Developments in Alcoholism*. New York: Plenum Press, 1985, pp 207–227.
95. Lishman WA, Jacobson RR, Acker C: Brain damage in alcoholism: Current concepts. *Acta Med Scand Suppl* 717:5–17, 1987.
96. Ron MA, Acker W, Shaw GK, et al: Computerized tomography of the brain in chronic alcoholism. *Brain* 105:497–514, 1982.
97. Butters N: Alcoholic Korsakoff's syndrome: Some unresolved issues concerning etiology, neuropathology, and cognitive deficits. *J Clin Exp Neuropsychol* 7:181–210, 1985.
98. Parkin AJ, Blunden J, Rees JE, et al: Wernicke-Korsakoff syndrome of non-alcoholic origin. *Brain Cogn* 15:69–82, 1991.
99. Brierly JB: Neuropathology of amnesic states, in Whitty C, Zangwill O (eds): *Amnesia*, 2d ed. Boston: Butterworths, 1977, pp 199–223.
100. Torvik A: Topographic distribution and severity of brain lesions in Wernicke's encephalopathy. *Clin Neuropathol* 6:25–29, 1987.
101. Mair WG, Warrington EK, Weiskrantz L: Memory disorder in Korsakoff's psychosis: A neuropathological and neuropsychological investigation of two cases. *Brain* 102:749–783, 1979.
102. Harding A, Halliday G, Caine D, et al: Degeneration of anterior thalamic nuclei differentiates alcoholics with amnesia. *Brain* 123:141–154, 2000.
103. Aggleton JP, Brown MW: Episodic memory, amnesia, and the hippocampal-anterior thalamic axis. *Behav Brain Sci* 22:425–489, 1999.
104. Mayes AR, Meudell PR, Mann D, et al: Location of lesions in Korsakoff's syndrome: Neuropsychological and neuropathological data on two patients. *Cortex* 24:367–388, 1988.
105. Arendt T, Bigl V, Arendt A, et al: Loss of neurons in the nucleus basalis of Meynert in Alzheimer's disease, paralysis agitans and Korsakoff's disease. *Acta Neuropathol* 61:101–108, 1983.
106. Charness ME, DeLaPaz RL: Mammillary body atrophy in Wernicke's encephalopathy: Antemortem identification using magnetic resonance imaging. *Ann Neurol* 22:595–600, 1987.
107. Shimamura AP, Jernigan TL, Squire LR: Korsakoff's syndrome: Radiological (CT) findings and neuropsychological correlates. *J Neurosci* 8:4400–4410, 1988.
108. Squire LR, Amaral D, Press G: Magnetic resonance imaging of the hippocampal formation and mammillary nuclei distinguish medial temporal lobe and diencephalic amnesia. *J Neurosci* 10:3106–3117, 1990.
109. Colchester A, Kingsley D, Lasserson D, et al: Structural MRI volumetric analysis in patients with organic amnesia: 1. Methods and comparative findings across diagnostic groups. *J Neurol Neurosurg Psychiatry* 71:13–22, 2001.
110. Visser PJ, Krabbendam L, Verhey FRJ, et al: Brain correlates of memory dysfunction in alcoholic Korsakoff's syndrome. *J Neurol Neurosurg Psychiatry* 67:774–778, 1999.
111. Sullivan EV, Lane B, Deshmukh A, et al: In vivo mammillary body volume deficits in amnesic and nonamnesic alcoholics. *Alcohol Clin Exp Res* 23:1629–1636, 1999.
112. Kril JJ, Halliday GM, Svoboda MD, et al: The cerebral cortex is damaged in chronic alcoholics. *Neuroscience* 79:983–998, 1997.
113. Hata T, Meyer JS, Tanahashi N, et al: Three-dimensional mapping of local cerebral perfusion in alcoholic encephalopathy with and without Wernicke-Korsakoff syndrome. *J Cereb Blood Flow Metab* 7:35–44, 1987.
114. Heiss W-D, Pawlik G, Holthoff V, et al: PET correlates of normal and impaired memory functions. *Cereb Brain Metab Rev* 4:1–27, 1992.
115. Perani D, Kartsounis LD, Costello A: Korsakoff's psychosis: A neuropsychological and positron emission tomography study of two cases, in Vallar G, Cappa SF, Wallesh C-W (eds): *Neuropsychological Disorders Associated with Subcortical Lesions*. Oxford, England: Oxford University Press, 1992, pp 169–180.
116. Eustache F, Desgranges B, Aupee A, et al: Functional neuroanatomy of amnesia: Positron emission tomography studies. *Microsc Res Techn* 51:94–100, 2000.
117. Hunter R, McLuskie J, Wyper D, et al: The pattern of function-related regional cerebral blood flow investigated by single photon emission tomography with 99mTc-HM-PAO in patients with presenile Alzheimer's disease and Korsakoff's psychosis. *Psychol Med* 19:847–855, 1989.
118. Paller KA, Acharya A, Richardson B, et al: Functional neuroimaging of cortical dysfunction in alcoholic Korsakoff's syndrome. *J Cogn Neurosci* 9:277–293, 1997.
119. McEntee WJ, Mair RG, Langlais PJ: Neurochemical pathology in Korsakoff's psychosis: Implications for other cognitive disorders. *Neurology* 34:648–652, 1984.

120. McEntee WJ, Mair RG: The Korsakoff syndrome: A neurochemical perspective. *Trends Neurosci* 13:340–344, 1990.
121. McEntee WJ, Mair RG: Memory impairments in Korsakoff's psychosis. A correlation with brain noradrenergic activity. *Science* 202:905–907, 1978.
122. McEntee WJ, Mair RG: Memory enhancement in Korsakoff's psychosis by clonidine: Further evidence for a noradrenergic deficit. *Ann Neurol* 7:466–470, 1980.
123. O'Carroll RE, Moffoot A, Ebmeier KP, et al: Korsakoff's syndrome, cognition and clonidine. *Psychol Med* 23:341–347, 1993.
124. Martin PR, Adinoff B, Lane E, et al: Fluvoxamine treatment of alcoholic amnestic disorder. *Eur Neuropsychopharmacol* 5:27–33, 1995.
125. Angunawela II, Barker A: Anticholinesterase drugs for alcoholic Korsakoff syndrome. *Int J Geriatr Psychiatry* 16:338–339, 2001.

Chapter 52

NEUROBEHAVIORAL ASPECTS OF VASCULITIS AND COLLAGEN VASCULAR SYNDROMES

Nancy N. Futrell
Clark H. Millikan

Collagen vascular and vasculitic diseases are overlapping categories of autoimmune diseases. Central nervous system (CNS) involvement with alterations in behavior may occur. Of these diseases, systemic lupus erythematosus (SLE) is most frequently encountered in neurologic or psychiatric practice. It has the widest spectrum of behavioral changes, with multiple etiologies for the CNS involvement. The vasculitic diseases most likely to involve the CNS are those that produce stroke, either from CNS vasculitis or from systemic involvement, which predisposes to cardiogenic embolism or a hypercoagulable state.

SYSTEMIC LUPUS ERYTHEMATOSUS

Background

Systemic lupus erythematosus was first reported as an erythematous skin disorder by von Hebra in 1845, with systemic manifestations described by Kaposi in 1872.[1] Kaposi reported disturbed consciousness, including stupor and coma, although some of these cases were complicated by major pulmonary infections, which are now well known to be associated with diffuse brain dysfunction.

The first report of focal brain dysfunction was made by Osler in 1904. After evaluating a lupus patient with repetitive episodes of right hemiparesis and aphasia, he postulated that vasculitis, similar to that seen in the skin, could produce focal neurologic abnormalities.[2] The first major neuropathologic autopsy study, done by Johnson and Richardson in 1968,[3] was remarkable for the rarity of true vasculitis in the brain. Subsequent studies by Devinsky and Petito in 1988[4] and Hanly in 1990[5] strengthened the evidence that vasculitis in lupus is rare, but cerebral infarcts from cardioembolic sources are relatively common. Although the word *cerebritis* has been used to describe CNS involvement in lupus, the only pathologically proven "cerebritis" has been caused by infectious agents.

A vast spectrum of neurologic involvement of both the central and peripheral nervous system has been described, including stroke,[6,7] seizure,[3] dementia,[8] psychosis,[9,10] coma,[11] peripheral neuropathy, and myositis.[12] This heterogeneous group of disorders is often referred to simply as *neuropsychiatric SLE*.[13,14] Although this term persists, there is increasing recognition of the need to accurately classify the neurologic abnormalities in each patient and to recognize both direct and indirect mechanisms of SLE-related damage to the nervous system.[15,16] Clearly, "CNS-SLE" is not a single disease[17] but includes a spectrum of neurologic disorders, each with different potential etiologies.[18]

Stroke

Stroke in SLE patients presents with the same constellation of behavioral changes that occur in other stroke patients. The major difference is the great propensity for multiple strokes,[7] producing variable combinations of aphasias, agnosias, and apraxias in addition to motor, sensory, and visual abnormalities. These patients are often misdiagnosed with either confusion or primary psychiatric disease and are sometimes labeled "lupus cerebritis." If a neurologic evaluation is done, multifocal abnormalities are present clinically and on imaging studies (Fig. 52-1).

The cause of stroke in SLE is generally cardiogenic embolism or a hypercoagulable state.[7]

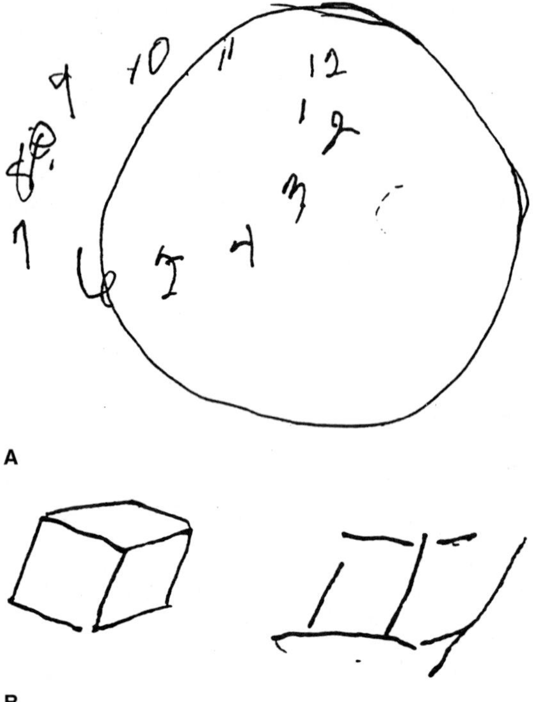

Figure 52-1
A 27-year-old woman with SLE and a history of five spontaneous abortions. The patient had a sudden onset of left hemiparesis and hemisensory deficit in her face, arm, and leg 5 months previously and was having episodic visual loss in the left eye of 5 to 30 min duration. The patient had a mild residual spastic hemiparesis with a Babinski sign on the left. The patient had been given a diagnosis of lupus cerebritis. A. *Clock face drawn by the patient.* B. *Three-dimensional box, examiner's example on the left, patient's attempt on the right. Over the next 18 months, the patient continued to have repeated cerebral infarcts, presenting with unilateral and bilateral visual field defects, visual agnosia, cognitive dysfunction, and multifocal motor and sensory deficits. Anticoagulant was started following a pulmonary embolus. Although recurrent focal neurologic episodes stopped abruptly, the patient was already severely debilitated.*

Transesophageal echocardiography is used to detect potential cardiac sources of emboli. A hypercoagulable state in lupus may present as stroke, multiple spontaneous abortions, or venous thrombosis without predisposing events. This coagulopathy is often associated with the lupus anticoagulant (LA) or antiphospholipid antibodies (APL). LA is diagnosed by an elevated partial thromboplastin time (PTT) that is not corrected with fresh frozen plasma or, alternatively, a Russell's viper venom time or a kaolin clotting time. Both LAs and APLs cause a hypercoagulable state by multiple mechanisms, including binding to endothelial cells[19] and inhibition of fibrinolysis.[20]

Patients with SLE face a very high risk of recurrent stroke, with over 50 percent of stroke patients having subsequent strokes. Preventive treatment with aggressive anticoagulant therapy is now generally accepted,[21,22] with an international normalized ratio (INR) of at least 3. Contraindications to anticoagulation–including thrombocytopenia, uncontrolled hypertension, history of GI bleeding, seizures, falls, dementia, and noncomplaince–are frequent in SLE patients and may limit preventive therapy. Steroids sometimes decrease APL titers[23] but do not reliably prevent strokes[21] and have serious long-term side effects. They can be used on a short-term basis in patients who have anticoagulant contraindications or who continue to have events on therapeutic anticoagulants.

Seizures

Behavioral changes associated with seizures must be differentiated from psychosis. Seizures are common in patients with SLE and are associated with anticardiolipin antibodies.[24] Seizures that manifest as primarily behavioral changes are uncommon but can occur in patient with a frontal or temporal lobe focus. We have seen inappropriate laughter, "gelastic" seizures, or another seizure where the patient screamed and ran down the hall. In each case the differentiation from psychosis was confirmed by normal interictal behavior and frontal or temporal epileptiform discharges on electroencephalography (EEG). Occasionally long-term EEG monitoring may be required.

Transient areas of high signal intensity on CT or T2-weighted magnetic resonance imaging (MRI) have been reported following seizures.[25] This has led to some confusion in the literature, with "resolution" of CT or MRI lesions in lupus patients attributed to immunosuppressive agents. As transient lesions can be caused by seizures and also by migraines,[26] which are also common with SLE patients, the improvement in images cannot automatically be interpreted as a reponse to a specific therapeutic agent. There is absolutely no evidence seizures in patients with lupus should be treated with immunosuppressive agents.

Encephalopathy and Psychosis

An acute or subacute diffuse encephalopathy occurs in SLE. The clinical presentation is highly variable, with confusion, disorientation, and often decreased consciousness. Absence of focal or multifocal abnormalities on neurologic examination and absence of infarcts on MRI are necessary to separate these patients from those with strokes.

Decreased consciousness is the most ominous symptom. It is often a manifestation of advanced infections in patients with SLE, and the prognosis is grim if the infection is not identified and treated quickly.[18] Pneumonia—with organisms including bacteria, fungi, and acid-fast bacilli (both *Mycobacterium* and *Nocardia*)—is the most frequent infection.[18] Patients with SLE may also present with abscesses, osteomyelitis, and CNS infections as well as viral, fungal, or bacterial meningitis.[27] Susceptibility to infection in SLE patients is increased[28]; however, the diagnosis may be delayed, as the infections often mimic active SLE. Such delays lead to a high rate of sepsis, which will produce encephalopathy in 70 percent of patients.[29]

Psychiatric disorders are common in SLE.[30] In our series of 91 patients located by consecutive hospital admissions, suicide attempts occurred in 6, generally during an acute psychotic outburst.[18] Clinical manifestations include hallucinations, paranoia, catatonia, mania, and major depressions.

The etiology of encephalopathy and psychiatric disorders is more difficult to sort out, in part due to the term *neuropsychiatric* lupus, which includes patients with focal and diffuse brain abnormalities of diverse etiologies.

It is clear that there is a category of patients with diffuse behavioral changes without strokes or seizures. Diffuse atrophy is often seen on computed tomography (CT) of the brain, and[31] the EEG may show diffuse slowing[32] and/or shifting asymmetry.[33] Earlier reports of associations with specific antibodies, such as antiribosomal P[34] and antineuronal antibodies,[35] appeared promising but have not been validated. Antiganglioside antibodies are a promising candidate for some types of CNS involvment.[36] SLE patients have abnormal production of cytokines.[37] Elevations of cytokines, namely interleukins IL-6 and IL-8, have been found in CSF in some patients with undefined "CNS" involvement. Concomitant increases CSF/serum IL-6 suggests CNS production of IL-6. [38] Abnormalities of cytokine levels have been found in mice with spontaneous lupus and cerebellar degeneration.[39]

The role of cytokines is an exciting new area with direct importance to patients with SLE. These patients begin with altered cytokine production,[40] which may be involved in both the pathogenesis of the disease and the predisposition to infections. Levels of cytokines and cytokine receptors may eventually be used as markers of disease activity and may be useful in determining the presence of systemic infections that may be altering brain activity.[41] Inhibition of specific cytokines offers the potential of more specific therapeutic intervention.[42]

At the time of this publication, the standard of care in SLE patients with acute neurologic disease other than stroke and seizure is a complete evaluation for infections, including lumbar puncture. Appropriate antimicrobial treatment is necessary. Antipsychotic and antidepressant agents are useful for psychosis and major depression. In patients without infection, steroids and immunosuppressive agents are often used, but their effectiveness has not been proven[43] and side effects can be serious. Use of these agents may best be guided by the activity of the systemic disease.

Cognitive Decline

Cognitive decline is common in patients with SLE, even in those without a history of clinical, neurologic, or psychiatric symptoms.[44] Visuospatial abnormalities are prominent.[45] Memory deficits, both recent and remote, fluctuate with activity of the systemic disease.[46] Other studies suggest that the chronic cognitive impairment is stable over time.[47]

The cause of this cognitive decline is unknown, but lymphocytotoxic antibodies are associated in several studies[45,48,49] Other secondary factors—such as uremia, hypertension, and metabolic abnormalities related to the systemic disease—may be important.[50]

There are no guidelines for treatment other than control of the systemic disease.

Vasculitis

Although focal and diffuse neurologic abnormalities in SLE are often attributed to "CNS vasculitis," autopsy studies suggest that this is rare.[3,4] Radiographic features, including diffuse white matter hyperintensity on T2-weighted MRI[51] (Fig. 52-2) or "beading" on angiography, are nonspecific.[52] If CNS vasculitis is suspected in a lupus patient, a biopsy should be performed, as immunosuppressive therapy would be given for confirmed vasculitis.

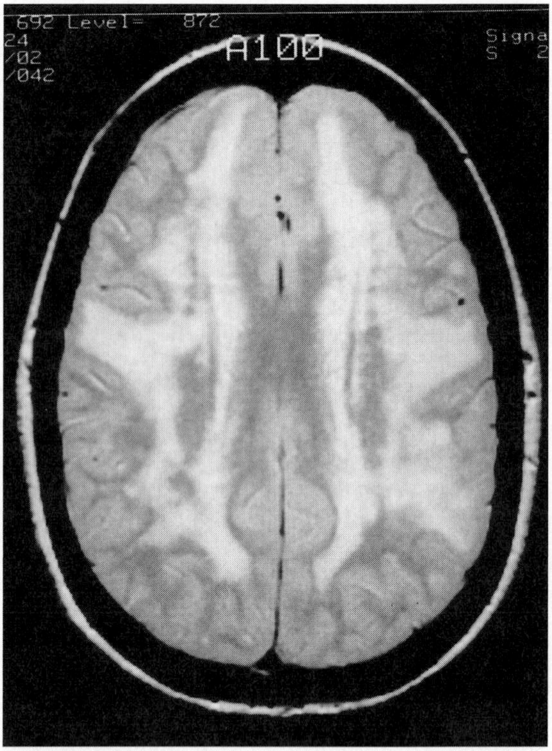

OTHER VASCULITIC DISEASES

The other vasculitic and collagen vascular diseases are listed in Table 52-1, including the tendency for CNS vasculitis and the general category of treatment for CNS involvement.

The primary APL syndrome presents as multiple systemic or cerebral thrombotic events, multiple spontaneous abortions, or livedo reticularis with a high titer of APLs.[53] This syndrome may be a forme fruste of SLE.[53] Patients with the primary APL syndrome are much like the SLE patients, presenting frequently with multiple cerebral infarcts.[54] Biopsy, when

Figure 52-2
A T-weighted MRI done on a 26-year-old woman with SLE who presented with "confusion," which was actually mild aphasia, and mild gait apraxia. The radiographic diagnosis was vasculitis. Brain biopsy revealed areas of normal tissue, areas of edema, and two areas with subacute infarcts. There was no vasculitis.

Table 52-1
Vasculitic diseases and treatment

Disorder	*Systemic vasculitis*	*CNS vasculitis*	*Treatment*
Systemic lupus erythematosus	+	−	S,AC
Primary antiphospholipid antibody syndrome	−	−	AC
Takayasu arteritis	++	+	S
Primary angiitis of the CNS	−	++	I
Rheumatoid arthritis	+	+	I
Periarteritis nodosa	++	+	I
Wegener granulomatosis	++	+	I
Scleroderma	±	−	S
Temporal arteritis, giant cell arteritis	++	+	S

Key: Presence of CNS vasculitis generally does not occur (−), occurs occasionally (+), occurs frequently (++); standard treatment with steroids (S), immunosuppressive agents (I), anticoagulants (AC).

done, reveals multiple thrombi rather than vasculitis.[55] Anticoagulation with warfarin with an INR of at least 3 is recommended.[56]

Patients with primary angiitis of the CNS may present with headache, dementia, or any combination of focal or multifocal neurologic abnormalities due to cerebral infarcts.[47–49] The diagnosis is suggested by pleocytosis in the CSF and beading or multiple vascular narrowings on angiography. In patients with suspected CNS vasculitis in association with primary angiitis of the CNS or SLE, biopsy should be obtained.[52] If CNS vasculitis is confirmed, immunosuppressive agents would be considered.[52] In systemic necrotizing vasculitides, such as periarteritis nodosa or Wegener's granulomatosis, which require immunosuppressive agents to treat the systemic disease, biopsy confirmation of CNS vasculitis as the etiology of CNS symptoms is not necessary.

REFERENCES

1. Kaposi MK: Neue Beiträge zur Kenntniss des Lupus erythematosus. *Arch Derm Syph* 4:36–78, 1872.
2. Osler W: On the visceral manifestations of the erythema group of skin diseases. *Am J Med Sci* 127:1–23, 1904.
3. Johnson RT, Richardson EP: The neurological manifestations of systemic lupus erythematosus: A clinical-pathological study of 24 cases and review of the literature. *Medicine (Baltimore)* 47:337–369, 1968.
4. Devinsky O, Petito CK, Alonso DR: Clinical and neuropathological findings in systemic lupus erythematosus: The role of vasculitis, heart emboli and thrombotic thrombocytopenic purpura. *Ann Neurol* 23:380–384, 1988.
5. Hanly JG, Walsh NMG, Sangalang V: Brain pathology in systemic lupus erythematosus. *J Rheumatol* 71:416–422, 1991.
6. Derksen RHWM, Bouma BN, Kater L: The association between the lupus anticoagulant and cerebral infarction in systemic lupus erythematosus. *Scand J Rheumatol* 15:179–184, 1986.
7. Futrell N, Millikan C: Frequency, etiology, and prevention of stroke in patients with systemic lupus erythematosus. *Stroke* 20:583–591, 1989.
8. Asherson RA, Mercey D, Phillips G, et al: Recurrent stroke and multi-infarct dementia in systemic lupus erythematosus: Association with antiphospholipid antibodies. *Ann Rheum Dis* 46:605–611, 1987.
9. Bonfa E, Glombek SJ, Kaufman LD, et al: Association between lupus psychosis and anti-ribosomal P protein antibodies. *N Engl J Med* 317:265–271, 1987.
10. Sergent JS, Lockshin MD, Klempner MS, Lipsky BA: Central nervous system disease in systemic lupus erythematosus: Therapy and prognosis. *Am J Med* 58:644–654, 1975.
11. Bennahum DA, Messner RP: Recent observations on central nervous system lupus erythematosus. *Semin Arthritis Rheum* 4:253–266, 1975.
12. Omdal R, Mellgran SI, Husby G: Clinical neuropsychiatric and neuromuscular manifestations in systemic lupus erythematosus. *Scand J Rheumatol* 17:113–117, 1988.
13. Denburg JA, Temesvari P: The pathogenesis of neuropsychiatric lupus. *Can Med Assoc J* 128:257–260, 1983.
14. Singer J, Denburg JA, ad hoc Neuropsychiatric Lupus Workshop Group: Diagnostic criteria for neuropsychiatric systemic lupus erythematosus: The results of a consensus meeting. *J Rheumatol* 17:1397–1402, 1990.
15. O'Connor P: Diagnosis of central nervous system lupus. *Can J Neurol Sci* 15:257–260, 1988.
16. Robbins ML, Kornguth SE, Bell CL, et al: Antineurofilament antibody evaluation in neuropsychiatric systemic lupus erythematosus. *Arthritis Rheum* 31:623–631, 1988.
17. Kaell AT, Shetty M, Lee BCP, Lockshin MD: The diversity of neurologic events in systemic lupus erythematosus. *Arch Neurol* 43:273–276, 1986.
18. Futrell N, Schultz LR, Millikan C: Central nervous system disease in patients with systemic lupus erythematosus. *Neurology* 42:1649–1657, 1992.
19. Vismara A, Meroni PL, Tincani A, et al: Relationship between anti-cardiolipin and anti-endothelial cell antibodies in systemic lupus erythematosus. *Clin Exp Immunol* 74:247–253, 1988.
20. Nilsson TK, Lofvenberg E: Decreased fibrinolytic capacity and increased von Willebrand factor levels as indicators of endothelial cell dysfunction in patients with lupus anticoagulant. *Clin Rheumatol* 8(1):58–63, 1989.
21. Futrell N, Millikan CH: Prevention of recurrent stroke in patients with systemic lupus erythematosus or lupus anticoagulant. *J Stroke Cerebrovasc Dis* 1:9–20, 1991.
22. Levine SR, Welch KMA: Neurological manifestations associated with antiphospholipid antibodies. *Ann Neurol* 22:161, 1987.
23. Derksen RHWM, Beisma D, Bouma BN, et al: Discordant effects of prednisone on anticardiolipin antibodies and the lupus anticoagulant [letter]. *Arthritis Rheum* 29:1295–1296, 1986.
24. Levine SR, Brey RL: Neurological aspects of antiphospholipid antibody syndrome. *Lupus* 5:347–353, 1996.

25. Sethi PK, Kumar BR, Madan VS, Mohan V: Appearing and disappearing CT scan abnormalities and seizures. *J Neurol Neurosurg Psychiatry* 48:866–869, 1985.
26. Jain S, Ahuja GK: Unusual transient high and low density CT lesion in migraine: A case report. *Headache* 26:19–21, 1986.
27. Al-Rasheed SA, Al-Fawaz IM: Cryptococcal meningitis in a child with systemic lupus erythematosus. *Ann Trop Paediatr* 10:323–326, 1990.
28. Yu CL, Chang KL, Chiu CC, et al: Defective phagocytosis, decreased tumour necrosis factor-alpha production, and lymphocyte hyporesponsiveness predispose patients with systemic lupus erythematosus to infections. *Scand J Rheumatol* 18:97–105, 1989.
29. Bolton CF, Young GB, Zochodne DW: The neurological complications of sepsis. *Ann Neurol* 33:94–100, 1993.
30. Hay EM, Huddy A, Black D, et al: A prospective study of psychiatric disorder and cognitive function in systemic lupus erythematosus. *Ann Rheum Dis* 53:298–303, 1994.
31. Gonzalez-Scarano F, Lisak RP, Bilaniuk LT, et al: Cranial computed tomography in the diagnosis of systemic lupus erythematosus. *Ann Neurol* 5:158–165, 1979.
32. Matsukawa Y, Sawada S, Hayama T, et al: Suicide in patients with systemic lupus erythematosus: A clinical analysis of seven suicidal patients. *Lupus* 3:31–35, 1994.
33. Ritchlin CT, Chabot RJ, Alper K, et al: Quantitative electroencephalography. *Arthritis Rheum* 35:1330–1342, 1992.
34. Teh LS, Hay EM, Amos N, et al: Anti-P antibodies are associated with psychiatric and focal cerebral disorders in patients with systemic lupus erythematosus. *Br J Rheumatol* 32:287–290, 1993.
35. Bluestein HG: Neuropsychiatric manifestations of systemic lupus erythematosus. *N Engl J Med* 317:309–311, 1987.
36. Galeazzi M, Annunziata P, Sebastiani GD, et al: Anti-ganglioside antibodies in a large cohort of European patients with systemic lupus erythematosus: Clinical, serological, and HLA class II gene associations. European Concerted Action on the Immunogenetics of SLE. *J Rheumatol* 27:135–141, 2000.
37. Mitamura K, Kang H, Tomita Y, et al: Impaired tumour necrosis factor-alpha (TNF-alpha) production and abnormal B cell response to TNF-alpha in patients with systemic lupus erythematosus (SLE). *Clin Exp Immunol* 85:386–391, 1991.
38. Trysberg E, Carlsten H, Tarkowski A: Intrathecal cytokines in systemic lupus erythematosus with central nervous system involvement. *Lupus* 9:498–503, 2000.
39. Tomita M, Holman BJ, Williams LS, Pang KC, Santoro TJ: Cerebellar dysfunction is associated with overexpression of proinflammatory cytokine genes in lupus. *J Neurosci Res* 64:26–33, 2001.
40. Swaak AJ, van den Brink HG, Aarden LA: Cytokine production (IL-6 and TNF alpha) in whole blood cell cultures of patients with systemic lupus erythematosus. *Scand J Rheumatol* 25:233–238, 1996
41. Gabay C, Cakir N, Moral F, et al: Circulating levels of tumor necrosis factor soluble receptors in systemic lupus erythematosus are significantly higher than in other rheumatic diseases and correlate with disease activity. *J Rheumatol* 24:303–308, 1997.
42. Aringer M, Steiner G, Graninger W, Smolen J: Role of tumor necrosis factor alpha and potential benefit of tumor necrosis factor blockade treatment in systemic lupus erythematosus: Comment on the editorial by Pisetsky. *Arthritis Rheum* 44:1721–1722, 2001.
43. Sibley JT, Olszynski WP, Decoteau WE, Sundaram MB: The incidence and prognosis of central nervous system disease in systemic lupus erythematosus. *J Rheumatol* 19:47–52, 1992.
44. Monastero R, Bettini P, Del Zotto E, et al: Prevalence and pattern of cognitive impairment in systemic lupus erythematosus patients with and without overt neuropsychiatric manifestations. *J Neurol Sci* 184:33–39, 2001.
45. Denburg SD, Behmann SA, Carbotte RM, Denburg JA: Lymphocyte antigens in neuropsychiatric systemic lupus erythematosus. *Arthritis Rheum* 37(3):369–375, 1994.
46. Martinez X, Tintore M, Montalban J, et al: Antibodies against gangliosides in patients with SLE and neurological manifestations. *Lupus* 1:299–302, 1992
47. Carlomagno S, Migliaresi S, Ambrosone L, et al: Cognitive impairment in systemic lupus erythematosus: A follow-up study. *J Neurol* 247:273–279, 2000
48. Denburg SD, Carbotte RM, Long AA, Denburg JA: Neuropsychological correlates of serum lymphocytotoxic antibodies in systemic lupus erythematosus. *Brain Behav Immunol* 2:222–234, 1988.
49. Denburg JA, Behmann SA: Lymphocyte and neuronal antigens in neuropsychiatric lupus: presence of an elutable, immunoprecipitable lymphocyte/neuronal 52 kd reactivity. *Ann Rheum Dis* 53:304–308, 1994.
50. Putterman C, Naparstek Y: Neuropsychiatric involvement in systemic lupus erythematosus. *Isr J Med Sci* 28:458–460, 1992.
51. Shintani S, Ono K, Hinoshita H, et al: Unusual neuroradiological findings in systemic lupus erythematosus. *Eur Neurol* 33:13–16, 1993.

52. Moore PM: Diagnosis and management of isolated angitis of the central nervous system. *Neurology* 39:167–173, 1989.
53. Asherson RA, Khamashta MA, Ordi-Ros J, et al: The "primary" antiphospholipid syndrome: Major clinical and serological features. *Medicine* 68:366–374, 1989.
54. Asherson RA, Merry P, Acheson JF, et al: Antiphospholipid antibodies: A risk factor for occlusive ocular vascular disease in systemic lupus erythematosus and the 'primary' antiphospholipid syndrome. *Ann Rheum Dis* 48:358–361, 1989.
55. Westerman EM, Miles JM, Backonja M, Sundstrom WR: Neuropathologic findings in multi-infarct dementia associated with anticardiolipin antibody. *Arthritis Rheum* 35:1038–1041, 1992.
56. Khamashta MA, Cuadrado MJ, Mujic F, et al: The management of thrombosis in the antiphospholipid-antibody syndrome. *N Engl J Med* 332:993–1027, 1995.

Chapter 53

NORMAL PRESSURE HYDROCEPHALUS

Thomas A. Krefft
Neill R. Graff-Radford

Doctors find the diagnosis and treatment of patients with normal pressure hydrocephalus (NPH), also called symptomatic hydrocephalus, particularly difficult. The reasons for this are as follows:

No combinations of the cardinal symptoms (gait difficulty, cognitive decline, and incontinence of urine) are pathognomonic for the diagnosis because each of the cardinal symptoms is common in the elderly[1–4] and may be caused by multiple disease processes.

Ventricle size increases with age[5] and in common dementing illnesses such as Alzheimer's disease (AD),[6] so that the finding of ventriculomegaly in an older population is common.

All of the diagnostic tests so far described give both false-positive and false-negative results.

The surgical treatment carries significant short- and long-term risks.

We do not know the cause or pathogenesis of many cases of NPH.

This chapter outlines the largely anecdotal evidence in the literature on which a diagnosis can be made and advice given regarding the risks and possible benefits of undergoing shunt surgery.

To do this, the following issues are addressed:

1. Findings in the history, clinical examination, and neuropsychological evaluation that are either reported to be associated with predicting surgical outcome or are important considerations in the management of the patient.
2. Radiologic evaluation, including computed tomography (CT), magnetic resonance imaging (MRI), cisternography, and single photon emission computed tomography (SPECT).
3. Special testing, including lumbar puncture, continuous cerebrospinal fluid (CSF) drainage, CSF absorption tests, and CSF pressure monitoring.
4. How to measure surgical outcome.
5. Surgical complications of shunt surgery.
6. Choice of a shunt.
7. Associations of idiopathic NPH that might have implications related to etiology.

A case illustrating the difficulties in diagnosis is illustrated in Figs. 53-1 through 53-4.

DIFFERENTIAL DIAGNOSIS, HISTORY, CLINICAL EXAMINATION AND NEUROPSYCHOLOGICAL EVALUATION

Differential Diagnosis

In evaluating a patient, one may keep in mind the important, but not exhaustive, differential diagnoses given in Table 53-1; the first three diagnoses may overlap.

Clinical Evaluation

General Factors The clinician should evaluate the patient's general medical health, because this may be important when surgery is being considered. Factors that theoretically could aggravate hydrocephalus include systemic hypertension (see later for association with hydrocephalus) and a recent head injury (which is particularly pertinent in individuals with gait difficulty). Evaluate for sleep apnea, congestive heart failure, and lung disease, all of which could increase jugular venous pressure and decrease CSF flow into the cerebral venous sinuses. If the patient is on long-term anticoagulants, such as warfarin for atrial fibrillation,

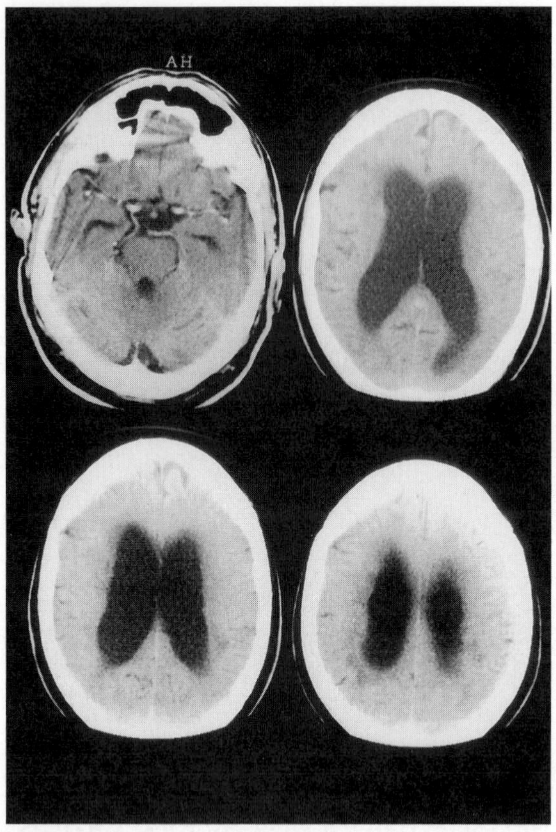

Figure 53-1
CT scan of a 71-year-old man with a diabetic peripheral neuropathy who presented with a 10-year history of difficulty walking. The scan shows hydrocephalus.

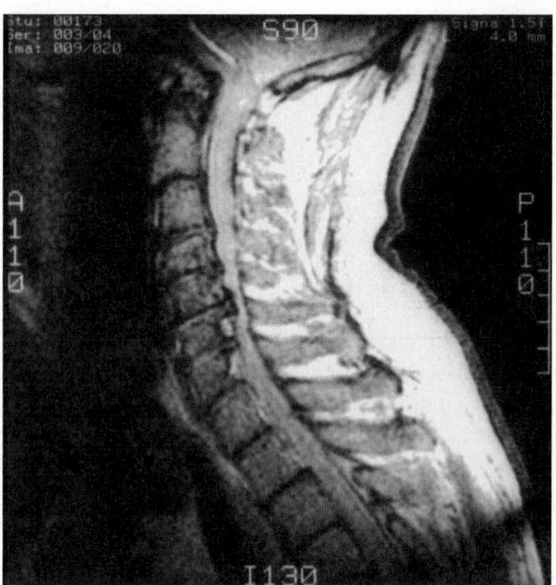

Figure 53-2
Examination of the patient in Fig. 53-1 revealed bilateral decreased biceps and brachioradialis reflexes with preservation of the triceps reflexes. Therefore an MRI of the cervical spine was performed, showing significant pressure on the cervical cord. The cervical cord was decompressed and the patient's gait improved, as documented on videotape.

take this into account for the theoretical increased risk of brain hemorrhage during and after surgery.

History There are several specific questions that should be asked in taking a history from these patients and their families.

Ask how long the patient has been demented. If this is more than 2 years, it is less likely that the patient will respond to surgery.[7,8] Note that the question is not how long the patient has had gait abnormality but how long the patient has been demented. In our series, this question predicted 5 of 7 unimproved and 21 of 23 improved patients[8] (see Table 53-2).

Ask which started first, gait abnormality or dementia. If the gait abnormality began before or at the same time as the dementia, there is a better chance for successful surgery; if dementia started before gait abnormality, shunting is less likely to help. This observation had been previously reported by Fisher.[9]

Ask if the patient abused alcohol, because alcohol abuse is a poor prognostic indicator.[10]

Ask if there are secondary causes for hydrocephalus, such as subarachnoid hemorrhage, meningitis, previous brain surgery, and head injury. If any of these are present, the chances of improvement with surgery are better.[7,10,11]

Ask if the patient has a large head size as evidenced by needing a large hat. This may indicate that the patient suffers from congenital hydrocephalus that has become symptomatic in later life.[12]

Examination On examination, the following issues should be addressed. Measure the head circumference. If greater than 59 cm in males or 57.5 cm in females (i.e., greater than the 98th percentile for head circumference), the patient could have congenital

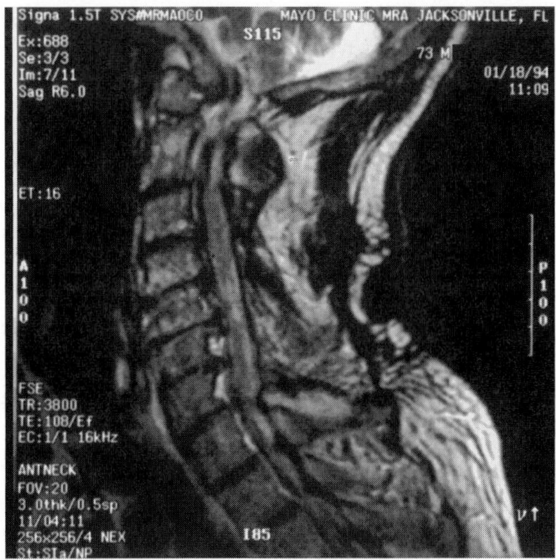

Figure 53-3
Three years later, the patient's gait again deteriorated. MRI of the cervical spine done at this time showed no cord compression.

hydrocephalus that has become symptomatic in later life.[12]

Look for signs of diseases that may mimic NPH, such as AD with extrapyramidal features; Parkinson's disease or parkinsonian syndromes; diffuse Lewy body disease; frontotemporal dementia; cervical spondylosis with spinal cord compression; phenothiazine use; multiple subcortical infarctions; arthritis of the hips, knees, or lumbar spine; or multiple sensory deprivation (as might occur in diabetics with peripheral neuropathy and visual impairment).

Neuropsychology

Look for evidence of aphasia. If there is such evidence (e.g., anomia), this is a poor prognostic indicator for surgical success[8,10] (see Table 53-2).

RADIOLOGIC EVALUATION

Computed Tomography (CT)

Since the advent of CT, the documentation of ventriculomegaly has become easier. This has had both advantages and disadvantages. There is a clear advantage of not having to subject patients to the uncomfortable procedure of air encephalography to diagnose hydrocephalus. However, physicians are often faced with the responsibility of knowing that a patient has ventriculomegaly when the scan may have been ordered for an unrelated indication.

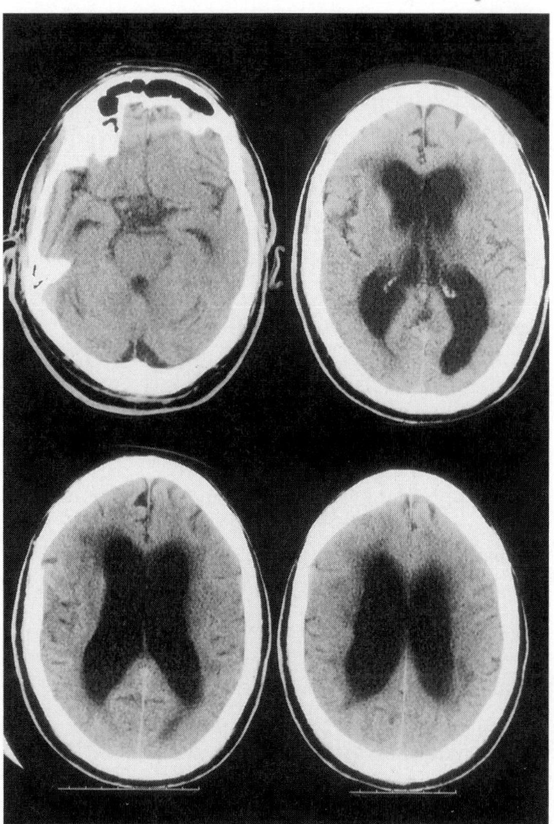

Figure 53-4
A repeat CT scan following the MRI confirmed the hydrocephalus. There was no improvement of gait after removal of CSF at lumbar puncture. The patient underwent shunt surgery and his gait improved to normal, again documented on videotape. This case shows that multiple etiologies may play a role in gait abnormality in the elderly.

A patient has ventriculomegaly (above the 95th percentile) when the modified Evans ratio is greater than 0.31.[13] The Evans ratio can be calculated on the axial CT slice where the frontal horns are largest. One measures the maximal diameter of the frontal horns

Table 53-1
Differential diagnosis of NPH

Alzheimer's disease with extrapyramidal features
Cognitive impairment in the setting of Parkinson's disease or parkinsonian syndromes; e.g., progressive supranuclear palsy, multiple system atrophy, and corticobasal ganglionic degeneration
Diffuse Lewy body disease
Frontotemporal dementia, which may have extrapyramidal symptoms; the scan may show caudate atrophy
Cervical spondylosis with cord compromise in the setting of degenerative dementia
Phenothiazine use
Multiple sensory deprivation syndrome (such as a diabetic with peripheral neuropathy and visual impairment)
Multiple infarction dementia, including the controversial entity subcortical ischemic encephalopathy or Binswanger's disease
Combination diseases such as
Alzheimer's disease, cervical spondylosis, and prostatism or stress incontinence
Alzheimer's disease, spinal stenosis, arthritis of the hips or knees, and prostatism or stress incontinence

and the inner table of the skull at the same level and then calculates the two measures as a ratio: the inner table of the skull/maximal diameter of the frontal horns. The ventricles normally enlarge with age,[5] a point to be taken into account in diagnosing hydrocephalus. There is slow ventricular enlargement to age 60 years and then the rate of enlargement increases. In Barron's study,[5] the mean ventricular size was 5.2 percent (percent of intracranial area) in the decade 50 to 59 years, 6.4 percent 60 to 69 years, 11.5 percent 70 to 79 years, and 14.1 percent 80 to 89 years.

If a patient has hydrocephalus without sulcal enlargement, this is a favorable surgical prognostic factor. However, if there is sulcal enlargement and hydrocephalus, patients can still improve with surgery. Borgesen and Gjerris[14] measured the largest sulcus in the high frontal or parietal region and found that if the cortical sulci were less than 1.9 mm, 17 of 17 patients shunted improved; if the sulci were 1.9 to 5 mm, 17 of 20 shunted improved; and if the sulci were 5 mm or more, 15 of 27 shunted improved.

Magnetic Resonance Imaging (MRI)

Detecting Congenital Hydrocephalus MRI is an excellent method for evaluating patients with possible symptomatic hydrocephalus and is the neuroimaging study of choice in NPH patients. It has the advantage of being able to visualize relevant structures in the posterior fossa, including cerebral aqueductal stenosis, cerebellar tonsillar herniation, and infarctions of the brainstem. Further, MRI can be used to obtain volumetric measures of mediotemporal lobe structures, a technique that has been shown to be useful in separating AD patients from normal elderly controls.[15]

At least 10 percent of elderly patients with symptomatic hydrocephalus may have congenital hydrocephalus that becomes symptomatic in later years.[12] A clinical clue to this is that the patient has a head circumference above the 98th percentile. On MRI, the ventricular enlargement shows no or little associated periventricular increased signal on T2-weighted imaging, indicating a chronic process. In addition, a cause for the congenital hydrocephalus may be found, such as an Arnold Chiari malformation.

White Matter Lesions and NPH Some report that the presence of transependymal flow may be related to a good surgical prognosis. In Borgesen and Gjerris's study,[14] 16 of 16 with periventricular hypodensity on CT improved with surgery, whereas in the study of Bradley and colleagues,[16] MR images were rated for deep white matter changes, and the presence or extent of these did not correlate with outcome. In 1996, Krauss and colleagues reported that the degree of improvement after shunt surgery depends on the extent and severity of white matter lesions[17]—i.e., the more extensive the white matter lesions, the less the improvement. In a subsequent report,[18] they compared the MRI findings in NPH to an age-matched control group and found that in both groups the periventricular white matter lesions (PVLs) correlated with the deep white matter lesions (DWMLs). In the control group, the white matter

Table 53-2
Variables predicting surgical outcome in symptomatic hydrocephalus

Variable	*No. of patients*	*Odds ratio*	*p value**	*95% confidence interval for odds ratio†*	*Correct classification unimproved*	*Correct classification improved*
Age	30	1.031	0.59	0.919–1.157		
Education	30	0.906	0.41	0.716–1.146		
Sex	30	4.615	0.215‡	0.423–2.330		
Gait abnormality (years)	30	1.133	0.51	0.789–1.626		
Incontinence (years)	30	1.441	0.402	0.614–3.408		
Dementia (years)	30	9.002	<0.001	1.542–5.256	5/7	21/23
Order of onset (gait versus dementia)	30	0	0.009‡	0–0.425	3/7	23/23
Percent time B waves present	28	0.969	0.04	0.937–1.001	2/6	22/22
Percent time pressure >15 mmHg	28	0.968	0.055	0.930–1.006	0/6	22/22
Percent time pressure 20 mmHg	28	0.979	0.23	0.940–1.020		
Visual naming	25	0.941	0.093	0.875–1.013	2/7	17/18
Visual naming pass/fail	25	8.750	0.058‡	0.887–1.133	5/7	14/18
Cerebral blood flow (anterior/posterior ratio slice 4)	30	1.120	<0.001	1.026–1.224	5/7	22/23
CSF conductance	23	0.254	0.956	0-infinity		
CSF conductance, 0.08 as cutoff value	23	1.071	1.00‡	0.065–67.354		

**p* Value based on likelihood ratio.
†Based on Wald test (which is slightly different from likelihood ratio test) and on Fisher exact test when this test was used.
‡*p* Value based on Fisher exact test.
Source: From Graff-Radford and Godersky,[12] with permission.

lesions correlated significantly with age and the anterior horn index (frontal horn width divided by the horizontal intracranial width). In contrast, in the NPH group, there was no correlation of white matter lesions with age and there was a significant negative correlation between the white matter lesions and the frontal horn index—i.e., the wider the frontal horns the less white matter lesions present. They argue that the white matter lesions do not cause the hydrocephalus but that the common link between the frequent coexistence of idiopathic NPH and vascular encephalopathy as (evidenced by white matter lesions) is arterial hypertension. See below for further discussion on the association of systemic hypertension and NPH.

In a postmortem MRI study of autopsied brains and the histologic analysis of the same brains, Munoz et al.[19] found that the white matter changes seen on MRI correlated with decreased density of axons and myelinated fibers, diffuse vacuolation of white matter (so-called spongiosis), and decreased density of glia. Infarctions were not common in these areas. While this study does not necessarily apply to the white matter changes seen in hydrocephalic patients, it does indicate that white matter MRI findings do not necessarily indicate irreversible periventricular infarctions, which would make shunt surgery unlikely to be effective.

MRI Differentiation of NPH and AD Traditionally the presence of ventriculomegaly without sulcal enlargement has been a radiologic finding felt to indicate NPH when accompanied by the typical clinical triad. However, Holodny[20] and Kitagaki[21] both have pointed out the occasional occurrence of focally dilated sulci over the convexity or medial surface of a hemisphere in NPH patients, unlike the diffuse sulcal enlargement seen in AD. Kitagaki also demonstrated significantly greater sylvian CSF volume in idiopathic NPH compared to AD patients. He felt this was a sign supportive of NPH indicating a "suprasylvian block."

Another area where MRI has the potential to be helpful prognostically is in volumetric measurements of certain structures in the temporal lobe. There is enlargement of the temporal horns of the lateral ventricles in both NPH and AD patients. Jack and colleagues[15] developed a technique for measuring the volumes of structures in the anterior temporal lobe and hippocampal formation. Holodny (in another paper[22]) measured the CSF volumes of the perihippocampal fissures (PHF), the lateral aspect of the transverse fissure of Bichat, and the choroidal and hippocampal fissures. He showed that the PHFs were significantly enlarged in AD patients compared to NPH patients. This was detectable both by visible inspection and computer volumetrics.

MR-based volumetric measurements of the hippocampal formation have been shown to be useful in discriminating between AD and normal elderly controls.[15] Though Golomb[23] found smaller hippocampal volumes in NPH patients compared to controls, Savolainen[24] found only a minor left-side decrease. However, Savolainen importantly detected significantly larger hippocampi in NPH patients compared to AD patients.

Flow Void on MRI as a Predictive Test of Surgical Outcome In 1991, Bradley and coworkers[16] retrospectively reviewed the MRI scans of 20 patients who had undergone ventriculoperitoneal shunt surgery for NPH. Bradley et al. rated initial surgical outcome as excellent, good, or poor and correlated this with the extent of flow void in the cerebral aqueduct. We should point out that the method of acquiring MR images may affect the flow void appearance. Bradley and coworkers used a 0.35-T MR imaging unit and a 128-by-128 acquisition matrix (1.7-mm spatial resolution), 7-mm section thickness with a 3-mm gap, a TR of 2.0 s, TEs of 28 and 56 ms, and four signal averages (17-min acquisition time). Bradley scored the extent (not signal loss per se) of flow void extension into the third and fourth ventricles on a scale of 0 to 4. Grade 0 meant no signal loss, grade 1 meant signal loss in the aqueduct that did not extend to the middle of the fourth ventricle, and grades 2, 3, and 4 demonstrated progressively more extensive signal loss, maximum being flow void extending from the posterior third ventricle through the entire fourth ventricle. A significant correlation ($p < 0.003$) was found between extent of increased aqueductal flow void and initial surgical outcome. More specifically, 8 out of 10 with an increased CSF flow-void score had an excellent or good response to surgery, whereas only

1 out of 9 who had a normal flow-void score improved with surgery.

In a subsequent study of 18 NPH patients, Bradley and colleagues[25] studied the CSF stroke volume (see Ref. 25 for methods) and the CSF flow-void score. The 12 patients with a CSF stroke volume of 42 mL all improved, but of those with a CSF stroke volume of less than 42 mL, 3 improved and 3 did not. Using the flow-void score, 4 of 15 improved patients had false-negative tests and 1 of 3 unimproved patients had a false-positive test.

Krauss and colleagues report that the flow void in the cerebral aqueduct of 37 idiopathic NPH patients was not significantly different to that in 37 age-matched controls.[26] Further, the extent of the flow void extension into the third, fourth, and lateral ventricles did not correlate with amount of improvement in these patients but rather correlated with the width of the ventricles. Unfortunately, this study does not confirm earlier reports that measures of CSF flow through the cerebral aqueduct can be used to predict surgical outcome.

Hakim and Black,[27] in a small study of 12 patients of whom 10 improved, found that the MRI-CSF flow studies were correct in 6, but 5 had false-negatives and 1 a false-positive. This casts further doubt on this diagnostic test.

Summary of Factors to Be Addressed in Looking at the CT or MRI

Hydrocephalus must be present. The modified Evans ratio (maximum width of the frontal horns/measure of the inner table at the same place) should be greater than 0.31.[13]

Is cortical atrophy prominent? If there is extensive cortical atrophy, this reduces but does not eliminate the chance of improvement with surgery.[14,17]

The pattern of atrophy may be useful diagnostically (e.g., does it involve the mediotemporal lobes, as in AD?). Although data on this point are lacking, it may be that prominent mediotemporal cortical atrophy decreases the chances for surgical improvement because these patients may have AD.[15,28]

Is there evidence of congenital hydrocephalus? For example, is there aqueductal stenosis or an Arnold Chiari malformation?[12,29]

Newer MRI techniques, such as cine-MRI, involving the analysis of a CSF flow void in the aqueduct of Sylvius, were first thought to be helpful,[16,25] but unfortunately they have not been found to be so in subsequent studies.[26,27]

Regional Cerebral Blood Flow (rCBF)

It has been reported that rCBF is decreased in the frontal areas in hydrocephalus[30] and in the parietotemporal areas in AD.[31] On the presumption that many of the nonimproved group have AD (which we had confirmed in two who came to autopsy and which Bech and colleagues have shown more recently[28]), we tried to differentiate those who will respond to shunt surgery from those who will not based on the pattern of preoperative regional CBF.[32] To do this, we calculated the ratio of frontal over posterior regional blood flow, expecting a lower frontal-posterior ratio in true symptomatic hydrocephalus and a higher ratio in pseudosymptomatic hydrocephalus patients who have AD. In fact, this has been a good method in predicting surgical outcome: the ratio predicted 5 of 7 unimproved and 22 of 23 improved patients in our series[8] (see Table 53-2).

Cisternography

Our experience with cisternography is limited, but the literature suggests that there are numerous cases with a positive test (radioisotope seen within the ventricles 48 to 72 h after being injected in the lumber area) who do not improve with surgery and patients with equivocal or negative tests who do improve. Further, the test itself may be difficult to interpret. Black[33] found the following: of 11 patients who had a positive test, 9 improved and 2 did not; of 6 patients who had mixed results, 3 improved and 3 did not; of 6 who had negative results, 4 improved and 2 did not. It was therefore suggested that a positive test is helpful but an equivocal or negative test is not. A more recent study by Vanneste et al.[34] reported that "cisternography did not improve the accuracy of combined clinical and computerized tomography in patients with presumed normal-pressure hydrocephalus." We do not use cisternography.

SPECIAL TESTING

CSF Drainage Procedures

If the patient's gait improves after removing a large quantity of CSF by lumbar puncture (30 to 50 mL, and this can be repeated daily), this person would be a good candidate for shunt surgery.[35,36]

A modification of this technique has also been reported; it is continuous CSF drainage via a catheter placed in the lumbar CSF space.[37,38] This involves placement of a thin subarachnoid catheter in the lumbar CSF space and leading it into a drainage bag. The height of the drainage bag is adjusted to allow drainage of 5 to 10 mL/h and yet avoid CSF hypotensive symptoms of headache. This is a closed system and allows an average of 150 mL drainage per day. The closed system helps prevent infection and the thin tube prevents rapid CSF drainage, cutting down the risk of subdural hemorrhage. There are other methods of doing this—e.g., Hanley et. al.[37] use a larger (16-gauge) catheter through which CSF pressure can also be monitored. They pay attention to the level of the drainage bag, aiming to drain 240 mL per day. To minimize infection, the drainage system is kept in for 2 to 5 days only. If symptoms of headache and nausea develop, one should be concerned that too much CSF is being drained.

Most recently Krauss and colleagues[39] reported their experience in removing CSF directly from the ventricles. They removed 15 to 18 mL at once from 20 patients and 24 mL over 6 h from 4 more patients. There were no complications. The 6 who showed a significant improvement with removal of the CSF and subsequently underwent shunt surgery had an excellent response to surgery. However, the 6 who had a moderate response to ventricular CSF removal had a more variable outcome.

There are shortcomings to these diagnostic tests. We have seen patients who eventually responded to shunt surgery but had no obvious improvement for the first postsurgical week. The drainage test could have given a falsely negative result in these patients. When doing the CSF drainage test, the patient may appear improved for the duration of the test (the placebo effect) but not maintain this response, leading to a false-positive result. In addition, meningitis and subdural hematoma are possible complications of the continuous CSF drainage procedures.

At this time our overall impression is that if either the LP or lumbar CSF drainage tests are strongly positive, this is a useful prognostic indicator; but if there is a mild response or the test is negative, one cannot accurately predict surgical outcome.

CSF Infusion Tests

Borgesen and Gjerris[14,40] described the CSF conductance test in which CSF absorption is measured at different CSF pressures. They reported in their series a greater than 90 percent accuracy in predicting short-term prognosis following shunt surgery and about an 85 percent accuracy in predicting long-term prognosis. The concept is that the greater the pressure needed to obtain an amount of absorption, the better the chances of that patient improving with shunt surgery. Absorption is calculated by infusing fluid through an LP (lumbar puncture) needle for a given time (5 min) while catching the overflow from a ventricular catheter. There is some evidence to show that the amount of CSF produced does not vary much at different CSF pressures and is about 0.4 mL/min. Because one knows how much is infused through the LP needle and how much overflow there is through the ventricular catheter, one can calculate the amount absorbed in this time period. The following equation gives absorption:

$$\begin{aligned}\text{Absorption} = {} & \text{infused (measured)} \\ & + \text{produced (assumed)} \\ & - \text{overflow (measured)}\end{aligned}$$

The overflow pressure for the ventricular catheter is then raised and absorption is then calculated at this new pressure. Between six and eight absorptions at different pressures are obtained in this way, and absorption is then plotted against pressure and the slope of the line calculated—i.e., absorption/pressure. The slope of this line is called the *conductance*. Borgesen and Gjerris reported that a conductance of < 0.08 predicted a favorable outcome. The inverse of the conductance gives the resistance to outflow (Rcsf). A conductance of 0.08 is equivalent to a resistance to outflow of 12.5 mmHg/mL/min.

Boon and colleagues[41] report the first multiple-center randomized study evaluating the predictive value for shunt surgery of measuring resistance to outflow of the CSF. They enrolled 101 patients and measured the Rcsf of CSF by infusing saline through a 19-gauge lumbar puncture needle at 1.4 to 1.6 mL/min until a stable pressure plateau was reached or the pressure exceeded 50 mmHg. The resistance to outflow was calculated as the difference between the plateau and the baseline pressure divided by the infusion rate. They randomized the patients to receive either low- or medium-pressure valves. Outcome measures were noted according to an NPH scale (sum of gait and dementia measures) and the modified Rankin scale. Follow-up was at 1, 3, 6, 9, and 12 months. Intention-to-treat analysis was performed on all 101 patients; 57 percent showed improvement in the NPH scale and 59 percent in the modified Rankin scale at 1 year. When all known serious events unrelated to NPH that clearly interfered with neurologic function were excluded, 95 patients were left. In these patients, 76 percent had a meaningful improvement on the NPH scale and 69 percent improved one grade on the modified Rankin scale.

Using a cutoff of the resistance to CSF outflow of <18 mmHg/mL/min, 20 of 59 patients had no improvement on the NPH scale. Above this cutoff, 3 of 36 had no improvement on the NPH scale.

The authors conclude that the Rcsf obtained by lumbar CSF infusion is a reliable method for selecting patients for shunt surgery if the Rcsf cutoff is 18 mmHg/mL/min or greater. Only patients with a Rcsf less than 18 mmHg/mL/min should undergo shunt placement when characteristic clinical features of NPH are present. Unfortunately, the majority of patients (>60 percent) under consideration for shunt surgery have a Rcsf of less than 18 mmHg/mL/min; therefore this diagnostic test is not helpful in this group.

CSF Pressure Monitoring

There have been reports of a significant relationship between measures of intracranial CSF pressure monitoring and surgical outcome for symptomatic hydrocephalus—e.g., in the Borgesen and Gjerris study[14] and in our study,[8] the greater the percentage of time B waves were present, the greater the chance of a good outcome (see Table 53-2).

Krauss and colleagues[42] have pointed out that there is a relationship of the quantity and type of B waves to the stage of sleep. Investigators should take into account the sleep stages when calculating the amount of time B waves are present on the recording.

Also, in our series, the longer the pressure was more than 15 mmHg, the better the chance of successful surgery (see Table 53-2). This implies that increased pressure may be pathogenic in symptomatic hydrocephalus.

These data raise the issue about what is meant by *normal pressure hydrocephalus*. Does it mean normal pressure at one spinal tap or does it imply the pressure remains normal all the time? We do not know what 24-h CSF pressure recordings in normal people show. It follows that we do not know if the pressure is normal or abnormal in those who respond to surgery but have CSF pressures greater than 15 mmHg for a percentage of time. For this reason, at present, we prefer the term *symptomatic hydrocephalus* to *normal pressure hydrocephalus* but recognize that, with the use of the latter term for more than two decades, it is unlikely to be replaced.

HOW TO ASSESS PATIENT IMPROVEMENT

Traditionally, patient improvement has been assessed on a five-point rating scale.[14,43] This may be problematic, because levels on the scale overlap and it is a subjective judgment into which level the patient falls. We have tried to develop more objective measures and use the following:

1. Serial videotaping of the patient's gait[8,44]
2. Katz Index of Activities of Daily Living[45]
3. Neuropsychological testing

The Katz scale rates the patient on six items: bathing, dressing, toileting, transferring, continence, and feeding. The worst score for each item is 3 and the best is 1. Thus the worst obtainable score is 18 and the best is 6. There is a written description for each score in each item. We regard a change of 2 or more in this index as significant. This allows measurements of small but functionally important changes. An example of a 2-point improvement on this index might be as follows:

a change from "occasional urinary accidents" to "controls urination and bowel movements completely by self" (1-point improvement) plus "moves in and out of bed or chair with assistance" to "moves in and out of bed as well as chair without assistance" (1-point improvement).

Finally, our patients receive a battery of neuropsychological tests before and 2 and 6 months after surgery.[8] These tests sample orientation, intelligence, verbal and visual memory, language, visuospatial functioning, and executive control. We judge the patient neuropsychologically improved when there has been a significant increase in the test scores in two or more neuropsychological areas evaluated, provided there is no decline in another area. Only about 50 percent of those responding to shunt surgery improve cognitively by the above criteria.

Other investigators have developed equally acceptable methods of evaluating surgical outcome objectively.[17,41,46]

SHUNT COMPLICATIONS

Shunt complications, both major and minor, unfortunately occur in 30 to 40 percent of patients.[7,43] These include intraoperative complications related to general anesthesia in an elderly population, intracranial hemorrhage from ventricular catheter placement, intra-abdominal injury (rare), and arrhythmias from incorrect ventriculoatrial distal catheter placement. Perioperative complications include infection (3 to 8 percent of cases), CSF hypotensive headaches, and the development of subdural effusions or hematomas. This last problem is more likely to occur in those with marked reduction in ventricular size postshunting and is more common when low-pressure valves are utilized for treatment. Depending on symptoms, conservative or surgical therapy may be indicated. Long-term complications are primarily related to shunt occlusion or catheter breakage. Infection after the first 2 months is unusual.

WHICH SHUNT TO RECOMMEND

The first randomized prospective study of NPH was completed in the Netherlands.[46] One of the questions addressed by this study was to compare the outcome after placement of low- or medium-pressure shunt valves in NPH patients. A total of 96 patients were randomized to receive low- or medium-pressure valves. Improvement was noted in 74 percent (marked to excellent in 45 percent) with low-pressure valves, whereas 53 percent (marked to excellent in 28 percent) improved with medium-pressure valves. The difference between the two groups was not quite significant ($p = 0.06$). Reduction in ventricular size was significantly greater in the low-pressure valve group ($p = 0.009$). However, subdural effusions occurred in 71 percent of the low-pressure group and in 34 percent of the medium-pressure group, most were transient but 32 percent were not. A total of 8 subdural effusions had to be drained. These authors advise the use of the low-pressure valve.

Other valves are in development, such as the dual-switch valve.[47] This valve has two parallel valve chambers in one device. One is blocked by a heavy tantalum ball in the upright position, avoiding overdrainage and the complication of slit ventricle syndrome (more common in children) and subdural hematomas (more common in adults). This may be a promising valve for this difficult problem and we await further information.

Yamashita et al.[48] reported their experience with the Codman Hakim programmable valve. This valve can have its opening pressure changed noninvasively with an externally applied programmer. The programmer transmits codified magnetic impulses. The opening pressure can be set from 30 to 180 mmH_2O in 18 steps. Settings can be verified with x-ray. There were no postoperative complications in their 85 NPH patients (20 were idiopathic). About 40 percent of the secondary NPH patients and 60 percent of the idiopathic NPH patients required reprogramming. In their total group of 168 patients, reprogramming was performed in 87 (50.6 percent) and symptoms or radiological findings (ventricular size) improved in 81 (93.1 percent). Because the valve is poorly resistant to magnetic fields, it is necessary to confirm opening pressure after every MR imaging procedure.

Mitchell and Mathew[49] obtained improvement in 3 of 4 NPH patients after performing third ventriculostomy. Interestingly this occurred despite pre- and postoperative ventricular pressure recordings that suggested the absence of improvement in ventricular pressures. He suggested third ventriculostomy relieves pulsatile tissue stress (from the waterhammer effect) by reducing the systolic transaqueductal pressure gradient.

ASSOCIATIONS OF IDIOPATHIC NPH THAT MIGHT HAVE IMPLICATIONS RELATED TO ETIOLOGY

Histopathology of Idiopathic NPH

In a unique study, Bech and colleagues[28] reported their experience with 38 consecutive patients with idiopathic NPH. They monitored and performed absorption tests on all, but most importantly, they performed brain biopsies on all. Of a total of 38 patients, 29 fulfilled hydrodynamic criteria for shunt surgery (resistance to outflow of 10 Hg/mL/min with or without B activity for more than 50 percent of the monitoring period). Of 29 individuals shunted, 27 had follow-up and of these 9 (33.3 percent) improved, 10 (37 percent) remained stable, and 8 (29.6 percent) deteriorated. These results are not necessarily representative of all series in which idiopathic NPH patients undergo shunt surgery—e.g., in our series, more than 70 percent improved[8] and in the series of Boon and colleagues,[46] 53 percent of the medium-pressure-valve group and 74 percent of the low-pressure-valve group improved. Nonetheless, the biopsy findings are of great interest and are shown in Table 53-3.

There was no significant association of the presence or absence of arachnoid fibrosis with the hydrodynamic measures.

The Bech study has some important implications. Of 38 patients who were thought clinically to possibly have NPH, 10 had biopsy-verified AD. The criteria used to diagnose AD were conservative—that is, 10 neuritic plaques per high-power field in the frontal lobe. It is possible that at autopsy several additional patients may have had AD. In a follow-up paper,[50] Bech found no correlation between clinical outcome after shunting NPH patients and the presence or absence of AD pathology. Further he also found that vascular disease and arachnoid fibrosis did not correlate with outcome. Golomb[51] found AD pathology in 23 of 56 (41 percent) biopsied NPH patients. The NPH patients with concomitant AD had more impairment of gait and cognition than the "pure" NPH patients. Only 18 percent of the patients with Global Deterioration Scores (GDSs) of 3 and below had AD-positive biopsies, whereas 75 percent of those with GDSs 6 or above were AD-positive. There was comparable improvement in gait velocity in NPH patients regardless of the presence of AD pathology. No consistent cognitive improvement occurred in either group after shunting. Savolainen[52] found concomitant AD pathology by biopsy in 31 percent of 51 consecutive NPH patients.

These three studies[50–53] show that AD pathology is frequent in patients diagnosed with idiopathic NPH. Further, some of these patients have gait improvement after shunting. The implication is that NPH and AD may occur simultaneously in the same patient and families should be made aware of this. Future studies should investigate if CSF markers, such as the amyloid β protein 1-42[53,54] and tau protein[53,54] may be helpful in these cases.

Table 53-3
Biopsy findings in 37 consecutive patients with idiopathic NPH

Arachnoid fibrosis	12 of 25 (not all biopsies had arachnoid tissue)
Normal parenchyma	17
Alzheimer's disease	8
Arteriosclerosis	4
Subrecent ischemic encephalomalacia	4
Alzheimer's disease and arteriosclerosis	1
Alzheimer's disease and encephalitis	1
Encephalitis	1
Nonspecific cortical degeneration	1
Cerebral hemorrhage, sequelae	1

Source: Adapted from Bech et al.,[50] with permission.

The Relationship of Idiopathic NPH and Systemic Hypertension

Several lines of evidence in the literature now point to a relationship between hydrocephalus and systemic hypertension.

Clinical and Autopsy Studies of NPH Patients

A number of postmortem examinations of NPH patients and case-control studies have reported the association of systemic hypertension and NPH.[55–59] In our own series,[44] a significantly higher prevalence of systemic hypertension was found in idiopathic NPH patients compared with matched, demented controls and to the published prevalence of hypertension in the U.S. population matched for age. A more recent, much larger case-control study[60] of 65 idiopathic NPH patients versus 70 matched control patients found a prevalence of 83 percent of systemic hypertension in the NPH patients compared to 36 percent in the control group. This was highly significant ($p < 0.001$).

Boon[61] showed that cerebrovascular risk factors (hypertension, diabetes mellitus, cardiac disease, peripheral vascular disease, male gender, and advancing age) did not influence outcome after shunt placement. However, the presence of cerebrovascular disease (history of stroke, cerebral infarction noted on CT, or moderate to severe white matter hypodense lesions on CT) was an important predictor of poor outcome. Nonetheless, even though 74 percent of those without concomitant cerebrovascular disease improved with shunting, 49 percent with it also improved. In fact, 4 of the 7 patients with the most severe white matter hypodense lesions responded favorably to shunting.

Sulfatide in the CSF correlates with the degree of white matter change.[62] However, the CSF level of sulfatide only showed a trend ($p = 0.09$) in its prediction of outcome with shunting.

At this time regarding hypertension, SAE, and NPH, we have more questions than answers. Are hypertension, white matter changes, and cerebrovascular disease merely frequent concomitants of NPH? Do NPH and SAE represent a spectrum (as suggested by Gallassi)?[63] Is one causative of the other?

Hydrocephalus following Subarachnoid Hemorrhage Another line of evidence showing that systemic hypertension and hydrocephalus may be related comes from the Cooperative Aneurysm Study.[64] In over 3000 patients with subarachnoid hemorrhage, it was found that a preoperative history of hypertension, the admission blood pressure measurement, and sustained hypertension during hospitalization after surgery all were highly significantly related to patients developing hydrocephalus.

Hypertension in Patients with Aqueductal Stenosis Greitz et al.[65] found a high prevalence of systemic hypertension in patients with hydrocephalus from aqueductal stenosis.

Hydrocephalus in the Spontaneously Hypertensive Rat The association of hypertension and hydrocephalus are corroborated by reports in the animal literature. Ritter and Dinh[66] showed that the spontaneously hypertensive rat develops hydrocephalus.

Experimental Models of Hydrocephalus, Ventricular Pulse Pressure, and Systemic Hypertension Portnoy et al.[67] showed, in dogs, that infusing dopamine and norepinephrine led to increased systemic blood pressure, which, in turn, resulted in an increased CSF pressure and pulse pressure. Experimentally creating an increased CSF pulse pressure with an inflatable balloon in the lateral ventricle of sheep leads to hydrocephalus within hours.[67] Bering and Salibi[68] performed seminal work on hydrocephalus in dogs. They tied off the jugular veins in the dogs and also measured the intraventricular pulse pressure. They concluded that the mechanism involved in the ventricular enlargement seemed to be a combination of at least two factors: "One was the possible failure of CSF absorption in the face of increased superior sagittal sinus venous pressure, and the other the increased intraventricular pulse pressure from the choroid plexus."

Thus, a body of information is accumulating that systemic hypertension and hydrocephalus are associated. It remains to be shown whether hypertension causes hydrocephalus or hydrocephalus causes hypertension, or both.

CONCLUSION

In working up with a patient with possible NPH, use the following systematic approach. Keeping in mind the differential diagnosis, look for pertinent factors in the history and examination and neuropsychological evaluation that have a bearing on diagnosis and surgical prognosis. On the MRI, look at the amount and pattern of atrophy and white matter changes. Perform between one and three spinal taps and evaluate the effect of this on the gait. Consider sending the CSF for AD markers (tau, amyloid protein 1-42, and neural thread protein). At this time you may wish to advise about surgery. If your center performs intracranial pressure monitoring, this may be helpful. The patient and family must be aware of both the possible benefits and the risks of the surgery (see Table 53-4). If they choose surgery, follow the patient carefully to see if there is improvement and to detect possible surgical complications. If you are uncertain whether the patient should undergo surgery or the family and patient choose that the patient should not undergo surgery, make sure you have established a baseline from which you can follow the patient. Ideally, this includes a video of gait, a brain MRI, and neuropsychological testing. Follow the patient at 3-month intervals with serial videotaping of gait. Stability or deterioration of the gait often helps both the family and doctor decide on further action.

Table 53-4
Factors related to shunt outcome

Factors favoring clinical improvement in NPH after shunting
Secondary NPH
Gait disturbance preceding cognitive impairment
Mild impairment in cognition
Short duration of cognitive impairment
Clinical improvement (usually in gait) following lumbar puncture or continuous lumbar CSF drainage
Resistance to CSF outflow of 18 mmHg/mL/min or greater during continuous lumbar CSF infusion test
Presence of B waves for 50% of the time or greater during continuous lumbar CSF monitoring
Factors weighing against clinical improvement after shunting
Moderate or severe cognitive impairment
Cognitive impairment preceding gait disturbance
Presence of aphasia
History of ethanol abuse
MRI with significant white matter involvement or diffuse cerebral atrophy
Factors of unproven significance
Long duration of gait disturbance
Absence of aqueductal flow void despite patent aqueduct (on MRI)
No clinical improvement after lumbar puncture
Cisternography
CBF measurements

REFERENCES

1. Graff-Radford NR: Normal pressure hydrocephalus. *Neurologist* 5:194–204, 1999.
2. Sudarsky L, Ronthal M: Gait disorders among elderly patients: A survey of 50 patients. *Arch Neurol* 40:740–743, 1983.
3. Evans DA, Funkenstein HH, Albert MS, et al: Prevalence of Alzheimer's disease in a community population of older persons higher than previously reported. *JAMA* 262:2551–2556, 1989.
4. Yarnell J, Leger A: The prevalence, severity and factors associated with urinary incontinence in a random sample of the elderly. *Age Ageing* 8:81–85, 1979.
5. Barron S, Jacobs L, Kinkel W: Changes in size of the normal lateral ventricles during aging determined by computerized tomography. *Neurology* 26:183–192, 1976.
6. Damasio H, Eslinger P, Damasio A: Quantitative computed tomographic analysis in the diagnosis of dementia. *Arch Neurol* 40:715–719, 1983.
7. Petersen RC, Mokri B, Laws ER Jr: Surgical treatment of idiopathic hydrocephalus in elderly patients. *Neurology* 35(3):307–311, 1985.
8. Graff-Radford NR, Godersky JC, Jones MP: Variables predicting surgical outcome in symptomatic hydrocephalus in the elderly. *Neurology* 39(12):1601–1604, 1989.
9. Fisher CM: The clinical picture in occult hydrocephalus. *Clin Neurosurg* 24:270–284, 1977.
10. De Mol J: Prognostic factors for therapeutic outcome in normal-pressure hydrocephalus. Review of the literature and personal study. *Acta Neurol Belg* 85(1):13–29, 1985.
11. Black PM, Ojemann RG, Tzouras A: CSF shunts for dementia, incontinence, and gait disturbance. *Clin Neurosurg* 32:632–651, 1985.

12. Graff-Radford NR, Godersky JC: Symptomatic congenital hydrocephalus in the elderly simulating normal pressure hydrocephalus. *Neurology* 39(12):1596–1600, 1989.
13. Gyldenstad C: Measurements of the normal ventricular system and hemispheric sulci of 100 adults with computerized tomography. *Neuroradiology* 14:183–192, 1977.
14. Borgesen S, Gjerris F: The predictive value of conductance to outflow of CSF in normal pressure hydrocephalus. *Brain* 105:65–86, 1982.
15. Jack C et al: MR-based hippocampal volume in the diagnosis of Alzheimer's disease. *Neurology* 42:183–188, 1992.
16. Bradley WG Jr et al: Marked cerebrospinal fluid void: indicator of successful shunt in patients with suspected normal-pressure hydrocephalus. *Radiology* 178(2):459–466, 1991.
17. Krauss JK et al: Cerebrospinal fluid shunting in idiopathic normal-pressure hydrocephalus of the elderly: Effect of periventricular and deep white matter lesions. *Neurosurgery* 39(2):292–299, discussion 299–300, 1996.
18. Krauss JK et al: White matter lesions in patients with idiopathic normal pressure hydrocephalus and in an age-matched control group: A comparative study. *Neurosurgery* 40(3):491–495, discussion 495–496, 1997.
19. Munoz D et al: Pathological correlates of increased signals of the centrum ovale on magnetic resonance imaging. *Arch Neurol* 50:492–497, 1993.
20. Holodny AI et al: Focal dilation and paradoxical collapse of cortical fissures and sulci in patients with normal-pressure hydrocephalus. *J Neurosurg* 89(5):742–747, 1998.
21. Kitagaki H et al: CSF spaces in idiopathic normal pressure hydrocephalus: morphology and volumetry. *A J N R* 19(7):1277–1284, 1998.
22. Holodny AI et al: MR differential diagnosis of normal-pressure hydrocephalus and Alzheimer disease: Significance of perihippocampal features. *A J N R* 19(5):813–819, 1998.
23. Golomb J et al: Hippocampal atrophy correlates with severe cognitive impairment in elderly patients with suspected normal pressure hydrocephalus. *J Neurol Neurosurg Psychiatry* 57(5):590–593, 1994.
24. Savolainen S et al: MR imaging of the hippocampus in normal pressure hydrocephalus: Correlations with cortical Alzheimer's disease confirmed by pathologic analysis. *A J N R* 21(2):409–414, 2000.
25. Bradley WG Jr et al: Normal-pressure hydrocephalus: evaluation with cerebrospinal fluid flow measurements at MR imaging. *Radiology* 198(2):523–529, 1996.
26. Krauss JK et al: Flow void of cerebrospinal fluid in idiopathic normal pressure hydrocephalus of the elderly: Can it predict outcome after shunting? *Neurosurgery* 40(1):67–73, discussion 73–74, 1997.
27. Hakim R, Black PM: Correlation between lumboventricular perfusion and MRI-CSF flow studies in idiopathic normal pressure hydrocephalus. *Surg Neurol* 49(1):14–19, discussion 19–20, 1998.
28. Bech RA et al: Frontal brain and leptomeningeal biopsy specimens correlated with cerebrospinal fluid outflow resistance and B-wave activity in patients suspected of normal-pressure hydrocephalus. *Neurosurgery* 40(3):497–502, 1997.
29. McHugh P: Occult hydrocephalus. *Q J Med* 130:297–308, 1964.
30. Jagust W, Friedland R, Budinger T: Positron emission tomography with (18F)-fluorodeoxyglucose differentiates normal pressure hydrocephalus from Alzheimer's dementia. *J Neurol Neurosurg Psychiatry* 48:1091–1096, 1985.
31. Foster N et al: Alzheimer's disease: Focal cortical changes shown by positron emission tomography. *Neurology* 33:961–965, 1983.
32. Graff-Radford NR et al: Regional cerebral blood flow in normal pressure hydrocephalus. *J Neurol Neurosurg Psychiatry* 50(12):1589–1596, 1987.
33. Black PM: Normal-pressure hydrocephalus: current understanding of diagnostic tests and shunting. *Postgrad Med* 71(2):57–61, 65–67, 1982.
34. Vanneste J et al: Shunting normal-pressure hydrocephalus: Do the benefits outweigh the risks? A multicenter study and literature review. *Neurology* 42(1):54–59, 1992.
35. Wikkelso C et al: The clinical effect of lumbar puncture in normal pressure hydrocephalus. *J Neurol Neurosurg Psychiatry* 45(1):64–69, 1982.
36. Wikkelso C et al: Normal pressure hydrocephalus. Predictive value of the cerebrospinal fluid tap-test. *Acta Neurol Scand* 73(6):566–573, 1986.
37. Hanley D, Borel C, Hedeman S: Normal-pressure hydrocephalus, in Johnson R (ed): *Current Therapy in Neurological Diseases.* Philadelphia: Decker, 1990, pp 305–309.
38. Haan J, Thomeer RT: Predictive value of temporary external lumbar drainage in normal pressure hydrocephalus. *Neurosurgery* 22(2):388–391, 1988.
39. Krauss JK, Regel JP: The predictive value of ventricular CSF removal in normal pressure hydrocephalus. *Neurol Res* 19(4):357–360, 1997.

40. Borgesen SE: Conductance to outflow of CSF in normal pressure hydrocephalus. *Acta Neurochir (Wien)* 71 (1–2):1–45, 1984.
41. Boon A et al: Dutch Normal-Pressure Hydrocephalus Study; prediction of outcome after shunting by resistance to outflow of cerebrospinal fluid. *J Neurosurg* 87:687–693, 1997.
42. Krauss JK et al: The relation of intracranial pressure B-waves to different sleep stages in patients with suspected normal pressure hydrocephalus. *Acta Neurochir (Wien)* 136 (3–4):195–203, 1995.
43. Black PM: Idiopathic normal-pressure hydrocephalus. Results of shunting in 62 patients. *J Neurosurg* 52(3): 371–377, 1980.
44. Graff-Radford NR, Godersky JC: Idiopathic normal pressure hydrocephalus and systemic hypertension. *Neurology* 37(5):868–871, 1987.
45. Kane R, Kane R: *Assessing the Elderly*. Lexington, MA: Lexington Books, 1981.
46. Boon AJ et al: Dutch Normal-Pressure Hydrocephalus Study: Randomized comparison of low- and medium-pressure shunts. *J Neurosurg* 88(3):490–495, 1998.
47. Sprung C et al: The importance of the dual-switch valve for the treatment of adult normotensive or hypertensive hydrocephalus. *Eur J Pediatr Surg* 7(Suppl 1):38–40, 1997.
48. Yamashita N, Kamiya K, Yamada K: Experience with a programmable valve shunt system. *J Neurosurg* 91(1):26–31, 1999.
49. Mitchell P, Mathew B: Third ventriculostomy in normal pressure hydrocephalus. *Br J Neurosurg* 13(4):382–385, 1999.
50. Bech RA et al: Shunting effects in patients with idiopathic normal pressure hydrocephalus; correlation with cerebral and leptomeningeal biopsy findings. *Acta Neurochir (Wien)* 141(6):633–639, 1999.
51. Golomb J et al: Alzheimer's disease comorbidity in normal pressure hydrocephalus: Prevalence and shunt response. *J Neurol Neurosurg Psychiatry* 68(6):778–781, 2000.
52. Savolainen S, Paljarvi L, Vapalahti M: Prevalence of Alzheimer's disease in patients investigated for presumed normal pressure hydrocephalus: A clinical and neuropathological study. *Acta Neurochir* (Wien) 141(8):849–853, 1999.
53. Arai H et al: Cerebrospinal fluid tau protein as a potential diagnostic marker in Alzheimer's disease. *Neurobiol Aging* 19:125–126, 1998.
54. Galasko D et al: High cerebrospinal fluid tau and low amyloid β 42 levels in the clinical diagnosis of Alzheimer's disease and relation to apolipoprotein E genotype. *Arch Neurol* 55:937–945, 1998.
55. Koto A et al: Syndrome of normal pressure hydrocephalus: possible relation to hypertensive and arteriosclerotic vasculopathy. *J Neurol Neurosurg Psychiatry* 40:73–79, 1977.
56. Earnest MP et al: Normal pressure hydrocephalus and hypertensive cerebrovascular disease. *Arch Neurol* 31(4):262–266, 1974.
57. Haidri N, Modri S: Normal pressure hydrocephalus and hypertensive cerebrovascular disease. *Dis Nerv Syst* 38:918–921, 1977.
58. Shukla D, Singh B, Strobos R: Hypertensive cerebrovascular disease and normal pressure hydrocephalus. *Neurology* 30:998–1000, 1980.
59. Casmiro M et al: Risk factors for the syndrome of ventricular enlargement with gait apraxia (idiopathic normal pressure hydrocephalus): A case-control study. *J Neurol Neurosurg Psychiatry* 52(7):847–852, 1989.
60. Krauss JK et al: Vascular risk factors and arteriosclerotic disease in idiopathic normal-pressure hydrocephalus of the elderly. *Stroke* 27(1):24–29, 1996.
61. Boon AJ et al: Dutch Normal-Pressure Hydrocephalus Study: The role of cerebrovascular disease. *J Neurosurg* 90(2):221–226, 1999.
62. Tullberg M et al: CSF sulfatide distinguishes between normal pressure hydrocephalus and subcortical arteriosclerotic encephalopathy. *J Neurol Neurosurg Psychiatry* 69(1):74–81, 2000.
63. Gallassi R et al: Binswanger's disease and normal-pressure hydrocephalus. Clinical and neuropsychological comparison. *Arch Neurol* 48(11):1156–1159, 1991.
64. Graff-Radford N et al: Factors associated with hydrocephalus after subarachnoid hemorrhage: A report of the Cooperative Aneurysm Study. *Arch Neurol* 46:744–752, 1989.
65. Greitz T, Levander B, Lopez J: High blood pressure and epilepsy in hydrocephalus due to stenosis of the aqueduct of Sylvius. *Acta Neurochir (Wien)* 24:201–206, 1971.
66. Ritter S, Dinh T: Progressive postnatal dilation of brain ventricles in spontaneously hypertensive rats. *Brain Res* 370:327–332, 1986.
67. Portnoy H, Chopp M, Branch C: Hydraulic model of myogenic autoregulation and the cerebrovascular bed: The effects of altering systemic blood pressure. *Neurosurgery* 13:482–498, 1986.
68. Bering RJ, Salibi B: Production of hydrocephalus by increased cephalic-venous pressure. *Arch Neurology Psychiatry* 81:693–698, 1959.

Chapter 54

COGNITIVE AND BEHAVIORAL ASPECTS OF EPILEPSY

Melanie Shulman
Orrin Devinsky

Except perhaps for stroke, the clinical paradigm of classic focal or disconnection syndromes in neurology, no other disorder has provided as fertile ground for the study of brain-behavior relationships as epilepsy. Derived from the Greek *epilepsia,* "grabbed hold of from above," the term itself attests to the dramatic paroxysmal behavioral manifestations that define the clinical syndrome. Several fundamental concepts of brain organization and function derive from epilepsy-based research and therapy. These include insights about the sensorimotor homunculus, plasticity of speech and language, hemispheric specialization, and perhaps most famously, the critical role of the hippocampal-temporal lobe complex in memory.[146] Indeed, epilepsy has served as a "natural laboratory" for the study of human memory.[188]

Epilepsy is associated with cognitive and behavioral changes that can occur in ictal, peri-ictal, and interictal states. The diversity of these changes reflects the heterogeneity of the patient population with epilepsy.[33,39,70,152,194] Specifically, cognitive and behavioral changes result from multifaceted and overlapping influences of genetics, neuropathology, seizure-related variables, antiepileptic drugs (AEDs), and psychosocial issues.[94,111,217] Most patients with epilepsy lead lives unencumbered by cognitive or psychiatric disturbances; however, neurobehavioral problems occur in a substantial minority.[44,156,208] Some patients develop significant cognitive deficits, especially in the domains of memory, attention, and motor speed.[47,90,185] Other patients develop psychiatric problems including aberrant personality traits, anxiety, depression, or even psychosis.[44,94,186]

Despite decades of investigation, our understanding of the nature of the relationship between epilepsy and neurobehavioral dysfunction remains fragmentary. Methodologic problems in the diagnosis of epilepsy, inadequate sampling procedures, small sample sizes, lack of adequate control groups, inadequate measures of behavioral phenomena, and conflating variables such as intelligence have yielded inconsistent findings in the literature.[119,194] These methodologic constraints notwithstanding, this field of study warrants renewed and intensified investigation. From a practical standpoint, the need to address the cognitive and behavioral manifestations of a common neurologic problem (the lifetime risk of developing epilepsy is approximately 3 percent) is obvious.[79] From a theoretical perspective, epilepsy remains a unique clinical opportunity to clarify the neural mechanisms underlying behavior, since it allows, as Geschwind (1979) pointed out, for direct correlation between specific aspects of affective behavior and localized dysfunction.[64]

CLASSIFICATION OF THE EPILEPSIES

Classification of the epilepsies is based on both anatomy and clinical manifestations. A "primary generalized seizure" affects the entire cortex at onset, whereas a "partial seizure" occurs as a result of a focal discharge in the brain. The designations *simple* and *complex* further connote whether or not a partial seizure affects consciousness. In simple partial seizures, a focal discharge remains localized and consciousness is not affected. In complex partial seizures, the discharge spreads beyond the focal area of onset and alters consciousness (as manifest by altered awareness, impaired responsiveness, or loss of memory for the event). Taken literally, however, the terms can be misleading. A "simple" partial seizure may be associated with complex experiential phenomena from déjà vu to autoscopy (the experience of seeing one's double or having an out-of-body experience) to fear and pleasure. "Complex" partial seizures may consist of a sudden isolated disruption without additional psychological phenomena. Approximately 60 percent of patients with epilepsy experience partial seizures, and nearly 60 percent of those fit the definitions of temporolimbic epilepsy (TLE).[78,79] However, many patients with TLE probably remain undiagnosed because their only symptoms are behavioral and difficult to capture.

The diverse phenomena of partial epilepsy have long captured the interest of clinicians and researchers studying brain-behavior relationships. The late 1930s was a crucial time for the future development of epileptology. Gibbs and colleagues (1937) gave a thorough description of the electroencephalographic (EEG) characteristics and phenomenology of psychomotor seizures and the critical involvement of the anterior temporal lobe.[66] They also proposed a link between psychomotor seizures and increased psychiatric risk. In that same year, Papez (1937) proposed a neuroanatomic basis for emotions.[150] The obvious overlap of psychomotor seizures and the anatomy of emotions generated a generation of clinical investigations of behavioral disturbances and psychiatric syndromes in patients with psychomotor seizures and, conversely, the prevalence of seizure disorders in psychiatric populations.

More recently, researchers emphasize the profound variability of the TLE syndrome, which contributes to the lack of consistent findings across different studies. Epilepsy of temporal lobe origin is characterized by considerable heterogeneity in clinical history, ictal symptoms, EEG characteristics, neuroimaging findings, neuropsychological features, and underlying neuropathologic condition.[151] A distinct syndrome has been proposed, namely mesial temporal lobe epilepsy, of which hippocampal sclerosis is a defining characteristic.[52,90,151] Clinically, mesial TLE is characterized by a history of an early febrile convulsion, particularly one that has been prolonged or complicated, followed by a seizure-free period for several years, and then the development of complex partial seizures in adolescence. Other features of the syndrome include affectively valenced seizure semiology, a lateralized EEG abnormality, characteristic magnetic resonance imaging (MRI) findings (hippocampal atrophy on T1-weighted images, increased mesial temporal signal on T2-weighted images), focal functional deficits, and a pattern of nonresponse to medications. Mesial temporal lobe epilepsy is usually associated with a particularly good outcome after anteromesial temporal lobectomy.[53]

The diverse spectrum of ictal and interictal behavioral phenomenology of patients with seizures emanating from the frontal lobes has received far less attention than that of patients with seizures of the temporal lobes. Several unique diagnostic dilemmas have historically complicated its study.[116] The EEG can be normal in either the ictal or interictal state.[224] Frontal lobe seizures spread widely and rapidly and have a tendency to manifest interictal discharges bilaterally, further complicating accurate localization of epileptiform foci.[159] The behavioral manifestations of frontal lobe seizures can be bizarre and are often mistaken for pseudoseizures.[172] Neuroimaging studies are often unrevealing. Neuropsychological batteries have been unable to distinguish frontal regional subgroups (based on EEG, seizure semiology, and neuroimaging) in frontal lobe epilepsy (FLE) populations.[83,214]

Epileptic syndromes considered under the rubric of *idiopathic generalized epilepsy* include juvenile myoclonic epilepsy, absence epilepsy, and tonic-clonic seizures upon wakening.[48,121] They are often associated with a family history of seizures but with normal neurologic development and normal neuroimaging studies. The interictal EEG may exhibit alterations that suggest a generalized origin of the seizures. The response to antiepileptic drug (AED) therapy is good: 80 to 90 percent of these patients will be seizure-free or nearly seizure-free with appropriate medical management.

ICTAL BEHAVIOR

A wide variety of behaviors correlate with the ictal discharge in temporal lobe epilepsy or electrical stimulation of temporal lobe regions. The majority of ictal behavioral changes result from seizure discharge involving the temporal lobe, both in its limbic and neocortical components. Whether an individual experiences only selected symptoms or a combination of these depends on the seizure's origin and ictal spread within the temporolimbic network.[71]

Auras immediately preceding a complex partial seizure are reportable, since memory is retained.[58]

Auras range from simple sensations easily described by patients to ineffable experiential phenomena. Auras provide unique access to investigate subjective experience in epilepsy and its anatomic substrate. Yet the relationship of seizure localization to the localization of auras remains controversial. Auras often persist after mediotemporal surgery even when the patients are rendered seizure-free.[57,189] This observation has raised the possibility that auras may be caused by a process distinct from that causing the seizure or that it may arise in a different location.

A brief summary of varied cognitive, experiential, and emotional ictal phenomena illustrating brain-behavior relationships is provided below.

Cognitive Ictal Phenomena

Ictal discharges in TLE can affect attention, language, and memory. Prolonged confusional and fugue states have been associated with ongoing seizure activity.[224] Aphasic disturbances related to left temporal discharges include speech arrest (most commonly) as well as varied paraphasic errors, comprehension deficits, anomia, and dysgraphia.[109] Epileptic discharges can elicit three different kinds of mnemonic phenomena: (1) an illusion of memory (i.e., déjà vu), (2) a memory flashback, or (3) interference with anterograde memory during the time of the seizure, later experienced as retrograde amnesia for the event.[71] Transient epileptic amnesia (TEA) mimics transient global amnesia, with transient amnesia as the sole manifestation of a temporal lobe seizure.[125,229] Episodes are typically brief, lasting less than 1 h, and recurrent, with a mean frequency of three a year. The question of whether TEA reflects ictal activity and/or a postictal state remains unresolved.

Experiential Phenomena

Experiential phenomena are described by patients in a way suggesting that their subjective quality of immediacy resembles that of personal experiences in everyday life.[71] They are extremely vivid and highly personalized. They usually occur in the very early stages of the seizure and are short-lived. Experiential phenomena include déjà vu or déjà vecu (already seen or experienced) phenomena, consisting of a sense that the events or location at the moment have been experienced or witnessed previously by the patient. Déjà vu can be described as an illusion of memory; that is, encountering a familiar person or place is normally associated with a cognitive component (memory of a specific experience) as well as an affective component (surprise, fear, pleasure). In déjà vu, the affective component is dissociated from the cognitive; the patient remains very much aware that the feeling is not commensurate with the experience.[71] Mullan and Penfield (1959) found that in most cases, the illusion of familiarity is elicited by right and not by left temporal lobe stimulation.[142] Jamais vu is the feeling that familiar things appear strange, foreign, or remote. Déjà entendu and jamais entendu are familiar or unfamiliar auditory experiences, respectively.

Other subjective mental states evoked by temporolimbic seizures are often complex and hard to describe. Autoscopy, the experience of seeing one's double or having an out-of-body experience, embarassment, religious experiences, and racing or involuntary thoughts can all occur; however, these events are rarely reported spontaneously by the patient.[27,36,37,42,70,139]

Emotional Phenomena

Ictal emotions mimic diverse normal experiences as well as psychiatric symptoms. Such paroxysmal waves of intense feeling typically arise spontaneously, but on occasion they may be triggered by an environmental stimulus, such as a particular odor or a piece of music. Emotional manifestations of ictal activity are most often negative in valence.[71,194] Ictal emotion can be isolated or associated with other ictal symptoms. The temporal duration of the paroxysm is often the key to distinguishing a partial seizure from a psychiatric disorder: seizures typically are of sudden onset and brief duration (10 s to 3 min), whereas panic attacks typically last longer than 10 min. Other helpful features of ictal fear that distinguish it from panic attacks include amnesia for the episode, childhood onset, and associated symptoms such as buccal automatisms.[16,35]

Fear and Anxiety Fear is the most frequent ictal emotion, occurring in approximately 20 percent of patients with temporal lobe epilepsy.[70,117,194] Ictal fear arises suddenly, out of context, and varies in intensity from slight anxiety to stark terror. Its duration can vary from several seconds to minutes.[16,44] Patients with partial epilepsy who have ictal fear are more likely than those without ictal fear to have frequent psychiatric hospitalizations, greater interictal anxiety, and increased scores for psychopathology on personality inventories.[44,76,87] Ictal fear does not have lateralizing value in most studies. Electrical stimulation studies have provided evidence that the amygdala is likely a critical structure in the induction of the fear response. Some epileptic patients' attacks of fear stopped after temporal lobectomy that included removal of portions of the amygdala.[129] Autonomic conditioned responses are reduced in patients having undergone temporal lobe with amygdala resections.[112]

Depression and Mania Pure ictal depression is uncommon.[194,199] The emotion may occur as an aura of the seizure, during the seizure, or immediately following the seizure. The duration is highly variable: it may be brief (several minutes) or prolonged (persisting for days), merging into the postictal state.[223] Electrical stimulation studies have not yielded a precise anatomic localization for induced feelings of sadness other than involvement of a temporolimbic discharge.[194] A mania-like state consisting of euphoria, hyperactivity, and social disinhibition has been reported in conjunction with ictal discharges originating from or spreading to orbitofrontal cortex.[204]

Laughter and Crying Ictal laughter (gelastic seizures) and ictal crying (dacrystic or quiritarian seizures) are seizures occurring with or without preserved consciousness or concomitant mood state, despite their apparent expression of emotion.[71,194,228] As in the case of pseudobulbar palsy, the dissociation of mood and affect reflects the anatomic dissociation of these behavioral functions in cortical and subcortical areas.[43]

Ictal laughter is rare, occurring in less than 0.2 percent of epilepsy patients.[194] The stereotypic attacks of ictal laughter usually last 5 to 120 s and occur spontaneously, without emotional or mental provocation.[228] Ictal laughter, often mechanical and staccato, may occur as part of either frontal or temporal seizures. It may also occur in deep midbrain lesions (often hypothalamic hamartomas) or diffuse encephalopathies; and, in those conditions, the laughter is described as distinctly unnatural.[71]

Ictal crying is extremely rare.[180] Right hemispheric lateralization has been suggested, but the few cases studied limit broad generalizations. Tearing and a sad mood may or may not accompany the facial motor and vocal changes.[123]

Aggression The existence of ictal aggression, whether associated with spontaneous temporal lobe discharge or electrical stimulation, has been the subject of intense study and debate.[194] Rigorously defined ictal aggression is a rare event. In a comprehensive study reported by Delgado and colleagues (1981), only 19 of 5400 patients (0.4 percent) whose seizures were studied on video-EEG monitoring displayed aggressive behavior.[32] In most of the cases, the aggressive behaviors were spontaneous, simple, nondirected stereotyped aggressive movements involving objects or persons. Although they appeared highly coordinated, the acts are associated with confusion. They do not occur in response to preictal provocation, nor are they premeditated.[207] The low frequency of ictal aggression in epilepsy centers may reflect bias (i.e., not admitting violent patients for hospitalization) as well as the hospital setting itself (i.e., not being environmentally conducive to violent reactions).[55] Aggressive behaviors have been correlated with electrophysiologic dysfunction in limbic structures, particularly the amygdala and hippocampus.[34,210]

POSTICTAL BEHAVIOR

Postictal behavioral symptoms offer clues to the lateralization and localization of the seizure onset. Postictal symptoms can last from minutes to days, but prolonged postictal symptoms (> 12 h) can often occur in patients with structural lesions such as tumors or stroke. A new postictal symptom suggests a more intense seizure or a recent structural change. Hypotheses regarding the mechanism underlying postictal dysfunction derive from the nineteenth century and remain relevant today: neuronal exhaustion or depletion of neurotransmitters (Todd-Jackson theory) and active inhibition (Gower's theory).[73,100,145]

Todd's Paralysis

Todd's paralysis, or "reversible hemiplegia after seizures," can affect cognitive and behavioral functions. Depending on seizure generalization, postictal reorientation times vary between 1 and 45 min.[80] Frontal lobe seizures do not influence postictal memory performance, but verbal and visual recognition memory are significantly decreased after temporal lobe seizures. Using subdural electrode recordings in TLE patients with left hemispheric language dominance, Devinsky et al. (1994) correlated the following behavioral phenomena with side of ictus and ictal spread: (1) impaired comprehension with fluent but unintelligible speech, as well as anomia, occurred after seizures arising from either temporal lobe; (2) postictal nonfluent or global aphasia exclusively followed seizures originating from the left temporal lobe; and (3) prolonged disorientation for place and flat affect were significantly more common after right temporal complex partial seizures (CPSs).[39]

Postictal Psychosis

Typical features of the postictal psychoses have been consistently reported in the literature.[33,120,205] They usually follow clusters of CPSs or secondary generalized seizures with a brief postictal interlude or "lucid interval" before the mental state deteriorates. The psychosis—frequently featuring mood alterations, delusional ideas, religious ideation, prolonged déjà vu, hallucinations, and aggressive behavior—may last for up to a week. The EEG may exhibit increased epileptiform activity or a slowed dominant rhythm. The episodes resolve spontaneously but often recur, usually with stereotyped phenomenology. Bilateral limbic lesions and bilateral seizure foci are risk factors.[33,213] Postictal psychotic patients report more seizure clustering and ictal fear.[169,213]

Postictal Aggression

Postictal aggression is the most common and best-documented form of aggressive behavior in epilepsy. Following a generalized tonic-clonic seizure or, less often, after a complex partial seizure, verbal or physical aggression can occur during the recovery period, when the patient is still confused. In this setting, physical restraint can provoke aggression, which almost always stops when the restraint is withdrawn.[55,164] Aggression may also be a prominent feature of postictal psychoses, particularly in patients with paranoid delusions and threatening hallucinations.[62]

INTERICTAL BEHAVIOR

Children and adults with epilepsy are more likely than normal persons and those with medical or other neurologic disorders to develop interictal cognitive and behavioral changes.[75,110,185,196,222,226] Classic psychiatric disorders such as depression, anxiety, psychosis, somatization, and dissociation are more frequent in epilepsy patients than in the general population.[5,44,61,94,186]

Cognitive and behavioral dysfunction in epilepsy fails to fit paradigms of behavioral neurology in the sense of the classic focal lesion or disconnection. The changes likely result from temporolimbic or neocortical disorders affected by various mechanisms (i.e., mesial temporal sclerosis, dysplasia, kindling, neurochemical or synaptic alterations) on complex distributed neural network activity.[187,208]

Interictal cognitive and behavioral disturbances present large intra- and interindividual variations. Hermann and colleagues (1984, 1999) proposed three potentially interactive categories to organize the multiplicity of risk factors for cognitive and behavioral changes in epilepsy: (1) neurobiological factors, including the neuropathology/etiology of the epileptic region, seizure variables, duration of epilepsy, seizure control, and interictal epileptiform activity; (2) psychosocial factors, including chronic illness-related and epilepsy-specific issues, both developmental and demographic; and (3) iatrogenic factors, including specific medication effects, mono- or polytherapy, alterations in brain neurotransmitter concentrations, and metabolic effects.[94,220]

Interictal Cognitive Manifestations

Intelligence Allowing for numerous methodologic constraints, several generalizations about cognitive function in epilepsy appear consistent in the literature.

Patients with well-controlled epilepsy rarely demonstrate significant impairment in general intellectual functioning as assessed by IQ tests.[19,155,185] However, numerous studies have confirmed greater cognitive impairments in patients with generalized (especially secondarily generalized) versus partial seizures, earlier onset and longer duration of epilepsy, greater seizure frequency, and episodes of status epilepticus.[46,47,178,185]

Although discrepancies in verbal-performance IQ on Wechsler Intelligence Scales can reflect laterality in some populations, these differences do not consistently reflect seizure laterality.[156] The Performance Scale is considered to be a more sensitive measure of general cerebral integrity than the Verbal Scale, and low performance IQ scores can be present in patients with either a right or a left seizure focus.

The VA Cooperative Study of Smith et al. (1986) controlled for medication effects by administering a neuropsychological test battery to 618 newly diagnosed epilepsy patients before the administration of any AED.[185] There was no significant difference in general intellectual ability between patients and controls. However, the patients with epilepsy did not perform as well as controls on measures of attention, psychomotor speed, and fluency. A recent Finnish study, however, recruited untreated patients with new-onset seizures and found no differences in terms of motor function, attention, or memory between individuals with partial versus generalized seizures; but all the patients scored worse than healthy controls.[157]

Memory Interictal memory deficits are frequently found in patients with generalized or complex partial seizures, especially with left or bilateral temporal onset.[15,31] Indeed, the study of epilepsy patients undergoing temporal lobectomy for control of intractable seizures led to a corpus demonstrating the critical role of the hippocampi and adjacent temporal lobe systems in memory.[140,146] Preoperative patients with left temporal lobe EEG foci have fixed long-term deficits on tests of verbal list learning, cued recall, and semantic encoding.[90,140,143] There has been much less consistency demonstrating nonverbal or visual memory impairment in presurgical patients with right temporal lobe EEG foci.[9,10,84,104] The lack of consensus raises complex theoretical and methodological issues about the nature of the right or "nondominant" hemisphere in nonverbal memory functioning.

Most of the epilepsy memory research has been performed in presurgical or surgical patients with the most severe impairment. In general practice, the degree of memory impairment in well-controlled patients is likely to be quite variable, with only a subset of well-controlled patients showing significant impairment.[156] A growing literature, however, is addressing the apparent weak association between neuropsychological measures and subjective memory complaints in patients with epilepsy.[49,81,171] This discrepancy may be due to the influence of a variety of factors (especially mood) on subjective reports of memory, or it may be due to an inadequacy in standard neuropsychology batteries to evaluate "everyday" memory problems.[17,81] Indeed, a subgroup of left-TLE patients show a form of accelerated forgetting characterized by normal retention of new information at standard 30-min delays but amnesia for information at intervals of days or weeks.[17] This accelerated forgetting is hypothesized to reflect the disruptive effects of seizures on the long-term consolidation of new information. Interictal memory impairment results from a combination of structural lesions, neuronal dysfunction or loss, interictal epileptiform discharges, recurrent seizures, and AEDs.[1,111,131,151,157]

Intellectual deterioration or dementia may complicate chronic TLE.[82,102] Specifically, concern has been raised as to whether the syndrome of mesial temporal lobe epilepsy may be associated with progressive damage to medial temporal lobe structures.[59,105,195] Earlier seizure onset and longer duration of epilepsy are associated with a higher risk of generalized cognitive impairment and progressive hippocampal atrophy; however, it remains unclear whether this is attributable to progressive epilepsy itself or rather to the additive effects of preexisting disease and physiologic aging.

Language Word-finding difficulties or even anomia can occur in patients with left temporal lobe seizures.[109,126] Anomia and other language deficits may account for some of the verbal memory deficits associated with left-TLE patients.[96,126] A recent positron emission tomography (PET) study found that the greatest metabolic depression in left-TLE patients was in the left inferior frontal and superior temporal regions (corresponding with Broca's and Wernicke's areas, respectively).[7] Language impairments correlated with metabolic deficits in the two regions. Several investigators have postulated that the "sticky" or "viscous" personality style recognized in TLE patients could arise from subtle interictal language disturbances.[126,158]

Executive Functions Specific executive function testing in undifferentiated epilepsy patients has found deficits in tasks of psychomotor speed, sequencing, and cognitive flexibility to mirror those of generalized intellectual impairment.[46]

The Wisconsin Card Sorting Test (WCST) assesses problem-solving, mental flexibility, and perseverative tendencies. It has been used in studying frontal lobe function in various epilepsy populations. A substantial proportion of patients with TLE (independent of hippocampal integrity) perform outside of normal limits on the WCST.[28,91,206] This finding has been used to bolster a "nociferous cortex" hypothesis, whereby executive dysfunction seen in TLE patients is not due to functional compromise of the epileptogenic temporal lobe or hippocampus but rather attributable to the noxious influence of epileptogenic cortex on extratemporal regions (the frontal lobes being particularly vulnerable).[91]

A single study comparing patterns of executive impairment in TLE versus frontal lobe epilepsy (FLE) found the former to be associated with impaired performance on tests of cognitive speed and attention and the latter to be associated with impaired performance on tests of motor programming and response inhibition.[83]

Medication Effects Numerous studies have investigated the cognitive effects of antiepileptic drugs (AEDs), and extensive reviews are available.[26,111,131,209] Controversial methodologic issues have surrounded many early reports of the adverse cognitive effects of these medications, including the conflation of various cognitive variables with motor performance and accuracy.[209] A series of well-controlled randomized double-blinded crossover studies in patients and healthy volunteers have demonstrated adverse cognitive effects (predominantly in concentration, attention, and psychomotor abilities) for all of the older AEDs tested but no clinically significant differences among phenytoin, carbamazepine, and valproic acid monotherapy.[22,67,130] The beneficial effects of reducing seizures largely offset the adverse cognitive effects. Factors that may increase the occurrence of cognitive side effects include increased AED dosage, higher AED blood levels, and polytherapy.

Data on the cognitive effects of the newer AEDs are still limited, but preliminary evidence suggests that gabapentin, tiagabine, vigabatrin, and lamotrigine have fewer cognitive side effects than the traditional AEDs.[26,111] Topiramate, however, may be a significant exception. Although it is one of the most potent of the new drugs, topiramate has the commonly reported side effects of impaired concentration and memory, slowed thinking, and word-finding difficulties.[182] Such cognitive effects might lessen over time and could perhaps be avoided by slower titration.[3]

Interictal Behavioral Manifestations

Psychosis The relationship between epilepsy and psychosis is laden with methodologic controversy due in part to variablity in definitions and classification systems. Attempts at determining the prevalence of psychosis in epilepsy have yielded rates between 3 and 7 percent (prevalence in the general population is 1 percent).[205] Most series report a higher frequency of psychosis in patients with temporal lobe epilepsy compared with generalized epilepsy.[21,137,183,211]

While the vast majority of patients with epilepsy do not develop psychosis, several risk factors for the development of psychosis in TLE have been described, including female gender, a left-sided temporal seizure focus, visible neuropathologic lesions at the seizure focus (particularly gangliogliomas), and lesions developing during the fetal or perinatal period.[56,161,165,200,211] The likelihood of psychosis is not related to seizure frequency; indeed, it often occurs when seizure frequency is declining.[205] Many variables related to the chronicity of epilepsy have been described as risk factors for the development of psychosis: duration of active epilepsy, young age of seizure onset, refractory epilepsy, and status epilepticus.[174] Chronicity may explain the average latency of 15 years between the onset of seizures and the onset of psychosis.[205]

Many studies have commented on the unique characteristics of the interictal psychoses: more preserved affect and personality, a predominance of visual rather than auditory hallucinations, less formal thought disorder, emotional withdrawal, and negative symptoms.[128,183] Other studies emphasize the phenomenologic similarities of the interictal psychoses and idiopathic schizophrenia.[21,153,205] Several authors have commented on the more favorable outcome among epilepsy patients with psychosis than those with schizophrenia, with less need for neuroleptics or institutionalization, but supportive, controlled studies are lacking.[153,181,183] Outcome may not be too different from that of late-onset schizophrenia.[165]

Forced normalization refers to the uncommon association between improved control of seizures or epileptiform activity and the onset or exacerbation of psychosis.[115] Forced normalization occurs with partial and generalized epilepsies, usually when seizures are controlled with AEDs or surgery.[149,160] When psychosis develops de novo after temporal lobectomy, it occurs more often after a right-sided resection.[25,50,124] Forced normalization remains controversial, and many investigators believe that it is rare.

Depression The actual incidence and prevalence of interictal depression in epilepsy remains unknown, despite numerous research studies addressing the issue.[113,168] Most studies have been criticized for being retrospective, for using biased hospital samples, for using questionnaires rather than clinical impression, or for conflating diagnostic categories. In general, depression is more common and/or more severe in patients with epilepsy than in patients with other neurologic or chronic medical conditions.[110,135,191] Interictal depression occurs at some time in up to two-thirds of patients, especially those with severe and/or frequent seizures.[113] The reported incidence of suicide in patients with epilepsy is four to five times that of the general population, and patients with TLE are at increased risk by a factor of up to 25.[11,77] Mendez et al. (1992) investigated this occurrence and found the risk more attributable to psychotic behaviors and borderline personality disorder than with depression or the psychosocial burden of epilepsy.[136] Most depressed epilepsy patients can be successfully treated with antidepressants without increasing the seizure frequency or severity.[29,74,147,162] Many observers have found a higher prevalence of depression among patients with left temporal seizure foci than among patients with right temporal seizure foci, but some reports are not supportive.[6,23,56,89,134,138,177] Recent functional imaging studies have helped to shed light on some of the complexities involved. For example, fluorodeoxyglucose (FDG)-PET and/or single photon emission computed tomography (SPECT) have demonstrated that, in patients with TLE, zones of hypometabolism can extend beyond the temporal regions, affecting frontal and subcortical regions most commonly.[85,98] Several studies have shown that left-temporal ictal onset and bifrontal hypometabolism or hypoperfusion are associated with high self-reported ratings of depression.[23,175] Thus, the combination of seizures from the left temporal lobe and frontal lobe dysfunction may form a potential neurobiologic substrate for depression in some patients with epilepsy.[220]

Psychosocial problems accompanying epilepsy can contribute to depression.[41] Several important themes in the literature regarding quality of life in epilepsy include (1) the mental health consequences of dealing with the fundamental paroxysmal nature of epilepsy (fear of loss of control); (2) social bias and stigma, leading to restrictions on employment, living situations, and companionship; and (3) disturbed family relations (e.g., dependency, overprotection, rejection, negative self-image), which act to reduce an individual's capacity to enjoy life and grow.[72,86,92,101]

Anxiety Despite methodologic obstacles regarding adequate patient and control populations, inconsistent psychiatric and neurologic diagnostic criteria, and sample selection bias, there are enough data to suggest a higher prevalence of anxiety symptoms in patients with epilepsy in both community and hospital studies than in controls.[176,201,218] Anxiety, panic, and phobic symptoms are most common among patients with limbic seizure foci, but patients with primary generalized epilepsy may also be at increased risk.[6,154,216]

The mechanisms mediating the development of anxiety disorders in epilepsy are complex and dependent on the interaction of multiple neurologic, pharmacologic, and psychosocial factors. The perception of seizure severity was found to be among the most significant predictors of anxiety in 100 patients with medication-refractory epilepsy.[186] Right-sided seizure foci may predispose to anxiety, but this has not been clearly established.[6,65,89] Interictal fear or anxiety can result from a simple reaction to worry about having a seizure or a response to the constellation of disruptions to quality of life created by epilepsy.[87]

Aggression With its medicolegal implications, interictal aggressiveness, like ictal aggression, has been a subject of intense study and controversy.[32,55,207] Several studies failed to demonstrate an increased incidence of interictal behavioral aggression between patients with TLE and those with other forms of epilepsy, neurologic disorders, or psychiatric disturbances (although the incidence of aggression among all the patient groups was higher than expected in the general population).[94,97,192] Interictal violence has a greater correlation with psychopathology and mental retardation than with epileptiform activity.[138] Several risk factors for aggression in epilepsy have been identified, including male sex, left-handedness, low socioeconomic status, focal or diffuse neurologic lesions, cognitive impairment, exposure to violence as a child, and medications such as barbiturates.[97,148,173,192,198]

In contrast, some clinical and animal research data do support a link between aggression and epilepsy. Almost 30 percent of epilepsy patients reported intense, paroxysmal irritability or moodiness during the interictal period, compared with 2 percent of normal controls or subjects with other neurologic disorders.[45] Extremely high rates of aggression (27 to 36 percent) have been reported in selected neurosurgical series of patients with TLE.[54,179,198] Case reports document interictal aggression after the development of a limbic seizure focus in patients without other risk factors for aggression.[34] Experimental temporal lobe seizure foci increase aggressive behavior in animal models.[194]

The neurobiology of aggressive behavior has increasingly focused on the amygdala, within the temporolimbic system, and on frontal lobe structures involved in impulse control.[51,108] A recent quantitative MRI has demonstrated no higher prevalence of amygdala sclerosis or atrophy among aggressive patients with TLE versus controls and nonaggressive patients with TLE.[215] Hippocampal sclerosis was significantly less common in patients with TLE and aggression. The patients with aggression, however, did have lower IQs and more psychopathology than controls. A follow-up study demonstrated a decrease of gray matter, most markedly in the left frontal lobe, compared with the control group and with nonaggressive TLE patients.[227]

Personality A vast and controversial literature has emphasized the association of specific personality traits with epilepsy, especially with temporal lobe epilepsy.[18,40,194] Waxman and Geschwind (1975) argued for the existence of a specific interictal personality syndrome in TLE, characterized by deepening of emotionality, guilt, hypermoralism, obsessionalism, "viscosity," sense of personal destiny, religiosity, and hypergraphia.[219] Emphasizing that the features were not necessarily negative or maladaptive, Waxman and Geschwind emphasized that the syndrome be described as that of a behavioral *change* in TLE rather than as a behavioral disorder. The symptoms can be grouped into three main divisions (Benson, 1986): (1) overinclusiveness in verbal output (circumstantiality), action (viscosity or stickiness), and writing (hypergraphia); (2) alteration of sexuality (usually hyposexuality); and (3) intensification of mental activities (philosophical, religious) and emotional behavior (depression, paranoia, irritability).[14] Although hyposexuality has been reported most often, case reports also document TLE patients with hypersexuality as well as fetishism, transvestism, and transsexualism.[40,63,141]

Based on a literature review, Bear and Fedio composed the Temporal Lobe Epilepsy Inventory, consisting of 18 traits, and found an increased frequency of all 18 traits in patients with TLE compared with normal controls or people with neuromuscular disease.[13] Laterality effects were also described. Patients with right temporal foci displayed more emotional traits and exhibited "denial" or "polished" their self-image, whereas those with left temporal foci exhibited more ideational traits and "tarnished" their self-images. Subsequent studies have not supported consistent lateralized personality changes in TLE.[40,88,163,194]

The Bear-Fedio Inventory (BFI) was criticized on numerous grounds: the small number of subjects studied (a total of 48 subjects in the two TLE and two control groups), the absence of a control group with other types of seizures, the refractoriness of the TLE patients studied, and the lack of AED information provided. Several cardinal signs of the syndrome, such as hyperreligiosity or hypergraphia, appear nonspecific.[93,144,170,212] Replication studies using the BFI have produced mixed results. In summary, the BFI reveals increased behavioral traits in patients with epilepsy (TLE as well as generalized epilepsy) compared with normal or nonbehavioral patient controls, but it does not distinguish patients with epilepsy (TLE or GE) from psychiatric patients.[20,88] Findings from TLE versus GE patient comparisons are inconsistent. Using invasive electrodes to localize seizure foci, Weiser (1986) found a nonsignificant increase in all behavioral traits on the BFI in patients with frontal lobe epilepsy compared with those with TLE.[221]

Theories regarding the pathogenesis of frequently observed behavioral changes in epilepsy have been postulated. Gastaut (1954) observed that some of the behavior changes in epilepsy patients were the converse of those seen in Kluver-Bucy syndrome (bitemporal hypofunction).[60] This led Bear (1979) to propose a sensory-limbic hyperconnection as a mechanistic explanation for the behaviors seen in TLE, whereby a chronic discharging focus involving temporal limbic structures might lead to extraneous sensory-emotional connections in response to overtly neutral stimuli.[12] Yet data are accumulating that interictal hypofunctionality and neuronal loss in TLE play a prominent role in cognitive (memory and language) and behavioral (depression) changes.[23,103,175] It is likely that in a given individual with epilepsy, behavioral changes may simultaneously result from hyperactivity in some systems, hypoactivity in other systems, and aberrant activity in still other systems.[40]

TREATMENT OF BEHAVIORAL AND COGNITIVE SYMPTOMS

When behavioral events are coincident with seizure activity, treatment is directed at rigorous seizure control. The primary therapeutic modality for control of seizures is AEDs. In refractory TLE patients, treatment of seizures by surgical approaches has yielded excellent results in selected populations (see Chap. 55). In general, control of ictal symptoms with AEDs is straightforward and beneficial, whereas management of interictal symptoms is often more challenging. These symptoms do not necessarily improve with seizure control. Further, AEDs are not proven to be effective in treating any behavioral disorder.

Postictal, Interictal Psychosis

The treatment for postictal psychosis is not well established. Some authors recommend dopamine blockers, and others advise the use of benzodiazepines and sedation with chloral hydrate for the time-limited condition.[107,114] The treatment of chronic interictal psychosis is similar to that of schizophrenia, with the additional caveat to avoid neuroleptics with a relatively greater tendency to lower seizure threshold, such as many of the phenothiazines and clozapine.[99,193] Molindone is a traditional neuroleptic that has been used successfully in treating both postictal and interictal psychoses.[122] The newer neuroleptics, such as risperidone, olanzapine, and quetiapine, which are active at serotoninergic and dopaminergic receptors, appear to carry a reduced risk for lowering seizure threshold. The results of several studies support the safety and efficacy of psychotropic medications, introduced slowly in low to moderate doses, in patients with epilepsy and comorbid psychopathology.[74,147]

Depression

Antidepressants are the mainstay of pharmacotherapy in epilepsy patients with depressive symptoms. Despite the large number of antidepressant agents available and the high frequency and severity of depression in epilepsy, there is only one double-blind, placebo-controlled study in the literature examining this issue to date.[162] Selective serotonin reuptake inhibitors (SSRIs) have become the first-line treatment in depressed patients without and with epilepsy. They have low epileptogenicity, are well tolerated in overdose, and have a favorable adverse-effects profile.[113,122,127] Citalopram and sertraline are widely used because of their minimal pharmacokinetic interactions with AEDs.

Among the AEDs, phenobarbital is notorious for producing depression as a side effect.[95] Primidone, tiagabine, vigabatrin, and felbamate are other AEDs known to cause symptoms of depression.[106] AEDs with mood-stabilizing properties, such as carbamazepine and valproate, occasionally cause depressive episodes, albeit with a lower frequency than the other AEDs.[127] Lamotrigine has been found to produce increased happiness and mastery (internal control) than placebo which was not dependent on a change in seizure frequency or severity.[184] Recent studies have found lamotrigine to be useful in the treatment of bipolar affective disorder.[190]

Supportive psychotherapy and cognitive-behavioral therapy can help ameliorate depression in epilepsy patients.[30,68] The multifactorial etiology of depression in patients with epilepsy lends itself to polymodal therapeutic options. Psychotherapy should be tailored to the patient's personality characteristics, coping skills, family support, educational level, and social environment. Patient and family education about the causes and course of depression in epilepsy will help to optimize treatment.

Cognition

AEDs are commonly implicated as partially responsible for cognitive complaints seen in patients with epilepsy, although recent studies on untreated epilepsy patients illustrate the drug-independent character of at least some aspects of cognitive impairment.[157] Nevertheless, since the introduction of the so-called new AEDs, consistent negative cognitive side effects have been demonstrated only for topiramate.[182] Otherwise the new AEDs appear to be safe with respect to memory, and a recent study on gabapentin in mice even showed an enhancement of retrieval.[2] In one study investigating vagal nerve stimulation, another therapeutic option for control of seizures, it has been demonstrated that stimulation administered after learning significantly enhances retention.[166]

No double-blind, placebo-controlled studies examining pharmacologic strategies for memory enhancement in epilepsy patients exists. The potential benefits of cholinesterase inhibitors and herbal preparations, such as ginkgo biloba, remain unexamined in epilepsy patients with cognitive dysfunction.

Evidence derived from neuropsychological testing correlated with functional imaging suggests a prominent role of frontal lobe dysfunction in patients with TLE.[98,103,151,203] In nonepilepsy populations, clear evidence of an association between depression and memory impairment exists: the association is stronger for self-reports of memory difficulties but remains substantial even on objective memory tests, with stronger effects being found in younger depressed patients and in inpatients relative to outpatients.[24] Thus attempts at improving cognitive function in epilepsy patients via demonstrated efficacy of stimulants and/or stimulating antidepressants in patients with complicated cognitive and behavioral profiles are plausible although unproven.

The past 20 years have seen a marked increase in cognitive rehabilitation publications addressing the real-life issues of patients with organic memory deficits.[225] Three major strands in memory rehabilitation in recent years include (1) environmental adaptations, (2) new technologies, and (3) the implementation of new strategies for improving learning.

CONCLUSION

The association of certain behavioral constellations with specific epilepsy syndromes remains uncertain. Alterations in cognitive and social functions, personality, affect, and drive-related behaviors like libido and aggression may develop in patients with partial and generalized epilepsies. The pathogenic roles of biologic factors such as brain disease, the epileptogenic process, site of the seizure focus, recurrent seizures, and family medical history, therapeutic factors, and psychosocial factors interact and vary among patients and for different disorders.

An insightful hypothesis, the "epileptogenic disorder of function," was offered four decades ago by Sir Charles Symonds (1962). Pondering the pathophysiologic origin of interictal psychosis in TLE patients, he stated:

> *If then neither the fits nor the temporal lobe damage can be held directly responsible for the psychosis, what is the link?... Epileptic seizures and epileptiform discharge in the EEG are epiphenomena. They may be regarded as occasional expressions of a fundamental and continuous disorder of neuronal function. The essence of this disorder is loss of the normal balance between excitation and inhibition at the synaptic junctions. From moment to moment there may be excess either of excitation or inhibition—or even both at the same time in different parts of the same neuronal system. The epileptogenic disorder of*

function may be assumed to be present continuously but with peaks at which seizures are likely to occur.[197]

The role of seizures in the progressive structural, cognitive, and behavioral changes in epilepsy patients remains controversial. In the search for the ideal balance between medication side effects and seizure control, physicians should heed Lennox's (1942) admonition that "many physicians in attempting to extinguish seizures only succeed in drowning the finer intellectual processes of their patients."[118]

REFERENCES

1. Aarts JHP, Bimmin CD, Smit AD, et al: Selective cognitive impairment during focal and generalized epileptiform EEG activity. *Brain* 107:293–308, 1984.
2. Acosta GB, Boccia MM, Baratti CM: Gabapentin, an epileptic drug, improves memory storage in mice. *Neurosci Lett* 279:173–176, 2000.
3. Aldenkamp AP, Baker G, Mulder OG, et al: A multicenter, randomized clinical study to evaluate the effect on cognitive function of topiramate compared with valproate as add-on therapy to carbamazepine in patients with partial-onset seizures. *Epilepsia* 41:1167–1178, 2000.
5. Alper K, Devinsky O, Perrine K, et al: Dissociation in epilepsy and conversion non-epileptic seizures. *Epilepsia* 38:991–997, 1997.
6. Altshuler LL, Devinsky O, Post RM, Theodore W: Depression, anxiety, and temporal lobe epilepsy: Laterality of focus and symptoms. *Arch Neurol* 47:284–288, 1990.
7. Arnold S, Schlaug G, Niemann H, et al: Topography of interictal glucose metabolism in unilateral mesiotemporal epilepsy. *Neurology* 46:1422–1430, 1996.
9. Barr WB, Chelune GJ, Hermann BP, et al: The use of figural reproduction tests as measures of nonverbal memory in epilepsy surgery candidates. *J Int Neuropsychol Soc* 3:435–443, 1997.
10. Barr WB: Examining the right temporal lobe's role in nonverbal memory. *Brain Cogn* 35:26–41, 1997.
11. Barraclough BM: The suicide rate of epilepsy. *Acta Psychiatr Scand* 76:339–345, 1987.
12. Bear DM: Temporal lobe epilepsy: A syndrome of sensory-limbic hyperconnection. *Cortex* 15:357–384, 1979.
13. Bear DM, Fedio P: Quantitative analysis of interictal behaviour in temporal lobe epilepsy. *Arch Neurol* 34:454–467, 1977.
14. Benson DF: Interictal behavior disorders in epilepsy. *Psychiatr Clin North Am* 9:283–292, 1986.
15. Bergin PS, Thompson PJ, Fish DR, et al: The effect of seizures on memory for recently learned material. *Neurology* 45:236–240, 1995.
16. Biraben A, Taussig D, Thomas P, et al: Fear as the main feature of epileptic seizures. *J Neurol Neurosurg Psychiatry* 70:186–191, 2001.
17. Blake RV, Wroe SJ, Breen EK, et al: Accelerated forgetting in patients with epilepsy: evidence for an impairment in memory consolidation. *Brain* 123:472–483, 2000.
18. Blumer D: Evidence supporting the temporal lobe epilepsy syndrome. *Neurology* 53 (suppl 2):S9–S12, 1999.
19. Bourgeois BFD, Prensky AL, Palkes HS, et al: Intelligence in epilepsy: A prospective study in children. *Ann Neurol* 14:438–444, 1983.
20. Brandt J, Seidman LJ, Kohl D: Personality characteristics of epileptic patients: A controlled study of generalized and temporal lobe cases. *J Clin Exp Neuropsychol* 7:25–38, 1985.
21. Bredkjaer SR, Mortensen PB, Parnas J: Epilepsy and non-organic non-affective psychosis: National epidemiologic study. *Br J Psychiatry* 172:235–238, 1998.
22. Brodie MJ, McPhail E, Macphee GJ, et al: Psychomotor impairment and anticonvulsant therapy in adult epileptic patients. *Eur J Clin Pharmacol* 31:655–660, 1987.
23. Bromfield EB, Altshuler LL, Leiderman DB, et al: Cerebral metabolism and depression in patients with complex partial seizures. *Arch Neurol* 49:617–623, 1992.
24. Burt DB, Zembar MJ, Niederehe G: Depression and memory impairment: A meta-analysis of the association, its pattern, and specificity. *Psychol Bull* 117:285–305, 1995.
25. Callender JS, Fenton GW: Psychosis de novo following temporal lobectomy. *Seizure* 6:409–411, 1997.
26. Chadwick DW: An overview of the efficacy and tolerability of new antiepileptic drugs. *Epilepsia* 38 (Suppl 1):S59–S62, 1997.
27. Cirignotta F, Todesco CV, Lugaresi E: Temporal lobe epilepsy with ecstatic seizures: So-called Dostoevsky epilepsy. *Epilepsia* 21:705–710, 1980.
28. Corcoran R, Upton D: A role for the hippocampus in card sorting? *Cortex* 29:293–304, 1993.

29. Curran S, de Pauw K: Selecting an antidepressant for use in a patient with epilepsy. *Drug Saf Concept* 18:125–133, 1998.
30. Davis GR, Armstrong HE, Donovan DM, Temkin NR: Cognitive-behavioural treatment of depressed affect amongst epileptics: preliminary findings. *J Clin Psychol* 4:930–935, 1984.
31. Delaney RC, Rosen AJ, Mattson RH, et al: Memory function in focal epilepsy: A comparison of nonsurgical, unilateral temporal lobe and frontal lobe samples. *Cortex* 16:103–117, 1980.
32. Delgado-Escueta AV, Mattson RH, King L, et al: Special report. The nature of aggression during epileptic seizures. *N Engl J Med* 305:711–716, 1981.
33. Devinsky O, Abramson H, Alper K, et al: Postictal psychosis: A case controlled series of 20 patients and 150 controls. *Epilepsy Res* 20:247–253, 1995.
34. Devinsky O, Bear D: Varieties of aggressive behavior in temporal lobe epilepsy. *Am J Psychiatry* 141:651–656, 1984.
35. Devinsky O, Cox C, Witt E, et al: Ictal fear in temporal lobe epilepsy. *J Epilepsy* 4:231–238, 1991.
36. Devinsky O, Feldmann E, Burrowes K, et al: Autoscopic phenomena with seizures. *Arch Neurol* 46:1080–1088, 1989.
37. Devinsky O, Hafler DA, Victor J: Embarassment as the aura of a complex partial seizure. *Neurology* 32:1284–1285, 1982.
39. Devinsky O, Kelley K, Yacubian EM, et al: Postictal behavior: A clinical and subdural electroencephalographic study. *Arch Neurol* 51:254–259, 1994.
40. Devinsky O, Najjar S: Evidence against the existence of the temporal lobe epilepsy syndrome. *Neurology* 53 (Suppl 2):S13–S25, 1999.
41. Devinsky O, Penry JK: Quality of life in epilepsy: The clinician's view. *Epilepsia* 34 (Suppl 4):S4–S7, 1993.
42. Devinsky O, Putnam F, Grafman J, et al: Dissociative states and epilepsy. *Neurology* 39:835–840, 1989.
43. Devinsky O: Emotion and the limbic system, in Devinsky O, D'Esposito M (eds): *Principles of Cognitive and Behavioral Neurology*. New York: Oxford University Press. In press.
44. Devinsky O: Interictal changes in behavior, in Devinsky O, Theodore WH (eds): *Epilepsy and Behavior*. New York: Wiley-Liss, 1991, pp 1–21.
45. Devinsky O: Fear and epilepsy, in Canger R, Saccheti E, Perini GI, Canevini MP (eds): *Carbamazepine: A Bridge between Epilepsy and Psychiatric Disorders*. Origio, Italy: Ciba-Geigy Edizione, 1990, pp 41–48.
46. Dikmen S, Matthews C, Harley J: The effect of early versus late onset of major motor epilepsy on cognitive-intellectual performance. *Epilepsia* 16:73–81, 1975.
47. Dodrill CB: Correlates of generalized tonic-clonic seizures with intellectual, neuropsychological, emotional, and social function in patients with epilepsy. *Epilepsia* 27:399–411, 1986.
48. Dreifuss FE. Classification of epileptic seizures and the epilepsies, in Shorvon S, Dreifuss FE, Fish D, Thomas D (eds): *The Treatment of Epilepsy*. London: Blackwell Science, 1996.
49. Elixhauser A, Leidy NK, Meador K, et al: The relationship between memory performance, perceived cognitive function, and mood in patients with epilepsy. *Epilepsy Res* 37:13–24, 1999.
50. Elwes RD, Dunn G, Binnie CD: Outcome following resective surgery for temporal lobe epilepsy: A prospective follow-up study of 102 consecutive cases. *J Neurol Neurosurg Psychiatry* 54:949–952, 1991.
51. Engel J, Caldecott-Hazard S, Bandler R: Neurobiology of behavior: Anatomic and physiologic implications related to epilepsy. *Epilepsia* 27(Suppl 2):S3–S13, 1986.
52. Engel J, Williamson PD: Mesial temporal lobe epilepsy, in Engel J, Pedley TA (eds): *Epilepsy: A Comprehensive Textbook*. Philadelphia: Lippincott-Raven, 1998, pp 2417–2426.
53. Engel J: Current concepts: surgery for seizures. *N Engl J Med* 334:647–652, 1996.
54. Falconer MA: Reversibility by temporal lobe resection of the behavioral abnormalities of temporal lobe epilepsy. *N Engl J Med* 289:451–455, 1973.
55. Fenwick P: Aggression in epilepsy, in Devinsky O, Theodore WH (eds): *Epilepsy and Behavior.* New York: Liss, 1991, pp 85–96.
56. Flor-Henry P: Psychosis and temporal lobe epilepsy: A controlled investigation. *Epilepsia* 10:363–395, 1969.
57. Fried I, Spencer DD, Spencer SS: The anatomy of epileptic auras: focal pathology and surgical outcome. *J Neurosurg* 83:60–66, 1995.
58. Fried I: Auras and experiential responses arising in the temporal lobe. *J Neuropsychiatry Clin Neurosci* 9:420–428, 1997.
59. Fuerst D, Shah J, Kupsky WJ: Volumetric MRI, pathological, and neuropsychological progression in hippocampal sclerosis. *Neurology* 57:184–188, 2001.
60. Gastaut H, Collomb K: Etude du comportement sexuel chez les epileptiques psychomoteurs. *Ann Med Psychol* 112:675–696, 1954.
61. Gates JR, Luciano D, Devinsky O: The classification and treatment of nonepileptic events, in Devinsky

O, Theodore WH (eds): *Epilepsy and Behavior*. New York: Wiley-Liss, 1991, pp 251–263.

62. Gerard ME, Spitz MC, Towbin JA, et al: Subacute postictal aggression. *Neurology* 50:384–388, 1998.
63. Geschwind N, Shader RI, Bear D, et al: Behavioral changes with temporal lobe epilepsy: assessment and treatment. *J Clin Psychiatry* 41:89–95, 1980.
64. Geschwind N: Behavioral changes in temporal lobe epilepsy. *Psychol Med* 9:217–219, 1979.
65. Ghadirian AM, Gauthier S, Bertrand S: Anxiety attacks in a patient with a right temporal lobe meningioma. *J Clin Psychiatry* 47:270–271, 1986.
66. Gibbs FA, Gibbs EL, Lenox WG: Epilepsy: A paroxysmal cerebral dysrhythmia. *Brain* 60:377–388, 1937.
67. Gillham RA, Williams N, Wiedmann KD: Cognitive function in adult epileptic patients established on anticonvulsant monotherapy. *Epilepsy Res* 7:219–225, 1990.
68. Gillham RA: Refractory epilepsy: an evaluation of psychological methods in outpatient management. *Epilepsia* 31:427–432, 1990.
70. Gloor P, Olivier A, Quensney LF, et al: The role of the limbic system in experiential phenomena in temporal lobe epilepsy. *Ann Neurol* 12:129–144, 1982.
71. Gloor P: Neurobiological substrates of ictal behavioral changes. *Adv Neurol* 55:1–34, 1991.
72. Goldstein J, Seidenberg M, Peterson R: Fear of seizures and behavioral functioning in adults with epilepsy. *J Epilepsy* 3:101–106, 1990.
73. Gowers WR: *Epilepsy and Other Chronic Convulsive Diseases: Their Causes, Symptoms, and Treatment.* London: Churchill, 1881.
74. Gross A, Devinsky O, Westbrook LE, et al: Psychotropic medication use in patients with epilepsy. *J Neuropsychiatry Clin Neurosci* 12:458–464, 2000.
75. Gundmundsson G: Epilepsy in Iceland: A clinical and epidemiological investigation. *Acta Neurol Scand* 43(Suppl 25):1–124, 1966.
76. Halgren E, Walter RD, Cherlow DG, et al: Mental phenomena evoked by electrical stimulation of the human hippocampal formation and amygdala. *Brain* 101:83–117, 1978.
77. Harris EC, Barraclough B: Suicide as an outcome for mental disorders: A meta-analysis. *Br J Psychiatry* 170:205–228, 1997.
78. Hauser WA, Annegers JF, Kurland LT: Prevalence of epilepsy in Rochester, Minnesota: 1940–1980. *Epilepsia* 32:429–445, 1991.
79. Hauser WA, Annegers JF, Kurland LT: Incidence of epilepsy and unprovoked seizures in Rochester, Minnesota: 1935–1984. *Epilepsia* 34:453–468, 1993.
80. Helmstaedter C, Elger CE, Lendt M: Postictal course of cognitive deficits in focal epilepsies. *Epilepsia* 35:1073–1078, 1994.
81. Helmstaedter C, Elger CE: Behavioral markers for self- and other attribution of memory: A study in patients with temporal lobe epilepsy and healthy volunteers. *Epilepsy Res* 41:235–243, 2000.
82. Helmstaedter C, Elger CE: The phantom of progressive dementia. *Lancet* 354:2133–2134, 1999.
83. Helmstaedter C, Kemper B, Elger CE: Neuropsychological aspects of frontal lobe epilepsy. *Neuropsychologia* 34:399–406, 1996.
84. Helmstaedter C, Pohl C, Hufnagel A, et al: Visual learning deficits in nonresected patients with right temporal lobe epilepsy. *Cortex* 27:547–555, 1991.
85. Henry TR, Mazziotta JC, Engel J: Interictal metabolic anatomy of mesial temporal lobe epilepsy. *Arch Neurol* 50:582–589, 1993.
86. Hermann BP, Wyler AR: Depression, locus of control and epilepsy surgery. *Epilepsia* 3:332–338, 1989.
87. Hermann BP, Chhabria S: Interictal psychopathology in patients with interictal fear: Examples of sensory-limbic hyperconnection. *Arch Neurol* 37:667–668, 1981.
88. Hermann BP, Reil P: Interictal personality and behavioral traits in temporal lobe and generalized epilepsy. *Cortex* 17:125–128, 1981.
89. Hermann BP, Seidenberg M, Haltiner A, et al: Mood state in unilateral temporal lobe epilepsy. *Biol Psychiatry* 30:1205–1218, 1991.
90. Hermann BP, Seidenberg M, Schoenfeld J, et al: Neuropsychological characteristics of the syndrome of mesial temporal lobe epilepsy. *Arch Neurol* 54:369–376, 1997.
91. Hermann BP, Seidenberg M: Executive system dysfunction in temporal lobe epilepsy: Effects of nociferous cortex versus hippocampal pathology. *J Clin Exp Neuropsychol* 17:809–819, 1995.
92. Hermann BP, Trenerry MR, Colligan RC: Learned helplessness, attributional style, and depression in epilepsy. *Epilepsia* 37:680–686, 1996.
93. Hermann BP, Whitman S, Arnston P: Hypergraphia in epilepsy: Is there a specificity to temporal lobe epilepsy? *J Neurol Neurosurg Psychiatry* 46:848–853, 1983.
94. Hermann BP, Whitman S: Behavioral and personality correlates of epilepsy: A review, methodological critique, and conceptual model. *Psychol Bull* 95:451–497, 1984.
95. Hermann BP, Whitman S: Psychosocial predictors of interictal depression. *J Epilepsy* 2:231–237, 1989.

96. Hermann BP, Wyler A, Steerman H, Richey ET: The inter-relationship between language function and verbal learning and memory performance in patients with complex partial seizures. *Cortex* 24:245–253, 1988.
97. Herzberg JL, Fenwick PBC: The aetiology of aggression in temporal-lobe epilepsy. *Br J Psychiatry* 153:50–55, 1988.
98. Homan RM, Paulman RG, Derons MD, et al: Cognitive function and regional cerebral blood flow in partial seizures. *Arch Neurol* 46:964–970, 1989.
99. Itil TM, Soldatos C: Epileptogenic side effects of psychotropic drugs: Practical recommendations. *JAMA* 244:1460–1463, 1980.
100. Jackson JH: *Selected Writings.* Taylor J (ed). New York: Basic Books, 1958, pp 6,15, 16, 34.
101. Jacoby A: Felt versus enacted stigma, a concept revisited: Evidence from a study of people with epilepsy. *Social Sci Med* 38:269–274, 1994.
102. Jokeit H, Ebner A: Long-term effects of refractory temporal lobe epilepsy on cognitive abilities: A cross-sectional study. *J Neurol Neurosurg Psychiatry* 67:44–50, 1999.
103. Jokeit H, Seitz A, Markowitsch HJ, et al: Prefrontal asymmetric interictal glucose hypometabolism and cognitive impairment in patients with temporal lobe epilepsy. *Brain* 120:2283–2294, 1997.
104. Jones-Gotman M: Right hippocampal excision impairs learning and recall of a list of abstract designs. *Neuropsychologia* 24:192–203, 1986.
105. Kalvainen R, Salmenpera T, Partanen K, et al: Recurrent seizures may cause hippocampal damage in temporal lobe epilepsy. *Neurology* 50:1377–1382, 1998.
106. Kanner AM, Rivas Nieto JC: Depressive disorders in epilepsy. *Neurology* 53(Suppl 2):S26–S32, 1999.
107. Kanner AM, Stagno S, Kotagal P, Morris HH: Postictal psychiatric events during prolonged video-electroencephalographic monitoring studies. *Arch Neurol* 53:258–263, 1996.
108. Kavoussi R, Armstead P, Coccaro E: The neurobiology of impulsive aggression. *Psychiatr Clin North Am* 20:395–403, 1997.
109. Koerner M, Laxer KD: Ictal speech, postictal language dysfunction, and seizure lateralization. *Neurology* 38:634–636, 1988.
110. Kogeorgos J, Fonagy P, Scott DF: Psychiatric symptom patterns of chronic epileptics attending a neurological clinic: A controlled investigation. *Br J Psychiatry* 140:236–243, 1982.
111. Kwan P, Brodie MJ: Neuropsychological effects of epilepsy and antiepileptic drugs. *Lancet* 357:216–222, 2001.
112. LaBar KS, LeDoux JE, Spencer DD, et al: Impaired fear conditioning following unilateral temporal lobectomy in humans. *J Neurosci* 15:6846–6855, 1995.
113. Lambert MV, Robertson MM: Depression in epilepsy: Etiology, phenomenology, and treatment. *Epilepsia* 40(Suppl 10):S21–S47, 1999.
114. Lancman ME, Craven WJ, Asconape JJ, Penry JK: Clinical management of recurrent postictal psychosis. *J Epilepsy* 7:47–51, 1994.
115. Landolt H: Serial electroencephalographic investigations during psychotic episodes in epileptic patients and during schizophrenic attacks, in de Hass L (ed): *Lectures on Epilepsy.* London: Elsevier, 1958, pp 91–133.
116. Laskowitz DT, Sperling MR, French JA, et al: The syndrome of frontal lobe epilepsy: characteristics and surgical management. *Neurology* 45:780–787, 1995.
117. LeDoux J: *The Emotional Brain.* New York: Simon & Schuster, 1996, p 172.
118. Lennox WG: Brain injury, drugs, and environment as causes of mental decay in epilepsy. *Am J Psychiatry* 99:174–180, 1942.
119. Levin R, Banks S, Berg B: Psychosocial dimensions of epilepsy: A review of the literature. *Epilepsia* 29:805–816, 1988.
120. Logsdail SJ, Toone BK: Post-ictal psychoses: A clinical and phenomenological description. *Br J Psychiatry* 52:246–252, 1988.
121. Loiseau P, Duche B, Loiseau J: Classification of epilepsies and epileptic syndromes in two different samples of patients. *Epilepsia* 32:303–309, 1991.
122. Luciano D, Alper K: Psychiatric aspects of seizures and epilepsy, in Standemire A, Fogel BS, Greenberg DB (eds): *Psychiatric Care of the Medical Patient,* 2d ed. New York: Oxford University Press, 2000, pp 635–651.
123. Luciano D, Devinsky O, Perrine K: Crying seizures. *Neurology* 43:2113–2117, 1993.
124. Manchanda R, Miller H, McLachlin RS: Post-ictal psychosis after right temporal lobectomy. *J Neurol Neurosurg Psychiatry* 56:277–279, 1993.
125. Manes F, Hodges JR, Graham KS, et al: Focal autobiographical amnesia in association with transient epileptic amnesia. *Brain* 124:499–509, 2001.
126. Mayeux R, Brandt J, Rosen J, et al: Interictal memory and language impairment in temporal lobe epilepsy. *Neurology* 30:120–125, 1980.
127. McConnell HW, Duncan D: Treatment of psychiatric comorbidity in epilepsy, in McConnell HW, Snyder PJ (eds): *Psychiatric Comorbidity in Epilepsy.*

Washington DC: American Psychiatric Press, 1998, pp 245–362.
128. McKenna PJ, Kane JM, Parrish K: Psychotic symptoms in epilepsy. *Am J Psychiatry* 142:895–904, 1985.
129. McLachlan RS, Blume WT: Isolated fear in complex partial status epilepticus. *Ann Neurol* 8:639–641, 1980.
130. Meador KJ, Loring DW, Moore EE, et al: Comparative cognitive effects of phenobarbital, phenytoin, and valproic acid in healthy adults. *Neurology* 45:1494–1499, 1995.
131. Meador KJ: Cognitive side effects of medications. *Neurol Clin* 16:141–155, 1998.
134. Mendez MF, Cummings JL, Benson DF: Depression in epilepsy: Significance and phenomenology. *Arch Neurol* 43:766–770, 1986.
135. Mendez MF, Doss RC, Taylor JL, et al: Depression and epilepsy: Relationship to seizures and anticonvulsant therapy. *J Nerv Ment Dis* 181:444–447, 1993.
136. Mendez MF, Doss RC: Ictal and psychiatric aspects of suicide in epileptic patients. *Int J Psychiatry Med* 22:231–237, 1992.
137. Mendez MF, Grau R, Doss RC, et al: Schizophrenia in epilepsy: Seizure and psychosis variables. *Neurology* 43:1073–1077, 1993.
138. Mendez MF, Doss RC, Taylor JL: Interictal violence in epilepsy: Relationship to behavior and seizure variables. *J Nerv Ment Dis* 181:566–569, 1993.
139. Mesulam MM: Dissociative states with abnormal temporal lobe EEG: Multiple personality and the illusion of possession. *Arch Neurol* 38:176–181, 1981.
140. Milner B: Disorders of learning and memory after temporal lobe lesions in man. *Clin Neurosurg* 19:421–466, 1972.
141. Morrell MJ: Sexual dysfunction in epilepsy. *Epilepsia* 32 (Suppl 6):S38–S45.
142. Mullan S, Penfield W: Illusions of comparative interpretation and emotion. *Arch Neurol Psychiatry* 81:269–284, 1959.
143. Mungas D, Ehlers C, Walton N, et al: Verbal learning differences in epileptic patients with left and right temporal lobe foci. *Epilepsia* 26:340–345, 1985.
144. Mungas D: Interictal behavior abnormality in temporal lobe epilepsy: A specific syndrome or nonspecific psychopathology. *Arch Gen Psychiatry* 39:108–111, 1982.
145. Newton MR, Berkovic SF, Austin MC, et al: Postictal switch in blood flow distribution and temporal lobe seizures. *J Neurol Neurosurg Psychiatry* 55:891–894, 1992.
146. Novelly RA: The debt of neuropsychology to the epilepsies. *Am Psychol* 47:1126–1129, 1992.
147. Ojemann LM, Baugh-Bookman C, Dudley DL: Effect of psychotropic medications on seizure control in patients with epilepsy. *Neurology* 37:1525–1527, 1987.
148. Ounstead C: Aggression and epilepsy: rage in children with temporal lobe epilepsy. *J Psychosom Res* 13:237–242, 1969.
149. Palkanis A, Drake ME, John K, et al: Forced normalization: Acute psychosis after seizure control in seven patients. *Arch Neurol* 44:289–292, 1987.
150. Papez JW: A proposed mechanism of emotion. *Arch Neurol Psych* 38:725–743, 1937.
151. Paradiso S, Hermann BP, Robinson RG: The heterogeneity of temporal lobe epilepsy: Neurology, neuropsychology, psychiatry. *J Nerv Ment Dis* 183:538–547, 1995.
152. Penfield W, Jasper H: *Epilepsy and the Functional Anatomy of the Human Brain*. Boston: Little Brown, 1954.
153. Perez MM, Trimble MR: Epileptic psychosis: Diagnostic comparison with process schizophrenia. *Br J Psychiatry* 137:245–249, 1980.
154. Perini GL, Mendius R: Depression and anxiety in complex partial seizures. *J Nerv Ment Dis* 172:287–290, 1984.
155. Perrine K, Gershenghorn J, Brown E: Interictal neuropsychological function in epilepsy, in Devinsky O, Theodore WH (eds): *Epilepsy and Behavior*. New York: Wiley-Liss, 1991, pp 181–194.
156. Perrine K, Kiolbasa T: Cognitive deficits in epilepsy and contribution to psychopathology. *Neurology* 53(Suppl 2):S39–S48, 1999.
157. Pullianen V, Kuikka P, Jokelainen M: Motor and cognitive functions in newly diagnosed adult seizure patients before antiepileptic medication. *Acta Neurol Scand* 101:73–78, 2000.
158. Rao SM, Devinsky O, Grafman J, et al: Viscosity and social cohesion in temporal lobe epilepsy. *J Neurol Neurosurg Psychiatry* 55:149–152, 1992.
159. Rasmussen T: Characteristics of a pure culture of frontal lobe epilepsy. *Epilepsia* 24:482–493, 1983.
160. Reutens DC, Savard G, Andermann F, et al: Results of surgical treatment in temporal lobe epilepsy with chronic psychosis. *Brain* 120:1929–1936, 1997.
161. Roberts GW, Done DJ, Bruton CJ, et al: A "mock-up" of schizophrenia: temporal lobe epilepsy and schizophrenia-like psychosis. *Biol Psychiatry* 28:127–143, 1990.
162. Robertson MM, Trimble MR: The treatment of depression in patients with epilepsy. *J Affect Disord* 9:127–136, 1985.

163. Rodin E, Schmaltz S: The Bear-Fedio personality inventory and temporal lobe epilepsy. *Neurology* 34:591–596, 1984.
164. Rodin EA: Psychomotor epilepsy and aggressive behavior. *Arch Gen Psychiatry* 28:210–213, 1973.
165. Sachdev P: Schizophrenia-like psychosis and epilepsy: The status of the association. *Am J Psychiatry* 155:325–336, 1998.
166. Sackheim HA, Clark KB, Naritoky DK, Smith DC, et al: Enhanced recognition memory following vagus nerve stimulation in human subjects. *Nat Neurosci* 2:94–98, 1999.
168. Salzberg MK, Vajda FJE: Epilepsy, depression, and antidepressant drugs. *J Clin Neurosci* 8:209–215, 2001.
169. Savard G, Andemann F, Olivier A, et al: Postictal psychosis after partial complex seizures: a multiple case study. *Epilepsia* 38:225–231, 1991.
170. Saver JL, Rabin J: The neural substrates of religious experience. *J Neuropsychiatry Clin Neurosci* 9:498–510, 1997.
171. Sawrie SM, Martin RC, Kuzniecky R, et al: Subjective versus objective memory change after temporal lobe epilepsy surgery. *Neurology* 53:1511–1517, 1999.
172. Saygi S, Katz A, Marks DA, et al: Frontal lobe partial seizures and psychogenic seizures: Comparison of clinical and ictal characteristics. *Neurology* 42:1274–1277, 1992.
173. Schachter SC: Aggressive behavior in epilepsy, in Ettinger AB, Kanner AM (eds): *Psychiatric Issues in Epilepsy: A Practical Guide to Diagnosis and Management.* Philadephia: Lippincott Williams & Wilkins, 2001, pp 201–213.
174. Schmitz B, Wolf P: Psychoses in epilepsy, in Devinsky O, Theodore WH (eds): *Epilepsy and Behavior*. New York: Wiley-Liss, 1991, pp 97–128.
175. Schmitz EB, Moriarty J, Costa DC, et al: Psychiatric profiles and patterns of cerebral blood flow in focal epilepsy: Interactions between depression, obsessionality, and perfusion related to the laterality of the epilepsy. *J Neurol Neurosurg Psychiatry* 62:458–463, 1997.
176. Scicutella A: Anxiety disorders in epilepsy, in Ettinger AB, Kanner AM (eds): *Psychiatric Issues in Epilepsy: A Guide to Diagnosis and Management.* Philadelphia: Lippincott Williams & Wilkins, 2001, pp 95–109.
177. Seidenberg M, Hermann B, Noe A, Wyler AR: Depression in temporal lobe epilepsy: Interaction between laterality of lesion and Wisconsin Card Sort performance. *Neuropsychiatry Neuropsychol Behav Neurol* 8:81–87, 1995.
178. Seidenberg M, O'Leary D, Berent S, et al: Changes in seizure frequency and test-retest scores on the Wechsler Adult Intelligence Scale. *Epilepsia* 22:75–83, 1981.
179. Serafetinides EA: Aggressiveness in temporal lobe epilepsy and its relationship to cerebral dysfunction and environmental factors. *Epilepsia* 6:33–42, 1965.
180. Sethi PK, Rao TS: Gelastic, quiritarian, and cursive epilepsy: A clinicopathological appraisal. *J Neurol Neurosurg Psychiatry* 39:823–828, 1976.
181. Sherwin I: Psychosis associated with epilepsy: Significance of the laterality of the epileptogenic lesion. *J Neurol Neurosurg Psychiatry* 44:83–85, 1981.
182. Shorvon SD: Safety of topiramate: Adverse events and relationship to dosing. *Epilepsia* 37(Suppl 2):S18–S22, 1996.
183. Slater E, Beard AW: The schizophrenia-like psychoses of epilepsy. *Br J Psychiatry* 109:95–150, 1963.
184. Smith D, Baker G, Davies G, et al: Outcomes of add-on treatment with lamotrigine in partial epilepsy. *Epilepsia* 34:312–322, 1993.
185. Smith DB, Craft BR, Collins J, et al: Behavioral characteristics of epilepsy patients compared with normal controls. *Epilepsia* 27:760–768, 1986.
186. Smith DF, Baker GA, Dewey M, et al: Seizure frequency, patient-perceived seizure severity and the psychosocial consequences of intractable epilepsy. *Epilepsy Res* 9:231–241, 1991.
187. Smith PF, Darlington CL: The development of psychosis in epilepsy: A re-examination of the kindling hypothesis. *Behav Brain Res* 75:59–64, 1996.
188. Snyder PJ: Epilepsy as a "natural laboratory" for the study of human memory. *Brain Cogn* 35:1–4, 1997.
189. Sperling MR, Lieb JP, Engel J, et al: Prognostic significance of independent auras in temporal lobe seizures. *Epilepsia* 30:322–331, 1989.
190. Sporn J, Sachs G: The anticonvulsant lamotrigine in treatment-resistant manic-depressive illness. *J Clin Psychopharmacol* 17:185–189, 1997.
191. Standage KF, Fenton GW: Psychiatric symptom profiles of patients with epilepsy: A controlled investigation. *Pyschol Med* 5:152–160, 1975.
192. Stevens JR, Hermann BP: Temporal lobe epilepsy, psychopathology, and violence: The state of the evidence. *Neurology* 31:1127–1132, 1981.
193. Stevens JR: Clozapine: The yin and yang of seizures and psychosis. *Biol Psychiatry* 37:425–426, 1995.
194. Strauss E: Ictal and interictal manifestations of emotions in epilepsy, in Boller F, Grafman J (eds): *Handbook of Neuropsychology*. Squire L, Gainotti G (eds): *Sec 6: Emotional Behavior and Its Disorders*. Amsterdam: Elsevier, 1989, vol 3, pp 315–344.

195. Sutula TP, Hermann BP: Progression in mesial temporal lobe epilepsy. *Ann Neurol* 45:553–556, 1999.
196. Swanson SJ, Rao SM, Grafman J, et al: The relationship between seizure type and interictal personality. Results from the Viet Nam Head Injury Study. *Brain* 118:91–103, 1995.
197. Symonds C: Discussion. *Proc R Soc Med* 55:315, 1962.
198. Taylor D: Aggression and epilepsy. *J Psychosom Res* 13:229–236, 1969.
199. Taylor DC: Lochery M: Temporal lobe epilepsy: Origin and significance of simple and complex auras. *J Neurol Neurosurg Psychiatry* 50:673–681, 1987.
200. Taylor DC: Factors influencing the occurrence of schizophrenia-like psychosis in patients with temporal lobe epilepsy. *Psychol Med* 5:249–254, 1975.
201. Taylor DC: Mental state and temporal lobe epilepsy: A correlative account of 100 patients treated surgically. *Epilepsia* 13:727–765, 1972.
203. Theodore WH, Fishbein D, Dubinsky R: Patterns of cerebral glucose metabolism in patients with partial seizures. *Neurology* 38:1201–1206, 1988.
204. Tishler PW, Holzer JC, Greenber M, et al: Psychiatric presentations of epilepsy. *Harvard Rev Psychiatry* 1:219–228, 1993.
205. Toone BK: The psychoses of epilepsy. *J Neurol Neurosurg Psychiatry* 69:1–3, 2000.
206. Trenerry MR, Jack CR: Wisconsin Card Sort Test performance before and after temporal lobectomy. *J Epilepsy* 7:313–317, 1994.
207. Trieman D: Epilepsy and violence: medical and legal issues. *Epilepsia* 27(Suppl 2):S77–S104, 1986.
208. Trimble MR, Mendez MF, Cummings JL: Neuropsychiatric symptoms from the temporolimbic lobes. *J Neuropsychiatry Clin Neurosci* 9:429–438, 1997.
209. Trimble MR, Ring HA, Schmitz B: Neuropsychiatric aspects of epilepsy, in Fogel BS, Schiffer RB, Rao SM (eds): *Neuropsychiatry*. Baltimore: Williams & Wilkins, 1996, pp 771–804.
210. Trimble MR, Van Elst LT: On some clinical implications of the ventral striatum and the extended amygdala: investigations of aggression. *Ann N Y Acad Sci* 877:638–644, 1999.
211. Trimble MR: *The Psychoses of Epilepsy*. New York: Raven Press, 1991.
212. Tucker DM, Novelly RA, Walker PJ: Hyperreligiosity in temporal lobe epilepsy: Redefining the relationship. *J Nerv Ment Dis* 175:181–184, 1987.
213. Umbricht D, Degreef G, Barr WB, et al: Postictal and chronic psychoses in patients with temporal lobe epilepsy. *Am J Psychiatry* 152:224–231, 1995.
214. Upton D, Thompson PJ: Epilepsy in the frontal lobes: Neuropsychological characteristics. *J Epilepsy* 9:215–222, 1996.
215. Van Elst LT, Woermann FG, Lemieux L, et al: Affective aggression in patients with temporal lobe epilepsy: A quantitative MRI study of the amygdala. *Brain* 123:234–243, 2000.
216. Vazquez B, Devinsky O, Luciano D, et al: Juvenile myoclonic epilepsy: Clinical features and factors related to misdiagnosis. *J Epilepsy* 6:233–238, 1993.
217. Vermeulen J, Aldenkamp AP: Cognitive side effects of chronic anti-epileptic drug treatment: A review of 25 years of research. *Epilepsy Res* 22:65–95, 1995.
218. Victoroff J: DSM-III-R psychiatric diagnoses in candidates for epilepsy surgery: Lifetime prevalence. *Neuropsychiatry Neuropsychol Behav Neurol* 7:87–97, 1994.
219. Waxman SA, Geschwind N: The interictal behavior syndrome of temporal lobe epilepsy. *Arch Gen Psychiatry* 32:1580–1586, 1975.
220. Weigartz P, Seidenberg M, Woodard A, et al: Comorbid psychiatric disorder in chronic epilepsy: Recognition and etiology of depression. *Neurology* 53(Suppl 2):S3–S8, 1999.
221. Weiser HG: Selective amygdalohippocampectomy: Indications, investigative technique and results. *Adv Tech Stand Neurosurg* 13:39–133, 1986.
222. Whitman S, Hermann BP, Gordon A: Psychopathology in epilepsy: How great is the risk? *Biol Psychiatry* 19:213–216, 1984.
223. Williams D: The structure of emotions reflected in epileptic experiences. *Brain* 79:29–67, 1956.
224. Williamson PD, Spencer DD, Spencer SS, et al: Complex partial seizures of frontal lobe origin. *Ann Neurol* 18:497–504, 1985.
225. Wilson BA, Evans JJ: Practical management of memory problems, in Berrios GE, Hodges JR (eds): *Memory Disorders in Psychiatric Practice*. Cambridge, England: Cambridge University Press, 2000, pp 291–310.
226. Wirrell EC, Camfield CS, Camfield PR: Long-term psychosocial outcome in typical absence epilepsy: Sometimes a wolf in sheep's clothing. *Arch Pediatr Adolesc Med* 151:152–158, 1997.
227. Woermann FG, Van Elst LT, Keopp MJ, et al: Reduction of frontal neocortical grey matter associated with affective aggression in patients with temporal lobe epilepsy: An objective voxel by voxel analysis of automatically segmented MRI. *J Neurol Neurosurg Psychiatry* 68:162–169, 2000.

228. Yamada H, Yoshida H: Laughing attack: a review and report of nine cases. *Folia Psychiatr Neurol Jpn* 31:129–137, 1977.
229. Zeman AZJ, Boniface SJ, Hodges JR: Transient epileptic amnesia: A description of the clinical and neuropsychological features in 10 cases and a review of the literature. *J Neurol Neurosurg Psychiatry* 64:435–443, 1998.
230. Camfield PR, Gates R, Ronen G, et al: Comparison of cognitive ability, personality profile, and school success in epileptic children with pure right versus left temporal lobe EEG foci. *Ann Neurol* 15:122–126, 1984.
231. Schneider SK, Nowack WJ, Fitzgerald JA, et al: WAIS performance in epileptics with unilateral EEG abnormalities. *J Epilepsy* 6:10–14, 1993.

Chapter 55

NEUROPSYCHOLOGICAL ASPECTS OF TEMPORAL LOBE EPILEPSY SURGERY

David W. Loring
Kimford J. Meador

The present chapter discusses neuropsychological aspects of temporal lobe epilepsy (TLE) and the effects of anterior temporal lobectomy (ATL) on cognitive abilities. We restrict our discussion to these patients since they represent the majority of individuals undergoing epilepsy surgery and are consequently the populations in whom the most clinical research has been performed. Corpus callosotomy is discussed elsewhere (see Chap. 34).

Behavioral measures in such patients may reflect physiologic disruption of normal neural function secondary to epileptic activity as well as subtle and not so subtle structural changes that are not always readily apparent with neuroimaging studies. Thus, behavioral measures assess the functional status of many regions to be affected by epilepsy surgery, which in turn, often provide a prognostic index of risk for significant postoperative neuropsychological deficits following epilepsy surgery as well as being related to postoperative seizure outcome.[1,2]

As a group, epilepsy patients tend to have poorer cognitive abilities than age- and education-matched controls,[3] although considerable intersubject variability exists. Most patients, however, have intelligence in the normal range. Many factors may affect cognition, including the etiology of the seizures; seizure type; age at seizure onset; seizure frequency, duration, and severity; intraictal and interictal physiologic dysfunction due to the seizures; structural cerebral damage due to repetitive or prolonged seizures; hereditary factors; psychosocial factors; and the cognitive side effects of antiepileptic drugs.[4,5]

The most consistent abnormal neuropsychological findings in patients with TLE are seen in those with seizure onset localized to the left temporal lobe; these findings include decreased memory function (primarily anterograde verbal memory) and poor confrontation naming. Reduced visual memory may be observed in patients with onset of right temporal seizures, although this finding is less consistent and less reliable. Similarly, the greatest cognitive morbidity risk following ATL selectively occurs following resection in the language-dominant hemisphere and includes a decline in confrontation naming and a decrease in recent memory. Neuropsychological changes following ATL in the non-language-dominant hemisphere may include a decline in visual memory, although this outcome generally has less clear-cut clinical significance.

Prior to the modern imaging techniques of computed tomography (CT), magnetic resonance imaging (MRI), positron emission tomography (PET), and single photon emission tomography (SPECT), preoperative Wada test (i.e., intracarotid amobarbital procedure) and neuropsychology results were often the only measures available whereby to identify patients at risk for significant postoperative memory impairment. In general, patients at risk for postoperative amnesia were those with bilateral mesial temporal lobe dysfunction; these patients were either excluded from surgery or a less extensive resection was performed. Developments and refinements in brain imaging, however, have provided additional tools with which to evaluate risk for postoperative memory decline. Consequently, neuropsychology and Wada testing are no longer the only measures with which to make probabilistic predictions of postoperative behavior change. Change in neuropsychological status, however, remains the primary outcome variable in examining potential cognitive risks for postoperative change.

In addition to assessing risk of significant memory decline following ATL, strong neuropsychological material-specific memory or Wada memory asymmetries may help in documenting seizure onset laterality in patients whose seizure localization has been suggestive but inconclusive. In these cases, a strong dissociation in material-specific recent memory deficits, or definite Wada memory asymmetry, may eliminate the need for invasive monitoring before surgery. Although not a primary goal of assessment, neuropsychological performance and Wada testing may also provide information regarding the likelihood of a patient becoming seizure-free following surgery.

General Intellectual Function

Full Scale IQ has previously been considered by some to be a factor in the decision-making process for ATL, since a low IQ may be interpreted as reflecting general cerebral impairment in which focal resection would less likely be beneficial. Patients with generalized or multifocal areas of dysfunction have poorer postoperative seizure control, although some mixed results have been reported.[6] Patients with good surgical outcomes reportedly have neuropsychological deficits that are more strongly lateralized and localized to the temporal lobe.[7] Although nonlateralized neuropsychological findings occur more frequently in poor-outcome groups, the concordance of the side of seizure onset and laterality of neuropsychological findings is not necessarily related to outcome.[8]

In a large multicenter study, ATL patients who continued to have seizures following surgery had statistically lower preoperative IQ scores than those who were seizure-free ($p < 0.009$), but only by 2.3 points.[9] Lower IQ is associated with early seizure onset in TLE patients,[10] although whether this reflects seizure-related effects, cognitive medication side effects over the course of learning, or other factors is not clear. Nevertheless, Full Scale IQ alone is rarely sufficient to exclude an otherwise good candidate from surgery. Comparison of Verbal IQ to Performance IQ sometimes provides a suggestion of lateralized cerebral impairment in other neurologic populations, but the use of these measures in ATL candidates is not generally informative.[11]

Language

Preoperative Performance Patients with seizure onset from the language-dominant temporal lobe often perform poorly on confrontation naming tasks.[12–14] Whether this reflects a specialized role of the mesial temporal lobe in confrontation naming, such as semantic degradation or access limitation, or simply reflects the lifetime of decreased verbal memory resulting in limited semantic memory acquisition is not known. Regardless, the relationship of poor preoperative naming ability in patients with left temporal lobe seizures indicates that reports relying solely on postoperative results have tended to overestimate the magnitude of postoperative decline. As a group, left TLE patients tend to display mild interictal naming deficits independent of any surgical effects.

Postictal Findings Postictal aphasia reflecting the cognitive equivalent of a Todd's paralysis may be present following seizures that originate in the language-dominant temporal lobe.[15–17] Thus, postictal aphasia may be a valuable sign to assist with seizure onset lateralization in patients with left cerebral language dominance. However, postictal aphasia may also be present in patients with bilateral or right cerebral language representation[18] and may be seen after seizures originating in the nondominant temporal lobe following seizure propagation to the contralateral left temporal lobe.[19]

Peri-ictal cognitive deficits may be present following right temporal lobe seizures, although they will be less obvious. These deficits may include tactile and visual extinction to double simultaneous stimulation, line bisection displacement to the right, hemi-inattention on cancellation tasks, hemidyslexia, hemispatial neglect in drawings, and anosognosia.[20]

Postoperative Performance A decline in naming ability following language-dominant ATL is a well-recognized surgical risk.[21] In general, however, other core linguistic functions such as fluency, repetition, and comprehension are not affected,[14] although language difficulty extending beyond naming may be seen in some left TLE patients.[22,23] Heilman[24] postulated that postoperative anomia may be related to age of seizure onset and, by extension, to cerebral plasticity.

Seizure onset before age 5 years, or the presence of a significant seizure risk factor before age 5 (e.g., febrile seizure, perinatal distress, etc.), is associated with a decreased risk of postoperative naming decline following dominant hemisphere ATL.[14,25] The presence of preoperative anomia, however, may be independent of early seizure risk factors.[14] Although Langfitt and Rausch[26] failed to observe a similar effect, this likely reflects a statistical artifact of their approach to data analysis. When separate analyses of left and right groups are performed (using an error term based solely upon the factors being evaluated), a statistically significant effect of early risk is present ($p < 0.05$), with the early-risk patients displaying a smaller naming decline (Langfitt 1996, personal communication). The increased risk of dysnomia with later seizure onset has been replicated in a large multicenter study.[27] The lower-risk postoperative naming decline in patients with early seizure risk factors is thought to result from functional reorganization of the networks involved in naming.

The vulnerability of specific items to the effects of surgery is related to the age at which the words were likely learned.[28] Object names learned in late childhood are more vulnerable than those acquired earlier, which is the pattern observed in patients with frank aphasia. There have been inconsistent reports on whether naming decline for living or nonliving items is more likely following ATL. In one report, naming of living objects was more vulnerable to the effects and anterior temporal lobe resection,[29] a finding favoring the hypothesis that the left anterior temporal region supports knowledge pertaining to living objects, whereas more posterior temporal regions play a critical role in naming nonliving things.[30] In another study, however, nonliving items were likely to decline following left ATL.[31] Nouns appear to be more difficult to name following left ATL than verbs, both for single-word productions and for comprehension tasks.[32]

Stimulation Language Mapping The risk of postoperative language decline provides the rationale for functional cortical speech mapping.[21] Although acute language deficits are common following temporal lobectomy,[33] they largely resolve over longer intervals. The benefit derived from stimulation language mapping is controversial and is not addressed here. Like the Wada test described below, however, the variability inherent in stimulation mapping across centers is typically not well appreciated. For example, verbal tasks employed across centers involve stimulation while repeating a nursery rhyme, during spontaneous speech, reading passages, or naming objects. Other centers have standard paradigms involving use of generative naming and formal assessment of diverse language functions. The degree to which one mapping procedure (e.g., nursery rhyme repetition) is consistent with another (e.g., object naming) is not known, and the impact of such variability on language outcome has not been determined. There is significant patient variability in the topography of language sites identified with stimulation mapping. Fewer sites are present in patients with higher IQ levels, and this inverse relationship is also observed for confrontation naming, verbal fluency, and verbal memory.[34] A larger spatial distribution of sites is also associated with earlier seizure onset (< 6 years).[35]

Few differences have been observed in language outcomes of ATL patients who received mapping as compared to those who did not. Pre- to postoperative naming change may be on the order of one-half of a standard deviation, suggesting that mapping may provide benefit in avoiding mild anomia.[36] In that study, however, patients who underwent surgery under general anesthesia had a better surgical outcome. This was attributed in part to better head positioning during surgery, which allows better use of the operating microscope and thus more complete hippocampal resection.[37] In a multicenter study, change in naming was observed regardless of whether language mapping was performed but was associated with a later age of seizure onset and more extensive resection of lateral temporal neocortex.[27]

Stimulation of the inferior temporal lobe may produce language impairment, and this region, which tends to be located on the fusiform gyrus, is called the basal temporal language area (BTLA).[38–40] Although BTLA is clearly involved with language, as revealed by both stimulation mapping studies as well as the presence of ictal aphasia when seizures are observed in this area,[41,42] BTLA resection is not necessarily associated with postoperative language impairment. Some patients with resection in this area, however, do display a persistent naming decline.[43]

Wada Testing The presence of language representation often determines the need for preoperative grid studies or intraoperative cortical mapping and may be considered when planning the extent of surgical resection. Preoperative identification of language is typically performed using the Wada test, although reliable language activation paradigms for functional MRI (fMRI) exist that potentially may be used as a noninvasive approach to establish cerebral language representation preoperatively.[44–47] With the Wada test, language dominance is usually easy to determine, since most patients initially become mute following left hemispheric injection and then display varying degrees of expressive and receptive language impairment as the medication effects recede.

The presence of language representation during the Wada test is more variable in patients with bilateral or asymmetrical (e.g., L > R) representation. Speech arrest, for example, may be present following right cerebral injection but is unrelated to language representation.[48–50] Right hemispheric language may also be observed without a corresponding shift in handedness and may be present in some dextral patients with either left[51] or right temporal seizure onset.[52] Given the differences in the criteria used to infer language representation,[53] it is not surprising that different frequencies of mixed and right cerebral language dominance have been reported. Most studies employing a comprehensive assessment of multiple language functions report mixed (or bilateral) language representation more frequently than exclusive right hemispheric language representation,[45,54,55] a finding that is consistent with fMRI results.[56]

Hippocampus and Naming The hippocampus appears to play a critical role not only in the acquisition of new memories but also in naming. Preoperative confrontation naming performance is poorer for left TLE patients with evidence of hippocampal sclerosis,[23,57] and patients without hippocampal atrophy experience a greater postoperative confrontation naming. Similar results have been observed in assessing the functional status of the hippocampus with magnetic resonance spectroscopy.[58,59]

The relationship between confrontation naming and verbal memory has long been recognized.[12,60] The distinction between the two is important on an applied basis. Often, patients will complain of having a memory deficit when they cannot "remember" names. However, the studies cited above relating both preoperative naming and postoperative changes in confrontation naming to pathologic status of the hippocampus indicate some overlap in the neuroanatomic substrates of memory and confrontation naming. It has been suggested that "the distinction between semantic and episodic memory could simply be in the strength and distribution of their connection within the temporal lobe memory system rather than separable anatomic memory sites."[59] While this may be an overstatement, research has implicated the hippocampus as part of a distributed neuroanatomic network of visual confrontation naming.

Memory

Preoperative Performance The roles of the left temporal lobe in verbal memory and the right medial temporal lobe in visual/nonverbal memory are well known,[61,62] and material-specific asymmetries may reveal cognitive deficits associated with the unilateral seizure focus in the temporal lobe. Compared to the robust relationship between the left temporal lobe and verbal memory, the association between right temporal lobe function and visuospatial memory is more variable, and the inference to right temporal lobe dysfunction is necessarily less reliable.[63–65] Consequently, when discordant or nonlateralizing neuropsychological findings are observed, they are typically associated with right temporal seizure onset.[66] Nevertheless, studies continue to demonstrate a relationship between right temporal impairment and visual memory (e.g., see Ref. 67). Correlations between spatial memory performance and MRI measures of hippocampal volume[68] suggest that part of the failure to observe reliable right temporal/spatial memory effects may be related to test characteristics.

Neuronal loss and MRI volume of the left temporal lobe and hippocampus are correlated with preoperative verbal memory,[69–73] and patients with hippocampal sclerosis perform more poorly on memory tasks than patients with sclerosis restricted to the amygdala.[74] Patients with right hippocampal sclerosis are more likely to display visual memory impairments than patients with a normal-appearing hippocampal structure.[68,75] Although the hippocampus is often discussed as the only critical temporal lobe structure contributing to memory, it does not work in isolation and is part of a network for memory acquisition that also involves neocortex[76,77] in addition to the thalamus and other brain structures.

Postictal Findings Patients who are tested immediately following a seizure display material-specific memory deficits that may not be seen during interictal testing,[78–80] and this impairment may last up to 1 h after the patient has become reoriented.[79] Because seizure onset lateralization by postictal memory testing is related to seizure onset laterality, this information offers confirmatory seizure onset information that is often of value during the preoperative evaluation. To date, however, there have been no reports relating lateralization and degree of postictal memory impairment to postsurgical neuropsychological outcome.

Postoperative Performance Although dysnomia is often exacerbated by left ATL, a significant decline in memory function interferes more greatly than mild dysnomia with vocational and social interactions and has the potential to greatly diminish quality of life. The ability to identify patients who are at risk for significant postoperative memory change is important, since there is substantial variability in patient outcome.[81,82] Issues surrounding what constitutes a significant or meaningful change are important considerations, and several approaches have been presented in great detail.[81,83–86] The use of Wada memory testing to predict postoperative memory performance is discussed in a separate section below.

The magnitude of postoperative memory decline following anterior temporal lobectomy depends upon the functional status of both the ipsilateral hippocampus/temporal lobe to be included in the resection *(functional adequacy)* and of the temporal lobe contralateral to the surgery that will be relied upon for the formation of new memory *(functional reserve)*.[87] Patients developing significant postoperative amnesia following unilateral temporal lobe resection have been shown to have a diseased and nonfunctional mesial temporal lobe contralateral to the surgery.[88,89] Thus, the contralateral temporal lobe possessed insufficient functional reserve to sustain new memory formation without the contribution of the resected temporal lobe.

The status of the contralateral temporal lobe may also be related to milder memory decline. Verbal memory following right ATL has been associated with left-sided abnormalities revealed by magnetic resonance spectroscopy or T2-weighted relaxometry.[90] Similarly, patients demonstrating a specific event-related potential to words recorded from the right hippocampus have better verbal memory outcomes following left ATL.[91]

The status of the ipsilateral temporal lobe to be included in the resection is also a factor associated with memory outcome. When tissue that is still functionally contributing to memory formation is resected *(functional adequacy)*, there is a risk of significant memory decline. The memory change is typically not global and does not produce a persistent postoperative amnesia. Several authors have demonstrated that the degree of verbal memory loss following left ATL appears to be inversely related to the degree of hippocampal pathology in the resected specimen.[69,92–95] Similarly, left ATL patients without significant PET or SPECT asymmetries in the left temporal lobe display greater verbal memory decline than those with hypometabolism associated with the left seizure onset.[96,97] The greater change present following resection of a relatively nonatrophic left hippocampus is sufficiently robust that it can be appreciated without formal neuropsychological testing.[98]

The relationship between right ATL and memory is less consistent, with some authors reporting a very modest relationship[69] and others reporting a decline in visual memory following resection of a relatively intact right hippocampus.[94] Although changes in visual memory following right anterior temporal lobectomy have not been consistently reported, this may reflect in part a limitation of standard visual and spatial memory tasks. Other tasks such as route learning[99] or object location memory[100,101] may be selectively impaired following right ATL.

Baseline memory assessment itself also poses a measure of risk to memory change following temporal lobectomy. High-functioning patients with intact verbal memory show the greatest declines in verbal memory declines postoperatively,[102–105] and this does not appear to be explained solely on the basis of statistical regression to the mean.[106] As described above, preoperative verbal memory generally reflects the pathologic status of the left hippocampus. Further, temporal lobe abnormalities reflected by T2-weighted relaxometry are associated with better verbal memory outcome independent of hippocampal atrophy revealed by MRI.[107] Even in the presence of hippocampal sclerosis, preoperative memory level is related to memory outcome.[105] Thus, the presence of atrophy on MRI does not negate the risk for memory decline in the presence of normal verbal memory. Patients with unilateral hippocampal MRI atrophy and poor baseline neuropsychological memory scores, however, do not appear to be at increased risk for postoperative amnesia,[108] although patients undergoing left ATL with bilateral hippocampal damage are at risk for postoperative memory decline.[109,110]

Patients who are not seizure-free following surgery are also more likely to show greater verbal memory impairments than those without postoperative seizures[111,112] and more likely to report subjective memory decline.[113,114] Other factors associated with a greater decline in verbal memory following left ATL include later age of seizure onset.[105,115] Subjective decline in memory also appears related to medication effects and depression and is poorly related to objective memory performance.

Wada Testing Probably the most research on the prediction of postoperative memory function has been conducted using Wada memory test results, since this was the approach developed by Milner in the early 1960s.[116] Wada memory testing was introduced to assess whether, to avoid postoperative amnesia, the hemisphere contralateral to a unilateral seizure focus could sustain memory function following temporal lobectomy *(functional reserve)*.[117,118] It is important to emphasize that as with Wada language assessment, there are multiple approaches to testing memory during the period of hemispheric anesthesia. Some of the variables include continuous stimulus recognition versus discrete item presentation,[119] different stimulus materials (e.g., words, designs, real objects),[120–123] timing of stimulus presentation,[124,125] medication dose,[126] and even whether both hemispheres are tested on a single day,[127] all of which may potentially affect results. Memory performance following injection of the language-dominant hemisphere is often slightly lower due to the effects of impairments in language or attention.[128–131]

Early efforts to validate the Wada test were limited, since Wada memory results were used as a selection criterion for surgery, thereby confounding the dependent and independent variables.[48] Thus, at least in certain circumstances, patients may "fail" the memory component of the Wada test yet successfully undergo ATL without the development of an amnesic syndrome.[132,133] Attempts to "validate" the procedure on other populations with memory impairment have not proven successful.[134]

Indirect approaches to Wada validation have demonstrated a relationship between Wada memory results and various hippocampal indices. Poor memory performance is more likely following injection contralateral to a seizure focus if there is significant hippocampal sclerosis,[135–139] and Wada memory performance is a better predictor of seizure onset laterality than traditional neuropsychological memory tests.[140] Wada memory performance is related to hippocampal structure as measured by MRI hippocampal volume asymmetries,[141] and Wada memory asymmetries are related to laterality of seizure onset.[120,130,140,142,145] Further, patients with a medial seizure focus are more likely to have asymmetrical Wada memory scores than those with a more lateral seizure onset.[146]

Another approach to indirect Wada memory validation has been to demonstrate a relationship to postoperative memory outcome.[147] Patients with verbal memory declines following left ATL tend to have symmetrical Wada memory scores[148] or have good Wada memory performance following right hemispheric injection, indicating that the functional adequacy of the tissue to be resected is inversely related to the likelihood of a postoperative decline in verbal memory.[149] Wada memory following left hemispheric injection is related to memory outcome, even in the presence of left hippocampal sclerosis.[105] The combination of Wada memory following left hemispheric injection and baseline memory performance may be even more predictive of postoperative memory outcome.[150]

Patients with significant volumetric MRI hippocampal asymmetries are more likely to have a good outcome following ATL,[151] and Wada memory asymmetries are also related to seizure outcome.[130,142,152] Patients with poor seizure outcomes rarely have asymmetrical Wada memory scores, although there does appear to be greater Wada performance variability in patients with good surgical results.[153]

Although the Wada test has been criticized because the posterior hippocampus is not directly supplied by the distribution of the internal carotid artery, EEG slowing in this region recorded from depth electrodes is seen following standard intracarotid amobarbital injection.[154] Wada memory performance is correlated with magnetic resonance spectroscopy (MRS)[155] as well as PET.[156] Patients with unilateral temporal lobe seizures who display bilateral hypometabolism by PET display poorer Wada memory performance and also have a longer disease duration.[157]

Just as fMRI may eventually replace Wada testing in the preoperative determination of language in most patients, fMRI holds the potential to provide a noninvasive alternative to Wada memory testing to assess the functional status of the mesial temporal lobe. To date, however, there have been few reports describing the association between fMRI temporal lobe asymmetries to seizure onset laterality,[158,159] and the relationship of these measures to cognitive outcome is not known.[160]

Surgical Variables The extent of resection has inconsistently been related to memory outcome. Corsi observed greater postoperative memory impairment with more extensive resections.[161] However, multiple attempts at replication have produced inconsistent results.[162–164] Ojemann and Dodrill reported that the verbal memory decline is associated with degree of lateral (but not medial) temporal resection.[76] Although a more limited resection may be performed with the goal of decreasing the likelihood of significant postoperative memory decline, the hippocampal remnant undergoes further volume loss over the first 3 postoperative months, and this change is related to postoperative memory change.[165]

Spatial memory may be related to the extent of resection of hippocampus and parahippocampal regions in right ATL patients.[166,167] However, in a small randomized trial, there was no increase in postoperative memory impairment associated with more extensive hippocampal resection.[168] It is likely that the degree of resection will be a positive predictor of memory change only in those patients with high functional adequacy of the ipsilateral temporal lobe.

CONCLUSIONS

Patients with partial complex seizures of left temporal lobe origin often present with focal neuropsychological deficits that include poor confrontation naming ability and decreased verbal learning and retention. Patients with right temporal lobe epilepsy may have poor visual learning ability, although this is a less consistent finding.

The pathologic status of the hippocampus appears to play a critical role, not only with regard to the preoperative presence of the naming and verbal memory deficits but also as to whether patients undergoing surgical resection of the temporal lobe are likely to display significant postoperative decline. In addition to the pathologic status of the hippocampus to be included in the resection, baseline memory performance is related to cognitive outcome. Patient with high preoperative verbal memory are at increased risk for postoperative memory decline. Thus, patients with good verbal memory in the presence of left hippocampal atrophy may still demonstrate significant change in verbal cognitive tasks. Finally, measures of hippocampal function (e.g., Wada test) provide additional information on the risk of postoperative cognitive deficits and are also predictive of seizure outcome.

REFERENCES

1. Engel J Jr, Rausch R, Lieb JP, et al: Correlation of criteria used for localizing epileptic foci in patients considered for surgical therapy of epilepsy. *Ann Neurol* 9(3):215–224, 1981.
2. Milner B: Psychological aspects of focal epilepsy and its neurosurgical management. *Adv Neurol* 8:299–321, 1975.
3. Smith DB, Craft BR, Collins J, et al: Behavioral characteristics of epilepsy patients compared with normal controls. *Epilepsia* 27(6):760–768, 1986.
4. Lennox WG: Brain injury, drugs and environment as causes of mental decay in epilepsy. *Am J Psychiatry* 99:174–180, 1942.
5. Lesser RP, Luders H, Wyllie E, et al: Mental deterioration in epilepsy. *Epilepsia* 27(Suppl 2):S105–123, 1986.
6. Dodrill CB, Hermann BP, Rausch R, et al: Neuropsychological testing for assessing prognosis following surgery for epilepsy, in Engel J (ed): *Surgical Treatment of the Epilepsies,* 2d ed. New York: Raven Press, 1993, pp 263–271.
7. Bengzon ARA, Rasmussen T, Gloor P, et al: Prognostic factors in the surgical treatment of temporal lobe epileptics. *Neurology* 18(8):717–731, 1968.

8. Dodrill CB, Wilkus RJ, Ojemann GA, et al: Multidisciplinary prediction of seizure relief from cortical resection surgery. *Ann Neurol* 20(1):2–12, 1986.
9. Chelune GJ, Naugle RI, Hermann BP, et al: Does presurgical IQ predict seizure outcome after temporal lobectomy? Evidence from the Bozeman Epilepsy Consortium. *Epilepsia* 39(3):314–318, 1998.
10. Glosser G, Cole LC, French JA, et al: Predictors of intellectual performance in adults with intractable temporal lobe epilepsy. *J Int Neuropsychol Soc* 3(3):252–359, 1997.
11. Hermann BP, Gold J, Pusakulich R, et al: Wechsler Adult Intelligence Scale—Revised in the evaluation of anterior temporal lobectomy candidates. *Epilepsia* 36(5):480–487, 1995.
12. Mayeux R, Brandt J, Rosen J, Benson DF: Interictal memory and language impairment in temporal lobe epilepsy. *Neurology* 30(2):120–125, 1980.
13. Hermann BP, Seidenberg M, Haltiner A, Wyler AR: Adequacy of language function and verbal memory performance in unilateral temporal lobe epilepsy. *Cortex* 28(3):423–433, 1992.
14. Saykin AJ, Stafiniak P, Robinson LJ, et al: Language before and after temporal lobectomy: Specificity of acute changes and relation to early risk factors. *Epilepsia* 36(11):1071–1077, 1995.
15. Koerner M, Laxer KD: Ictal speech, postictal language dysfunction, and seizure lateralization. *Neurology* 38(4):634–636, 1988.
16. Privitera MD, Morris GL, Gilliam F: Postictal language assessment and lateralization of complex partial seizures. *Ann Neurol* 30(3):391–396, 1991.
17. Gabr M, Luders H, Dinner D, et al: Speech manifestations in lateralization of temporal lobe seizures. *Ann Neurol* 25(1):82–87, 1989.
18. Privitera M, Kohler C, Cahill W, Yeh HS: Postictal language dysfunction in patients with right or bilateral hemispheric language localization. *Epilepsia* 37(10):936–941, 1996.
19. Ficker DM, Shukla R, Privitera MD: Postictal language dysfunction in complex partial seizures: Effect of contralateral ictal spread. *Neurology* 56(11):1590–1592, 2001.
20. Meador KJ, Moser E: Negative seizures. *J Int Neuropsychol Soc* 6(6):731–733, 2000.
21. Penfield W, Roberts L: *Speech and Brain Mechanisms.* Princeton, NJ: Princeton University Press, 1959.
22. Hermann BP, Wyler AR: Effects of anterior temporal lobectomy on language function: A controlled study. *Ann Neurol* 23(6):585–588, 1988.
23. Seidenberg M, Hermann B, Wyler AR, et al: Neuropsychological outcome following anterior temporal lobectomy in patients with and without the syndrome of mesial temporal lobe epilepsy. *Neuropsychology* 12(2):303–316, 1998.
24. Heilman KM, Wilder BJ, Malzone WF: Anomic aphasia following anterior temporal lobectomy. *Trans Am Neurol Assoc* 97:291–293, 1972.
25. Stafiniak P, Saykin AJ, Sperling MR, et al: Acute naming deficits following dominant temporal lobectomy: Prediction by age at first risk for seizures. *Neurology* 40(10):1509–1512, 1990.
26. Langfitt JT, Rausch R: Word-finding deficits persist after left anterotemporal lobectomy. *Arch Neurol* 53(1):72–76, 1996.
27. Hermann BP, Perrine K, Chelune GJ, et al: Visual confrontation naming following left anterior temporal lobectomy: A comparison of surgical approaches. *Neuropsychology* 13(1):3–9, 1999.
28. Bell BD, Davies KG, Hermann BP, Walters G: Confrontation naming after anterior temporal lobectomy is related to age of acquisition of the object names. *Neuropsychologia* 38(1):83–92, 2000.
29. Strauss E, Semenza C, Hunter M, et al: Left anterior lobectomy and category-specific naming. *Brain Cogn* 43(1–3):403–406, 2000.
30. Damasio H, Grabowski TJ, Tranel D, et al: A neural basis for lexical retrieval. *Nature* 380:499–505, 1996.
31. Tippett LJ, Glosser G, Farah MJ: A category-specific naming impairment after temporal lobectomy. *Neuropsychologia* 34(2):139–146, 1996.
32. Glosser G, Donofrio N: Differences between nouns and verbs after anterior temporal lobectomy. *Neuropsychology* 15:39–47, 2001.
33. Loring DW, Meador KJ, Lee GP: Effects of temporal lobectomy on generative fluency and other language functions. *Arch Clin Neuropsychol* 9:364–367, 1994.
34. Devinsky O, Perrine K, Hirsch J, et al: Relation of cortical language distribution and cognitive function in surgical epilepsy patients. *Epilepsia* 41(4):400–404, 2000.
35. Schwartz TH, Devinsky O, Doyle W, Perrine K: Preoperative predictors of anterior temporal language areas. *J Neurosurg* 89(6):962–970, 1998.
36. Hermann BP, Wyler AR: Comparative results of dominant temporal lobectomy under general or local anesthesia: Language outcome. *J Epilepsy* 1:127–134, 1988.
37. Wyler AR, Hermann BP: Comparative results of temporal lobectomy under local or generalized anesthesia: Seizure outcome. *J Epilepsy* 1:121–125, 1988.

38. Luders H, Lesser RP, Hahn J, et al: Basal temporal language area demonstrated by electrical stimulation. *Neurology* 36(4):505–510, 1986.
39. Burnstine TH, Lesser RP, Hart J Jr, et al: Characterization of the basal temporal language area in patients with left temporal lobe epilepsy. *Neurology* 40(6):966–970, 1990.
40. Luders H, Lesser RP, Hahn J, et al: Basal temporal language area. *Brain* 114(Pt 2):743–754, 1991.
41. Abou-Khalil B, Welch L, Blumenkopf B, et al: Global aphasia with seizure onset in the dominant basal temporal region. *Epilepsia* 35(5):1079–1084, 1994.
42. Kirshner HS, Hughes T, Fakhoury T, Abou-Khalil B: Aphasia secondary to partial status epilepticus of the basal temporal language area. *Neurology* 45(8):1616–1618, 1995.
43. Krauss GL, Fisher R, Plate C, et al: Cognitive effects of resecting basal temporal language areas. *Epilepsia* 37(5):476–483, 1996.
44. Brockway JP: Two functional magnetic resonance imaging (fMRI) tasks that may replace the gold standard, Wada testing, for language lateralization while giving additional localization information. *Brain Cogn* 43(1–3):57–59, 2000.
45. Binder JR, Swanson SJ, Hammeke TA, et al: Determination of language dominance using functional MRI: A comparison with the Wada test. *Neurology* 46(4):978–984, 1996.
46. Lehericy S, Cohen L, Bazin B, et al: Functional MR evaluation of temporal and frontal language dominance compared with the Wada test. *Neurology* 54(8):1625–1633, 2000.
47. Benson RR, FitzGerald DB, LeSueur LL, et al: Language dominance determined by whole brain functional MRI in patients with brain lesions. *Neurology* 52(4):798–809, 1999.
48. Loring DW, Meador KJ, Lee GP, King DW: *Amobarbital Effects and Lateralized Brain Function: The Wada Test*. New York: Springer-Verlag, 1992.
49. Oxbury SM, Oxbury JM: Intracarotid amytal test in the assessment of language dominance. *Adv Neurol* 42:115–123, 1984.
50. Benbadis SR, Binder JR, Swanson SJ, et al: Is speech arrest during Wada testing a valid method for determining hemispheric representation of language? *Brain Lang* 65(3):441–446, 1998.
51. Rausch R, Walsh GO: Right-hemisphere language dominance in right-handed epileptic patients. *Arch Neurol* 41(10):1077–1080, 1984.
52. Loring DW, Meador KJ, Lee GP, et al: Crossed aphasia in a patient with complex partial seizures: evidence from intracarotid amobarbital testing, functional cortical mapping, and neuropsychological assessment. *J Clin Exp Neuropsychol* 12(2):340–354, 1990.
53. Snyder PJ, Novelly RA, Harris LJ: Mixed speech dominance in the intracarotid sodium amytal procedure: Validity and criteria issues. *J Clin Exp Neuropsychol* 12(5):629–643, 1990.
54. Loring DW, Meador KJ, Lee GP, et al: Cerebral language lateralization: Evidence from intracarotid amobarbital testing. *Neuropsychologia* 28(8):831–838, 1990.
55. Helmstaedter C, Kurthen M, Linke DB, Elger CE: Right hemisphere restitution of language and memory functions in right hemisphere language-dominant patients with left temporal lobe epilepsy. *Brain* 117(Pt 4):729–737, 1994.
56. Springer JA, Binder JR, Hammeke TA, et al: Language dominance in neurologically normal and epilepsy subjects: A functional MRI study. *Brain* 122(Pt 11):2033–2046, 1999.
57. Davies KG, Bell BD, Bush AJ, et al: Naming decline after left anterior temporal lobectomy correlates with pathological status of resected hippocampus. *Epilepsia* 39(4):407–419, 1998.
58. Martin RC, Sawrie S, Hugg J, et al: Cognitive correlates of 1H MRSI-detected hippocampal abnormalities in temporal lobe epilepsy. *Neurology* 53(9):2052–2058, 1999.
59. Sawrie SM, Martin RC, Gilliam FG, et al: Visual confrontation naming and hippocampal function: A neural network study using quantitative (1)H magnetic resonance spectroscopy. *Brain* 123(Pt 4):770–780, 2000.
60. Hermann BP, Wyler AR, Steenman H, Richey ET: The interrelationship between language function and verbal learning/memory performance in patients with complex partial seizures. *Cortex* 24(2):245–253, 1988.
61. Milner B: Disorders of learning and memory after temporal lobe lesions in man. *Clin Neurosurg* 19:421–446, 1972.
62. Hermann BP, Wyler AR, Somes G, et al: Declarative memory following anterior temporal lobectomy in humans. *Behav Neurosci* 108(1):3–10, 1994.
63. Barr WB, Chelune GJ, Hermann BP, et al: The use of figural reproduction tests as measures of nonverbal memory in epilepsy surgery candidates. *J Int Neuropsychol Soc* 3(5):435–443, 1997.
64. Barr WB: Examining the right temporal lobe's role in nonverbal memory. *Brain Cogn* 35(1):26–41, 1997.

65. Ivnik RJ, Sharbrough FW, Laws ER Jr: Anterior temporal lobectomy for the control of partial complex seizures: Information for counseling patients. *Mayo Clin Proc* 63(8):783–793, 1988.
66. Williamson PD, French JA, Thadani VM, et al: Characteristics of medial temporal lobe epilepsy: II. Interictal and ictal scalp electroencephalography, neuropsychological testing, neuroimaging, surgical results, and pathology. *Ann Neurol* 34(6):781–787, 1993.
67. Abrahams S, Pickering A, Polkey CE, Morris RG: Spatial memory deficits in patients with unilateral damage to the right hippocampal formation. *Neuropsychologia* 35(1):11–24, 1997.
68. Baxendale SA, Thompson PJ, Van Paesschen W: A test of spatial memory and its clinical utility in the pre-surgical investigation of temporal lobe epilepsy patients. *Neuropsychologia* 36(7):591–602, 1998.
69. Hermann BP, Wyler AR, Somes G, et al: Pathological status of the mesial temporal lobe predicts memory outcome from left anterior temporal lobectomy. *Neurosurgery* 31(4):652–656, discussion 656–657, 1992.
70. Lencz T, McCarthy G, Bronen RA, et al: Quantitative magnetic resonance imaging in temporal lobe epilepsy: Relationship to neuropathology and neuropsychological function. *Ann Neurol* 31(6):629–637, 1992.
71. Miller LA, Munoz DG, Finmore M: Hippocampal sclerosis and human memory. *Arch Neurol* 50(4):391–394, 1993.
72. Rausch R, Babb TL: Hippocampal neuron loss and memory scores before and after temporal lobe surgery for epilepsy. *Arch Neurol* 50(8):812–817, 1993.
73. Sass KJ, Spencer DD, Kim JH, et al: Verbal memory impairment correlates with hippocampal pyramidal cell density. *Neurology* 40(11):1694–1697, 1990.
74. Hudson LP, Munoz DG, Miller L, et al: Amygdaloid sclerosis in temporal lobe epilepsy. *Ann Neurol* 33(6):622–631, 1993.
75. Gleissner U, Helmstaedter C, Elger CE: Right hippocampal contribution to visual memory: A presurgical and postsurgical study in patients with temporal lobe epilepsy. *J Neurol Neurosurg Psychiatry* 65(5):665–669, 1998.
76. Ojemann GA, Dodrill CB: Verbal memory deficits after left temporal lobectomy for epilepsy. Mechanism and intraoperative prediction. *J Neurosurg* 62(1):101–107, 1985.
77. Perrine K, Devinsky O, Uysal S, et al: Left temporal neocortex mediation of verbal memory: Evidence from functional mapping with cortical stimulation. *Neurology* 44(10):1845–1850, 1994.
78. Andrewes DG, Puce A, Bladin PF: Post-ictal recognition memory predicts laterality of temporal lobe seizure focus: Comparison with post-operative data. *Neuropsychologia* 28(9):957–967, 1990.
79. Helmstaedter C, Elger CE, Lendt M: Postictal courses of cognitive deficits in focal epilepsies. *Epilepsia* 35(5):1073–1078, 1994.
80. Pegna AJ, Qayoom Z, Gericke CA, et al: Comprehensive postictal neuropsychology improves focus localization in epilepsy. *Eur Neurol* 40(4):207–211, 1998.
81. Martin RC, Sawrie SM, Roth DL, et al: Individual memory change after anterior temporal lobectomy: A base rate analysis using regression-based outcome methodology. *Epilepsia* 39(10):1075–1082, 1998.
82. Phillips NA, McGlone J: Grouped data do not tell the whole story: Individual analysis of cognitive change after temporal lobectomy. *J Clin Exp Neuropsychol* 17(5):713–724, 1995.
83. Chelune GJ, Naugle RI, Lüders H: Individual change after epilepsy surgery: Practice effects and base-rate information. *Neuropsychology* 7(1):41–52, 1993.
84. Hermann BP, Seidenberg M, Schoenfeld J, et al: Empirical techniques for determining the reliability, magnitude, and pattern of neuropsychological change after epilepsy surgery. *Epilepsia* 37(10):942–950, 1996.
85. Sawrie SM, Chelune GJ, Naugle RI, Lüders HO: Empirical methods for assessing meaningful neuropsychological change following epilepsy surgery. *J Int Neuropsychol Soc* 2(6):556–564, 1996.
86. Bruggemans EF, Van de Vijver FJ, Huysmans HA: Assessment of cognitive deterioration in individual patients following cardiac surgery: Correcting for measurement error and practice effects. *J Clin Exp Neuropsychol* 19(4):543–559, 1997.
87. Chelune GJ: Hippocampal adequacy versus functional reserve: Predicting memory functions following temporal lobectomy. *Arch Clin Neuropsychol* 10:413–432, 1995.
88. Penfield W, Mathieson G: Memory: Autopsy findings and comments on the role of the hippocampus in experimental recall. *Arch Neurol* 31:145–154, 1974.
89. Warrington EK, Duchen LW: A re-appraisal of a case of persistent global amnesia following right temporal lobectomy: A clinico-pathological study. *Neuropsychologia* 30(5):437–450, 1992.
90. Incisa della Rocchetta A, Gadian DG, Connelly A, et al: Verbal memory impairment after right temporal lobe surgery: Role of contralateral damage as revealed by 1H magnetic resonance spectroscopy and T2 relaxometry. *Neurology* 45(4):797–802, 1995.

91. Grunwald T, Lehnertz K, Helmstaedter C, et al: Limbic ERPs predict verbal memory after left-sided hippocampectomy. *Neuroreport* 9(15):3375–3378, 1998.
92. Sass KJ, Westerveld M, Buchanan CP, et al: Degree of hippocampal neuron loss determines severity of verbal memory decrease after left anteromesiotemporal lobectomy. *Epilepsia* 35(6):1179–1186, 1994.
93. Seidenberg M, Hermann BP, Dohan FC Jr, et al: Hippocampal sclerosis and verbal encoding ability following anterior temporal lobectomy. *Neuropsychologia* 34(7):699–708, 1996.
94. Baxendale SA, Van Paesschen W, Thompson PJ, et al: Hippocampal cell loss and gliosis: relationship to preoperative and postoperative memory function. *Neuropsychiatry Neuropsychol Behav Neurol* 11(1):12–21, 1998.
95. Trenerry MR, Jack CR Jr, Ivnik RJ, et al: MRI hippocampal volumes and memory function before and after temporal lobectomy. *Neurology* 43(9):1800–1805, 1993.
96. Griffith HR, Perlman SB, Woodard AR, et al: Preoperative FDG-PET temporal lobe hypometabolism and verbal memory after temporal lobectomy. *Neurology* 54(5):1161–1165, 2000.
97. Grunwald F, Durwen HF, Bockisch A, et al: Technetium-99m-HMPAO brain SPECT in medically intractable temporal lobe epilepsy: A postoperative evaluation. *J Nucl Med* 32(3):388–394, 1991.
98. Hermann BP, Seidenberg M, Dohan FC Jr, et al: Reports by patients and their families of memory change after left anterior temporal lobectomy: relationship to degree of hippocampal sclerosis. *Neurosurgery* 36(1):39–44, discussion 44–45, 1995.
99. Worsley CL, Recce M, Spiers HJ, et al: Path integration following temporal lobectomy in humans. *Neuropsychologia* 39(5):452–464, 2001.
100. Pigott S, Milner B: Memory for different aspects of complex visual scenes after unilateral temporal- or frontal-lobe resection. *Neuropsychologia* 31(1):1–15, 1993.
101. Milner B, Johnsrude I, Crane J: Right medial temporal-lobe contribution to object-location memory. *Philos Trans R Soc Lond Ser B Biol Sci* 352(1360):1469–1474, 1997.
102. Szabo CA, Wyllie E, Stanford LD, et al: Neuropsychological effect of temporal lobe resection in preadolescent children with epilepsy. *Epilepsia* 39(8):814–819, 1998.
103. Chelune GJ, Naugle RI, Luders H, Awad IA: Prediction of cognitive change as a function of preoperative ability status among temporal lobectomy patients seen at 6–month follow-up. *Neurology* 41(3):399–404, 1991.
104. Davies KG, Bell BD, Bush AJ, Wyler AR: Prediction of verbal memory loss in individuals after anterior temporal lobectomy. *Epilepsia* 39(8):820–828, 1998.
105. Bell BD, Davies KG, Haltiner AM, Walters GL: Intracarotid amobarbital procedure and prediction of postoperative memory in patients with left temporal lobe epilepsy and hippocampal sclerosis. *Epilepsia* 41(8):992–997, 2000.
106. Hermann BP, Wyler AR, VanderZwagg R, et al: Predictors of neuropsychological change following anterior temporal lobectomy: Role of regression toward the mean. *J Epilepsy* 4:139–148, 1991.
107. Wendel JD, Trenerry MR, Xu YC, et al: The relationship between quantitative T2 relaxometry and memory in nonlesional temporal lobe epilepsy. *Epilepsia* 42(7):863–868, 2001.
108. Baxendale SA, Van Paesschen W, Thompson PJ, et al: The relation between quantitative MRI measures of hippocampal structure and the intracarotid amobarbital test. *Epilepsia* 38(9):998–1007, 1997.
109. Martin RC, Sawrie SM, Knowlton RC, et al: Bilateral hippocampal atrophy: Consequences to verbal memory following temporal lobectomy. *Neurology* 57(4):597–604, 2001.
110. Trenerry MR, Jack CR Jr, Cascino GD, et al: Bilateral magnetic resonance imaging-determined hippocampal atrophy and verbal memory before and after temporal lobectomy. *Epilepsia* 37(6):526–533, 1996.
111. Novelly RA, Augustine EA, Mattson RH, et al: Selective memory improvement and impairment in temporal lobectomy for epilepsy. *Ann Neurol* 15(1):64–67, 1984.
112. Rausch R, Crandall PH: Psychological status related to surgical control of temporal lobe seizures. *Epilepsia* 23(2):191–202, 1982.
113. McGlone J, Wands K: Self-report of memory function in patients with temporal lobe epilepsy and temporal lobectomy. *Cortex* 27(1):19–28, 1991.
114. Sawrie SM, Martin RC, Kuzniecky R, et al: Subjective versus objective memory change after temporal lobe epilepsy surgery. *Neurology* 53(7):1511–1517, 1999.
115. Hermann BP, Seidenberg M, Haltiner A, Wyler AR: Relationship of age at onset, chronologic age, and adequacy of preoperative performance to verbal memory change after anterior temporal lobectomy. *Epilepsia* 36(2):137–145, 1995.
116. Milner B, Branch C, Rasmussen T: Study of short-term memory after intracarotid injection of sodium Amytal. *Trans Am Neurol Assoc* 87:224–226, 1962.

117. Jones-Gotman M: Commentary: Psychological evaluation; testing hippocampal function, in Engel JJ (ed): *Surgical Treatment of the Epilepsies*. New York: Raven Press, 1987.
118. Snyder PJ, Harris LJ: The intracarotid amobarbital procedure: An historical perspective. *Brain Cogn* 33(1):18–32, 1997.
119. Dodrill CB, Ojemann GA: An exploratory comparison of three methods of memory assessment with the intracarotid amobarbital procedure. *Brain Cogn* 33(2):210–223, 1997.
120. Loring DW, Hermann BP, Perrine K, et al: Effect of Wada memory stimulus type in discriminating lateralized temporal lobe impairment. *Epilepsia* 38(2):219–224, 1997.
121. Glosser G, Deutsch GK, Cole LC, et al: Differential lateralization of memory discrimination and response bias in temporal lobe epilepsy patients. *J Int Neuropsychol Soc* 4(5):502–511, 1998.
122. Rouleau I, Robidoux J, Labrecque R, Denault C: Effect of focus laterlization on memory assessment during the intracarotid amobarbital procedure. *Brain Cogn* 33(2):224–241, 1997.
123. Perrine K, Gershengorn J, Brown ER, et al: Material-specific memory in the intracarotid amobarbital procedure. *Neurology* 43(4):706–711, 1993.
124. Loring DW, Meador KJ, Lee GP, et al: Stimulus timing effects on Wada memory testing. *Arch Neurol* 51(8):806–810, 1994.
125. Carpenter K, Oxbury JM, Oxbury S, Wright GD: Memory for objects presented early after intracarotid sodium Amytal: A sensitive clinical neuropsychological indicator of temporal lobe pathology. *Seizure* 5(2):103–108, 1996.
126. Loring DW, Meador KJ, Lee GP: Amobarbital dose effects on Wada memory testing. *J Epilepsy* 5:171–174, 1992.
127. Grote CL, Wierenga C, Smith MC, et al: Wada difference a day makes: Interpretive cautions regarding same-day injections. *Neurology* 52(8):1577–1582, 1999.
128. Meador KJ, Loring DW, Lee GP, et al: Level of consciousness and memory during the intracarotid sodium amobarbital procedure. *Brain Cogn* 33(2):178–188, 1997.
129. Glosser G, Cole LC, Deutsch GK, et al: Hemispheric asymmetries in arousal affect outcome of the intracarotid amobarbital test. *Neurology* 52(8):1583–1590, 1999.
130. Perrine K, Westerveld M, Sass KJ, et al: Wada memory disparities predict seizure laterality and postoperative seizure control. *Epilepsia* 36(9):851–856, 1995.
131. Breier JI, Thomas AB, Plenger PM, et al: Asymmetries in the effect of side of seizure onset on recognition memory following intracarotid amobarbital injection. *Epilepsia* 38(11):1209–1215, 1997.
132. Loring DW, Lee GP, Meador KJ, et al: The intracarotid amobarbital procedure as a predictor of memory failure following unilateral temporal lobectomy. *Neurology* 40(4):605–610, 1990.
133. Kubu CS, Girvin JP, McLachlan RS, et al: Does the intracarotid amobarbital procedure predict global amnesia after temporal lobectomy? *Epilepsia* 41(10):1321–1329, 2000.
134. McGlone J, Black SE, Evans J, et al: Criterion-based validity of an intracarotid amobarbital recognition-memory protocol. *Epilepsia* 40(4):430–438, 1999.
135. Rausch R, Babb TL, Engel J Jr, Crandall PH: Memory following intracarotid amobarbital injection contralateral to hippocampal damage. *Arch Neurol* 46(7):783–788, 1989.
136. Sass KJ, Lencz T, Westerveld M, et al: The neural substrate of memory impairment demonstrated by the intracarotid amobarbital procedure. *Arch Neurol* 48(1):48–52, 1991.
137. O'Rourke DM, Saykin AJ, Gilhool JJ, et al: Unilateral hemispheric memory and hippocampal neuronal density in temporal lobe epilepsy. *Neurosurgery* 32(4):574–580, discussion 580–581, 1993.
138. Davies KG, Hermann BP, Foley KT: Relation between intracarotid amobarbital memory asymmetry scores and hippocampal sclerosis in patients undergoing anterior temporal lobe resections. *Epilepsia* 37(6):522–525, 1996.
139. Davies KG, Bell BD, Dohan FC, et al: Prediction of presence of hippocampal sclerosis from intracarotid amobarbital procedure memory asymmetry scores and epilepsy on set age. *Epilepsy Res* 33(2–3):117–123, 1999.
140. Kneebone AC, Chelune GJ, Luders HO: Individual patient prediction of seizure lateralization in temporal lobe epilepsy: A comparison between neuropsychological memory measures and the Intracarotid Amobarbital Procedure. *J Int Neuropsycho Soc* 3(2):159–168, 1997.
141. Loring DW, Murro AM, Meador KJ, et al: Wada memory testing and hippocampal volume measurements in the evaluation for temporal lobectomy: *Neurology* 43(9):1789–1793, 1993.
142. Sperling MR, Saykin AJ, Glosser G, et al: Predictors of outcome after anterior temporal lobectomy. The intracarotid amobarbital test. *Neurology* 44(12):2325–2330, 1994.

143. Kim H, Yi S, Kim J, Son EI: Lateralizing value of the Wada memory test in non-western patients with temporal lobe epilepsy. *Epilepsy Res* 33(2–3):125–131, 1999.
144. Wyllie E, Naugle R, Chelune G, et al: Intracarotid amobarbital procedure: II. Lateralizing value in evaluation for temporal lobectomy. *Epilepsia* 32(6):865–869, 1991.
145. Roman DD, Beniak TE, Nugent S: Memory performance on the intracarotid amobarbital procedure as a predictor of seizure focus. *Epilepsy Res* 25(3):243–248, 1996.
146. Hamberger MJ, Walczak TS, Goodman RR: Intracarotid amobarbital procedure memory performance and age at first risk for seizures distinguish between lateral neocortical and mesial temporal lobe epilepsy. *Epilepsia* 37(11):1088–1092, 1996.
147. Wyllie E, Naugle R, Awad I, et al: Intracarotid amobarbital procedure: I. Prediction of decreased modality-specific memory scores after temporal lobectomy. *Epilepsia* 32(6):857–864, 1991.
148. Loring DW, Meador KJ, Lee GP, et al: Wada memory asymmetries predict verbal memory decline after anterior temporal lobectomy. *Neurology* 45(7):1329–1333, 1995.
149. Kneebone AC, Chelune GJ, Dinner DS, et al: Intracarotid amobarbital procedure as a predictor of material-specific memory change after anterior temporal lobectomy. *Epilepsia* 36(9):857–865, 1995.
150. Jokeit H, Ebner A, Holthausen H, et al: Individual prediction of change in delayed recall of prose passages after left-sided anterior temporal lobectomy. *Neurology* 49(2):481–487, 1997.
151. Jack CR Jr, Sharbrough FW, Cascino GD, et al: Magnetic resonance image-based hippocampal volumetry: Correlation with outcome after temporal lobectomy. *Ann Neurol* 31(2):138–146, 1992.
152. Loring DW, Meador KJ, Lee GP, et al: Wada memory performance predicts seizure outcome following anterior temporal lobectomy. *Neurology* 44(12):2322–2324,1994.
153. Lancman ME, Benbadis S, Geller E, Morris HH: Sensitivity and specificity of asymmetric recall on WADA test to predict outcome after temporal lobectomy. *Neurology* 50(2):455–459, 1998.
154. Bouwer MS, Jones-Gotman M, Gotman J: Duration of sodium Amytal effect: Behavioral and EEG measures. *Epilepsia* 34(1):61–68, 1993.
155. Ferrier CH, Alarcon G, Glover A, et al: *N*-Acetylaspartate and creatine levels measured by (1)H MRS relate to recognition memory. *Neurology* 55(12):1874–1883, 2000.
156. Salanova V, Markand O, Worth R: Focal functional deficits in temporal lobe epilepsy on PET scans and the intracarotid amobarbital procedure: Comparison of patients with unitemporal epilepsy with those requiring intracranial recordings. *Epilepsia* 42(2):198–203, 2001.
157. Koutroumanidis M, Hennessy MJ, Seed PT, et al: Significance of interictal bilateral temporal hypometabolism in temporal lobe epilepsy. *Neurology* 54(9): 1811–1821, 2000.
158. Detre JA, Maccotta L, King D, et al: Functional MRI lateralization of memory in temporal lobe epilepsy. *Neurology* 50(4):926–932, 1998.
159. Bellgowan PS, Binder JR, Swanson SJ, et al: Side of seizure focus predicts left medial temporal lobe activation during verbal encoding. *Neurology* 51(2):479–484, 1998.
160. Killgore WD, Glosser G, Casasanto DJ, et al: Functional MRI and the Wada test provide complementary information for predicting post-operative seizure control. *Seizure* 8(8):450–455, 1999.
161. Corsi P: *Human Memory and the Medial Temporal Region of the Brain*. Montreal: McGill University, 1972.
162. Loring DW, Lee GP, Meador KJ, et al: Hippocampal contribution to verbal recent memory following dominant-hemisphere temporal lobectomy. *J Clin Exp Neuropsychol* 13(4):575–586, 1991.
163. Frisk V, Milner B: The role of the left hippocampal region in the acquisition and retention of story content. *Neuropsychologia* 28(4):349–359, 1990.
164. Wolf RL, Ivnik RJ, Hirschorn KA, et al: Neurocognitive efficiency following left temporal lobectomy: Standard versus limited resection. *J Neurosurg* 79(1):76–83, 1993.
165. Baxendale SA, Thompson PJ, Kitchen ND: Postoperative hippocampal remnant shrinkage and memory decline: A dynamic process. *Neurology* 55(2):243–249, 2000.
166. Nunn JA, Polkey CE, Morris RG: Selective spatial memory impairment after right unilateral temporal lobectomy. *Neuropsychologia* 36(9):837–848, 1998.
167. Nunn JA, Graydon FJ, Polkey CE, Morris RG: Differential spatial memory impairment after right temporal lobectomy demonstrated using temporal titration. *Brain* 122(Pt 1):47–59, 1999.
168. Wyler AR, Hermann BP, Somes G: Extent of medial temporal resection on outcome from anterior temporal lobectomy: A randomized prospective study. *Neurosurgery* 37(5):982–990, 1995.

Part 8

EMOTIONAL DISORDERS

Chapter 56

EMOTION AND THE BRAIN: AN OVERVIEW*

Kevin S. LaBar
Joseph E. LeDoux

The psychological and neuroscientific investigation of the nature of emotion has a long and varied history. While fundamental questions regarding the concept of emotion continue to be debated,[1] interest in emotion and the brain has reemerged in recent years. Significant progress has already been made in identifying brain regions involved in certain domains of emotional behavior, particularly fear. Most of this advance in knowledge has come from animal models of emotion, although extensions of this work into human populations have begun to be established. The purpose of this chapter is to provide an overview of research aimed at understanding the neural basis of emotion. We begin with a review of early pioneering studies linking emotion and the brain. We then present current conceptualizations of emotional information processing networks and propose directions for future research. Because of the vastness of this topic, certain aspects of emotional processing are not emphasized. Below, we focus on the neural systems mediating the acquisition and retention of fearful and defensive behaviors.

HISTORICAL PERSPECTIVE

William James[2] was among the late-nineteenth-century thinkers to postulate a specific relationship between brain-body function and emotional states. His feedback hypothesis stated that peripheral physiologic changes in the body determined emotional experience by their influence on sensory and motor areas in the neocortex. This view, shared to a large extent by Lange,[3] suggested that emotion can be differentiated on the basis of internal monitoring of autonomic and somatic changes and that a specialized brain network regulating emotion need not exist.

The James-Lange theory was soon challenged by physiologists examining autonomic function and brain localization of emotion. Studies in decorticate animals showed that transection of the cerebral cortex left intact mechanisms of emotional expression, particularly elicitation of "sham rage,"[4] but that midbrain transection eliminated integrated emotional reactions.[5,6] Thus, emotional expression appeared to be mediated by diencephalic structures, including the thalamus and hypothalamus, located below the cortex but above the midbrain.[7,8] In addition, the diffuse sympathetic arousal in the periphery seemed to be too undifferentiated to determine distinct emotional states.[9] According to the Cannon-Bard formulation, sensory input reaching the diencephalon simultaneously produced emotional expression by projections to peripheral organs and emotional experience by projections to the neocortex. In contrast to the James-Lange theory, this hypothesis suggested that structures specialized in emotional processing were present in the brain and that bodily feedback was not required to produce emotional feeling.

Papez[10] incorporated the notions of Cannon and Bard into an anatomic framework. His emotional circuit consisted of the hypothalamus, anterior thalamus, cingulate gyrus, and hippocampal formation. Papez viewed the cingulate gyrus as the cortical area for emotional experience, whereas the hypothalamus imbued incoming sensory signals with affective coloration. At the same time, Klüver and Bucy[11,12] reported a

* **ACKNOWLEDGMENT:** This work was supported in part by a Young Investigator Award from the National Alliance for Research on Schizophrenia and Depression and National Institute of Health grant DA14094.

behavioral deficit in monkeys with bilateral temporal lobe lesions. The syndrome consisted of an emotional tameness or hypoemotionality, increased oral tendencies, visual agnosia ("psychic blindness"), and altered feeding habits and sexual behavior. This constellation of behaviors indicated that the monkeys lacked the ability to evaluate the affective significance of objects in their environment, which Klüver and Bucy attributed to the destruction of the hippocampus, the medial temporal lobe component of Papez's model.

The Papez circuit was subsequently incorporated by MacLean[13,14] into an influential *limbic system* theory of emotion. MacLean expanded upon Papez's neuroanatomic model by incorporating such areas as the amygdala, orbitofrontal cortex, septum, and portions of the basal ganglia to form a "visceral brain" engaged in emotion and survival functions (see Fig. 56-1). The centerpiece of this conceptualization was the hippocampal formation, which was viewed as playing a key evaluative role in combining external stimuli and internal states into conscious emotional experience. According to this theory, the hippocampus, rather than the cingulate gyrus, was the cortical seat of emotional feeling.

CONTEMPORARY CHALLENGES TO THE LIMBIC SYSTEM CONCEPT

The limbic system concept was an important and persuasive development toward understanding the neural correlates of emotional processing. At the time of its development, very little was known about the anatomy and physiology of the structures contained within the limbic forebrain, and subsequent research on emotion was inspired and guided by this conceptual framework. Recently, however, the limbic system theory has been challenged on both anatomic[15,16] and functional[17,18] grounds. Anatomically, a consistent set of inclusion criteria for the classification of structures into this system has not been substantiated. In addition, it is now clear that some of the regions originally contained within this system primarily serve functions other than those related to emotion. In particular, the hippocampus, the cornerstone of the limbic system concept, has been primarily linked to cognitive functions, such as declarative memory,[19] spatial cognition,[20,21] and contextual/configural/relational processes.[22–24] Importantly, selective lesions of the amygdala, and not the hippocampus, produce the emotional disturbances

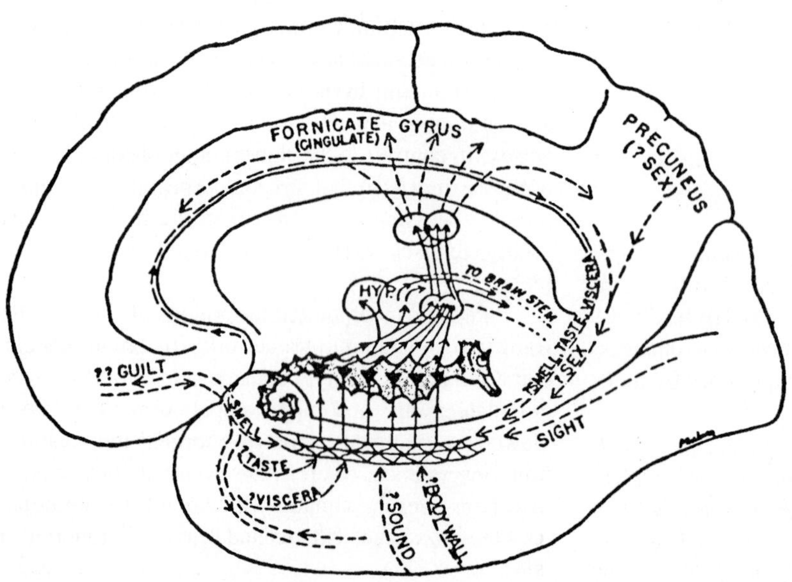

Figure 56-1
MacLean's visceral brain, the foundation of the limbic system theory of emotion. According to this theory, the hippocampus, or "seahorse," played a central role in emotional experience. (From MacLean,[13] with permission.)

constituting the Klüver-Bucy syndrome in monkeys.[25] Subsequent work has primarily implicated the amygdala in emotional processing.[26] Thus, the inclusion of the amygdala by MacLean may explain the longstanding survival of the limbic system concept as a model for emotional processing in the brain.

EMOTION AND BRAIN: A REFORMULATION

Recent advances in understanding brain function have been made by decomposing global behavioral constructs into subdomains. This approach has led to the discovery of parallel processing streams in vision[27] and multiple brain systems supporting memory.[28–30] We believe that this strategy holds great promise for identifying neural systems involved in emotion and that a renewed neuropsychological theory of emotion(s) can emerge from this line of inquiry. Insights gained from such brain studies should complement psychological investigations and may help constrain current debates, such as the influence of peripheral feedback on emotional states[31,32] and the relation between emotion and cognition.[33–37] Progress in this direction has already been made for some emotions, most notably fear. Next, we review the functional anatomy of fear as revealed by animal studies and consider the role of these brain regions in the generation of human fear and anxiety.

FEAR CONDITIONING: A MODEL SYSTEMS APPROACH

Background and Definitions

Threatening stimuli produce a variety of species-typical defensive responses, such as changes in autonomic activity (e.g., heart rate, arterial pressure, skin conductance, pupillary dilation), endocrine function ("stress"), behavioral reactions (cessation of movement, or "freezing"), reflex modulation (fear-potentiated startle), and pain sensitivity. This repertoire of fear reactivity is largely biologically innate; however, through learning, novel stimuli can come to control these responses through their association with threatening stimuli.[38] One way in which emotional learning can be achieved in the laboratory is through classical conditioning procedures.[39,40] In classical fear conditioning, an emotionally neutral stimulus, such as a tone, is presented in association with an aversive event, such as the presentation of a mild electric shock. The tone is called a conditioned stimulus (CS), and the shock is called an unconditioned stimulus (US). The US elicits a set of unconditioned defensive responses (URs); over several CS-US pairings, conditioned fear responses (CRs) develop in reaction to the CS itself.[44]

Through this experimental arrangement, fear conditioning paradigms provide a controlled method to investigate how emotional significance is attached to novel stimuli. The innocuous tone acquires aversive signaling properties through its predictive affiliation with the shock. As the animal learns the relationship between these stimuli, species-typical defensive responses come under the control of the CS. Conditioned fear responses develop very quickly (within one trial if the US is sufficiently intense[42]) and are long-lasting.[43] Because the sensory stimuli and motor/autonomic responses involved are relatively simple and stereotyped, it has been possible to pinpoint the central neural pathways mediating this type of emotional learning. More complex aspects of emotional processing have also been assessed within this model, such as the establishment and retention of emotional reactions to contextual cues[44–46] and control of emotional responses involving higher-order interactions of the CS-US contingency.[47,48] Finally, extinction of emotional learning has been examined by repeatedly presenting a CS without reinforcement after a CR has already been acquired.[49–52] A schematic depiction of the experimental parameters in a typical fear conditioning procedure is given in Fig. 56-2.

Animal Studies Reveal the Neural Circuitry

Using modern neuroanatomic, behavioral, and electrophysiologic recording techniques, researchers have begun to uncover the neural circuits involved in emotional learning and memory as measured by fear conditioning. Across many species and paradigms, the amygdala has emerged as a brain region critical for the learning of conditioned fear associations.[53–56] Pretraining lesions or reversible inactivation of the amygdala during

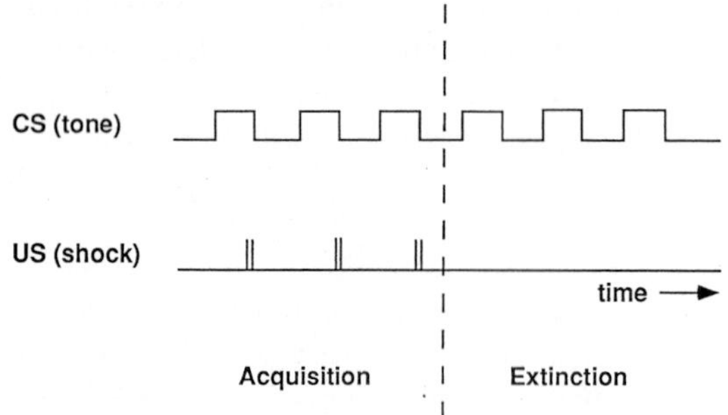

Figure 56-2
Schematic diagram of a typical fear conditioning experiment. CS = conditioned stimulus, US = unconditioned stimulus. During the acquisition phase, the CS (e.g., a tone) is presented several times in association with a noxious US (e.g., a mild electric shock). During the extinction phase, the CS is repeatedly presented alone.

training disrupts the development of CRs on a variety of fear indices, some of which are illustrated in Fig. 56-3.[57–61] The firing patterns of neuronal subpopulations within the basolateral amygdala and sensory neocortex change during conditioning,[62–67] implicating learning-induced plasticity within amygdalocortical circuits. A number of pharmacologic agents with anxiolytic properties used in the treatment of human anxiety disorders reduce conditioned fear in both humans[68,69] and animals.[70,71] Some of these drug effects have been localized to action sites within the amygdala.[70–72]

The fear conditioning pathways by which sensory information reaches the amygdala have been detailed, particularly in the auditory domain. Auditory CS transmission to the amygdala occurs by both a direct thalamoamygdala projection and an indirect thalamocorticoamygdala loop.[58,73] The direct route is faster than the indirect route, but it provides cruder information regarding stimulus features. The direct pathway may function to prime the amygdala to respond quickly to danger, leaving more intricate analysis of the incoming signal for the cortical pathway. This neurobiologic warning signal can grant organisms an evolutionary advantage by rapidly communicating the existence of potentially threatening environmental stimuli. Either of these transmission routes is sufficient to mediate conditioned fear to single auditory cues,[73] but the cortical pathway may be necessary to process more complex auditory associations.[74]

These parallel input pathways converge in the lateral nucleus of the amygdala, which serves as a sensory interface to the region.[58] Neurons in the lateral nucleus that respond to acoustic input are also sensitive to somatosensory stimulation.[75] The lateral nucleus thus functions as a site of CS-US integration, a place where emotional associations can be formed and directed to output pathways regulating emotional responses. Synaptic plasticity through the induction of long-term potentiation (LTP) has been observed in the thalamoamygdala, corticoamygdala, and hippocampoamygdala pathways.[76–84] LTP in the lateral amygdala is accompanied by concurrent enhancement of auditory evoked responses.[81] Fear conditioning and LTP produce similar changes in amygdalar processing of sensory cues and are sensitive to the same stimulus contingencies.[82,84] Synaptic transmission is also facilitated in amygdalar slices from animals that have been previously conditioned.[85] Although the relationship between LTP and memory processes remains tenuous,[86] these studies provide strong links between LTP mechanisms in the amygdala and behavioral indices of emotional learning.

Once incoming sensory information is processed by the lateral nucleus, it is relayed by intraamygdalar connections[87–89] to the central nucleus, the main output station of the amygdala. Target zones of central nucleus innervation in the brainstem and diencephalon are critical for the generation of emotional responses, although the efferent structures exert specialized control over particular facets of emotional expression. For example, central nucleus projections to the dorsal motor nucleus of the vagus nerve mediate parasympathetic responses[53]; projections to the lateral hypothalamus are implicated in sympathetic regulation[90,91]; projections to the central gray region are crucial for conditioned freezing responses and conditioned analgesia[54,91]; and projections to the pons are important for fear-potentiated startle.[55] Lesions to these efferent target sites disrupt the generation of individual conditioned emotional responses, leaving others intact.[91] However, ablation of the central nucleus itself produces global deficits in CR production regardless of response modality.[53–57] The central nucleus of the amygdala therefore serves to coordinate divergent emotional response output during aversive fear conditioning. This nucleus also directs

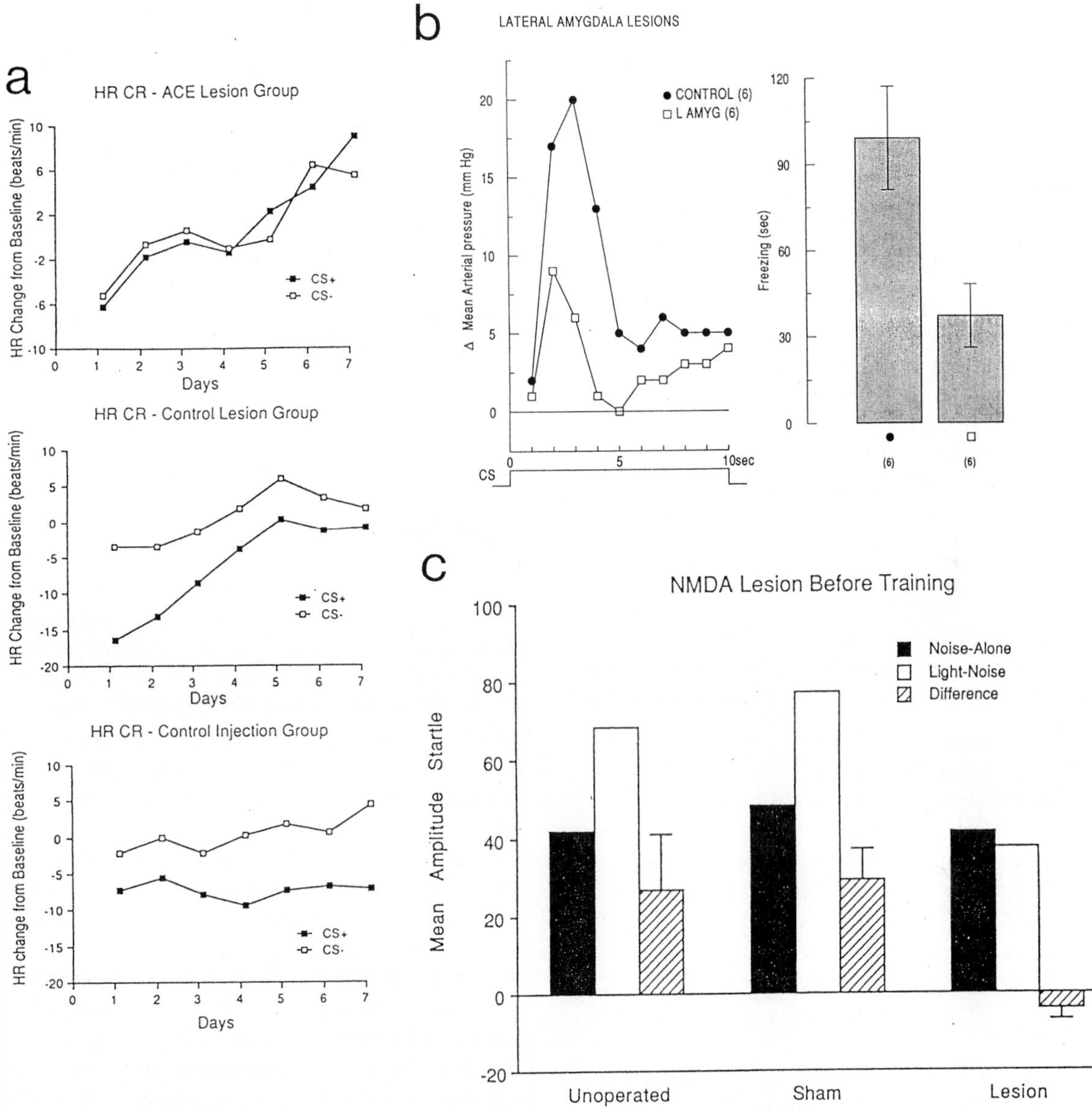

Figure 56-3

Some examples of the effects of amygdalar lesions on indices of conditioned fear. A. *Ibotenic acid lesions of the central nucleus (ACE) block differential heart rate conditioned responses (HR CR), measured as a difference in HR changes over baseline to one tone paired with a periorbital shock (CS+) and another tone presented alone (CS-). (From McCabe et al.,[59] with permission.)* B. *Electrolytic lesions of the lateral nucleus (L AMYG) disrupt both conditioned arterial pressure responses and conditioned freezing duration. (From LeDoux et al.,[91] with permission.)* C. *NMDA lesions of the lateral/basolateral nuclei block fear-potentiated startle, measured as a difference in startle amplitude evoked by the auditory startle stimulus presented alone and the startle stimulus presented in the presence of a visual conditioned stimulus. (From Sananes and Davis,[57] with permission.)*

attentional orienting systems during appetitive conditioning tasks.[92]

Contribution of Other Brain Structures

While it is clear that the amygdala plays a central role in the computation of emotional stimulus value, other brain regions make important contributions to the acquisition and retention of fear responses. For example, the integrity of the hippocampus is not essential for conditioning to simple phasic cues but is critical for conditioning to spatial contextual stimuli.[44–46,80] The effect of hippocampal lesions on the retention of contextual fear is shown in Fig. 56-4. These findings are consistent with cognitive theories regarding the role of the hippocampus in processing spatial and relational information.[20–24] (See Chaps. 37 and 38.) This contextual information may be important in allowing organisms to learn and remember the environmental subtexts in which threatening stimuli occur. The hippocampus may be exerting its influence via anatomic interactions with the amygdala.[93] These connections provide a neural passageway by which higher-order cognitive and mnemonic processes can trigger and shape emotional experience, and vice versa.

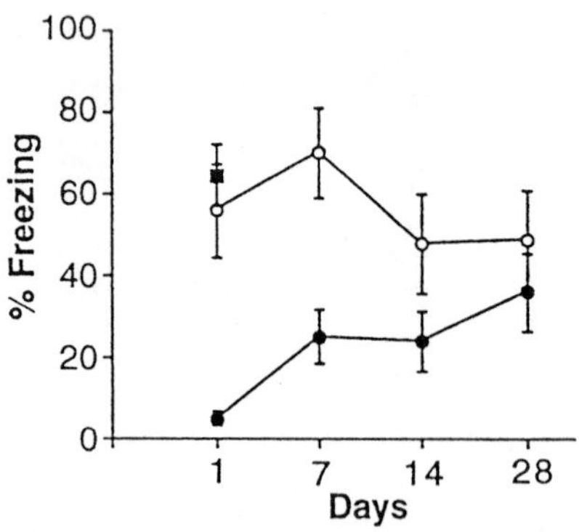

Figure 56-4
Effect of electrolytic hippocampal lesions on retention of contextual fear. Lesions were made either 1, 7, 14, or 28 days after training. The hippocampus has an important but time-limited role in conditioned fear memories elicited by contextual stimuli, as measured by the percentage of time spent freezing to the context following training. ○ = control; ● = hippocampal lesions; ■ = cortex lesions. (From Kim and Fanselow,[45] with permission.)

Lesions of the ventromedial prefrontal cortex selectively prolong the extinction or suppression of acquired fear responses after they are acquired.[49–52] These findings are the emotional equivalent of perseveration found in patients with frontal lobe damage (see Chaps. 32 and 33).[94,95] Extinction involves active brain processing[96] that is likely regulated by prefrontal-amygdalar projections.[97,98] The neural traces laid down in amygdala neurons during emotional learning are relatively indelible, and their suppression requires neocortical input.[99] If extended into human populations, these results may have relevance for understanding the neurobiology of affective disorders characterized by persistent, contextually inappropriate emotional responses.

Fear Conditioning in Humans

Figure 56-5 summarizes a current model of the neural circuitry involved in the emotional processing of conditioned fear. As this model becomes refined through animal studies, it is important to address whether these structures perform similar functions in humans. Human subjects do exhibit reliable conditioned fear responses,[100,101] although these responses may be influenced by certain personality characteristics[102,103] and cognitive processes.[104] Despite its success in animal research, fear conditioning has not been widely used in the neuropsychological assessment of human brain function. Recent studies have shown that neurologic patients with amygdalar damage are impaired at forming conditioned fear associations, as measured by skin conductance (Fig. 56-6).[105–108] The extent of impairment increases when the amygdala is compromised bilaterally, similar to that observed in rats.[109] Since the patients generate intact URs to eliciting stimuli, the deficits are not due to impaired autonomic function per se. This stands in contrast to patients with damage to the ventromedial prefrontal cortex, who show more general problems with autonomic response control.[110] Interestingly, the deficit is also unrelated to declarative knowledge of the CS-US contingency. Patients whose damage excludes the hippocampus bilaterally can state the proper relations among the stimuli even on discrimination tasks where more than one CS is used.[105–107] Declarative knowledge of the predictive relationship

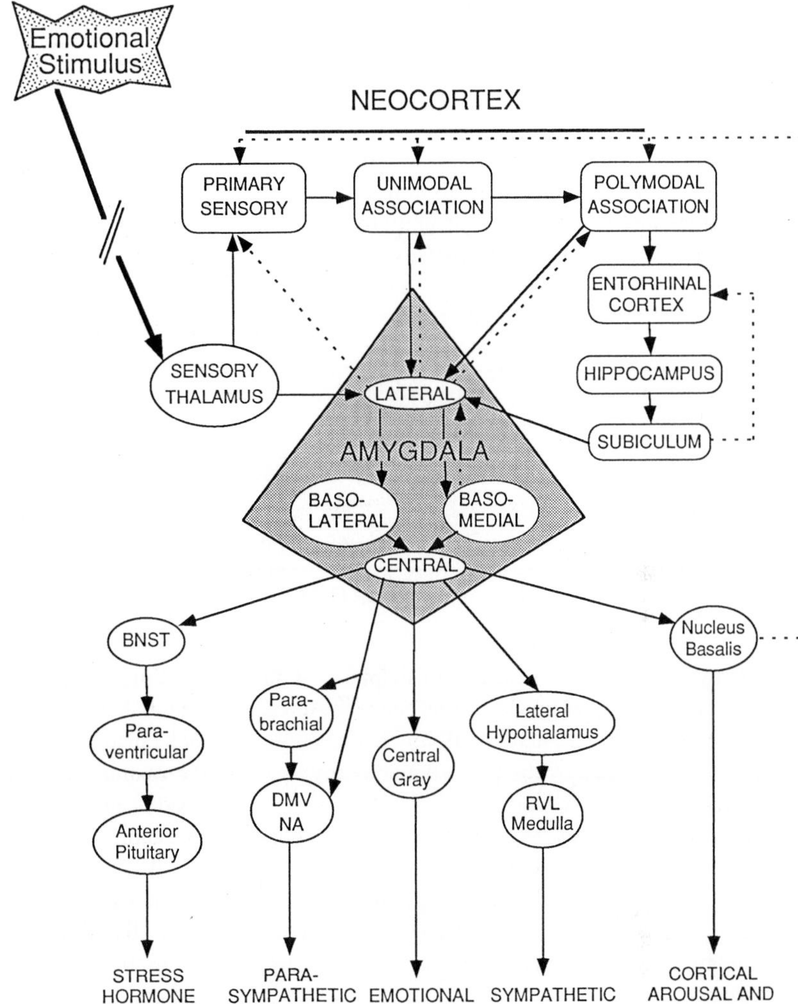

Figure 56-5
An emotional processing network based on studies of conditioned fear. Increasingly complex information transmitted by parallel afferent projections to the lateral nucleus of the amygdala is integrated and sent via intraamygdalar connections to the central nucleus of the amygdala, which functions to coordinate diverse effector systems to produce appropriate emotional responses. Feedforward projections are indicated by solid lines, while feedback projections are indicated by dashed lines. Additional outputs of the central nucleus are not shown. BNST = bed nucleus of the stria terminalis, DMV = dorsal motor nucleus of the vagus, NA = nucleus ambiguus, RVL medulla = rostral ventrolateral nuclei of the medulla.

between the CS and US is thus insufficient for generating conditioned fear.[111]

In contrast, amnesic patients without amygdalar damage show the opposite pattern. They acquire conditioned fear responses on simple tasks but fail to gain explicit knowledge regarding the stimulus contingencies.[105,111,112] These results demonstrate a double dissociation between the role of the amygdala and hippocampus relative to implicit and explicit memory during fear conditioning tasks. Amnesics who implicitly acquire conditioned fear, however, fail to recover their CRs when the fearfulness of the spatial context is reinstated after extinction.[112] Thus, as in other species, the hippocampus may relay information regarding the appropriateness of fear responses based on spatial contextual cues.[44–46,80]

The role of the amygdala in human fear conditioning has been confirmed in functional neuroimaging studies.[113–115] Amygdalar activation is found during the acquisition and extinction phases of fear conditioning, but the responses are maximal during the early stages of learning, when the CS-US contingencies are initially changed. Rapid signaling of changes in emotional significance is also characteristic of subpopulations of lateral amygdalar neurons in the rat.[66,67] Activation of the human amygdala is even

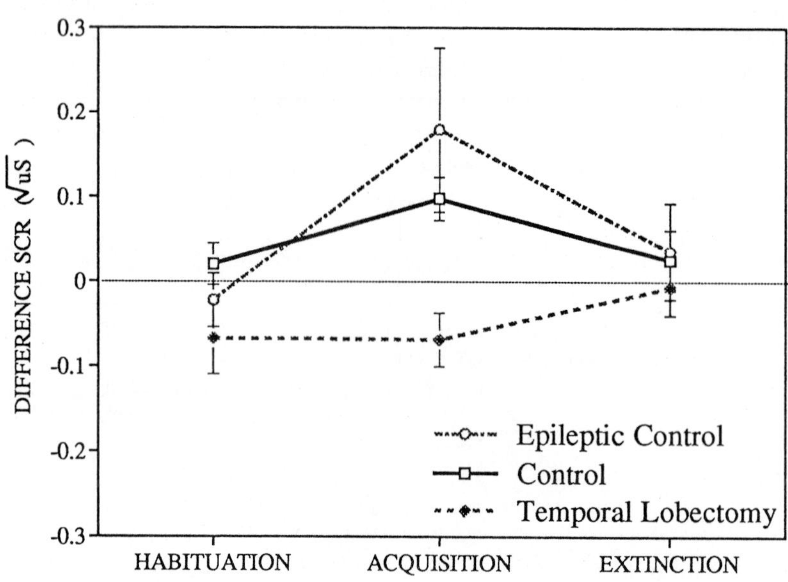

Figure 56-6
Impaired fear conditioning in human epileptic patients following medial temporal lobe resection, including the amygdala. Data from each experimental phase are collapsed across trials. Difference skin conductance responses (SCR) above zero reflect intact discrimination performance during the acquisition phase, with relatively greater conditioning to a tone paired with a loud noise unconditioned stimulus compared to another tone presented alone. μs = microsiemens. (From LaBar et al.,[106] with permission.)

elicited by subliminal (unconscious) displays of facial affect that were previously conditioned.[116] Across species, conditioning-related plasticity in the amygdala is partly mediated by the direct thalamoamygdala pathway.[66,67,117]

Fear conditioning paradigms have also been proposed as a model system for studying emotional processing in clinical populations with affective and traumatic memory disorders.[118,119] The clinical symptomatology of human anxiety shares many markers with measures of conditioned fear in animals.[55] In general, anxious patients show enhanced fear conditioning.[120,121] Schizophrenic patients tend to exhibit decreased fear conditioning,[122,123] although they must be divided into subgroups based on overall electrodermal reactivity.[124] Consistent with biologic preparedness theory,[125] fear conditioning with phobic CSs produces greater resistance to extinction than does conditioning with nonphobic stimuli.[126] Behavioral therapies based on conditioning principles have been largely successful in the treatment of phobias,[127] although remission is sometimes observed after systematic desensitization or counterconditioning. Spontaneous remission and renewal of fears are currently being studied as contextual effects in animal models of conditioning,[43] with important implications for work in clinical settings.[128] Finally, conditioning interpretations have been postulated to account for initial attack episodes in patients with panic disorder, although the maintenance of panic disorder once it has developed is guided by other factors.[129] Cognitive appraisal mechanisms, vicarious learning, and coping strategies are also crucial to the development and maintenance of other anxiety disorders.[130] Behavioral therapies for these disorders have evolved to incorporate contemporary theories of conditioning, instrumental learning, and cognition.[131]

TOWARD AN INTEGRATED VIEW OF THE EMOTIONAL BRAIN

Fear conditioning paradigms have influentially shaped our current understanding of how emotionally significant events are learned and remembered. As outlined above, the model systems approach is beginning to bridge the gap in emotion research aimed at various levels of nervous system organization, from molecular/genetic studies to behavioral/computational models and clinical applications. This is a major step toward the integration of disparate research domains across experimental techniques and species.

Other aspects of fear and anxiety are also mediated by this circuitry. For example, amygdala-lesioned patients have difficulty interpreting the degree of arousal associated with displays of facial affect, particularly fearful ones,[132] and fearful facial expressions elicit amygdalar activation in healthy subjects.[133,134] Gray[135] has proposed that the septohippocampal axis constitutes a behavioral inhibition system important for cognitive monitoring and coping strategies involved in anxiety and stress. This model shows how cognitive factors influence emotional networks and complements the investigation of the role of the hippocampus in more complex (contextual) aspects of conditioned fear. Ultimately, maladaptive evaluation of danger and safety signals leads to risky, inflexible decision making and inappropriate social interactions. These functions have been linked to the ventromedial prefrontal cortex,[110] extending its role from studies of conditioned fear extinction.

Thus, particular structures of the limbic forebrain differentially contribute to affective processing in ways that relate to their functions outside of the emotional domain. Another good example is the role of the insula in mediating disgust-related emotions. This brain region contains primary gustatory cortex and has been implicated in both taste aversion learning and evaluation of facial displays of disgust.[136,137] Of the structures comprising MacLean's limbic system hypothesis, the amygdala has been most consistently linked to the assessment of emotional salience, a function originally attributed to the hypothalamus by previous theorists (see "Historical Perspective," above). The amygdala's involvement in other emotions, including appetitive ones,[92,138–141] and other cognitive processes, such as memory consolidation,[142–144] remain to be detailed.

To conclude, the greatest advances in affective neuroscience to date have been made in discrete domains of emotional behavior tested through experimentally controlled and well-defined paradigms. As exemplified by the discussion of fear conditioning in the present chapter, such studies have yielded an emerging view of the emotional brain with much greater specificity than previously possible. Significant knowledge has been gained from animal models, but with the advent of more refined brain mapping techniques, human research will become increasingly informative in characterizing and localizing emotional functions. Future research should expand upon the breadth of existing behavioral paradigms to provide a more complete account of the range, complexity, and subtlety of emotional experience. Combining efforts across multiple levels of analysis and experimental preparations will provide the foundation for a more integrated view of emotional processing in the brain.

REFERENCES

1. Ekman P, Davidson RJ: *The Nature of Emotion.* New York: Oxford University Press, 1994.
2. James W: What is an emotion? *Mind* 9:188–205, 1884.
3. Lange CG: *Über Gemuthsbewegungen.* Leipzig: Thomas, 1887.
4. Cannon WB, Britton SW: Pseudoaffective medulloadrenal secretion. *Am J Physiol* 72:283–294, 1925.
5. Woodworth RS, Sherrington CS: A pseudoaffective reflex and its spinal path. *J Physiol (Lond)* 31:234–243, 1904.
6. Bazett HC, Penfield WG: A study of the Sherrington decerebrate animal in the chronic as well as the acute condition. *Brain* 45:185–265, 1922.
7. Cannon WB: The James-Lange theory of emotions: A critical examination and an alternative theory. *Am J Psychol* 39:106–124, 1927.
8. Bard P: A diencephalic mechanism for the expression of rage with special reference to the sympathetic nervous system. *Am J Physiol* 84:490–515, 1928.
9. Cannon WB: *Bodily Changes in Pain, Hunger, Fear, and Rage,* 2d ed. New York: Appleton, 1929.
10. Papez JW: A proposed mechanism of emotion. *Arch Neurol Psychiatry* 79:217–224, 1937.
11. Klüver H, Bucy PC: "Psychic blindness" and other symptoms following bilateral temporal lobectomy in rhesus monkeys. *Am J Physiol* 119:352–353, 1937.
12. Klüver H, Bucy PC: Preliminary analysis of functions of the temporal lobes in monkeys. *Arch Neurol Psychiatry* 42:979–1000, 1939.
13. MacLean PD: Psychosomatic disease and the visceral brain: Recent developments bearing on the Papez theory of emotion. *Psychosom Med* 11:338–353, 1949.
14. MacLean PD: Some psychiatric implications of physiological studies on frontotemporal portion of limbic system (visceral brain). *Electroencephalogr Clin Neurophysiol* 4:407–418, 1952.
15. Brodal A: *Neurological Anatomy.* New York: Oxford University Press, 1982.

16. Swanson LW: The hippocampus and the concept of the limbic system, in Seifert W (ed): *Neurobiology of the Hippocampus.* London: Academic Press, 1983, pp 3–19.
17. Kotter R, Meyer N: The limbic system: A review of its empirical foundation. *Behav Brain Res* 52:105–127, 1992.
18. LeDoux JE: Emotion and the limbic system concept. *Concepts Neurosci* 2:169–199, 1991.
19. Squire LR: Mechanisms of memory. *Science* 232:1612–1619, 1987.
20. O'Keefe J, Nadel L: *The Hippocampus as a Cognitive Map.* Oxford, England: Clarendon Press, 1978.
21. Nadel L: Hippocampus and space revisited. *Hippocampus* 1:221–229, 1991.
22. Hirsh R: The hippocampus and contextual retrieval of information from memory: A theory. *Behav Biol* 12:421–444, 1974.
23. Sutherland RJ, Rudy JW: Configural association theory: The role of the hippocampal formation in learning, memory, and amnesia. *Psychobiology* 17:129–144, 1989.
24. Wallenstein GV, Eichenbaum H, Hasselmo ME: The hippocampus as an associator of discontiguous events. *Trends Neurosci* 21:317–323, 1998.
25. Weiskrantz L: Behavioral changes associated with ablation of the amygdaloid complex in monkeys. *J Comp Physiol* 49:381–391, 1956.
26. LeDoux JE: Emotion and the amygdala, in Aggleton JP (ed): *The Amygdala: Neurobiological Aspects of Emotion, Memory, and Mental Dysfunction.* New York: Wiley-Liss, 1992, pp 339–352.
27. Ungerleider LG, Mishkin M: Two cortical visual systems, in Ingle DJ, Goodale MA, Mansfield RJW (eds): *Analysis of Visual Behavior.* Cambridge, MA: MIT Press, 1982.
28. Tulving E, Schacter DL: Priming and human memory systems. *Science* 247:301–306, 1990.
29. Weiskrantz L: Problems of learning and memory: One or multiple memory systems? *Phil Trans R Soc Lond B* 329:99–108, 1990.
30. Squire LR, Knowlton B, Musen G: The structure and organization of memory. *Annu Rev Psychol* 44:453–495, 1993.
31. Levenson RW: Emotion and the autonomic nervous system: A prospectus for research on autonomic specificity, in Wagner H (ed): *Social Psychophysiology and Emotion: Theory and Clinical Applications.* London: Wiley, 1988, pp 17–42.
32. Izard CE: *The Psychology of Emotions.* New York: Plenum Press, 1991.
33. Schacter S, Singer JE: Cognitive, social, and physiological determinants of emotional state. *Psychol Rev* 69:379–399, 1962.
34. Lazarus RS: On the primacy of cognition. *Am Psychol* 39:124–129, 1984.
35. Zajonc RB: On the primacy of affect. *Am Psychol* 39:117–123, 1984.
36. Leventhal H, Scherer K: The relationship of emotion to cognition: A functional approach to a semantic controversy. *Cogn Emot* 1:3–28, 1987.
37. LeDoux JE: Cognitive-emotional interactions in the brain. *Cogn Emot* 3:267–289, 1989.
38. Blanchard DC, Blanchard RJ: Innate and conditioned reactions to threat in rats with amygdaloid lesions. *J Comp Physiol Psychol* 81:281–290, 1972.
39. Pavlov IP: *Conditioned Reflexes.* New York: Dover, 1927.
40. Estes WK, Skinner BF: Some quantitative properties of anxiety. *J Exp Psychol* 29:390–400, 1941.
41. McAllister WR, McAllister DE: Behavioral measurement of conditioned fear, in Brush FR (ed): *Aversive Conditioning and Learning.* New York: Academic Press, 1971, pp 105–179.
42. Fanselow MS: Conditional and unconditional components of postshock freezing. *Pavlov J Biol Sci* 15:177–182, 1980.
43. Bouton ME: Context, ambiguity, and classical conditioning. *Curr Dir Psychol Sci* 3:49–53, 1994.
44. Selden NRW, Everitt BJ, Jarrads LE, Robbins TW: Complementary roles for the amygdala and hippocampus in aversive conditioning to cues and contextual cues. *Neuroscience* 42:335–350, 1991.
45. Kim JJ, Fanselow MS: Modality-specific retrograde amnesia of fear. *Science* 256:675–677, 1992.
46. Phillips RG, LeDoux JE: Differential contribution of amygdala and hippocampus to cued and contextual fear conditioning. *Behav Neurosci* 106:274–285, 1992.
47. Rickert EJ, Bennett TL, Lane PL, French J: Hippocampectomy and the attenuation of blocking. *Behav Biol* 22:147–160, 1978.
48. Kaye H, Pearce JM: Hippocampal lesions attenuate latent inhibition of a CS and of a neutral stimulus. *Psychobiology* 15:293–299, 1987.
49. Morgan MA, Romanski LM, LeDoux JE: Extinction of emotional learning: Contribution of medial prefrontal cortex. *Neurosci Lett* 163:109–113, 1993.
50. Morgan MA, LeDoux JE: Differential contribution of dorsal and ventral medial prefrontal cortex to the acquisition and extinction of conditioned fear in rats. *Behav Neurosci* 109:681–688, 1995.

51. Gewirtz MA, Falls WA, Davis M: Normal conditioned inhibition and extinction of freeing and fear-potentiated startle following electrolytic lesions of medial prefrontal cortex in rats. *Behav Neurosci* 111:712–726, 1997.
52. Quirk GJ, Russo GK, Barron JL, Lebron K: The role of ventromedial prefrontal cortex in the recovery of extinguished fear. *J Neurosci* 20:6225–6231, 2000.
53. Kapp BS, Whalen PJ, Supple WF, Pascoe JP: Amygdaloid contributions to conditioned arousal and sensory information processing, in Aggleton JP (ed): *The Amygdala: Neurobiological Aspects of Emotion, Memory, and Mental Dysfunction.* New York: Wiley-Liss, 1992, pp 229–254.
54. Fendt M, Fanselow MS: The neuroanatomical and neurochemical basis of conditioned fear. *Neurosci Biobehav Rev* 23:743–760, 1999.
55. Davis M: The role of the amydgala in conditioned and unconditioned fear and anxiety, in Aggleton JP (ed): *The Amygdala: A Functional Analysis,* 2d ed. New York: Oxford University Press, 2000, pp 213–288.
56. LeDoux JE: Emotion circuits in the brain. *Annu Rev Neurosci* 23:155–184, 2000.
57. Sananes CB, Davis M: *N*-Methyl-D-aspartate lesions of the lateral and basolateral nuclei of the amygdala block fear-potentiated startle and shock sensitization of startle. *Behav Neurosci* 106:72–80, 1992.
58. LeDoux JE, Cicchetti P, Xagoraris A, Romanski LM: The lateral amygdaloid nucleus: Sensory interface of the amygdala in fear conditioning. *J Neurosci* 10:1062–1069, 1990.
59. McCabe PW, Gentile CG, Markgraf CG, et al: Ibotenic acid lesions in the amygdaloid central nucleus but not in the lateral subthalamic area prevent the acquisition of differential Pavlovian conditioning of bradycardia in rabbits. *Brain Res* 580:155–163, 1992.
60. Helmstetter FJ, Bellgowan PS: Effects of muscimol applied to the basolateral amygdala on acquisition and expression of contextual fear conditioning in rats. *Behav Neurosci* 108:1005–1009, 1994.
61. Muller J, Corodimas KP, Fridel Z, LeDoux JE: Functional inactivation of the lateral and basal nuclei of the amygdala by muscimol infusion prevents fear conditioning to an explicit CS and to contextual stimuli. *Behav Neurosci* 111:683–691, 1997.
62. Applegate CD, Frysinger RC, Kapp BS, Gallagher M: Multiple unit activity recorded from amygdala central nucleus during Pavlovian heart rate conditioning in the rabbit. *Brain Res* 238:457–462, 1982.
63. Pascoe JP, Kapp BS: Electrophysiological characteristics of amygdaloid central nucleus neurons during Pavlovian fear conditioning in the rabbit. *Behav Brain Res* 16:117–133, 1985.
64. Cruikshank SJ, Weinberger NM: Receptive-field plasticity in the adult auditory cortex induced by Hebbian covariance. *J Neurosci* 16:861–875, 1996.
65. Quirk GJ, Repa JC, LeDoux JE: Fear conditioning enhances short-latency auditory responses of lateral amygdala neurons: Parallel recordings in the freely behaving rat. *Neuron* 15:1029–1039, 1995.
66. Quirk GJ, Armony JL, LeDoux JE: Fear conditioning enhances different temporal components of tone-evoked spike trains in auditory cortex and lateral amygdala. *Neuron* 19:613–624, 1997.
67. Repa JC, Muller J, Apergis J, et al: Two different lateral amygdala cell populations contribute to the initiation and storage of memory. *Nat Neurosci* 4:724–731, 2001.
68. Molander L: Effect of melperone, chlorpromazine, haloperidol, and diazepam on experimental anxiety in normal subjects. *Psychopharmacology* 77:109–113, 1982.
69. Hensman R, Guimarães FS, Wang M, Deakin JFW: Effects of ritanserin on aversive classical conditioning in humans. *Psychopharmacology* 104:220–224, 1991.
70. Fanselow MS, Helmstetter FJ: Conditional analgesia, defensive freezing, and benzodiazepines. *Behav Neurosci* 102:233–243, 1988.
71. Davis M: Pharmacological and anatomical analysis of fear conditioning. *NIDA Res Monogr* 97:126–162, 1990.
72. Gallagher M, Kapp BS, McNall CL, Pascoe JP: Opiate effects in the amygdala central nucleus on heart rate conditioning in rabbits. *Pharmacol Biochem Behav* 14:497–505, 1981.
73. Romanski LM, LeDoux JE: Equipotentiality of thalamo-amygdala and thalamo-cortico-amygdala projections as auditory conditioned stimulus pathways. *J Neurosci* 12:4501–4509, 1992.
74. Jarrell TW, Gentile CG, Romanski LM, et al: Involvement of cortical and thalamic auditory regions in retention of differential bradycardia conditioning to acoustic conditioned stimuli in rabbits. *Brain Res* 412:285–294, 1987.
75. Romanski LM, Clugnet MC, Bordi F, LeDoux JE: Somatosensory and auditory convergence in the lateral nucleus of the amygdala. *Behav Neurosci* 107:444–450, 1993.
76. Chapman PF, Kairiss EW, Keenan CL, Brown TH: Long-term synaptic potentiation in the amygdala. *Synapse* 6:271–278, 1990.
77. Clugnet MC, LeDoux JE: Synaptic plasticity in fear conditioning circuits: Induction of LTP in the lateral

nucleus of the amygdala by stimulation of the medial geniculate body. *J Neurosci* 10:2818–2824, 1990.

78. Chapman PF, Bellevance LL: NMDA receptor-independent LTP in the amygdala. *Synapse* 11:310–318, 1992.
79. Gean P-W, Chang F-C, Hung C-R: Use-dependent modification of a slow NMDA receptor-mediated synaptic potential in rat amygdalar slices. *J Neurosci Res* 34:635–641, 1993.
80. Maren S, Fanselow MS: Synaptic plasticity in the basolateral amygdala induced by hippocampal formation stimulation in vivo. *J Neurosci* 15:7548–7564, 1995.
81. Rogan MT, LeDoux JE: LTP is accompanied by commensurate enhancement of auditory-evoked responses in a fear conditioning circuit. *Neuron* 15:1–20, 1995.
82. Rogan MT, Staubli U, LeDoux JE: Fear conditioning induces associative long-term potentiation in the amygdala. *Nature* 390:604–607, 1997.
83. Huang YY, Kandel ER: Postsynaptic induction and PKA-dependent expression of LTP in the lateral amygdala. *Neuron* 21:169–178, 1998.
84. Bauer EP, LeDoux JE, Nader K: Fear conditioning and LTP in the lateral amygdala are sensitive to the same stimulus contingencies. *Nat Neurosci* 4:687–688, 2001.
85. McKernan MG, Shinnick-Gallagher P: Fear conditioning induces a lasting potentiation of synaptic currents in vitro. *Nature* 390:607–611, 1997.
86. Martin SJ, Grimwood PD, Morris RGM: Synaptic plasticity and memory: An evaluation of the hypothesis. *Annu Rev Neurosci* 23:649–711, 2000.
87. McDonald AJ: Cell types and intrinsic connections of the amygdala, in Aggelton JP (ed): *The Amygdala: Neurobiological Aspects of Emotion, Memory, and Mental Dysfunction.* New York: Wiley-Liss, 1992, pp 67–96.
88. Pare D, Smith Y, Pare JF: Intra-amygdaloid projections of the basolateral and basomedial nuclei in the cat: *Phaseolus vulgaris*–leucoagglutinin anterograde tracing at the light and electron microscopic level. *Neuroscience* 69:567–583, 1995.
89. Pitkänen A, Stefanacci L, Farb CR, et al: Intrinsic connections of the rat amygdaloid complex: Projections originating in the lateral nucleus. *J Comp Neurol* 356:288–310, 1995.
90. Smith OA, Astley CA, Devito JL, et al: Functional analysis of hypothalamic control of the cardiovascular responses accompanying emotional behavior. *Fed Proc* 39:2487–2494, 1980.
91. LeDoux JE, Iwata J, Cicchetti P, Reis DJ: Different projections of the central amygdaloid nucleus mediate autonomic and behavioral correlates of conditioned fear. *J Neurosci* 8:2517–2529, 1988.
92. Gallagher M, Holland PC: The amygdala complex: Multiple roles in associative learning and attention. *Proc Natl Acad Sci USA* 91:11771–11776, 1994.
93. Canteras NS, Swanson LW: Projections of the ventral subiculum to the amygdala, septum, and hypothalamus: a PHAL anterograde tract-tracing study in the rat. *J Comp Neurol* 324:180–194, 1992.
94. Janowsky JS, Shimamura AP, Kritchevsky M, Squire LR: Cognitive impairment following frontal lobe damage and its relevance to human amnesia. *Behav Neurosci* 103:548–560, 1989.
95. Freedman M, Black S, Ebert P, Binns M: Orbitofrontal function, object alternation and perseveration. *Cereb Cortex* 8:18–27, 1998.
96. Falls WA, Miserendino MJD, Davis M: Extinction of fear-potentiated startle: Blockade by infusion of an NMDA antagonist into the amygdala. *J Neurosci* 12:854–863, 1992.
97. Amaral DG, Price JL, Pitkänen A, Carmichael ST: Anatomical organization of the primate amygdaloid complex, in Aggleton JP (ed): *The Amygdala: Neurobiological Aspects of Emotion, Memory, and Mental Dysfunction.* New York: Wiley-Liss, 1992, pp 1–66.
98. Garcia R, Vouimba R-M, Baudry M, Thompson RF: The amygdala modulates prefrontal cortex activity relative to conditioned fear. *Nature* 402:294–296, 1999.
99. LeDoux JE, Romanski LM, Xagoraris AE: Indelibility of subcortical emotional memories. *J Cogn Neurosci* 1:238–243, 1989.
100. Grillon C, Ameli R, Woods SW, et al: Fear-potentiated startle in humans: Effects of anticipatory anxiety on the acoustic blink reflex. *Psychophysiology* 28:588–595, 1991.
101. Fredrickson M, Annas P, Georgiades A, et al: Internal consistency and temporal stability of classically conditioned skin conductance responses. *Biol Psychol* 35:153–163, 1993.
102. Eysenck HJ: The conditioning model of neurosis. *Behav Brain Sci* 2:155–199, 1979.
103. Guimarães FS, Hellewell J, Hensman R, et al: Characterization of a psychophysiological model of classical fear conditioning in healthy volunteers: Influence of gender, instruction, personality and placebo. *Psychopharmacology* 104:231–236, 1990.
104. Davey G (ed): *Cognitive Processes and Pavlovian Conditioning in Humans.* Chichester, England: Wiley, 1987.
105. Bechara A, Tranel D, Damasio H, et al: Double dissociation of conditioning and declarative knowledge relative to the amygdala and hippocampus in humans. *Science* 269:1115–1118, 1995.

106. LaBar KS, LeDoux JE, Spencer DD, Phelps EA: Impaired fear conditioning following unilateral temporal lobectomy in humans. *J Neurosci* 15:6846–6855, 1995.
107. Phelps EA, LaBar KS, Anderson AK, et al: Specifying the contribution of the human amygdala to emotional memory: A case study. *Neurocase* 4:527–540, 1998.
108. Bechara A, Damasio H, Damasio AR, Lee GP: Different contributions of the human amygdala and ventromedial prefrontal cortex to decision-making. *J Neurosci* 19:5473–5481, 1999.
109. LaBar KS, LeDoux JE: Partial disruption of fear conditioning in rats with unilateral amygdala damage: Correspondence with unilateral temporal lobectomy in humans. *J Neurosci* 15:6846–6855, 1996.
110. Tranel D, Bechara A, Damasio AR: Decision making and the somatic marker hypothesis, in Gazzaniga MS (ed): *The New Cognitive Neurosciences.* Cambridge, MA: MIT Press, 2000, pp 1047–1064.
111. LaBar KS, Disterhoft JF: Conditioning, awareness, and the hippocampus. *Hippocampus* 8:620–626, 1996.
112. O'Connor KJ, LaBar KS, Phelps EA: Impaired contextual fear conditioning in amnesics. *J Cogn Neurosci* 11 (Suppl S):19, 1999.
113. Büchel C, Morris J, Dolan RJ, Friston KJ: Brain systems mediating aversive conditioning: An event-related fMRI study. *Neuron* 20:947–957, 1998.
114. LaBar KS, Gatenby JC, Gore JC, et al: Human amygdala activation during conditioned fear acquisition and extinction: A mixed-trial fMRI study. *Neuron* 20:937–945, 1998.
115. Büchel C, Dolan RJ, Armony JL: Amygdala-hippocampal involvement in human trace fear conditioning: An event-related functional magnetic resonance imaging study. *J Neurosci* 19:10869–10876, 1999.
116. Morris JS, Öhman A, Dolan RJ: Conscious and unconscious emotional learning in the human amygdala. *Nature* 393:467–470, 1998.
117. Morris JS, Öhman A, Dolan RJ: A subcortical pathway to the right amygdala mediating "unseen" fear. *Proc Natl Acad Sci USA* 96:1680–1685, 1999.
118. Öhman A: Fear-relevance, autonomic conditioning, and phobias: A laboratory model. In Sjöden PO, Bates S, Dockens WS (eds): *Trends in Behavior Therapy.* New York: Academic Press, 1979, pp 107–133.
119. Charney DS, Deutch AY, Krystal JH, et al: Psychobiologic mechanisms of posttraumatic stress disorder. *Arch Gen Psychiatry* 50:294–305, 1993.
120. Ashcroft K, Guimarães FS, Wang M, Deakin JFW: Evaluation of a psychophysiological model of classical fear conditioning in anxious patients. *Psychopharmacology* 104:215–219, 1991.
121. Pitman RK, Orr SP: Test of the conditioning model of neurosis: Differential aversive conditioning of angry and neutral facial expressions in anxiety disorder patients. *J Abnorm Psychol* 95:208–213, 1986.
122. Ax AF, Banford JL, Beckett PGS, et al: Autonomic conditioning in chronic schizophrenia. *J Abnorm Psychol* 76:140–154, 1970.
123. Gorham IC, Novelly RA, Ax A, Frohman CE: Classically conditioned autonomic discrimination and tryptophan uptake in chronic schizophrenia. *Psychophysiology* 15:158–164, 1978.
124. Öhman A: Electrodermal activity and vulnerability to schizophrenia: A review. *Biol Psychol* 12:87–145, 1981.
125. Seligman MEP: Phobias and preparedness. *Behav Ther* 2:307–320, 1971.
126. Marks I, Tobena A: Learning and unlearning fear: A clinical and evolutionary perspective. *Neurosci Biobehav Rev* 14:365–384, 1989.
127. Masters JC, Burish TG, Hollon SD, Rimm DC: *Behavior Therapy: Techniques and Empirical Findings,* 3d ed. New York: Harcourt Brace Jovanovich, 1987.
128. Bouton ME, Schwartzentruber D: Sources of relapse after extinction in Pavlovian and instrumental learning. *Clin Psychol Rev* 11:123–140, 1991.
129. Wolpe J, Rowan VC: Panic disorder: A product of classical conditioning. *Behav Res Ther* 26:441–450, 1988.
130. Carr AT: The psychopathology of fear, in Sluckin W (ed): *Fear in Animals and Man.* New York: Van Nostrand Reinhold, 1979, pp 199–235.
131. Thorpe GL, Olson SL: *Behavior Therapy: Concepts, Procedures, and Applications.* Boston: Allyn & Bacon, 1990.
132. Adolphs R, Tranel D, Hamann S, et al: Recognition of facial emotion in nine individuals with bilateral amygdala damage. *Neuropsychologia* 37:1111–1117, 1999.
133. Breiter HC, Etcoff NL, Whalen PJ, et al: Response and habituation of the human amygdala during visual processing of facial expression. *Neuron* 17:875–887, 1996.
134. Morris JS, Frith CD, Perrett DI, et al: A differential neural response in the human amygdala to fearful and happy facial expressions. *Nature* 383:812–815, 1996.
135. Gray JA: *The Psychology of Fear and Stress,* 2d ed. Cambridge, England: Cambridge University Press, 1987.
136. Yamamoto T, Shimura T, Sako N, et al: Neural substrates for conditioned taste aversion in the rat. *Behav Brain Res* 65:123–137, 1994.
137. Phillips ML, Young AW, Scott AJ, et al: Neural responses to facial and vocal expressions of fear and disgust. *Proc R Soc Lond B* 83:1809–1817, 1998.

138. Hamann SB, Ely TD, Grafton ST, Kilts CS: Amygdala activity related to enhanced memory for pleasant and unpleasant stimuli. *Nat Neurosci* 2:289–293, 1999.
139. Johnsrude IS, Owen AM, White NM, et al: Impaired preference conditioning after anterior temporal lobe resection in humans. *J Neurosci* 20:2649–2656, 2000.
140. LaBar KS, Gitelman DR, Parrish TB, et al: Hunger selectively modulates corticolimbic activation to food stimuli in humans. *Behav Neurosci* 115:293–500.
141. Easton A, Gaffan D: Amygdala and the memory of reward: The importance of fibres of passage from the basal forebrain, in Aggleton JP (ed): *The Amygdala: A Functional Analysis,* 2d ed. New York: Oxford University Press, 2000, pp 569–586.
142. Cahill L, McGaugh JL: Mechanisms of emotional arousal and lasting declarative memory. *Trends Neurosci* 21:294–298, 1998.
143. LaBar KS, Phelps EA: Arousal-mediated memory consolidation: Role of the medial temporal lobe. *Psychol Sci* 9:527–540, 1998.
144. Nader K, Schafe GE, LeDoux JE: The labile nature of consolidation theory. *Nat Rev Neurosci* 1:216–219, 2000.

Chapter 57

EMOTIONAL DISORDERS IN RELATION TO UNILATERAL BRAIN DAMAGE

Guido Gainotti

The hypothesis of hemispheric specialization for emotions and affect is a recent one in the history of neuropsychology. This hypothesis was advanced only 40 years ago, a century after the discovery of left hemispheric dominance for language,[1,2] on the basis of clinical observations independently made during pharmacologic inactivation of the right and left hemispheres[3–5] and during observation of the emotional behavior of unilaterally brain-damaged patients.[6,7] The interest of these early clinical studies does not reside only in the fact that they called the attention of neuropsychologists to a problem that had been previously substantially neglected. It also stems from the fact that the theoretical models proposed by those who made these clinical observations later served to orient most of the experimental studies devised to clarify the links between emotions and hemispheric specialization.

THE FIRST CLINICAL STUDIES AND THE CORRESPONDING THEORETICAL MODELS

Those who observed the emotional behavior of patients submitted to the Wada test found that a "depressive-catastrophic" reaction is often noted after the injection of sodium Amytal into the left carotid artery, whereas a "euphoric-maniacal" reaction is observed after pharmacologic inactivation of the right hemisphere. Taking implicitly as a reference point the biological model of the bipolar maniac-depressive psychosis, these authors considered the depressive-catastrophic reaction to be a form of endogenous depression, resulting from inactivation of a "center for positive emotions" located in the left hemisphere. Analogously, they considered the euphoric-maniacal reaction to be a hypomanic state resulting from inactivation of a "center for negative emotions" located in the right hemisphere.

The clinical observations made by Gainotti[6,7] while studying the emotional behavior of right- and left-brain-damaged patients were at first similar to those made by previous authors during the Wada test. Patients with left brain damage typically showed a "catastrophic reaction" (i.e., increasing signs of anxiety and/or sudden bursts of tears) in the face of their difficulties of verbal communication, whereas those with right brain damage showed a strange "indifference reaction" toward failures and disabilities. However, clinical considerations concerning the typical context of catastrophic reactions and the qualitative features of indifference reactions led Gainotti[7–10] to reject the interpretation linking the former to an endogenous depression and the latter to a manic state. Gainotti noticed that catastrophic reactions were usually triggered by frustrating, repeated attempts at verbal expression. He therefore suggested that catastrophic reactions should be considered a dramatic but psychologically appropriate form of reaction to a catastrophic event rather than a biologically based form of depression. He also noticed that, from the qualitative point of view, the indifference reactions of right-brain-damaged patients did not show the features of excitement and euphoric mood typical of a manic state but rather consisted of a heterogeneous and rather paradoxical set of emotional abnormalities. A first set of features, which could properly be grouped under the heading of *indifference,* included overt expressions of unawareness or of minimization of the disease, an obvious lack of concern for the disability, and an attitude of indifference toward failures met during the neuropsychological examination. A second pattern of behavior, which could be labeled *verbal disinhibition,* consisted of a tendency to joke in a fatuous, ironic, or sarcastic manner, which sometimes gave an impression of childish euphoria but at other times that of black humor. A last set of behavioral patterns seemed to suggest an implicit attitude of denial of illness and of rejection of the paralyzed limbs. This set included delusions about the paralyzed limbs (somatoparaphrenia), which were felt as unattached to the patient's body and were attributed to someone else[11,12]; confabulations of denial,[13] consisting of a marked tendency to tell stories that, although not explicitly concerning the paralyzed limbs, were clearly inconsistent with the patient's disease; and expressions of hatred toward the paralyzed limbs (misoplegia), usually couched in grotesque, exaggerated, or sarcastic language[14] (see also Chaps. 29 and 30). All these patterns of behavior are reported here in some detail because they are surprising and paradoxical and represent the emotional disturbances more frequently observed in patients with right brain damage. Gainotti noticed that they are, in any case, much more abnormal and less psychologically appropriate than the catastrophic reactions of left-brain-damaged patients. He therefore proposed that the difference between the emotional behavior of left- and right-brain-damaged patients could be better explained by the contrast between "appropriate" and "inappropriate" forms of emotional reaction than by the opposition between depression and euphoria. According to this interpretation, the right hemisphere might play a critical role in emotions and affects. When this hemisphere is intact (as in left-brain-damaged patients), the emotional reaction may be dramatic but psychologically appropriate. When, on the contrary, the lesion impinges upon right hemispheric structures crucially involved in emotional behavior, a composite set of abnormal emotional responses (grouped for the sake of simplicity under the heading of *indifference reactions*) would usually ensue.

COMPREHENSION AND EXPRESSION OF EMOTIONS IN RIGHT- AND LEFT-BRAIN-DAMAGED PATIENTS

Since the exact nature of the emotional modifications observed after right and left brain injury remained controversial, a large series of investigations were undertaken to clarify this issue by means of experiments with both normal subjects and patients with unilateral hemispheric damage. Although these investigations have explored various aspects of emotional behavior, the attention of neuropsychologists has been focused mainly on the most cognitive components of emotions, namely the comprehension of emotional stimuli and the (facial or vocal) expression of emotions. This was partly due to the assumption that the type of information processing typical of the right hemisphere (and characterized by a syncretic and holistic rather than by a sequential and analytic style) may be particularly suited to the treatment of emotional information.[15] Since a critical review of investigations conducted in normal subjects obviously exceeds the scopes of this chapter, it will be limited to giving some details about studies conducted on patients with unilateral brain injury and to summarizing results of research conducted on normal subjects.

The methodology of investigations conducted on patients with focal brain injury has consisted of matching the capacity of right- and left-brain-damaged patients to comprehend and/or express emotions at the facial level or through the tone of voice. Following this research strategy, several authors have shown that right-brain-damaged patients are consistently impaired in recognizing emotions expressed through tone of voice,[16–21] in the identification of facial emotional expressions,[19,22–25] and in the ability to express emotions through facial movements[25–27] or with the prosodic contours of speech.[17,19,28,29] On the other hand, investigations conducted on normal subjects have allowed a better control of the hypothesis assuming a different specialization of the right and left hemispheres for negative and positive emotions, respectively. Even if some studies have supported the hypothesis of an interaction between hemisphere and positive or negative emotional valence, most have failed to confirm it (see Refs. 9, 10, and 30 to 32 for surveys). On the contrary, the great majority of these investigations have substantially confirmed the hypothesis of a general superiority of the right hemisphere for functions of emotional comprehension and expression.

This fact has led some authors to hypothesize that right hemispheric dominance for emotions may mainly concern the communicative aspects of emotional behavior rather than other, more basic components of emotions. This line of thought has been developed in particular by Ross (Refs. 18, 28, and Chap. 59 in this volume), who has suggested that disorders of nonverbal communication might be the primary defect of right-brain-damaged patients and that emotional disturbances usually observed in these patients may simply be a consequence of their basic inability to comprehend and express emotions. According to this viewpoint, the indifference reaction of right-brain-damaged patients should not be considered as an inappropriate form of emotional behavior but simply the consequence of a basic inability to correctly evaluate emotional signals and to express an otherwise intact emotional experience. Three main objections can be addressed to this interpretation of the indifference reaction of right-brain-damaged patients. The first refers to the heterogeneity of the patterns of behavior grouped under the general heading of *indifference reaction.* As we have seen in discussing the clinical aspects of the emotional behavior of right- and left-brain-damaged patients, different behavioral patterns are grouped under this heading. Some of them, namely those considered as indifference proper, could more easily be interpreted as a consequence of a reduced ability to communicate an otherwise intact emotional experience. Other behavioral patterns, however—namely, those considered as manifestations of a verbal disinhibition and, even more, those suggesting an attitude of denial of the disability and of rejection of the paralyzed limbs—are inconsistent with this interpretation and point to a deeper emotional disorder. The second objection refers to the fact that several investigations have failed to confirm a significant difference between right- and left-brain-damaged patients in the capacity to express and comprehend emotional signals. Thus, in research conducted at the expressive level, no difference has been found between right- and left-brain-damaged patients in the facial expressions elicited by positive, neutral, and strongly negative emotional movies[33]; in the ability to produce posed rather than spontaneous facial emotional expressions[34,35]; or in the capacity to express emotions through emotional contours of speech.[36,37]

Analogously, in studies conducted at the receptive level, no difference between right- and left-brain-damaged patients has been found on tasks requiring the identification of facial emotional expressions[10,38–40] or the recognition of the emotion expressed through the prosodic components of speech.[36,37] All these data suggest that right hemispheric dominance for functions of emotional communication has probably been overemphasized in previous studies and that the emotional indifference of right-brain-damaged patients cannot simply be considered the consequence of a defect of emotional communication.

AUTONOMIC COMPONENTS AND EXPERIENCE OF EMOTIONS IN PATIENTS WITH RIGHT HEMISPHERIC DAMAGE

The third objection that can be raised to the hypothesis considering as apparent the emotional indifference of right-brain-damaged patients consists in the fact that this hypothesis is at variance with results obtained in studies that have investigated the autonomic components of emotions in right- and left-brain-damaged patients. As a matter of fact, if one accepts that the autonomic components of emotion play an important role in the generation (or, in any case, in determining the intensity and duration) of the emotional experience,[41–43] then these components of emotions should be intact in right-brain-damaged patients if their apparent indifference is basically due to an inability to express an otherwise intact emotional experience. This prediction, however, is at variance with results of investigations that have studied the electrodermal responses (or other indices of autonomic activation) in right- and left-brain-damaged patients submitted to presentation of emotional stimuli. Thus several authors have observed in right- but not in left-brain-damaged patients a flattened galvanic skin response to painful stimuli applied to the hand ipsilateral to the damaged hemisphere,[44] to emotion-provoking slides,[45–47] and to emotionally arousing movies.[48,49] Other authors have observed that right-brain-damaged patients fail to show the normal cardiac deceleration not only in response to emotional stimuli[48,49] but also during a nonemotional attention-demanding task.[50] This observation has suggested that the right hemisphere might play a critical role in vegetative functions and that this hemispheric asymmetry might express itself in emotional and nonemotional activities that require the activation of the autonomic system. If this hypothesis is correct, then in patients with right brain damage we should observe, on one hand, a greater incidence of properly autonomic disorders and, on the other hand, a state of emotional indifference resulting from a reduced vegetative response to emotionally laden stimuli.

The first prediction is supported by studies that have investigated possible hemispheric asymmetries in the autonomic control of the heart. Thus, some authors[51] have shown that sympathetic effects, such as tachycardia and increased blood pressure, elicited by electrical stimulation of the insular cortex, are provoked more by right than by left stimulations. Other authors [52,53] have made the complementary observation that in patients submitted to a unilateral Wada test, an increased heart rate (considered as physiologically due to the stress provoked by the unilateral brain inactivation) is observed after injection of sodium Amytal into the left but not into the right carotid artery. Still other authors have shown that the physiologic variability in heart rate observed during the circadian cycle[54] or in response to increased respiratory activity [55] is reduced more by right than by left hemispheric lesions. The pathologic nature of this reduced variability in heart rate is demonstrated by its association with an increased risk of sudden death in patients with and without a history of myocardial infarction [56,57] and by the recent observation [58] that stroke in the region of the right insula leads to decreased heart rate variability and to an increased incidence of sudden death.

The second prediction, assuming that the emotional indifference of right-brain-damaged patients may be due at least in part to a reduced capacity to react to emotionally laden stimuli with an appropriate autonomic response is supported by an unexpected observation made by Mammucari and coworkers[33] while studying, in right- and left-brain-damaged patients, the facial expression of emotions elicited by the presentation of emotional movies.

These authors noticed that during the presentation of a very unpleasant emotional film, normal subjects and left-brain-damaged patients tended to divert their gaze from the screen, whereas similar avoidance eye movements were not shown by right-brain-damaged patients. The investigators argued that normal subjects and left-brain-damaged patients diverted their gaze from the screen because they were emotionally distressed by the crude scenes of the film, whereas right-brain-damaged patients did not look away from the screen because they were much less emotionally involved. This interpretation is supported by experimental data obtained by Caltagirone and associates[49] studying, in the same subjects, the relationships between modifications of heart rate and presence of the avoidance eye movements. In normal subjects and in left-brain-damaged patients, heart rate deceleration was much greater in those who watched the entire film sequence than in those who displayed avoidance eye movements, whereas in right-brain-damaged patients, heart rate changes were very mild, regardless of the presence or absence of avoidance eye movements.

Data consistent with the hypothesis of a leading role of the right hemisphere in the generation of the autonomic components of the emotions and of the concomitant emotional experience have also recently been obtained by Wittling and Roscmann[59,60] during lateralized presentation of emotionally laden films to normal subjects. These authors found that both the increase of diastolic and systolic blood pressure and the subjective rating of the intensity of the emotional experience were higher during presentation of the film to the right rather than to the left hemisphere. In conclusion, results of investigations conducted both in patients with unilateral brain damage and in normal subjects, by means of different experimental procedures, seem to show that the right hemisphere subserves not only the communicative but also the autonomic components and therefore the inner experience of emotions.

THE RELATIONSHIP BETWEEN POSTSTROKE DEPRESSION AND LESION OF LEFT FRONTAL CORTEX

We have seen above that investigations of the communicative aspects of emotions have failed to support the hypothesis of a different specialization of the right and left hemispheres for negative and positive emotions, respectively. In order to circumvent these negative results, some authors have tried to reformulate the original theory in slightly different terms. In particular, Davidson [61–63] has proposed that the specialization of the left hemisphere for positive emotions and of the right hemisphere for negative emotions may account only for the expressive but not for the evaluative aspects of emotions. Even if the experimental evidence supporting this theory consists mostly of data obtained with psychophysiologic procedures in normal subjects (see Refs. 61 to 63 and 64 and 65 for contrasting viewpoints on this subject), a series of anatomoclinical studies conducted by Robinson and coworkers[66–69] on patients with poststroke depression seems consistent with Davidson's hypothesis. These studies are discussed here in some detail, since they are quite relevant to the scope of the present volume. In their papers, Robinson and coworkers have distinguished, on the basis of DSM-III[70] diagnostic criteria, two different types of poststroke depression (PSD): a major form, considered as an endogenous (psychotic) depression, and a minor form, considered as a dysthymic (neurotic or reactive) depression. According to these authors, the former should result from interruption of the monoaminergic pathways linking the brainstem to the cerebral cortex and should usually be due to left frontal lesions, whereas the latter should be caused by less specific (psychological) mechanisms and show no relationship with a specific locus of lesion. Now, even if the neurochemical mechanism proposed by Robinson and coworkers cannot be easily reconciled with the hypothesis of a "center for positive emotions" located in the left frontal cortex, the observation that a form of major depression results from injury to the left frontal lobe could be consistent with Davidson's theory.

During the last few years, however, some methodologic and empiric objections have been addressed to the claim that a form of "major" depression undistinguishable from the clinico-symptomatological point of view from the endogenous forms of major depression[68] may be specifically caused by left frontal lesions. From the methodologic point of view, it has been argued that the criteria suggested by DSM-III to make a diagnosis of "major" depression cannot be valid for patients with an organic form of depression. According to this manual, in fact, a diagnosis of major depression can be made if, in addition to a depressed mood, the patient presents at least five symptoms out of a series of eight that include, among others, sleep disorders, loss of weight and/or appetite, fatigue, apathy, and concentration disorders. The objection that, in a stroke patient, some of these symptoms may be due to the brain injury per se has been therefore advanced and a new scale (the "Post-Stroke Depression Rating Scale") specifically devised by having in mind symptoms and problems of depressed stroke patients has been constructed.[71,72] This scale has been used to check Robinson's claim that the major form of PSD may be undistinguishable from the symptomatological point of view from the endogenous forms of major depression. With this aim in mind, the symptomatological profiles of patients classified (on the basis of DSM-III diagnostic criteria) as minor or major PSD or as major functional depression have been compared. Contrary to the predictions based on Robinson's model, the symptomatological profiles of patients classified as having major PSD were more similar to those of patients with minor PSD than to those of subjects with endogenous major depression. Furthermore, the unmotivated aspects of depression prevailed in patients with endogenous depression, whereas the motivated (reactive) aspects prevailed in patients with a (major or minor) form of PSD, suggesting that this form of depression is mostly due to the psychological reaction of the patient to handicaps and disabilities provoked by the lesion. Finally, the assumption of a strong link between left frontal lesions and major PSD has not been confirmed by further investigations. In particular, almost all of the recent studies conducted on this subject[73–76] have failed to confirm the relationship between PSD and left hemisphere (or left frontal) lesions (see Refs.77 and 78 for recent reviews), whereas some studies[74,79,80] have found that patients with anterior lesions are more depressed than those with posterior lesions irrespective of the hemispheric side of injury. These findings can, perhaps, be reconciled with Robinson's hypothesis, assuming that the PSD may be due to a disruption of pathways providing the monoaminergic input to the neocortex. They are, however, clearly inconsistent with Davidson's theory, assuming a different lateralization of structures subserving the expression of positive and negative emotions at the level of the left frontal lobes.

THE SIDE OF LESION IN CONTENT-SPECIFIC DELUSIONS SECONDARY TO BRAIN DAMAGE

In addition to the phenomenological and anatomoclinical data contrasting with the model of PSD proposed by Robinson and coworkers, some recent observations concerning other forms of psychopathology secondary to brain damage are also consistent with the hypothesis of a right hemispheric dominance for various aspects of emotional behavior. We refer here in particular to content-specific delusions of the kind reviewed in Chap. 31, involving the reduplication or the misidentification of persons (Capgras's syndrome) or of places (environmental reduplications). In the Capgras's syndrome, the patient maintains that a person well known to him or her (usually a family member) has been replaced by an impostor or by a double and that there are two versions of this person. In the environmental reduplications (or reduplicative paramnesia) the patient maintains that there are two or more versions of a particular place (or room or building), the present place being usually closer to home than it is in fact the case. Several authors have recently shown that in these forms of content-specific delusions secondary to brain damage, lesions are usually bilateral or restricted to the right hemisphere.[81–83] Furthermore, the relationship between content-specific delusions and right hemisphere dysfunction has been recently confirmed by Staff et al.[84] using single photon emission computed tomography (SPECT) to study the neuroanatomic correlates of these delusions in Alzheimer's disease patients. These authors have, indeed, clearly shown that content-specific delusions are associated with hypoperfusion of the right hemisphere frontotemporal limbic structures. Even if some authors have attributed these findings to specific aspects of the right hemisphere cognitive functions, it is important not to neglect the emotional disturbances that certainly play an important role in the pathophysiology of the delusional misidentification syndromes. The selective involvement of the right hemisphere in these forms of content-specific delusions is, therefore, also consistent with the hypothesis of a right hemispheric dominance for emotional functions.

CONCLUDING REMARKS

Taken together, results of investigations conducted in patients with unilateral brain damage and in normal subjects seem more consistent with the hypothesis assuming a general dominance of the right hemisphere for various aspects of emotional behavior than with the alternative hypothesis assuming a different specialization of the right and left hemispheres for opposite aspects of the mood. It is also possible that the difference between the right and left hemispheres in the regulation of emotions may be qualitative rather than simply quantitative and that the two sides of the brain may play complementary roles in emotional behavior. The author has, in fact, hypothesized elsewhere[64,65] that the right hemisphere might be involved mainly in the more basic and automatic aspects of emotions (namely in the generation of the autonomic components of the emotional response, in the correlative subjective experience, and in the spontaneous expression of emotions), whereas the left hemisphere might play a more important role in control functions, particularly in the intentional control of the emotional expressive apparatus.

Obviously, this is not the place to dwell upon this rather speculative issue. However, it is worthwhile to stress the fact that emotions are based on a highly complex and articulated system, which can be fractionated according to different criteria. Two of these criteria, namely the emotional valence (i.e., the positive or negative polarity of the emotional experience) and the functional subcomponents of the emotional system (i.e., communicative aspects, autonomic response, and subjective experience of emotions) have been taken into account in the present survey. Other criteria, however—such as, for example, the automatic or controlled level of the emotional behavior—could be relevant to the problem of the relationships between emotions and hemispheric specialization.

REFERENCES

1. Broca P: Sur la faculté du langage articulé. *Bull Soc Antropol* 6:377–393, 1865.
2. Dax M: Lésions de la moité gauche de l'encéphale coincidant avec l'oubli des signes de la pensée. *Gax Hebd Med Chir* 2:259–260, 1865.
3. Terzian H, Cecotto C: Determinazione e studio della dominanza emisferica mediante iniezione intracarotide di Amytal sodico nell'uomo: I. Modificazioni cliniche. *Boll Soc Ital Biol Sper* 35:1623–1626, 1959.
4. Alema G, Donini G: Sulle modificazioni cliniche ed elettroencefalografiche da introduzione intracarotidea di isoetil-barbiturato di sodio nell'uomo. *Boll Soc Ital Biol Sper* 36:900–904, 1960.

5. Perria L, Rosadini G, Rossi GF: Determination of side of cerebral dominance with amobarbital. *Arch Neurol* 4:173–181, 1961.
6. Gainotti G: Réaction "catastrophiques" et manifestations d'indifferénce au cours des atteintes cérébrales. *Neuropsychologia* 7:195–204, 1969.
7. Gainotti G: Emotional behavior and hemispheric side of the lesion. *Cortex* 8:41–55, 1972.
8. Gainotti G: Laterality of affect: the emotional behavior of right and left brain-damaged patients, in Myslobodsky MS (ed): *Hemisyndromes: Psychobiology, Neurology, Psychiatry.* New York: Academic Press, 1983, pp 175–192.
9. Gainotti G: Disorders of emotional behavior and of autonomic arousal resulting from unilateral brain damage, in Ottoson D (ed): *The Dual Brain.* London: Macmillan, 1987, pp 161–179.
10. Gainotti G: The meaning of emotional disturbances resulting from unilateral brain injury, in Gainotti G, Caltagirone C (eds): *Emotions and the Dual Brain.* Heidelberg: Springer-Verlag, 1989, pp 147–167.
11. Gestmann J: Problem of imperception of disease and of impaired body territories with organic lesions: Relation to body scheme and its disorders. *Arch Neurol Psychiatry* 48:890–913, 1942.
12. Nathanson M, Bergman PS, Gordon GG: Denial of illness: Its occurrence in one hundred consecutive cases of hemiplegia. *Arch Neurol Psychiatry* 68:380–387, 1952.
13. Gainotti G: Confabulations of denial in senile dementia. *Psychiatr Clin* 8:99–108, 1975.
14. Critchley M: Personification of paralysed limbs in hemiplegics. *Br Med J* 30:284–286, 1955.
15. Tucker DM: Neural substrates of thought and affective disorders, in Gainotti G, Caltagirone C (eds): *Emotions and the Dual Brain.* Heidelberg: Springer-Verlag, 1989, pp 225–234.
16. Heilman KM, Scholes R, Watson RT: Auditory affective agnosia. *J Neurol Neurosurg Psychiatry* 38:69–72, 1975.
17. Tucker DM, Watson RT, Heilman KM: Discrimination and evocation of affectively intoned speech in patients with right parietal disease. *Neurology* 27:947–950, 1977.
18. Ross ED: The aprosodias. *Arch Neurol* 38:561–569, 1981.
19. Benowitz LI, Bear DM, Rosenthal R, et al: Hemispheric specialization in nonverbal communication. *Cortex* 19:5–11, 1983.
20. Heilman KM, Bowers D, Speedie L, Coslett HB: Comprehension of affective and nonaffective prosody. *Neurology* 34:917–921, 1984.
21. Blonder LX, Bowers D, Heilman KM: The role of the right hemisphere in emotional communication. *Brain* 114:1115–1127, 1991.
22. Cicone M, Wapner W, Gardner H: Sensitivity to emotional expression and situations in organic patients. *Cortex* 16:145–158, 1980.
23. DeKosky S, Heilman KM, Bowers D, Valenstein E: Recognition and discrimination of emotional faces and pictures. *Brain Lang* 9:206–214, 1980.
24. Bowers D, Bauer RM, Coslett HB, Heilman KM: Processing of faces by patients with unilateral hemisphere lesions: Dissociation between judgments of facial affect and facial identity. *Brain Cogn* 4:258–272, 1985.
25. Borod JC, Koff E, Perlman-Lorch M, Nicholas M: The expression and perception of facial emotion in brain-damaged patients. *Neuropsychologia* 24:169–180, 1986.
26. Blonder LX, Burns A, Bowers D, et al: Right hemisphere facial expressivity during natural conversation. *Brain Cogn* 21:44–56, 1993.
27. Buck R, Duffy RJ: Nonverbal communication of affect in brain-damaged patients. *Cortex* 16:351–362, 1980.
28. Ross ED: Right hemisphere's role in language, affective behavior, and emotion. *Trends Neurosci* 7:342–346, 1984.
29. Gorelick PB, Ross ED: The aprosodias: further functional-anatomical evidence for the organization of affective language in the right hemisphere. *J Neurol Neurosurg Psychiatry* 50:553–560, 1987.
30. Etcoff NL: Recognition of emotions in patients with unilateral brain damage, in Gainotti G, Caltagirone C (eds): *Emotions and the Dual Brain.* Heidelberg: Springer-Verlag, 1989, pp 168–186.
31. Borod JC: Cerebral mechanisms underlying facial, prosodic and lexical emotional expression: A review of neuropsychological studies and methodological issues. *Neuropsychology* 7:445–463, 1993.
32. Borod JC, Zgaljardic D, Tabert MH, Koff E: Asymmetries of emotional perception and expression in normal adults, in Gainotti G (ed): *Handbook of Neuropsychology,* 2d ed. *Emotional Behavior and Its Disorders.* Amsterdam: Elsevier, 2001, vol 5, pp 181–205.
33. Mammucari A, Caltagirone C, Ekman P, et al: Spontaneous facial expression of emotions in brain-damaged patients. *Cortex* 24:521–533, 1988.
34. Caltagirone C, Ekman P, Friesen W, et al: Posed emotional expression in unilateral brain damaged patients. *Cortex* 25:653–663, 1989.
35. Weddel RA, Moller DJ, Trevarthen C: Voluntary emotional facial expression in patients with focal cerebral lesions. *Neuropsychologia* 28:43–60, 1990.

36. Bradvik B, Dravins C, Holtas S, et al: Do single right hemisphere infarcts or transient ischemic attacks result in aprosody? *Acta Neurol Scand* 81:61–70, 1990.
37. Cancelliere AEB, Kertesz A: Lesion localization in acquired deficits of emotional expression and comprehension. *Brain Cogn* 13:133–147, 1990.
38. Weddel RA: Recognition memory for emotional facial expressions in patients with focal cerebral lesions. *Brain Cogn* 11:1–17, 1989.
39. Young AW, Newcombe F, De Haan EHF, et al: Face perception after brain injury. *Brain* 116:941–959, 1993
40. Peper M, Irle E: The decoding of emotional concepts in patients with focal cerebral lesions. *Brain Cogn* 34:360–387, 1997.
41. Hohmann G: Some effects of spinal cord lesions on experimental emotional feelings. *Psychophysiology* 3:143–156, 1966.
42. Schachter S: Cognition and peripheralist-centralist controversies in motivation and emotion, in Gazzaniga MS, Blakmore C (eds): *Handbook of Psychobiology.* New York: Academic Press, 1975, pp 529–564.
43. Le Doux JE: Cognitive-emotional interactions in brain. *Cogn Emotion* 3:267–289, 1989.
44. Heilman KM, Schwartz H, Watson RT: Hypoarousal in patients with the neglect syndrome and emotional indifference. *Neurology* 28:229–232, 1978.
45. Morrow L, Vrtunsky PB, Kim Y, Boller F: Arousal responses to emotional stimuli and laterality of lesion. *Neuropsychologia* 20:77–81, 1982.
46. Zoccolotti P, Scabini D, Violani V: Electrodermal responses in patients with unilateral brain damage. *J Clin Neuropsychol* 4:143–150, 1982.
47. Meadows ME, Kaplan RF: Dissociation of autonomic and subjective responses to emotional slides in right hemisphere damaged patients. *Neuropsychologia* 32:847–856, 1994.
48. Zoccolotti P, Caltagirone C, Benedetti N, Gainotti G: Perturbation des réponses végétatives aux stimuli émotionnels au cours des lésions hémisphériques unilatérales. *Encéphale* 12:263–268, 1986.
49. Caltagirone C, Zoccolotti P, Originale G, et al: Autonomic reactivity and facial expression of emotions in brain-damaged patients, in Gainotti G, Caltagirone C (eds): *Emotions and the Dual Brain.* Heidelberg: Springer-Verlag, 1989, pp 204–221.
50. Yokoyama K, Jennings R, Ackles P, et al: Lack of heart rate changes during an attention demanding task after right hemisphere lesions. *Neurology* 37:624–630, 1987.
51. Oppenheimer SM, Gelb A, Girvin JP, Hachinski VC: Cardiovascular effects of human insular cortex stimulation. *Neurology* 42:1727–1732, 1992.
52. Rosen AD, Gur RC, Sussman N, et al: Hemispheric asymmetry in the control of heart rate. *Abstr Soc Neurosci* 8:917, 1982.
53. Zamrini EY, Meador KJ, Loring DW, et al: Unilateral cerebral inactivation produces differential left/right heart rate responses. *Neurology* 40:1408–1411, 1990.
54. Sander D, Klingelhofer J: Changes of circadian blood pressure patterns and cardiovascular parameters indicate lateralization of sympathetic activation following hemispheric brain infarction. *J Neurol* 242:313–318, 1995.
55. Naver HK, Blomstrand C, Wallin G: Reduced heart rate variability after right-sided stroke. *Stroke* 27:247–251, 1996.
56. Kleiger RE, Miller P, Bigger JT, Moss AJ: Multicenter post-infarction group: Decreased heart rate variability and its association with increased mortality after acute myocardial infarction. *Am J Cardiol* 59:256–262, 1987.
57. Johnson RH, Robinson BJ: Mortality in alcoholics with autonomic neuropathy. *J Neurol Neurosurg Psychiatry* 51:476–480, 1988.
58. Tokgozoglu SL, Batur MK, Topçuoglu MA, et al: Effects of stroke location on cardiac autonomic balance and sudden death. *Stroke* 30:1307–1311, 1999.
59. Wittling W: Psychophysiological correlates of human brain asymmetry: Blood pressure changes during lateralized presentation of an emotionally laden film. *Neuropsychologia* 28:457–470, 1990.
60. Wittling W, Roscmann R: Emotion-related hemisphere asymmetry: Subjective emotional response to laterally presented films. *Cortex* 29:431–448, 1993.
61. Davidson RJ: *Affect, Cognition and Behavior.* Cambridge, England: Cambridge University Press, 1984.
62. Davidson RJ: Cerebral asymmetry and emotion: Conceptual and methodological conundrums. *Cogn Emotion* 7:115–138, 1993.
63. Davidson RJ: Affective style and affective disorders: Perspectives from affective neuroscience. *Cogn Emotion* 12:307–330, 1998.
64. Gainotti G, Caltagirone C, Zoccolotti P: Left/right and cortical/subcortical dichotomies in the neuropsychological study of human emotions. *Cogn Emotion* 7:71–93, 1993.
65. Gainotti G : Neuropsychology of emotions, in Denes GF, Pizzamiglio L (eds): *Handbook of Clinical and Experimental Neuropsychology.* Hove, UK: Psychology Press, 1999, pp 613–633.
66. Robinson RG, Kubos KL, Starr LB, et al: Mood changes in stroke patients: Relationship to lesion location. *Comp Psychiatry* 24:555–566, 1983.

67. Robinson RG, Kubos KL, Starr LB, et al: Mood disorders in stroke patients: Importance of location of lesion. *Brain* 107:81–93, 1984.
68. Lipsey JR, Spencer WC, Rabins PV, Robinson RG: Phenomenological comparison of post-stroke depression and functional depression. *Am J Psychiatry* 143:527–529, 1986.
69. Starkstein SE, Robinson RG: Affective disorders and cerebrovascular disease. *Br J Psychiatry* 154:170–182, 1989.
70. American Psychiatric Association: *Diagnostic and Statistical Manual of Mental Disorders,* 3d ed (DSM-III). Washington, DC: American Psychiatric Press, 1980.
71. Gainotti G, Azzoni A, Lanzillotta M, et al: Some preliminary findings on a new scale for the assessment of depression and related symptoms in stroke patients. *Ital J Neurol Sci* 16:439–451, 1995.
72. Gainotti G, Azzoni A, Razzano C, et al: The Post-Stroke Depression Rating Scale: A test specifically devised to investigate affective disorders of stroke patients. *J Clin Exp Neuropsychol* 19:340–356, 1987.
73. Andersen G, Vestergaard K, Ingeman-Nielsen M, Lauritzen L: Risk factors for post-stroke depression. *Acta Psychiatr Scand* 92:193–198, 1995.
74. Gainotti G, Azzoni A, Gasparini F: Relation of lesion location to verbal and nonverbal mood measures in stroke patients. *Stroke* 28:2145–2149, 1997.
75. Gainotti G, Azzoni A, Marra C: Frequency, phenomenology and anatomical-clinical correlates of major post-stroke depression. *Brit J Psychiatry* 175:163–167, 1999.
76. Hermann N, Black SE, Lawrence J, et al: The Sunnybrook Stroke Study: A prospective study of depressive symptoms and functional outcome. *Stroke* 29:618–624, 1998.
77. Agrell B, Dehlin O: Depression in stroke patients with left and right hemisphere lesion: A study in geriatric rehabilitation in-patients. *Aging Clin Exp Res* 6:49–56, 1994.
78. Carson AJ, MacHale S, Allen K, et al: Depression after stroke and lesion location: A systematic review. *Lancet* 356:122–126, 2000.
79. Sinyor D, Jacques P, Kaloupek DG, et al: Poststroke depression and lesion location: An attempted replication. *Brain* 109:537–546, 1986.
80. House A, Dennis M, Warlow C, et al: Mood disorders after stroke and their relation to lesion location. *Brain* 113:1113–1129, 1990.
81. Feinberg TE, Shapiro RM: Misidentification-reduplication and the right hemisphere. *Neuropsychiatry Neuropsychol Behav Neurol* 2:39–48, 1989.
82. Malloy P, Cimino C, Westlake R: Differential diagnosis of primary and secondary Capgras delusions. *Neuropsychiatry Neuropsychol Behav Neurol* 5:83–96, 1992.
83. Murai T, Toichi M, Sengoku A, et al: Reduplicative paramnesia in patients with focal brain damage. *Neuropsychiatry Neuropsychol Behav Neurol* 10:190–196, 1997.
84. Staff RT, Shanks MF, Macintosh L, et al: Delusions in Alzheimer's disease: SPECT evidence of right hemisphere dysfunction. *Cortex* 35:549–560, 1999.

Chapter 58

EMOTIONAL DISORDERS IN RELATION TO NONFOCAL BRAIN DYSFUNCTION

Elizabeth S. Ochoa
Hulya M. Erhan
Todd E. Feinberg

Diffuse brain damage that causes widespread, generalized disruption of brain functions frequently produces emotional and behavioral disturbances. (For a discussion of the effects of focal brain pathology on emotion, see Chap. 57). In this chapter we discuss the emotional and behavioral consequences of diffuse brain dysfunction associated with several conditions, including degenerative brain disorders, anoxia, and closed head injury.

ALZHEIMER'S DISEASE

Alzheimer's disease (AD) is characterized by cortical changes that include the accumulation of senile plaques and neurofibrillary tangles, synaptic and dendritic reduction, neuronal loss, and alteration of several neurotransmitter systems[1,2] (see Chaps. 44 to 46). Loss of cholinergic neurons in the substantia innominata, locus ceruleus, medial septal nuclei, and the diagonal band of Broca is also observed.[1] Alteration in several neurotransmitter systems—including acetylcholine, serotonin, dopamine, norepinephrine and gamma—aminuobutyric acid—has been documented in AD, as well as reductions in concentrations of glutamate, somatostatin, substance P, and cholecystokinin.[1,2] The contribution of these specific changes to alterations in the diagnosed individuals' emotional and behavioral functioning is not well understood.

Emotional and behavioral changes associated with AD include depression, anxiety, agitation, delusions, and hallucinations.[3–11] For example, Teri and Wagner[6] reported that 30 percent of individuals diagnosed with AD met criteria for clinical depression. Migliorelli et al. reported that 28 percent of patients with probable AD met DSM-III-R criteria for dysthymia and 23 percent met criteria for major depression.[7,8] Chemerinski et al.[9] reported that the symptom profile of depression in individuals with AD was similar to that in age-matched individuals with major depression who did not have dementia. Starkstein et al.[8] have suggested that dysthymia may be a short-term response to cognitive deterioration—unlike major depression which may reflect a more pervasive condition.

Reports of Generalized Anxiety Disorder (GAD) in association with AD have ranged from 0 to 5 percent.[12,13] Mega et al.[14] noted anxiety in 48 percent of 50 individuals with AD of varying severity, suggesting that while the anxiety experienced by those with AD may not be severe enough to warrant a clinical diagnosis of anxiety disorder, it is often present. Agitation, unlike GAD, is a common behavioral feature of AD.[15] The reported prevalence of agitation has ranged from 24 to 66 percent.[11] While some studies have reported increased agitation with greater severity of dementia, others have not.[16] In an investigation that examined agitation in a series of AD outpatients, Aarsland et al.[16] noted that physical aggression appeared to be associated with hallucinations, while verbal aggression was associated with the presence of delusions.

The percentage of AD patients suffering from delusions is reported to range from of 30 to 55 percent. Delusions have been found to be more common in women than men and to occur most in the middle stage of the disease.[3–5] Delusional jealousy, paranoid delusions, and delusional misidentification have been described in AD. Paranoid delusions have been reported to be more common in the early phase of the disorder, while other types of delusions, such as misidentification, tend to occur in the moderate to severe phases of the disease.[5] Visual, auditory and multimodal hallucinations have been reported in 3 to 49 percentof individuals diagnosed with AD.[3,4] Visual hallucinations have been noted to occur more frequently than other types of hallucinations.[3] In a 4-year follow up of a large cohort of individuals with AD, hallucinations were noted in about 70 percent of participants.[4]

HUNTINGTON'S CHOREA

Huntington's chorea is a movement disorder characterized by choreiform movements and progressive cognitive decline. Neuropathologic degeneration in HD occurs in the caudate nuclei and putamen and is characterized by neuronal loss, accumulation of fibrous astrocytes, dendritic reduction in spiny neurons, and reduction in myelinated fibers.[17] There is accompanying atrophy in the frontal and temporal gyri[1] (see Chap. 48). Neurotransmitter system changes include increased sensitivity of dopamine receptors in the striatal region, increased norepinephrine, decreased gamma—aminobutyric acid and decreased acetylcholine in the area of the striatum and lateral pallidum.[1] Alterations in the function of pathways from the medial aspect of the caudate nucleus to the orbitofrontal cortex as well as to the cingulate gyrus have been identified as contributing to the development of emotional or behavioral difficulties.[18]

Emotional disturbances may be the most prominent feature of this disorder in individuals who suffer from HD with early onset, between 15 to 40 years of age, who subsequently develop movement and cognitive difficulties. Individuals with late onset HD, between 55 and 60 years of age, tend to develop the movement and cognitive symptoms initially and simultaneously. Emotional changes noted in HD patients include the development of depression, irritability, impulsivity, apathy, and hallucinations.[1,18–21] While 30 to 50 percent of individuals with HD experience some form of affective disorder, only about 10 to 25 percent demonstrate features of bipolar disorder.[19–21] In a review of a series of eight studies, the prevalence of depression was from 9 to 44 percent, with the mean frequency of 23 percent.[22] The incidence of suicidal ideation or suicidal behaviors ranges between less than 1 to 29.5 percent, with the suicide rate reported generally as more than 5 percent.[19–22] Irritability was noted in 18 to 50 percent of a total of 702 individuals with HD.[22] Irritability may take the form of being difficult to get along with, emotional lability, and temper outbursts in response to minor incidents.[22]

The occurrence of delusions and hallucinations, obsessive-compulsive disorder, and alterations in sexual functioning have also been noted. A study of 134 patients in the United Kingdom reported that less than 5 percent of HD patients exhibited hallucinations or delusions[19]; however, a prevalence of 10 to 12 percent has been reported elsewhere.[21–23] Mendez noted that five studies reported the prevalence of changes in sexuality, from 2.5 to 29.4 percent, with the average of 10.8 percent.[22] Craufurd et al.[19] noted sexually demanding behavior in 5 percent of their sample and disinhibited and inappropriate sexual behavior in 6 percent. They also noted that hyposexuality was much more commonly reported than hypersexuality, the former occurring in 62 percent of their sample.

PARKINSON'S DISEASE

Parkinson's disease (PD) is accompanied by a variety of changes in behavior and emotional functioning (see Chap. 48). Brain characteristics associated with idiopathic PD include degeneration of neurons in the substantia nigra and the presence of Lewy bodies.[24] Cellular changes that occur in the substantia nigra and locus ceruleus include loss of dendritic length, reduction in dendritic spines, and decreased arborization. Lewy bodies have been identified in several regions of the cerebral cortex, diencephalon, midbrain, pons, and medulla.[24]

Depression is the predominant emotional difficulty in patients with PD, with prevalence rates varying from 2.7 to 90 percent. Recently reported prevalence rates range between 20 and 40 percent.[25–28] Depression occurs most frequently in the early and late stages of the disease.[26,28] Individuals may meet criteria for major depression or dysthymia.[27,28] The depression in PD differs from primary major depression by the less frequent occurrence of suicide, guilt feelings, sense of failure, and self-blame.[26] Between 15 and 25 percent of individuals with PD may present with depression prior to the manifestation of motor symptoms by 1 or more years.[25,27,28]

Another feature associated with PD is psychosis. Hallucinations and delusions had been reported prior to the advent of dopaminergic or anticholinergic treatments in PD; however, the reported frequency of these symptoms has increased since the introduction of these pharmacologic agents.[29,30] In one cohort of PD patients, 25.5 percent had experienced vivid dreams (thought to be harbinger of psychosis), 9.8 percent had experienced hallucinations with insight, and 6.0 percent had experienced psychosis with hallucinations or delusions within the 1-week period prior to their assessment.[29,30] Aarsland et al.[29] found that 22.9 percent of PD individuals residing in nursing homes or senior residences reported hallucinations with insight, while 18.8 percent were found to have psychosis—a figure that is consistent with other reports in the literature.[25,29] Lower scores on the Mini-Mental State Exam, greater likelihood of meeting criteria for dementia, and greater symptoms of depression were noted in those individuals who experienced hallucinations or delusions than in those who did not.[29,30] Hallucinations experienced in PD are more commonly visual.

Anxiety disorders and sleep disturbances are frequent in PD, with up to 40 percent of patients described as anxious.[25,31,32] Anxiety may develop into phobias, including fear of falling, of being alone, or of being in open spaces or crowds.[25] Sleep difficulties that are reported in PD and described by patients include difficulty staying asleep, with frequent, sometimes long periods of awakening. This is confirmed by polysomnographic studies that show lower amounts of rapid-eye-movement (REM) sleep and increased REM sleep latency in PD patients.[32]

ANOXIA

The human brain receives approximately 15 percent of total cardiac output.[33] The terms *anoxia, hypoxia,* or *hypoxia-ischemia* are often used interchangeably in the literature to refer to states of oxygen deprivation, although subtle differences in meaning exist.[33,36] When brain oxygenation is insufficient (hypoxia) or absent (anoxia) due to a sustained reduction of circulating arterial oxygen or failed perfusion (ischemia), diffuse brain damage and encephalopathy can result.[33–35] (For review, see Caine and Watson).[33]

Acute oxygen deprivation usually results from cardiac or respiratory failure.[34,36] Common causes of hypoxic-ischemic encephalopathy include myocardial infarct, ventricular arrhythmia, hemorrhage, suffocation, carbon monoxide poisoning, anesthesia-related complications, diseases that paralyze the respiratory muscles, and conditions that cause diffuse brain damage (traumatic brain injury, vascular disorders, epilepsy, pediatric encephalopathies).[34]

The extent of brain damage is a function of several factors, including the severity of the anoxia, its duration, and its etiology.[34,37] Anoxia and severe hypoxia produce acute brain damage, while mild hypoxia has been associated with brain damage if the hypoxic condition continues or is recurrent.[36] Adams and colleagues[34] have suggested that, in general, if there is no loss of consciousness, a hypoxic condition will not produce permanent neurologic damage. When acute oxygen deprivation lasts longer than 4 to 8 min, cerebral infarction and disseminated cell death result.

Brain regions are differentially vulnerable to the effects of oxygen deprivation,[33,34,38,39] and anoxia or sustained hypoxia may produce diffuse brain damage, with superimposed focal damage.[34,35] For example, the hippocampus is susceptible to anoxic injury, with the pyramidal neurons of the CA1 zone being most likely affected.[33,35,40] The basal ganglia, cerebellum, "border zone" regions of the parietotemporal cortex, and the thalamus have been found to be as vulnerable to anoxic effects as the hippocampus.[33–35]

In a review of 67 individual case studies, Caine and Watson[33] found that approximately half (46 percent) of individuals had changes in personality or executive functioning following anoxic injury. Impaired affect regulation (either emotional lability or apathy) was the most frequently described personality change.[33,37,41,42] Emotional lability was characterized by various investigators as depression, anxiety, hysterical behavior, intolerance to suggestion or criticism, hyperactivity, or uncontrollable emotional expressions and regression in mental and emotional behavior.[33,41,43,44]

CARBON MONOXIDE POISONING

Carbon monoxide is a colorless, odorless gas that is found in the environment.[45] It is produced as an oxidation product of methane and from incomplete combustion (i.e., burning of waste materials, emissions, ovens and blast furnaces, and tobacco smoke).[45] Approximately 10,000 cases of carbon monoxide poisoning are reported in the United States each year, with 40 percent of the resultant 3800 deaths being attributed to accidental causes and 60 percent to suicide.[45]

Acute, high-level carbon monoxide exposure is toxic to the brain and heart and may be fatal. Carbon monoxide interferes with cellular respiration by displacing oxygen from hemoglobin and restricting available oxygen.[45] The combination of hypoxia from hemoglobin binding and the ischemia from systemic hypotension and acidosis has been implicated in white matter demyelination[45,46]

Investigators generally concur that the development of neurologic and psychiatric symptoms in carbon monoxide poisoning correlates with the percentage of carbon monoxide that is bound to blood hemoglobin(COHb).[45] Severe symptoms emerge as COHb levels rise.[45] Severe carbon monoxide exposure causes diffuse brain damage in addition to focal damage to the frontal lobes, hippocampus, cerebellum, or basal ganglia.[36,45] The globus pallidus of the basal ganglia is particularly vulnerable to the effects of carbon monoxide poisoning.[36,46]

Brief exposure to carbon monoxide and low COHb levels (<20 percent) do not appear to cause significant brain dysfunction in healthy individuals, although those who have compromised brain or cardiac function might experience adverse effects even at low levels.[45,47] Severe carbon monoxide poisoning occurs with levels of COHb of greater than 50 percent. Cortical and subcortical dysfunction may occur, and persistent effects include dementia, apraxias, agnosias, and cortical blindness as well as movement disorders such as parkinsonism.[36,45] Up to half of patients who experience severe effects have persistent memory impairment. Psychosis and depression have been reported.[45,47] Personality changes involve lability, instability, and impulsivity.[36] Escalona et al.[48] described the case of a man who developed obsessive-compulsive disorder following bilateral globus pallidus infarction secondary to carbon monoxide poisoning.

After patients appear to have recovered adequately, delayed encephalopathy can occur in 10 to 30 percent within 2 to 4 weeks of acute, high-level carbon monoxide exposure.[36] Min[49] reported that 11 percent of 738 patients developed delayed-onset encephalopathy and that almost all of these individuals had been initially unconscious. During this delayed-onset phase, significant white matter damage may occur, along with bilateral damage to the globus pallidus, hippocampus, and focal cortical areas.[45]

Neurologic and psychiatric features associated with delayed encephalopathy may include apathy, incontinence, gait disturbance, mutism with frontal release signs, masked facies, dementia, and hypokinesia.[36,45,49] Irritability and distractibility also was described by Min.[49] Mendez and Doss[50] reported a case of delayed encephalopathy in a 28-year-old woman who developed a frontal lobe syndrome, visuoperceptual impairment, and diffuse white matter lesions in the context of an otherwise normal neurologic examination.

CLOSED HEAD INJURY

Personality and behavioral changes following closed head injury have been described in the literature since the sixteenth century.[51] The particular effects of diffuse brain damage on emotional regulation and behavior following closed head injury are complicated by heterogeneous patient characteristics including the following: premorbid personality, premorbid psychiatric history, contribution of focal lesion locations when present, and the severity (length of coma) and etiology of injury.[52] Risk factors for the development of psychiatric illness after head injury include premorbid personality predisposition,[55,56] history of psychiatric illness,[56] cognitive impairment,[56] and fewer years of formal education.[56] In general, the neuropsychiatric effects of diffuse brain damage secondary to closed head injury are related to the degree of diffuse axonal injury (DAI)[53] and the presence and extent of DAI is a strong predictor of outcome and recovery.[51,53]

DAI results from the rapid acceleration/deceleration and rotational movement of the brain within the skull.[36,51] Microscopic axonal injuries typically are found in cortical white matter and subcortical pathways as well as the basal ganglia, periventricular regions, corpus callosum, upper brainstem, and cerebellum.[36,53,54] White matter changes are marked by the deterioration of myelin and scarring, and small hemorrhages may be found throughout the brain.[36]

Acute posttraumatic psychosis following head injury has been observed in patients who are confused and stuporous or who are emerging from coma.[51] Subtypes of psychosis that have been reported, include schizophrenic-like, Korsakoff's, depressive, manic-depressive, paranoid, and reactive psychoses. Auditory, visual, or tactile hallucinations may be noted.[51]

Affective disturbances are common in the head-injured population, with mood disturbances ranging from mania to depressive symptoms.[57] Some investigators[36,52,54,58,59] have noted that emotional and behavioral disturbances may be expressed as either an exaggeration (disinhibition) or a flattening (decreased initiation and apathy) of emotional reactivity and responsiveness.[52] Mania, anxiety, depression, paranoia, and negative symptoms (flat affect, suspiciousness, and social withdrawal) along with obsessive-compulsive behavior, and interpersonal sensitivity,[36,52,58,60–65] posttraumatic stress disorder,[66] and personality dysfunction[66–68] have been found to result from head injury. Suicidality has also been reported, particularly among individuals who experience emotional disturbance and neuropsychological deficits.[69,70]

Behavioral manifestations of damage to the temporolimbic system include episodic temper flare-ups or dysphoric mood.[36] Mapou[54] has suggested that in the absence of focal brain lesions, diffuse damage to the efferent and afferent frontal lobe pathways can partially account for the emergence of behavioral and emotional disorders after head injury. Fontaine et al.[71] suggested that decreased cortical metabolism in the mesial prefrontal and cingulate cortex were correlated with behavioral disorders of patients following severe head trauma.

Social isolation is common among head-injured individuals because of deficits in social skills, or poor interpersonal relatedness,[36] or diminished relationships following severe head injury.[72] Alcohol and polysubstance abuse can predispose an individual to engage in behaviors that risk head injury and hamper recovery.[62,73] Sexual dysfunction, including decreased libido, may also occur.[74]

REFERENCES

1. Adams RD, Victor M, Ropper AH: *Principles of Neurology,* 6th ed. New York: McGraw-Hill, 1997, pp 1046–1107.
2. Nixon SJ: Alzheimer's disease and vascular dementia, in Adams RL, Oscar AP, Culbertson JL, Nixon SJ (eds): *Neuropsychology for Clinical Practice: Etiology, Assessment and Treatment of Common Neurological Disorders.* Washington, DC: American Psychological Association, 1996, pp 65–105.
3. Mega MS, Lee L, Dinov ID, et al: Cerebral correlates of psychotic symptoms in Alzheimer's disease. *J Neurol Neurosurg Psychiatry* 69(2):167–171, 2000.
4. Robert RS, Gilley DW, Bennett DA, et al: Hallucinations, delusions, and cognitive decline in Alzheimer's disease. *J Neurol Neurosurg Psychiatry* 69(2):172–177, 2000.
5. Geroldi C, Akkawi NM, Galluzzi S, et al: Temporal lobe asymmetry in patients with Alzheimer's disease with delusions. *J Neurol Neurosurg Psychiatry* 69(2):187–191, 2000.
6. Teri L, Wagner A: Alzheimer's disease and depression. *J Consult Clin Psychol* 60(3):379–391, 1992.
7. Miglorelli R, Teson A, Sabe L, et al: Prevalence and correlates of dysthymia and major depression among patients with Alzheimer's disease. *Am J Psychiatry* 152(1):37–44, 1995.
8. Starkstein SE, Chemerinski E, Sabe L, et al: Prospective longitudinal study of depression and anosognosia in Alzheimer's disease. *Br J Psychiatry* 171(7):47–52, 1997.
9. Chemerinski E, Petracca G, Sabe L, et al: The specificity of depressive symptoms in patients with Alzheimer's disease. *Am J Psychiatry* 158(1):68–72, 2001.
10. Lopez OL, Zivkovic S, Smith G, et al: Psychiatric symptoms associated with cortical-subcortical dysfunction in Alzheimer's disease. *J Neuropsychiatry Clin Neurosci* 13(1):56–60, 2001.
11. Borson S, Raskind M: Clinical features and pharmacologic treatment of behavioral symptoms of Alzheimer's disease. *Neurology*, 45(5 Suppl 6):17S–24S,1997.

12. Chemerinski E, Petracca G, Manes F, et al: Prevalence and correlates of anxiety and Alzheimer's disease. *Depression Anxiety* 7(4):166–170, 1998.
13. Bungener C, Jouvent R, Derouesne C: Affective disturbances in Alzheimer's disease. *J Am Geriatr Soc* 44(9):1066–1071, 1996.
14. Mega MS, Cummings JL, Fiorello T, Gornbein J: The spectrum of behavioral changes in Alzheimer's disease. *Neurology* 46(1):130–135, 1996.
15. Cohen-Mansfield J, Deutsch LH: Agitation: Subtypes and their mechanisms. *Semin Clin Neuropsychiatry* 1(4):325–339, 1996.
16. Aarsland D, Cummings JL, Yenner G, Miller B: Relationship of aggressive behavior to other neuropsychiatric symptoms in patients with Alzheimer's disease. *Am J Psychiatry* 153(2):243–247, 1996.
17. Hersch SM, Ferrante RJ: Neuropathology and pathophysiology of Huntington's Disease, in Watts RL, Koller WC (eds): *Movement Disorders: Neurologic Principles and Practice*. New York: McGraw-Hill, 1997, pp 503–518.
18. Zappacosta B, Monza D, Meoni C, et al: Psychiatric symptoms do not correlate with cognitive decline, motor symptoms, or CAG repeat length in Huntington's disease. *Arch Neurol* 53(6):493–497, 1996.
19. Craufurd D, Thompson JC, Snowden JS: Behavioral changes in Huntington disease. *Neuropsychiatry Neuropsychol Behav Neurol* 14(4):219–226, 2001.
20. Ross CA, Margolis RL, Rosenblatt A, et al: Huntington disease and the related disorder, dentatorubral pallidoluysian atrophy. *Medicine* 76(5):305–338, 1997.
21. Marshall FJ, Shoulson I: Clinical features and treatment of Huntington's disease, in Watts RL, Koller WC (eds): *Movement Disorders: Neurologic Principles and Practice*. New York: McGraw-Hill, 1997, pp 491–502.
22. Mendez MF: Huntington's disease: Update and review of neuropsychiatric aspects. *Int J Psychiatry Med* 24(3):189–208, 1994.
23. Watt DC, Seller A: A clinico-genetic study of psychiatric disorder in Huntington's chorea, *Psychol Med* Suppl 23:1–46, 1993.
24. Fearnley J, Lees AJ: Parkinson's disease: neuropathology, in Watts RL, Koller WC (eds): *Movement Disorders: Neurologic Principles and Practice*. New York: McGraw-Hill, 1997, pp 263–278.
25. Melamed E: Neurobehavioral abnormalities in Parkinson's disease, in Watts RL, Koller WC (eds): *Movement Disorders: Neurologic Principles and Practice*. New York: McGraw-Hill, 1997, pp 257–262.
26. Brooks D, Doder M: Depression in Parkinson's disease. *Curr Opin Neurol* 14(4), 465–470, 2001.
27. Rao SM, Huber SJ, Bornstein RA: Emotional changes in multiple sclerosis and Parkinson's disease. *J Consult Clin Psychol* 60(3):369–378, 1992.
28. Poewe W, Luginger E: Depression in Parkinson's disease: Impediments to recognition and treatment options. *Neurology* 52(7 Suppl 3):S2–S6, 1999.
29. Arsland D, Larsen JP, Cummings JL, Laake K: Prevalence and clinical correlates of psychotic based symptoms in Parkinson disease: A community-based study. *Arch Neurol* 56(5):595–601, 1999.
30. Barnes, J, David AS: Visual hallucinations in Parkinson's disease: A review and phenomenological survey. *J Neurol Neurosurgery Psychiatry* 70(6):727–833, 2001.
31. Lieberman A: Managing the neuropsychiatric symptoms of Parkinson' disease. *Neurology* 50(suppl 6):S33–S38, 1998.
32. Poewe W, Hogl B: Parkinson's disease and sleep. *Curr Opin Neurol* 13(4):423–426, 2000.
33. Caine D, Watson JDG: Neuropsychological and neuropathological sequelae of cerebral anoxia: A critical review. *J Int Neuropsychol Soc* 6(1):86–99, 2000.
34. Adams RD, Victor M, Ropper AH: Acquired metabolic disorders of the nervous system, in *Principles of Neurology,* 6th ed. New York: McGraw-Hill, 1997, pp 1108–1113.
35. Bigler ED, Alfano M: Anoxic enoephalopathy: Neurological and neuropsychological findings. *Arch Clin Neuropsychol* 3(4):383–396, 1988.
36. Lezak MD: *Neuropsychological Assessment.* Portland, OR: Oregon Health Sciences University and Veterans Administration Hospital, 1995.
37. Steegmann, AT: *Clinical Aspects of Cerebral Anoxia in Man.* Kansas City, KS: University of Kansas School of Medicine, 1951, pp 261–274.
38. Brierley JB, Graham DI: Hypoxia and vascular disorders of the central nervous system, in Blackwood W, Corsellis JAN (eds): London: Edwin Arnold, 1984, pp 125–207.
39. Myers RE: A unitary theory of causation of anoxic and hypoxic brain pathology, in Fahn S et al (eds): *Advances in Neurology*. New York: Raven Press, 1979, pp 195–213.
40. Zola-Morgan S, Squire LR, Amural, DG: Human amnesia and the medial temporal region: Enduring memory impairment following a bilateral lesion limited to field CA1 of the hippocampus. *J Neurosci* 6:2950–2967, 1986.

41. Fletcher DE: Personality disintegration incident to anoxia: Observations with nitrous oxide anesthesia. *J Nerv Ment Dis* 102:392–403, 1945.
42. Armengol CG: Acute oxygen deprivation: Neuropsychological profiles and implications for rehabilitation. *Brain Injury* 14(3):237–250, 2000.
43. Pation S. Medical studies in aviation: Effects of low oxygen pressure on the personality of the aviator. *Aviat Space Environ Med* 60(12):1225–1226, 1989.
44. Bouwer C, Stein D: Panic disorder following torture by suffocation is associated with predominantly respiratory symptoms. *Psychol Med* 29(1):233–236, 1999.
45. Hartman DE: *Neuropsychological Toxicology: Identification and Assessment of Human Neurotoxic Syndromes,* 2nd ed. New York: Plenum Press, 1995, pp 356–362.
46. Ginsberg MD: Carbon monoxide intoxication: Clinical features, neuropathology, and mechanisms of injury. *Clin Toxicol* 23(4–6):281–288, 1985.
47. Jaeckle RS, Nasrallah HA: Major depression and carbon monoxide-induced parkinsonism: Diagnosis, computerized axial tomography, and response to 1–dopa. *J Nerv Ment Dis* 173(8):503–508, 1985.
48. Escalona RP, Adair JC, Roberts BB, Graeber, DA: Obsessive-compulsive disorder following bilateral globus pallidus infarction. *Biol Psychiatry* 42(5):410–412, 1997.
49. Min SK: A brain syndrome associated with delayed neuropsychiatric sequelae following acute carbon monoxide intoxication. *Acta Psychiatr Scand* 73(1):80–86, 1986.
50. Mendez MF, Doss RC: Neurobehavioral aspects of the delayed encephalopathy of carbon monoxide intoxication: Case report and review. *Behav Neurol* 8(1):47–52, 1995.
51. Levin HS, Benton AL, Grossman RG: *Neurobehavioral Consequences of Closed Head Injury*. New York: Oxford University Press, 1982.
52. Prigatano GP: Personality disturbances associated with traumatic brain injury. *J Consult Clin Psychol* 60(3):360–368, 1992.
53. Jallo JI, Narayan RK: Craniocerebral trauma, in Bradley WG, Daroff RB, Fenichel GM, et al (eds): *Neurology in Clinical Practice*. Boston: Butterworth Heinemann, 2000, vol III, pp 1066–1087.
54. Mapou RL: Neuropathology and neuropsychology of behavioral disturbances following traumatic brain injury, in Long CJ, Ross LK (eds): *Handbook of Head Trauma*. Memphis, TN: Memphis State University and University of Tennessee Center for the Health Sciences, 1992, pp 75–89.
55. Gasquoine PG: Affective state and awareness of sensory and cognitive effects after closed head injury. *Neuropsychology* 6(3):187–196, 1992.
56. Deb S, Lyons I, Koutzoukis C: Neuropsychiatric sequelae one year after minor head injury. *J Neurol Neurosurg Psychiatry* 65(6):899–902, 1998.
57. Silver JM, Kramer R, Greenwald S, Weissman MA: The association between head injuries and psychiatric disorders: Findings from the New Haven NIMH Epidemiologic Catchment Area Study. *Brain Inj* 15(11):935–945, 2001.
58. Butler RW, Satz P: Individual psychotherapy with head injured adults. *Profess Psychol* 19(5):536–541, 1988.
59. Al-Adawi S, Powel JH, Greenwood RJ: Motivational deficits after brain injury. *Neuropsychology* 12(1):115–124, 1998.
60. DiCesare A, Parente R, Anderson-Parente JK: Personality change after traumatic brain injury: Problems and solutions. *Cogn Rehabi* 8(2):14–18, 1990.
61. Fann JR, Katon WJ, Uomoto JM, Esselman PC: Psychiatric disorders and functional disabilities in outpatients with traumatic brain injuries. *Am J Psychiatry* 152(10):1493–1499, 1995.
62. Hibbard MR, Uysal S, Kepler K, et al: Axis I psychopathology in individuals with traumatic brain injury. *J Head Trauma Rehabil* 13(4):24–39, 1998.
63. Van Reekum R, Cohen T, Wong J: Can traumatic brain injury cause psychiatric disorders? *J Neuropsychiatry Clin Neurosci* 12(3):316–327, 2000.
64. Berthier ML, Kulisevsky J, Gironell A, Lopez OL: Obsessive-compulsive disorder and traumatic brain injury: Behavioral, cognitive, and neuroimaging findings. *Neuropsychiatry Neuropsychol Behav Neurol* 14(1):23–31, 2001.
65. Perino C, Rago R, Cicolin A, et al: Mood and behavioural disorders following traumatic brain injury: Clinical evaluation and pharmacological management. *Brain Inj* 15(2):139–149, 2001.
66. Parker RS, Rosenblum A: IQ loss and emotional dysfunctions after mild head injury in a motor vehicle accident. *J Clin Psychol* 52(1):32–43, 1996.
67. Franulic A, Horta E, Maturana R, et al: Organic personality disorder after traumatic brain injury: cognitive, anatomic and psychosocial factors. *Brain Inj* 14(5):431–439, 2000.
68. Hibbard MR, Bogdany J, Uysal S, et al: Axis II psychopathology in individuals with traumatic brain injury. *Brain Inj* 14(1):45–61, 2000.
69. Tate R, Simpson G, Flanagan S, Coffey M: Completed suicide after traumatic brain injury. *J Head Trauma Rehabil* 12(6):16–28, 1997.

70. Carrion JL, Serdio-Arias ML, Murillo Cabezas F, et al: Neurobehavioural and cognitive profile of traumatic brain injury patients at risk for depression and suicide. *Brain Inj* 15(2):175–181, 2001.
71. Fontaine A, Azouvi P, Remy P, et al: Functional anatomy of neuropsychological deficits after severe traumatic brain injury. *Am Acad Neurol* 53(9):1963–1968, 1999.
72. Elsass L, Kinsella G: Social interaction following severe closed head injury. *Psychol Med* 17(1):67–78, 1987.
73. Weinstein D, Martin P: Psychiatric implications of alcoholism and traumatic brain injury. *Am J Addict* 4(4):285–296, 1995.
74. Kreuter M, Dahlloef AG, Gudjonsson G, et al: Sexual adjustment and its predictors after traumatic brain injury. *Brain Inj* 12(5):349–369, 1998.

Chapter 59

THE APROSODIAS*

Elliott D. Ross

Communication is a multifaceted behavior whereby organisms exchange information through various mediums and sensory systems, such as olfaction, vocalization, and posturing. In lower animals, much of the communication takes place through species-specific displays that are relatively hard-wired and organized, at the lowest level, by the mesencephalic periaqueductal gray, with higher-order control furnished by the hypothalamus and limbic system.[1–4] In humans and to a far lesser degree in higher-order primates, communication in the form of language is organized predominantly by the neocortex and is no longer constrained by the innate and nonflexible demands of species-specific displays. This has allowed language to evolve as a graded, infinitely variable behavior.

The fundamental discoveries of Broca[5] and Wernicke[6] that focal lesions in the left hemisphere cause spectacular deficits in many aspects of language have led to the widely held belief that human language is a dominant and highly lateralized function of the left hemisphere, with the right hemisphere being relegated to a "minor" or "nondominant" role in language, communication, and overall control of behavior.[7,8] Over the last two and a half decades, however, considerable evidence has accrued to support the thesis that communication functions are distributed between the hemispheres.[9–37]

The left hemisphere is primarily concerned with lexical and syntactic processing and related functions such as pantomime, pragmatics, denotation, and the linguistic and dialectal aspects of prosody. The right hemisphere is primarily concerned with affective prosody, gestures, and certain related functions such as connotation, thematic inference, and comprehension of nonliteral phrases and complex linguistic relations. Numerous functional neuroimaging studies have established an active role for the right hemisphere in language.[11,38–40] The most intensively analyzed right hemisphere function has been affective prosody and gestures.

ELEMENTS OF LANGUAGE AND COMMUNICATION

Language and communication are characterized by four major constituents: the lexicon (vocabulary), syntax (grammar), prosody, and kinesics. The segment is the smallest articulated feature of a language which, in nontechnical terms, is most closely allied with the syllable.[41,42] Segments, therefore, are the primary building blocks for creating words which form the lexicon. Words, in turn, are concatenated into grammatical relationships to form phrases, sentences, and discourse. It is the segmentally related or verbal-propositional features of language that are primarily disrupted by focal left brain injury that cause aphasic syndromes.

Prosody is a nonverbal or suprasegmental feature of language that conveys various levels of information to the listener, including linguistic, affective (attitudinal and emotional), dialectal, and idiosyncratic data.[31,42–45] The acoustic features underlying prosody include pitch, intonation, melody, cadence, loudness, timbre, tempo, stress, accent, and pauses. Although the preeminence of the propositional aspects of language is well accepted, developmental studies have established that the earliest building blocks of language are prosodic-intonational rather than verbal-segmental features.[46–50] As children acquire the verbal-segmental features of language, prosodic phenomena eventually become embedded and carried by the articulatory line.

Kinesics refers to the limb, body, and facial movements associated with language and communication.[51] Movements that are used for semiotic purposes,

* **ACKNOWLEDGMENT:** This work was supported in part by grants from the Merit Review Board, Medical Research Service, Department of Veterans Affairs, Washington, DC, and OCAST, Oklahoma City, Oklahoma, to Dr. Ross.

such as the "V for victory" sign, are classified as pantomime, since they convey specific semantic information; whereas movements used to color, emphasize, and embellish speech are classified as gestures.[51,52] Most spontaneous kinesic activity associated with discourse usually blends gestures and pantomime into a single movement.

Neurology of Prosody

The first in-depth inquiry into the neurology of prosody was initiated by Monrad-Krohn.[44,53] During World War II he cared for a native Norwegian woman who sustained a shrapnel wound to the left frontal area, causing an acute Broca's aphasia. The woman made an excellent recovery except for a lingering accent, which caused her great emotional distress during the Nazi occupation, since she was consistently mistaken for being German and was, consequently, socially ostracized. Her speech was reported to have preserved melody, as evidenced by her ability to sing, intone, and emote. The acquired foreign accent was due to inappropriate application of stresses and pauses to the articulatory line.

On the basis of this patient and others, Monrad-Krohn[44] divided prosody into three major components as indicated by the italicized words. *Intrinsic* (linguistic) prosody provides the means for using nonverbal features to enhance the linguistic functions of a language; for example, raising the intonation at the end of a statement to indicate a question, changing the stress and timing on certain segments of a phrase to clarify meaning [e.g., "the Redcoats are coming" (British regulars) versus "the red coats are coming" (red-colored coats)], or changing the stress on certain words and altering the pause structure to clarify potentially ambiguous syntax [e.g., "The man . . . and woman dressed in black . . . came to visit" (only the woman was dressed in black) versus "The man and woman dressed in black . . . came to visit" (both were dressed in black)].[31,43,45] Dialectal and idiosyncratic prosody are also to some degree subsumed by the term *intrinsic prosody* and refer to regional and individual differences in speech quality. *Intellectual* prosody imparts attitudinal information to discourse that may drastically alter meaning. For example, if the sentence "He is clever" is emphatically stressed on *is,* it becomes a resounding acknowledgment of the person's ability; whereas if the emphatic stress resides on *clever,* with a terminal rise in intonation, sarcasm becomes apparent. *Emotional* prosody injects primary types of emotions into speech, such as happiness, sadness, fear, and anger. The term *affective prosody* refers to the combination of attitudinal and emotional prosody. *Inarticulate* prosody is the use of certain paralinguistic nonverbal elements, such as grunts and sighs, to embellish discourse.

Monrad-Krohn[44] also described various clinical disorders of prosody. *Dysprosody* is a change in voice quality that gives rise to a foreign accent syndrome. Since it is encountered primarily in patients with fairly good recovery from motor types of aphasia, it is associated with left hemisphere lesions that alter the patient's dialectal and idiosyncratic aspects of prosody. *Aprosody* is the general lack of prosody encountered in Parkinson's disease as part of the akinesia, masked facies, and soft monotone voice. *Hyperprosody* refers to the excessive use of prosody observed in mania or in patients with Broca's aphasia who have very few words at their disposal but use them to their utmost to convey attitudes and emotions. Although Monrad-Krohn did not describe prosodic disorders from focal right brain damage, he did predict that disorders of prosodic comprehension should also be encountered in brain-damaged patients.

Recent clinical studies have shown that focal right brain damage may seriously impair, in various combinations, the production, comprehension, and repetition of the affective-prosodic elements of language without disrupting its propositional elements (see below).[8–10,12,13,16,17,19,22–25,27–30,35,37] These affective-prosodic components, when coupled with gestures, impart vitality to discourse and, in many instances, are far more important than the verbal-linguistic message. Various studies have shown that if a statement contains an affective-prosodic message that is at variance with its verbal-linguistic meaning, the prosodic message normally takes precedence in adults and to a lesser degree in children.[12,54–57] For example, if the sentence "I had a really great day" is spoken using irony it will be understood as communicating a meaning that is actually opposite to its linguistic content.

Neurology of Kinesics

Disturbances in the production and comprehension of pantomimal kinesics have been firmly linked to left brain damage.[57,58] Goodglass and Kaplan[59] proposed that pantomimal disorders in aphasics with significant comprehension deficits can be attributed to their general inability to comprehend symbols, whereas pantomimal disorders in aphasics without significant comprehension deficits can be attributed to ideomotor apraxia. Other investigators, however, have not shown such tight correlation of a specific pantomimal disturbance with a specific linguistic disturbance,[60–62] although all studies to date have found that disorders of pantomime are almost always the result of left hemisphere damage resulting in aphasic disturbances.[59–63]

Gestural kinesics, on the other hand, has not been well studied neurologically, although occasionally clinical researchers have mentioned that gestural activity is often preserved in aphasic patients.[51,52] The first paper to specifically address the possible relationship of gestures to right brain damage and loss of affective prosody was published in 1979 by Ross and Mesulam.[8] They observed that lesions of the right frontal operculum may cause complete loss of spontaneous gestural activity in the nonparalyzed right face and limbs without any disturbance in praxis. The suggestion was made, therefore, that gestural behavior as opposed to pantomime was a dominant function of the right hemisphere. Since then a number of studies have lent further support to this hypothesis by showing that the right hemisphere is not only specialized for producing gestures but also for comprehending their meaning.[9,22,27,64–67]

THE APROSODIAS

Although Hughlings-Jackson[52] suggested almost a hundred years ago that the right hemisphere may have a dominant role in emotional communication, the first clinical study of affective prosody was published in 1975 by Heilman et al.[24] They assessed the ability of patients with right and left hemisphere strokes in the posterior sylvian distribution to recognize the affective content of verbally neutral statements that were spoken with various emotional intonations. Patients with right brain damage were markedly impaired on the task when compared to normals and (mildly) aphasic patients with left brain damage. In a follow-up study, Tucker et al.[30] found that patients with right but not left brain damage also had great difficulty in inserting affective variation into verbally neutral sentences on request and on a repetition task.

In 1979, Ross and Mesulam[8] described two patients with infarctions of the right anterior suprasylvian region verified by computed tomography (CT). Neither patient was aphasic or apraxic, but both complained bitterly of their almost total inability to insert affective variation into their speech and gestural behavior. Both patients seemed to have no difficulty perceiving affective displays in others and both insisted that they could feel and experience emotions inwardly. Based on these patients and the previous publications by Heilman and associates,[24,30] it was hypothesized that (1) the right hemisphere was dominant for organizing the affective-prosodic components of language and gestural behavior and (2) the functional/anatomic organization of affective language in the right hemisphere was analogous to the organization of propositional language in the left hemisphere. An issue not resolved in the paper, however, was whether the prosodic deficits from right brain damage also involved the linguistic aspects of prosody. Subsequent studies by Weintraub et al.,[35] Heilman et al.,[23] and Danly et al.[68,69] have looked more carefully at this issue in both right and left brain–damaged patients. The composite data indicate that the linguistic features of prosody may be impaired by either right or left brain damage but that the affective components seem to be disrupted exclusively by right brain damage.

In 1981, Ross[27] approached the issue of whether the anatomic organization of affective language in the right hemisphere was, in fact, similar to the organization of propositional language in the left hemisphere. Ten patients with focal right brain damage, localized by CT, underwent a bedside assessment of their ability to modulate affective prosody and gestures in a manner similar to methods utilized for propositional language. Thus, the patients were examined qualitatively for (1) spontaneous use of affective prosody and gesturing during conversation, (2) ability to repeat verbally neutral sentences with affective variation, (3) ability to auditorily comprehend affective prosody, and (4) ability to visually comprehend gestures. All patients who had lesions bordering the right sylvian fissure had some disorder of affective language. Because specific combinations of affective-prosodic deficits occurred following circumscribed lesions in the right hemisphere, which were analogous to the functional-anatomic clustering of aphasic deficits observed after focal left brain damage,[7] these particular syndromes were called

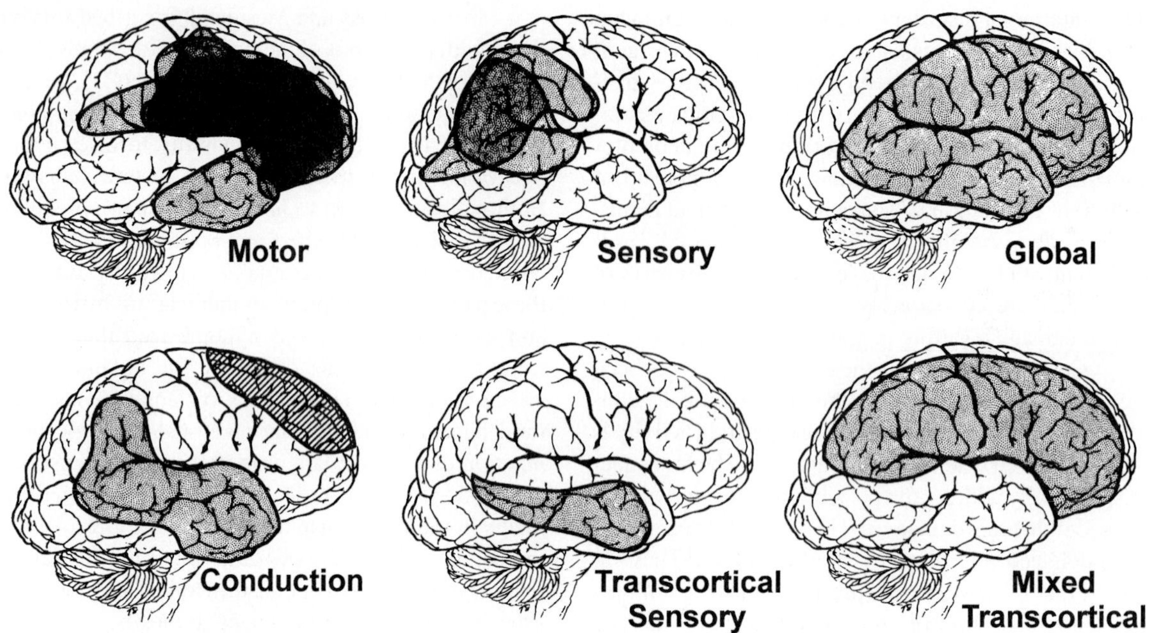

Figure 59-1

Composite cortical distribution of published CT scan lesions associated with various aprosodias[22,27] projected onto a lateral template of the right hemisphere. Stippled areas represent ischemic infarctions except for the patient with transcortical sensory aprosodia, who had a discrete hemorrhage without edema. Although the stippled lesion causing conduction aprosodia should have produced a sensory aprosodia, an analogous lesion in the left hemisphere may occasionally cause conduction rather than Wernicke's (sensory) aphasia[7,108,109]; the patient represented by the hatchmarked lesion in the lower left panel had a mild conduction aprosodia that evolved from an initial motor-type aprosodia.[27]

aprosodias and the same modifiers were applied for classification purposes as those used in the aphasias (Fig. 59-1, Table 59-1).[27] In a follow-up study, using blinded evaluations of affective language, Gorelick and Ross[22] corroborated that patients with focal right brain lesions display various deficits in affective language that corresponded with the aprosodic classifications and localizations published previously. They also reported that the prevalence of aprosodia following right brain damage was equal to the prevalence of aphasia following left brain damage, thus underscoring that the aprosodias are common rather than esoteric syndromes.

Although quantitative acoustic and neuropsychological testing paradigms exist for assessing affective prosody and communication,[26,28,29] clinicians can, with some practice and familiarization, readily incorporate an assessment of aprosodia into their bedside neurologic examination much as one assesses patients for aphasia.

Spontaneous Affective Prosody and Gesturing During the interview, observations are made as to whether the patient gestures and imparts affect into his or her spontaneous conversation, especially when asked emotionally loaded questions about current illness or about past emotional experiences. Overall, loudness or softness of speech should be ignored, with attention paid to intonational variation in voice and gesturing to determine if emotional information appropriate to the situation under discussion is incorporated into the patient's discourse.

Repetition of Affective Prosody A declarative sentence, void of emotional words, is used to test

Table 59-1
The aprosodias

Type of aprosodia	*Spontaneous affective prosody and gesturing*	*Affective prosodic repetition*	*Affective prosodic comprehension*	*Gestural comprehension*
Motor*	poor	poor	good	good
Sensory*	good	poor	poor	poor
Conduction	good	poor	good	good
Global*	poor	poor	poor	poor
Transcortical motor	poor	good	good	good
Transcortical sensory*	good	good	poor	poor
Agesic†	good	good	good	poor
Mixed transcortical	poor	good	poor	poor

*Indicates aprosodias having anatomic correlations to right hemisphere lesions that are analogous to left hemisphere lesions resulting in similar types of aphasia (see Fig. 59-1).

†Agesic aprosodia is analogous to anomic aphasia,[7] initially described by Bowers and Heilman.[107]

affective repetition. After producing a token sentence using, for example, a happy, sad, tearful, disinterested, angry, or surprised tone of voice, the examiner immediately asks the patient to repeat the sentence. Repetition should be judged on how well the patient imitates the affective prosody of the examiner; raising or lowering the overall loudness of voice, slightly raising the voice at the end of a statement to indicate a question rather than surprise, or producing an incorrect emotion should not be considered a correct response.

Comprehension of Affective Prosody A declarative statement, void of emotional words, is used. The examiner injects the sentence with different affects and asks the patient to either verbally identify the emotion or choose the correct answer from a verbal list of five choices. Standing behind the patient during this assessment avoids giving the patient visual clues through gestural behaviors.

Comprehension of Gestures This is accomplished by standing in front of the patient and conveying a particular affective state using only gestural activity involving the face and limbs. As with affective-prosodic comprehension, the patient is asked to either identify the emotion verbally or, if necessary, choose the correct answer from a verbal list of five choices.

Using the bedside evaluation outlined above, aprosodias may be identified and subtyped as shown in Table 59-1. CT correlates of aprosodias involving a predominantly cortical-subcortical distribution are presented in Fig. 59-1. For detailed clinical descriptions of the aprosodias, the indicated references should be consulted.[22,27,37]

To date, aprosodias resulting from predominantly cortical lesions, assessed early poststroke (2 to 8 weeks), before long-term recovery of deficits occurs, appear to have a functional-anatomic organization in the right hemisphere analogous to aphasias caused by left hemisphere injury (see Figs. 59-1 and 59-2).[16,17,22,25,27,70,71] Other researchers, however, have not confirmed this observation. Some, such as Baum and Pell,[72,73] have studied patients approximately 1 to 4 years poststroke, which probably confounds their data because of long-term recovery mechanisms, much like what has been reported in the aphasia literature.[74] Others, such as Bradvik et al.,[75] have studied patients with predominantly lacunar-type infarctions that were assessed many months poststroke (mean of 13.5 months). In addition, some of the recovery patterns observed in patients with aprosodia[27] are similar to those described with aphasias,[7,76] and subcortical lesions in the right hemisphere may produce aprosodias,[22,27,37,77] just as subcortical lesions in the left hemisphere may produce aphasias.[78–80] There have also been case reports of crossed aprosodia, in which a strongly right-handed patient becomes aprosodic but not aphasic following a left hemisphere stroke, similar to cases of crossed aphasia in which a strongly right-handed patient becomes aphasic following a

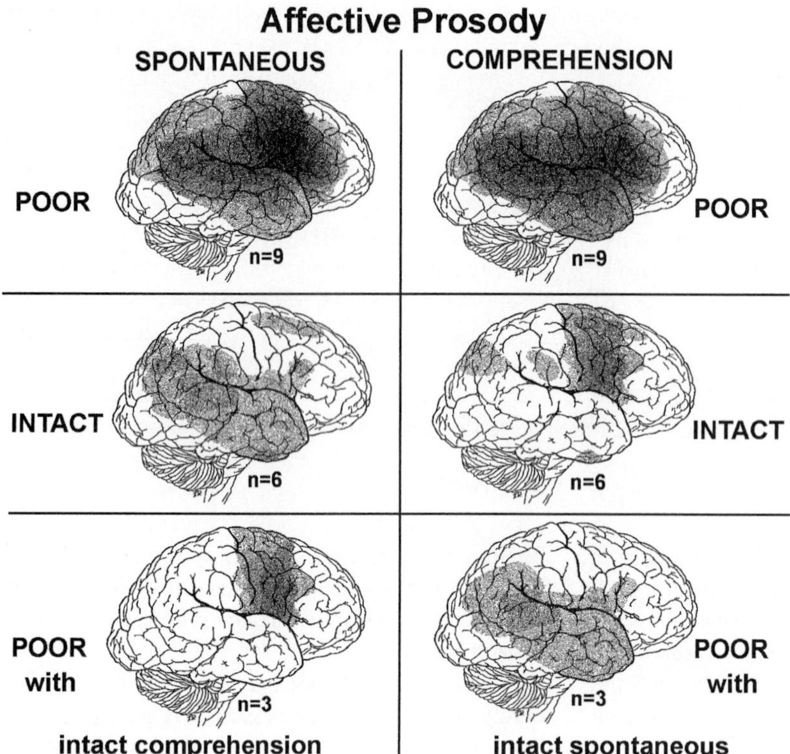

Figure 59-2 *Cortical distributions of ischemic strokes observed on MRI scan in 22 patients with right unilateral brain damage[71] classified by affective-prosodic performance on the Aprosodia Battery[96] based on spontaneous affective prosody and affective-prosodic comprehension. As in the case of aphasic deficits from left hemisphere lesions,[7] injury to the right inferior frontal region causes loss of spontaneous affective prosody in speech (analogous to aphasic nonfluency), whereas injury to the posterosuperior temporal lobe causes loss of affective-prosodic comprehension (analogous to aphasic loss of comprehension).*

right hemisphere stroke.[81] Last, acquired aprosodias in children[82] and developmental disorders of affective prosody associated with aberrant psychosocial development resulting from early right brain damage[83–85] have been published that are comparable to the syndromes of acquired aphasia in children and with developmental dyslexia.

Hemispheric Lateralization of Affective Prosody

The terms *dominant* and *lateralized* are used interchangeably in the literature to describe brain function, even though they have overlapping but somewhat different neurologic implications. A brain function is considered dominant if a unilateral lesion produces a behavioral deficit that subtends both sides of space,[86,87] a criterion easily met by the various aphasic and aprosodic syndromes. For a function to be strongly lateralized, however, it must also be shown that the behavioral deficit does not occur following lesions of the opposite hemisphere. In this regard, it is of historic interest that, soon after his initial discovery that damage to the foot of the left third frontal convolution caused loss of articulate speech,[5] Broca[88] reported that right hemisphere lesions did not result in the loss of articulate speech, thus establishing that articulation was both a dominant and highly lateralized function of the left hemisphere.[89] Unlike the aphasias, however, the degree of lateralization of affective prosody has not been established, since various publications have documented affective-prosodic disturbances in aphasic patients with left hemisphere strokes. In some instances authors have assumed incorrectly that all prosodic systems—intrinsic, affective, idiolectal, and dialectal, rather than just affective prosody—are modulated by the right hemisphere.[90,91] Nevertheless, certain publications[92–94,95] have reported considerable disturbances in the production and comprehension of affective prosody in left brain–damaged patients with severe aphasias, suggesting that affective prosody may not be strongly lateralized to the right hemisphere even though it appears to be a dominant function of that hemisphere.

De Bleser and Poeck[92] examined prosodic intonation in severe global aphasics whose speech output was restricted to one or two recurring syllables. Their intonations tended to be very stereotypic, bringing into question the original observations by Hughlings-Jackson[52] that severely aphasic patients are able to communicate through emotional channels. Schlanger et al.[93] reported affective-prosodic comprehension deficits in aphasics in opposition to the original studies by Heilman et al.[24] On reviewing the data published by both groups, it would appear that the discrepancy is most likely attributable to the distribution and severity of aphasic deficits; Heilman et al.[24] used patients with relatively preserved comprehension, whereas Schlanger et al.[93] used patients with significant deficits in verbal comprehension. More importantly, however, when Schlanger et al.[93] sorted their patients into "low-verbal" and "high-verbal" groups, the low-verbal aphasics were significantly more impaired on the emotional comprehension task than the high-verbal aphasics. Similarly, Seron et al.[94] also reported a significant positive correlation between scores of affective performance and verbal comprehension in aphasic patients. This would suggest, therefore, that verbal impairments per se rather than a primary defect in affective processing underlie deficient performances on affective comprehension tasks in aphasic patients.

To further address this issue, Ross and colleagues[96] developed an Aprosodia Battery to assess affective prosody in a series of right and left brain–damaged (RBD, LBD) patients using a quantitative testing paradigm in which the verbal-articulatory demands were progressively reduced by using token sentences in which various emotions are carried by words, a repeated monosyllable ("ba ba ba ba ba ba"), and an asyllabic articulation ("aaaaaahhhhhhh"). In the LBD patients, reducing the verbal-articulatory load caused statistically robust improvement in their ability to comprehend affective prosody and to produce affective prosody on a repetition task, whereas no improvement occurred in the RBD patients (Fig. 59-3). Interestingly, the performance of LBD patients was not correlated with the presence, severity, or type of aphasic deficit(s).

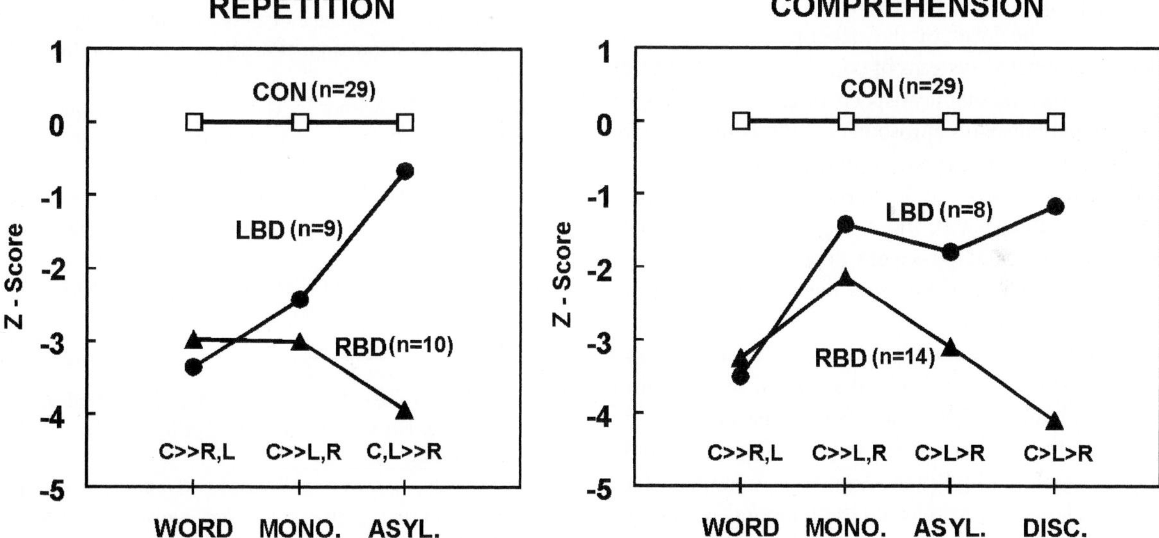

Figure 59-3
Patterns of deficits found on the Aprosodia Battery[96] in 22 RBD and 21 LBD patients with unilateral ischemic strokes compared to 29 controls.[71] Only LBD and RBD patients who had Z-scores of < -1.64, compared to controls on any repetition subtask or any comprehension subtask were included in the figure to focus attention on abnormal performance. Mono. = monosyllabic; Asyl. = asyllabic; Disc. = discrimination subtasks; C = Controls; R = RBD; and L = LBD with post hoc statistical relations for each subtask (alpha = 0.01) shown just above the abscissa. (See text and Ross et al.[96] for details about construction of the Aprosodia Battery and reasons for testing subjects under reduced verbal-articulatory demands.)

Based on functional-anatomic correlations for both spontaneous affective prosody and affective-prosodic repetition, deep white matter lesions located below the supplementary motor area that disrupt interhemispheric connections coursing through the midrostral corpus callosum seem to contribute to affective-prosodic deficits that are both additive and independent of any aphasic deficits. These findings, therefore, sustain the hypothesis that affective prosody is both a dominant and a lateralized function of the right hemisphere and lend strong support to research by Blonder et al.[10] and Bowers et al.[12,13] suggesting that RBD causes loss of affective-communicative representations as the theoretical basis for the aprosodias, similar to LBD causing the loss of verbal-syntactic representations as the theoretical basis for the aphasias.[96]

Neurology of Emotions

The aprosodias represent disturbances of graded emotional behavior encompassing both affective prosody and gestures. These behaviors are organized predominantly at the level of the neocortex as part of the language-related systems of communication. Since the experiential and display aspects of emotions are available to patients with aprosodia,[27,97,98] seemingly paradoxical behaviors may occur during clinical and social interactions. The most dramatic examples reported to date are patients with motor-types of aprosodia who are also experiencing severe depression. Because of their aprosodia, they exhibit a flat affective demeanor even when discussing highly emotional issues, such as suicide.[97,98] Consequently, their verbal reports of emotional distress can easily be discounted by both clinicians and family. Other patients may verbally deny depression but have vegetative indicators of melancholia that respond readily to antidepressant treatment. Current evidence has implicated the temporal limbic system, in particular the amygdala, as the nodal point of a neuroanatomic network for experiencing emotions and related phenomena.[99–103] Patients with motor or global aprosodia may also be observed to display extremes of emotions during very sad, happy, or angry situations despite their otherwise affectively flat demeanor.[22,27,97,98] These displays tend to be all or none, uncontrollable, and socially embarrassing, giving them the quality of pathologic regulation of affect, similar to behaviors encountered in patients with pseudobulbar palsy.[7,104,105] Thus, the organization of emotional displays must also be modulated by areas outside the right neocortical motor system. The critical areas seem to reside in the temporal limbic system and basal forebrain, which have descending connections to alpha motor neurons through hypothalamus, periaqueductal gray, locus ceruleus, subceruleus, and the median raphe,[98,106] since lesions and epileptic discharges in these regions are known to induce sham emotional displays that usually take the form of pathologic regulation of affect.[104] For a more complete review of the neurology of emotions, the reader is referred to Chaps. 56 and 57 in this book and a recent article by Ross et al.[102] addressing the differential hemispheric lateralization of emotions and related behaviors based on the concept that emotions may be classified as having either primary or social properties.

REFERENCES

1. Bandler R, Keay KA: Columnar organization in the midbrain periaqueductal gray and the integration of emotional expression. *Prog Brain Res* 107:285–300, 1996.
2. Jurgens U, Zwirner P: The role of the periaqueductal grey in limbic and neocortical vocal fold control. *Neuroreport* 7:2921–2923, 1996.
3. Davis PJ, Zhang SP, Winkworth A, Bandler RJ: Neural control of vocalization: Respiratory and emotional influences. *J Voice* 10:23–38, 1996.
4. Jurgens U: Neural pathways underlying vocal control. *Neurosci Biobehav Rev* 26:235–258, 2002.
5. Broca P: Remarques sur le siege de la faculte du langage articule, suives d'une observation d'aphemie. *Bull Soc Anthropol Paris* 6:330–337, 1861. (Translated in von Bonin G: *The Cerebral Cortex*. Springfield, IL: Charles C Thomas, 1960.)
6. Wernicke C: *Der Aphasische Symptomencomplex. Eine Psychologische Studie auf Anatomischer Basis.* Breslau: Cohn & Weigert, 1874. (Translated in Eggert GH: *Wernicke's Works on Aphasia: Sourcebook and Review*. The Hague: Mouton, 1977.)
7. Benson DF: *Aphasia, Alexia and Agraphia*. Edinburgh: Churchill Livingstone, 1979.
8. Ross ED, Mesulam MM: Dominant language functions of the right hemisphere? Prosody and emotional gesturing. *Arch Neurol* 36:144–148, 1979.
9. Benowitz LI, Bear DM, Rosenthal R, et al: Hemispheric specialization in nonverbal communication. *Cortex* 19:5–14, 1983.

10. Blonder LX, Bowers D, Heilman KM: The role of the right hemisphere in emotional communication. *Brain* 114:1115–1127, 1991.
11. Bottini G, Corcoran R, Sterzi R, et al: The role of the right hemisphere in the interpretation of figurative aspects of language: A positron emission tomography activation study. *Brain* 117:1241–1253, 1994.
12. Bowers D, Coslett HB, Bauer RM, et al: Comprehension of emotional prosody following unilateral hemispheric lesions: Processing defect versus distraction defect. *Neuropsychologia* 25:317–328, 1987.
13. Bowers D, Bauer RM, Heilman KM: The nonverbal affect lexicon: Theoretical perspectives from neuropsychological studies of affect perception. *Neuropsychology* 7:433–444, 1993.
14. Brownell HH, Potter HH, Bihrle A: Inference deficits in right brain-damaged patients. *Brain Lang* 29:310–321, 1986.
15. Brownell HH, Potter HH, Michelow D, Gardner H: Sensitivity to lexical denotation and connotation in brain-damaged patients: A double dissociation? *Brain Lang* 22:253–265, 1984.
16. Darby DG: Sensory aprosodia: A clinical clue to lesions of the inferior division of the right middle cerebral artery? *Neurology* 34:567–572, 1993.
17. Denes G, Caldognetto EM, Semenza C, et al: Discrimination and identification of emotions in human voice by brain damaged subjects. *Acta Neurol Scand* 69:154–162, 1984.
18. Edmondson JA, Ross ED, Chan JL, Seibert GB: The effect of right-brain damage on acoustical measures of affective prosody in Taiwanese patients. *J Phonet* 15:219–233, 1987.
19. Ehlers L, Dalby M: Appreciation of emotional expressions in the visual and auditory modality in normal and brain-damaged patients. *Acta Neurol Scand* 76:251–256, 1987.
20. Emmorey K: The neurologic substrates for the prosodic aspects of speech. *Brain Lang* 30:305–320, 1987.
21. Foldi NC: Appreciation of pragmatic interpretations of indirect commands: Comparison of right and left brain-damaged patients. *Brain Lang* 31:88–108, 1987.
22. Gorelick PB, Ross ED: The aprosodias: Further functional-anatomic evidence for the organization of affective language in the right hemisphere. *J Neurol Neurosurg Psychiatry* 50:553–560, 1987.
23. Heilman KM, Bowers D, Speedie L, Coslett HB: Comprehension of affective and nonaffective speech. *Neurology* 34:917–921, 1984.
24. Heilman KM, Scholes R, Watson RT: Auditory affective agnosia: Disturbed comprehension of affective speech. *J Neurol Neurosurg Psychiatry* 38:69–72, 1975.
25. Hughes CP, Chan JL, Su MS: Aprosodia in Chinese patients with right cerebral hemisphere lesions. *Arch Neurol* 40:732–736, 1983.
26. Kent RD, Rosenbeck JC: Prosodic disturbances and neurologic lesion. *Brain Lang* 15:259–291, 1982.
27. Ross ED: The aprosodias: Functional-anatomic organization of the affective components of language in the right hemisphere. *Arch Neurol* 38:561–569, 1981.
28. Ross ED, Edmondson JA, Seibert GB, Homan RW: Acoustic analysis of affective prosody during right-sided Wada test: A within-subjects verification of the right hemisphere's role in language. *Brain Lang* 33:128–145, 1987.
29. Shapiro B, Danly M: The role of the right hemisphere in the control of speech prosody in propositional and affective contexts. *Brain Lang* 25:19–36, 1985.
30. Tucker DM, Watson RT, Heilman KM: Discrimination and evocation of affectively intoned speech in patients with right parietal disease. *Neurology* 27:947–950, 1977.
31. Van Lancker D: Cerebral lateralization of pitch cues in the linguistic signal. *Int J Hum Commun* 1980; 13:201–277.
32. Van Lancker D: The neurology of proverbs. *Behav Neurol* 3:169–187, 1990.
33. Van Lancker D, Kempler D: Comprehension of familiar phrases by left- but not right-hemisphere damaged patients. *Brain Lang* 32:256–277, 1987.
34. Wapner W, Hamby S, Gardner H: The role of the right hemisphere in the apprehension of complex linguistic materials. *Brain Lang* 14:15–33, 1981.
35. Weintraub S, Mesulam MM, Kramer L: Disturbances in prosody. *Arch Neurol* 38:742–744, 1981.
36. Winner E, Gardner H: The comprehension of metaphor in brain-damaged patients. *Brain* 100:717–729, 1977.
37. Wolfe GI, Ross ED: Sensory aprosodia with left hemiparesis from subcortical infarction. Right hemisphere analogue of sensory-type aphasia with right hemiparesis? *Arch Neurol* 44:661–671, 1987.
38. Meyer M, Alter K, Friederici AD, et al: fMRI reveals brain regions mediating slow prosodic modulations in spoken sentences. *Hum Brain* 17:73–88, 2002.
39. Ferstl E, von Cramon D: The role of coherence and cohesion in text comprehension: An event-related fMRI study. *Cogn Brain Res* 11:325–340, 2001.
40. Bookheimer S: Functional MRI of language. *Ann Rev Neurosci* 25:151–188, 2002.
41. Ladefoged P: *A Course in Phonetics*. New York: Harcourt Brace Jovanich, 1975.
42. Kent RD, Read C: *The Acoustic Analysis of Speech*. San Diego, CA: Singular Publishing Group, 1992.

43. Crystal D: *The English Tone of Voice.* New York: St Martin's Press, 1975.
44. Monrad-Krohn GH: The third element of speech: Prosody and its disorders, in Halpern L (ed): *Problems in Dynamic Neurology.* Jerusalem: Hebrew University Press, 1963, pp 101–118.
45. Van Lancker D, Canter GJ, Terbeek D: Disambiguation of ditropic sentences: Acoustic and phonetic cues. *J Speech Hear Res* 24:330–335, 1981.
46. Crystal D: Non-segmental phonology in language acquisition: Review of the issues. *Lingua* 32:1–45, 1973.
47. Lewis A: *Infant Speech: A Study of the Beginnings of Language.* New York: Harcourt Brace, 1936.
48. Werker JF, Tees RC: Cross-language speech perception: Evidence for perceptual reorganization during the first year of life. *Infant Behav Devel* 7:49–63, 1984.
49. Moon C, Cooper RP, Fifer WP: Two-day-old infants prefer their native language. *Infant Behav Dev* 16:495–500, 1993.
50. Dehaene-Lambbertz G, Houston G: Faster orientation latencies toward native language in two-month-old infants. *Lang Speech* 41:21–43, 1998.
51. Critchley M: *The Language of Gesture.* London: Edward Arnold, 1939.
52. Hughlings-Jackson J: On affectations of speech from diseases of the brain. *Brain* 38:106–174, 1915.
53. Monrad-Krohn GH: Dysprosody or altered "melody of language." *Brain* 70:405–415, 1948.
54. Ackerman BP: Form and function in children's understanding of ironic utterances. *J Exp Child Psychol* 35:487–508, 1983.
55. Bolinger D (ed): *Intonation.* Hardmondsworth: Penguin Press, 1972.
56. De Groot A: Structural linguistics and syntactic laws. *Word* 5:1–12, 1949.
57. De Renzi E, Motti F, Nichelli P: Imitating gestures: A quantitative approach to ideomotor apraxia. *Arch Neurol* 37:6–10, 1980.
58. Gainotti G, Lemmo M: Comprehension of symbolic gestures in aphasia. *Brain Lang* 3:451–460, 1976.
59. Goodglass H, Kaplan E: Disturbance of gesture and pantomime in aphasia. *Brain* 86:703–720, 1963.
60. Cicone M, Wapner W, Foldi N, et al: The relationship between gesture and language in aphasic communication. *Brain Lang* 8:324–349, 1979.
61. Delis D, Foldi NS, Hambe S, et al: A note on temporal relations between language and gestures. *Brain Lang* 8:350–354, 1979.
62. Feyereisen P, Seron X: Nonverbal communication and aphasia: A review (in 2 parts; I. Comprehension, II. Expression). *Brain Lang* 16:191–212, 213–236, 1982.
63. Seron X, Van der Kaa MA, Remitz A, Van der Linden M: Pantomime interpretation and aphasia. *Neuropsychologia* 17:661–668, 1979.
64. Borod JC, Koff E, Lorch MP, Nicholas M: Channels of emotional communication in patients with unilateral brain damage. *Arch Neurol* 42:345–348, 1985.
65. Borod JC, Koff E, Perlman M, et al: The expression and perception of facial emotion on focal lesion patients. *Neuropsychologia* 24:169–180, 1986.
66. Cicone M, Wapner W, Gardner H: Sensitivity to emotional expressions and situations in organic patients. *Cortex* 16:145–158, 1980.
67. DeKosky ST, Heilman KM, Bowers D, Valenstein E: Recognition and discrimination of emotional faces and pictures. *Brain Lang* 9:206–214, 1980.
68. Danly M, Cooper WE, Shapiro B: Fundamental frequency, language processing, and linguistic structure in Wernicke's aphasia. *Brain Lang* 19:1–24, 1983.
69. Danly M, Shapiro B: Speech prosody in Broca's aphasia. *Brain Lang* 16:171–190, 1982.
70. Starkstein SE, Federoff JP, Price TR, et al: Neuropsychological and neuroradiologic correlates of emotional prosody comprehension. *Neurology* 44:515–522, 1994.
71. Ross ED, Orbelo DM, Burgard M, Hansel S: Functional-anatomic correlates of aprosodic deficits in patients with right brain damage. *Neurology* 50(suppl 4):A363, 1998.
72. Baum SR, Pell MD: Production of affective and linguistic prosody by brain-damaged patients. *Aphasiology* 11:177–198, 1997.
73. Pell MD, Baum SR: The ability to perceive and comprehend intonation in linguistic and affective contexts by brain-damaged patients. *Brain Lang* 57:80–99, 1997.
74. Goodglass HG: *Understanding Aphasia.* New York: Academic Press, 1993, chap. 3.
75. Bradvik B, Dravins C, Holtas S, et al: Disturbances of speech prosody following right hemisphere infarcts. *Acta Neurol Scand* 84:114–126, 1991.
76. Kertesz A: *Aphasia and Associated Disorders.* New York: Grune & Stratton, 1979.
77. Ross ED, Harney JH, de Lacoste C, Purdy P: How the brain integrates affective and propositional language into a unified brain function. Hypotheses based on clinicopathological correlations. *Arch Neurol* 38:745–748, 1981.
78. Alexander MP, LoVerme SR: Aphasia after left hemispheric intracerebral hemorrhage. *Neurology* 30:1193–1202, 1980.
79. Damasio AR, Damasio H, Rizzo M, et al: Aphasia with nonhemorrhagic lesions in the basal ganglia and internal capsule. *Arch Neurol* 39:15–20, 1982.

80. Naeser MA, Alexander MP, Helm-Estabrooks N, et al: Aphasia with predominantly subcortical lesion sites: Description of three capsular/putaminal aphasia syndromes. *Arch Neurol* 39:2–14, 1982.
81. Ross ED, Anderson B, Morgan-Fisher A: Crossed aprosodia in strongly dextral patients. *Arch Neurol* 46: 206–209, 1989.
82. Bell WL, Davis DL, Morgan-Fisher A, Ross ED: Acquired aprosodias in children. *J Child Neurol* 5:19–26, 1989.
83. Weintraub S, Mesulam MM: Developmental learning disabilities of the right hemisphere: Emotional, interpersonal, and cognitive components. *Arch Neurol* 40:463–468, 1983.
84. Manaoch DS, Sandson TA, Weintraub S: The developmental social-emotional processing disorder is associated with right hemisphere abnormalities. *Neuropsychiatr Neuropsychol Behav Neurol* 8:99–105, 1995.
85. Voeller KKS: Right hemisphere deficit syndrome in children. *Amer J Psychol* 143:1004–1009, 1986.
86. Denny-Brown D, Banker BQ: Amorphosynthesis from left parietal lesion. *Arch Neurol Psychiatry* 71:302–313, 1954.
87. Denny-Brown D, Meyer JS, Horenstein S: The significance of perceptual rivalry resulting from parietal lesion. *Brain* 75:433–471, 1952.
88. Broca P: Du siege de la faculte du langage articule. *Bull Soc Anthropol Paris* 6:337–393, 1865.
89. Lecours AR, Lhermitte F: Historical review: From Franz Gall to Pierre Marie, in Lecours AR, Lhermitte F, Bryans B (eds): *Aphasiology.* London: Baillière Tindall, 1983, pp 12–14.
90. Ryalls J: Concerning right-hemisphere dominance for affective language. *Arch Neurol* 45:337–338, 1988.
91. Ross ED: Prosody and brain lateralization: Fact vs fancy or is it all just semantics? *Arch Neurol* 45:338–339, 1988.
92. de Bleser R, Poeck K: Analysis of prosody in the spontaneous speech of patients with CV-recurring utterances. *Cortex* 21:405–416, 1985.
93. Schlanger BB, Schlanger P, Gerstmann LJ: The perception of emotionally toned sentences by right hemisphere-damaged and aphasic subjects. *Brain Lang* 3:396–403, 1976.
94. Seron X, van der Kaa MA, van der Linden M, et al: Decoding paralinguistic signals: Effect of semantic and prosodic cues on aphasic comprehension. *J Commun Disord* 15:223–231, 1982.
95. Cancelliere AEB, Kertesz A: Lesion localization in acquired deficits of emotional expression and comprehension. *Brain Lang* 13:133–147, 1990.
96. Ross ED, Stark RD, Yenkosky JP: Lateralization of affective prosody in brain and the callosal integration of hemispheric language functions. *Brain Lang* 56:27–54, 1997.
97. Ross ED, Rush AJ: Diagnosis and neuroanatomical correlates of depression in brain-damaged patients: Implications for a neurology of depression. *Arch Gen Psychiatry* 38:1344–1354, 1981.
98. Ross ED, Stewart R: Pathological display of affect in patients with depression and right focal brain damage: An alternative mechanism. *J Nerv Ment Dis* 175:165–172, 1978.
99. Gloor P: Experiential phenomena of temporal lobe epilepsy: Facts and hypothesis. *Brain* 113:1673–1694, 1990.
100. Gloor P, Olivier A, Quesney LF, et al: The role of the limbic system in experiential phenomena of temporal lobe epilepsy. *Ann Neurol* 12:129–144, 1982.
101. LeDoux JE: Emotion and the amygdala, in Aggleton JP (ed): *The Amygdala: Neurobiological Aspects of Emotion, Memory, and Mental Dysfunction.* New York: Wiley-Liss, 1992, pp 339–351.
102. Ross ED, Homan RW, Buck R: Differential hemispheric lateralization of primary and social emotions: Implications for developing a comprehensive neurology for emotion, repression, and the subconscious. *Neuropsychiatr Neuropsychol Behav Neurol* 7:1–19, 1994.
103. Zola-Morgan S, Squire LR, Alvarez-Royo P, Clower RP: Independence of memory functions and emotional behavior: Separate contributions of the hippocampal formation and the amygdala. *Hippocampus* 1:207–220, 1991.
104. Poeck K: Pathophysiology of emotional disorders associated with brain damage, in Vinken PJ, Bruyn GW (eds): *Handbook of Clinical Neurology.* Amsterdam: North-Holland, 1969, vol 3, pp 343–367.
105. Wilson SAK: Some problems in neurology: II. Pathological laughing and crying. *J Neurol Psychopathol* 4:299–333, 1924.
106. Kuypers HGJM: A new look at the organization of the motor system. *Prog Brain Res* 57:381–403, 1982.
107. Bowers D, Heilman KM: Dissociation between the processing of affective and nonaffective faces: A case study. *J Clin Neuropsychol* 6:367–379, 1984.
108. Benson DF, Sheremata WA, Bouchard R, et al: Conduction aphasia: A clinicopathologic study. *Arch Neurol* 28:339–346, 1973.
109. Damasio H, Damasio AR: The anatomical basis of conduction aphasia. *Brain* 103:337–350, 1980.

Chapter 60

VIOLENCE AND THE BRAIN

Jonathan M. Silver
Karen E. Anderson
Stuart C. Yudofsky

Explosive and violent behavior has long been associated with neuropsychiatric disorders. These episodes range in severity from mild irritability to severe outbursts that result in damage to property or assaults on others. A full discussion of the neuropsychiatry of violent behavior and the assessment and treatment of aggression is beyond the scope of this chapter (see Refs. 1 to 4 for a review of unusual organic causes of violent behavior). In this chapter, the authors review several of the major neuropsychiatric conditions associated with aggressive and violent behavior, summarize the major neurobiologic findings, and outline treatment procedures.

SELECT MEDICAL CONDITIONS ASSOCIATED WITH VIOLENT BEHAVIOR

Dementia

Alzheimer's disease, the most common type of dementia, often causes behavioral changes along with memory loss. Among a sample of outpatients with Alzheimer's disease, Reisberg and coworkers[5] reported that 48 percent exhibited agitation, 30 percent violent behavior, and 24 percent verbal outbursts, which together accounted for the most common behavioral problems in this population. Devanand et al.[6] followed a sample of mild to moderate Alzheimer's disease patients over 5 years to look at persistence of behavioral disturbances. Over 90 percent of these patients lived at home. The investigators found that agitation was the most common and persistent symptom; agitation and physical aggression were both likely to increase in prevalence over time. In a recent nursing home study, over 80 percent of residents displayed activity disturbances or aggression, and these symptoms were often associated with psychosis or depression.[7]

Traumatic Brain Injury

Aggression is highly prevalent in both the acute and chronic recovery stages from traumatic brain injury. In the acute recovery period, 35 to 96 percent of patients are reported to have exhibited agitated behavior. After the acute recovery phase, irritability or bad temper is common. In follow-up periods ranging from 1 to 15 years after injury, these behaviors occurred in 31 to 71 percent of patients who had experienced severe traumatic brain injury.[1] A small study of death row inmates found that 75 percent had a history of traumatic brain injury.[8] Prediction of which patients will become aggressive after brain injury is challenging. Risk factors may include irritability, impulsivity, and a premorbid history of aggression; neuropsychological test performance does not consistently predict propensity toward violence in brain-injured patients.[9]

Epilepsy

Studies of the emotional and psychiatric syndromes associated with epilepsy have documented an increase in hostility, irritability, and aggression interictally.[10] In a retrospective survey of aggressive and nonaggressive patients with temporal lobe epilepsy, Herzberg and Fenwick[11] found that aggressive behavior was associated with early onset of seizures, a long duration of behavioral problems, and male gender. A study in a residential facility of severely impaired epileptic patients found that 27 percent were aggressive in the course of 1 year.[12] Younger age was a predictor of violent behavior. Psychosis occurred in some cases of violence but was not a major predictor. Other factors such as disease duration, intellectual impairment, abnormalities noted on magnetic resonance imaging (MRI), mobility, and seizure frequency were not predictive of aggression in these patients.

Mental Retardation

Those patients who have mental retardation and require institutionalization frequently exhibit aggressive behaviors. In a group of severely to profoundly mentally retarded individuals, approximately 33 percent were irritable and 20 percent were injurious to themselves.[13] In a survey of patients in community residences or institutions for the mentally retarded, 30 to 40 percent of the residents showed either disruptive behaviors or injury to self, others, or property.[14] An English regional total population study of behavioral problems in people with mental retardation found aggression in 7 percent of mentally retarded individuals and destructive behavior in over 4 percent.[15]

EVALUATION

Characteristics of Outbursts

Aggressive outbursts that result from organic brain dysfunction have typical characteristics.[16] These include the reactive, nonreflective, nonpurposeful nature of the outbursts. Incidents are explosive and periodic. The diagnostic category in the fourth edition of the APA's *Diagnostic and Statistical Manual* (DSM-IV) is "Personality Change Due to a General Medical Condition."[17] Patients with aggressive behavior would be specified as "Aggressive Type."

Differential Diagnosis

Patients who exhibit aggressive behavior require a thorough assessment. It is important to assess systematically the presence of concurrent neuropsychiatric disorders, since this may guide subsequent treatment. Thus, the clinician must be prepared to diagnose psychosis, depression, mania, mood lability, or anxiety. Evaluation for intellectual impairment and learning disabilities using neuropsychological testing can be helpful. Seizure disorders should also be considered, and a sleep-deprived electroencephalogram (EEG) may be helpful in more subtle cases. Other concurrent neurologic conditions—including dementia, central nervous system neoplasms, traumatic brain injury, cerebrovascular disease, Huntington's disease, epilepsy, infectious conditions with central nervous system involvement (e.g., human immunodeficiency virus), endocrine conditions (e.g., hypothyroidism, hypo- and hyperadrenalcorticalism), and autoimmune conditions with central nervous system involvement (e.g., systemic lupus erythematosus)—should also be ruled out.[2,4,10]

Medication Effects

Drug effects and side effects commonly result in disinhibition or irritability.[1,2] By far the most common drug associated with aggression is alcohol, during both intoxication and withdrawal. Stimulating drugs—such as cocaine and amphetamines, as well as the stimulating antidepressants—may produce severe anxiety and agitation in patients with or without brain lesions. Antipsychotic medications often increase agitation through anticholinergic side effects, and agitation and irritability usually accompany severe akathisia. Many other drugs may produce confusional states, especially anticholinergic medications that cause agitated delirium.[18]

Psychosocial Aspects

Psychosocial factors are important in the expression of aggressive behavior. Certain brain-injured patients become aggressive only in specific circumstances, as in the presence of particular family members. This suggests that the patient maintains some level of control over aggressive behaviors and that the level of control may be modified by behavioral therapeutic techniques. Most families require professional support to adjust to the impulsive behavior of a violent relative with organic dyscontrol of aggression.

NEUROBIOLOGY OF AGGRESSION

Neuroanatomy

Hypothalamus Many areas of the brain are involved in the production and mediation of aggressive behavior, and lesions at different levels of neuronal organization can elicit specific types of aggressive behavior.[19,20] Regulation of the neuroendocrine and autonomic response is controlled by the hypothalamus, which is involved in "flight or fight" reactions.

Investigations in animals have shown that lesions in the hypothalamus in animals who have undergone cortical ablation result in nondirected rage with stereotypic behavior (i.e., scratching, biting, etc.)[21]

It was then shown that stimulation of only the posterior lateral hypothalamus in decorticate animals induced "sham rage" episodes of fierce behavior with no external provocation.[22] Stimulation of the ventromedial hypothalamus may lead to inhibition of aggression, although some animals may assume defensive posturing.[23] Similarly, humans with hypothalamic tumors can exhibit aggressive behavior.[24]

Limbic System The limbic system, especially the amygdala, is responsible for mediating between impulses from the prefrontal cortex and hypothalamus; it adds emotional content to cognition and associates biological drives with specific stimuli (i.e., searching for food when hungry).[25] Activation of the amygdala, which can occur in seizure-like states or in kindling, may result in enhanced emotional reactions, such as outrage at personal slights. Damage to the amygdaloid area has resulted in violent behavior.[26] Injury to the anterior temporal lobe, which is a common site for contusions, has been associated with the "dyscontrol syndrome." Some patients with temporal lobe epilepsy exhibit emotional lability, impairment of impulse control, and suspiciousness.[27]

Neocortex The most recent region of the brain to evolve, the neocortex, coordinates timing and observation of social cues, often prior to the expression of associated emotions. Lesions in this area give rise to disinhibited anger after minimal provocation, characterized by an individual showing little regard for the consequences of the affect or behavior. Patients with violent behavior have been found to have a high frequency of frontal lobe lesions.[28] A recent review of the literature concluded that injury to the orbitofrontal region may put an individual at a particularly high risk for the commission of violent acts.[29] Frontal lesions may result in the sudden discharge of limbic and/or amygdala-generated affects, which are no longer modulated, processed, or inhibited by the frontal lobe. In this condition, the patient overresponds with rage and/or aggression to thoughts or feelings that would ordinarily have been modulated, inhibited, or suppressed. In summary, prefrontal damage may cause aggression by a secondary process involving lack of inhibition of the limbic areas.

Neurochemistry

Overview of Neurotransmitters Many neurotransmitters are involved in the mediation of aggression; this area has been reviewed in detail by Eichelman.[30] Among the neurotransmitter systems, serotonin, norepinephrine (NE), dopamine, acetylcholine, and the gamma aminobutyric acid (GABA) systems have prominent roles in influencing aggressive behavior.

Norepinephrine Animal studies suggest that NE enhances aggressive behavior, including sham rage, affective aggression, and shock-induced fighting.[30] Higley and coworkers[31] found an association between aggression in free-ranging rhesus monkeys and cerebrospinal fluid (CSF) norepinephrine. Humans who exhibit aggressive or impulsive behavior have been shown to have increased levels of the NE metabolite 5-hydroxy-3-methoxyphenyleneglycol (5-MHPG).[32] Stimulation of the amygdala produces sham rage and is associated with decrease in brainstem levels of NE (indicative of NE release).[33] The major NE tracts in the brain start in the locus ceruleus and the lateral tegmental system and course to the forebrain; they are thus vulnerable to traumatic injury.[34] $Beta_1$-adrenergic receptors are located in the limbic forebrain and cerebral cortex, areas known to be involved in the mediation of aggressive behavior.[35] As discussed in the treatment section below, blockade of the beta-adrenergic system in humans has been shown to help treat violent behavior.[36]

Serotonin Lowered levels of serotoninergic activity have been associated with increased aggression in a number of studies, including studies of predatory aggression and shock-induced fighting in rats[30] and in a study of free-ranging rhesus monkeys.[31] Clinical studies have confirmed the role of decreased serotonin in the expression of aggressiveness and impulsivity in humans,[37,38] particularly as it applies to self-destructive acts. Some studies have shown an increase in 5-HT_2 receptor binding in the frontal cortex of suicide victims,[39] although not all results are consistent with these findings.[40] A link between the gene for tryptophan hydroxylase and levels of CSF 5-hydroxyindoleacetic acid (5-HIAA) in impulsive aggressive individuals has been reported.[41] Olivier and colleagues[42] suggest that serotonin-specific drugs with putative antiaggressive properties bind to the 5-HT_{1B} subtype of the serotonin receptor, which can be found in the neocortex and hypothalamus among other brain regions. Interestingly, 5-HT_2 receptor antagonists, including antipsychotic drugs, have antiaggressive properties.[43] Other work looking at receptor subtypes in rats found multifaceted relationships between serotonin receptor type and aggression. Only 5-HT_2 agonists decreased defensive aggression. but agonists at 5-HT_{1A}, 5-HT_{1B}, and 5-HT_2 all reduced offensive aggression.[44] It has been reported that deleting the 5-HT_{1B} gene increases aggression.[45]

Dopamine Increases in dopamine may lead to aggression in several animal models,[30] and agitation is a common symptom in schizophrenia, often treated with antidopaminergic medications. L-Dopa has been shown to cause aggression in animals, and personality changes in Parkinson's disease patients treated with this medication have also been reported.[46,47] Some work has also shown reduction in the dopaminergic metabolites of patients who have attempted suicide.[48,49]

Other Neurotransmitters Acetylcholine has been reported to increase aggressive behaviors.[30] However, use of acetylcholinesterase inhibitors has been suggested as a treatment for disruptive patients with Alzheimer's disease.[50] Increasing GABA, via benzodiazepines, results in reduced aggressive behavior in animals,[30] but GABA agonists such as the benzodiazepines have been reported to be associated with paradoxical rage attacks.[51,52]

Neurophysiology of Aggression

Kindling Aggressive behavior may result from neuronal excitability of limbic system structures. For example, subconvulsive stimulation (i.e., kindling) of the amygdala leads to permanent changes in neuronal excitability.[53] Epileptogenic lesions in the hippocampus in cats, induced by the injection of the excitotoxic substance kainic acid, result in interictal defensive rage reactions.[54] When the cat experiences partial seizures, it exhibits heightened emotional reactivity and lability. In addition, defensive reactions can be elicited by excitatory injections to the midbrain periaqueductal gray region. Hypothalamus-induced rage reactions can be modulated by amygdaloid kindling.[55]

TREATMENT

Aggressive and agitated behaviors may be treated in a variety of settings, including the acute brain injury unit in a general hospital, a "neurobehavioral" unit in a rehabilitation facility, a nursing home, a residential facility for mentally retarded individuals, an outpatient environment, and the home setting. A multifactorial, multidisciplinary, collaborative approach to treatment is necessary in most cases. The continuation of family treatments and psychopharmacologic interventions, as well as insight-oriented psychotherapeutic approaches, are often required. We have reviewed the treatment of aggressive behavior in detail elsewhere.[1,2] Therefore only the more important general principles of treatment are reviewed here.

Documentation of Aggressive Episodes Before therapeutic intervention to treat violent behavior is initiated, the clinician should document the baseline frequency of these behaviors.[56,57] It is essential that the clinician establish a treatment plan which utilizes objective documentation of aggressive episodes to monitor the efficacy of interventions and to designate specific time frames for the initiation and discontinuation of pharmacotherapy of acute episodes as well as the initiation of pharmacotherapy for chronic aggressive behavior.

The Overt Aggression Scale (OAS) is an operationalized instrument of proven reliability and validity that can be used to rate, easily and effectively, aggressive behavior in patients with a wide range of disorders.[56–58] The OAS comprises items that assess verbal aggression, physical aggression against objects, physical aggression against self, and physical aggression against others. Aggressive behavior can be monitored by staff or by family members utilizing this instrument.

Pharmacotherapy

Although no drug is approved by the U.S. Food and Drug Administration (FDA) specifically for the management of acute or chronic aggression, medications are widely used (and commonly misused) for this purpose. After diagnosis and treatment of underlying causes of aggression and evaluation and documentation of aggressive behaviors, the use of pharmacologic interventions can be considered in two categories: (1) the use of the sedating effects of medications, as required in acute situations, so that the patient does not harm self or others, and (2) the use of nonsedating antiaggressive medications to treat for chronic aggression when necessary. The clinician must be aware that patients may not respond to just one medication but may require combination treatment, as is done in the pharmacotherapy of refractory depression. We suggest utilizing the consensus guidelines for the treatment of agitation in the elderly with dementia as a framework for the assessment and management of agitation and aggression.[59]

Acute Aggression and Agitation In the treatment of agitation and for treating acute episodes of aggressive behavior, medications that are sedating, such as antipsychotic drugs or benzodiazepines, may be indicated. However, as these drugs are not specific in their ability to inhibit aggressive behaviors; there may be detrimental effects on arousal and cognitive function. In addition, due to the potential for interference with respiration and temperature regulation, these drugs should be administered only under careful medical supervision. Therefore, the use of sedation-producing medications must be time-limited to avoid the emergence of seriously disabling side effects ranging from oversedation to tardive dyskinesia.

Chronic Aggression If a patient continues to exhibit periods of agitation or aggression beyond several weeks, the use of specific antiaggressive medications should be initiated to prevent these episodes from occurring. The choice of medication may be guided by the underlying hypothesized mechanism of action (i.e., effects on serotonin system, adrenergic system, kindling, etc.) or in consideration of the predominant clinical features. Since no medication has been approved by the FDA for the treatment of aggression, the clinician must use medications that may be antiaggressive but that have been approved for other uses (i.e., for seizure disorders, depression, anxiety, mood stabilization, hypertension, etc.).

Summary of Treatments Table 60-1 summarizes our recommendations for the utilization of various classes of drugs in the treatment of aggressive disorders. In treating aggression, the clinician, where possible, should diagnose and treat underlying disorders, and utilize, where possible, antiaggressive agents specific for those disorders. When there is a partial response after a therapeutic trial with a specific medication, adjunctive treatment with a medication with a different mechanism of action should be instituted. For example, a patient with a partial response to beta blockers may show further improvement with the addition of an anticonvulsant or a serotoninergic antidepressant.

Behavioral Treatment

It is clear that aggression can be caused and influenced by a combination of environmental and biological factors. Because of the dangerous and unpredictable nature of aggression, caretakers, both in institutions and at home, have intense and sometimes unjudicious reactions to aggression when it occurs. Behavioral treatments have been shown to be highly effective in treating patients with organic aggression and may be useful when combined with pharmacotherapy. Behavioral strategies—including a token economy, aggression replacement strategies, and decelerative techniques—may reduce aggression in the inpatient setting and can be combined effectively with pharmacologic treatment. A review of this subject is found in Ref. 60.

CONCLUSION

Aggressive behavior in the presence of brain damage is common and can be highly disabling. Neuroanatomic, neurochemical, and neurophysiologic factors may have an etiologic or mediating role in the production of violence. After appropriate evaluation and assessment of possible etiologies, treatment begins with the documentation of the aggressive episodes. Psychopharmacologic strategies may be divided into those intended

Table 60-1
Psychopharmacologic treatment of chronic aggression

Agent	*Indications*	*Special clinical considerations*
Propranolol (and other beta blockers)	Chronic or recurrent aggression	May require usual clinical doses
Antipsychotics and benzodiazepines	Psychotic and anxiety symptoms	Oversedation, multiple side effects, paradoxical rage, cardiac arrhythmias, agranulocytosis, seizures with clozapine Consider atypical neuroleptics if chronic use is indicated, since the incidence of side effects is lower.
Anticonvulsants Carbamazepine (CBZ) Valproic acid (VPA) Gabapentin (preliminary studies are promising)	Seizure disorder	Bone marrow suppression (CBZ) and hepatotoxicity (CBZ and VPA)
Lithium	Manic excitement or bipolar disorder	Neurotoxicity and confusion
Buspirone	Persistent, underlying anxiety and/or depression	Delayed onset of action
Propranolol (and other beta blockers)	Chronic or recurrent aggression	Latency of 4 to 6 weeks
Serotoninergic antidepressants Selective serotonin reuptake inhibitors (SSRIs), trazodone	Depression or mood lability with irritability, anxiety	May require higher than usual doses if obsessive/compulsive symptoms are part of the reason for aggressive behavior

Source: Adapted from Yudofsky et al.,[16] with permission.

to treat acute aggression and those intended to prevent episodes in the patient with chronic aggression. While the treatment of acute aggression involves the judicious use of sedation, the treatment of chronic aggression is guided by underlying diagnoses and symptomatologies. Behavioral strategies remain an important component in the comprehensive treatment of aggression.

REFERENCES

1. Silver JM, Yudofsky SC: Aggressive disorders, in Silver JM, Yudofsky SC, Hales RE (eds): *Neuropsychiatry of Traumatic Brain Injury.* Washington, DC: American Psychiatric Press, 1994.
2. Yudofsky SC, Silver JM, Hales RE: Treatment of aggressive disorders, in Schatzberg A, Nemeroff C (eds): *American Psychiatric Press Textbook of Psychopharmacology*. Washington, DC: American Psychiatric Press, 1995, pp 735–751.
3. Volavka J: *Neurobiology of Violence*. Washington, DC: American Psychiatric Press, 1995.
4. Anderson K, Silver J: Neurological and medical diseases, in Tardiff K (ed): *Medical Management of the Violent Patient*. New York: Marcel Dekker, 1999, pp 87–124.
5. Reisberg B, Borenstein J, Salob SP, et al: Behavioral symptoms in Alzheimer's disease. Phenomenology and treatment. *J Clin Psychiatry* 48 (5, suppl): 9–15, 1987.
6. Devanand DP, Jacobs DM, Tang MX, et al: The course of psychopathologic features in mild to moderate Alzheimer disease. *Arch Gen Psychiatry* 54 (3):257–263, 1997.
7. Brodaty H, Draper B, Saab D, et al: Psychosis, depression and behavioural disturbances in Sydney nursing home

residents: Prevalence and predictors. *Int J Geriatr Psychiatry* 16:504–512, 2001.

8. Freedman D, Hemenway D: Precursors of lethal violence: A death row sample. *Soc Sci Med* 50 (12):1757–1770, 2000.
9. Greve KW. Sherwin E, Stanford MS, et al: Personality and neurocognitive correlates of impulsive aggression in long-term survivors of severe traumatic brain injury. *Brain Injury* 15 (3):255–262. 2001.
10. Robertson MM, Trimble MR, Townsend HRA: Phenomenology of depression in epilepsy. *Epilepsia* 28:364–372, 1987.
11. Herzberg JL, Fenwick PBC: The aetiology of aggression in temporal-lobe epilepsy. *Br J Psychiatry* 153:50–55, 1988.
12. Bogdanovic MD, Mead SH, Duncan JS: Aggressive behaviour at a residential epilepsy centre. *Seizure* 9 (1):58–64, 2000.
13. Reid AH, Ballinger BR, Heather BB, et al: The natural history of behavioral symptoms among severely and profoundly mentally retarded patients. *Br J Psychiatry* 145:289–293, 1984.
14. Hill BK, Balow EA, Bruininks RH: A national study of prescribed drugs in institutions and community residential facilities for mentally retarded people. *Psychopharmacol Bull* 21:279–284, 1985.
15. Emerson E, Kiernan C, Alborz A, et al: The prevalence of challenging behaviors: A total population study. *Res Dev Disabil* 22:77–93, 2001.
16. Yudofsky SC, Silver JM, Hales RE: Pharmacologic management of aggression in the elderly. *J Clin Psychiatry* 51 (10, suppl):22–28, 1990.
17. American Psychiatric Association: *Diagnostic and Statistical Manual of Mental Disorders*, 4th ed. Washington, DC: American Psychiatric Association, 1994.
18. Beresin E: Delirium in the elderly. *J Geriatr Psychiatry Neurol* 1:127–143, 1988.
19. Ovsiew F, Yudofsky SC: Aggression: A neuropsychiatric perspective, in Roose S, Glick RD (eds): *Rage, Power, and Aggression*. New Haven, CT: Yale University Press, 1993.
20. Garza-Trevino E: Neurobiological factors in aggressive behavior. *Hosp Commun Psychiatry* 45:690–699, 1994.
21. Valzelli L: *Psychobiology of Aggression and Violence*. New York: Raven Press, 1981.
22. Bard P: A diencephalic mechanism for the expression of rage with special reference to the sympathetic nervous system. *Am J Physiol* 84:490–515, 1928.
23. Roberts WW: Escape learning without avoidance learning motivated by hypothalamic stimulation in cats. *J Comp Physiol Psychol* 51:391–399, 1958.
24. Malamud N: Psychiatric disorder with intracranial tumors of the limbic system. *Arch Neurol* 17:113–123, 1967.
25. Halgren E: Emotional neurophysiology of the amygdala within the context of human cognition, in Aggleton JP (ed): *The Amygdala: Neurobiological Aspects of Emotion, Memory, and Mental Dysfunction*. New York: Wiley-Liss, 1992, pp 191–228.
26. Tonkonogy TM: Violence and temporal lobes lesion: Head CT and MRI data. *J Neuropsychiatry Clin Neurosci* 3:189–196, 1991.
27. Garyfallos G, Manos N, Adamopoulou A: Psychopathology and personality characteristics of epileptic patients: Epilepsy, psychopathology and personality. *Acta Psychiatr Scand* 78:87–95, 1988.
28. Heinrichs RW: Frontal cerebral lesions and violent incidents in chronic neuropsychiatric patients. *Biol Psychiatry* 25:174–178, 1989.
29. Brower MC, Price BH: Neuropsychiatry of frontal lobe dysfunction in violent and criminal behaviour: A critical review. *J Neurol Neurosurg Psychiatry* 71:720–726, 2001.
30. Eichelman B: Neurochemical and psychopharmacologic aspects of aggressive behavior, in Meltzer HY (ed): *Psychopharmacology: The Third Generation of Progress*. New York: Raven Press, 1987, pp 697–704.
31. Higley JD, Mehlman PT, Taum DM, et al: Cerebrospinal fluid monoamine and adrenal correlates of aggression in free-ranging rhesus monkeys. *Arch Gen Psychiatry* 49:436–441, 1992.
32. Brown GL, Goodwin FK, Ballenger JC, et al: Aggression in humans correlates with cerebrospinal fluid amine metabolites. *Psychiatry Res* 1:131–139, 1979.
33. Reis DJ: The relationship between brain norepinephrine and aggressive behavior. *Res Publ Assoc Res Nerv Ment Dis* 50:266–297, 1972.
34. Cooper JR, Bloom FE, Roth RH: *The Biochemical Basis of Neuropharmacology*, 6th ed. New York: Oxford University Press, 1991.
35. Alexander RW, Davis JN, Lefkowitz RJ: Direct identification and characterization of beta-adrenergic receptors in rat brain. *Nature* 258:437–440, 1979.
36. Silver JM, Yudofsky SC, et al: Propranolol treatment of chronically hospitalized aggressive patients. *J Neuropsychiatry Clin Neurosci* 11:328–335, 1999.
37. Kruesi MJP, Hibbs ED, Zahn TP, et al: A 2-year prospective follow-up study of children and adolescents with disruptive behavior disorders: Prediction by cerebrospinal fluid 5-hydroxyindoleacetic acid, homovanillic acid, and autonomic measures? *Arch Gen Psychiatry* 49:429–435, 1992.

38. Linnoila VMI, Virkkunen M: Aggression, suicidality, and serotonin. *J Clin Psychiatry* 53 (10, suppl):46–51, 1992.
39. Arango V, Ernsberger P, Marzuk P, et al: Autoradiographic demonstration of increased serotonin $5HT_2$ and beta-adrenergic binding sites in the brains of suicide victims. *Arch Gen Psychiatry* 47:1038–1047, 1990.
40. Cheetham S, Crompton M, Katona C, et al: Brain $5\text{-}HT_2$ receptors binding sites in depressed suicide victims. *Brain Res* 443:271–280, 1988.
41. Nielsen DA, Goldman D, Virkkunen M, et al: Suicidality and 5-hydroxyindoleacetic acid concentration associated with a tryptophan hydroxylase polymorphism. *Arch Gen Psychiatry* 51:34–38, 1994.
42. Olivier B, Mos J, Rasmussen DL: Behavioural pharmacology of the serenic, eltoprazine. *Drug Metab Drug Interact* 8:31–38, 1990.
43. Mann JJ: Violence and aggression, in Bloom FE, Kupfer DJ (eds): *Psychopharmacology: The Fourth Generation of Progress*. New York: Raven Press, 1995, pp 1919–1928.
44. Muehlencamp F, Lucion A, Vogel WH: Effects of selective serotonin agonists on aggressive behavior in rats. *Pharmacol Biochem Behav* 50 (4):671–674, 1995.
45. Hen R, Boschert U, Lemeur M, et al: $5\text{-}HT_{1B}$ receptor "knockout": Pharmacological and behavioral consequences. *Soc Neurosci Abstr* 19:632, 1993.
46. Lammers AJJC, Van Rossum JM: Bizarre social behavior in rats induced by a combination of a peripheral decarboxylase inhibitor and dopa. *Eur J Pharmacol* 5:103–106, 1968.
47. Saint-Cyr JA, Taylor AE, Lang AE: Neuropsychological and psychiatric side effects in the treatment of Parkinson's disease. *Neurology* 43 (suppl 6):S47–S52, 1993.
48. Traskman L, Asberg M, Bertilsson L, et al: Monoamine metabolites in CSF and suicidal behavior. *Arch Gen Psychol* 38:631–636, 1981.
49. Roy A, Argen H, Pickar D et al: Reduced CSF concentrations of homovanillic acid and homovanillic acid to 5-hydroxyindoleacetic acid ratios in depressed patients: relationship to suicidal behavior and dexamethasone suppression. *Am J Psychol* 143:1539–1545, 1986.
50. Kaufer D, Cummings JL, Christine D: Differential neuropsychiatric symptom responses to tacrine in Alzheimer's disease: Relationship to dementia severity. *J Neuropsychiatry Clin Neurosci* 10(1):55–63, 1998.
51. Salzman C, Kochansky GE, Shader RI, et al: Chloridazepoxide-induced hostility in a small group setting. *Arch Gen Psychiatry* 31:401–405, 1974.
52. Yudofsky SC, Silver JM, Hales RE: Treatment of agitation and aggression, in Schatzberg AF, Nemeroff CB (eds): *American Psychiatric Press Textbook of Psychopharmacology*, 2d ed. Washington, DC: American Psychiatric Press, 1998, pp 881–900.
53. Post RM, Uhde TW, Putnam FE, et al: Kindling and carbamazepine in affective illness. *J Nerv Ment Dis* 170: 717–731, 1982.
54. Engel J Jr, Bandler R, Griffith NC, et al: Neurobiological evidence for epilepsy-induced interictal disturbances, in Smith D, Treiman D, Trimble M (eds): *Advances in Neurology: Neurobehavioral Problems in Epilepsy*. New York: Raven Press, 1991, vol 55.
55. Adamec RE, Stark-Adamec C: Kindling and interictal behavior: An animal model of personality change. *Psychiatr J U Ottawa* 10:220–230, 1985.
56. Silver JM, Yudofsky SC: Documentation of aggression in the assessment of the violent patient. *Psychiatr Ann* 17:375–384, 1987.
57. Silver JM, Yudofsky SC: The Overt Aggression Scale: Overview and clinical guidelines. *J Neuropsychiatry Clin Neurosci* 3:S22–S29, 1991.
58. Yudofsky SC, Silver JM, Jackson W, et al: The Overt Aggression Scale for the objective rating of verbal and physical aggression. *Am J Psychiatry* 143:35–39, 1986.
59. Alexopoulos GS, Silver JM, Kahn DA, et al: The expert consensus guideline series: treatment of agitation in older persons with dementia. *Postgrad Med Special Report*. April 1998.
60. Corrigan PW, Yudofsky SC, Silver JM: Pharmacological and behavioral treatments for aggressive psychiatric inpatients. *Hosp Commun Psychiatry* 44:125–133, 1993.

Part 9

NEUROBEHAVIORAL DISORDERS IN CHILDREN

Chapter 61

THE NEUROBEHAVIORAL EXAMINATION FOR CHILDREN*

Martha Bridge Denckla†

The first large difference between mental status examination in adult acquired and child/developmental contexts is that, in the latter, one must memorize or carry around for reference normative data arranged according to age expectations. This author was inspired to construct and norm a developmental neuromotor examination by the experience of having, in a weekly clinic, to ask a pediatric neurologist such questions as, "Should a 4-year-old child be able to hop on her nonpreferred foot?" Although the evolution of research on aging and dementia has increased awareness in all behavioral neurologists that all adults do not, decade by decade, perform across tasks at a uniform level of expectation, those who see children must have an annualized normative frame of reference and a sense of when each neurodevelopmental domain spurts steeply and then enters a plateau (temporary or ultimate). Thus, with minor exceptions, the developmental neurobehavioral examination relies on tests or tasks with norms, requires scoring, and demands additional "behind the scenes" time for looking up age-referenced expectations for performance before a profile can be described and/or diagnostic decisions reached.

Apart from such tests or tasks themselves, for each of which there is a rationale, there is an aspect of evaluation that goes beyond the term *examination* and is indispensable to developmental "mental status"; this is the history and description of the patient by parents and teachers. Of course, this is shared with all of behavioral neurology, since the literal confines of *examination* cannot sample complex social, vocational, and communal behaviors relevant to any patient's mental status. For the developmental clinic, however, the need to collect and interpret parent- and teacher-derived data relates with urgency to decisions about certain diagnostic "entities" that are shared by professional colleagues in psychiatry and education. Whatever our neurologically based intellectual qualms about some of these "diagnoses," service to the patients demands that data considered to be the basis of these "entities" be included in the neurobehavioral assessment (see Table 61-1).

Above and beyond these "formal" diagnosis-oriented obligations, there is a genuine need for the

* **ACKNOWLEDGMENTS:** This work was supported by grant #P50 HD25806 from the National Institutes of Health. The author wishes to acknowledge Pamula D. Yerby for her help in the preparation of this manuscript.

† The title of this chapter could as well be "The Mental Status Examination in a Developmental Context," with the added qualification, "with Special Emphasis on the Interface between Motor Functions and Cognition." The reader of this chapter will benefit from the knowledge that the author thereof was, in the beginning, a behavioral neurologist trained to examine adults with aphasia or dementia; construction of a neurobehavioral examination for children (and adults with disorders of development) was approached by this author in apprenticeship to pediatric neurologists and developmental neuropsychologists. Through the didactic generosity of the pediatric neurologists then (1968–1976) at the Neurological Institute (Columbia University's College of Physicians and Surgeons) and the late Rita G. Rudel, to all of whom this author is deeply indebted, this chapter was made possible. Through a subsequent brief but intense growth period experienced in Boston (with the authors of the chapter that follows) this chapter was further facilitated. The author makes no clear line of demarcation other than that dictated by custom or convenience between the "neurobehavioral" and "neuropsychological" examination of children; neuropsychologists may use the timed motor exam and behavioral neurologists use digit span. Long ago, Rita G. Rudel came to the conclusion that these were the boundaries; neuropsychologists could not use the neurologist's reflex hammer or other physical examination instruments, while neurologists could not trepass upon the subtests used to compute IQ.

Table 61-1
Rating scales and questionnaires for use in conjunction with history

Broad-band mental health dimensional screening
(externalizing, internalizing, somaticizing, socializing)
Sources: Parent
Child/adolescent
Teacher

ADHD-oriented checklists and rating scales
1. For hyperactivity/impulsivity
2. For inattention/disorganization
Sources: Parent
Teacher(s)
Self (if adolescent or adult)
"Significant other" (if adult)

Autistic spectrum questionnaires
1. For communication level
2. For socialization level
3. For range of activities (versus restricted repertoire)
4. For unusual sensory responsivity (hyper- or hyporeactivity)
Sources: Parent
Teacher(s)

developmental neurobehavioral assessment to include descriptions and illustrative anecdotes of how the patient functions in the home, the family, the classroom, and in extracurricular activities. These situations of environmental complexity and social dynamics reveal aspects of "mental status" that no clinical "examination" can approximate. The historical perspective is particularly important, because the record of when skills and capacities became evident is itself part of the diagnostic formulation; for example, disproportionate delay in speech/language "milestones" (compared with normal or precocious emergence of motor skills) would fit with and convergently validate an examination data set in which the same profile is apparent. Yet it is even more urgent to fill in the "social mental status" and the "self-regulatory" or broader "executive function" mental status from history taking alone; we are at the mercy of the history to assess the capacity to delay gratification, to accept limits set by parents and teachers, to attend to and process nonverbal social/interpersonal cues from others (particularly peers), and to organize space/plan time. It is naive to expect to sample or elicit such naturally occurring behaviors in a clinic. In examining an individual patient in the one-on-one clinical setting, the developmental behavioral neurologist typically provides an adult authoritative structure that, while facilitating collection of data about many domains of importance in the mental status examination, effectively bypasses the self-regulatory, the social, and the executive. Many are the adorably compliant examinees whose history of oppositional-defiant behaviors comes as a shock to clinicians or physician-assistant colleagues (see below) who test "blind" to history.

A "parallel assessment" format evolved for the most pragmatic of reasons—this author's goals of (1) no child sitting alone in a waiting area and (2) two visits per family, only one of which involves the child and the second of which is a parent informing/interpreting/advising session. In addition, because schools are the major settings for the "treatment" of most developmental disorders (and even of the less numerous referrals for chronic states following closed head injury or brain tumor survival), an educator (preferably a special educator) was the chosen professional for a specialized physician-assistant colleague who (blind to history) directly tests/examines in parallel during the time that the neurologist looks over the questionnaires, rating scales, and report cards and does the formal history-oriented interview of the parent(s) or (as more adults are being evaluated) of the adult patient's "significant other." The special educator/neuropsychological colleague is trained to write down qualitative observations and impressions and then score (from raw to age-referenced norms) as much as possible during the second half of the evaluation visit, during which the neurologist (who is not blind to history but at this point blind to whatever aspects of the direct examination were done by the assistant) examines the patient. In the week usually intervening between the evaluation visit and the conference visit, the neurologist meets with his or her colleague; together, they generate a profile, a diagnostic formulation, and a set of recommendations. Most of the time, the assistant (whose unique contribution is the educator's perspective) joins the conference, which itself serves as another opportunity for expanding and refining the history, because frequently the other parent (or some professional already involved with the patient) attends the conference. The conference also serves as a dress rehearsal for report preparation. Reports have to serve many purposes; it takes quite a bit of experience and art to produce *one* report that addresses referring physicians, parents, teachers, and sometimes other agencies, in language appropriate for diverse "subcultures."

As is the case with the ultimate report, what is included in the evaluation is multidetermined. To be unkind, one could call the "menu" of what is included a "hodgepodge"; to be generous, one could call it eclectic and pragmatic. It is not a fixed battery; it changes with conceptual and data driven shifts in the current relevant literatures. For example, as there emerged convergent consensus that phonologic coding skills are the basis for reading acquisition, the inclusion of direct norm-referenced measures of phoneme segmentation, phonologic memory, and reading (decoding) nonsense words became standard in the "learning disability"–oriented workup. Depending on the chief complaint, which varies somewhat from patient to patient and age group to age group, only a "core" is invariant; but a certain set of mental status constructs is assessed flexibly, on an individualized basis. As Rita G. Rudel so aptly warned, "Don't assault (patients) with your battery."

It will be perfectly obvious and recognizable to any professional trained to engage in the mental status examination that the developmentalist surveys language, attention, memory, visual perception, and (emphatically) motor skills. In the approach that this author has adopted, only the history (of all domains) and motor skills are exclusively the responsibility of the neurologist. The other domains are divided up between the neurologist and the colleague (the person with a neuropsychoeducational background). At the beginning of the partnership, it is best to allocate to the colleague (assuming at least minimal neuropsychological training in his or her background) those aspects of the neuropsychological tests requiring the least qualitative appraisal; specifically, multiple-choice tests of "perception" or recognition memory can be done while, simultaneously, the neurologist is interviewing parents and taking the history. Even at the beginning, however, the colleague should be exhorted to write down observations of every aspect of *how* the patient does the multiple-choice task. Impulsive or perseverative choices, wandering eyes (off task), and an obbligato of chatter are extremely useful clinical data. The neurologist will assess those tasks requiring spoken or graphomotor output, because the nature of errors and quality of responses will have major implications well beyond the quantitative level of performance. As the colleague in clinical practice becomes more sophisticated (usually because he or she participates in the informing/interpreting sessions), the colleague and the neurologist may decide to alter the pattern of "who does what" so as to avoid habituation or downright boredom. Table 61-2 lists a proposed division of labor for a $2\frac{1}{2}$-h visit; the reader is cautioned against taking this 1995 "menu" as "carved in stone."

It should also be taken into consideration that this system of evaluation is based upon the assumption that IQ and academic testing are carried out elsewhere, with the results made available for integration with the neurobehavioral examination. It should also be noted that, were the author of this chapter working in a setting alongside the authors of the next chapter, the neurobehavioral visit would be shortened and reshaped to take into consideration the particularly enriched offerings of that environment. Similarly, pragmatic constraints may alter the format; scheduling and reimbursement strictures may rule out the luxury of a $2\frac{1}{2}$-h initial evaluation visit followed by a $1\frac{1}{2}$-h visit informing, interpreting, and advising patients and/or families. There is no universal "usual and customary" format, just as there is no "battery" of tests.

The most "neurologic" core of the developmental mental status examination is located at the interface where motor control is adjacent to cognitive control. An eye-movement examination would, in fact, be the most elegant instance of such assessment; in fact, getting the equipment and neurooptalmologic training to do a "saccade battery" is a good plan for the future. At present, however, the neurodevelopmental general motor examination is the most practical and relevant one to emphasize.

The reader may be puzzled by the lack of emphasis on "higher cortical sensory" portions of the neurobehavioral examination. Certainly, it goes without saying that vision and hearing should have been elsewhere assessed and, if need be, corrected. Basic pain, temperature, vibration, and touch sensations are not considered part of the mental status examination or often enough relevant to chief complaints to warrant time spent on examining them. Problems with the intuitively relevant "higher-order" sensory functions are that (1) task demands, such as keeping eyes closed and responding

Table 61-2
A model for the developmental neurobehavioral examination

Neurologist	*Colleague (EdD, PhD)*
History/interview	Multiple-choice tests
Questionnaires	Visual "what" perception
Rating scales	Visual "where" perception
Review other reports	Visual recognition memory (what, where)
	Design copying
	Target search
	Simple/choice reaction time
	Go/no go with reaction time
	Receptive language (sentence level)
	Word fluency
	Basic reading
	Nonsense
	Real words
	Basic calculations
Confrontation naming	
Complex design copying	
Word-list learning	
Neurodevelopmental motor[a]	
Praxis	

[a]Described in Table 61-3.

with good attention to each stimulus, are frequently not met, due to deficits in the youngsters being evaluated, and (2) the significance of "finger agnosia" or "graphesthesia" failures is even less clear in a developmental context than in adult acquired cases, as attachment of some name, numbering, or "mapping" system to a sensory input is not necessarily "sensory" in any meaningful way. Little is known about firmness of association between mental image or visual memory of a letter, the name of the letter, and the dynamic-tactile experience of "graphesthesia," especially in children. To put it bluntly, one may waste a lot of time on "higher cortical sensation" and come up with little meaningful nonredundant data about the patient.

By contrast, the motor examination—even as it transcends the basics of strength, tone, and reflexes—gives the neurologist information that is both directly and indirectly relevant. For greater detail about the motor function examination, the reader is referred to Denckla and Roeltgen (Table 61-3).[1]

The directly relevant items most often bear upon "excuse slips" for gym or, more commonly, for handwriting. Sometimes a child's balance—hopping, tandem, and tone—are so much below age expectation that playground and athletic accommodations are advisable. Far more commonly, the examination elicits characteristics that lead to a recommendation that handwriting be minimized and, where unavoidable, be deemphasized in the teacher's attitude or grading/marking responses. The two most common handwriting-relevant findings are, in order of frequency, (1) choreiform movements and (2) slowness of finger sequencing (successive tapping against thumb of index, middle, ring, and little fingers). Choreiform movements are elicited by instructing the patient to stand with eyes closed, holding arms extended in front and all fingers extended and abducted. Rather than describe these as "involuntary movements," it is useful to describe them to parents and teachers as lapses in postural stability. Indeed, one can see the consequences of choreiform lapses, as recorded on design-copying tasks, in wobbly line quality and excessive pressure. Thus, there is cross-validation of choreiform postural instability between the neurologic manuever for elicitation and the design-copying elicitation of the abnormality. The patient's unconscious compensatory maneuver of

Table 61-3
Motor function: Neurodevelopmental examination

Observations
Hand and eye (gaze) preference
Pencil grasp
Choreiform movements
Extraneous overflow movements
Semiquantified tasks[a]
Heel, toe, outside-of foot gaits (10 steps)
Tandem gait (10 steps forward, 10 steps backward—if age >10)
Unipedal balance (to limit 30 s)
Tandem balance (to limit 20 s)
Hop (to limit 50 times)
Quantified "time to do 20 movements"
Tongue wiggles
Finger repetitive, finger sequential taps
Hand pats, hand pronation-supination
Foot taps, foot heel-toe alternations

[a]Physical and Neurological Examination for Subtle Signs (PANESS).

Source: From Denckla,[2] with permission.

excessive pen/pencil pressure, while somewhat corrective of the irregular jerks and jiggles caused by the choreiform syndrome, leads to fatigue during handwriting and gradual aversive conditioning toward tasks involving handwriting.

Slow finger sequencing correlates with poor handwriting;[3] in that sense it is not as direct a causal link to poor handwriting as is the choreiform syndrome, because it is by the adjacent neural substrate for sequence-of-pencil-moves (graphomotor praxis) that slow/poor finger sequencing bears directly on handwriting. In the original normative studies of timed motor coordination,[4,5] 5 percent of boys in kindergarten could not even perform finger sequencing; subsequent clinical experience has shown that illegible "dyspraxic" handwriting correlates with such nonperformance. Drawing unconstrained, self-generated pictures does not correlate with finger sequencing, while precise copying of designs does serve as a "surrogate" for handwriting in 5- and 6-year-olds.

The timed motor coordination examination [revised and itself a part of the revision of the National Institute of Mental Health–initiated Physical and Neurological Examination for Subtle (Soft) Signs][2] is a source of evidence of finger slowing. Motor speeds may also reveal or unmask subtle left/right differences of "classic" lateralizing significance. As youngsters are followed over years, changes in motor speed can be used to track their age-expected development or, in the shorter run, medication effects (for better or for worse) of stimulants, psychotropics, or anticonvulsants.

Of indirect relevance, as markers of the development of control processes in whose brain neighborhood they reside, are those aspects of the neurodevelopmental examination with which child neurologists are most familiar; these are the extraneous or overflow movements normally seen early in development and expected to disappear in an orderly, "milestone"-like fashion.[6] It is presumed that this disappearance reflects the maturation of inhibitory pathways. When bilaterally symmetrical, such extraneous movements as "feet-to-hands overflow" are markers of developmental failure to meet milestones; had the child been younger, the "imitative"-looking (but actually uninhibited) hand postures accompanying heel walking or outsides-of-feet walking would have been expected. When unilateral or asymmetrical, extraneous overflow movements may have subtle classic lateralizing significance. In children less than 10 years old with recovering congenital hemiparesis, mirror movements of the intact hand are elicited by the formerly hemiplegic hand's performance of a unimanual task. In these same children, when they are older than 10 years, the intact hand's mirroring decreases but a mild degree of mirroring is seen bilaterally in such tasks as finger sequencing that normally (up to age 13 years) elicit subtle mirror overflow. (For an in-depth explanation and discussion, the reader is referred to Nass.[7]) The meaning of the prominence and distribution of extraneous overflow must be derived from an integrated history and examination. As "archaeology" of the brain's anterior control systems, this part of the examination can make a surprising contribution to the assessment of adults presenting with questions about having residual signs and symptoms of attention deficit hyperactivity disorder. The deficit in age-appropriate motor inhibition can be quite striking and diagnostically helpful when the clinical problem concerns the origin of disinhibited adult behavior. To quote Norman Geschwind's clinical teaching maxim, "where we are so ignorant, we cannot afford to throw out information." Findings that implicate motor control/inhibition deficits in adults are like "laboratory data" that help to confirm the neurodevelopmental origins of certain persistent cognitive problems, especially when (as is far from uncommon) there are comorbid depressive or anxious states.

Pencil grasp is another observable motor characteristic of interest. Each grasp reflects the degree to which there is deviation from the ideal mature pencil control, that which allows movements from the distal phalanges of thumb and forefinger. Stability (not movement or pressure) is contributed by the middle finger and the ulnar "cushion" of the hand. Common deviations are depicted in Fig. 61-1 as (1) "one plus," (2) "two plus," and (3) "three plus" inefficient, reflecting movement (respectively) from (1) proximal portions of fingers, (2) too many fingers, and (3) hand muscles. Not depicted (because so rarely seen) is the truly primitive ulnar (also called simian) grasp that reflects forearm movement.

Interpretation of pencil grasp is not as straightforward as is noting its practical effect on handwriting, in terms of lack of ease or frank fatigue. A pencil grasp, like a regional accent, is a hard-to-change early-acquired motor habit; some individuals may show inefficient pencil grasps as residual indicators of the state of maturation of their motor system at the time they began to use a pencil. Sometimes it is far from easy to obtain this history of the chronological age at which pencil use began. Hence, pencil grasp does not clearly "stigmatize" the patient's *current* motor repertoire but may be like an old snapshot of past status during the period of motor skill learning.

Hand and eye preference (the latter actually a surrogate for "gaze" preference) are standard neurologic observations; rarely are they in any way diagnostic or clinically applicable. However, as research data someday to be proven relevant to understanding variations in underlying brain organization patterns of motor preference, these observations may well prove their worth, as Geschwind taught. There is one clinical situation in which the neurologist can use the observation of left-handedness or right-hand/left-"eye" preference (although "eye" is really gaze preference): this is to reassure parents whose 5- or 6-year-olds "mirror-write." This is easily corrected by explicit teaching and is not a predictor of any kind of reading or learning disability unless other risk factors coexist.

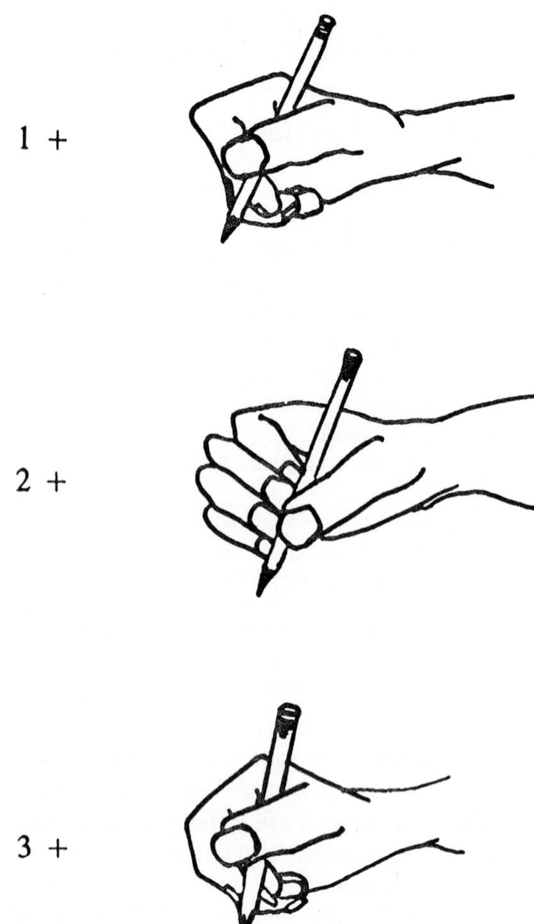

Figure 61-1
Pencil grasp as an indicator of motor control. "One plus" reflects movement from proximal portions of fingers, "two plus" from too many fingers, and "three plus" from hand muscles—all common deviations from normal.

Finally, the neurodevelopmental motor examination must be integrated with other mental status findings. As is true in all behavioral neurology, certain clusters occur in a way that confirms the existence of recognizable syndromes (convergent validity). These do not conform well to official educational, legal, and mental health syndromes but do at least overlap with the constructs, reviewed later in this section, of "reading disability," "nonverbal learning disability," and the subtypes (preponderantly inattentive and/or preponderantly hyperactive-impulsive) of attention deficit hyperactivity disorder (ADHD; see Chaps. 64–66). For example, the prototypical case of "reading disability" (RD), while not conforming exactly to the neurologic construct of "developmental dyslexia," will show phonologic coding deficits, with confrontation naming and word memory recall being deficits that occur outside of the reading task per se; and on the timed motor exam, the "dyslexic" person often shows slow tongue wiggling and finger sequencing. Significant "negatives" for the pure RD patient are executive control tasks of search and choice, visuospatial and visual memory, and nongraphomotor visuoconstructive skills.

By contrast, the pure ADHD case (more likely to visit a neurologist if ADHD is of the preponderantly inattentive type) usually shows variability or some discrepantly low scores *within* the verbal or visuospatial domain in proportion to the executive control demands of such tasks (e.g., poor letter/word fluency despite excellent confrontation naming and reasonably average semantic word fluency), looks worst in terms of speed and consistency of reaction time, disorganized on target search tasks (the simpler the worse!), and shows much "young-for-age" motor overflow and incoordination. Visual-motor design-copying tasks are also poorly done by most patients with ADHD, and qualitatively the appearance of the copy products differs from that of the patient with RD. Copying standard designs is thus a very sensitive but, unless evaluated qualitatively, nonspecific screening test for those "at risk" developmentally.

Beyond attempts to document "syndromes" that overlap entities recognizable to the schools and clinics where treatment is carried out, the neurobehavioral examination is free to describe the strengths and weaknesses of each patient. Rarely is "localization" or classic brain-behavior correlation the purpose of the evaluations. Explanation of the cluster of deficits or the profile, consistent with established knowledge of brain organization, helps to legitimize educational approaches or accommodations. Sometimes brain-based explanations even serve to clarify prognosis. (Further discussion of goals and methods can be found in Refs. 8 and 9.) At the very least, brain-based explanations usually help to avoid irrational or harmful treatments and, for those patients mature enough to attempt to understand themselves, self-knowledge and insight are the not inconsiderable benefits.

REFERENCES

1. Denckla MB, Roeltgen DP: Disorders of motor function and control, in Rapin I, Segalowitz SJ (vol eds). Boller F, Grafman J (series eds): *Handbook of Neuropsychology:* vol 6. *Child Neuropsychology.* Amsterdam: Elsevier, 1992, pp 455–476.
2. Denckla MB: Revised neurological examination for subtle signs. *Psychopharm Bull* 21:773–779, 1985.
3. Berninger VW, Rutberg J: Relationship of finger function to beginning writing: Application to diagnosis of writing disabilities. *Dev Med Child Neurol* 34:198–215, 1992.
4. Denckla MB: Development of speed in repetitive and successive finger movements in normal children. *Dev Med Child Neurol* 15:635–645, 1973.
5. Denckla MB: Development of motor coordination in normal children. *Dev Med Child Neurol* 16:729–741, 1974.
6. Wolff PH, Gunnoe CE, Cohen C: Associated movements as a measure of developmental age. *Dev Med Child Neurol* 25:417–429, 1983.
7. Nass R: Mirror movement asymmetries in congenital hemiparesis: The inhibition hypothesis revisited. *Neurology* 35:1059–1062, 1985.
8. Pennington BF: *Diagnosing Learning Disorders: A Neuropsychological Framework.* New York: Guilford, 1991, pp vii–x, 32–34.
9. Touwen BCL: Examination of the child with minor neurological dysfunction, in *Clinical Developmental Medicine,* No. 71, 2d ed. London: MacKeith, 1979.

Chapter 62

PEDIATRIC NEUROPSYCHOLOGICAL ASSESSMENT

Jane Holmes Bernstein
Deborah P. Waber

Neuropsychological assessment is a complex clinical activity that cannot be reduced to the simple application of psychological tests (see also Chap. 3),[1,2] although, especially in the pediatric context, it has been notably shaped by the availability of such tests. Assessment is better conceptualized as the clinical process whose goals are to determine a diagnosis as well as to guide the development and implementation of a management plan.[3,4] Given these goals, the theoretical context that drives the assessment process is as important as patterns of assets and deficits revealed by test scores. It is the model that is derived from theory that renders the test scores relevant to the child and to interventions that are meaningful for the child's well-being and adjustment.

The neuropsychological assessment of children, like that of adults, typically utilizes one of two broad strategies, which can be characterized primarily by the way in which psychological tests are utilized. "Fixed battery" approaches are highly regimented; they consist of menus of well-normed psychological tests and associated statistical procedures that provide the basis for assigning a diagnosis.[5–8] The theoretical basis for these approaches to neuropsychological assessment is typically rooted more in statistical considerations than in neuroscience. "Flexible" approaches, by contrast, are more eclectic in terms of test instruments and allow for a more flexible response to expectable variation from child to child.[4,9–12] These approaches typically involve both a consistent set of measures that is routinely administered to all patients and selected tasks that address specific referral questions, findings elicited by the core measures, symptoms characteristic of given disorders, and/or potential models of intervention strategies. Integration of the various components of the evaluation depends on the particular theoretical framework brought to bear by the assessor. Although there is typically no a priori algorithm for arriving at a diagnosis, as is the case for the fixed battery approaches, there are principles that guide the diagnostic formulation.[4,13–19] These principles are theory-driven, based on an appreciation of processes of neurobehavioral development in the child. The choice of a particular strategy can be based on a number of considerations, including the setting in which it is applied, the qualifications of the examiner, the fit between the examiner's preferred style of assessment and the format of different approaches, and the demands of the clinical practice in which the method is applied.

Each of the approaches has obvious advantages and disadvantages. Fixed approaches are sturdy in a variety of settings. Because reliability and validity are well established (assuming that the tests are administered in the prescribed fashion), they are less vulnerable to variations in the training or the biases of the examiner, to variations in the manner of administration of tests, or to subtle social variables that may impinge on the test situation. Disadvantages are primarily related to clinical utility. The fixed approaches are structured primarily to provide for group discrimination (e.g., normal versus abnormal) but are less effective at providing the more descriptive information that can be most valuable for intervention (e.g., learning style, social/personality variables, developmental context). The more flexible approaches have the obvious disadvantage of limited reliability and validity. These can be far more dependent on the skill of "experts" who may or may not provide useful diagnostic information, depending on their training, experience, and theoretical sophistication.[8] Advantages, however, include the ability to assimilate a broad range of information (including but not limited to test scores), to provide extensive descriptive information that is valuable in intervention, and to draw conclusions and make predictions that are based on a developmental context.

In the present chapter, we review specific considerations entailed in the neuropsychological assessment of children; these should inform any approach that is employed. We then provide a conceptual description of our own approach, which is flexible, but also—and importantly—"systemic." The goal of this approach is to integrate developmental principles, viewed in a systemic perspective, more formally into the assessment process. Each of these discussions would obviously be worthy of much lengthier treatment. In the present format, significant issues are outlined relatively briefly in order to provide an overview of the major issues involved.

CONSIDERATIONS IN THE NEUROPSYCHOLOGICAL ASSESSMENT OF CHILDREN

Pediatric neuropsychology emerged largely as a derivative of adult neuropsychology. Early efforts to assess children with neurologic impairment were derived to a great extent from adult models. Such models, however, proved to have significant limitations when applied in the pediatric setting. In a defining paper published in 1984,[15] Fletcher and Taylor outlined four basic fallacies in the application of adult methods and models to pediatric neuropsychology: "... differential sensitivity, similar skills, special sign, and brain-behavior isomorphism." Although their critique led to reexamination of practices and of (especially) data interpretation, the points they raised then are not always accorded adequate consideration.

Perhaps the most significant problem with reliance on adult-derived models of brain-behavior relationships is that the adult models cannot accommodate the defining characteristic of the child—that is, development.[20] One response to this problem has been to characterize as "developmental" test batteries that bring together instruments that show systematic, generally monotonic age-related variation. Such solutions, however, continue to be vulnerable to the problems of downward extension from adult psychology and neuropsychology, as pointed out by Fletcher and Taylor. Furthermore, approaches that rely only or primarily on linear trajectories of psychological test scores do not accurately reflect developmental processes, which are better characterized by organization and reorganization of functions. Bernstein[3,21] has argued that psychological tests should not be the primary indices of behavioral function in neuropsychological assessment. The concept of development should be incorporated into clinical assessment from the top down. If the assessment is conceptualized as an N-of-1 clinical experiment, developmental principles are integral to the design of the experiment and can shape the methodology. Structured psychological instruments, along with other techniques for eliciting and observing behavior (such as dynamic interviewing strategies, clinical limit testing, behavioral questionnaires, and so forth), can be employed within this framework. Other relevant considerations are presented here.

Focal versus Nonfocal Neural Substrates

Clinicoanatomic correlation of brain lesions and behavior as seen in adults form a basis for such fundamental neuropsychological principles as hemispheric specialization, the differential functions of prefrontal and frontal cortex, substrates for motor coordination, and so forth. More recent analyses of the neural substrates for behavioral functions have highlighted the importance of functional networks (see Chaps. 4 and 10).[22] This perspective has been increasingly elaborated with advances in functional neuroimaging techniques such as positron emission tomography (PET) and especially functional magnetic resonance imaging (fMRI) as described in Chap. 7. Nonetheless, studies of individuals with focal lesions or specific forms of neuropathology continue to occupy a prominent position in adult neuropsychology.

Focal lesions, however, are relatively rare in children, and the literature on functional neuroimaging in children is sparse. When focal lesions do occur in children, their behavioral correlates are not nearly as straightforward to interpret as are those seen in adults. Although some of the same principles of functional organization appear to be common for children and adults, the functional neural architecture presumably undergoes transformation during childhood, prior to achieving the mature adult form.[23] The prevalent forms of childhood neuropathology, which form the basis for correlative neurodevelopmental studies, tend to be more diffuse (e.g., periventricular lesions associated with prematurity, structural correlates of neurogenetic disorders, congenital brain malformations, effects of lead intoxication and other environmental hazards, consequences of systemic disease and its treatment). Furthermore, a substantial subset of the children who present for neuropsychological assessment have a disorder of presumed developmental origin (e.g., learning disability, developmental delay) with as yet no clearly defined neural correlates. In this developmental context, the functional network is a far more salient concept than the focally organized deficit.

Modularity versus Nonmodularity

A related issue is the architecture of cognition. In the adult, specific cognitive functions, it can be argued, assume a modular structure[24]; that is, cognitive functions can be understood as "packaged" in modules. Focal brain injury can thus result in alteration of such a behavioral module with relative sparing of other functions. However, the nature of such modules and the processes by which neurobehavioral development might result in a modular structure is currently a matter of spirited debate.[25–29] Empirically, it appears that, in children, cognition has not yet assumed the adult modular architecture but is more global, dynamic, and systemically integrated. Indeed, one of the hallmarks of cognitive development is progressive differentiation of functions (and increasing limitations in terms of plasticity and recovery of function; see Chap. 5). Hence, in children, even focal brain injury will not necessarily result in relatively isolated impairment of a specific cognitive function, but is likely to have more wide-ranging effects as the impact of the injury comes to be integrated within the powerful processes of development.

More generally, the issue of modularity presents a challenge for theories of neurobehavioral development.[25–29] The best approximation of the truth is most likely to be a combination of modular and connectionist (developmental process) approaches with different functions assuming a more or less modular form in the course of development. What is clear is that (1) the character of the behavioral changes associated with acquired lesions in children is quite different from that seen in adults; (2) forces of development are crucial in the evolution of outcomes of brain injury in children; and (3) development is a lifelong process and that theoretical formulations of brain-behavior relationships in both children and adults can learn from, and inform, each other.

For the clinical neuropsychological assessment, different perspectives on the modularity issue potentially have implications for intervention. Is the goal of the assessment to identify, and "fix," a broken module? In that case, the focus of intervention is likely to be remedial. If the goal is adaptation, that is, maximizing the child-world "fit," the emphasis will favor compensatory strategy development. In addition, different views of the trajectory of module development can be expected to influence the clinical answer to the question: Which approach should be used, and when?

Stability versus Developmental Change

Although changes in neural structure and function occur throughout the life span,[30] such changes are most dramatic in children, especially young children. In children, both pathologic changes and normative developmental differences are rooted in the ontogenetic forces that shape cognitive and affective development in childhood.[31] Psychological tests are constructed so that changes will be manifest empirically as an apparently linear accretion of knowledge or skill. Developmental psychology, however, has consistently demonstrated that these apparently linear changes actually represent the sequential organization and reorganization of cognitive functions, presumably reflecting the complex interplay between maturational changes and experiential influences. Thus, developmental progress may appear linear but is in fact nonlinear.[32,33] Cognitive function is thus transformed in response to the developmental mandates that organize ongoing behavioral change. These transformations will lead to recovery or compensation in some instances and the emergence of seemingly new problems in others. Diagnosis and, in particular, prediction must therefore be undertaken with cognizance of the developmental context and its significance.

In the clinical setting, deficits that are apparent during one developmental period may have little predictive role in the management of a child at a later stage. Problems will be defined by the brain-world interaction, with the particular *demand* on the child at any given point determining the functional problem.[3,34] For example, children who have difficulty with processing higher-order language can appear to be good readers in the early grades because their decoding skills are adequate but then show difficulty in later years, developing an unexpected reading problem as the complexity of the language within the material increases. At the later stage, the higher-order language problem can present as comprehension and memory problems.

Pathognomonic Signs versus Developmental Normality

One of the most fascinating challenges for pediatric neuropsychology is the extent to which signs or behaviors that are clearly pathologic in adults can be normative (at certain ages), of equivalent pathologic significance, or pathognomonic—but of different systems—in children. For example, when copying and/or recalling the Rey-Osterrieth Complex Figure,[35,36] young children are very likely to rotate the whole figure 90 degrees counterclockwise. Such dramatic rotations, which are normal during certain stages of development, can prompt diagnoses of focal brain pathology in adults. Similarly, a failure to draw the figure from left to right is of potential diagnostic significance in adults but typical in young children. Indeed, it is not until approximately 9 years of age that the majority of children proceed from left to right and only at 13 that better than 90 percent do so.[35] The overriding consideration in the assessment of children is thus the normal developmental context, not a specific deficit—unless, of course, the deficit-causing lesion is catastrophic! The effects of even a very circumscribed and localized lesion will become incorporated into the ongoing flow of normal developmental forces, modifying them certainly, but typically remaining subservient to them. Thus, assessment of the child needs to be guided by an appreciation of developmental psychology and developmental neurobiology.

Neurobehavioral Deficits versus Environmental Expectations

In adult neuropsychology, the complaint that brings an individual to evaluation is most frequently apparent or suspected loss of function, presumably referable to some underlying pathologic process. For children, the issues are typically quite different. Acquired lesions of childhood most frequently occur in the pre- or perinatal period. The primary consequence of these early insults is that the impairment itself, as noted above, becomes integrated into the broader developmental process. This developmental perspective has important implications for the diagnostic process, shifting the focus from measuring the child's functional repertoire at the time of assessment to analyzing the behavioral outcome of the child's developmental course to date and predicting the future course in the context of ongoing developmental processes.[3]

Most children who present for neuropsychological assessment do so because of functional problems that do not have an identifiable neural substrate. The issue, then, is not that a previously acquired function has been lost. Rather, the child's problems stem from the fact that the functional repertoire does not comfortably meet normative expectations for adaptation and achievement. To address this, the task of the pediatric assessment is not primarily (or optimally) to identify impairments (as in the adult) but to analyze the child's complement of developing skills (both current and future) in relation to environmental demands (the *child-world system*[4]), with the aim of improving the "fit" between the two. These demands will not only be general, referenced to expectable developmental challenges for the general population, but also specific, referenced to the demands placed on a particular child in a particular setting.[37] A child with a particular neuropsychological profile might encounter significant functional problems in one setting but appear reasonably well adapted in another. By the same token, opportunities for remediation and accommodation can be expected to differ from setting to setting. Although the ideal may be that there is some objective diagnostic "truth" that can be attached to a child, the reality is that local ecologic forces play a significant role in the formulation of both diagnosis and management.

THE SYSTEMIC APPROACH TO PEDIATRIC NEUROPSYCHOLOGICAL ASSESSMENT

The foregoing discussion highlights the importance of integrating developmental principles into pediatric neuropsychological assessment. In the systemic approach to assessment, which derives from the systemic tradition of Luria and Vygotsky,[38,39] observed and reported behaviors are scrutinized within the *brain-context-development* matrix.[3] The primary goal of the assessment is thus not the specification or even diagnosis of deficits within the child but delineation of the transaction between the developing child and the ecologic context (the *child-world system*[3,4]). The fundamental premise of this approach, much like that of structuralist psychology (e.g., Piaget), is that there is an essential neuropsychological diagnostic profile that evolves developmentally. This profile is framed in neuroanatomic terms (at a heuristic level), thus organizing observations of behavioral adaptation across functional domains. Such a description may reflect damage or dysfunction; it may also reflect naturally occurring individual differences. The diagnostic formulation evaluates this heuristically derived behavioral profile against a general knowledge of the potential disorders of children and their outcomes. The goal of the assessment is thus not simply to formulate a diagnosis but also to describe the child's profile, to analyze how well it fits with environmental demands and expectations, to thus determine the child's "risk,"[3] and to then outline a comprehensive management plan that includes recommendations for reorganizing the system so as to minimize the impact of the risk.

The Assessment: Diagnostic Method

The diagnostic process integrates models from medicine and behavioral neurology with those of neuropsychology. The clinician reviews neurobehavioral systems with the goal of identifying a diagnostic behavioral cluster,[4] attempting to establish both convergent validity (behaviors that should go together do so) and discriminant validity (behaviors that should not be present are not). Relevant behaviors are manifest in the context of specific systemic interactions in both the natural environment and in the testing situation and are referenced to the developmental status of the child. The relevant data come from the family history; from the child's developmental, medical, and educational history; from detailed observations of the child's behavioral repertoire in a variety of contexts; and from performance on selected psychological tests. Although it is well recognized that any behavioral datum is "neuropsychological" to the extent that it is used systematically by a trained clinician to make inferences about the central nervous system,[40,41] historic and observational data have most frequently been conceptualized as moderator variables, which influence the diagnostic inferences drawn from test performance but do not themselves contribute directly to the diagnosis. In contrast, the systemic approach assigns equivalent weight to historic, observation, and test-based sources of data. Indeed, we have demonstrated empirically that it is possible, largely on the basis of historic and observational aspects of the assessment, to derive biologically relevant behavioral profiles that may be invisible on the basis of test scores.[42]

This does not mean that a valid assessment can or should be accomplished without psychological testing or that tests should not be administered rigorously in the standard fashion. Psychological tests are an essential component of the systemically based assessment, and valid, norm-referenced scores should be generated. However, testing of limits—that is, determining systematically what modifications can facilitate successful performance—provides invaluable data for the diagnostic formulation and especially for intervention. Such testing must be done in a way that preserves the integrity of the tests themselves and allows for standardized use. In addition, assembling test protocols that are used on a relatively routine basis, with provision for flexibility to evaluate specific issues as needed, provides for consistency across children and enhances observational analyses as it becomes possible to build an experiential base of knowledge about the range of responses that children will demonstrate given the same set of challenges.

Forecasting the Future

The pediatric neuropsychologist is typically expected not only to evaluate current status but also to render predictions about the future. These predictions can be based not only on results of tests that measure specific functions (e.g., visuomotor skill) but can also be derived from the *brain-context-development* matrix as applied to this particular child. The neuropsychological diagnostic profile, its developmental context, and environmental expectations are all essential considerations. Children often will manifest difficulties in one skill area at a specific developmental stage and difficulties in a different skill area later on. Such "time-referenced symptoms"[43] are as much a function of academic and curricular demands as they are of the child.[44]

For example, a language-impaired child who has demonstrated consistent strength in mathematics in the early grades may unexpectedly encounter major difficulty in the upper grades. Strict adherence to test findings would not have predicted this problem, since in the general population of children a strong score on a mathematics achievement test typically predicts subsequent success. Closer examination might reveals, however, that the difficulty emerged in response to a change in the language demands of the mathematics curriculum. While underlying conceptual strengths may continue to be present, production and achievement can falter as the child struggles to manage the more complex verbal demands of a particular topic or indeed of a whole curriculum. In the systemic formulation, this would have been predicted directly—as a result of the child's neuropsychological profile interacting with demands that are guided by anticipated developmental change in the normally developing peer cohort. For this type of student, the recommendation would not necessarily be to institute math support but to emphasize certain elements of the curriculum over others or modify the language demands of the existing curriculum.

Formulating an Intervention Strategy

Within the systemic model, the goal of intervention strategies cannot be confined to remediation of the deficit; it is, as if not more, important to improve the fit between the child's complement of skills and specific environmental demands. The approach is thus twofold. Specific remediation can facilitate development in skill areas, classroom management techniques can facilitate performance, or social skills instruction or psychotherapy may address social and emotional issues. The ultimate goal of intervention, however, is not to normalize every child to the same level of performance but to maximize each child's developmental potential and adaptation, given an underlying neuropsychological profile that is most likely going to be relatively stable (albeit through various developmental transformations). To this end, analysis and modification of environmental demands so that they are more appropriate for the child's neuropsychological endowment must be central to any management plan.

Reporting the Findings

The feedback session(s) and written report form the basis for the interpretive or informing process, the latter also constituting a record of the assessment itself. Although formal communication of findings is an essential component of any psychological assessment, it takes on added importance in the pediatric setting. Children come to evaluation at the behest of adults and are dependent on parents and teachers for support of their development. The goal of the pediatric neuropsychological assessment is not simply to evaluate the child but also to institute a process of change in a system that is not functioning optimally. Parents and teachers, who are the major potential agents of change in the child's world, are central to any plan to modify the child-world system. Providing parents and teachers with information that enables them to better understand both the child's complement of skills now and the risk(s) posed for that child by changing environmental demands and expectable developmental challenges in the future is thus integral to the assessment process.

Consequently, the feedback session(s) and written report should not be viewed as a simple statement of findings and recommendations. Rather, they constitute a crucial opportunity to reframe models of attribution, to assign responsibility more appropriately, and to provide all involved with a working model of the child. Engaging parents (and teachers where possible) in a process of face-to-face dialogue is thus imperative. The assessment process is not complete without the interpretive feedback session. Although specific recommendations are always helpful, in the systemic context the feedback and report help adults to understand the diagnostic formulation as well as to assimilate its significance so that they can respond to the child more effectively on a day-to-day basis in "on line" situations.

To take an example, children who present with apparent attentional problems are often found on evaluation to have difficulties in processing language. Reframing the "attentional problem" in terms of an underlying language-processing problem can have a profound influence on the child-world system. Instead of viewing inattention as a "deficit" that needs to be remediated, teachers can be encouraged to view inattention as a signal that the child has not effectively processed the language and is, as a consequence, confused and distracted. The appropriate intervention in this context is to facilitate comprehension and ensure that the child is engaged with the classroom discussion or activity. Should the attentional failure represent a true disorder of attention, alternative strategies, both behavioral and pharmacologic, may be more successful.

CONCLUSION

Pediatric neuropsychology is a rapidly evolving discipline in which clinicians and researchers engage in a dialogue to elucidate the nature of brain-behavior relationships in the child. Clinicians contribute to this dialogue via the practice of assessment. Assessment is not a set of techniques learned once and for all by clinicians in training. It is itself a developmental process undertaken in the context of a theoretical framework that must be informed by the changing knowledge base in the developmental sciences, both clinical and research. Assessment is an integral component of the search for new knowledge, a process to be constantly reviewed in light of new information. Differences in approach to the neuropsychological assessment of children reflect differences in the training and expertise of clinicians, in the populations assessed, in the types of neuropathology or behavioral disorders addressed, and in the goals of intervention and management. Differing approaches to assessment are not, however, exclusive; each contributes in complementary ways to extend our understanding of neurobehavioral development.

REFERENCES

1. Vanderploeg RD: Interview and testing: The data-collection phase of neuropsychological evaluations, in Vanderploeg RD (ed): *Clinician's Guide to Neuropsychological Assessment.* Hillsdale, NJ: Erlbaum, 1994, pp 1–41.
2. Matarazzo JD: Psychological assessment versus psychological testing. *Am Psychol* 45:999–1017, 1990.
3. Bernstein JH: Developmental neuropsychological assessment, in Yeates KO, Ris D, Taylor HG (eds): *Pediatric Neuropsychology: Research, Theory and Practice.* New York: Guilford Press, 2000, pp 405–438.
4. Holmes-Bernstein JM, Waber DP: Developmental neuropsychological assessment: The systemic approach, in Boulton AA, Baker GB, Hiscock M (eds): *Neuromethods: Neuropsychology.* Clifton, NJ: Humana Press, 1990, vol 17, pp 311–371.
5. Golden CJ: The Luria-Nebraska Children's Battery: Theory and formulation, in Hynd GW, Obrzut JE (eds): *Neuropsychological Assessment and the School-Age Child.* New York: Grune & Stratton, 1981, pp 277–302.
6. Reed HB, Reitan RM, Klove H: Influence of cerebral lesions on psychological test performances of older children. *J Consult Psychol* 29:247–251, 1965.
7. Reitan RM: Psychological effects of cerebral lesions on children of early school age, in Reitan RM, Davison LA (eds): *Clinical Neuropsychology: Current Status and Applications.* Washington, DC: Hemisphere, 1974, pp 53–89.
8. Rourke BP, Fisk J, Strang JD: *Neuropsychological Assessment of Children.* New York: Guilford Press, 1986.
9. Taylor HG, Fletcher JM: Neuropsychological assessment of children, in Goldstein G, Hersen M (eds): *Handbook of Psychological Assessment,* 2d ed. New York: Pergamon Press, 1990, pp 228–255.
10. Hartlage LC, Telzrow C: *Neuropsychological Assessment and Intervention with Children and Adolescents.* Sarasota, FL: Professional Resource Exchange, 1986.
11. Pennington BF: *Diagnosing Learning Disorders.* New York: Guilford Press, 1991.
12. Wilson BC: The neuropsychological assessment of the preschool child: A branching model, in Rapin I, Segalowitz SJ (eds): *Handbook of Neuropsychology: Child Neuropsychology.* Amsterdam: Elsevier, 1992, vol 6, pp 377–394.

13. Christensen AL: *Luria's Neuropsychological Investigation.* New York: Spectrum, 1975.
14. Fennell EB, Bauer RM: Modes of inference in evaluating brain-behavior relationships in children, in Reynolds CR, Fletcher-Janzen E (eds): *Handbook of Clinical Child Neuropsychology.* New York: Plenum Press, 1989, pp 167–177.
15. Fletcher JM, Taylor HG: Neuropsychological approaches to children: towards a developmental neuropsychology. *J Clin Neuropsychol* 6:39–56, 1984.
16. Morris RD, Fletcher JM, Francis DJ: Conceptual and psychometric issues in the neuropsychologic assessment of children: Measurement of ability discrepancy and change, in Rapin I, Segalowitz SJ (eds): *Handbook of Neuropsychology: Child Neuropsychology.* Amsterdam: Elsevier, 1992, vol 6, pp 341–352.
17. Rourke BP: Brain-behavior relationships in children with learning disabilities: A research program. *Am Psychol* 30:911–920, 1975.
18. Waber DP: Rate and state: A critique of models underlying the assessment of learning disabled children, in Zelazo PR, Barr RG (eds): *Challenges to Developmental Paradigms: Implications for Theory, Assessment and Treatment.* Hillsdale, NJ: Erlbraum, 1988, pp 29–41.
19. Wilson BC, Finucci DA: A model for clinical-quantitative classification: Application to language-disordered preschool children. *Brain Lang* 27:282–309, 1986.
20. Tramontana MG, Hooper SR: Child neuropsychological assessment: Overview of current status, in Tramontana MG, Hooper SR (eds): *Assessment Issues in Child Neuropsychology.* New York: Plenum Press, 1988, pp 3–38.
21. Bernstein JH, Weiler M: "Pediatric neuropsychological assessment" examined, in Goldstein G, Hersen M (eds): *Handbook of Psychological Assessment,* 3rd ed. New York: Pergamon Press, 2000, pp 263–300.
22. Mesulam M-M: Large scale neurocognitive networks and distributed processing for attention, language and memory. *Ann Neurol* 28:597–613, 1990.
23. Bates E: Plasticity, localization and language development, in Broman SH, Fletcher JM (eds): *The Changing Nervous System: Neurobehavioral Consequences of Early Brain Lesions.* New York: Oxford University Press, 1999, pp 214–253.
24. Fodor J: *Modularity of Mind.* Cambridge, MA: MIT Press, 1983.
25. Pinker S: *How the Mind Works.* New York: Norton, 1997.
26. Cosmides L, Tooby J: Origins of domain specificity: The evolution of functional organization, in Hirschfeld LA, Gelman SA (eds): *Mapping the Mind: Domain Specificity in Cognition and Culture.* New York: Cambridge University Press, 1994, pp 85–116.
27. Elman J, Bates E, Johnson M, et al: *Rethinking Innateness: A Connectionist Perspective on Development.* Cambridge, MA: MIT Press/Bradford Books, 1996.
28. Buller DJ, Hardcastle VG: Evolutionary psychology, meet developmental neurobiology: Against promiscuous modularity. *Brain Mind* 1:307–325, 2000.
29. Quartz SR, Sejnowski TJ: The neural basis of cognitive development: a contructivist manifesto. *Behav Brain Sci* 20:537–596, 1997.
30. Benes FM, Turtle M, Khan Y, et al: Myelination of a key relay zone in the hippocampal formation occurs in the human brain during childhood, adolescence, and adulthood. *Arch Gen Psychiatry* 51:477–484, 1994.
31. Segalowitz SJ, Hiscock M: The emergence of a neuropsychology of normal development: Rapprochement between neuroscience and developmental neuropsychology, in Rapin I, Segalowitz SJ (eds): *Handbook of Neuropsychology:Child Neuropsychology.* Amsterdam: Elsevier, 1992, vol 6, pp 45–71.
32. Sameroff AJ: Developmental systems: Contexts and evolution, in Mussen PH (ed): *Handbook of Child Psychology,* 4th ed. *History, Theory, and Methods.* New York: Wiley, 1983, vol 1, pp 237–294.
33. Fischer KW, Bidell TR: Dynamic development of psychological structures in action and thought, in Lerner RM (ed): Damon W (ed): *Handbook of Child Psychology* 5th ed. *Theoretical Models of Human Development.* New York, Wiley, 1998, vol 1, pp 467–561.
34. Rudel RG, Holmes JM, Pardes JR: *Assessment of Developmental Learning Disorders: A Neuropsychological Approach.* New York: Basic Books, 1988.
35. Waber DP, Holmes JM: Assessing children's copy productions of the Rey-Osterrieth Complex Figure. *J Clin Exp Neuropsychol* 7:264–280, 1985.
36. Waber DP, Holmes JM: Assessing children's memory productions of the Rey-Osterrieth Complex Figure. *J Clin Exp Neuropsychol* 8:563–580, 1986.
37. Gottlieb G: Experiential canalization of behavioral development: Theory. *Dev Psychol* 27:4–13, 1991.
38. Luria AR: *The Working Brain.* New York, Basic Books, 1973.
39. Vygotsky LS: *Mind in Society: The Development of Higher Psychological Functions.* Cambridge, MA: Harvard University Press, 1978.
40. Mattis S: Neuropsychological assessment of school-aged children, in Rapin I, Segalowitz SJ (eds): *Handbook of Neuropsychology: Child Neuropsychology.* Amsterdam: Elsevier, 1992, vol 6, pp 395–415.

41. Taylor HG: Neuropsychological testing: Relevance of assessing children's learning disabilities. *J Consult Clin Psychol* 56:795–800, 1988.
42. Waber DP, Bernstein JH, Kammerer BL, et al: Neuropsychological diagnostic profiles of children who received CNS treatment for acute lymphoblastic leukemia: Neurodevelopmental implications. *Dev Neuropsychol* 8:1–28, 1992.
43. Rudel RG: Residual effects of childhood reading disabilities. *Bull Orton Soc* 31:89–102, 1981.
44. Holmes JM: Natural histories in learning disabilities: Neuropsychological difference/environmental demand, in Ceci SJ (ed): *Handbook of Cognitive, Social and Neuropsychological Aspects of Learning Disabilities.* Hillsdale, NJ: Erlbaum, 1987, vol 2, pp 303–319.

Chapter 63

ACQUIRED DISORDERS OF LANGUAGE IN CHILDREN*

Maureen Dennis

Childhood-acquired language disorder, or *childhood-acquired aphasia,* refers to language impairment that is evident after a period of normal language acquisition and that is precipitated by, or associated with, an identified form of brain insult. It differs from language acquisition disorders without clearly established brain pathology and from language deficits that emerge during or after initial language acquisition in children with neurodevelopmental brain disorders (see Chaps. 61, 62, 67, and 68).

In an earlier research era, acquired language disorders in children were referenced to adult aphasic syndromes. It was concluded that, compared to adults, children showed fewer aphasic symptoms (especially comprehension symptoms), more transient aphasic deficits, and fewer focal and lateralized precipitating brain insults.[1,2]

A more recent view of childhood-acquired aphasia has been shaped by the explosion of empirical studies; the publication of benchmarks, assessment instruments, and theoretical models of normal language development; and the availability of structural and functional imaging techniques to identify the brain correlates of aphasic disorders. It has also been shaped by developmental neuropsychological models of childhood brain disorders, which have proposed that functional outcome, including language, represents the effects of the biology of the brain injury, the age and development of the child, the time since onset of injury, and the available cognitive and psychosocial reserve.[3]

Any advantage for an earlier onset of acquired aphasia is short-lived and concerns the faster abatement of acute-stage aphasic symptoms. In the long term, children with acquired aphasia continue to exhibit language impairment. Age at aphasia-producing brain injury has proved to be less predictive of aphasic symptoms but more relevant to long-term language function than was previously thought. Given a similar brain injury, children and adults exhibit similar aphasic symptoms in the acute stage of acquired aphasia; however, while children show a faster resolution of aphasic symptoms than adults, their long-term language function may sometimes be poorer. These conclusions have emerged from studies conducted over the last 20 years, which have questioned many of the features once considered to define childhood-acquired aphasia—namely, fewer language symptoms, faster rate of recovery, less focal and lateralized lesions.

Nonfluent Characteristics of Childhood-Acquired Aphasia

Historically, childhood-acquired aphasia was characterized by nonfluent and impoverished spontaneous speech,[4–6] ranging in severity from mutism to articulatory difficulties, as well as by nonfluent language, often with simplified syntax, telegraphic speech, and word-finding difficulties (see Chap. 11 for a discussion of these aphasic signs). Dysfluency has been reported in both older[7–9] and more recent[10] studies of childhood-acquired aphasia.

Symptoms of adult fluent aphasia (logorrhea, verbal stereotypies, perseverations, neologisms, jargon, and paraphasias; see Chap. 11) would once have been thought to be rare in children with acquired language disorders.[8] More recently, studies have shown that children with acquired aphasia show fluent aphasia[11] that includes phonemic jargon, neologisms,

* **ACKNOWLEDGMENTS:** The author's research described in this paper was supported by project grants from the Ontario Mental Health Foundation and the Physicians' Services Incorporated Foundation and by NINDS Grant 2R01NS 21889-16, "Neurobehavioral Outcome of Head Injury in Children."

and paraphasias[12] and also that aphasic symptoms in children are quite varied.[13] Moreover, a number of adult aphasic syndromes have been described in children: jargon aphasia[12,14]; Wernicke's aphasia and transcortical sensory aphasia[15]; conduction aphasia[16]; transcortical sensory aphasia[11,17]; anomic aphasia[18]; and alexia without agraphia.[19,20] In short, most adult aphasic syndromes can be observed in children, albeit with different base frequencies.[21]

From its first description in 1957, the Landau-Kleffner syndrome (LKS),[22] whose defining feature is a severe and long-lasting verbal auditory agnosia for words and for sounds, became the paradigm of childhood-acquired aphasia.[23] Comprehension deficits are features of the long-term language function in other childhood-acquired aphasic conditions and may even be more pronounced than in adults; for example, global aphasia from a childhood left middle cerebral artery infarct may resolve to a transcortical sensory aphasia characterized by poorer language comprehension than in comparable adult cases.[24]

Recent research has not supported the traditional view that comprehension, especially auditory comprehension, is preserved in childhood-acquired aphasia. Instead, it has shown comprehension deficits to be central to childhood-acquired aphasic disorders.

Transient Nature of Childhood-Acquired Aphasia

Recovery of aphasic symptoms in cases of childhood-acquired aphasia is often rapid,[25] although some 25 to 50 percent of cases still show residual aphasia 1 year later. Recent long-term follow-up studies, which have focused on recovery of language function rather than on abatement of aphasic symptoms, show that childhood-acquired aphasia is long-lasting, with effects that extend in time beyond the disappearance of aphasic symptoms.[23] Although clinical signs of aphasia somewhat similar to those in the adult occur in the acute phase of childhood-acquired aphasia, long-term language outcome may be poor even after aphasic symptoms have resolved,[26] especially for pragmatic language.[27,28]

Functional outcomes that require intact language skills, such as academic achievement, continue to be poor beyond the period of clinical aphasia recovery,[29–31] and problems in new academic learning[17] may even become exacerbated over time, perhaps because of the escalating demands of academic work in the higher grades.[32]

Nonfocal Brain Bases of Childhood-Acquired Aphasia

Early study groups of children with acquired aphasia had an overrepresentation of traumatic and infectious etiologies.[7] At that time, techniques for determining lesion lateralization involved principally clinical status, such as the presence of hemiplegia, which meant that actual lesions might have been bilateral or unilateral.[14] As a result of these limitations, the view arose that childhood-acquired aphasia involved nonfocal brain insult.

Child and adult aphasia–producing lesions may have different long-term effects on the brain. Some early lesions may leave little focal residual change,[33] with the result that the brain does not show characteristic gliotic changes but rather tissue shrinkage, so that even with an initially focal insult, brain lesions in childhood may involve decreased brain volume.[34]

Nonlateralized Brain Bases of Childhood-Acquired Aphasia

It was once assumed that the lateralization of language was incremental over the first decade of life, but the question then arose of a left hemisphere bias for language development (discussed in Refs. 21 and 35). Recent empirical studies have not only challenged the idea that aphasia after right-sided lesions is more common in children than in adults[14] but have shown that the risk of acquired aphasia after left hemisphere damage in right-handers is approximately the same in children and adults,[25,36,37] leading to the conclusion that, given a unilateral lesion to the dominant hemisphere, childhood aphasia is no more uncommon than adult aphasia.[38]

Even the characteristics of the aphasia are similar in children and adults. Left-sided lesions to the classic adult language areas in childhood produce a fluent aphasia with many neologisms and paraphasias.[39]

Recovery from childhood-acquired aphasia depends on the integrity of the left posterior language areas,[30] which suggests that a lateralized and focal language representation is well established by middle childhood and also that recovery from childhood-acquired aphasia may engage intact areas of the left hemisphere.[40]

Age-Related versus Etiologic Differences in Adult- and Childhood-Acquired Aphasia

In earlier studies, child and adult differences in outcome after acquired aphasia have been attributed to the younger age of the child (and to the putative plasticity of the brain for which the younger age was a marker). Early research selected study groups on the basis of aphasia and combined heterogeneous pathologies in assessing outcome.[7]

However, differences in age at aphasia onset are correlated with differences in etiology. Relative to an adult group, a child group studied because of aphasic symptoms will have an overrepresentation of traumatic and convulsive etiologies and an underrepresentation of vascular disorders. Because inferences about acquired aphasia are based on data from the etiology most frequently reported, views about adult-acquired aphasia have been shaped from parallels with arteritic stroke while those for childhood-acquired aphasia have been understood in terms of head injury and convulsive disorders.

Child and adult acquired aphasias typically differ in both age and etiology,[31] and recent studies have addressed the question of etiologic differences in childhood-acquired aphasia.[2,41] Recovery, both short- and long-term, varies with etiology.[26]

PRINCIPAL ETIOLOGIES OF CHILDHOOD-ACQUIRED APHASIA

This section reviews the characteristics of the principal etiologies of childhood-acquired aphasia. For each etiology, some general issues are discussed; where sufficient evidence is available, cross-etiology comparisons are facilitated by Tables 63-1 through 63-4.

Seizure and Seizure-Related Disorders: The Landau-Kleffner Syndrome (LKS)

Seizure disorders affect cognition and language,[42] and language symptoms have been observed both as part of clinical seizures and as part of ictal speech automatisms. Recurrent generalized seizures and medication may have diffuse effects that can confound the interpretation of otherwise focal lesions. The most fully studied aphasia-producing seizure disorder, however, is the LKS,[22] the characteristics of which are reviewed in Table 63-1.

Vascular Disorders

Vascular disorders involve interruptions to the blood supply within the brain as a result of occlusion (ischemic stroke) or rupture (hemorrhagic stroke). Most vascular diseases observed in the adult also occur in children, albeit with different base frequencies. Degenerative disorders like atherosclerosis are common in the middle-aged and elderly but rare in children, while vascular disorders associated with congenital heart disease occur more commonly in childhood[68] and may produce strokes by an embolism from the heart, from complications of heart surgery, or from hypoperfusion from prolonged hypotension. The characteristics of childhood-acquired aphasia from vascular diseases are reviewed in Table 63-2.

Traumatic Disorders

Traumatic head injury is a common cause of childhood-acquired aphasia. Children exhibit a range of aphasic symptoms and language disturbances after head injury.[76] The characteristics of childhood-acquired aphasia from traumatic disorders are reviewed in Table 63-3.

Brain Tumors

Brain tumors in children may be associated with language disturbances.[11,79,95] Language disturbances after tumors above the tentorium have been described, although studies are not numerous. Posterior fossa tumors occur with relatively high frequency in children,

Table 63-1
Childhood-acquired aphasia and the Landau-Kleffner syndrome

Definition

Landau-Kleffner syndrome (LKS) involves acquired aphasia with convulsive disorder[22] occurring in normal children who acutely or progressively lose previously acquired language ability.

A variety of typologies have been proposed.[43]

It was originally claimed that pregnancy, birth, and early development were normal in LKS,[44] and that, classically, LKS occurs after some period of normal language development. More recently, however, it has been found that a history of language pathology may precede the onset of language deterioration and loss,[45] with some 75 percent of patients exhibiting language disturbance before the aphasia.[46]

Loss of language is associated with either clinical seizures (generalized, partial, partial complex, or absence) or with an electroencephalogram (EEG) showing unilateral or paroxysmal activity, sometimes more prominent in slow-wave sleep.[47]

It has been argued that LKS overlaps with other epileptic conditions: rolandic epilepsy, electrical status epilepticus during sleep (ESES), and autistic regression and disintegrative disorder associated with unilateral or bilateral centrotemporal spike/spike-wave discharges.[21]

Core Features

A severe comprehension defect[48] occurs, characteristically with severe verbal auditory agnosia, which may involve both common sounds (such as a dog barking or a doorbell ringing) and words.[2,49]

Epileptic seizures occur in 70 to 75 percent of patients.[50]

Severe behavior disturbances occur in 75 percent of patients.[50] Long-term (≥7 years) follow-up studies have reported mild behavior disturbance (hyperactivity, impulsivity, and oppositional behavior) that is chronologically linked with the language disturbances and follows their fluctuations.[51]

Oral expression is typically poorer than written expression,[52,53] although severe impairment of written language and mathematical skills has been reported.[48]

Neurologic examination is reported to be normal.[54]

Nonverbal intelligence appears to be well preserved.[55]

Half the published cases present first with comprehension disorder, the other half with seizures.[50]

Most LKS patients have a mild form of epilepsy that responds to drug therapy.[56]

There is a correlation between the aphasia and the seizure disorder, although both may fluctuate out of phase,[56] so that the relation is not obvious.[57]

Epidemiology, Demography, and Risk Factors

Some 200 cases have been reported from 1957 to 1995.[50]

The male:female ratio is 2:1.[50]

There are currently no epidemiologic data in regard to geography, infectious disease, toxins, nutrition, or environmental exposures.[58]

Age-Related Factors

Onset occurs from 3 to 8 years of age in 50 percent of cases.[50]

Onset is rare after 8 years of age, although several cases have been reported with loss of language after age 9. Later-onset cases are more likely to have a primarily expressive aphasia with dysfluency and word-finding difficulties.[59]

An age-prognosis relationship has been proposed, such that the younger the child, the poorer the recovery from the acquired aphasia—the reasoning being that newly acquired language skills are particularly vulnerable to bilateral brain pathology.[44] However, age-prognosis effects, such as the claim that recovery is worse with a diagnosis before age 5,[60] have not been replicated with more clearly defined case selection criteria.[51]

Table 63-1 (*Continued*)

Time-Related Factors

Language impairments in LKS persist for months or even years.[49]

Long-term language outcome is often poor. When studied 10 to 28 years after onset of acquired aphasia, more than half of an LKS sample continued to show language disorder.[47] In a long-term follow-up of at least 7 years—into the adolescent years—no individual with LKS fully recovered language.[51]

Typically, seizures remit before adulthood and the aphasia subsides, although not necessarily in parallel.[44]

The long-term outcome of the aphasia has been considered to be unpredictable with respect to medical history features,[47] despite the fact that both epilepsy and EEG abnormalities improve.[61] There is an unpredictable prognosis on an individual case basis, with a fluctuating course of remissions and exacerbations of both aphasia and EEG abnormalities.

In a long-term (2- to 15-year) follow-up of LKS cases, it was found that, even when the EEG normalized in the long term, few individuals achieved normal language, and, further, that no individual with persisting EEG abnormalities recovered normal or near normal language.[46] Thus, persisting EEG abnormalities appear to be a risk factor for continuing aphasia.

Neuropathologic Substrate

Initially, it was unclear whether the language disturbances in LKS was functional or due to an identifiable brain lesion. Proposals for the brain basis of LKS have ranged widely.

It has been suggested that LKS might involve focal subclinical epileptogenic discharges involving the language areas. In this view, aphasic symptoms arise because persistent epileptic discharges cause functional ablation of the primary cortical language areas.[62]

Because the course of the aphasia in LKS may be linked to the appearance and disappearance of ESES,[61] LKS has been considered related to ESES. However, few children with ESES have specific language disorders, and the characteristic EEG of ESES is infrequently found in LKS.[56]

The mild to moderate elevation of cerebrospinal fluid proteins in some LKS cases[47,63] has been used to suggest a low-grade focal inflammation of the brain as the mechanism of LKS aphasia.[64]

Cortical biopsies in some LKS cases have shown changes indicative of a slow virus infection, implying that a subacute viral encephalitis might produce both aphasia and seizures, either from a low-grade selective encephalitis[55] or a subchronic viral encephalitis affecting both hemispheres.[44]

The finding of a positive autoimmune reaction to myelin during clinical deterioration of language in LKS patients has been used to suggest a disorder of myelin metabolism and to account for the positive effect of corticosteroids as immunosuppressive therapy.[65]

Computed tomography and structural magnetic resonance imaging are typically normal.[64]

Angiography has shown isolated arteritis of some branches of the carotid arteries, which implies that focal cerebral vasculitis may be involved in the pathogenesis of LKS.[64]

Positron emission tomography has shown abnormal glucose utilization during sleep, with lower metabolic rates in subcortical than in cortical areas.[66]

Treatment

There is no convincing evidence of empirically effective therapy.[58]

Various drug treatments (antiepileptics, corticosteroids) have been tried, with success on an individual-case basis.

Based on the view that focal vasculitis is responsible for LKS, calcium channel blockers have been proposed as a possible therapy.[64]

Subpial resection has been proposed as therapy in some cases of LKS.

Speech and language therapy has long been used in the rehabilitation of individuals with LKS, but there has been controversy about whether therapy should involve enhancing the residue of oral language; intensive training in the visual domain (gestures, communication boards, signing, computers); brief training in the visual domain with rapid transfer to oral language; or a more pragmatic, multimodal approach. A recent review[67] suggests that no single therapy program will work, that LKS patients are not like deaf individuals, and that any therapy will likely take several years to be effective.

Table 63-2
Language disturbances from vascular etiologies

Definition

Acquired aphasia may be precipitated by a vascular brain lesion occurring in children who acutely or progressively lose previously acquired language skills.

Brain localization depends on the pathophysiology of the stroke. In children, most strokes are secondary to intracranial occlusive disease and are localized in the basal ganglia;[69] however, cortical vascular lesions in the left temporoparietal lobe that produce aphasia have been reported to occur from cerebral arteritis[39] and ruptured arteriovenous malformations.[70]

Core Features

The type of aphasia depends on the localization of the lesion. Aphasia is fluent in form with lesions to the posterior left hemisphere cortical language areas[71] but nonfluent with predominantly subcortical pathology.[72,73]

In the fluent form of aphasia, anomia, word-finding deficits, paraphasias, and circumlocutions occur.[39,70]

Reading and spelling may be relatively preserved with cortical lesions in the left hemispheric posterior language areas, despite anomia,[39,70] which suggests poor phonologic representation of target words.

Reading and writing disorders are common in both the acute and chronic stages of subcortical vascular lesions.[73]

Epidemiology, Demography, and Risk Factors

Few cases have been reported.[71]

Age-Related Factors

Onset at any point throughout childhood.

Time-Related Factors

There is significant recovery from aphasic symptoms after vascular lesions,[73] although naming and word-finding problems persist into the chronic stage of recovery.[39,70]

Neuropathologic Substrate

The laterality and localization of cortical lesions are similar to those of anomic aphasia in adults; damage occurs to the posterior left hemisphere cortical language areas.[39,70]

Most subcortical vascular aphasias of childhood also appear to accord with the clinical-radiologic correlation observed in adults with subcortical aphasias.[72,73]

Lesion laterality may be related to the pattern of impaired language comprehension. In a mixed group of brain-injured children—many with acquired lesions from vascular etiologies—children with left-sided lesions were unable to integrate pragmatic knowledge with syntactic constraints,[74] whereas those with right-sided lesions showed impairments in lexical-semantic and pragmatic knowledge.[74,75]

Treatment

None specific.

Table 63-3
Language disturbances from head injury

Definition

Acquired aphasia may occur after a head injury, typically a closed head injury.

The aphasia is precipitated by injury to the brain, which includes both immediate-impact injury (contusions, diffuse axonal damage) and secondary brain damage involving intracranial events (hematomas, brain swelling, infections, subarachnoid hemorrhages, hydrocephalus) and extracranial factors (hypoxia, hypotension).

Focal brain contusions are common in the frontal and temporal lobes after head injury, whether or not the head has been struck in these particular regions.[77]

Core Features

Children with acquired aphasia from head injury show a variety of aphasic symptoms in the acute stage.[7,78,79]

Frank aphasia and adult-like aphasic syndromes occur infrequently.[76]

Mutism or reduced verbal output and anomia are common in the short term after head injury.[76,80,81]

Epidemiology, Demography, and Risk Factors

Head injury is the leading cause of childhood death in North America,[82] with an incidence of 200 per 10,000 per year.[83] Eighty percent of survivors of severe childhood head injury have learning difficulties, including problems in language-related skills.[84]

Age-Related Factors

Onset can occur at any point throughout childhood.

An earlier age at onset may be associated with more deficits in reading decoding and reading comprehension.[85]

Injury before age 7 versus injury at an older age is associated with more long-term difficulties in understanding the linguistic-symbolic nature of facial expressions, in metalinguistic awareness, and in comprehension monitoring.[86,87]

Time-Related Factors

Aphasic symptoms resolve over time in children with acquired aphasia from head injury.[7,78,79]

Anomia and reduced verbal fluency are consistent deficits after childhood head injury even 18 months postinjury.[37,88–90]

One group of persisting problems for children after head injury involve what have been termed *nonaphasic language disorders* with nonliteral language, discourse, and inferencing.[91] In the long term, head-injured children show a variety of discourse deficits, not so much in the gross aspects of communication[92,93] as in telling a story,[27] using and understanding idiomatic or ambiguous statements, making inferences, and producing speech acts appropriate to particular contexts.[28,94]

In the long term, children with head injury have difficulty in comprehension—monitoring tasks requiring them to evaluate statements that violate semantic selection rules, grammatical structures, or pragmatic constraints.[86]

In the long term, children who have had a head injury at a younger rather than an older age are poor at referential communication tasks requiring them to judge the relevance of an instruction, suggesting poor metacognitive function.[86]

Children with head injury have long-term difficulties in understanding how language is used to serve social-communicative goals that include emotional deception. These children have difficulty understanding the linguistic-symbolic nature of facial displays, such as those involved in the deceptive expression of emotion (e.g., they have difficulty selecting a neutral or happy expression when told that a story character is feeling sad but has a reason for hiding that feeling from another character).[87]

Academic abilities in language-related areas are poor in the long-term after childhood head injury.[80,81]

Vocabulary tests may deteriorate with increasing time, because head-injured children are unable to acquire new language-based knowledge at an age-appropriate rate.[29]

Table 63-3 (*Continued*)

Neuropathologic Substrate
The degree of residual language impairment appears to be related to the severity of the head injury,[5,81] and children with mild head injury recover functional language faster than do children with more severe injuries.[90]
The clinical-pathologic correlation of language disorders in childhood head injury is poorly understood, particularly as it concerns contusional damage to the frontal and temporal lobes. However, it is known that frontal contusions and left-sided contusions in children and adolescents with head injury are variously associated with problems in understanding the linguistic-symbolic nature of facial expressions, in metalinguistic awareness, and in oral comprehension monitoring.[86,87]
Early frontal lobe injury particularly affects nonaphasic discourse disorders in the long term after a childhood head injury,[86,87] which is consistent with the importance of an intact frontal lobe system for the development of social awareness and social cognition.
Treatment
None specific.

and studies of cerebellar medulloblastomas, astrocytomas, and ependymomas have provided the principal source of information about childhood brain tumors and language.[96] The features of childhood-acquired aphasia from posterior fossa tumors are reviewed in Table 63-4.

Cancer Treatments

Radiotherapy and chemotherapy are often part of the treatment for childhood cancers such as acute lymphoblastic leukemia. Central nervous system (CNS) prophylaxis is known to cause structural and functional damage to the brain.[108] Children treated for cancer show cognitive deficits[109] and a variety of impairments in speech and language,[110] including mutism, expressive aphasia, anomia, and problems with academic skills. These speech and language deficits are not fully understood with respect to the relations between degree of language impairment and prophylactic dose, the specificity of the language disorders within particular conditions, and the correlation between language function and neuropathology.

Infectious Conditions

Infectious diseases of the brain may involve viral, bacterial, spirochetal, and other microorganisms that infect the meninges (meningitis) and/or the brain (encephalitis; see Chap. 50). Infectious conditions, which have long-term cognitive effects,[111] are reported to produce childhood-acquired aphasia,[112] either as a primary effect of CNS involvement in conditions like herpes simplex encephalitis or as a secondary effect of sensorineural hearing loss in conditions such as bacterial meningitis or toxoplasmosis.

Studies of the effects of meningitis on language function have not provided clear information. While some studies have suggested that deficits in communication are an effect of meningitis, others have not.[112] Differences in research methods and assessment procedures for language may be responsible for the apparent inconsistency in results in studies of meningitis and language.

Aphasia is often part of the morbidity of herpes simplex encephalitis,[15,29,40,113] although antiviral medication in recent years has reduced the mortality associated with this condition. There is an acute-stage comprehension defect that is similar to that seen in global aphasia following an initial period of mutism and that involves a fluent aphasia with neologisms, semantic and phonemic paraphasias, stereotypies, and perseverations.[15,29] That a fluent form of aphasia is associated with herpes simplex encephalitis appears consistent with the fact that the herpesvirus has a tropism for the temporal lobes.[2]

Recovery from aphasia appears to be especially poor after herpes simplex encephalitis.[112] Children with aphasia from encephalitis exhibit long-term paraphasias, word-finding problems, and severe

Table 63-4
Language disturbances after posterior fossa brain tumors

Definition

Acquired aphasia occurs secondary to astrocytomas, medulloblastomas, and ependymomas of the cerebellum, fourth ventricle, and/or brainstem, occurring in children who acutely or progressively lose previously acquired language skills.

Core Features

Mutism occurs commonly in acute-stage cerebellar lesions of childhood.[97,98]

The mutism is not tumor-specific in that it involves various tumor pathologies.[97]

A syndrome of mutism and subsequent dysarthria (MSD) has been identified[99]; it is not obviously related to cerebellar ataxia but characterized by a complete but transient loss of speech resolving into dysarthria.

Analysis of the dysarthria of posterior fossa tumors in children suggests that it shares some of the features of adult dysarthria—namely, imprecise consonants, articulatory breakdowns, prolonged phonemes, prolonged intervals, slow rate of speech, lack of volume control, harsh voice, pitch breaks, variable pitch, and explosive onsets.[100–103]

There appears to be no adult-like pattern of fluent or nonfluent aphasia in children treated for posterior fossa tumors. However, children with treated posterior fossa tumors, including medulloblastomas, show mild language impairments in oral expression and auditory comprehension.[101]

Epidemiology, Demography, and Risk Factors

As of 1994, a total of 36 cases of MSD have been reported.[99]

In children with posterior fossa tumors, risk factors for the development of MSD are hydrocephalus at the time of tumor presentation, ventricular localization of the tumor, and postsurgical edema of the pontine tegmentum.[99]

Age-Related Factors

Some 90 percent of MSD patients are less than 10 years of age, and the condition has been described in children as young as age 2.[99]

Time-Related Factors

In cases of MSD, recovery of dysarthria to normal speech seems to be related to the recovery of complex movements of the mouth and tongue.[99]

A range of short- and long-term intellectual, neuropsychological, and academic difficulties have been identified in children with posterior fossa tumors,[95] including language-related difficulties. Academic failure occurs frequently in survivors of posterior fossa tumors; the rate is higher in survivors of medulloblastoma than in survivors of cerebellar astrocytomas.[104–106]

Neuropathologic Substrate

Mutism may occur with a midline location of the tumor combined with postoperative complications that involve destruction of the midline roof structures and penetration of the peduncles and/or lateral wall or ventricular floor parenchyma.[97]

Mutism occurs particularly with posterior fossa tumors located in the midline or vermis of the cerebellum and with tumors invading both cerebellar hemispheres or the deep nuclei of the cerebellum.[97,98]

Table 63-4 (*Continued*)

Isolated lesions in cerebellar structures are not sufficient to produce MSD. An additional ventricular location of the tumor and adherence to the dorsal brainstem are necessary—an idea supported by the frequent occurrence of pyramidal and eye-movement signs in children with MSD.[99]

Localization of the brainstem dysfunction in MSD appears to be rostral to the medulla oblongata and caudal to the mesencephalon.[99]

It has been proposed that the mutism of MSD is related to bilateral involvement of the dentate nuclei and that the subsequent dysarthric speech represents a recovering cerebellar mechanism.[105]

Treatment

None specific to the language disorders, only the appropriate course of tumor treatment.

comprehension deficits.[15,29] The poor outcome may be related to the bilateral effects of brain infections,[33] and also to the necrotic brain lesions and significant neurologic sequelae associated with herpesvirus infections.[114]

Hypoxic Disorders

Anoxia is a state in which the oxygen levels in the body fall below physiologic levels because of depleted oxygen supply. Anoxia can come about from various causes—including severe hypotension, cardiac arrest, carbon monoxide poisoning, near-drowning, and suffocation—that involve a drop in the level of cerebral blood flow or the oxygen content of the blood. In turn, this results in cerebral anoxia, a prolonged period of which will produce permanent brain damage or anoxic encephalopathy, which is associated with a range of neurologic disorders, including language deficits.[115]

Anoxic encephalopathy affects short- and long-term language function. An initial mutism resolves into a variety of forms of language disorder, ranging from dysarthria, increased speech rate, problems initiating speech movements, and anomia.[29,116] Children who suffer a near-drowning episode show speech and language disorders that appear to recover in the longer term,[117,118] although that subset of children who initially present as comatose after a near-drowning episode may continue to be at risk for language disorders.[115]

The neuropathology of cerebral anoxia is fairly well known, although there have been few research studies in children that correlate language status and patterns of anoxic brain damage. In one study, subcortical lesions resulting from anoxic encephalopathy in adolescence have been related to motor speech disorders involving a progression from mutism to dysarthria.[116]

Metabolic Disorders

Systemic metabolic disorders that result in the accumulation of metabolites in the bloodstream cause brain disruption and cognitive impairments[119] that may include speech and language deficits. Some of the inborn errors of metabolism that have been shown to affect speech and language include phenylketonuria (an absence of the liver enzyme phenylalanine), galactosemia (an inability to utilize the sugars galactose and lactose because of disordered carbohydrate metabolism), and Wilson's disease (a progressive degenerative disorder of the brain and liver resulting from inability to process dietary copper). Congenital hypothyroidism also affects intellectual functions, including language. Other hereditary metabolic diseases such as homocystinuria, a disorder of amino acid metabolism, may cause vascular occlusive disease when enzyme deficiencies damage blood vessels, leading to thrombosis and ischemic stroke.[68] The specificity of speech and language disorders and the relation between language and neuropathology are poorly understood in these various metabolic conditions.

CONCLUSIONS AND ONGOING DIRECTIONS

Recent studies of the acquired aphasias of childhood have provided the basis of more systematic knowledge about these conditions—specifically about language symptoms and type of aphasia, demographic and incidence, and the course of resolution of language symptoms.

Children show a wide range of acquired aphasic features. There is no single profile of language loss in the acquired aphasic conditions of childhood. Various profiles of language loss are associated with different etiologies of childhood-acquired aphasias, ranging from the mutism of cerebellar lesions through the impairments in pragmatic and social discourse commonly observed in the long term after childhood head injury.

The symptoms manifest in the acute phase of childhood-acquired aphasia often differ according to etiology, although some acquired aphasic symptoms are common to a range of etiologies while others occur in only a few conditions. For example, many types of childhood-acquired aphasia[120] resolve to anomic and word-finding deficits, while the severe auditory agnosia of LKS is distinctive.

Age-Related Issues: Similarities and Differences between Children of Different Ages and between Children and Adults

One age-related issue concerns the difference among children with acquired aphasia in relation to age at onset of language disorder. Language disturbances involving the use and understanding of mental states and social discourse are more common with an earlier rather than a later age at head injury.[86,87]

A second age-related issue concerns the consequences for language-related skills of the developmental timing of brain injury. If the onset of epilepsy coincides with beginning to read and write, it will impair the acquisition of written language.[42] The profile of reading outcome varies with the timing of childhood head injury with respect to phonologic skills.[85] Compared to later prophylaxis, earlier treatment for childhood acute lymphoblastic leukemia results in poorer phonemic awareness.[121] These data suggest that actively developing but unconsolidated skills are highly vulnerable to disruption by brain damage.

Aphasic mutism is of interest under the above model of heightened vulnerability for skills that are in the course of acquisition but not yet automatized. Mutism occurs more commonly in children than in adults, variously from a range of etiologies that include the acute phase of vascular, epileptogenic, traumatic, tumorigenic, and infectious conditions. The ubiquity of aphasic mutism in childhood-acquired aphasia over the age range of childhood suggests that the initiation of speech is a volatile and imperfectly automatized language function during childhood.

An important age-related issue concerns similarities and differences between childhood- and adulthood-acquired aphasia. Children and adults show more similarities in aphasic patterns than was earlier recognized. This is not to argue, however, that the aphasic symptoms and patterns are identical in children and adults; for one reason, the base frequencies of symptoms like mutism are higher in children than in adults, whereas the base frequencies of symptoms like neologisms are lower in children than in adults.

The neuroanatomy of childhood-acquired aphasia is both similar to and different from that of adulthood-acquired aphasia.[17] When the same etiology is compared in childhood and in adulthood, a number of language deficits prove to be similar. In children as well as in adults, a lesion in the left hemispheric posterior cortical language areas produces a fluent aphasia and impaired comprehension[124]; specifically, the correlation between lesion site and aphasia in children duplicates the anatomic-clinical correlation in adults.[17] Further, age does not predict recovery from aphasic symptoms when etiology is constant.[30]

To be sure, aphasic symptoms are not identical in children and adults with the same brain damage. Unlike adults, for example, children do not suffer speech disturbances from damage to the superior paravermal cortical regions associated with posterior fossa tumors.[99] Differences in base rate and frequency of aphasic symptoms may be associated with different underlying neuropathologic substrates in children and adults.

The differences between acquired aphasia in children and in adults, once thought to concern short-term aphasic symptoms, now appear to relate more to long-term language function. With increasing time since aphasia, adult language improves, albeit at variable rates. Time does not always improve language function after childhood-acquired aphasia. Children with aphasia may show an increasing inability to accrue a new verbal knowledge base, which results in chronic problems in reading and vocabulary development.[29,73]

Time-Related Issues and Their Importance for Theoretical Accounts and Taxonomies of Childhood-Acquired Aphasia

The time course of aphasic symptoms and resolution of language seems to discriminate among different etiologies of childhood-acquired aphasia. Aphasic symptoms arising from head injury resolve more quickly than do symptoms from infectious and vascular etiologies. Granted that abatement of symptoms varies according to etiology,[26] a continuing task in understanding childhood-acquired aphasia is to specify the time course of symptoms within conditions.

A better understanding of the time course and pattern of preserved and disrupted language skills is essential to establishing a more theoretically grounded account of childhood-acquired aphasia. This is also relevant to the question of the taxonomy of these conditions.

At present, there are few plausible theories of the language disturbances underlying the principal forms of childhood-acquired aphasia. Certainly no single theory is likely to account for every manifestation of childhood aphasia. Even within a particular etiology, any theory must account for the vagaries of symptoms throughout the time course of the aphasia. For example, central receptive deficits have been proposed to be primary in LKS,[60] but a closer analysis of the time course in LKS patients with more slowly developing symptoms reveals a predominantly motor aphasia evident during a language deterioration phase,[45] which seems inconsistent with the idea of a core disorder that is exclusively receptive. By understanding patterns of language deficits that change over time, it will be possible to provide a theoretically motivated account of what distinguishes impaired from preserved language skills in childhood-acquired aphasia.

The neuroanatomy of symptom patterns over time is likely to provide important clues to the underlying mechanisms of language loss and hence to be part of any theory of acquired aphasia. It has been claimed that subcortical lesions in children may have long-term effects similar to those of cortical lesions; for example, one interpretation of the mutism from subcortical vascular lesions is that it arises from a transient frontal diaschisis secondary to subcortical damage. Correlations between language and neuroimaging to allow a detailed comparison of cortical and subcortical lesions producing acquired aphasia have not yet been reported.

It is likely that the same acquired aphasic symptom may be produced by more than one mechanism. In support of this, the time course of resolution of aphasic mutism appears to be different with supratentorial and subtentorial lesions. In the case of posterior fossa tumors, the mutism resolves to dysarthria; with vascular subcortical lesions, however, the resolution of the mutism does not appear to include dysarthric symptoms.[72] This is consistent with the developmental role of the cerebellum in a range of functions, including motor timing and speech production.[102,103,122]

Without a theory of language disruption grounded in the time course of symptoms and long-term language function, there can be no workable taxonomy for childhood-acquired aphasia and its symptom patterns. For the most part, the loose descriptive taxonomy that exists among etiologies is based simply on frequency of reporting and aphasic symptoms for particular etiologies, with a condition like LKS somewhat overrepresented in publications on childhood-acquired aphasia in relation to its frequency of occurrence.[2]

Neither the classic adult taxonomy of aphasia nor existing childhood language classification systems appear adequate to describe childhood-acquired aphasia. When such cases are coded according to a taxonomy of adult aphasia,[123] some 30 to 50 percent of cases cannot be classified.[124,125] Most children with acquired aphasia cannot be classified in either the adult taxonomy or a taxonomy devised for pediatric conditions.[126]

A productive approach to the issue of taxonomy would be one that used theory-driven paradigms of normal language development rather than a priori taxonomies. In recent reviews of childhood-acquired aphasia, there has been a more explicit awareness of the need for paradigms of normal language development.[54] At the same time, it has become apparent that any such paradigms must be complex and expressed as patterns of acquisition over very long time spans, because there are wide individual differences in the rate, strategy, and style of language acquisition in normally developing children, and brain damage affects language acquisition patterns in a number of different ways.[127]

Neuropathology of Language Disorders

One reason for the dearth of workable taxonomies of childhood-acquired aphasic conditions must be the limited number of clinical-pathologic correlations that would allow comparisons of patterns of neuropathology underlying language disorders. An important objective in studies of childhood-acquired aphasia has been to contrast the pathologic processes that produce acquired aphasia with those that do not.[33] Only noninvasive forms of neuroimaging make possible this endeavor; in recent years, structural and functional neuroimaging has provided information about the temporal and spatial extent of brain pathology and hence about the neuropathologic substrates of childhood-acquired aphasia. Of direct relevance are findings from functional neuroimaging studies suggesting what had long been suspected, that areas of brain dysfunction are much larger than the areas of structural lesion in some forms of aphasia-producing childhood vascular lesions.[128]

Studies that correlate language status with neuroimaging are able to identify the factors that produce poor recovery of language. Three such factors have been suggested: an infectious etiology, poor verbal comprehension, and involvement of Wernicke's area.[30] As a larger database of such studies is accrued, it will become easier to understand the mechanism of recovery in cases of childhood-acquired aphasia.[10]

Structural and functional neuroimaging studies have enormous value in shaping taxonomies of childhood-acquired aphasia. The correlation between language symptoms and brain pathology will inform any taxonomy of childhood-acquired aphasic conditions, which must also be grounded in developmental models of language.

REFERENCES

1. Collignon R, Hécaen H, Angelergues R: A propos de 12 cas d'aphasie acquise de l'enfant. *Acta Neurol Belg* 68:245–277, 1968.
2. Paquier P, Van Dongen HR: Current trends in acquired childhood aphasia: An introduction. *Aphasiology* 7:421–440, 1993.
3. Dennis M: Childhood medical disorders and cognitive impairment: Biological risk, time, development, and reserve, in Yeates KO, Ris MD, Taylor HG (eds): *Pediatric Neuropsychology: Research, Theory, and Practice.* New York: Guilford Press, 2000, pp 3–22.
4. Freud S: *Infantile Cerebral Paralysis* (1897). Russin LA (trans). Coral Gables, FL: University of Miami, 1968.
5. Assal G, Campiche R: Aphasie et troubles du langage chez l'enfant apres contusion cerebrale. *Neurochirurgie* 19(Suppl 4):399–406, 1973.
6. Byers RK, McLean WT: Etiology and course of certain hemiplegias with aphasia in childhood. *Pediatrics* 29:376–383, 1962.
7. Guttmann E: Aphasia in children. *Brain* 65:205–219, 1942.
8. Alajouanine TH, Lhermitte F: Acquired aphasia in children. *Brain* 88:653–662, 1965.
9. Hécaen H: Acquired aphasia in children and the ontogenesis of hemispheric functional specialization. *Brain Lang* 3:114–134, 1976.
10. Satz P: Symptom pattern and recovery outcome in childhood aphasia: A methodological and theoretical critique, in Martins IP, Castro-Caldas A, Van Dongen HR, Van Hout A (eds): *Acquired Aphasia in Children.* Dordrecht, The Netherlands: Kluwer, 1991, pp 95–114.
11. Van Dongen HR, Paquier P: Fluent aphasia in children, in Martins IP, Castro-Caldas A, Van Dongen HR, Van Hout A (eds): *Acquired Aphasia in Children.* Dordrecht, The Netherlands: Kluwer, 1991, pp 125–141.
12. Visch-Brink EG, Van de Sandt-Koenderman M: The occurrence of paraphasias in the spontaneous speech of children with an acquired aphasia. *Brain Lang* 23:258–271, 1984.
13. Van Hout A: Characteristics of language in acquired aphasia in children, in Martins IP, Castro-Caldas A, Van Dongen HR, Van Hout A (eds): *Acquired Aphasia in Children.* Dordrecht, The Netherlands: Kluwer, 1991, pp 117–124.
14. Woods BT, Teuber HL: Changing patterns of childhood aphasia. *Ann Neurol* 3:273–280, 1978.

15. Van Hout A, Evrard P, Lyon G: On the positive semiology of acquired aphasia in children. *Dev Med Child Neurol* 27:231–241, 1985.
16. Van Dongen HR, Loonen MCB, Van Dongen KJ: Anatomical basis for acquired fluent aphasia in children. *Ann Neurol* 17:306–309, 1985.
17. Cranberg LD, Filley CM, Hart EJ, Alexander MP: Acquired aphasia in childhood: Clinical and CT investigations. *Neurology* 37:1165–1172, 1987.
18. Dennis M: Dissociated naming and locating of body parts after left temporal lobe resection: An experimental case study. *Brain Lang* 3:147–163, 1976.
19. Makino A, Soga T, Obayashi M, et al: Cortical blindness caused by acute general cerebral swelling. *Surg Neurol* 29:393–400, 1988.
20. Paquier P, Saerens J, Parizel PM, et al: Acquired reading disorder similar to pure alexia in a child with ruptured arteriovenous malformation. *Aphasiology* 3:667–676, 1989.
21. Rapin I: Acquired aphasia in children. *J Child Neurol* 10:267–270, 1995.
22. Landau WM, Kleffner FR: Syndrome of acquired aphasia with convulsive disorder in children. *Neurology* 7:523–530, 1957.
23. Paquier P, Van Dongen HR: Acquired childhood aphasia: A rarity? *Aphasiology* 7(Suppl 5):417–419, 1993.
24. Ikeda M, Tanabe H, Yamada K, et al: A case of acquired childhood aphasia with evolution of global aphasia into transcortical sensory aphasia. *Aphasiology* 7 (Suppl 5):497–502, 1993.
25. Satz P, Bullard-Bates C: Acquired aphasia in children, in Sarno MT (ed): *Acquired Aphasia.* San Diego, CA: Academic Press, 1981, pp 399–426.
26. Loonen MCB, Van Dongen HR: Acquired childhood aphasia: Outcome one year after onset, in Martins IP, Castro-Caldas A, Van Dongen HR, Van Hout A (eds): *Acquired Aphasia in Children.* Dordrecht, The Netherlands: Kluwer, 1991, pp 185–200.
27. Chapman SB, Culhane KA, Levin HS, et al: Narrative discourse after closed head injury in children and adolescents. *Brain Lang* 43:42–65, 1992.
28. Dennis M, Barnes MA: Knowing the meaning, getting the point, bridging the gap, and carrying the message: Aspects of discourse following closed head injury in childhood and adolescence. *Brain Lang* 3:203–229, 1990.
29. Cooper JA, Flowers CR: Children with a history of acquired aphasia: Residual language and academic impairments. *J Speech Hear Disord* 52:251–262, 1987.
30. Martins IP, Ferro JM: Recovery of acquired aphasia in children. *Aphasiology* 6(Suppl 4):431–438, 1992.
31. Van Hout A: Outcome of acquired aphasia in childhood: Prognosis factors, in Martins IP, Castro-Caldas A, Van Dongen HR, Van Hout A (eds): *Acquired Aphasia in Children.* Dordrecht, The Netherlands: Kluwer, 1991, pp 163–169.
32. Cross JA, Ozanne AE: Acquired childhood aphasia: Assessment and treatment, in Murdoch BE (ed): *Acquired Neurological Speech/Language Disorders in Childhood.* London: Taylor & Francis, 1990, pp 66–123.
33. Woods BT: Patient selection in studies of aphasia acquired in childhood, in Martins IP, Castro-Caldas A, Van Dongen HR, Van Hout A (eds): *Acquired Aphasia in Children.* Dordrecht, The Netherlands: Kluwer, 1991, pp 27–34.
34. Taveras JM, Wood EH: *Diagnostic Neuroradiology,* 2d ed. Baltimore: Williams & Wilkins, 1976, vol 1.
35. Seron X: L'aphasie de l'enfant. *Enfance* 24:249–270, 1977.
36. Carter RL, Hohenegger MK, Satz P: Aphasia and speech organization in children. *Science* 218:797–799, 1982.
37. Hécaen H: Acquired aphasia in children: Revisited. *Neuropsychologia* 21:581–587, 1983.
38. Satz P, Lewis R: Acquired aphasia in children, in Blanken G, Dittmann J, Grimm H, et al. (eds): *Linguistic Disorders and Pathologies: An International Handbook.* Berlin: Walter de Gruyter, 1993, pp 646–659.
39. Dennis M: Strokes in childhood: I. Communicative intent, expression, and comprehension after left hemisphere arteriopathy in a right-handed nine-year-old, in Rieber R (ed): *Language Development and Aphasia in Children.* New York: Academic Press, 1980, pp 45–67.
40. Martins IP, Ferro JM: Recovery from aphasia and lesion size in the temporal lobe, in Martins IP, Castro-Caldas A, Van Dongen HR, Van Hout A (eds): *Acquired Aphasia in Children.* Dordrecht, The Netherlands: Kluwer, 1991, pp 171–184.
41. Murdoch BE: *Acquired Speech and Language Disorders: A Neuroanatomical and Functional Neurological Approach.* London: Chapman & Hall, 1990.
42. Williams J, Sharp GB: Epilepsy, in Yeates KO, Ris MD, Taylor HG (eds): *Pediatric Neuropsychology: Research, Theory, and Practice.* New York: Guilford Press, 2000, pp 47–73.
43. Deonna T, Beaumanoir A, Gaillard F, Assal G: Acquired aphasia in childhood with seizure disorder: A heterogeneous syndrome. *Neuropadiatrie* 8:263–273, 1977.
44. Lou HC, Brandt S, Bruhn P: Aphasia and epilepsy in childhood. *Acta Neurol Scand* 56:46–54, 1977.

45. Marien P, Saerens J, Verslegers W, et al: Some controversies about type and nature of aphasic symptomatology in Landau-Kleffner's syndrome: A case study. *Acta Neurol Belg* 93:183–203, 1993.
46. Soprano AM, Garcia EF, Caraballo R, Fejerman N: Acquired epileptic aphasia: Neuropsychologic follow-up of 12 patients. *Pediatr Neurol* (Suppl 3):230–235, 1994.
47. Mantovani JF, Landau WM: Acquired aphasia with convulsive disorder. *Neurology* 30:524–529, 1980.
48. Papagno C, Basso A: Impairment of written language and mathematical skills in a case of Landau-Kleffner syndrome. *Aphasiology* 7:451–461, 1993.
49. Cooper JA, Ferry PC: Acquired auditory verbal agnosia and seizures in childhood. *J Speech Hear Disord* 43:176–184, 1978.
50. Appleton RE: The Landau-Kleffner syndrome. *Arch Dis Child* 72:386–387, 1995.
51. Dugas M, Gerard CL, Franc S, Sagar D: Natural history, course and prognosis of the Landau and Kleffner syndrome, in Martins IP, Castro-Caldas A, Van Dongen HR, Van Hout A (eds): *Acquired Aphasia in Children.* Dordrecht, The Netherlands: Kluwer, 1991, pp 263–277.
52. Aicardi J: Syndrome of acquired aphasia with seizure disorder: Epileptic aphasia, Landau-Kleffner syndrome, and verbal auditory agnosia with convulsive disorder, in Aicardi J (ed): *Epilepsy in Children.* New York: Raven Press, 1986, pp 176–182.
53. Dugas M, Masson M, Le Heuzey MF, Regnier N: Aphasie "acquise" de l'enfant avec epilepsie (syndrome de Landau et Kleffner): Douze observations personnelles. *Rev Neurol* 138:755–780, 1982.
54. Martins IP: Introduction, in Martins IP, Castro-Caldas A, Van Dongen HR, Van Hout A (eds): *Acquired Aphasia in Children.* Dordrecht, The Netherlands: Kluwer, 1991, pp 3–12.
55. Worster-Drought C: An unusual form of acquired aphasia in children. *Dev Med Child Neurol* 13:563–571, 1971.
56. Genton P, Guerrini R: The Landau-Kleffner syndrome or acquired aphasia with convulsive disorder. *Arch Neurol* 50:1009, 1993.
57. Van Dongen HR, De Wijngaert E, Wennekes MJ: The Landau-Kleffner syndrome: Diagnostic considerations, in Martins IP, Castro-Caldas A, Van Dongen HR, Van Hout A (eds): *Acquired Aphasia in Children.* Dordrecht, The Netherlands: Kluwer, 1991, pp 253–261.
58. Landau WM: Landau-Kleffner syndrome. *Arch Neurol* 49:353, 1992.
59. Gerard C-L, Dugas M, Valdois S, et al: Landau-Kleffner syndrome diagnosed after 9 years of age: Another Landau-Kleffner syndrome? *Aphasiology* 7:463–473, 1993.
60. Bishop DVM: Age of onset and outcome in "acquired aphasia with convulsive disorder." *Dev Med Child Neurol* 27:705–712, 1985.
61. Paquier PF, Van Dongen HR, Loonen CB: The Landau-Kleffner syndrome or "acquired aphasia with convulsive disorder." *Arch Neurol* 49:354–359, 1992.
62. Shoumaker RD, Bennett DR, Bray PF, Curless RG: Clinical and EEG manifestations of an unusual aphasic syndrome in children. *Neurology* 24:10–16, 1974.
63. McKinney W, McGreal DA: An aphasic syndrome in children. *Can Med Assoc J* 110:637–639, 1974.
64. Pascual-Castroviejo I, Lopez Martin VL, Martinez Bermejo AM, Perez Higueras AP: Is cerebral arteritis the cause of the Landau-Kleffner syndrome? Four cases in childhood with angiographic study. *Can J Neurol Sci* 19:46–52, 1992.
65. Nevsimalova S, Tauberova A, Doutlik S, et al: A role of autoimmunity in the etiopathogenesis of Landau-Kleffner syndrome? *Brain Dev* 14:342–345, 1992.
66. Maquet P, Hirsch E, Dive D, et al: Cerebral glucose utilization during sleep in Landau-Kleffner syndrome: A PET study. *Epilepsia* 31:778–783, 1990.
67. De Wijngaert E, Gommers K: Language rehabilition in the Landau-Kleffner syndrome: Considerations and approaches. *Aphasiology* 7(Suppl 5):475–480, 1993.
68. Ozanne AE, Murdoch BE: Acquired childhood aphasia: Neuropathology, linguistic characteristics and prognosis, in Murdoch BE (ed): *Acquired Neurological Speech/Language Disorders in Childhood.* London: Taylor & Francis, 1990, pp 1–65.
69. Zimmerman RA, Bilaniuk LT, Packer RJ, et al: Computed tomographic-arteriographic correlates in acute basal ganglionic infarction in childhood. *Neuroradiology* 24:241–248, 1983.
70. Hynd GW, Leathem J, Semrud-Clikeman M, et al: Anomic aphasia in childhood. *J Child Neurol* 10:189–293, 1995.
71. Klein SK, Masur D, Farber K, et al: Fluent aphasia in children: Definition and natural history. *J Child Neurol* 7:50–59, 1992.
72. Aram DM, Rose DF, Rekate HI, Whitaker HA: Acquired capsular/striatal aphasia in childhood. *Arch Neurol* 40:614–617, 1983.
73. Martins IP, Ferro JM: Acquired childhood aphasia: A clinicoradiological study of 11 stroke patients. *Aphasiology* 7(Suppl 5):489–495, 1993.
74. Eisele JA: Selective deficits in language comprehension following early left and right hemisphere damage, in Martins IP, Castro-Caldas A, Van Dongen HR, Van Hout

A (eds): *Acquired Aphasia in Children.* Dordrecht, The Netherlands: Kluwer, 1991, pp 225–238.
75. Eisele JA, Aram DM: Differential effects of early hemisphere damage on lexical comprehension and production. *Aphasiology* 7:513–523, 1993.
76. Jordan FM: Speech and language disorders following childhood closed head injury, in Murdoch BE (ed): *Acquired Neurological Speech/Language Disorders in Childhood.* London: Taylor & Francis, 1990, pp 124–147.
77. Gennarelli TA, Graham DI: Neuropathology of the head injuries. *Semin Clin Neuropsychiatry* 3:160–175, 1998.
78. Van Dongen HR, Loonen MCB: Factors related to prognosis of acquired aphasia in children. *Cortex* 13:131–136, 1977.
79. Loonen MCB, Van Dongen HR: Acquired childhood aphasia: Outcome one year after onset. *Arch Neurol* 47:1324–1328, 1990.
80. Ewing-Cobbs L, Brookshire B, Scott MA, Fletcher JM: Children's narratives following traumatic brain injury: Linguistic structure, cohesion, and thematic recall. *Brain Lang* 61:395–419, 1998.
81. Ewing-Cobbs L, Fletcher JM, Levin HS, Eisenberg HM: Language functions following closed head injury in children and adolescents. *J Clin Exp Neuropsychol* 5:575–592, 1987.
82. Adelson PD, Kochanek PM: Head injury in children. *J Child Neurol* 13:2–15, 1998.
83. Kraus JF: Epidemiological features of brain injury in children: Occurrence, children at risk, causes and manner of injury, severity, and outcomes, in Broman SH, Michel ME (eds): *Traumatic Head Injury in Children.* New York: Oxford University Press, 1995, pp 22–39.
84. Ewing-Cobbs L, Fletcher JM, Levin HS, et al: Academic achievement and academic placement following traumatic brain injury in children and adolescents: A two-year longitudinal study. *J Clin Exp Neuropsychol* 20:769–781, 1998.
85. Barnes MA, Dennis M, Wilkinson M: Reading after closed head injury in childhood: Effects on accuracy, fluency, and comprehension. *Dev Neuropsychol* 15:1–24, 1999.
86. Dennis M, Barnes MA, Donnelly RE, et al: Appraising and managing knowledge: Metacognitive skills after childhood head injury. *Dev Neuropsychol* 12:77–103, 1996.
87. Dennis M, Barnes MA, Wilkinson M, Humphreys RP: How children with head injury represent real and deceptive emotion in short narratives. *Brain Lang* 61:450–483, 1996.
88. Jordan FM, Ozanne AE, Murdoch BE: Long-term speech and language disorders subsequent to closed head injury in children. *Brain Inj* 2:179–185, 1988.
89. Jordan FM, Ozanne AE, Murdoch BE: Performance of closed head injury children on a naming task. *Brain Inj* 4:27–32, 1990.
90. Jordan FM, Murdoch BE: A prospective study of the linguistic skills of children with closed-head injuries. *Aphasiology* 7:503–512, 1993.
91. Dennis M, Barnes MA: Speech acts after mild or severe childhood head injury. *Aphasiology* 14:391–405, 2000.
92. Dennis M, Purvis K, Barnes MA, Wilkinson M: Understanding of literal truth, ironic criticism, and deceptive praise following childhood head injury. *Brain Lang* 78:1–16, 2001.
93. Dennis M, Barnes MA: Comparison of literal, inferential, and intentional text comprehension in children with mild or severe closed head injury. *J Head Trauma Rehab* 16:456-468, 2001.
94. Barnes MA, Dennis M: Knowledge-based inferencing after childhood head injury. *Brain Lang* 76:253–265, 2001.
95. Dennis M, Spiegler B, Riva D, MacGregor DL: Neurocognitive outcomes after treatment for childhood brain tumors, in Walker D, Perilongo G, Punt J, Taylor R (eds): *Brain and Spinal Tumors of Childhood.* London: Arnold, 2002.
96. Hudson LJ: Speech and language disorders in childhood brain tumours, in Murdoch BE (ed): *Acquired Neurological Speech/Language Disorders in Childhood.* London: Taylor & Francis, 1990, pp 245–268.
97. Humphreys RP: Mutism after posterior fossa tumor surgery. *Concepts Pediatr Neurosurg* 9:57–64, 1989.
98. Rekate HL, Grubb RL, Aram DL, et al: Muteness of cerebellar origin. *Arch Neurol* 42:697–698, 1985.
99. Van Dongen HR, Catsman-Berrevoets CE, Van Mourik M: The syndrome of "cerebellar" mutism and subsequent dysarthria. *Neurology* 44:2040–2046, 1994.
100. Hudson LJ, Murdoch BE, Ozanne AE: Posterior fossa tumours in childhood: Associated speech and language disorders post-surgery. *Aphasiology* 3:1–18, 1989.
101. Hudson LJ, Murdoch BE: Language recovery following surgery and CNS prophylaxis for the treatment of childhood medulloblastoma: A prospective study of three cases. *Aphasiology* 6:17–28, 1992.
102. Huber-Okrainec J, Dennis M, Bradley K, Spiegler BJ: Motor speech deficits in long-term survivors of childhood cerebellar tumors: Effects of tumor type, radiation, age at diagnosis, and survival years (abstr). *Neurooncology* 3:371, 2001.

103. Huber-Okrainec J, Dennis M, Bradley K, Spiegler BJ: *Cerebellar tumor resection in childhood followed by transient cerebellar mutism: An investigation of residual speech deficits in long-term survivors.* (Retrieved January 7, 2002 from http://cnshome.org/abstracts/search.html.)
104. Dennis M, Spiegler BJ, Hetherington CR, Greenberg ML: Neuropsychological sequelae of the treatment of children with medulloblastoma. *J Neurooncol* 29:91–101, 1996.
105. Hirsch JF, Reiner D, Czernichow P, et al: Medulloblastoma in childhood: Survival and functional results. *Acta Neurochir* 48:1–15, 1979.
106. Johnson DL, McCabe MA, Nicholson HS, et al: Quality of long-term survival in young children with medulloblastoma. *J Neurosurg* 80:1004–1010, 1994.
107. Ammirati M, Mirzai S, Samii M: Transient mutism following removal of a cerebellar tumour: A case report and review of the literature. *Childs Nerv Syst* 5:12–14, 1989.
108. Withers HR: Biological basis of radiation therapy for cancer. *Lancet* 339:156–159, 1992.
109. Dropcho EJ: Central nervous system injury by therapeutic irradiation. *Neurol Clin* 9:969–988, 1991.
110. Hudson LJ, Buttsworth DL, Murdoch BE: Effect of CNS prophylaxis on speech and language function in children, in Murdoch BE (ed): *Acquired Neurological Speech/Language Disorders in Childhood.* London: Taylor & Francis, 1990, pp 269–307.
111. Smyth V, Ozanne AE, Woodhouse LM: Communicative disorders in childhood infectious diseases, in Murdoch BE (ed): *Acquired Neurological Speech/Language Disorders in Childhood.* London: Taylor & Francis, 1990, pp 148–176.
112. Paquier P, Van Dongen HR: Two contrasting cases of fluent aphasia in children. *Aphasiology* 5:235–245, 1991.
113. Van Hout A, Lyon G: Wernicke's aphasia in a 10-year-old boy. *Brain Lang* 29:268–285, 1986.
114. Kleiman MB, Carver DH: Central nervous system infections, in Black P (ed): *Brain Dysfunction in Children: Etiology, Diagnosis, and Management.* New York: Raven Press, 1981, pp 79–107.
115. Murdoch BE, Ozanne AE: Linguistic status following acute cerebral anoxia in children, in Murdoch BE (ed): *Acquired Neurological Speech/Language Disorders in Childhood.* London: Taylor & Francis, 1990, pp 177–198.
116. Murdoch BE, Chenery HJ, Kennedy M: Aphemia associated with bilateral striato-capsular lesions subsequent to cerebral anoxia. *Brain Inj* 3:41–49, 1989.
117. Pearn JM, DeBuse P, Mohay M, Golden M: Sequential intellectual recovery after near-drowning. *Med J Aust* 1:463–464, 1979.
118. Reilly K, Ozanne AE, Murdoch BE, Pitt WR: Linguistic status subsequent to childhood immersion injury. *Med J Aust* 149:225–228, 1988.
119. Ozanne AE, Murdoch BE, Krimmer HL: Linguistic problems associated with childhood metabolic disorders, in Murdoch BE (ed): *Acquired Neurological Speech/Language Disorders in Childhood.* London: Taylor & Francis, 1990, pp 199–215.
120. Dennis M: Word finding after brain-injury in children and adolescents. *Top Lang Disord* 13:66–82, 1992.
121. Kleinman SN, Waber DP: Neurodevelopmental bases of spelling acquisition in children treated for acute lymphoblastic leukemia. *Cogn Neuropsychol* 9:403–425, 1992.
122. Schmahmann JD: An emerging concept: The cerebellar contribution to higher function. *Arch Neurol* 48:1178–1186, 1991.
123. Goodglass H, Kaplan E: *The Assessment of Aphasia and Related Disorders.* Philadelphia: Lea & Febiger, 1972.
124. Marshall JC: The description and interpretation of aphasic language disorder. *Neuropsychologia* 24:5–24, 1986.
125. Martins IP, Ferro JM: Acquired conduction aphasia in a child. *Dev Med Child Neurol* 29:529–540, 1987.
126. Lees JA: Differentiating language disorder subtypes in acquired childhood aphasia. *Aphasiology* 7(Suppl 5):481–488, 1993.
127. Bates E, Thal D, Janowsky JS: Early language development and its neural correlates, in Boller F, Grafman J (eds): *Handbook of Neuropsychology.* Amsterdam: Elsevier, 1992, vol 7, pp 69–110.
128. Shahar E, Gilday DL, Hwang PA, et al: Pediatric cerebrovascular disease: Alterations of regional cerebral blood flow detected by TC 99m–HMPAO SPECT. *Arch Neurol* 47:578–584, 1990.

Chapter 64

DEVELOPMENTAL READING DISORDERS*

Maureen W. Lovett
Roderick W. Barron

HISTORICAL BACKGROUND

For more than a century, it has been recognized that a sizable minority of otherwise intelligent, healthy children unexpectedly fail to learn to read. In 1895, Hinshelwood[1,2] described these specific reading acquisition failures as *visual word blindness* and Morgan[3] suggested a parallel between cases of acquired (alexia) and developmental reading disorders (dyslexia). The most influential early student of reading disability was Samuel Orton,[4,5] who described a condition he labeled *strephosymbolia,* proposing that it was caused by developmental delay in specialization of the left hemisphere for language. Orton's work formed the basis for a number of early educational therapies for the disorders,[6,7] some of which continue to be popular.[8]

In 1968, the World Federation of Neurology defined specific developmental dyslexia by exclusionary criteria as "a disorder manifested by difficulty in learning to read despite conventional instruction, adequate intelligence, and sociocultural opportunity." The disorder was attributed to "fundamental cognitive disabilities which are frequently of constitutional origin."[9] In 1979, Denckla offered a more specific definition that connected developmental dyslexia to speech and language disorders; she described it as the "index symptom of a developmental language disorder too subtle to lead to referral of the child in preschool life",[10] a view reiterated by other investigators since that time.[11–15]

Exclusionary definitions of dyslexia fostered diagnostic approaches based on a discrepancy between reading achievement and intellectual potential as measured by standardized psychometric tests. The working assumption was that higher-IQ disabled readers have a more specific form of dyslexia characterized by a uniquely deviant pattern of development in reading-related cognitive processes, while lower-IQ disabled readers were handicapped by developmental lags in many reading-related and reading-unrelated cognitive processes.[16] Some authors considered the IQ-discrepant group more purely dyslexic, with different etiology, than the IQ-consistent group of *"garden-variety"* poor readers.[17] Discrepancy-based definitions have dominated clinical practice and research for decades and have been legislated into eligibility requirements for special education services in many parts of the United States and Canada.[18,19]

CURRENT DEFINITIONS

Recent research, however, has demonstrated that disabled readers with and without discrepancies between aptitude (IQ) and reading achievement have similar profiles on the phonologically based information processing subskills that underlie word identification[20,21];

* **ACKNOWLEDGMENTS:** Preparation of this chapter was supported by a National Institute of Child Health and Human Development Grant (HD30970–01A1) to Georgia State University, Tufts University, and The Hospital For Sick Children/University of Toronto. The remediation research reported here was supported, in addition, by operating grants to the authors from the Ontario Mental Health Foundation, the Velleman Foundation, and the Social Sciences and Humanities Research Council of Canada. We gratefully acknowledge the conceptual contributions of our collaborators and colleagues over the years, particularly those of Robin Morris and Maryanne Wolf. We also gratefully acknowledge the intellectual contributions of senior members of the Learning Disabilities Research Program at The Hospital for Sick Children— Nancy J. Benson, Karen A. Steinbach, Maria De Palma, Jan C. Frijters, Léa Lacerenza, and the whole LDRP staff who have contributed so much to past and current intervention studies.

there is no support for greater specificity of cognitive deficits in relation to IQ-based discrepancies.[22,23] The current view is that reading disability is dimensional, like hypertension or obesity, and on the lower end of a normal distribution that includes both reading-disabled individuals and those with normal reading ability. An assessment of intellectual potential, while useful in practice, is not essential to the definition of developmental reading disorders; instead, the defining features of these disorders are found in the domain of language, particularly in impairments associated with phonological processing.[24]

The prevalence of developmental reading disorders is dictated by how they are defined. Some 4 to 10 percent of school-aged children in the United States are regarded as reading-disabled when an IQ-achievement discrepancy definition is used and 17 to 20 percent when the definition involves just low achievement.[25,26] These differences in prevalence have implications for educational practice, funding, and access to special education services. Research is required to determine reliable cutoffs for access to treatment that involve precise measurement of achievement in reading and reading-related skills.[23] Developmental reading disability is a chronic disorder that persists into adulthood,[27] and girls are as likely as boys to be identified when classroom-wide objective screening measures rather than teacher referrals are employed.[25]

The prevalence of developmental reading disorders varies across countries, with 1 percent reported in China and Japan to over 30 percent in Venezuela.[28] Although cultural values, educational practices, and opportunities for literacy experiences influence these differences, there is also evidence that the relationship between orthography and phonology in a language plays a significant role. In alphabetic languages such as Italian, Spanish, and German, the mapping between spelling and sound is relatively consistent and orthography tends to represent phonology almost directly. These phonologically shallow orthographies contrast with phonologically deep orthographies such as English, Danish, and French, where the consistency is much lower because the mapping between sequences of letters and phonemes is complex and permissible sequences are constrained by etymology and morphology as well as phonology.[29] As a result, the reported prevalence of developmental reading disorders in countries with shallow orthographies tends to be lower than that of countries with deep orthographies. Nevertheless, there is increasing agreement that deficiencies in phonological processes constitute the underlying basis of the disorders across different orthographies.[30]

WORD RECOGNITION AND PHONOLOGICAL PROCESSES

The most reliable indicator of developmental reading disorders is difficulty in acquiring rapid, context-free word-reading skill.[24,31–33] Many of the inconsistent results in this area of research can be traced to studies in which reading-disabled individuals were defined by criteria other than their ability to read aloud individual words that have been isolated from the context of a phrase or sentence.[12] Decoding nonwords, such as *nersh,* is a very sensitive measure for identifying problems in word reading.[34] Although disabled readers experience problems with comprehension when reading connected text, the correlation between nonword decoding and comprehension is high ($r = 0.79$), indicating that a substantial portion of the variability in comprehension performance can be attributed to print-to-sound decoding skill.[35]

Developmental reading disorders are accompanied by associated deficits in speech and language processing. Evidence accumulated over the past three decades indicates that deficient phonological awareness is a core linguistic deficit characterizing developmental reading disorders[12,20,21,24,36–38]; this deficit persists into adulthood even among individuals with childhood diagnoses of dyslexia who have attained reasonable standards of literacy as adults.[39]

The phonemes making up a syllable are coarticulated, resulting in a representation with considerable overlap in the acoustic and articulatory information for individual phonemes. Phonemes are not physically discrete units; they are embedded in syllables. Children have difficulty accessing phonemes as separate mental objects that can be associated with letters in the course of learning grapheme-phoneme correspondences.[40] The word *steep,* for example, consists of four phonemes: /s/,/t/,/i/,/p/.

Phonological awareness is demonstrated in oral language tasks in which the individual phonemes are matched, deleted, categorized, counted, *blended,* and reordered. Phonological awareness task performance is a unique and independent predictor of word reading in grades 1 through 5 even when the influence of the autocorrelated variable of word reading skill in previous grades is controlled statistically.[41] Phonological awareness tasks are memory-demanding, and verbal working memory is related to reading skill[42]; however, phonological awareness accounts for variability in reading skill when verbal working memory is controlled statistically. Results from longitudinal studies indicate that verbal working memory is not a unique predictor of reading skill in comparison to phonological awareness.[41]

Speed in naming sequences of familiar letters, numbers, objects, and colors is also a strong predictor of word reading skill.[43–45] Performance on these rapid serial naming tasks (also referred to as *rapid automatized naming tasks,* or RAN[46]) is a unique predictor of word reading skill, particularly early in the course of reading acquisition.[41] Naming speed is more strongly associated with measures of comprehension, fluency, and orthographic processing than phonological awareness performance.[47,48]

Phonological awareness and rapid serial naming, along with verbal working memory and oral vocabulary, have been conceptualized as a core set of processing skills which involve accessing, maintaining, and using precise phonological representations of verbal information.[21,24,38,49,50] Word reading and nonword decoding utilize core phonological processing skills extensively.[51] Deficiencies in these skills are the primary neurocognitive signature for the phenotype of developmental reading disorders[12,20,21,52] in studies of underlying brain and genetic bases of reading skill.[29,30,53–56] These deficiencies also are the focus of efforts to improve reading skill through early intervention and remediation.[57–68]

SUBTYPES

Developmental reading disorders have long been regarded as heterogeneous and subtypes have been reported to exist within the phenotype; hence the use of the term *disorders* rather than *disorder*.[69] In an influential study involving over 200 children, Morris and colleagues[70] assessed core phonological processing measures (phonemic awareness, verbal working memory, serial naming tasks) as well as language (vocabulary and speech production tasks) and nonverbal skill measures identified as being associated with reading disorders (visuospatial, visual attention, and nonverbal memory tasks). Nine subtypes were identified: two subgroups were not disabled and two conformed to the profile of lower-IQ garden-variety poor readers.[16] Four of the remaining subtypes were deficient in phonological awareness, with different patterns of strength and weakness in verbal working memory and rapid serial naming as well as language and nonverbal processing. The ninth subtype was characterized by weakness in verbal and nonverbal rate of processing measures and relative strength on language measures. Consistent with a model of deficits in core phonological processes,[16,21] the most central finding was that of a pervasive deficit in phonological awareness across the four specific reading disability subtypes and the two garden-variety subtypes.

Two of the specific reading-disabled subtypes had deficiencies in phonemic awareness and rapid serial naming, whereas the other two were characterized by just one deficiency: phonemic awareness or rapid serial naming. This profile of results is consistent with Wolf and Bowers' double deficit hypothesis, in which it is proposed that children can be deficient in rapid serial naming or phonological awareness or they can also have a more serious double deficit that involves impairments in both.[44,45,71,72]

The dual-route model of word recognition as well as research on acquired dyslexia, both discussed in Chap. 14, provide the framework for another theoretically motivated subtyping scheme. Children were identified who fit the pattern of surface dyslexics because they were more impaired in exception (e.g., *have*) than nonword reading (e.g., *nersh*). *Have* is an exception word because it is pronounced differently from most _ave words. Other children fit the pattern of phonological dyslexics because they were more impaired in nonword than exception word reading.[73] Subsequent research, however, indicated that children in the surface dyslexia subtype could not be distinguished from younger normal readers who had less reading experience and therefore less opportunity to acquire the unique orthographic patterns characterizing exception words.[74,75] Consistent with evidence that nonword decoding is a primary impairment associated with developmental reading disorder,[12,34] the phonological dyslexics emerged as a robust subtype—a finding that is consistent with a deficit rather than a developmental delay pattern over time.[76]

Children classified as phonological dyslexics have a pattern of impairment in core phonological processing skills similar to that reported by Morris and colleagues for most of their subtypes.[70,74,75] The S-shaped function characteristic of categorical speech perception was markedly deviant for some of these children, even though their phonological awareness performance was very similar to other phonological dyslexics with normal categorical speech functions.[77] Furthermore, children who were impaired in both phonological awareness and speech perception were also impaired in morphological processing, a measure of language processing,[78] indicating that some children with developmental reading disorders may have comorbid language disorders that may warrant different approaches to treatment.[79]

VISUAL AND AUDITORY TEMPORAL PROCESSES

Developmental reading disorders involve deficits in phonological processing—a fundamental component of the language system. These phonological deficits cannot be further decomposed and understood as more basic deficits in sensory processing.[13,14,80] Despite this well-established theoretical perspective, there remains continuing interest in the visual and auditory foundations of developmental reading disorders.[81,82] Word recognition is initially visual, and basic neural mechanisms of vision are engaged during the act of reading[83,84] as well as eye movement control systems.[85] Visually based deficits tend to persist in the clinical profiles of disabled readers[86] and are associated with their word-reading performance.[87]

Compared to normal readers, dyslexic readers have been reported to have impaired contrast sensitivity in discriminating low-spatial-frequency grating patterns and in detecting flicker at high temporal frequencies; they are also characterized as having longer visible persistence for low-spatial-frequency patterns.[88–90] Dyslexic children performed worse than normal reading controls on motion-detection tasks, with motion-detection measures related to word and nonword reading performance.[87,91–94] Dyslexic adults had lower levels of activation on functional magnetic resonance imaging (fMRI) in the extrastriate visual area V5/MT on motion-detection tasks than normal reading controls, but the two groups did not differ in activation in areas V1/V2 when processing stationary patterns.[95]

The distinction between the magnocellular and parvocellular pathways in vision has been used to interpret these findings.[81,82,96] Magno cells have relatively large cell bodies as well as dendrites that are dense and heavily myelinated; they are associated with fast conduction times and short response latencies. Magno cells ultimately project to the posterior parietal cortex and provide information about movement and coarse-grained information about form. Parvo cells are smaller, more numerous, and densely packed, with slower conduction times and longer latencies. Parvo cells ultimately project to the inferotemporal cortex and provide information about color and fine-grained information about form. Unlike magno cells, parvo cells give optimal responses to high luminance, spatial frequency, and contrast stimuli as well as to stimuli that are stationary (low-temporal-frequency) and chromatic.

The magnocellular system is involved in reading through eye-movement control; it inhibits the parvocellular system during a saccade and prevents visible persistence from the previous fixation from degrading a new fixation. The inhibitory capabilities of the magnocellular system are hypothesized to be deficient for dyslexic readers, resulting in less efficient reading. Evidence consistent with this hypothesis is mixed,[81,82,97–100] however, and it does not address the fact that reading words in isolation rather than in connected text is the primary area of difficulty for dyslexic readers.[101]

Two preliminary hypotheses have been proposed about how a deficient magnocellular system might influence individual word recognition. One is that the magnocellular system is involved in attentional allocation and it does not effectively inhibit the parvocellular system during the letter-to-letter shifts in attention that are involved in serial nonword decoding.[94] The other is that the magnocellular system prevents effective compensation for retinal slips (unintended eye movements) when fixating small targets such as letters in a word.[102,103] The retinal slip problem is increased with binocular perception. Stein and colleagues have reported that occluding the left eye tends to stabilize the binocular control of dyslexic children and increase their word-reading performance compared to a control (no occlusion) or those who were unable to achieve binocular stability.[104] These findings should be interpreted with considerable caution, however, because visual rather than reading problems may have been the primary basis for inclusion in this study, and direct comparisons were not made with phonologically based procedures for improving reading skill.

Specific language-impaired (SLI) children are reported to have an auditory temporal processing deficit for stimuli that is brief in duration, has a brief interstimulus interval, or is changing rapidly.[105] Tallal and Merzenich have shown that intensive training can improve the linguistic and nonlinguistic temporal processing deficits of these children,[106] and that their speech discrimination and language comprehension skills can be improved when the intensity and duration of critical speech cues (e.g., consonant format transitions) is increased online using computer speech algorithms.[107]

This interpretation of specific language impairment continues to be controversial, with evidence that is both consistent[108,109] and inconsistent.[110–113] Evidence for a connection between auditory temporal processing and developmental reading disorders is also very controversial, with positive results being reported for temporal order and same-different judgment tasks and for psychophysical tasks that involve thresholds for frequency and amplitude modulation.[94,114–116] Negative results have centered on failures to replicate and reports that reading-disabled children who differ in categorical speech perception do not differ when the stimuli are nonspeech analogues.[117,118] Although many of these studies indicate that auditory temporal processing measures are related to literacy and phonological processing, they do not address whether these sensory measures contribute uniquely to variance in word reading once the variance contributed by core linguistic processes, such as phonological awareness and rapid serial naming, have been controlled statistically.

Magno cells in the auditory relay nucleus of the thalamus (medial geniculate nucleus) are responsive to changes in frequency and amplitude, and postmortem evidence indicates that these cells, particularly on the side projecting to the left hemisphere, may be disordered in the brains of some dyslexic individuals.[119,120] Stein has hypothesized that visual and auditory magno cells may be similar and therefore both susceptible to influences that might alter their characteristics during the course of early brain development.[81,82] Recently, investigators have reported that measures of visual and auditory sensory processes index different aspects of developmental reading disorder; specifically, visual motion detection was correlated with orthographic processing and auditory temporal processing was correlated with phonological processing in the same individuals.[93,115,116]

These neuroanatomic and behavioral findings are consistent with the hypothesis of a more general temporal processing deficit.[55,81,82] Such a general deficit may also involve impaired motor development, which co-occurs with developmental dyslexia,[121] as well as functions of the cerebellum, which is the recipient of substantial magnocelluar input.[122] Although these speculations have the potential to push research on developmental reading disorders further into the mainstream of neuroscience research, the evidence for a nonlinguistic sensorimotor basis for developmental reading disorders continues to be preliminary and highly controversial. Even regarding visual, auditory, and motor deficits as different subtypes is inconsistent with current evidence indicating that virtually all subtypes associated with developmental reading disorders are characterized by deficits in linguistically based core phonological processes.[70]

GENETICS

Reading disabilities run in families, and family history is a critical risk factor for developmental reading disorders. Some 40 percent of boys and 18 percent of girls with an affected parent have been estimated to exhibit reading disability profiles.[123] Approximately 31 percent of the children in whom one or two of the parents were dyslexic were identified by their school as having difficulty learning to read by the end of second grade, and this prevalence doubled when their reading was assessed by psychometric tests.[29,124,125]

Comparison of monozygotic (MZ or identical) and dizygotic (DZ or fraternal) twins provides another methodology for exploring genetic contributions to reading orders. Using the Colorado Twin Study database, the unbiased concordance rate of reading disorder for MZ twins has been estimated at 68 percent and at 38 percent for DZ twins, providing evidence that reading disorder has significant genetic etiology.[126] In a subsequent study, reading performance was reported to be highly heritable for both disabled (0.82) and normal reader (0.66) groups while shared environmental influences were low (0.01 and 0.18, respectively). Both phonological and orthographic reading–related measures also appear highly heritable.[127,128]

Linkage analysis is currently used to assess "whether heritable variations at two loci (genetic positions on chromosomes) are transmitted together in relatives at a rate that is greater than would be expected by chance" (see Ref. 129, p. 513). A significant linkage to chromosome 15 was reported in a subset of nine multigenerational families in the first report of a genetic linkage to reading disorder.[130] This finding was not initially replicated with other families,[131–133] but recent evidence is consistent with a linkage to chromosome 15 involving reading[134] and spelling disability.[135]

Siblings can share several alleles or no alleles for a particular DNA marker. If those siblings who share more alleles also happen to have similar scores on a quantitative measure of a trait such as word reading (e.g., both scores are low), then it is possible to infer that a quantitative trait locus (QTL) linkage exits. This technique is more powerful when one of the siblings is selected because he or she has a very low score on the quantitative trait under investigation. Cardon and colleagues used interval mapping of genetic data from two independent samples of sibling pairs (fraternal twins and siblings) and identified a quantitative trait locus (QTL) for reading disability on chromosome 6 within the same area as the human leukocyte antigen (HLA) region.[132] This part of chromosome 6 had attracted interest because of a hypothesis about an association between autoimmune disorders and reading.[136] Although this hypothesis has not been supported,[137] the association of the HLA region on the short arm of chromosome 6 with reading disability has been a productive area of research.[53,138,139]

Grigorenko and colleagues reported loci for different components of reading disorder on chromosomes 6 and 15.[53] A phenotype related to single word-reading difficulties was linked to a marker on chromosome 15, and a correlated phenotype related to phonological awareness difficulties was linked to markers on the short arm of chromosome 6. The linkage findings implicating chromosome 6 and chromosome 15 in reading disability have been replicated, particularly the results for chromosome 6.[138,139] The distinction between the phonological awareness and word-reading phenotypes has not been replicated, however, possibly because the measures that identify them are highly correlated.

Initially, Grigorenko's results were interpreted as indicating that different components of reading skill might be linked to different genes. Pennington pointed out, however, that QTLs which appear to be localized to regions on chromosomes 6 and 15 should not be regarded as evidence that there are specific genes for reading ability or reading disability.[140] Instead, these and other genes may disrupt brain development in a way that eventually alters the developmental process of reading acquisition. Similarly, Plomin has argued that molecular biological techniques may not be productive when applied to the study of cognition and behavior if it is assumed that one or two major genes are responsible for genetic variation in complex behavioral traits and disorders. A more productive strategy would involve identifying multiple genes, each accounting for a relatively small amount of variance. Both genetic and environmental influences may be equally important in accounting for variation in the pheneotype according to this perspective.[141,142]

Fisher and colleagues[143] have recently published a complete genome scan for reading disorders that involved two reading-disabled families with a previously established genetic linkage to chromosome 6p. The most significant single point finding was for markers on chromosome 18p, with evidence of linkage at this locus for measures of single-word identification as well as orthographic and phonological processing skill. It is possible that a number of reading-related processes may be associated with this locus, and it may represent a more general risk factor for reading disability because it may influence several reading-related skills.[144]

Additional loci for reading disability have been reported, including a region on chromosome 2.[145,146]

While these linkage findings are encouraging, current evidence suggests that at least six different genes potentially influence reading disability,[147] and it is likely that more will be identified. Other developmental learning disorders that are frequently comorbid with developmental reading disorders may overlap genetically—such as attention deficit hyperactivity disorder (ADHD),[148,149] specific language impairment,[150] and mathematical learning disorders[151]—although the evidence to date is very preliminary. Recognition of the heterogeneity of both genetic and environmental contributions to the development of reading disorders has provided a more realistic and sophisticated perspective on the complexities involved in understanding these disorders.

NEUROBIOLOGICAL FOUNDATIONS

The neurobiological bases of reading disorder have been a topic of scientific interest since the first reports of visual word blindness over a century ago. Interest has been increasing and has been particularly strong in the past two decades.[29,55,152,153] Galaburda has provided unique neuroanatomic evidence for reading disorder in a series of postmortem investigations of individuals with a childhood history of dyslexia.[154,155] He reported that the planum temporale, which is located in the posterior aspect of the superior temporal lobe and is involved in language, was symmetrical in all seven of the dyslexic brains investigated.[156–158] In contrast, asymmetry is typical of normal readers, with the left side being larger in approximately 65 percent of the cases, and it may be a structural prerequisite for normal phonological development. Galaburda's finding reflects an unexpected increase in the size of the right planum in dyslexic individuals rather than a smaller left planum, a pattern interpreted as arising from reduced cell death during fetal brain development.[154,155]

Cortical malformations (ectopias, dysplasia, vascular micromalformations) in the frontal and language areas were also reported,[156–158] and Galaburda speculated that genetic factors may influence neuronal migration and contribute to establishing abnormal neuronal circuits in brain areas typically devoted to language functions. The result is that the dyslexic brain may have too many neurons in the posterior language areas, particularly in the right hemisphere, rather than too few.[154,155]

These autopsy investigations have been criticized, however, for the small sample of brains studied, the heterogeneity of the dyslexic symptoms, and comorbidity with other disorders. It is possible that symmetrical plana temporale may reflect a different pattern of early brain development common to several neurolinguistic disorders rather than just developmental reading disorder.[12,159] In addition, there is considerable variability in the planum temporale within the general population, and measurement problems prevent accurate comparisons across studies.[152,160,161]

Large samples of dyslexic and control twins have been investigated with quantitative MRI analyses in Colorado studies on the genetics of size variations in brain structure in dyslexia.[162] Individuals with reading disorders had the largest operculum, temporal, and posterior parietal/occipital regions and smaller bilateral insula and frontal cortex; there were no differences in subcortical structure volumes (e.g., basal ganglia, thalamus). Filipek[152] suggests that these findings provide evidence for developmental structural anomalies among individuals with developmental reading disorder in areas of the brain involved in receptive language. Despite progress in this area, there is relatively little evidence of substantial differences in anatomic brain structure between dyslexic and nondyslexic individuals but small sample sizes, measurement, and phenotype definition issues contribute to the conflicting evidence.[12,29,56] Nevertheless, this research is valuable because it encourages the hypothesis that developmental reading disorders are the result of anomalies in neural development arising from an event or sequence of events that occur in utero and may produce different patterns of brain development.[29,81,82]

Recent advances in functional brain imaging methods such as positron emission tomography (PET), functional MRI (fMRI), and magnetic source imaging (MSI) allow examination of the underlying neural systems involved in performing reading and reading-related tasks.[83,84] Using a subtraction paradigm common to fMRI studies (see Chap. 7), S. E. Shaywitz,

B.A. Shaywitz, and colleagues at Yale University[54] administered five tasks that varied the level of phonological/linguistic coding required: (1) visuospatial processing (do (\\\/) and (\\\/) match?), (2) orthographic processing (do *bbBb* and *bbBb* match?), (3) simple phonological analysis (do *T* and *V* rhyme?), (4) phonological assembly (do *leat* and *jete* rhyme?), and (5) lexical-semantic processing (are *corn* and *rice* in the same category?). As the phonological demands of print-to-sound mapping increased, adult disabled readers failed to increase activation within a large posterior cortical system that included the posterior superior temporal gyrus (Wernicke's area), the angular gyrus, and the striate cortex. Instead, these readers demonstrated overactivation in anterior areas, including the inferior frontal gyrus (Broca's area), on phonological tasks.

These data suggest disruption of a posterior cortical system that involves both visual and language processing areas as well as part of the association cortex. The association cortex includes the angular gyrus, which is thought to be recruited in the cross-modal processing involved in print-to-sound mapping during reading. S.E. Shaywitz, B.A. Shaywitz, and colleagues regard a pattern of relative *under*activation of posterior areas combined with relative *over*activation of anterior areas as "a neural signature for the phonologic difficulties characterizing dyslexia" (see Ref. 54, p. 2640).

Subsequent research by the Yale group[163] indicated that when task performance did not require phonological assembly (tasks 1 to 3), functional connectivity correlations between the angular gyrus and related posterior cortical areas relevant to reading were similar for dyslexic and nondyslexic readers. In contrast, functional connectivity correlations for the left hemisphere were weak on the word and nonword reading tasks (tasks 4 to 5) for the dyslexic readers because they require phonological assembly. When left hemisphere functional connectivity correlations were low for dyslexic readers on phonological assembly tasks, strong correlations were obtained at the corresponding right hemisphere homologues, suggesting that reading disabled individuals may be overly reliant on right hemisphere systems in performing phonologically demanding tasks.

Dorsal (temporoparietal circuit) and ventral (occipitotemporal circuit) left hemisphere systems are hypothesized to be associated with different functions in the normally developing reader's brain and in different phases of reading acquisition.[153] These two left hemisphere posterior systems and their functional connectivity are deviant in the brains of dyslexic readers. Individuals with reading disorders are characterized by increased reliance on the inferior frontal gyrus (Broca's area) during reading, possibly because it supports control and sequencing of articulatory recoding that may be recruited in response to phonological processing demands. These readers also show increased activation in the right hemisphere homologues of the impaired left hemisphere posterior systems. This right hemisphere shift may support word identification learning through nonphonological, visual-semantic pattern recognition processes.

The dorsal system includes the angular gyrus, the supermarginal gyrus in the inferior parietal lobule, and the posterior aspect of the superior temporal gyrus (Wernicke's area), and it is hypothesized to be dominant early in development. This system involves mapping visual units of print (graphemes) onto phonological units of language (phonemes) as well as analytic processing of the morphological and lexical semantic components of printed words. The ventral system predominates later in development and includes the lateral extrastriate areas and the left inferior occipitotemporal area. It involves rapid word identification, which is associated with the automatic, fluent word identification abilities of mature, skilled readers.[153]

Development of the ventral (occipitotemporal) system within the left hemisphere posterior reading system depends upon tight integration of the neural representations of the orthographic, phonological, and lexical-semantic information about words. Achieving this level of integration crucially depends upon first having an intact and functioning dorsal (temporoparietal) system. Deficits within the dorsal system, which supports the initial acquisition of word reading skill, preclude the subsequent development of the rapid ventral word-identification system.

Impaired temporoparietal circuitry, with its signature phonological processing deficits, disrupts the developmental trajectory of reading acquisition for children with developmental reading disorder by preventing them from developing a fast, ventral-occipital word-identification system. Activation of the inferior frontal gyrus and a shift to right hemisphere posterior processing by these readers is regarded as a response to the demands of word recognition and results in relatively inaccurate and nonfluent reading. This model of the course of reading development provides an initial characterization of both reading skill and reading disorder within the context of developmental cognitive neuroscience and provides a framework for understanding both the phonological decoding failures of struggling readers (impaired temporoparietal circuit) and their subsequent difficulty in attaining fluent and automatic word identification (impaired ventral-occipital circuit).[153]

The cross-linguistic nature of developmental reading disorders was examined by comparing cognitive and neuroimaging data on dyslexic and nonimpaired adult readers from three countries with alphabetic writing systems that varied in the depth of their orthographies.[30] Dyslexic Italian readers, who have a shallow orthography, were relatively better performers on literacy and phonological processing tasks than dyslexic French and English readers, whose orthographies are regarded as more complex (deep). PET brain scans taken during explicit and implicit reading activities revealed a common profile of reduced activation in the left middle, inferior, and superior temporal cortex and in the middle occipital gyrus for the dyslexic adult readers from all three countries. The nonimpaired control readers from each country showed a significantly greater activation in this large region of left cortex.

These results are consistent with the view that dyslexia is characterized by a universal neurocognitive profile in the brain that occurs regardless of whether the orthography is deep or shallow and is associated with characteristic phonological processing deficits. The depth of an orthography influences the extent to which the phonological deficits will impair the acquisition of reading skill and limit reading performance, but associated brain activation profiles during reading are similar across alphabetic languages regardless of their orthographic depth.

TREATMENT

Evidence indicates that reading ability improves with age and intervention for most reading-disordered children when adolescent and adult outcome data are examined. Core phonological deficits persist into adulthood, however, particularly among individuals who are severely impaired. Even in cases where the literacy outcome is good and educational success is achieved, phonological processing problems persist, as well as problems with spelling accuracy, word-recognition speed, and reading rate, particularly in the reading of technical expository text.[27,39,164,165] Dyslexic individuals who had pursued college education had the highest word-recognition achievement among a sample of adult dyslexics, but they were only at the 32nd percentile on a standardized word identification test. Standardized reading comprehension scores were higher, providing further evidence that aspects of word identification are the major area of difficulty for these individuals.[27,39]

Based on data from the Connecticut Longitudinal Study, children identified as reading-disabled in grades 2 through 6 continued to exhibit deficits in phonological coding in adolescence and to demonstrate continuing problems in reading, spelling, and reading rate compared to normally developing children with average and superior reading skills in the same grades. Children with persistent reading problems remained inferior readers relative to other students in high school despite having access to special education services during their schooling.[164] These findings are generally consistent with a deficit rather than a developmental lag model of reading disorder.[76]

There were no differences between good and poor readers in reports of legal problems, or use of alcohol or tobacco, or in the prevalence of conduct or attention problems in the Connecticut Longitudinal data.[164] Although there are differences in the composition of the different study samples, these results from the Connecticut Longitudinal Study appear inconsistent with other reports that adolescents with learning disorders have a threefold increase in their risk for substance abuse and elevated risk for adverse outcomes, including lower family socioeconomic status, IQ scores, and educational and occupational achievement.[166,167]

Many approaches to treating reading disorders have been advocated and attempted, but reports of reliable evidence from well-controlled studies on the efficacy of different interventions have emerged only since the mid- to late-1980s.[168] The absence of scientific evidence over so many decades led to inevitable questions about whether it is possible to treat these disorders successfully.[65,67,169] Within the last several years, a number of controlled and comparative research studies have been reported that have assessed the efficacy of different instructional approaches to remediating problems in reading acquisition in the early elementary grades.[57,64,170,171] Controlled intervention studies that focus on the core phonological and word-identification deficits of reading-disabled children in later grades have also been reported with positive results.[60–62,172–174]

These studies indicate that significant improvement can be achieved on speech-based and phonological reading measures for both young children at risk for reading disability and older children who are reading-disabled.[57,61,63,64,175,176] Furthermore, even with the most severely impaired readers drawn from a clinical sample, evidence from controlled intervention studies indicates that focused and systematic intervention, concentrated on remediating core deficits, results in measurable progress in learning phonological reading skills throughout the elementary school years.[59,72,172]

Remedial gains do not reliably generalize to other aspects of reading acquisition when children improve in phonologically based word attack and decoding skills. Although reading-disabled children could, after intervention, "sound out" new words or nonwords, they were not always improved in word recognition, text reading, or reading comprehension skills relative to a comparison group.[177] Generalization of remedial gains has been a substantial problem for many intervention methods evaluated in the literature[61,176] and for methods assessed in initial remediation studies we have conducted at The Hospital for Sick Children in Toronto.[178–180]

Generalization problems in these treatment studies may reflect the severity and complexity of the processing impairments exhibited by some disabled readers and the fact that the core processing deficits of many disabled readers extend beyond the realm of phonological awareness. Deficits in both phonological awareness and naming speed constitute a risk factor far more severe than either deficit alone.[45,72] There is also evidence that disabled readers have difficulty in specific aspects of executive functioning and strategy learning that are independent of their phonological processing impairments.[181–183] Many of the generalization failures may be due to difficulty in acquiring effective, flexible word-identification strategies and monitoring the effectiveness of strategy implementation.[60] It should be noted, however, that generalization and transfer-of-learning difficulties for disabled readers are specific to printed language learning; transfer occurs readily in learning tasks that have similar cognitive demands but do not require phonological processing.[184,185]

Difficulties children have in generalizing the gains they make following remedial instruction have motivated some of our most recent research with severely reading-disabled children referred to our laboratory classrooms at The Hospital for Sick Children in Toronto. Children with severe reading disorders were assigned randomly to one of two remedial reading programs or to a control treatment that dealt with classroom survival skills and consisted of instruction on study, organizational, and problem-solving skills.[59,72,172] Each reading program targeted generalization of treatment gains in word-identification learning but involved different instructional approaches and different levels of print-to-sound segmentation during training.

The PHAB/DI (Phonological Analysis and Blending/Direct Instruction) Program involves lessons from the direct instructional programs developed by Engelmann and colleagues; it trains phonological analysis, phonological blending, and letter-sound association skills in the context of word recognition and decoding instruction (see Reading Mastery I/II Fast Cycle, and Corrective Reading Programs).[186–188] The WIST (Word Identification Strategy Training) Program has a strong metacognitive focus in which children are taught how to use and monitor the application of four metacognitive decoding strategies. WIST was developed in our laboratory classrooms at The Hospital for Sick Children and is partially based on the original Benchmark School Word Identification/Vocabulary Development Program.[189] The dialogue structure for strategy instruction, the keywords, and the compare/contrast strategy (a strategy of word identification by analogy) were adapted from the Benchmark Program. WIST also includes, however, a direct training focus on the subskills necessary for strategy implementation, a metacognitive "Game Plan" for training flexibility in strategy choice and evaluating the success of those choices, and three additional word-identification strategies (Peeling Off,

Vowel Variations, and Spy). In summary, PHAB/DI focuses on grapheme-phoneme spelling-to-sound units while WIST trains recognition of larger subsyllabic units, particularly the rime. PHAB/DI promotes generalization of word-identification learning by intensive systematic remediation of basic sound analysis and sound blending deficits, while WIST involves teaching a set of flexible word-identification strategies as well as the specific skills and content required to implement them.

PHAB/DI and WIST proved much more effective than our previous interventions in achieving generalization of remedial gains.[178–180] PHAB/DI- and WIST-trained children were significantly improved on several standardized and experimental reading measures and showed evidence of generalization on a set of word-reading measures including words that varied in their spelling-to-sound similarity (distance) to the target words instructed in the PHAB/DI and WIST lessons. While both approaches were associated with large positive effects compared to the alternative treatment control condition (Classroom Survival Skills), different patterns of transfer were observed. PHAB/DI, with its emphasis on grapheme-phoneme analysis and blending, yielded broader-based and deeper generalization on speech- and print-based measures of phonological skill. WIST, with its strategy training focus, produced broader-based generalization for exceptions as well as regular words. These results indicated that children who were severely reading-disabled could learn phonological skills and letter-sound correspondences after extensive training, and they could generalize their word-identification skills to a range of uninstructed words. Furthermore, these effects could be obtained with relatively late intervention in grades 5 and 6.

The phonological processing and reading deficits of these children were not ameliorated after 35 h of intervention, but their speech- and print-based phonological skills were improved significantly and moved closer to age-appropriate levels; they showed substantially improved letter-sound knowledge, decoding abilities, and word-identification skills. These severely disabled readers were incorrectly identifying one-syllable words like *way, left,* and *put* before remedial intervention. Following PHAB/DI or WIST lessons, however, many were able to decode accurately, though often slowly, multisyllable words like *unintelligible*, *mistakenly*, and *disengaged.*

In a recent sequential crossover design involving 70 h of instruction, PHAB/DI and WIST were combined and compared to longer-term intervention, with each approach separately as well as with an alternative treatment control group (Classroom Survival Skills to Mathematics).[60] Generalized treatment effects were obtained on standardized measures of word identification, nonword reading, and passage comprehension, confirming the effectiveness of PHAB/DI and WIST on multiple indices of reading skill. The most important results, however, were the superior outcomes and steeper learning curves for children who had the sequential combination of PHAB/DI and WIST (PHAB/DI to WIST; WIST to PHAB/DI) compared to either intervention alone (PHAB/DI $\times$ 2; WIST $\times$ 2) on a variety of measures of word reading skill including nonword reading, letter-sound knowledge, keywords, near and far transfer words, and multisyllabic challenge words.

These results are important because they indicate that phonologically based approaches alone are not sufficient for achieving optimal remedial outcomes with reading disabled children. Phonologically based interventions appear necessary to achieve remedial gains, but generalization of those gains is more likely with a broader-based approach that combines direct and dialogue-based instructional methods, with children being taught different levels of subsyllabic segmentation and effective use of multiple decoding strategies. These results highlight the critical importance of strategy instruction and the promotion of a flexible approach to word-identification and text reading contexts.

Recent findings from a meta-analysis of the treatment outcome literature on learning disabilities are consistent with this conclusion. The optimal approach in instructing children with learning disabilities, according to a review of 180 intervention studies, is a combination of direct and strategy instruction methods. This combined approach appeared particularly effective in remedial reading interventions when the outcome measures required reading comprehension and text reading.[190]

We have begun to integrate these approaches into a single intervention program called the PHAST Track Reading Program (PHAST for Phonological and Strategy Training). It begins with PHAB/DI's program of phonological remediation and uses it as a foundation for introducing and scaffolding each of the four WIST strategies.[191] PHAST attempts to build context-free word identification skills and strategies to facilitate achieving the goal of reading connected text for meaning and is intended to be situated in a linguistically enriched and literature-based balanced literacy program. The dialogue structure of the PHAST Program and its metacognitive instructional focus are compatible with dialogue-based approaches to text comprehension and writing training. It could be implemented in the classroom as part of an integrated approach to reading, spelling, and writing instruction to allow intense instruction in spelling-to-sound and sound-to-spelling analysis at the subsyllabic, lexical, and connected text levels.

In a recent study, Torgesen and colleagues found significant improvements in generalized reading skills that were sustained over 2 years following intensive, phonologically based remediation programs (67.5 h).[62] These programs had little impact, however, on the disabled readers' impairment in reading speed. On average, children scored within the age-appropriate range on measures of word identification and passage comprehension 2 years after intervention, but they were two standard deviations below age norms on measures of reading rate despite increasing the number of words they could read per minute. There has been growing recognition that different models of remedial intervention will be required if disabled readers are to make gains in phonological processing skills, word identification and text reading accuracy, as well as in word-identification speed and text reading fluency.

RAVE-O is an experimental reading intervention program developed by Wolf that is designed to facilitate the acquisition of fluency.[192] It is to be taught in combination with a systematic phonologically based intervention program that provides instruction in letter-sound knowledge, decoding, and word-identification skills with the goal of improving speech-based phonological deficits in disabled readers. RAVE-O (Retrieval, Automaticity, Vocabulary Elaboration, Engagement with language, and Orthography) is designed to facilitate accuracy and automaticity in reading subskills and component processes and to develop fluency in word identification, word attack, and text reading and comprehension processes. RAVE-O encourages children to learn to play with their language and it employs animated computer games[193] as well as minute-mystery stories, word webs, and word-retrieval strategies during instruction.

The PHAST Track Reading Program described above[191] and the RAVE-O Program[192] in conjunction with the previously described PHAB/DI Program[59,186–188] are being evaluated against both an alternative treatment control program (Classroom Survival Skills + Math)[60] and a phonological treatment control program (PHAB/DI + Classroom Survival Skills) in a large multisite intervention study funded by the National Institute of Child Health and Human Development.

Substantial increases in evidence-based treatment approaches to developmental reading disorder now allow more refined research questions to be posed about the combination of treatment components that are most effective, the characteristics of optimal treatment delivery, and mediators and moderators of long-term treatment outcome. New questions have also emerged about potential neurobiological correlates of the gains in performance that accompany effective intervention. Do the neurobiological substrates for reading behavior change with behavioral evidence of improvements in reading skill? And, if that is the case, what are the characteristics and limitations to the functional circuitry that underlie these newly acquired literacy skills?

Recent findings using magnetic source imaging (MSI) address some of these issues.[194] Eight dyslexic children (range 7 to 17 years of age, with a mean age of 11.4 years) received 80 h of intense, individualized, phonologically based remediation. They were given an MSI scan before and after the intervention while they performed a visual nonword rhyme-detection task (e.g., do *yoat* and *wote* rhyme?) which requires grapheme-phoneme decoding of each nonword. Eight normal readers were also scanned while they performed the rhyming task on two separate occasions 2 months apart, and no significant changes were observed in their activation profiles. Before the intervention, the dyslexic readers had limited activation in the left superior temporal gyrus as well as strong activation in the corresponding right hemisphere areas. After the intervention, the investigators reported that the brain activation profiles of the children were normalized, with an increase in the activation in the left superior temporal gyrus and a decrease in the right superior temporal gyrus.[194] These changes in activation were accompanied by behavioral evidence that the postintervention reading scores of the disabled readers had moved into the normal range. For the majority of dyslexic subjects, the postintervention brain activation profiles were indistinguishable from those of the age-matched normal readers, suggesting that the intervention had the effect of normalizing brain function rather than creating a compensatory reorganization. These findings, which require replication with larger samples and other measures, provide evidence that intense, phonologically based reading intervention procedures can alter the functional organization of the brains of developmentally reading-disordered children, even in adolescence.

REFERENCES

1. Hinshelwood J: Word blindness and visual memories. *Lancet* 2:1566–1570, 1895.
2. Hinshelwood J: *Congenital Word Blindness*. London: Lewis, 1917.
3. Morgan WP: A case of congenital word-blindness. *Bri Med J* 2:1378, 1896.
4. Orton ST: "Word-blindness" in school children. *Arch Neurol Psychiatry* 14:581–615, 1925.
5. Orton ST: Specific reading disability—Strephosymbolia. *JAMA* 90:1095–1099, 1928.
6. Gillingham A, Stillman BW: *Remedial Training for Children with Specific Disability in Reading, Spelling, and Penmanship*. Cambridge, MA: Educators Publishing Service, 1960.
7. Orton ST: *Reading, Writing, and Speech in Children*. New York: Norton, 1937.
8. Ansara A: The Orton-Gillingham approach to remediation, in Malatesha RN, Aaron PG (eds): *Reading Disorders: Varieties and Treatment*. New York: Academic Press, 1982, pp 409–433.
9. Critchley M: *The Dyslexic Child*. Springfield, IL: Charles C Thomas, 1970.
10. Denckla MB: Childhood learning disabilities, in Heilman KM, Valenstein E (eds): *Clinical Neuropsychology*. New York: Oxford University Press, 1979, p 550.
11. Bishop DVM, Adams C: A prospective study of the relationship between specific language impairment, phonological disorders and reading retardation. *J Child Psychol Psychiatry* 31:1027–1050, 1990.
12. Fletcher JM: Foorman BR, Shaywitz SE, et al: Conceptual and methodological issues in dyslexia research: A lesson for developmental disorders, in Tager-Flusberg, H (ed): *Neurodevelopmental Disorders*. Cambridge, MA: MIT Press, 1999, pp 271–305.
13. Liberman A: How theories of speech affect research on reading and writing, in Blachman, B (ed): *Foundations of Reading Acquisition and Dyslexia*. Mahwah, NJ: Erlbaum, 1997, pp 3–19.
14. Mann, V: Language problems: The key to early reading problems, in Wong B (ed): *Learning About Learning Disabilities*. San Diego, CA: Academic Press, 1998, pp 163–201.
15. Scarborough, HS: Early identification of children at risk for reading disabilities, in Shapiro BK, Acardo PJ, Capute AJ (eds): *Specific Reading Disability: A View of the Spectrum*. Timonium, MD: York Press, 1998, pp 75–119.
16. Stanovich, KE: Explaining the differences between dyslexic and garden-variety poor reader: The phonological core variable difference model. *J Learn Disabil* 21:590–604, 1988.
17. Gough PB, Tunmer WE: Decoding, reading, and reading disability. *Remed Spec Educ* 7:6–10, 1986.
18. Frankenberger W, Fronzaglio K: A review of state's criteria and procedures for identifying children with learning disabilities. *J Learn Disabil* 24:495–500, 1991.
19. Mercer CD, Jordan L, Allsop DH, et al: Learning disabilities definition and criteria used by state education departments. *Learn Disabil Q* 19:217–232, 1996.
20. Fletcher JM, Shaywitz SE, Shankweiler DP, et al: Cognitive profiles of reading disability: Comparisons of discrepancy and low achievement definitions. *J Educ Psychol* 86:6–23, 1994.
21. Stanovich KE, Siegel LS: Phenotypic performance profile of children with reading disabilities: A regression-based test of the phonological-core variable-difference model. *J Educ Psychol* 86:24–53, 1994.
22. Hoskyn M, Swanson HL: Cognitive processing of low achievers and children with reading disabilities: A selective meta-analytic review of the published literature. *School Psychol Rev* 29:102–119, 2000.
23. Stuebing KK, Fletcher JM, LeDoux JM, et al: Validity of IQ-discrepency classifications of reading disabilities: A meta-analysis. *Am Educ Res J*. 39:469–518, 2002.
24. Share DL, Stanovich KE. Cognitive processes in early reading development: Accommodating individual differences into a model of acquisition. *Issues Educ Contrib Educ Psychol* 1:1–57, 1995.

25. Shaywitz SE, Shaywitz BA, Fletcher JM, et al: Prevalence of reading disability in boys and girls: Results of the Connecticut Longitudinal Study. *JAMA* 264:998–1002, 1990.
26. Shaywitz SE, Fletcher JM, Shaywitz BA: A conceptual model and definition of dyslexia: Findings emerging from the Connecticut Longitudinal Study, in Beitchman JH, Cohen NJ, Konstantareas MM, et al (eds): *Language, Learning, and Behavior Disorder*. New York: Cambridge University Press, 1996.
27. Bruck M: Outcomes of adults with childhood histories of dyslexia, in Hulme C, Joshi RM (eds), *Reading and Spelling: Development and Disorders*. Mahwah, NJ: Erlbaum, 1998, pp 179–200.
28. Tarnapol L, Tarapol M: *Comparative Reading Difficulties*. Lexington, KY: Lexington Books, 1981.
29. Grigorenko E: Developmental dyslexia: An update on genes, brains, and environments. *J Child Psychol Psychiatry* 42:91–125, 2001.
30. Paulesu E, Demonet JF, Fazio F, et al: Dyslexia: Cultural diversity and biological unity. *Science* 291:2165–2167, 2001.
31. Stanovich KE: Toward an interactive-compensatory model of individual differences in the development of reading fluency. *Read Res Q* 16:32–71, 1980.
32. Stanovich KE: Matthew effects in reading: Some consequences of individual differences in the acquisition of literacy. *Read Res Q* 21:360–407, 1986.
33. Perfetti CA: *Reading Ability*. New York: Oxford University Press, 1985.
34. Rack JP, Snowling M, Olson RK: The nonword reading deficit in developmental dyslexia: A review. *Read Res Q 27*:28–53, 1992.
35. Shankweiler D, Lundquist E, Katz L, et al: Comprehension and decoding: Patterns of association in children with reading difficulties. *Sci Stud Read 3*:69–94, 1999.
36. Bradley L, Bryant PE: Categorizing sounds and learning to read—a causal connection. *Nature* 301:419–421, 1983.
37. Wagner RK, Torgesen JK: The nature of phonological processing and its causal role in the acquisition of reading skills. *Psychol Bull* 101:192–212, 1987.
38. Wagner RK, Torgesen JK, Rashotte CA: Development of reading-related phonological processing abilities: New evidence of bidirectional causality from a latent variable longitudinal study. *Dev Psychol* 30:73–87, 1994.
39. Bruck M: Persistence of dyslexics' phonological awareness deficits. *Dev Psychol* 28:874–886, 1992.
40. Bryne B: *Foundations of Literacy: The Child's Acquisition of the Alphabetic Principle*. Hove, East Sussex, UK: Psychology Press, 1998.
41. Wagner RK, Torgesen JK, Rashotte CA, et al: Changing relations between phonological processing abilities and word-level reading as children develop from beginning to skilled readers: A five year longitudinal study. *Dev Psychol* 33:468–479, 1997.
42. Brady SA: The role of working memory in reading disability, in Brady SA, Shankweiler D (eds): *Phonological Processes in Literacy: A Tribute to Isabelle Y. Liberman*. Hillsdale, NJ: Erlbaum, 1991, pp 128–152.
43. Wolf M, Bally H, Morris R: Automaticity, retrieval processes, and reading: A longitudinal study in average and impaired readers. *Child Dev* 57:988–1000, 1986.
44. Wolf M, Bowers PG: The double-deficit hypothesis for the developmental dyslexias. *J Educ Psychol* 91:415–438, 1999.
45. Wolf M, Bowers, PG, Biddle K: Naming-speed processes, timing, and reading: A conceptual review. *J Learn Disabil* 33:387–407, 2000.
46. Denckla MB, Rudel RG: Rapid 'automatized' naming (RAN): Dyslexia differentiated from other learning disabilities. *Neuropsychologia* 14:471–479, 1976.
47. Bowers PG, Sunseth K, Golden J: The route between rapid naming and reading progress. *Sci Stud Read* 3:31–53, 1999.
48. Manis FR, Seidenberg MS, Doi L: See Dick RAN: Rapid naming and the longitudinal prediction of reading subskills in first and second graders. *Sci Stud Read* 3:129–157, 1999.
49. Goswami U, Bryant PE: *Phonological Skills and Learning to Read*. Hove, East Sussex: Erlbaum, 1990.
50. Stanovich KE: Early acquisition and the causes of reading difficulty: The contributions to research on phonological processing, in Stanovich KE (ed): *Progress in Understanding Reading: Scientific Foundations and New Frontiers*. New York: Guilford Press, 2000, pp 57–79.
51. Share DL: Phonological recoding and self-teaching. Sine qua non of reading acquisition. *Cognition* 55:151–218, 1995.
52. Bradley L, Bryant PE: Difficulties in auditory organization as a possible cause of reading backwardness. *Nature* 271:746–747, 1978.
53. Grigorenko EL, Wood FB, Meyer MS et al.: Susceptibility loci for distinct components of developmental dyslexia on chromosomes 6 and 15. *Am J Hum Genet* 60:27–39, 1997.
54. Shaywitz SE, Shaywitz BA, Pugh KR: Functional disruption in the organization of the brain for reading in dyslexia. *Proc Natl Acad Sci U S A* 95:2636–2641, 1998.
55. Habib M: The neurological basis of developmental dyslexia: An overview and working hypothesis. *Brain* 123:2373–2399, 2000.

56. Pennington BF: Dyslexia as a neurodevelopmental disorder, in Tager-Flusberg H (ed): *Neurodevelopmental Disorders*. Cambridge, MA: MIT Press, 1999, pp 307–330.
57. Foorman BR, Francis DJ, Fletcher, JM, et al: The role of instruction in learning to read: Preventing reading failure in at-risk children. *J Educ Psychol* 90:37–55, 1998.
58. Hatcher PJ, Hulme C, Ellis AW: Ameliorating early reading failure by integrating the teaching of reading and phonological skills: The phonological linkage hypothesis. *Child Dev* 65:41–57, 1994.
59. Lovett MW, Borden SL, DeLuca T, et al: Treating the core deficits of developmental dyslexia: Evidence of transfer-of-learning following phonologically- and strategy-based reading training programs. *Dev Psychol* 30:805–822, 1994.
60. Lovett MW, Lacerenza L, Borden SL, et al: Components of effective remediation for developmental reading disabilities: Combining phonological and strategy-based instruction to improve outcomes. *J Educ Psychol* 92:263–283, 2000.
61. Olson RK, Wise B, Ring J, et al: Computer-based remedial training in phoneme awareness and phonological decoding: Effects on the posttraining development of word recognition. *Sci Stud Read* 1:235–254, 1997.
62. Torgesen JK, Alexander AW, Wagner RK, et al: Intensive remedial instruction for children with severe reading disabilities: Immediate and long-term outcomes from two instructional approaches. *J Learn Disabil* 34: 33–58, 2001.
63. Torgesen, JK, Wagner RK, Rashotte CA et al: Preventing reading failure in young children with phonological processing disabilities: Group and individual responses to instruction. *J Educ Psychol* 91:579–593, 1999.
64. Vellutino FR, Scanlon DM, Sipay ER, et al: Cognitive profiles of difficult-to-remediate and readily remediated poor readers: Early intervention as a vehicle for distinguishing between cognitive and experiential deficits as basic causes of specific reading disability. *J Educ Psychol* 88:601–638, 1996.
65. Lovett MW, Barron RW: The search for individual and subtype differences in reading disabled children's response to remediation, in Molfese DL, Molfese VJ (eds): *Developmental Variations in Learning: Applications to Social, Executive Function, Language, and Reading Skills*. Mahwah, NJ: Erlbaum, 2002, pp 309–337.
66. Lovett MW, Barron RW: Neuropsychological perspectives on reading development and reading disorders, in Segalowitz SJ, Rapin I (eds): *Handbook of Neuropsychology:* Child Neuropsychology, 2d ed., New York: Elsevier, 2003, vol. 8, part II, pp 255–300.
67. Lovett MW, Barron RW, Benson NJ: Effective remediation of word identification and decoding difficulties in school-age children with reading disabilities, in Swanson HL, Harris K, Graham S (eds): *Handbook of Learning Disabilities*. New York: Guilford. In press.
68. Swanson HL, Hoskyn M: Experimental intervention research on students with learning disabilities: A meta-analysis of treatment outcomes. *Rev Educ Res* 68: 277–321, 1998.
69. Fletcher JM, Morris RD: Classification of disabled learners: Beyond exclusionary definitions. in Ceci S (ed): *Handbook of Cognitive, Social, and Neuropsychological Aspects of Learning Disabilities*. Hillsdale, NJ: Erlbaum,1986, pp 55–80.
70. Morris RD, Stuebing KK, Fletcher JM et al: Subtypes of reading disability: Variability around a phonological core. *J Educ Psychol* 90:1–27, 1998.
71. Wolf M, Goldberg A, Gidney C, et al: The second deficit: An investigation of the independence of phonological and naming-speed deficits in developmental dyslexia. *Read Writing Interdiscip J* 15:43–72, 2002.
72. Lovett MW Steinbach KA, Frijters JC: Remediating the core deficits of developmental reading disability: A double deficit perspective. *J Learn Disabil* 33:334–358, 2000.
73. Castles A, Coltheart M: Varieties of developmental dyslexia. *Cognition* 47:149–180, 1993.
74. Manis FR, Seidenberg, MS, Doi LM, et al: On the basis of two subtypes of developmental dyslexia. *Cognition* 58:157–195, 1996.
75. Stanovich KE, Siegel LS, Gottardo A: Converging evidence for phonological and surface subtypes of reading disability. *J Educ Psychol* 89:114–127, 1997.
76. Francis DJ, Shaywitz SE, Stuebing KK, et al: Developmental lag versus deficit models of reading disability: A longitudinal, individual growth curves analysis. *J Educ Psychol* 88:3–17, 1996.
77. Manis FR, McBride-Chang C, Seidenberg MS, et al: Are speech perception deficits associated with developmental dyslexia? *J Exp Child Psychol* 66:211–235, 1997.
78. Joanisse MF, Manis FR, Keating P, et al: Language deficits in dyslexic children: Speech perception, phonology, and morphology. *J Exp Child Psychol* 77:30–60, 2000.
79. Bishop DVM, Adams C: A prospective study of the relationship between specific language impairment, phonological disorders and reading retardation. *J Child Psychol Psychiatry* 31:1027–1050, 1990.

80. Studdert-Kennedy M, Mody M: Auditory temporal deficits in the reading impaired: A critical review of the evidence. *Psychonom Bulletin Rev* 2:508–514, 1995.
81. Stein JF: The neurobiology of reading difficulties, in Wolf M (ed): *Dyslexia, Fluency, and the Brain*. Baltimore, MD: York Press, 2001, pp 3–21.
82. Stein JF: The sensory basis of reading problems. *Dev Neuropsychol* 20:509–534, 2001.
83. Joseph J, Noble K, Eden G: The neurobiological basis of reading. *J Learn Disabil* 34:566–579, 2001.
84. Demb JB, Poldrack RA, Gabrieli JDE: Functional neuroimaging of word processing in normal and dyslexic readers, in Klein RM, McMullen PM (eds): *Converging Method for Understanding Reading and Dyslexia*. Cambridge, MA: MIT Press, 1999, pp 245–304.
85. Rayner K: Eye movements in reading and information processing: 20 years of research. *Psychol Bull* 124:372–422, 1998.
86. Willows DM, Terepocki M: The relation of reversal errors to reading disabilities, in Willows DM, Kruk RS, Corcos E (eds): *Visual Processes in Reading and Reading Disabilities*. Hillsdale, NJ: Erlbaum, 1993, pp 31–56.
87. Cornelissen PL, Hansen PC, Hutton JL et al: Magnocellular visual function and children's single word reading. *Vis Res* 38:471–482, 1998.
88. Lovegrove WJ, Bowling A, Badcock D, et al: Specific reading disability: Differences in contrast sensitivity as a function of spatial frequency. *Science* 210:439–440, 1980.
89. Lovegrove WJ, Garzia RP, Nicholson SB: Experimental evidence for a transient system deficit in specific reading disability. *J Am Optom Assoc* 61:137–146, 1990.
90. Lovegrove WJ, Martin F, Slaghuis W: A theoretical and experimental case for a visual deficit in specific reading disability. *Cogn Neuropsychol* 3:225–267, 1986.
91. Cornelissen PL, Richardson AJ, Mason AJ, et al: Contrast sensitivity and coherent motion detection measured at photopic luminance levels in dyslexics and controls. *Vis Res* 35:1483–1494, 1995.
92. Cornelissen PL, Hansen PC, Gilchrist I, et al: Coherent motion detection and letter position encoding. *Vis Res* 38:2181–2191, 1998.
93. Witton C, Talcott JB, Hansen PC, et al: Sensitivity to dynamic auditory and visual stimuli predicts nonword reading ability in both dyslexic and normal readers. *Curr Biol* 8:791–797, 1998.
94. Cestnick L, Coltheart M: The relationship between language-processing and visual-processing deficits in developmental dyslexia. *Cognition* 71:231–255, 1999.
95. Eden GF, VanMeter JW, Rumsey JM, et al: Abnormal processing of visual motion in dyslexia revealed by functional brain imaging. *Nature* 382:66–69, 1996.
96. Stein JF, Walsh V: To see but not to read: The magnocellular theory of dyslexia. *Trends Neurosci* 20:147–152, 1997.
97. Hayduk S, Bruck M, Cavanagh P: Low-level visual processing skills of adults and children with dyslexia. *Cogn Neuropsychol* 13:975–1016, 1996.
98. O'Brien BA, Mansfield JS, Legge GE: The effect of contrast on reading speed in dyslexia. *Vis Res* 40:1921–1935, 2000.
99. Skottun BC, Parke LA: The possible relationship between visual defcits and dyslexia: Examination of a critical assumption. *J Learn Disabil* 32:2–5, 1999.
100. Skottun BC: The magnocellular deficit theory of dyslexia: The evidence from contrast sensitivity. *Vis Res* 40:111–127, 2000.
101. Hulme C: The implausibilty of low-level visual deficits as a cause of children's reading difficulties. *Cogn Neuropsychol* 5:369–374, 1986.
102. Stein JF, Fowler S: Visual dyslexia. *Trends Neurosci* 4:77–80, 1981.
103. Eden GF, Stein JF, Wood HM: Differences in eye movements and reading problems in dyslexic and normal children. *Vis Res* 34:1345–1358, 1995.
104. Stein JF, Richardson AJ, Fowler MS: Monocular occlusion can improve binocular control and reading in dyslexics. *Brain* 123:164–170, 2000.
105. Tallal P: An experimental investigation of the role of auditory temporal processing in normal and disordered language development, in Caramazza A, Zurif EB (eds): *Language Acquisition and Language Breakdown*. Baltimore, MD: Johns Hopkins University Press, 1978, pp 25–61.
106. Merzenich MM, Jenkins WM, Johnston P, et al: Temporal processing deficits of language-learning impaired children ameliorated by training. *Science* 271:77–81, 1996.
107. Tallal P, Miller SL, Bedi G, et al: Language comprehension in language-learning impaired children improved with acoustically modified speech. *Science* 271:81–84, 1996.
108. Habib M, Espesser R, Ray V, et al: Training dyslexics with acoustically modified speech: Evidence of improved phonological performance. *Brain Cogn* 40:143–146, 1999.
109. Wright BA, Lombardino LJ, King WM, et al: Defcits in auditory temporal and spectral resolution in language-impaired children. *Nature* 387:176–178, 1997.

110. Bishop DVM, Bishop SJ, Bright P, et al: Different origin of auditory and phonological processing problems in children with language impairment: Evidence from a twin study. *J Speech Lang Hear Res* 42:155–168, 1999.
111. Bishop DVM, Carlyon RP, Deeks JM, et al: Auditory temporal processing impairment: Neither necessary nor sufficient for causing language impairment in children. *J Speech Lang Hear Res* 42:1295–1310, 1999.
112. Bradlow AR, Kraus N, Nicol T, et al: Effects of lengthened format transitions duration on discrimination and neural representation of synthetic CV syllables by normal and learning disabled children. *J Acoust Soc Am* 106:2086–2096, 1999.
113. Nittrouer S: Do temporal processing deficits cause phonological processing problems? *J Speech Lang Hear Res* 42:925–942, 1999.
114. Tallal P: Auditory temporal perception, phonics and reading disabilities in children. *Brain Lang* 9:182–198, 1980.
115. Booth JR, Perfetti CA, MacWhinney B, et al: The association of rapid temporal perception with orthographic and phonological processing in children and adults with reading impairment. *Sci Stud Reading* 4:101–132, 2000.
116. Talcott JB, Witton C, McLean MF, et al: Dynamic sensory sensitivity and children's word decoding skills. *Proc Natl Acad Sci USA* 97:2952–2957, 2000.
117. Mody M, Studdert-Kennedy M, Brady S: Speech perception deficits in poor readers: Auditory processing or phonological coding? *J Exp Child Psychol* 64:199–231, 1997.
118. Studdert-Kennedy M: Deficits in phoneme awareness do not arise from failures in rapid auditory processing. *Read Writing* 15:5–14, 2002.
119. Galaburda AM, Livingstone M: Evidence for a magnocellular defect in developmental dyslexia. *Ann NY Acad Sci* 68:70–82, 1993.
120. Galaburda AM, Menard MT, Rosen GD: Evidence for aberrant auditory anatomy in developmental dyslexia. *Proc Natl Acad Sci U S A* 91:8010–8013, 1994.
121. Nicholson RI, Fawcett AJ, Berry EL, et al: Motor learning difficulties and abnormal cerebellar activation in dyslexic children. *Lancet* 353:43–47, 1999.
122. Irvy RB, Justus TC, Middleton C: The cerebellum, timing, and language, in Wolf M (ed): *Dyslexia, Fluency, and the Brain*. Timonium, MD: York Press, 2001 pp 189–211.
123. Pennington BF, Smith SD: Genetic influences on learning disabilities: An update. *J Consult Clin Psychol 56:*817–823, 1988.
124. Finucci JM, Gottfredson L, Childs B: A follow-up study of dyslexic boys. *Ann Dyslexia* 35:117–136, 1985.
125. Wood FB, Grigorenko EL: Emerging issues in the genetics of dyslexia: A methodological review. *J Learn Disabil* 34:503–511, 2001.
126. DeFries JC, Alarcón M: Genetics of specific reading disability. *Ment Retard Dev Disabil Res Rev* 2:39–47, 1996.
127. Hohnen B, Stevenson J: Genetic effects in orthographic ability: A second look. *Behav Genet* 25:271, 1995.
128. Gayán J, Olson RK: Reading disability: Evidence for a genetic etiology. *Eur Child Adolesc Psychiatry* 8: 52–55, 1999.
129. Smith SD, Kelley PM, Askew JW, et al: Reading disability and chromosome 6p21.3: Evaluation of MOG as a candidate gene. *J Learn Disabil* 34:512–519, 2001.
130. Smith SD, Kimberling WJ, Pennington BF, et al: Specific reading disability: Identification of an inherited form through linkage analysis. *Science* 219:1345–1347, 1983.
131. Bisgaard ML, Eiberg H, Moller N, et al: Dyslexia and chomosome 15 heteromorphism: negative lod score in a Danish material. *Clin Gene* 32:118–119, 1987.
132. Cardon LR, Smith SD, Fulker FW, et al: Quantitative trait locus for reading disability on chromosome 6. *Science* 266: 276–279, 1994.
133. Lubs HA, Duara R, Levin B, et al: Dyslexia subtypes: Genetics, behavior, and brain imaging, in Duane DD, Gray DB (eds), *The Reading Brain: The Biological Basis of Dyslexia*. Parkton, MD: York Press, 1991, pp 89–118.
134. Morris DW, Robinson L, Turic D, et al: Family-based association mapping provides evidence for reading disability on chromosome 15q. *Hum Mol Genet* 9:843–848, 2000.
135. Schulte-Körne G, Brimm T, Nöthen MM, et al: Evidence for linkage of spelling disability to chromosome 15. *Am J Med Genet Neuropsychol Genet* 74:661, 1997.
136. Geshwind N, Behan PO: Laterality, hormones, and immunity, in Geshwind N, Galaburda A (eds): *Cerebral Dominance*. New York: MIT Press, pp 211–224.
137. Gilger JW, Pennington BF, Harbeck RJ, et al: A twin and family study of the association between immune system dysfunction and dyslexia using blood serum immunoassay and survey data. *Brain Cogn* 26:310–333, 1998.
138. Fisher SE, Marlow AJ, Lamb J, et al: A quantitative-trait locus on chromosome 6p influences different aspects of developmental dyslexia. *Am J Hum Genet* 64: 146–156, 1999.
139. Gayán J, Smith SD, Cherny SS, et al: Quantitative-trait locus for specific language and reading deficits on chromosome 6p. *Am J Hum Genet* 64: 157–164, 1999.

140. Pennington BF: Using genetics to dissect cognition. *Am J Hum Genet* 60: 13–16, 1997.
141. Plomin R, Crabbe J: DNA. *Psychol Bull* 126:806–828, 2000.
142. Plomin R, Rutter M: Child development, molecular genetics, and what to do with genes once they are found. *Child Dev* 69:1221–1240.
143. Fisher SE, Francks C, Marlow AJ, et al: Independent genome-wide scans identify a chromosome 18 quantitative-trait locus influencing dyslexia. *Nat Genet* 30: 86–91, 2002.
144. Barr CL, Wigg K, Feng Y, et al: Linkage study of reading disabilities and attention-deficit hyperactivity disorder in the chromosome 6p region. American Society of Human Genetics 51st Annual Meeting, San Diego, CA. *Am J Human Genet* 69: 544, 2001.
145. Fagerheim T, Raeymaekers P, Tonnessen FE, et al: A new gene (DYX3) for dyslexia is located on chromosome 2. *J Med Genet* 36:664–669, 1999.
146. Petryshen, TL, Kaplan BJ, Hughes ML, et al: Supportive evidence for the DYX3 dyslexia susceptibility gene in Canadian families. *J Med Genet 39*(2):125–126, 2000.
147. Barr CL: Personal communication.
148. Willcutt EG, Pennington BF: Comorbidity of reading disability and attention-deficit / hyperactivity disorder: Differences by gender and subtype. *J Learn Disabil* 33: 179–191, 2000.
149. Willcutt EG, Pennington BF, DeFries JC: Etiology of inattention and hyperactivity/impulsivity in a community sample of twins with learning difficulties. *J Abnorm Child Psychol* 28:149–159, 2000.
150. SLI Consortium: A genomewide scan identifies two novel loci involved in specific language impairment. *Am J Hum Genet* 70:384–398, 2001.
151. Light JG, DeFries JC: Comorbidity of reading and mathematics disabilities: Genetic and environmental etiologies. *J Learn Disabil* 28:96–106, 1995.
152. Filipek PA: Neuroimaging in the developmental disorders: The state of the science. *J Child Psychol Psychiatry* 40:113–128, 1999.
153. Pugh KR, Mencl WE, Jenner AJ, et al: Functional neuroimaging studies of reading and reading disability (developmental dyslexia). *Ment Retard Dev Disabil Rev* 6:207–213, 2000.
154. Galaburda AM: Neurology of developmental dyslexia. *Curr Opin in Neurobiology* 3:237–242, 1993.
155. Galaburda AM: Developmental dyslexia and animal studies: At the interface between cognition and neurology. *Cognition* 50:133–149, 1994.
156. Galaburda, AM Kemper, TL: Cytoarchitectonic abnormalities in dyslexia: A case study. *Ann Neurol* 6: 94–100, 1979.
157. Galaburda AM, Sherman GF, Rosen GD, et al: Developmental dyslexia: Four consecutive patients with cortical anomalies. *Ann Neurol* 18:222–233, 1985.
158. Humphreys P, Kaufman WE, Galaburda AM: Developmental dyslexia in women: Neuropathological finding in three patients. *Ann Neurol* 28:727–738, 1990.
159. Morgan AE, Hynd GW: Dyslexia, neurolinguistic ability, and anatomical variation of the planum temporale. *Neuropsychol Rev* 8:79–93, 1998.
160. Filipek PA: Neurobiological correlates of developmental dyslexia: What do we know of how dyslexics' brains differ from those of normal readers? *J Child Neurol* 10: 62–69, 1995.
161. Westbury CF, Zatorre RJ, Evans AC: Quantifying variability in the palnum temporale: A probability map. *Cereb Cortex* 9:382–405, 1999.
162. Pennington BF., Filipek PA, Churchwell J, et al: Brain morphometry in reading-disabled twins. *Neurology* 53: 723–729, 1999.
163. Pugh KR, Mencl WE, Shaywitz BA, et al: The angular gyrus in developmental dyslexia: Task-specific differences in functional connectivity within posterior cortex. *Psychol Sci* 11:51–59, 2000.
164. Shaywitz SE, Fletcher JM, Holahan JM, et al: Persistence of dyslexia: The Connecticut Longitudinal Study at adolescence. *Pediatrics* 104:1351, 1999.
165. Scarborough HS: Continuity between childhood dyslexia and adult reading. *Br J Psychol* 75:329–348, 1984.
166. Beitchman JH, Wilson B, Douglas L, et al.: Substance use disorders in young adults with and without LD: Predictive and concurrent relationships. *J Learn Disabil* 34:317–332, 2001.
167. Beitchman JH, Wilson B, Johnson CJ, et al: Fourteen-year follow-up of speech/language-impaired and control children: Psychiatric outcome. *J Am Acad Child Adolesc Psychiatry* 40:75–82, 2001.
168. Lovett MW: Developmental dyslexia, in Rapin I, Segalowitz SJ (eds): *Handbook of Neuropsychology: Child Neuropsychology*. Amsterdam: Elsevier 1992, vol 7, pp 163–185.
169. Lovett MW: Defining and remediating the core deficits of developmental dyslexia: Lessons from remedial outcome research with reading disabled children, in Klein R, McMullen P (eds): *Converging Methods for Understanding Reading and Dyslexia*. Cambridge, MA: MIT Press, 1999, pp 111–132.

170. Foorman BR, Francis DJ, Winikates D, et al: Early interventions for children with reading disabilities. *Sci Stud Reading* 1:255–276, 1997.
171. Scanlon DM, Vellutino FR: A comparison of the instructional backgrounds and cognitive profiles of poor, average, and good readers who were initially identified as at risk for reading failure. *Sci Stud Reading* 1:191–216, 1997.
172. Lovett MW, Steinbach KA: The effectiveness of remedial programs for reading disabled children of different ages: Is there decreased benefit for older children? *Learn Disabil Q* 20:189–210, 1997.
173. Wise BW, Olson RK: Computer-based phonological awareness and reading instruction. *Ann Dyslexia* 45: 99–122, 1995.
174. Wise BW, Ring J, Olson RK: Training phonological awareness with and without explicit attention to articulation. *J Exp Child Psychol* 72:271–304, 1999.
175. Wise BW, Ring J, Sessions L, et al: Phonological awareness with and without articulation: A preliminary study. *Learn Disabil Q* 20:211–225, 1997.
176. Torgesen JK, Wagner RK, Rashotte CA: Approaches to the prevention and remediation of phonologically-based reading disabilities, in Blachman BA (ed), *Foundations of Reading Acquisition and Dyslexia: Implications for Early Intervention*. Mahwah, NJ: Erlbaum, 1997, pp. 287–304.
177. Moats LC, Foorman BR: Components of effective reading instruction. *Sci Stud Reading* 1:187–189, 1997.
178. Lovett MW, Ransby MJ, Barron RW: Treatment, subtype, and word type effects in dyslexic children's response to remediation. *Brain Lang* 34:328–349, 1988.
179. Lovett MW, Ransby MJ, Hardwick N, et al: Can dyslexia be treated? Treatment-specific and generalized treatment effects in dyslexic children's response to remediation. *Brain Lang* 37:90–121, 1989.
180. Lovett MW, Warren-Chaplin PM, Ransby MJ, et al: Training the word recognition skills of reading disabled children: Treatment and transfer effects. *J Educ Psychol* 82:769–780, 1990.
181. Levin BE: Organizational deficits in dyslexia: Possible frontal lobe dysfunction. *Dev Neuropsychol* 6:95–110, 1990.
182. Swanson HL: Reading comprehension and working memory in learning-disabled readers: Is the phonological loop more important than the exdecutive system? *J Exp Child Psychol* 72:1–31, 1999.
183. Swanson HL, Alexander JE: Cognitive processes as predictors of word recognition and reading comprehension in learning-disabled and skilled readers: Revisiting the specificity hypothesis. *J Educ Psychol* 89:128–158, 1997.
184. Benson NJ: Analysis of specific deficits: Evidence of transfer in disabled and normal readers following oral-motor awareness training. *J Educ Psychol* 92:646–658, 2000.
185. Benson NJ, Lovett MW, Kroeber CL: Training and transfer-of-learning effects in disabled and normal readers: Evidence of specific deficits. *J Exp Child Psychol* 64:343–366, 1997.
186. Engelmann S, Bruner EC: *Reading Mastery I/II Fast Cycle: Teacher's Guide*. Chicago: Science Research Associates, 1988.
187. Engelmann S, Carnine L, Johnson G: *Corrective Reading: Word Attack Basics, Decoding A*. Chicago: Science Research Associates, 1988.
188. Engelmann S, Johnson G, Carnine L, et al: *Corrective Reading: Decoding Strategies, Decoding B1*. Chicago: Science Research Associates, 1988.
189. Gaskins IW, Downer MA, Gaskins RW: *Introduction to the Benchmark School Word Identification/Vocabulary Development Program*. Media, PA: Benchmark School, 1986.
190. Swanson HL, Hoskyn M: Experimental intervention research on students with learning disabilities: A meta-analysis of treatment outcomes. *Rev Educ Res* 68:277–321, 1998.
191. Lovett MW, Lacerenza L, Borden SL: Putting struggling readers on the PHAST track: A program to integrate phonological and strategy-based remedial reading instruction and maximize outcomes. *J Learn Disabil* 33:458–476, 2000.
192. Wolf M, Miller L, Donnelly K: Retrieval, automaticity, vocabulary elaboration, orthography (RAVE-O): A comprehensive, fluency-based reading intervention program. *J Learn Disabil* 33:375–386, 2000.
193. Wolf M, Goodman G: Speed wizards [computerized reading program]. Tufts University Boston, and Rochester Institute of Technology, Rochester, NY, 1996.
194. Simos PG, Fletcher JM, Bergman E, et al: Dyslexia-specific brain activation profile becomes normal following successful remedial training. *Neurology*. In press.

Chapter 65

NONVERBAL, SOCIAL, AND EMOTIONAL LEARNING DISABILITIES

Kytja K. S. Voeller

WHAT ARE NONVERBAL, SOCIAL, AND EMOTIONAL LEARNING DISABILITIES?

Nonverbal social-emotional learning disabilities (NVLD) refers to a group of disorders characterized by chronic difficulties in social relationships accompanied by deficits in visuospatial and arithmetic skills that first appear in childhood. Children with NVLD are usually highly verbal, not at all aggressive, and have the best of social intentions. They wish to make friends but lack the ability to do so. Their social obtuseness and odd behaviors lead other children to consider them "weird" and to avoid them. This chapter focuses heavily on the social behaviors of these children.

THE COGNITIVE NEUROLOGY OF NVLD

Children and adults with NVLD are impaired in processing the visual and prosodic signals that convey social-emotional information as well as having deficits in higher-order social cognition. They often appear hypoaroused, indifferent to emotional stimuli, and inattentive.

Deficits in Processing Social-Emotional Information at a Perceptual and Motor Level

Children and adults with NVLD have difficulty identifying faces (prosopagnosia) and comprehending emotional gestures of the face and limbs as well as vocal intonational patterns.[1–4] They seem remote and disinterested in others and develop a self-image and way of interacting that persists into adulthood.[5] Although some may become aware of their difficulty in this sphere by the time they are adolescents or young adults, many never develop this insight.

Their difficulty in the motor sphere—the timing and generation of affective face and limb gestures and prosody that are appropriately integrated into social interactions—results in a restricted array of emotional expressions and speech that is monotonous and robotic.[1–4] Eye contact is poor and they do not use gaze in a reciprocal, socially communicative fashion. Their timing in interactions is off. They often violate societal rules of distance by standing too close and impinging on the social space of the person they are talking to. They may also be inappropriately familiar, overly affectionate, and "sticky." All of these features contribute to their oddness.

The neural system involved in the processing of faces travels in the ventral stream (see Chaps. 17 and 19): it originates in the striate cortex and moves through a series of increasingly complex associational cortices (superior temporal sulcus, inferior temporal gyrus, and amygdala); the highly processed information from these areas then flows into inferior frontal cortex.[6,7] The fusiform face area (FFA) serves as an important node in the processing of face information. It is not clear whether the FFA is specifically "hard wired" for face processing[8] or can be trained by repeated exposure to objects within a specific class.[9]

Functional magnetic resonance imaging (fMRI) studies of face processing in high-functioning subjects with autistic disorder and/or Asperger's disorder have demonstrated an atypical pattern of activation of the face-processing pathway (see Chap. 68). Although studies have not been conducted in the NVLD population, it is likely that there are some common features in the pathophysiology of all three entities. Critchley et al.[10] reported that high-functioning adults with autism did not activate the fusiform gyrus, cerebellum, insula, amygdalohippocampal junction, putamen, or middle temporal gyrus to the same extent as controls. Schultz et al.[11] observed that high-functioning subjects with autistic disorder and Asperger's disorder used the right inferior temporal gyrus for face processing rather than the right FFA. Since the left inferior temporal gyrus was activated in both groups when the task involved object recognition, it was suggested that these subjects used an area typically activated with object recognition for face recognition. Pierce et al.[12] studied carefully selected high-functioning autistic subjects and reported that each individual used a unique area of cortex other than FFA for face processing. At this point, it is not clear whether this anomalous face processing results from miswiring, a lack of exposure to faces (autistic children seem less fascinated with faces than normal children), or a combination of factors.

Only a few functional neuroimaging studies have been conducted with regard to the processing of prosodic information, but it appears that the right hemisphere and frontal cortex are involved (see Chap. 59). Buchanan et al.[13] examined normal adult males in an f MRI study. The discrimination of prosodic utterances and initial phonemes evoked bilateral activity. Emotional prosody activated the right inferior frontal lobe and right auditory cortex, in contrast to phonemic discriminations which activated homologous left hemisphere structures. The amygdala does not appear to play a role in the processing of prosody as it does in face processing.[14] The production of emotional intonation is also impaired in patients with right hemisphere damage.[15]

Deficits in Social Cognition

Theory of Mind (ToM) refers to the awareness that other persons may have perceptions and motivations that differ from one's own, and that one's perceptions and beliefs can be valid or invalid.[16] In normal children this concept begins to emerge around the age of 3 or 4 years. By age 6 to 7, the child begins to understand that others may have incorrect perceptions and beliefs, and by age 9 to 11 they develop the concept of the faux pas.[17] ToM deficits are a prominent feature of autistic disorder, even high-functioning autistic disorder. In contrast, persons with Asperger's disorder have difficulty only on the more subtle and complex ToM tasks, such as the faux pas questions.[17] Older children and adults with NVLD rarely have difficulty on the first- and second-order ToM tasks, but they have trouble understanding deceit and are strikingly lacking in tact and prone to making disastrous faux pas. Their inability to understand when they are being deceived or manipulated often gets them into trouble. One patient, a high school student, who had for many years borne the brunt of teasing and ostracism by peers, was brought up on sexual harassment charges because he touched a girl's breasts after being encouraged by his male classmates, who told him that "she would like it." Children and adults with NVLD often have deficits in the pragmatic use of language: they have difficulty modifying verbal output to meet the needs of their conversational partners and are often oblivious to their listeners' interests. Deficits in executive function (EF), particularly with regard to social behaviors, are quite prominent in persons with NVLD.

There has been considerable controversy regarding the relationship of ToM and prefrontal EF (see Chap. 33). Some feel that ToM is not a specific prefrontal function but rather just another manifestation of EF (both require what might be called "cognitive multitasking"—integrating multiple pieces of information and drawing correct inferences from that information). Others feel that it represents a specific and localizable prefrontal function[16] or, possibly—depending on the nature of the task—several different functions. In interpreting studies of ToM and EF, the issue of the linguistic load of the tasks needs to be considered. The ToM tasks are often presented in the form of stories that require both right hemisphere resources (in terms of making inferences and understanding what the examiner is asking)[18] and left frontal resources,[19] which may reflect demands on auditory working memory and syntax–processing,[20] although some studies have failed to show that left hemisphere lesions affect performance on ToM tasks.[21]

Several conclusions can be drawn from studies dealing with the relationship of EF and ToM (relevant articles are summarized in Table 65-1). The first is that although ToM requires EF,[22] ToM can be intact in the presence of damage to the prefrontal area and significant executive dysfunction.[23] Second, ToM may well be a specific frontal function, most likely instantiated in medial prefrontal cortex, probably on the right[22,24] Third, one cannot ignore evidence that

Table 65-1
The relationship of theory of mind and prefrontal executive function

Subjects/lesions	*Tasks*	*Results*	*References*
17 RHD, 11LHD	2 types of false-belief task: one requiring comprehension of implications of story, other did not require grasp of implications	When requirements for making inferences are decreased, Ss with RH lesions perform better on ToM stories	18
LFD ($n = 5$) and bilateral OMPFC/anterior temporal ($n = 5$)	Graded series of ToM tasks (1st and 2nd order) and faux pas	No ToM deficits in L frontal; OMPFC/anterior temporal group made more errors on faux pas task.	21
Single case study: adult with dysplastic L amygdala tumor since childhood, DX: Asperger's? schizophrenia	ToM and EF	Severe ToM deficits in presence of normal EF.	25
Ss with lesions (RH=21; LH=10) (anterior/posterior) & controls.	ToM and EF	Ss with L anterior lesions had problems comprehending stories—made nonliteral interpretations and more errors on EF tasks than other groups.	20
Normal Ss	PET scan; story comprehension tasks: (1) ToM-type, (2) "physical" stories not requiring mental state attribution, (3) unlinked sentences	Only ToM task activated L medial frontal gyrus (BA 8) and also activated posterior cingulate to a greater extent than "physical" stories.	19
RFD ($n = 15$) and LFD ($n = 16$) and controls ($n = 31$)	ToM (and EF tasks)	Both lesioned groups manifested impairment in EF and ToM, but pattern of impairment suggested that they were independent.	24
RFD ($n = 4$); LFD ($n = 8$); BFD ($n = 7$); RNFD ($n = 5$); LNFD ($n = 8$); Control ($n = 14$)	Graded ToM tasks (visual perspective taking requiring inference) and deception	RFD associated with higher error rates on visual-perspective taking tasks; R frontal medial lesions associated with higher error rate on deceit task.	22
Single case study of adult with lesions of bilateral OMPFC, L temporal lobe, and L amygdala, with severe behavioral dyscontrol, hyporesponsive autonomic responses, and impaired emotional face processing	ToM	Patient had severe EF deficits but performed well on advanced ToM tasks.	23

Key: BFD = bilateral frontal lesion; EF = executive function; L = left; LFD = left frontal lesion; LHD = left hemisphere lesion; LNFD = left nonfrontal lesion; OMPFC = orbitomedial prefrontal cortex; R = right; RFD = right frontal lesion; RHD = right hemisphere lesion; RNFD = right nonfrontal lesion; ToM = theory of mind.

congenital lesions of the amygdala can also impair ToM performance and produce a clinical picture resembling Asperger's disorder.[25] However, it is possible that early lesions of the amygdala exert a remote effect on the connectivity of orbitomedial prefrontal cortex because of the strong reciprocal relationship that exists between orbitomedial prefrontal cortex and the amygdala. Fourth, patients with frontal lesions are less severely impaired on ToM tasks than high-functioning autistic subjects who manifest serious impairment.

Hypoarousal and Inattention

Many children with NVLD also have striking attentional dysfunction. They appear inattentive, disorganized, and apathetic and have difficulty regulating arousal, reminiscent of adults with right frontal lesions.[25] They are rarely hyperactive.

ETIOLOGIC FACTORS

Acquired Brain Lesions

It has been well established that right hemisphere lesions occurring in adulthood result in impairment of a broad spectrum of social-emotional behaviors.[26,27] Older children who have sustained right hemisphere injury also present with a similar array of symptoms (Refs. 1 to 5; see Ref. 28 for a review). However, lesions in some specific areas have more profound effects on social-emotional behaviors than those in others. For example, Weniger and Irle[29] observed that the heteromodal cortices serve as a conduit for information to limbic structures. In a study comparing various lesion sites, they showed that lesions affecting heteromodal cortex are more likely to produce severe deficits in social-emotional behaviors than lesions of limbic/paralimbic cortices alone or in unimodal or primary motor and sensory cortices. Cerebellar lesions produce a "cognitive affective" syndrome in both adults and children, possibly because of the strong connectivity between cerebellum and prefrontal cortex. Following tumor resections in the cerebellum, children present with loss of normal prosody, avoidance of eye contact, and difficulty with other aspects of social interaction.[30]

Neuromigrational Anomalies and Lesions in the Prenatal Period

Neuronal migration disorders have been reported in children with atypical social behaviors. These include partial agenesis of the anterior corpus callosum[31] and an area of anomalous neuronal migration in prefrontal cortex.[32] In some children, there is no history of an encephalopathic event and no evidence of any lesions on MRI, but morphometric measurements reveal that structures in the right hemisphere are significantly smaller than average.[5] This would also suggest a subtle disturbance of neuronal migration.

Although an NVLD-like picture is more likely to occur following a right hemisphere lesion, a few cases have been reported of *developmental crossed aprosodia,* analogous to the crossed aprosodias described in adults.[4,33] In these situations, patients present with anomalous dominance, atypical social development, and evidence of left hemisphere dysfunction. A possible alternative explanation has been suggested: that is, that lesions of the left hemisphere in early childhood may result in shifting language processing to the right hemisphere, resulting in *crowding*. This leads to a situation in which the neural substrates of the right hemisphere are taken up with language processing and do not have the capacity to compute social-emotional information.[4]

There is little doubt that brain lesions occurring early in development may also affect social behaviors, but in a very complex manner. Moreover, the impact of such lesions may not become apparent until adolescence or adulthood. Studies on nonhuman primates indicate that the outcome of brain injury early in development depends on multiple factors—such as the timing, location and size of the lesion and the sex of the fetus.[34,35] In addition, postnatal experience has a potent effect.[36] Early lesions of the amygdala produce marked disturbances of social behaviors as the animal matures.[37] Fine et al.[25] described an adult who had a dysplastic embryonic tumor of the left amygdala. He had severely impaired social-emotional behaviors and reclusiveness (he was in prison for murder). This case contrasts with that of the 30-year-old described by Lê et al.[38] who sustained bilateral damage to the ventral pathway (particularly posteriorly) as the result of meningoencephalitis at the age of 3 years. He was alexic, achromotopsic, and unable to identify faces or recognize emotional expressions. Functions related to the dorsal pathway were intact and he appeared to have relatively appropriate social behaviors, although these were not described in detail. This would suggest that lesions to limbic areas early in development have a much more severe impact on later social behaviors than lesions occurring in nonlimbic areas. In this case, too, social development was normally stimulated during the first 3 years of life.

Genetic Factors

Genetic factors are likely to play the most important role in the etiology of NVLD, as many affected individuals do not have any history of encephalopathic events and have family members with similar problems.[2–4] In reviewing family histories, it is not unusual to find that some relatives are odd and socially remote but functioning in society and would be labeled as merely eccentric or reclusive.

Some of the neuromigrational lesions described above are likely secondary to a genetic process that disrupts normal brain development. The case described of the patient with an area of anomalous neuronal migration in the frontal lobe[32] is of particular interest in this regard because the mother also had a left temporal macrogyrus.

Certain genetic syndromes are associated with impaired social behaviors. Thus, female fragile-X carriers often manifest NVLD-like difficulties.[39] Girls with Turner's syndrome can also manifest social deficits, but inconsistently so.[40] It has been observed that females with Turner's syndrome who inherit the X chromosome from their mothers are at greater risk for impaired EF and dysfunctional social behaviors than those whose X chromosome is inherited from their fathers.[41] These investigators suggest that there is a genetic locus for social cognition that is imprinted and is not expressed from the maternally derived X chromosome. Thus, males whose single X chromosome is inherited from their mothers are at greater risk for neurodevelopmental disorders than normal females. Velocardiofacial syndrome has been reported to be associated with social-emotional deficits, but there is a long list of other neuropsychological deficits.[42] Prader-Willi syndrome is also associated with ToM deficits.[43] However, at this time there is no genetic syndrome that appears to be consistently associated with NVLD. With further work on the human genome project, it is entirely possible that a specific genetic anomaly will ultimately be defined.

WORKUP AND DIAGNOSTIC EVALUATION

The diagnosis of NVLD requires a careful psychiatric and neurologic history, with particular attention to the patient's developmental history.[44] In addition to standard assessments of intelligence and academic achievement, a neuropsychological/neurobehavioral evaluation focusing on executive function, ToM, attention, memory, language (particularly the pragmatic/semantic aspects of language), praxis, and visuospatial ability should be conducted. In the course of the interview and examination, observation of the patient's social behaviors and ability to engage in reciprocal social interaction should be carefully assessed. Does the patient manifest social anxiety, inability to maintain eye contact, aprosodia, constricted affect? The patient's internal social-emotional experiences and social judgment must be explored: what makes him or her happy? Sad? Angry? Frightened? (The examiner must also evaluate the affect generated in the course of this discussion.) Assessment of the ability to interpret facial and prosodic signals should be carried out. Does the patient have an adequate vocabulary of words to describe emotions and internal states? Can these patients soothe themselves? (Self-soothing implies some awareness of one's own internal emotional states and the ability to develop a strategy for calming oneself.) How much insight does the patient have? How well does the patient appear to understand the perceptions and motivations of others? The neurologic examination often supplies important evidence of lateralizing signs suggesting subtle right hemispheric dysfunction (e.g., growth asymmetries of the face and extremities, posturing of the left upper extremity with stress gait, left-sided hyperreflexia, left parietal sensory deficits). Patients should be carefully screened for evidence of a subclinical seizure disorder. Neurophysiologic and neuroimaging examinations may contribute valuable information to the clinical picture. However, a standard clinical examination of the MRI may not be as valuable as careful morphometric measurements. The adult with developmental prosopagnosia described by Laeng and Caviness[4] had a "normal" MRI, but morphometric measurements revealed that volumes of right neocortex, hippocampus, and pallidum were more than one standard deviation below that of controls.

DIFFERENTIAL DIAGNOSIS

The diagnosis of NVLD is separate from the nosology of the *Diagnostic and Statistical Manual of Mental Disorders*[45] or the *International Statistical Classification of Diseases and Related Health Problems.*[46] Historically, children with NVLD were described as being a specific subgroup of learning-disabled children who presented with atypical social behaviors associated with an arithmetic learning disability.[47] Rourke[48] expanded the diagnosis of these children with NVLD and conducted a detailed analysis of their neuropsychological profile, which included motor and visuospatial deficits. Denckla[1] recognized the similarity of NVLD to right hemisphere deficits in adults and noted the left-sided signs on neurologic examination. A number of terms, such as *right hemisphere deficit syndrome,* have also been applied to NVLD. Children with NVLD have visuoperceptual and an associated arithmetic learning disability, as well as the characteristic social deficits. However, some children have significant deficits in the social sphere and yet perform well academically, even in arithmetic.

There is a marked overlap between NVLD and psychiatric pathology. Children and adults with NVLD are often first seen by psychiatrists. The major differential diagnosis involves autistic disorder and Asperger's disorder, but NVLD is somewhat milder and more subtle. There are two areas in which children with NVLD can be differentiated on a clinical basis from those with autistic disorder and Asperger's disorder. To meet DSM-IV diagnostic criteria for autistic disorder, a language deficit needs to be present and stereotypies are typically present. Children with Asperger's disorder and NVLD do not have an obvious language disorder, although they may have significant pragmatic difficulties. Stereotypies are a feature of both autistic disorder and Asperger's disorder, but children with NVLD do not have prominent motor stereotypies although they may have obsessional ruminations, which can be considered a "cognitive" stereotypy and likely involves a similar pathophysiology. Although children with NVLD do not present with the dramatically constricted intellectual interests that sometimes characterize Asperger's disorder (such as an encyclopedic knowledge of all the subway cars in New York City) they often manifest highly focused interests in certain areas of their environment.

Several other psychiatric diagnostic labels are applied to children with NVLD. A frequently encountered comorbid condition is anxiety disorder and sometimes social phobia (patients with NVLD are often shy, inhibited, and socially anxious). Other psychiatric diagnoses, such as obsessive-compulsive disorder (usually more obsessional than compulsive) are sometimes applied to children with NVLD. Diagnoses such as schizoid/schizotypal are not frequently applied to adults. Many of these children also meet criteria for attention hyperactivity disorder, predominantly inattentive type (they rarely meet criteria for the hyperactive/impulsive or combined types). Adolescents and adults with NVLD frequently present with depression, sometimes associated with suicidality.

TREATMENT

The treatment of NVLD has yet to be developed; therefore the following suggestions should be considered only possible strategies for dealing with these patients.

1. Evaluate for and treat a subclinical seizure disorder if found to be present. Manoach and coworkers[5] reported that one of their patients improved significantly in mood, eye contact, social interaction, and prosody following treatment with anticonvulsant medication.
2. Evaluate and treat for comorbid psychiatric symptoms—attention deficit hyperactivity disorder, predominantly inattentive type; impulsivity; depression; symptoms of obsessive-compulsive disorder. Great caution should be used in prescribing neuroleptics, as they enhance emotional flatness and interfere with EF.
3. Not every patient with NVLD presents with all the features; it is sometimes possible to identify

islands of strength and use them as an infrastructure on which to build more appropriate behaviors. Thus, in the course of the initial history and evaluation, it is possible to note (a) dissociations between the expression and comprehension of affective signals, (b) whether the deficit is modality-specific or not, (c) the degree to which Theory of Mind is intact, (d) if the patient shows some awareness of his or her deficits, (e) if the patient is able to use social-emotional information in any context to guide behavior, and (f) how well the patient can regulate his or her behavior. For example, patients who are aprosodic, with a constricted array of affective expression, may or may not be as severely impaired in processing incoming social signals. Some of these patients will benefit from focused training of motor behaviors such as eye contact, maintaining appropriate social distance, and diminishing social "stickiness." Computer programs have been developed to provide feedback to adults with Parkinson's disease to enhance intonational contour, and these might be useful in training patients with NVLD. Patients who cannot "read" visual or prosodic social signals can sometimes be taught either to utilize an intact pathway or ask for verbal information about the emotional state of others. It is much more difficult to work with patients who "don't know they don't know" or who are extremely impulsive and have difficulty regulating motor behaviors. These patients usually require a great deal of structure and use of "environmental prostheses." For the young child, an understanding teacher who can structure social interactions in a positive fashion and provide specific behavioral cues to the child with NVLD is extremely helpful. For the young adult, a job coach who can train appropriate behaviors can often contribute to effective functioning in the workplace.

4. For patients with some degree of meta-awareness and concomitant distress about their social difficulties, recasting these deficits as a neurologically based disability is often helpful. Since they are typically viewed as having a mental disorder, they perceive themselves as "weird" or "crazy." Developing a specific cognitive rehabilitation program is often helpful. One can utilize videotaping with instant replay for this purpose.

5. Youngsters with NVLD benefit from external structuring of their social environment and from modeling of appropriate social behaviors. Therapy situations in which they are intensively and consistently prompted to display correct behaviors can be helpful. The goal should be to reduce the "odd" behaviors to the minimum and program appropriate social behaviors that will get these children through some of their social interactions. Although these patients may not be able to spontaneously select the correct social motor program 100 percent of the time, even modest improvements in appropriateness improve their chances of surviving in the community. Although "social skills" programs are available, these are not often helpful to children with NVLD. Such training programs are typically conducted in group settings and are directed at children with behavioral problems in the realm of oppositional defiant disorder/conduct disorder and aggression; they therefore focus heavily on self-control issues. Because most children with oppositional defiant/conduct disorder usually do not have deficits in social perception, this issue is not addressed with the intensity that would be appropriate for a child with NVLD.

6. Older patients in the job market will benefit from a realistic appraisal of their cognitive strengths and assistance with finding an appropriate work environment. Having a supportive job coach is extremely beneficial.

REFERENCES

1. Denckla MB: Minimal brain dysfunction, in Chall J, Mirsky A (eds): *Education and the Brain.* Chicago: National Society for the Study of Education and the University of Chicago Press, 1978, p 223.
2. Weintraub S, Mesulam MM: Developmental learning disabilities of the right hemisphere: Emotional, interpersonal and cognitive components. *Arch Neurol* 40:463, 1983.
3. Voeller KKS: Right hemisphere deficit syndrome in children. *Am J Psychiatry* 143:1004, 1986.
4. Manoach DS, Sandson TA, Weintraub S: The developmental social-emotional processing disorder is associated with right hemisphere abnormalities. *Neuropsychiatry Neuropsychol Behav Neurol* 8:99, 1995.
5. Laeng B, Caviness VS: Prosopagnosia as a deficit in encoding curved surface. *J Cogn Neurosci* 13:556, 2001.
6. Iidaka T, Omori M, Murata T, et al: Neural interaction of the amygdala with the prefrontal and temporal cortices in the processing of facial expressions as revealed by fMRI. *J Cogn Neurosci* 13:1035, 2001.

7. Scalaidhe SPO, Wilson FAW, Goldman-Rakic PS: Areal segregation of face-processing neurons in prefrontal cortex. *Science* 278:1135, 1997.
8. Kanwisher N, Stanley D, Harris A: The fusiform face area is selective for faces not animals. *Neuroreport* 10:183, 1999.
9. Tarr MJ, Gauthier I: FFA—a flexible fusiform area for subordinate-level processing automated by expertise. *Nat Neurosci* 3:764, 2000.
10. Critchley HD, Daly EM, Bullmore ET, et al: The functional neuroanatomy of social behaviour. Changes in cerebral blood flow when people with autistic disorder process facial expressions. *Brain* 123:2203, 2000.
11. Schultz RT, Gauthier I, Klin A, et al: Abnormal ventral temporal cortical activity during face discrimination among individuals with autism and Asperger syndrome. *Arch Gen Psychiatry* 57:331, 2000.
12. Pierce K, Müller R-A, Ambrose J, et al: Face processing occurs outside the fusiform "face area" in autism: Evidence from fMRI. *Brain* 124:2059, 2001.
13. Buchanan TW, Lutz K, Mirzazade S, et al: Recognition of emotional prosody and verbal components of spoken language: An fMRI study. *Brain Res Cogn Brain Res* 9:227, 2000.
14. Adolphs R, Tranel D: Intact recognition of emotional prosody following amygdala damage. *Neuropsychologia* 37:1285, 1999.
15. Tucker DM, Watson RT, Heilman KM: Discrimination and evocation of affectively intoned speech in patients with right parietal disease. *Neurology* 27:947, 1977.
16. Frith CD, Frith U: Interacting minds–biological basis. *Science* 286:1692, 1999.
17. Baron-Cohen S, O'Riordan M, Stone V, et al: Recognition of faux pas by normally developing children and children with Asperger syndrome or high-functioning autism. *J Autism Dev Disord* 29:407, 1999.
18. Siegal M, Carrington J, Radel M: Theory of mind and pragmatic understanding following right hemisphere damage. *Brain Lang* 53:40, 1996.
19. Fletcher PC, Happe E, Frith U, et al: Other minds in the brain: A functional imaging study of "theory of mind" in story comprehension. *Cognition* 57:109, 1995.
20. Channon S, Crawford S: The effects of anterior lesions on performance on a story comprehension test: Left anterior impairment on a theory of mind-type task. *Neuropsychologia* 38:1006, 2000.
21. Stone VE, Baron-Cohen S, Knight RT: Frontal lobe contributions to theory of mind. *J Cogn Neurosci* 10:640, 1988.
22. Stuss DT, Gallup GG, Alexander MP: The frontal lobes are necessary for "theory of mind." *Brain* 124:279, 2001.
23. Blair RJR, Cipoletti L: Impaired social response reversal. A case of acquired "sociopathy." *Brain* 123:1122, 2000.
24. Rowe AD, Bullock PR, Polkey CE, Morris RG: "Theory of mind" impairments and their relationship to executive functioning following frontal lobe excisions. *Brain* 124:600–616, 2001.
25. Fine C, Lumsden J, Blair RJR: Dissociation between "theory of mind" and executive functions in a patient with early left amygdala damage. *Brain* 124:287, 2001.
26. Heilman KM, Schwartz HD, Watson RT: Hypoarousal in patients with the neglect syndrome and emotional indifference. *Neurology* 28:229–232, 1978.
27. Heilman KM, Bowers D, Speedie L, et al: Comprehension of affective and nonaffective prosody. *Neurology* 34:917–921, 1984.
28. Semrud-Clikeman M, Hynd GW: Right hemispheric dysfunction in nonverbal learning disabilities: Social, academic, and adaptive functioning in adults and children. *Psychol Bull* 107:196, 1990.
29. Weniger G, Irle E: Impaired facial affect recognition and emotional changes in subjects with transmodal cortical lesions. *Cereb Cortex* 12:258, 2002.
30. Levisohn L, Cronin-Golomb A, Schmahmann JD: Neuropsychological consequences of cerebellar tumor resection in children: Cerebellar cognitive affective syndrome in a paediatric population. *Brain* 123:1041, 2000.
31. David AS, Wacharasindhu A, Lishman WA: Severe psychiatric disturbance and abnormalities of the corpus callosum: Review and case series. *J Neurol Neurosurg Psychiatry* 56:85, 1993.
32. Berthier ML, Starkstein SE, Leiguarda IR: Developmental cortical anomalies in Asperger's syndrome: Neuroradiological findings in two patients. *J Neuropsychiatry Clin Neurosci* 2:197, 1990.
33. Sandson TA, Manoach DS, Price BH, et al: "Right hemisphere learning disability" associated with left hemisphere dysfunction: Anomalous dominance and development. *J Neurol Neurosurg Psychiatry* 57:1129, 1994.
34. Clark AS, Goldman-Rakic PS: Gonadal hormones influence the emergence of cortical function in nonhuman primates. *Behav Neurosci* 103:1287, 1991.
35. Goldman-Rakic PS, Rakic P: Experimental modification of gyral patterns, in Geschwind N, Galaburda AM (eds): *Cerebral Dominance: The Biological Foundations.* Cambridge, MA: Harvard University Press, 1985, p 179.
36. Goldman PS, Mendelson MJ: Salutary effects of early experience on deficits caused by lesions of frontal association cortex in developing rhesus monkeys. *Exp Neurol* 57:588, 1977.

37. Bachevalier J: Medial temporal lobe structures and autism: A review of clinical and experimental findings. *Neuropsychologia* 32:627, 1994.
38. Lê S, Cardebat K, Boulanouar K, et al: Seeing since childhood without ventral stream. *Brain* 125:44, 2002.
39. Reiss AL, Hagerman RJ, Vinogradov S, et al: Psychiatric disability in female carriers of the fragile X chromosome. *Arch Gen Psychiatry* 45:25–30, 1988.
40. McCauley E, Kay T, Ito J, Treder R: The Turner syndrome: Cognitive deficits, affective discrimination, and behavior problems. *Child Dev* 58:464, 1987.
41. Skuse DH, James RS, Bishop DV, et al: Evidence from Turner's syndrome of an imprinted X-linked locus affecting cognitive function. *Nature* 387:705, 1997.
42. Swillen A, Vandeputte L, Cracco J, et al: Neuropsychological, learning and psychosocial profile of primary school aged children with the velo-cardio-facial syndrome (22q11 deletion): Evidence for a nonverbal learning disability? *Neuropsychol Dev Cogn Sect C Child Neuropsychol* 5:230, 1999.
43. Tager-Flusberg H, Boshart J, Baron-Cohen S: Reading the windows to the soul: Evidence for domain-specific sparing in William's syndrome. *J Cogn Neurosci* 10:631, 1998.
44. Voeller KKS: Techniques for measuring social competence in children, in Lyon GR (ed): *Frames of Reference for the Assessment of Learning Disability: New Views on Measurement Issues.* Baltimore: Brooks, 1994, p 523.
45. American Psychiatric Association: *Diagnostic and Statistical Manual of Mental Disorders,* 4th ed (DSM-4). Washington, DC: American Psychiatric Association, 1994.
46. World Health Organization: *International Statistical Classification of Diseases and Related Health Problems.* Geneva: WHO, 1992.
47. Johnson DJ, Myklebust HR: *Learning Disabilities.* New York: Grune & Stratton, 1971.
48. Rourke BP, Finlayson MAJ: Neuropsychological significance of variations in patterns of academic performance: Verbal and visual-spatial abilities. *J Abnorm Child Psychol* 6:121, 1978.

Chapter 66

ATTENTION DEFICIT HYPERACTIVITY DISORDER*

Bruce F. Pennington
Nomita Chhabildas

A syndrome involving hyperactivity in children was first described over 150 years ago by Heinrich Hoffman,[1] a German physician, who wrote a humorous poem describing the antics of "fidgety Phil who couldn't sit still." Somewhat later, Still[2] described the main problem in this syndrome as a deficiency in "volitional inhibition" or "a defect in moral control." As we will see, problems with inhibition continue to be central to current conceptions of ADHD. However, much work remains to be done to determine whether inhibition deficits can truly account for symptom presentation in ADHD or whether other deficits are at the core of the disorder.

Whether there is brain dysfunction in ADHD and how to characterize it have been confusing and controversial issues in the history of ADHD research. The notion that childhood hyperactivity was a brain disorder was promoted by Strauss and Lehtinen,[3] based on similarities with the behavior of children who had suffered brain damage because of encephalitis. Unfortunately, this analogy led to some muddled terminology, whereby children with hyperactivity were described as having "minimal brain damage" or "minimal brain dysfunction." These terms are misleading for several reasons: (1) the large majority of children with ADHD have a developmental disorder, not acquired brain damage; (2) the damage or dysfunction to the brain implied in these labels was not documented directly but only inferred from behavioral symptoms that could have many different causes; (3) many children with acquired brain damage do not have hyperactivity[4]; and (4) these terms were vague and overinclusive and thus impeded progress in delineating distinct neuropsychological syndromes affecting learning and behavior in childhood. As detailed below, there is now much more direct evidence that ADHD is related to brain dysfunction that is substantially heritable, although we are still learning about the neurobiology of ADHD.

ADHD is now more clearly defined and better understood than it once was, yet it remains a somewhat broad and controversial diagnosis. Over half of children who meet diagnostic criteria for ADHD qualify for a comorbid diagnosis,[5] and the list of comorbid disorders includes conduct disorder, depression, anxiety, Tourette's disorder, dyslexia, and bipolar disorder. Moreover, children with autism, schizophrenia, and mental retardation frequently exhibit the symptoms of ADHD, although the DSM-IV stipulates that their more serious primary diagnosis excludes an ADHD diagnosis. So more research is needed to understand the basis of these comorbidities and to define purer subtypes of ADHD.

DEFINITION

DSM-IV[6] defines ADHD with two distinct but correlated dimensions of symptoms, those involving *inattention* (e.g., making careless mistakes and not paying close attention to details, forgetfulness, difficulty organizing tasks and activities, and failure to begin or complete tasks that require sustained mental effort) and those comprising *hyperactivity-impulsivity* (e.g., excessive fidgeting, locomotion, or talking; interrupting or intruding in conversations, games, and other situations). With two dimensions, there are thus three possible subtypes of ADHD: a predominantly inattentive subtype, a predominantly hyperactive-impulsive subtype, and a combined subtype. Someone who meets the

* **ACKNOWLEDGMENTS:** This work was supported by NICHD grants HD27802 and HD04024, an NIMH grant, MH38820, as well as by the second author's NRSA fellowship, MH12017.

diagnostic cutoff (six of nine symptoms) for a single dimension qualifies for that subtype; someone who meets this cutoff on both dimensions qualifies for the combined subtype. Additional requirements for the diagnosis include that the symptoms (1) must cause a clinically significant impairment in adaptive functioning, (2) are inconsistent with developmental level (e.g., not just secondary to mental retardation), (3) have been present for at least 6 months with an onset of some symptoms before age 7, (4) are present in two or more settings, and (5) are not better accounted for by another mental disorder (pervasive developmental disorder, psychosis, or a mood, anxiety, dissociative, or personality disorder). As pointed out below, there is more empirical support for the construct validity of the inattentive and combined subtypes than for the hyperactive-impulsive subtype.

EPIDEMIOLOGY

Attention deficit hyperactivity disorder (ADHD) is one of the most common chronic disorders of childhood, with a 6-month prevalence of 3 to 5 percent among school-aged children according to recent epidemiologic studies.[7] Of course, prevalence depends on definition and definitions vary in how pervasive they require the ADHD symptoms to be. In a careful epidemiologic study that required pervasiveness across three different reporters—parents, teachers, and a physician—the prevalence was only 1.2 percent.[8] Sex ratios in referred samples have been reported to be as high as 9:1 (males:females), but an epidemiologic study found a sex ratio of 3:1.[9] Thus, as in other disorders such as reading disability (RD), males are more likely to be referred than females. Because much of the research on ADHD has relied on referred samples, we currently know much more about ADHD in males than in females.

ADHD has been found across social classes and cultures. There are higher rates of ADHD in lower social classes, but these differences are no longer found once comorbid conditions, such as conduct disorder, are controlled for (see review, Ref. 10). Roughly comparable rates of ADHD have been found in studies in the United States, Japan, and India, with a somewhat higher rate in Germany.[10] At times, there can be dramatic differences in prevalence even between very similar cultures (i.e., the United States and the United Kingdom) simply due to differences in diagnostic criteria and practice.[7]

In terms of natural history, the age of onset is usually in toddlerhood, with a peak age of onset between ages 3 and 4.[11] Symptoms of ADHD may appear earlier, even in utero. It is becoming clearer that ADHD is a chronic disorder across the life span[12] and that many of the tasks of adult development are disrupted by ADHD because sustained effort, planning, and organization are central to many adult responsibilities.

ETIOLOGY

The exact etiology of ADHD is still unknown. However, recent progress in understanding the genetics of developmental disorders (see Chap. 69), as well as developmental cognitive neuroscience more generally, has taught us a fair amount about genes and brain pathways that may be involved in the disorder. Thus, ADHD represents a success story for a neuroscience approach to understanding psychopathology. This section comprises a review of evidence that ADHD is familial, moderately heritable, and may be influenced by two genes that affect dopamine neurotransmission. Environmental influences on ADHD are also discussed.

Familiality

The rate of ADHD in families of ADHD male probands has been found to be over seven times the rate of the disorder in nonpsychiatric control families[13]; a later study reported a similar increase in risk among relatives of female probands.[14,15]

Heritability

Stevenson[16] found a heritability of 0.76 for ADHD in his twin study, and numerous other twin studies have found similar results, both for the diagnosis of ADHD as well as for individual differences in ADHD symptomatology.[17–24] Although extreme scores on both the defining dimensions of ADHD, inattention (IA) and hyperactivity-impulsivity (HI), are moderately heritable, this appears to *not* be the case for the

HI dimension once the correlation between the two dimensions is accounted for.[23] That is, extreme scores on the IA dimension are moderately heritable regardless of the level of HI symptoms in the proband (i.e., both the inattentive and combined subtypes of ADHD are moderately heritable). However, extreme scores on the HI dimension were *not* significantly heritable ($h^2g = 0.08$) when probands were not also extreme on IA. These results suggest the etiology of the HI subtype is largely nongenetic and differs from the etiology of the other two subtypes.

Mode of Transmission There has been one segregation analysis of ADHD,[15] which found autosomal dominant transmission with considerably reduced penetrance of the hypothesized major gene. Although this suggests that there may be loci of sizable effect, the genetic etiology of ADHD is very unlikely to be due to just one gene.

Gene Locations Efforts to identify specific genes influencing ADHD illustrate the potential power of the candidate gene association approach. This approach usually depends on a hypothesis derived from an understanding of the neurobiology of the disorder. We know that the primary drug used to treat ADHD, methylphenidate (Ritalin), is a dopamine agonist, and that it achieves this effect by blocking the dopamine transporter, a receptor on the presynaptic neuron involved in the reuptake of dopamine in the synapse. Hence, blocking reuptake increases the dopamine available in the synapse. Since receptors are coded for by genes, a gene for a dopamine transporter or genes for other dopamine receptors are reasonable candidate genes in ADHD.

Molecular genetic research on ADHD has focused on dopamine genes, particularly a dopamine transporter gene (DAT1) and DRD4, one of the dopamine receptors. Since both of these dopamine genes are polymorphic (they have frequently occurring allelic variations), they could be tested as candidates in association studies.

The 10-copy allele of DAT1 was significantly associated with ADHD in a study of 53 families.[25] This finding has now been replicated in two separate samples,[26,27] although it is not significant in all samples.[28–30]

An allele of the DRD4 gene that contains a seven-repeat base-pair sequence was shown to be significantly associated with novelty-seeking behavior, which prompted the hypothesis that it might also be linked to impulsive behavior seen in ADHD.[31,32] Indeed, numerous studies have now found an association between the DRD4 allele and ADHD,[33–37] although again this result is not significant in all studies.[28,38]

A recent metanalysis of all available studies of the association between ADHD and DRD4[39] concluded that the association between the two is indeed real, although small in magnitude.

Although these are exciting findings, there are complications that still need to be resolved. Counterintuitively, the risk allele of the DAT1 gene is *more* frequent than the nonrisk allele in the general population, a result that may well hold for many alleles associated with psychopathology. Second, the effect size of each of these risk alleles is small. Finally, as discussed further on, one study[40] found that presence of the DRD4 risk allele was *not* associated with the neuropsychological deficits that characterize ADHD.

In sum, there will likely be other risk alleles that influence ADHD, and this influence may vary by ADHD subtype, whether these be DSM-IV subtypes or those defined by comorbidities.

Other evidence for genetic influence on ADHD or its symptoms comes from their association with known genetic syndromes, including Turner's syndrome (45, X) in females; 47, XYY in males; fragile X syndrome; neurofibromatosis; and early treated PKU (reviewed in Ref. 41).

Environmental Influences

There are several known bioenvironmental correlates of ADHD, including fetal alcohol exposure, environmental lead, and pediatric head injury (reviewed in Ref. 41). Since that review, it has become clear that maternal smoking in pregnancy is associated with an increased risk of ADHD in offspring (see review in Ref. 10). However, exposure to these bioenvironmental risk factors is not randomly assigned and, for some of them, we have evidence that exposure is correlated with ADHD in the parent or child, which may be genetically mediated. At the same time, it seems implausible that the dramatic ADHD symptoms observed clinically in fetal alcohol syndrome or pediatric head injury can be entirely explained by such a confound. Instead, it might be better to conceptualize at least some of these bioenvironmental risk factors as examples of gene-environment correlations: the presence of the ADHD genotype increases exposure to environmental risk factors that exacerbate the ADHD phenotype.

We do not have evidence that the social environment, in particular parenting practices, can directly cause ADHD. At the same time, there is no doubt that the social environment influences the course of ADHD, in particular whether ADHD develops into another disruptive behavior disorder.

BRAIN MECHANISMS

The hypothesis of frontal lobe dysfunction in ADHD has been advanced by several researchers[42–47] based on the observation that frontal lesions in both experimental animals and human patients sometimes produce hyperactivity, distractibility, and/or impulsivity, alone or in combination.[48–50] Of course, lesions in other parts of the brain can also produce these symptoms. The evidence that supports frontal-striatal dysfunction in ADHD is reviewed below.

Structural Studies

With regard to brain structure, earlier work[51,52] found no evidence of structural differences in computed tomography (CT) studies of ADHD children and colleagues. Hynd and colleagues,[53] however, using magnetic resonance imaging (MRI), did find absence of the usual R>L frontal asymmetry in ADHD children. They contrasted ADHD subjects with both dyslexics and controls; the frontal finding was present in both clinical groups but did not differentiate between them, even though the dyslexic group was selected to be non-ADHD. There is an association between the right frontal lobe and measures of sustained attention, so this neuroanatomic difference has theoretical relevance to ADHD. This lack of frontal asymmetry in ADHD has been replicated in two other studies.[54,55] Abnormalities of caudate volume have also been found across numerous studies of ADHD.[54–57] In addition, the globus pallidus has been found to be significantly smaller in those with ADHD.[54,58,59] These structural studies support developmental differences in frontal-striatal structures known to be important in action selection.

The hypothesis that these structural differences were related to deficits in action selection was tested in a study by Casey et al.[60] They correlated performance on three separate inhibition tasks with measures of prefrontal cortex and basal ganglia volume. The three inhibition tasks, which were designed to tap response inhibition at different stages of attentional processing, were all impaired in the children with ADHD when compared to controls. Furthermore, prefrontal cortex, caudate, and globus pallidus volumes correlated significantly with task performance. Of course, this correlation does not prove cause. Such a finding could be a *result* of ADHD or just a correlate of ADHD.

However, brain structure differences in ADHD are not exclusively in the prefrontal cortex and basal ganglia. Decreased areas in different regions of the corpus callosum have been observed in several studies,[53,54,61–63] as well as smaller total cerebral volume and a smaller cerebellum.[54]

Functional Studies

In terms of brain function, electrophysiologic measures have supported the hypothesis of CNS underarousal in at least a subgroup of hyperactive children.[64] Likewise, Lou and coworkers,[65] using regional cerebral blood flow, found decreased blood flow to the frontal lobes in ADHD children, which increased after the children received methylphenidate. This treatment also decreased blood flow to the motor cortex and primary sensory cortex, "suggesting an inhibition of function of these structures, seen clinically as less distractibility and decreased motor activity during treatment" (Ref. 65, p. 829). These investigators replicated this result in an expanded sample[66]; in this second report they emphasize the basal ganglia as the locus of reduced blood flow in ADHD. Zametkin et al.[67] used positron emission tomography (PET) to study the parents of ADHD children, who themselves had residual-type ADHD. They found an overall reduction in cerebral glucose utilization, particularly in right frontal areas, but increased utilization in posterior medio-orbital areas. A second study by this group[68] investigating teenagers with

ADHD replicated some but not all of those findings. This second study found significant reductions in the ADHD group in normalized glucose metabolism in 6 of 60 brain regions, including the left anterior frontal lobe. Metabolism in that region correlated inversely with ADHD symptom severity across the combined sample of patients and controls. Since hyperfrontality of blood flow is characteristic of the normal brain, hypofrontality in ADHD could explain the low central arousal found in the electrophysiologic studies.

Other studies have demonstrated decreased blood flow in ADHD subjects both in prefrontal regions and the striatum.[69] More recently, functional magnetic resonance imaging (fMRI) has demonstrated similar results, showing hypoperfusion in the right caudate nucleus, which was ameliorated after treatment with methylphenidate.[70]

Neurochemical Studies

In terms of brain biochemistry, Shaywitz and colleagues[71] found lower levels of homovanillic acid (HVA—the main dopamine metabolite) in the cerebrospinal fluid of ADHD children compared to controls. This could also lend support to a frontal theory of ADHD, as dopamine has a preponderant distribution in the frontal regions of the cortex. Moreover, a well-validated animal model of ADHD involves dopamine depletion.[52]

In summary, one plausible theory of brain mechanisms in ADHD is as follows. The symptoms of ADHD are caused by functional hypofrontality, which in turn is caused by either structural and/or biochemical changes in the prefrontal lobes and striatum and is detectable as reduced frontal blood flow. Biochemically, the cause would be low dopamine levels, which methylphenidate treatment reverses at least in part.

Unfortunately, the story is not that simple. One study found that some dopamine agonists were not effective in treating hyperactive children,[72] whereas certain dopamine *antagonists* did have unexpected beneficial effects in children with ADHD.[47] Both of these results are opposite to what would be predicted by the dopamine depletion hypothesis. So the neurochemical mechanisms may be more complex, although the ubiquitous problem of heterogeneity in ADHD samples is another explanation.

Zametkin and Rapoport[47] argue that no single neurotransmitter is exclusively involved in the pathogenesis of ADHD, both because stimulant medications always affect more than one neurotransmitter and because of the multiple interrelations among specific catecholamines and their precursors and metabolites. They and Oades[73] both argue that the combined action of dopaminergic and noradrenergic systems should be considered in the biology of ADHD.

Obviously, much more research is needed, preferably using familial samples that are as phenotypically homogeneous as possible. The associations between ADHD and the DAT1 and DRD4 alleles will begin to allow neurobiologic research to focus on genetic subtypes of ADHD.

NEUROPSYCHOLOGY

There is a fairly extensive literature on cognitive processes in ADHD, which has become more explicitly neuropsychological in the hypotheses tested. Virginia Douglas has been a pioneer in this area, establishing that there is a distinctive cognitive phenotype in ADHD that needs to be explained. She and others have found that children with ADHD are impaired on tasks requiring vigilance, systematic search, and motor control and inhibition but are unimpaired on tasks tapping basic verbal and nonverbal memory functions.[74]

Neuropsychological studies of ADHD have mainly focused on the frontal lobe or executive function (EF) hypothesis, for reasons discussed earlier. A number of researchers have proposed an EF deficit theory of ADHD.[41,75–79]

We recently reviewed published studies of EFs in ADHD.[80] We found that 15 of 18 studies found a significant difference between ADHD subjects and controls on one or more EF measures. A total of 60 EF measures were used across studies; for 40 of these (67 percent), there was significantly worse performance in the ADHD group. In contrast, *none* of the 60 measures was significantly better in the ADHD group. The most consistently impaired domain of EF was inhibition; in contrast, children with ADHD were less likely to be impaired at set-shifting or working memory. In addition, children with ADHD in these studies were generally unimpaired on measures of verbal memory, other verbal processes, or visuospatial processing. They were fairly consistently impaired on measures of vigilance (GDS) and perceptual speed (Coding and Digit Symbol), but these measures would be expected to be influenced by an inhibitory deficit.

Although there are many different meanings of the term *inhibition* in psychology, inhibition in this case is "intentional motor inhibition,"[81] which requires consciously restraining a dominant or prepotent motor response. The inhibitory process is thought to be primarily mediated by higher cognitive processes and thus is thought to require prefrontally mediated executive function.

The most widely researched measure of this type of inhibition in the domain of ADHD is the stop signal paradigm.[82] In this paradigm, a subject is taught a particular response and then later told to inhibit the very same response on the subset of trials signaled by a beep. The paradigm allows for the computation of the stop signal reaction time (SSRT), or the time it takes to inhibit a response. In a recent meta-analysis of studies using the stop task,[83] consistent deficits were demonstrated in groups with ADHD, providing evidence that children with ADHD are impaired in their ability for response inhibition. Nigg[84] also recently demonstrated inhibitory deficits in children with ADHD combined type using the stop signal paradigm. Deficits on the task were specific to ADHD and not associated with comorbid reading or behavior problems. Furthermore, a study by Aman and coworkers[85] demonstrated that deficits of children with ADHD on the stop task were normalized when the children had taken methylphenidate.

These findings that children with ADHD consistently have slower SSRTs than control children, that this deficit is specific to ADHD, and that it is reversed by stimulant medication are all consistent with the hypothesis that ADHD is caused by a slow inhibitory process. However, this interpretation is clouded by the fact that children with ADHD often have slower "go" reaction times as well. Some researchers (e.g., Ref. 86 and Swanson, personal communication) suggest that rather than a specific inhibitory deficit, ADHD is characterized by slower and more variable reaction times, which would produce the pattern of performance observed in groups with ADHD on the stop task and on a variety of other tasks.

More generally, although the executive or inhibitory deficit theory of ADHD has considerable support, there are nonetheless several important threats to its validity. Perhaps the most important threat is the amount of variance in ADHD symptoms that EF measures can account for. The most sensitive measures of EF with regard to ADHD, as discussed previously, tend to be those that tap inhibition, such as the stop task and continuous performance tasks.[87–89] However, when comparing performance of those with ADHD and controls, even these measures produce effect sizes that are relatively small, ranging from about .5 to 1.5.[80,84,90] This effect is much smaller than the effect size of the typical difference in symptoms of ADHD between the two groups, which is usually in the range of 2.5 to 3.5. In addition, correlations between behavior ratings of attention and impulsivity do not correlate highly with EF measures, typically being in the range of 0.15 to 0.30.[91] These limited correlations mean that an EF deficit, as currently measured, cannot totally account for the symptoms that define the disorder.

There are several competing explanations to account for these relatively small effect sizes. One possibility is that children with ADHD are a substantially heterogeneous group, and some but not all have primary deficits in inhibition. In addition, differences within or among samples in ADHD subtype, age, gender, and prevalence of comorbid disorders could also affect the findings.

A second possibility is that EF deficits are not the primary deficit in ADHD but instead are just a correlate of the actual, underlying deficit. There are a number of competing motivational and arousal theories of ADHD, and they all argue that the primary deficit in ADHD is not a cognitive one. For instance, Sonuga-Barke et al.[92] argue that the underlying difference in ADHD is not a deficit of inhibition but rather a preference to shorten delay. Other competing theories of ADHD argue that state regulation, regulation of arousal, or motivation may truly be the critical deficit in children with ADHD.[93–96] These authors view the inhibition deficit as being secondary to a more primary difficulty in another area. Therefore, in the appropriate circumstances, children with ADHD should be able to inhibit responses. A recent study by Kuntsi and associates[97] compared performance of children with ADHD and control children on tasks of inhibition, working memory, and delay aversion. Children with ADHD performed more poorly than control children on some of the working memory measures and on the delay aversion task. In contrast, this study found no group differences on the inhibition measures from the stop signal paradigm. However, on the stop signal task, children with ADHD had slower "go" reaction times. The authors suggest these results could be consistent with a state-regulation theory of ADHD,[86] as this response style could reflect a lack of consistent effort.

Yet a third possibility is that there are two (or more) primary deficits in ADHD, which may interact. In this case, each deficit by itself would account for a relatively small proportion of the variance in ADHD symptoms.

Another threat to the validity of an EF theory of ADHD comes from a recent study relating molecular measures to executive measures in ADHD.[40] Since the seven-repeat allele of the DRD4 receptor is significantly associated with ADHD, the next link in an EF theory of ADHD would be to test whether this gene is linked to the hypothesized underlying psychological deficit in ADHD, the EF deficit. Such a finding would provide a comprehensive explanation of symptom presentation in ADHD using an EF framework: Variations in dopamine genes lead to reduced dopaminergic function in the prefrontal cortex and basal ganglia, thereby impairing executive functions, particularly inhibition, and thus producing the behavioral symptoms of ADHD. So, from an EF framework, the presence of the seven-repeat allele should be significantly associated not only with ADHD but also with deficits in EF.

To test this theory, Swanson and colleagues compared subgroups of ADHD children with and without the seven-repeat allele on a series of EF tasks. Directly *opposite* to prediction, only children in the seven-absent group were impaired on EF tasks, whereas those with the DRD4 risk allele performed very similarly to controls on all EF measures in the study. This finding is inconsistent with an EF theory of ADHD or is at least inconsistent with the hypothesis that the DRD4 receptor mediates the EF deficits.

However, this study had a relatively small sample size (with 13 children in the seven-present group and 19 children in the seven-absent group) and needs to be replicated. In addition, the presence of the DRD4 seven-repeat allele is not necessary for a diagnosis of ADHD and is clearly not the only genetic locus contributing to the phenotype of ADHD. It is possible that EF deficits in ADHD are instead related to another genetic locus, such as the DAT1 allele or to an interaction among several alleles. It is also possible that the DRD4 receptor is significantly related only to a particular subtype of ADHD, the inattentive subtype. A recent study[35] found that the seven-repeat allele of DRD4 was associated more strongly with the predominantly inattentive subtype rather than the combined subtype of ADHD. In the study of Swanson et al., however, only children with the combined subtype of ADHD were studied.

Another study used a behavioral genetic approach to examine the relationship between ADHD and EF deficits and obtained some support for a state-regulation conceptualization of ADHD.[98] This study tested whether hyperactivity shared common genetic factors with underlying psychological processes found to be related to ADHD in previous work.[98] Since ADHD is highly heritable, a primary psychological deficit accounting for symptom presentation would be expected to be coheritable with the ADHD diagnosis. The study only found significant evidence of shared genetic factors between hyperactivity and variability of response time, whereas there was not evidence of shared genetic influence on measures of working memory, inhibition, or delay aversion. These results do not support an EF theory but could support a state-regulation account of ADHD.

In sum, despite converging evidence in support of an EF theory of ADHD, there are several important threats to the validity of this theory, including the low effect sizes obtained in studies using inhibition paradigms, competing explanations for the underlying deficit (such as motivational, delay aversion, and state-regulation perspectives), and the inconsistent genetic findings just discussed.[40,98]

TREATMENT

The treatment of ADHD has recently been reviewed.[7] Here, the main points of that review are summarized. The use of psychostimulant drugs such as methylphenidate (Ritalin), dextroamphetamine (Dexedrine), and pemoline (Cylert) to treat ADHD is the most thoroughly researched application of psychopharmacology in child psychiatry. The efficacy and safety of these drugs in treating ADHD has now been well established. About 75 to 90 percent of children with ADHD show a favorable treatment response with psychostimulant medication. The side effects of psychostimulants are generally mild, especially compared to other psychopharmacologic treatments, and usually abate with time and changes in dose. These side effects include decreased sleep and appetite, jitteriness, stomachaches, and headaches.

There are ongoing public controversies about the diagnosis and treatment of ADHD, not all of which are supported by research. Earlier concerns about growth retardation, precipitation of a tic disorder, psychostimulants becoming drugs of abuse, overdiagnosis of ADHD, or overprescription of psychostimulant drugs have not been supported by research, but some of these concerns could become real problems in the future. There is nonetheless valid concern about the misdiagnosis of ADHD. Not all practitioners prescribing stimulant medication for ADHD have the time or the training to make this demanding differential diagnosis accurately.

Psychosocial treatments for ADHD mainly consist of behavioral intervention techniques for parents and teachers to help them better manage these children, who can be very disruptive in a classroom or family. Such treatments are particularly important for children who do not respond to medication or whose parents prefer not to use medication. In general, the efficacy of psychosocial treatments for improving ADHD symptoms is (1) less than that of psychostimulants[99] and (2) greater for teachers than parents.

The question naturally arises as to whether the combination of psychostimulant and behavioral interventions would be more efficacious than either alone. A recent large study funded by the National Institute of Mental Health addressed this question. This 3-year multimodal treatment of ADHD study[100] compared four treatment conditions: medication alone, behavioral intervention alone, a combination of the two, and no treatment beyond what is already typically provided in the community. The behavioral intervention was intensive, involving parent training, school intervention, and summer treatment in a camp setting. The medication management was more intensive than what would typically be provided in a community setting. Subjects were randomly assigned to one of the four conditions, treated for 14 months, and followed for 22 months after that. There was a large main effect of medication treatment on ADHD symptoms, for which the addition of the behavioral intervention produced no added benefit. However, the behavioral intervention did improve outcome in some nonsymptom areas.

There are also several nonconventional therapies for ADHD, including the Feingold diet and EEG biofeedback, which have not been supported by careful treatment studies.

REFERENCES

1. Hoffman H: *Der Struwelpeter: Oder lustige Geschichten und drollige Bilder*. Leipzig: Insel-Verlag, 1845.
2. Still GF: Some abnormal psychical conditions in children. *Lancet* 1:1008–1012, 1163–1168, 1077–1082, 1902.
3. Strauss A, Lehtinen L: *Psychopathology and Education of the Brain-Injured Child*. New York: Grune & Stratton, 1947.
4. Rutter M, Quinton, D: Psychiatric disorders: Ecological factors and concepts of causation, in McGurk H (ed): *Ecological Factors in Human Development*. Amsterdam: North-Holland, 1977, pp 173–187.
5. Biederman J, Faraone, SV, Keenan K, et al: Further evidence for family-genetic risk factors in attention deficit hyperactivity disorder. Patterns of comorbidity in probands and relatives in psychiatrically and pediatrically referred samples. *Arch Gen Psychiatry* 49:728–738, 1992.
6. *Diagnostic and Statistical Manual of Mental Disorders*, 4th ed (DSM-IV). Washington, DC: American Psychiatric Association, 1994.
7. Satcher D: *Mental Health: A Report of the Surgeon General*. http://www.mentalhealth.org/specials/surgeongeneralreport, 1999.
8. Spreen O, Tupper D, Risser A, et al: *Human Developmental Neuropsychology*. New York: Oxford University Press, 1984.
9. Szatmari P, Offord DR, Boyle M: Correlates, associated impairments, and patterns of service utilization of children with attention deficit disorders: Findings from the Ontario Child Health Study. *J Child Psychol Psychiatry* 30:205–217, 1989.
10. Barkley RA: Attention-deficit/hyperactivity disorder, in Mash EJ, Barkley RA (eds): *Child Psychopathology*. New York: Guilford Press, 1996; pp 63–112.
11. Palfrey JS, Levine MD, Walker DK, et al: The emergence of attention deficits in early childhood: A

prospective study. *J Dev Behav Pediatr* 6:339–348, 1985.

12. Gittleman R, Mannuzza S, Shenker R, et al: Hyperactive boys almost grown up. *Arch Gen Psychiatry* 42:937–947, 1985.
13. Biederman J, Faraone SV, Keenan K, et al: Family-genetic and psychosocial risk factors in DSM III attention deficit disorder. *J Am Acad Child Adolesc Psychiatry* 29:526–533, 1990.
14. Faraone S, Biederman J, Keenan K, et al: A family genetic study of girls with DSM-III attention deficit disorder. *Am J Psychiatry* 148:112–117, 1991.
15. Faraone S, Biederman J, Chen WJ, et al: Segregation analysis of attention deficit hyperactivity disorder: Evidence for single major gene transmission. *Psychiatr Genet* 2:257–275, 1992.
16. Stevenson J: Evidence for a genetic etiology in hyperactivity in children. *Behav Genet* 2:337–344, 1992.
17. Eaves L, Silberg J, Meyer J, et al: Genetics and developmental psychopathology: 2. The main effects of genes and environment on behavioral problems in the Virginia Twin Study of Adolescent Behavioral Development. *J Child Psychol Psychiatry* 38:965–980, 1997.
18. Gillis JJ, Gilger JW, Pennington BF, et al: Attention deficit disorder in reading-disabled twins: Evidence for a genetic etiology. *J Abnorm Child Psychol* 20(3):303–331, 1992.
19. Gjane H, Stevenson J, Sundet J: Genetic influence on parent-reported attention-related problems in a Norwegian general population twin sample. *J Am Acad Child Adolesc Psychiatry* 35:588–596, 1996.
20. Levy F, Hay D, McStephen M, et al: Attention-deficit hyperactivity disorder: A category or a continuum? A genetic analysis of a large-scale twin study. *J Am Acad Child Adolesc Psychiatry* 36:737–744, 1997.
21. Sherman D, lacono W, McGue M: Attention-deficit/hyperactivity disorder dimensions: A twin study of inattention and impulsivity/hyperactivity. *J Am Acad Child Adolesc Psychiatry* 36:745–753, 1997.
22. Thapar A, McGuffin P: Are anxiety symptoms in childhood heritable? *J Child Psychol Psychiatry*, 36:439–447, 1995.
23. Willcutt EG, Pennington BF, DeFries JC: A twin study of the etiology of comorbidity between reading disability and attention-deficit/hyperactivity disorder. *Am J Med Genet* (*Neuropsychiatr Gene*) 96:293–301, 2000.
24. Willerman L: Activity level and hyperactivity in twins. *Child Dev* 44:288–293, 1973.
25. Cook EH, Stein MA, Krasowski MD, et al: Association of attention deficit disorder and the dopamine transporter gene. *Am J Hum Genet* 56:993–998, 1995.
26. Gill M, Daly G, Heron S, et al: Confirmation of association between attention deficit hyperactivity disorder and a dopamine transporter polymorphism. *Mol Psychiatry* 2:311–313, 1997.
27. Waldman ID, Rowe DC, Abramowitz A, et al: Association of the dopamine transporter gene (DAT1) and attention deficit hyperactivity disorder in children (abstr). *Am J Hum Genet* 59:A25, 1996.
28. Asherson P, Virdee V, Curran S, et al: Association of DSM-IV attention deficit hyperactivity disorder and monoamine pathway genes. *Am J Med Genet* 81:549, 1998.
29. LaHoste G, Wigal S, Glabe C, et al: Dopamine related genes and attention deficit hyperactivity disorder. Paper presented at the annual meeting of the Society for the Neurosciences, San Diego, CA, November 1995.
30. Poulton K, Holmes J, Hever T, et al: A molecular genetic study of hyperkinetic disorder/attention deficit hyperactivity disorder. *Am J Med Gen* 81:458, 1998.
31. Benjamin J, Li L, Patterson C, et al: Population and family association between the D4 dopamine receptor gene and measures of novelty seeking. *Nat Genet* 12:81–84, 1996.
32. Ebstein R, Novick O, Umansky R, et al: Dopamine D4 receptor (DRD4) exon III polymorphism associated with the human personality trait of novelty seeking. *Nat Gene* 12:78–80, 1996.
33. Faraone SV, Biederman J, Weiffenbach B, et al: Dopamine D4 gene 7-repeat allele and attention-deficit hyperactivity disorder. *Am J Psychiatry* 156:768–770, 1999.
34. LaHoste GJ, Swanson JM, Wigel SB, et al: Dopamine D4 receptor gene polymorphism is associated with attention deficit hyperactivity disorder. *Mol Psychiatry* 1(2):121–124, 1996.
35. Rowe DC, Stever G, Giedinghagen LN, et al: Dopamine DRD4 receptor polymorphism and attention deficit hyperactivity disorder. *Mol Psychiatry* 3:419–426, 1998.
36. Smalley SL, Bailey JN, Palmer GG, et al: Evidence that the dopamine D4 receptor is a susceptibility gene in attention deficit hyperactivity disorder. *Mol Psychiatry* 3:427–430, 1998.
37. Swanson J, Sunhora GA, Kennedy JL, et al: Association of the dopamine receptor D4 (DRD4) gene with a refined phenotype of attention deficit hyperactivity disorder (ADHD): A family based approach. *Mol Psychiatry* 3:38–41, 1998.
38. Castellanos FX, Lau E, Tayebi N, et al: Lack of an association between a dopamine-4 receptor polymorphism and attention-deficit/hyperactivity disorder:

Genetic and brain morphometric analyses. *Mol Psychiatry* 3:431–434, 1998.

39. Faraone SV, Doyle AE, Mick E, et al: Meta-analysis of the association between the 7-repeat allele of the dopamine D4 receptor gene and attention deficit hyperactivity disorder. *Am J Psychiatry* 158:1052–1057, 2001.
40. Swanson J, Oosterlaan J, Murias M, et al: Attention deficit/hyperactivity disorder children with a 7-repeat allele of the dopamine receptor D4 gene have extreme behavior but normal performance on critical neuropsychological tests of attention. *Proc Natl Acad Sci U S A* 97:4754–4759, 2000.
41. Pennington BF: *Diagnosing Learning Disorders: A Neuropsychological Framework*. New York: Guilford Press, 1991.
42. Gualtieri CT, Hicks RE: Neuropharmacology of methylphenidate and a neural substrate for childhood hyperactivity. *Psychiatr Clin North Am* 6:875–892, 1985.
43. Mattes JA: The role of frontal lobe dysfunction in childhood hyperkinesis. *Comp Psychiatry* 21:358–369, 1989.
44. Pontius AA: Dysfunctional patterns analogous to frontal lobe system and caudate nucleus syndromes in some groups of minimal brain dysfunction. *J Am Med Women Assoc* 28:285–292, 1973.
45. Rosenthal RH, Allen TW: An examination of attention, arousal and learning dysfunctions of hyperkinetic children. *Psychol Bull* 85:689–715, 1978.
46. Stamm JS, Kreder SV: Minimal brain dysfunction: Psychological and neuropsychological disorders in hyperkinetic children, in Gazzaniga MS (ed), *Handbook of Behavioral Neurology: Neuropsychology*. New York: Plenum Press, 1979, vol 2, pp 119–150.
47. Zametkin AJ, Rapoport JL: The pathophysiology of attention deficit disorders, in Lahey BB, Kadzin AE (eds): *Advances in Clinical Child Psychology*. New York: Plenum Press, 1986. pp 177–216.
48. Fuster JM: *The Prefrontal Cortex: Anatomy, Physiology and Neuropsychology of the Frontal Lobe*, 2d ed. New York: Raven Press, 1989.
49. Levin HS, Eisenberg HM, Benton AL: *Frontal Lobe Function and Dysfunction*. New York: Oxford University Press, 1991.
50. Stuss DT, Benson DF: *The Frontal Lobes*. New York: Raven Press, 1986.
51. Harcherick DF, Cohen DJ, Ort S, et al: Computed tomographic brain scanning in four neuropsychiatric disorders of childhood. *Am J Psychiatry* 142:731–737, 1985.
52. Shaywitz SE, Shaywitz BA, Cohen DJ, et al: Monoaminergic mechanisms in hyperactivity, in Rutter M (ed): *Developmental Neuropsychiatry*. New York: Guilford Press, 1983.
53. Hynd GW, Semrud-Clikeman M, Lorys AR, et al: Brain morphology in developmental dyslexia and attention deficit disorder/hyperactivity. *Arch Neurol* 47:919–926, 1990.
54. Castellanos FX, Giedd JN, Marsh WL, et al: Quantitative brain magnetic resonance imaging in attention-deficit/hyperactivity disorder. *Arch Gen Psychiatry* 53:607–616, 1996.
55. Filipek PA, Semrud-Clikeman M, Steingard RJ, et al: Volumetric MRI analysis comparing attention deficit hyperactivity disorder with normal controls. *Neurology* 48:589–601, 1997.
56. Hynd GW, Hern KL, Novey ES, et al: Attention deficit hyperactivity disorder and asymmetry of the caudate nucleus. *J Child Neurol* 8:339–347, 1993.
57. Mataro M, Garcia-Sanchez C, Junque C, et al: Magnetic resonance imaging measurement of the caudate nucleus in adolescents with attention-deficit hyperactivity disorder and its relationship with neuropsychological and behavioral measures. *Arch Neurol* 54:963–968, 1997.
58. Aylward EH, Reiss AL, Reader MJ, et al: Basal ganglia volumes in children with attention-deficit hyperactivity disorder. *J Child Neurol* 11:112–115, 1996.
59. Singer HS, Reiss AL, Brown JE, et al: Volumetric MRI changes in basal ganglia of children with Tourette's syndrome. *Neurology* 43:950–956, 1993.
60. Casey BJ, Castellanos FX, Giedd JN, et al: Implication of right frontostriatal circuitry in response inhibition and attention deficit hyperactivity disorder. *J Am Acad Child Adolesc Psychiatry* 36:374–383, 1997.
61. Baumgardner TL, Singer HS, Denckla MB, et al: Corpus callosum morphology in children with Tourette syndrome and attention deficit hyperactivity disorder. *Neurology* 4:477–482, 1996.
62. Giedd JN, Castellanos FX, Casey BJ, et al: Quantitative morphology of the corpus callosum in attention deficit hyperactivity disorder. *Am J Psychiatry* 151:665–669, 1994.
63. Semrud-Clikeman M, Filipek PA, Biederman J, et al: Attention-deficit hyperactivity disorder: Magnetic resonance imaging morphometric analysis of the corpus callosum. *J Am Acad Child Adolesc Psychiatry* 33:875–881, 1994.
64. Ferguson HB, Rappaport JL: Nosological issues and biological validation, in Rutter M (ed): *Developmental*

Neuropsychiatry. New York: Guilford Press, 1993, pp 369–384.

65. Lou HC, Henriksen L, Bruhn P: Focal cerebral hypoperfusion in children with dysphasia and/or attention deficit disorder. *Arch Neurol* 41:825–829, 1984.
66. Lou HC, Henriksen L, Bruhn P: Striatal dysfunction in attention deficit and hyperkinetic disorder. *Arch Neurol* 46:48–52, 1989.
67. Zametkin AJ, Nordahl TE, Gross M, et al: Cerebral glucose metabolism in adults with hyperactivity of childhood onset. *N Engl J Med* 323:1361–1366, 1990.
68. Zametkin AJ, Liebenauer LL, Fitzgerald GA, et al: Brain metabolism in teenagers with attention-deficit hyperactivity disorder. *Arch Gen Psychiatry* 50:333–340 1993.
69. Amen DG, Paldi JH, Thisted RA: Brain SPECT imaging. *J Am Acad Child Adolesc Psychiatry* 32:1080–1081, 1993.
70. Teicher MH, Polcari A, English CD, et al: Dose-dependent effects of methylphenidate on activity, attention, and magnetic resonance imaging measures in children with ADHD (abstr). *Society Neurosci Abstr* 22:1191, 1996.
71. Shaywitz BA, Cohen DJ, Bowers MB: CSF monoamine metabolites in children with minimal brain dysfunction: Evidence for alteration of brain dopamine. *J Pediatr* 90:67–71, 1977.
72. Mattes JA, Gittelman R: A pilot trial of amantadine in hyperactive children. Paper presented at the NCDEU meeting, Key Biscayne, FL, 1979.
73. Oades RD: Attention deficit disorder with hyperactivity: The contribution of catecholaminergic activity. *Prog Neurobiol* 29:365–391, 1987.
74. Douglas VI: Cognitive deficits in children with attention deficit disorder with hyperactivity, in Bloomingdale LM, Sergeant J (eds): *Attention Deficit Disorder: Criteria, Cognition, Intervention.* Elmsford, NY: Pergamon Press, 1988.
75. Barkley RA: *Attention-Deficit Hyperactivity Disorder: A Handbook for Diagnosis and Treatment*. New York: Guilford Press, 1990.
76. Barkley RA: Behavioral inhibition, sustained attention, and executive functions: Constructing a unifying theory of ADHD. *Psychol Bull* 121:65–94, 1997.
77. Conners CK, Wells KC: *Hyperkinetic Children: A Neuropsychological Approach*. Beverly Hills, CA: Sage, 1986.
78. Douglas VI: Attention and cognitive problems, in Rutter M (ed): *Developmental Neuropsychiatry*. New York: Guilford Press, 1983, pp 280–329.
79. Schachar RJ, Tannock R, Logan G: Inhibitory control, impulsiveness, and attention deficit hyperactivity disorder. *Clin Psychol Rev* 13:721–739, 1993.
80. Pennington BF, Ozonoff S: Executive functions and developmental psychopathology. *J Child Psychol Psychiatry* 37:51–87, 1996.
81. Nigg JT: On inhibition/disinhibition in developmental psychopathology: Views from cognitive and personality psychology and a working inhibition taxonomy. *Psychol Bull* 126:1–27, 2000.
82. Logan GD, Cowan WB, Davis KA: On the ability to inhibit simple and choice reaction time responses: A model and a method. *J Exp Psychol Hum Percept Perform* 10:276–291, 1984.
83. Oosterlaan J, Sergeant JA: Response inhibition in ADHD, CD, comorbid ADHD + CD, anxious and normal children: A meta-analysis of studies with the stop task. *J Child Psych Psychiatry* 39:411–426, 1998.
84. Nigg JT: The ADHD response inhibition deficit as measured by the stop task: Replication with DSM-IV combined type, extension, and qualification. *J Abnor Child Psychol* 27:391–400, 1999.
85. Aman CJ, Roberts RJ, Pennington BF: A neuropsychological examination of the underlying deficit in attention deficit hyperactivity disorder: Frontal lobe versus right parietal lobe theories. *Dev Psychol* 34:956–969, 1998.
86. Van der Meere J: The role of attention, in Sandberg S (ed): *Hyperactivity Disorders of Childhood.* Cambridge, England: Cambridge University Press, 1996, pp 111–148.
87. Barkley RA, Grodzinsky G, DuPaul G: Frontal lobe functions in attention deficit disorder with and without hyperactivity: A review and research report. *J Abnorm Child Psychol* 20:163–188, 1992.
88. Halperin J, Wolfe L, Pascualvaca D, et al: Differential assessment of attention and impulsivity in children. *J Am Acad Child Adolesc Psychiatry* 27:326–329, 1988.
89. Losier B, McGrath P, Klein R: Error patterns on the continuous performance test in non-medicated and medicated samples of children with and without ADHD: A meta-analytic review. *J Child Psychol Psychiatry* 37:971–987, 1996.
90. Chhabildas N, Pennington BF, Willcutt EG: A comparison of the cognitive deficits in the DSM-IV subtypes of ADHD. *J Abnorm Child Psychol* 29:529–540, 2001.
91. Nigg JT, Hinshaw SP, Carte E, et al: Neuropsychological correlates of childhood attention deficit hyperactivity disorder: Explainable by comorbid disruptive behavior or reading problems? *J Abnorm Psychol* 107:468–480, 1998.

92. Sonuga-Barke EJS, Taylor E, Sembi S, et al: Hyperactivity and delay aversion: I. The effect of delay on choice. *J Child Psychol Psychiatry* 33:387–398, 1992.
93. Borger N, van der Meere JJ, Ronner, A, et al: Heart rate variability and sustained attention in ADHD. *J Abnorm Child Psychol* 27:25–33, 1999.
94. Douglas VI: Can Skinnerian theory explain attention deficit disorder? A reply to Barkley, in Bloomingdale LM, Sergeant JA (eds): *Attention Deficit Disorder: Current Concepts and Emerging Trends in Attentional and Behavioral* Disorders of Childhood. Elmsford, NY: Pergamon Press, 1989, pp 235–254.
95. Sanders AF: Towards a model of stress and performance. *Acta Psychol* 53:61–97, 1983.
96. Sergeant JA, van der Meere JJ: Convergence of approaches in localizing the hyperactivity deficit, in Lahey BB, Kazdin AE (eds): *Advancements in Clinical Child Psychology*. New York: Plenum Press, 1990; vol 13, pp 207–245.
97. Kuntsi J, Oosterlaan J, Stevenson J: Psychological mechanisms in hyperactivity: I. Response inhibition deficit, working memory impairment, delay aversion, or something else? *J Child Psychol Psychiatry* 42:199–210, 2001.
98. Kuntsi J, Stevenson J: Psychological mechanisms in hyperactivity: II. The role of genetic factors. *J Child Psychol Psychiatry* 42:211–219, 2001.
99. Pelham WE Jr, Wheeler T, Chronis A: Empirically supported psychosocial treatments for attention deficit hyperactivity disorder. *J Clin Child Psychol* 27:190–205, 1998.
100. MTA Cooperative Group: A 14- month randomized clinical trial of treatment strategies for attention-deficit/hyperactivity disorder. *Arch Gen Psychiatry* 56:1073–86, 1999.

Chapter 67

MENTAL RETARDATION

Kytja K. S. Voeller

Mental retardation (MR) as defined by the American Association of Mental Retardation (AAMR) comprises an array of clinical syndromes with onset before age 18 years, "...characterized by significantly subaverage intellectual functioning, existing concurrently with related limitations in two or more of the following applicable adaptive skill areas: communication, self-care, home living, social skills, community use, self-direction, health and safety, functional academics, leisure and work."[1]

Examining each component of this definition, "significantly subaverage" implies that general cognitive ability, measured by an individually administered, standardized test, falls below a specific point. Although previously set at –2 standard deviations (SDs) below the mean, the cutoff point was raised in the 1992 AAMR definition from 70 to 75. Sattler[2] points out that it is also important to take into consideration the statistical properties of the specific test that is used. That is, "below −2 standard deviations" (SD) in tests with an SD of 15 (e.g., the Wechsler series) results in an IQ of 69 or less, whereas those with an SD of 16 (e.g., the Stanford-Binet) will result in an IQ of 67 or less.

The severity of MR is not specified in the AAMR definition, but the American Psychiatric Association (APA) identifies four levels of severity (Mild, IQ 50 or 55 to 70; Moderate 35 or 40 to 50 to 55, Severe 20 or 25 to 35 to 40, Profound < 20 to 25) and a "severity unspecified" category, indicating a strong presumption of MR, but the patient cannot be tested in a formal manner.[3]

Although intelligence is determined by a combination of genetic and environmental factors, recent studies that control statistically for effects of intrafamilial environments strongly support the notion that genetic factors have a profound influence on cognition and behavior.[4,5] Genetic effects on regional brain volumes have been demonstrated in a study of monozygotic (MZ) and dizygotic (DZ) twin pairs. Thompson et al. demonstrated that gray matter volumes and cortical volumes in frontal association areas and those subserving language (including Broca's and Wernicke's areas) appear to be under a greater degree of genetic control than sensorimotor and parietal association cortices.[6] Correlations in MZ twins for frontal and language association cortices were in the range of 95 to 100 percent ($p < 0.0001$), in contrast to more a modest 60 to 70 percent ($p < 0.05$) correlations in DZ twins. These authors were able to demonstrate a highly significant correlation between frontal gray matter and Spearman's g ($p < 0.0044$) after controlling for other factors.

NEUROBIOLOGICAL FACTORS IN MENTAL RETARDATION

The majority of cases of MR result from a perturbation of early brain development that is influenced to a variable and usually modest extent by environmental factors. With the exception of brain injury occurring either pre- or postnatally, most cases of MR result from genetic anomalies.

How do various genetic syndromes result in MR? There are many different specific causes of MR, but they can be grouped into two general classes: (1) a disruption of neuronal migration and/or (2) "dysgenetic dendrites" or "sick synapses."* Disorders of neuronal

* A special subclass of structural brain malformations are associated with inborn errors of metabolism. For example, hypoplastic temporal lobes are found in association with glutaric aciduria (both type 1 and type 2). Dysplasia of the corpus callosum is a very common anomaly, being found in maternal phenylketonuria, Menkes' syndrome, and numerous other metabolic disorders. (This subject was reviewed in detail by Nissenkorn A, Michelson M, Ben-Zeev B, et al.: Inborn errors of metabolism: A cause of abnormal brain development. *Neurology* 56:1265, 2001.)

differentiation and migration often result in structural malformations that are visible to the naked eye, whereas disruption of the proliferation of dendrites and synapses may result in anomalies that are more subtle and obvious only with morphometric measurements or histologic techniques.

Dendritic spines receive the bulk of the excitatory glutamatergic inputs that regulate synaptic plasticity, a process that underlies not only early in brain development but also learning and memory throughout life. Although dendrites were originally viewed as relatively immutable structures, the notion that they moved ("twitched") was proposed by Crick in 1982[7] and confirmed by direct observation somewhat later.[8] Dendrites turn out to be remarkably plastic structures, and dendritic spines and associated synapses can be remodeled in a matter of seconds.[9] These changes are dependent on the polymerization and depolymerization of actin in the spines, which is regulated by small GTPases from the Rho family that are highly expressed in neurons. For example, one of these GTPases, RacV12, increases spine density, reduces spine size, and may facilitate development of new spines; another–RhoAV14–reduces spine density and length and may block spine formation and maintenance, suggesting that density and spine size are independent.[10] Neurotransmitters also play an important role in regulating brain growth during early development and then, postnatally, are involved in neural transmission.[11] Thus, any disruption of the genes governing these multiple processes that are involved in building a brain is likely to result in some form of cognitive dysfunction if not frank MR. Thus, it is not surprising that Golgi studies have revealed a number of abnormalities in both the morphology and branching patterns of dendrites in a number of MR syndromes.[12] Moreover, in some cases, the brain is subjected to a double whammy in the sense that not only is the initial connectivity disrupted but the ability to learn new information is severely compromised by the same process. A challenge in this area is to be able to link the genetic perturbation to the specific pattern of cognitive dysfunction.

In the pages that follow, I will briefly describe a limited number of common MR syndromes and discuss relevant neurobehavioral and neurobiologic features.

LISSENCEPHALY

Lissencephaly reflects a disturbance of migration early in brain development, so that neurons do not reach their normal ultimate positions in the brain. There are four cortical layers, and the brain is smooth and lacks normal sulcal and gyral markings. Affected children are microcephalic; they have severe spasticity, profound MR, intractable seizures, and usually die at an early age. There are two forms, one involving the *LIS1* gene located on chromosome 17p13.3.[13] Although the precise role of LIS1 is unclear, this is a highly conserved protein that likely is involved in neuroblast proliferation, migration, and dendritic development.[14] Mild forms of lissencephaly—at least one with an IQ in the average range—present with pachygyria restricted to posterior cortical regions. These are associated with missense mutations of the *LIS1* gene.[15] The other—*double cortin—(DCX or XLIS)* gene—is located at Xq22.3-q23.[16] Few male fetuses survive. Carrier females have a highly variable phenotype, presumably due to X-inactivation, with some 20 percent having average-range intelligence, with mild to severe MR in the remaining 80 percent.[17] Seizures are very common. The brain has a relatively normal external appearance, with six cortical layers, but there is a band of heterotopic gray matter lying between the ventricles and the cortex (the "double cortex") or subcortical band heterotopia. The DCX protein is expressed from 9 to 20 gestational weeks, most intensely during the period of neuronal migration, and plays a critical role in stabilizing microtubule formation and nucleokinesis.[18]

RETT'S SYNDROME

Rett's syndrome (RS) is an X-linked disorder with a prevalence of 1 in 10,000 to 15,000 females. Only about 1 percent of RS cases are familial. Most cases (70 to 80 percent) arise from de novo mutations of the methyl-CpG-binding protein 2 (MECP2) gene, which has been mapped to Xq28.[19] Mutations, which mainly occur in the paternal germ line,[20] involve nonsense, missense, and frameshift mutations.

It was originally believed that RS occurred almost exclusively in females. In the classic situation, the affected girl is normal at birth and develops normally until 3 to 4 months, when a deceleration of head growth becomes apparent. Delayed somatic growth, followed by loss of milestones and language, emerges around 6 and 18 months. A characteristic hand-washing stereotypy appears, with ataxia as well as gait and limb apraxia. Affected girls are typically severely retarded and without language; they have severe seizures and periods of hyperpnea as well as impaired somatic growth and often present an autistic façade. However, it is now known that the phenotypic spectrum is much broader than previously imagined and encompasses males as well as females, with preserved language or only mild learning problems. In these females, X-inactivation may play an important role in the clinical phenotype. Males who have the MECP2 mutation and Klinefelter's syndrome (XXY) or whose mothers are mosaic for the mutation often present with a clinical picture similar to that of the more classic RS phenotype.[21]

What is the pathophysiology of RS? The early deceleration of head growth coupled with neuroimaging studies suggest a failure of the normal exuberant growth of the neuropil in early childhood. The MECP2 gene is a highly conserved gene that is expressed in both fetal and brain and is involved in transcriptional silencing of genes restricting synaptic proliferation.[22] Johnston et al.[23] have suggested that since these restrictive genes are not inhibited, normal synaptic expansion does not occur.

RUBINSTEIN-TAYBI SYNDROME

RTS is a syndrome characterized by severe MR, growth retardation, a characteristic facial appearance, broad thumbs and toes, and cardiac abnormalities. Behaviors reminiscent of bipolar disorder have been reported in RTS.[24] The RTS gene has been localized to 16p13.3. The gene encoding cAMP response element-binding binding protein (CREBBP) (a ubiquitously expressed transcriptional coactivator and histone acetyl transferase which regulates the expression of numerous other genes) is localized to this region. Impaired synaptic proliferation in RTS appears to result from a mutation in CREBBP. CREB also plays an important role in long term memory (LTM) formation, a process that has many similarities to synaptic plasticity.[25] Although yet to be demonstrated in human subjects with RTS, a mouse model has been shown to be deficient in LTM but not STM storage.[26]

CRETINISM

Cretinism results from a lack of thyroid hormone (TH) during early brain development. Although rare in the United States, there are endemic pockets of cretinism around the world where iodine deficiency leads to the full-blown syndrome. Cretins have IQs in the 20 to 40 range, impaired somatic growth, sensorineural hearing loss, deaf-mutism, spasticity and hyperreflexia (particularly in the lower extremities), and retained primitive reflexes. Even in cases of equivalent iodine deficiency, the clinical severity can vary. It has been suggested that the presence of the APOE $\varepsilon 4$ allele, which has TH-binding properties, is a risk factor for iodine-deficient cretinism.[27] When cretinism is treated early and vigorously, brain development and ultimate intellectual function can be normal but usually somewhat below that of siblings. The IQ often declines with age. Visuospatial and attentional deficits are noted, with relative preservation of verbal ability. Those receiving early treatment often perform within the average range in reading and spelling but often experience greater difficulty with arithmetic.[28]

TH regulates the transcription and the rate of gene expression during brain development both by direct effects on specific genes and indirect effects on "downstream" genes. TH impacts neuronogenesis, neuronal migration, dendritic and synaptic proliferation (in part through effects on the small GTPase system[29]), and myelinization. Although all these processes ultimately do occur, even in the brain deprived of TH, and the gross morphology of the brain is not anomalous, the normal timing of brain development is disrupted.[30]

NONSYNDROMIC X-LINKED MENTAL RETARDATION

Boys with nonsyndromic X-linked MR (XMR) have no characteristic somatic features except for MR. They represented something of an enigma in the past, but at this point at least seven genes have been cloned, all of which play an important role in dendritic proliferation and synapse formation through either direct or indirect effects on the Rho GTPases and the actin cytoskeleton.[31] MECP2 has been identified as one of the genes.[32]

DOWN'S SYNDROME

Down's syndrome (DS) (trisomy 21) is the most common genetic cause of MR, occurring in 1 out of every 700 live births. In women aged 45 to 49 years, the prevalence increases to 5 per 100. The DS phenotype is characterized by a small, brachycephalic head, epicanthic folds, upward-slanting palpebral fissures, Brushfield spots, protruding tongue, and transverse palmar creases. Persons with DS are at increased risk for congenital heart disease, duodenal atresia, seizures, and immunologic and hematologic problems (particularly leukemia).

The IQ of children with DS ranges from <40 to the average range. The mean IQ of children with trisomy is generally lower (52 ± 14.6) compared to those with mosaic DS (67 ± 13.8).[33] Language (particularly syntax)[34] and verbal memory[35] are typically impaired, with relative strengths in the visuospatial and social areas. Children with DS are typically friendly and sociable. They perform relatively well on Theory of Mind tasks.[36] Compared to an age- and IQ-matched group of boys with fragile-X syndrome, boys with DS performed somewhat better on tasks requiring visual attentional control and inhibition, although relative to a normal IQ group their performance was impaired.[37]

Alzeheimer's dementia (AD) is a significant risk in adults with DS: the average age of onset of dementia is in the range of 50 to 55 years. By age 40, the DS brain has neurofibrillary tangles and senile plaques similar to those seen in AD. Atrophy of the medial temporal lobe can be observed before the onset of clinically apparent memory loss.[38] However, amyloid deposition starts earlier and is much more widespread in DS than AD[39] and can be observed even in the 21-week-old fetus.[40] The APOE $\varepsilon 4$ genotype represents an additional and independent risk factor.[41]

The brain in DS is small, with disproportionately small cerebellar, brainstem, frontal lobe, and hippocampal volumes and atrophy of the superior temporal gyrus.[42,43] In children with DS, amygdalar volume, when corrected for total brain volume, did not differ from that of controls, but hippocampal volumes were significantly smaller.[44]

Although DS is one of the oldest and best-studied of the MR syndromes, the pathophysiology has yet to be worked out. The mouse trisomy 16 model, which shares many of the genes with human trisomy 21, has been helpful in elucidating the underlying pathophysiology. Current information points to a restriction of dendritic proliferation starting in midgestation. By 22 weeks of gestation in the human fetus, anomalies of cortical lamination are noted.[45] One possible explanation is that cytokines resulting from amyloid deposition during fetal brain development disrupt the process of dendritic expansion. Another is that nerve growth factor transfer is deficient, resulting in degeneration of cholinergic input to the basal forebrain.[46]

FRAGILE-X SYNDROME

Fragile-X syndrome (FRAX) occurs in 1 out of every 2000 to 5000 live births and is the most common form of inherited MR. Adult males with FRAX have a characteristic long, narrow face, large dysmorphic ears, a prominent jaw, and macroorchidism. The neuropsychiatric phenotype is characterized by hyperactivity, impaired social relatedness, social anxiety, gaze avoidance, and stereotypies that appear "autistic." These behavioral and physical attributes are not as prominent in young boys. IQ ranges from normal to profound MR and declines in early puberty.[47]

Carrier females have few somatic features and a milder cognitive phenotype but manifest deficits in working memory as well as impaired visuospatial and prefrontal executive function. Social anxiety, hyperarousal, attention problems, and stereotypic movements are often seen. IQ is variable.[48]

Neuroimaging studies reveal an enlarged fourth ventricle, with decrease in size of the cerebellar vermis (especially lobules VI and VII), and enlarged caudate nuclei.[49] In each case, these measurements are most striking in FRAX males, with carrier females falling in an intermediate status between affected males and controls. There is an association between decreased vermis size and IQ.[50]

FRAX results from an expansion of an unstable CGG trinucleotide repeat,[51] which causes transcriptional silencing of the FMR1 gene (located at Xq27.3) by methylation. Silencing occurs when the number of CGG trinucleotide repeats within the initial (5′) untranslated portion of the gene reaches 200 or more. The average person has no more than 50 CGG repeats, whereas in persons with FRAX, CGG repeats range from 200 to over 1000. The FMR1 gene regulates the production of FMR protein (FMRP), a protein found in many cells, FMRP, which is prominently expressed in neurons and plays a critical role in the transport and regulation of mRNA. FMRP increases rapidly in the normal synapse in response to neuronal stimulation.[52] Histologic studies of the brains of humans with FRAX and of *fmr-1* knockout mice reveal abnormal dendritic spine morphology.[53] In the developing brain, decreased or absent FMRP results in impaired synaptic plasticity; in the adult, learning and memory are disrupted.

In carrier females, there is a relationship between IQ and CGG repeats. The mean group IQ of those with CGG repeats greater than 200 was 89.4 in comparison to a mean IQ of 107 in those with CGG repeats below 200. Dyer-Friedman et al. studied the relationship of home environment to genetic factors and found that mean parental IQ contributed strongly to the variance of the cognitive outcome, particularly verbal and attentional abilities in girls with FRAX, whereas in males the mean parental IQ contributed only to the performance IQ and processing scale scores. Surprisingly, they could not demonstrate a strong correlation between FMRP and cognitive outcomes in either males or females.[54] Kwon et al. studied female FRAX carriers and demonstrated that there was a correlation between neural activation in the middle frontal gyrus on a visuospatial working memory task and the level of FMRP expression and activation of various areas of the frontal lobe, suggesting that FMRP may play a dynamic role in modulating brain activation in response to working memory load.[55]

PRADER-WILLI SYNDROME

Prader-Willi syndrome (PWS) has a prevalence of 1 in 10,000 to 1 in 25,000. Persons with PWS are of short stature and severely obese; they have small hands and feet, almond-shaped eyes, and hypogonadism. IQ can range from the retarded to low-average range, but language is often particularly impaired. At birth, children with PWS are hypotonic and undergrown. Around age 2, they develop a voracious appetite and gain weight rapidly. As they mature, it becomes increasingly hard for their care providers to limit food intake. Older children and adults are prone to display tantrums, OCD-spectrum behaviors, and skin-picking.[56] PWS results from an absence of expression of paternally active genes in 15q11-q13 ("PWS critical region"). In 70 percent of the cases this is the result of a deletion on paternal chromosome 15. In 30 percent of the cases both chromosomes come from the mother, a case of *uniparental disomy* (UPD).

ANGELMAN'S SYNDROME

Children with Angelman's syndrome (AS) appear normal at birth, but their subsequent development is severely delayed and many children with AS never speak. They are often microcephalic and hypopigmented relative to other members of their families. There is prominent motor dysfunction, hyperactivity, hyperarousability, and a seizure disorder that is hard to control. Because patients with AS smile almost continuously, AS has been dubbed the "happy puppet" syndrome. AS involves the same deletion at 15q11-q13 as PWS, but it is due to an absence of expression of maternally active genes. Four distinct genetic mechanisms have been identified: paternal UPD, an imprinting defect, a large insterstitial deletion of 15q11-q13, and a mutation in the E3ubiquitin protein ligase gene. A fifth type does not have any identifiable genetic mechanisms. Deletion patients are the most severely affected, while those with a mutation of the ubiquitin gene or an imprinting defect have a milder phenotype and do not differ substantially from one another.[57]

TURNER'S SYNDROME

Turner's syndrome occurs in about 1 out of every 5000 live female births. Babies with TS have a short, webbed neck, low hairline, low-set ears, ptosis, micrognathia, a high-arched palate, and an atypical facies. Older girls and women are short, and a percentage have ovarian failure. There is an increased incidence of coarctation of the aorta. IQ ranges from normal to mild MR. Verbal skills are typically a strength, and there is often a verbal > performance gap.[58] These children typically manifest both visuospatial and executive function deficits, characterized by inattention and impulsivity. This pattern is reminiscent of dysfunction of the frontal-parietal system (the "where" system). Arithmetic skills are often poor. Neither estrogen nor normal hormonal function improves cognitive performance, and cognitive deficits remain stable into adulthood.

There are a variety of different genotypic patterns in TS. About 50 percent of TS have an absent X chromosome (45XO) and 10 to 15 percent are XO/XX mosaics. TS is rarely inherited, but this does occur.[59]

Reiss and colleagues reported a particularly instructive study of twins discordant for TS.[60] Both twins had superior full-scale IQs and the verbal IQs were within 3 points of each other, but there was a 25 point V>P discrepancy in the XO twin. The Perceptual Organization index of the XO twin was 21 points lower than that of the unaffected twin, with impaired performance on visuospatial, attentional, and executive function tasks relative to the normal twin. Mild atrophy with decreased gray matter was noted on the XO twin's MRI.

CHROMOSOME 22q11.2–DELETION SYNDROME

The chromosome 22q11.2–deletion syndrome (Chr 22q11.2) includes velocardiofacial syndrome, DiGeorge syndrome, and conotruncal face syndrome; it involves a spectrum of serious cardiovascular malformations as well as immunologic and endocrinologic disorders. Most patients have a characteristic facial appearance, with abnormalities of the palate and ears, but some do not. It is quite common, occurring in 1 in 2000 to 4000 live births. IQ ranges from mild MR to normal but there is a high incidence of learning disabilities and borderline IQ, with a pattern of declining IQ scores with maturation. In a group of 4-year-olds, the mean IQ obtained on the Stanford-Binet IQ was 87; it was 84 on the Leiter International Performance Test. On the WISC-R, 8-year-olds obtained a mean verbal IQ of 76 and a mean Performance IQ of 79; this IQ was about the same in a group of 13-year-olds. Young children often present with speech and language problems,[61,62] but deficits in the visuospatial domain, including memory, are prominent. Impaired reading comprehension and arithmetic are often noted.[63]

Chr 22q11.2 is overrepresented in psychiatric samples—there is a higher incidence of ADHD, OCD, and bipolar disorder[64] as well as schizophrenia (in fact, Chr 22q11.2 appears to be the highest known risk factor for schizophrenia).[65] Interestingly, the 22q11 deletion includes the catechol O-methyltransferase (COMT) gene. COMT inactivates catecholamine neurotransmitters. A common polymorphism (the COMT108^{met} variant) leads to a reduction of COMT activity. Patients who are homozygous for the COMT108^{met} variant or have Chr 22q11.2 and the COMT108^{met} variant on the allele that is not deleted have reduced levels of COMT, with a resulting increase in circulating catecholamines. This group is at very high risk for neuropsychiatric disorders. A knockout mouse model shows defective sensorimotor gating as well as learning and memory defects.[66] Graf et al.[67] reported that treatment with metyrosine, a competitive inhibitor of tyrosine hydroxylase that reduces brain dopamine and subsequent stages of the catecholamine pathway, resulted in modest improvements in the neuropsychiatric status of these patients.

MRI morphometric studies have revealed reduced total brain volume and reduced volumes of left parietal lobe and right cerebellum.[68] A high incidence of midline anomalies (cavum vergae) and atrophy were reported in schizophrenics.[69] Polymicrogyria have also been noted.[70] These markers for disturbed neuronal migration may reflect the impact of the disordered catecholamine levels during early brain development.

This syndrome has been mapped to a deletion on chromosome 22q11.2, involving some 30 genes. Eliez et al. have reported that patients who inherit the deletion on the maternal chromosome have reduced gray matter volumes compared to normal controls and those inheriting the deletion from their fathers.[71]

WILLIAMS' SYNDROME

Williams' syndrome (WS) is a rare type of MR, with an incidence of 1 in 25,000. Hypercalcemia and supravalvular stenosis are often detected in the neonatal period. Early motor and language development is delayed. As they mature, persons with WS acquire sophisticated vocabularies and elaborate syntactic structures and often demonstrate average range performance on language tasks. Social skills are relatively intact—they are gregarious (if not overly friendly), and object recognition and face-processing are cognitive strengths.[72] WS is associated with significantly impaired visuospatial function and prefrontal deficits—characterized by impulsivity and impaired attention. IQs range from 40 to 100 with a mean of about 60.[73]

On gross examination and MRI morphometric studies, the brain in WS is only slightly reduced in size (13 percent) compared to that of controls. The shape of the brain is unusual, with a marked reduction in the volume of the parieto-occipital area, and a decrease in the size of the splenium. The cerebellum is normal in size except for some enlargement of the vermis.[74,75] The gyral pattern is generally normal, but the central sulcus and some gyri in the dorsal area are anomalous.[76] Microscopic examination reveals a normal cytoarchitectonic structure with subtle changes—diminished neuronal cell packing density and increased glia. Columnar organization is reduced, particularly in the posterior region.[77] The difference between the relatively normal structure of the ventral, perisylvian, and anterior regions of the brain and the subtle anomalies observed in dorsal and posterior areas is consistent with the symmetry in cognitive function in WS. That is, functions of the ventral pathway are relatively intact whereas those subserved by the dorsal pathway are defective.

The genetic anomaly has been identified as a submicroscopic deletion on chromosome 7q11.23[78] Several genes in this region are expressed in the brain and play prominent roles in brain development. These are LIM kinase-1 (a protein tyrosine kinase), STX1-A (involved in synaptic development), and FZD9 (previously known as FZD3—the human homologue of the drosophila "frizzled" gene). It has been suggested that these genes may be related to the cognitive and morphologic features of WS, but subsequent reports have shown that the typical WS cognitive phenotype occurs in persons with small deletions that do not include these genes.[79,80]

SUMMARY

This brief review of some of the MR syndromes has attempted to portray the remarkable variety of the neurocognitive profiles which are seen in these syndromes and discuss the pathophysiology with particular attention to some of the neurogenetic aspects. In the next decade we can look forward to dramatic advances in our understanding of how these genetic anomalies result in differences in cognitive profile, brain structure, and behavior. However, it is apparent that there is considerable variability in the genetic aspect of these syndromes and one cannot predict the outcome in most cases from the genotype. Thus, clinicians need to conduct detailed neurocognitive examinations in order to define the cognitive strengths and weaknesses of these patients. For the clinician, the challenge is to be aware of the genetic features of these syndromes but at the same time understand the functional abilities of the specific patient. This will enable the clinician to provide the patient with appropriate and carefully tailored adaptive and cognitive strategies and to control adverse environmental factors so that persons with MR can function at an optimal level.

REFERENCES

1. American Association on Mental Retardation: *Mental Retardation: Definition, Classification, and Systems of Supports,* 9th ed.Washington DC: AAMR, 1992.
2. Sattler JM: *Assessment of Children. Behavioral and Clinical Applications,* 4th ed. San Diego, CA: Jerome M. Sattler, 2002.
3. American Psychiatric Association: *Diagnostic and Statistical Manual of Mental Disorders: Text Revision,* 4th ed. (DSM-IV-TR). Washington, DC: American Psychiatric Association, 2000.
4. McClearn GE, Johansson B, Berg S, et al: Substantial genetic influence on cognitive abilities in twins 80 or more years old. *Science* 276:1560:1997.
5. Tramo MJ, Loftus WC, Stukel TA, et al: Brain size, head size, and intelligence quotient in monozygotic twins. *Neurology* 50:1246, 1998.
6. Thompson PM, Cannon, TD, Narr KL, et al: Genetic influences on brain structure. *Nat Neurosci* 4:1253, 2001.
7. Crick F: Do spines twitch? *Trends Neurosci* 5:44, 1982.

8. Dunaevsky A, Tashiro A, Majewska A, et al: Developmental regulation of spine motility in mammalian CNS. *Proc Natl Acad Sci U S A* 96:13438, 1999.
9. Fischer M, Kaech S, Knutti D, et al: Rapid actin-based plasticity in dendritic spines. *Neuron* 20:847, 1998.
10. Tashiro A, Minden A, Yuste R: Regulation of dendritic spine morphology by the rho family of small GTPases: Antagonistic roles of rac and rho. *Cereb Cortex* 10:927, 2000.
11. Levitt P, Harvey JA, Friedman E, et al: New evidence for neurotransmitter influences on brain development. *Trends Neurosci* 20:269, 1997.
12. Marín-Padilla M: Structural abnormalities of the cerebral cortex in human chromosomal aberrations. A Golgi study. *Brain Res* 44:625, 1972.
13. Lo Nigro C, Chong SS, Smith ACM, et al: Point mutations and an intragenic deletion in *LIS1,* the lissencephaly causative gene in isolated lissencephaly sequence and Miller-Dieker syndrome. *Hum Mol Genet* 6:157:1997.
14. Liu Z, Steward R, Luo L: Drosophila *Lis1* is required for neuroblast proliferation, dendritic elaboration and axonal transport. *Nat Cell Biol* 2:776, 2000.
15. Leventer RJ, Cardoso C, Ledbetter DH, et al: *LIS1* missense mutations cause milder lissencephaly phenotypes including a child with normal IQ. *Neurology* 57:416, 2001.
16. Ross ME, Allen KM, Srivastava AK, et al: Linkage and physical mapping of X-linked lissencephaly/SBH *XLIS*: A gene causing neuronal migration defects in human brain. *Hum Mol Genet* 6:555, 1997.
17. Dobyns WB, Andermann E, Andermann F, et al: X-linked malformations of neuronal migration. *Neurology* 47:331, 1996.
18. Qin J, Mizuguchi M, Itoh M, et al: Immunohistochemical expression of doublecortin in the human cerebrum: Comparison of normal development and neuronal migration disorders. *Brain Res* 863:225, 2000.
19. Amir RE, Van den Veyver IB, Wan M, et al: Rett syndrome is caused by mutations in X-linked MeCP2, encoding methyl-CpG-binding protein 2. *Nat Genet* 23:185, 2001.
20. Girard M, Couvert P, Carrié A, et al: Parental origin of de novo MECP2 mutations in Rett syndrome. *Eur J Hum Genet* 9:231, 2001.
21. Schanen C: Rethinking the fate of males with mutations in the gene that causes Rett syndrome. *Brain Dev* 23:S144, 2001.
22. Nan X, Ng HH, Johnson CA, et al: Transcriptional repression by the methyl-CpG-binding protein MeCP2 involves a histone deacetylase complex. *Nature* 393:386, 1998.
23. Johnston MV, Jeon O-H, Pevsner J, et al: Neurobiology of Rett syndrome: A genetic disorder of synapse development. *Brain Dev* 23:S206, 2001.
24. Hellings JA, Hossain S, Martin JK, et al: Psychopathology, GABA, and the Rubinstein-Taybi syndrome: A review and case study. *Am J Med Genet* 8:114, 2001.
25. Wang HY, Zhang FC, Cao JJ, et al: Apolipoprotein E is a genetic risk factor for fetal iodine deficiency disorder in China. *Mol Psychiatry* 5:363, 2000.
26. Oike Y, Hata A, Mamiya T, et al: Truncated CBP protein leads to classical Rubinstein-Taybi syndrome phenotypes in mice: Implications for a dominant-negative mechanism. *Hum Mol Genet* 8:387, 1999.
27. Wang HY, Zhang FC, Cao JJ, et al: Apolipoprotein E is a genetic risk factor for fetal iodine deficiency disorder in China. *Mol Psychiatry* 5:363:2000.
28. Rovet J: Congenital hypothyroidism, in Rourke BP (ed): *Syndrome of Nonverbal Learning Disabilities: Neurodevelopmental Manifestations*. New York: Guilford Press, 1995; pp 255–281.
29. Vargiu P, Morte B, Manzano J, et al: Thyroid hormone regulation of rhes, a novel Ras homolog gene expressed in the striatum. *Brain Res Mol Brain Res* 94:1, 2000.
30. Madeira MD, Paula-Barbosa MM: Reorganization of mossy fiber synapses in male and female hypothyroid rats: A stereological study. *J Comp Neurol* 337:334, 1993.
31. Ramakers GJA: Rho proteins, mental retardation and the cellular basis of cognition. *Trends Neurosci* 25:191, 2002.
32. Couvert P, Bienvenu T, Aquaviva C, et al: ME CP2 is highly mutated in X-linked mental retardation. *Hum Mol Genet* 10:941, 2001.
33. Fishler K, Koch R, Donnell GN: Comparison of mental development in individuals with mosaic and trisomy 21 Down's syndrome. *Pediatrics* 58:744, 1976.
34. Bellugi U, Bihrle A, Jernigan T, et al: Neuropsychological, neurological, and neuroanatomical profile of Williams syndrome. *Am J Hum Genet Suppl* 6:115, 1990.
35. Brugge KL, Nichols SL, Salmon DP, et al: Cognitive impairment in adults with Down's syndrome: Similarities to early cognitive changes in Alzheimer's disease. *Neurology* 44:232, 1994.
36. Baron-Cohen S, Leslie AM, Frith U: Does the autistic child have a "theory of mind"? *Cognition* 21:37, 1985.
37. Wilding J, Cornish K, Munir F: Further delineation of the executive deficit in males with fragile-X syndrome. *Neuropsychologia* 40, 1343, 2002.
38. Krasuski JS, Alexander GE, Horwitz B, et al: Relation of medial temporal lobe volumes to age and memory function in nondemented adults with Down's syndrome:

Implications for the prodromal phase of Alzheimer's disease. *Am J Psychiatry* 159:74–81, 2002.

39. Hof PR, Couras C, Perl DP, et al: Age-related distribution of neuropathologic changes in the cerebral cortex of patients with Down's syndrome: Quantitative regional analysis and comparison with Alzheimer's disease. *Arch Neurol* 52:379, 1995.
40. Teller JK, Russo C, DeBusk LM, et al: Presence of soluble amyloid beta-peptide precedes amyloid plaque formation in Down's syndrome. *Nat Med* 2:93, 1996.
41. Hyman BT, West HL, Rebeck GW, et al: Neuropathological changes in Down's syndrome hippocampal formation. *Arch Neurol* 52:373, 1995.
42. Kemper TL: Down syndrome, in Peters A, Jones EG (eds): *Cerebral Cortex. IX: Normal and Altered States of Function*. New York: Plenum Press, 1991, vol 9, p 511.
43. Pinter JD, Eliez S, Schmitt JE, et al: Neuroanatomy of Down's syndrome: A high-resolution MRI study. *Am J Psychiatry* 158:1659, 2001.
44. Pinter JD, Brown WE, Eliez S, et al: Amygdala and hippocampal volumes in children with Down syndrome: A high resolution MRI study. *Neurology* 56:972, 2001.
45. Schmidt-Sidor B, Wisniewski KE, Shepard T, et al: Brain growth in Down syndrome subjects 15 to 22 weeks of gestational age and birth to 60 months. *Clin Neuropathol* 9:181, 1990.
46. Cooper JD, Salehi A, Delcroix JD, et al: Failed retrograde transport of NGF in a mouse model of Down's syndrome: Reversal of cholinergic neurodegenerative phenotypes following NGF infusion. *Proc Natl Acad Sci U S A* 98:10439, 2001.
47. Hodapp RM, Dykens EM, Hagerman R, et al: Developmental implications of changing trajectories of IQ in males with fragile X syndrome. *J Am Acad Child Adolesc Psychiatry* 29:214, 1990.
48. Rousseau F, Heitz D, Tarleton J, et al: A multicenter study on genotype-phenotype correlations in the fragile X syndrome, using direct diagnosis with probe StB123.3: The first 2,253 cases. *Am J Hum Genet* 55:225, 1994.
49. Eliez S, Blasey CM, Freund LS, et al: Brain anatomy, gender and IQ in children and adolescents with fragile X syndrome. *Brain* 124:1610, 2001.
50. Mostofsky SH, Mazzocco MMM, Aakalu G, et al: Decreased cerebellar posterior vermis size in fragile X syndrome. Correlation with neurocognitive performance. *Neurology* 50:121, 1998.
51. Oberlé I, Rousseau F, Heitz D, et al: Instability of a 550-base pair DNA segment and abnormal methylation in fragile X syndrome. *Science* 252:1097, 1991.
52. Weiler IJ, Irwin SA, Klintsova AY, et al: Fragile X mental retardation protein is translated near synapses in response to neurotransmitter activation. *Proc Natl Acad Sci U S A* 94:5395, 1997.
53. Nimchinsky EA, Oberlander AM, Svoboda K: Abnormal development of dendritic spines in FMR1 knock-out mice. *J Neurosci* 21:5139, 2001.
54. Dyer-Friedman J, Glaser B, Hessi D, et al: Genetic and environmental influences on the cognitive outcomes of children with fragile X syndrome. *J Am Acad Child Adolesc Psychiatry* 41:237, 2002.
55. Kwon H, Menon V, Eliez S, et al: Functional neuroanatomy of visuospatial working memory in fragile X syndrome: Relation to behavioral and molecular measures. *Am J Psychiatry* 158:1040, 2001.
56. Dimitropoulos A, Feurer ID, Butler MG, et al: Emergence of compulsive behavior and tantrums in children with Prader-Willi syndrome. *Ment Retard* 106:39, 2001.
57. Lossie AC, Whitney MM, Amidon D, et al: Distinct phenotypes distinguish the molecular classes of Angelman syndrome. *J Med Genet* 38:834, 2001.
58. Temple CM, Carney RA: Intellectual functioning of children with Turner syndrome: A comparison of behavioural phenotypes. *Dev Med Child Neurol* 35:691, 1993.
59. Leichtman D, Schmickel R, Gelehrntner T, et al: *Ann Intern Med* 89:473, 1978.
60. Reiss AL, Freund L, Plotnick L, et al: The effects of X monosomy on brain development: Monozygotic twins discordant for Turner's syndrome. *Ann Neurol* 34:95, 1993.
61. Solot CB, Knightly C, Handler SD, et al: Communication disorders in the 22q11.2 microdeletion syndrome. *J Commun Disord* 33:187, 2000.
62. Bearden CE, Woodin MR, Wang PP, et al: The neurocognitive phenotype of the 22q11.2 deletion syndrome: Selective deficit in visual-spatial memory. *J Clin Exp Neuropsychol* 23:447, 2001.
63. Golding-Kushner KJ, Weller G, Shprintzen RJ: Velo-cardio-facial syndrome: Language and psychological profiles. *J Craniofac Genet Dev Biol* 5:259, 1985.
64. Papolos DR, Faedda GL, Veit S, et al: Bipolar spectrum disorders in patients diagnosed with velo-cardio-facial syndrome: Does a hemizygous deletion of chromosome 22q11 result in bipolar affective disorder? *Am J Psychiatry* 153:1541, 1996.
65. Murphy KC, Jones LA, Owen NH: High rates of schizophrenia in adults with velo-cardio-facial syndrome. *Arch Gen Psychiatry* 56:940–945, 1999.
66. Paylor R, McIlwain KL, McAninch R, et al: Mice deleted for the DiGeorge/velocardiofacial syndrome region show abnormal sensorimotor gating and learning and memory impairments. *Hum Mol Genet* 20:2645, 2001.

67. Graf WD, Unis AS, Yates CM, et al: Catecholamines in patients with 22q11.2 deletion syndrome and the low-activity COMT polymorphism. *Neurology* 57:410, 2001.
68. Eliez S, Schmitt JE, White CD, et al: Children and adolescents with velocardiofacial syndrome, a volumetric MRI study. *Am J Psychiatry* 157:409, 2000.
69. Chow EW, Mikulis DJ, Zipursky RB, et al: Qualitative MRI findings in adults with 22q11 deletion syndrome and schizophrenia. *Biol Psychiatry* 157:409, 1999.
70. Cramer SC, Schaefer PW, Krishnamoorthy KS: Microgyria in the distribution of the middle cerebral artery in a patient with DiGeorge syndrome. *J Child Neurol* 11:494, 1996.
71. Eliez S, Antonarakis SE, Morris MA, et al: Parental origin of the deletion 22qll.2 and brain development in velocardiofacial syndrome. *Arch Gen Psychiatry* 58:64, 2001.
72. Tager-Flusberg H, Boshart J, Baron-Cohen S: Reading the windows to the soul: Evidence for domain-specific sparing in William's syndrome. *J Cogn Neurosci* 10:631, 1998.
73. Bellugi U, Lictenberger L, Mills D, et al.: Bridging cognition, the brain and molecular genetics: Evidence from Williams syndrome. *Trends Neurosci* 22:197, 1999.
74. Wang PP, Hesselink JR, Jernigan TL, et al: Specific neurobehavioral profile of Williams' syndrome is associated with neocerebellar hemispheric preservation. *Neurology* 42:1999, 1992.
75. Schmitt JE, Eliez S, Warsofsky IS, et al: Enlarged cerebellar vermis in Williams syndrome. *J Psychiatr Res* 35:225, 2001.
76. Galaburda AM, Schmitt JE, Atlas SW, et al: Dorsal forebrain anomaly in Williams syndrome. *Arch Neurol* 58:1865, 2001.
77. Galaburda AM, Wang PP, Bellugi U, et al: Cytoarchitectonic anomalies in a genetically based disorder. Williams syndrome. *Neuroreport* 5:753, 1994.
78. Ewart AK, Morris CA, Atkinson D, et al: Hemizygosity at the elastin locus in a developmental disorder. Williams syndrome. *Nat Genet* 5:11, 1993.
79. Botta A, Novelli G, Mari A, et al: Detection of an atypical 7q11.23 deletion in Williams syndrome patients which does not include the STX1A and FZd3 genes. *J Med Genet* 36:478, 1999.
80. Tassabehji M, Metcalfe K, Karmiloff-Smith A, et al: Williams syndrome: use of chromosomal microdeletions as a tool to dissect cognitive and physical phenotypes. *Am J Hum Gen* 64:118, 1999.

Chapter 68

THE PERVASIVE DEVELOPMENTAL DISORDERS: AUTISM AND RELATED CONDITIONS

Nancy J. Minshew
Jessica A. Meyer

INTRODUCTION

Classification

The diagnostic category of Pervasive Developmental Disorders (PDD) refers to autism and related disorders whose features share qualities referred to as autistic-like. These disorders are now commonly referred to as Autism Spectrum Disorders (ASD) because this term is more meaningful, but the term PDD is entrenched in legislation and educational policy and so is likely to remain in official use. These terms are used interchangeably and both were chosen to encompass the full range of intellectual functioning associated with these disorders, from severe and profound mental retardation to IQ scores in the superior range. Even "mild" forms have by definition a severe impact on adaptive function.

The PDDs are diagnosed clinically by abnormalities in social reciprocity, verbal and nonverbal language and its use for communication, imaginative play, and restricted and repetitive behavioral patterns and interests. The current diagnostic classification for PDD in the *Diagnostic and Statistical Manual for Mental Disorders*, 4th ed, Text Revision (DSM-IV-TR),[1] includes Autistic Disorder, Asperger's Disorder, Pervasive Developmental Disorder Not Otherwise Specified (PDDNOS), Childhood Disintegrative Disorder (CDD), and Rett's Disorder.

Rett's disorder presents with regression or global neurologic deterioration in the first or second year of life, which is the sole basis for its potential confusion with autism. It is otherwise a very different disorder, being characterized by decelerating head growth, microcephaly, loss of voluntary hand movements and walking if acquired, periodic breathing, and difficulty swallowing. It is also a disorder of females. Childhood disintegrative disorder is defined by regression or neurologic deterioration between 2 and 12 years of age, typically after sentence language has been established. Given the wide age span of these cases, CDD is likely to be related to diverse neurologic degenerative disorders, the most commonly now recognized of which is adrenoleukodystrophy. Because of these key differences from the other PDDs, clinical discussions of PDD usually refer to autistic disorder, Asperger's disorder, and PDDNOS only.

There are two diseases that produce the syndrome of autism above chance association—tuberous sclerosis and fragile-X syndrome; autistic symptoms are common among those with these diseases. A third condition, the Nonverbal Learning Disabilities Syndrome (NLD) or the Syndrome of the Developmental Learning Disabilities of the Right Hemisphere, is probably a subset of the PDDs rather than a separate syndrome, but it was originally described on the basis of a neuropsychological profile of right hemisphere deficits. Social dysfunction was described as part of this syndrome but was not well characterized.

A diverse and large group of diseases has been associated with cases of autism. Within each disease, autism is a rare occurrence. These cases account for less than 10 percent of autism, and the percentage is directly related to the stringency of the diagnostic criteria used.

Prevalence

The prevalence of autism is substantially higher than in the past. In 1980, the prevalence of the PDDs—e.g., autism and PDDNOS—was estimated at 20 per 10,000. Three studies in the last 2 years have estimated the prevalence of Autistic Disorder, Asperger's Disorder, and PDDNOS at 58, 63, and 67/10,000.[2–4] This corresponds to 1 per 150 to 1 per 170 births. Although it has been suggested that this increase is due to overdiagnosis, these studies were conducted by internationally acknowledged autism experts using state-of-the-art research diagnostic instruments. A second explanation proposed for this increase is that autism was previously underdiagnosed. The correction of the underdiagnosis of the past is not, however, sufficient to account for the tremendous increase in cases that is being seen internationally. The exact timing of the rise in prevalence is unknown but appears to be about a decade old. There is an overall ratio of 3 or 4 to 1 in terms of male:female predominance for the PDDs, but the male predominance is much higher at the higher-IQ end of the spectrum, approaching 15 to 1.

Genetics

Autism is now generally acknowledged to be a polygenetic disorder resulting from three or four interacting liability genes, with the particular genes differing between cases and thus complicating their identification.[5] It is estimated that as many as 20 autism liability genes exist. Heritability is estimated at 90 percent. The recurrence risk is about 6 percent, though both lower and higher numbers are proposed. Approximately 1 to 4 percent of cases have identifiable chromosome 15 abnormalities.[6,7] Genome-wide linkage studies of sibling pair families have provided support for involvement of chromosomes 7q, 2q, and 16p.[8]

CLINICAL SYNDROME

Clinical distinctions between the PDDs are largely defined in terms of deviations from autism. Most of the distinctions, other than the absence of developmental language delay in Asperger's disorder, are based on less severe symptoms than those expected for an individual of the same age and IQ with autism. Such clinical distinctions are not reliably attainable outside of a research setting and are not clinically important. The clinical emphasis should be on whether the person has a PDD, because it is the quality of the symptoms that necessitates an entirely different approach to intervention from that used in any other disability. The diagnostic evaluation should focus on defining deficits and skill levels in social, language, communication, play, and reasoning, along with challenging behaviors. A practice parameter for the screening and diagnosis of children with autism and PDD has been published and provides excellent guidelines for practice.[9]

The clinical signs and symptoms of autism are the most severe in early childhood, but the course diverges dramatically thereafter, with a wide range of outcomes. Approximately one-half of autistic children make no developmental progress. The remainder makes small to large gains between 3 and 8 years of age. Thus, the manifestations of autism change substantially with age and the natural history is one of substantial improvement by school age in many children. With the increase in prevalence, a much higher percentage of children with PDD are now nonretarded at diagnosis, likely changing the natural history and developmental trajectories of autism and the PDDs in ways that are difficult to assess with the nearly universal intensive intervention.

Onset

In the majority of children, symptoms emerge in the form of developmental delays in the second year of life, though first-birthday videotapes have demonstrated impairments earlier. Early symptoms involve delayed language development, diminished or odd social contact, odd play with toys or preference for objects over people, and irritability related to change. Children with Asperger's disorder will not have the language abnormalities and in fact will often read early but will have the social oddities, the odd intense interests, and the unusual memory for facts. The social impairment in these high-functioning children may not be apparent until preschool, when they are first exposed to group social situations and it becomes apparent that they do not have group social etiquette and do not relate to other children. These children may be considered affectionate in terms of accepting or giving hugs,[9] and this should not preclude consideration of a diagnosis of PDD.

About 25 percent of children with PDD present with regression and loss of acquired language, social, and play skills, with the emergence of autistic behavior between 12 and 24 months. This usually takes place over a few months at most.

Social

The essential quality of the social deficit involves the lack of coordination or reciprocity. Social reciprocity requires the capacity to accurately judge and predict the reactions of others, to clearly grasp social situations and understand social cause and effect, and to subtly influence social interaction patterns. All of the components comprising social reciprocity are seriously impaired in autism. In its most severe form, it is expressed as a complete lack of comprehension of the social behavior of others and a profound incapacity for social responses. In moderate forms, the individual has a very rudimentary comprehension of common social situations and one- or two-step ways of interacting, such as repeating a few rote or canned phrases upon encountering and leaving people. In its least severe form, social exchanges are more extensive, involving conversation, but are actually no better coordinated. These children typically make off-topic comments, deliver monologues on their obsession, and make odd comments reflecting the disturbance in abstract reasoning. Their understanding of social situations is partial; as a result, they are extremely naïve, prone to being socially "exploited" and, at the same time, liable unwittingly to violate social conventions and infringe on the social rights of others. They are typically characterized as strange, odd, or weird. Persistent difficulties are present in peer relationships. They lack a best friend and do not establish close interpersonal connections based on a history of shared emotions and experiences. The level of social emotional function is often severely overestimated in these individuals and can range in adults from 18 months of age to 10 or 12 years. The developmental social-emotional level should be carefully assessed in every high-functioning individual with PDD.[10,11]

One of the key contributions to the understanding of the cognitive basis of the social deficit in autism was the discovery of the *theory of mind* deficit. This is the capacity for knowing that others have different thoughts from one's own and for automatically making inferences about what those thoughts are. This capacity is the basis for social reciprocity, empathy, understanding the motives and intentions of others, manipulation, and lying, none of which are within the repertoire of autistic individuals, although the most able individuals may develop some elementary capacity for empathy.

Verbal Language

The verbal language deficit in ASD is characterized by wide-ranging differences in the acquisition of spoken language and at times loss of language through regression, failure to compensate for verbal language deficits with nonverbal language, deviant language development, abnormalities in the use of all forms of language for social communication, and substantial residual deficits despite developmental progress. Parallel deficits are also present in language comprehension. Individuals with Asperger's disorder often have precocious language abilities, talking and reading early.

In its most severe form, neither expressive or receptive language abilities develop in autistic children, nor can they repeat. Unlike children with expressive and receptive language disorders, however, autistic children fail to compensate with alternate forms of communication, such as gesture, facial expression, eye contact, and body language. With some developmental progress, autistic children develop the capacity to repeat without the capacity to comprehend or speak using original language, resulting in echolalia, which can follow immediately after hearing the source or be delayed. With additional developmental progress, the child is able to associate the echolalia with an outcome and the echolalia is used to attain needs and thus is called functional. With further developmental progress, sufficient language comprehension is attained and correct grammar emerges. In the cases with the best outcome, grammatically correct complex sentence language is achieved between 5 and 6 years of age. Comprehension, though, remains below expressive language level, in that metaphoric and idiomatic language does not emerge automatically but must be taught. Use of language for communication is also abnormal in that at each level these individuals may have language but do not use it to ask for needs or to be social. Early on they do not know the basic elements of conversational etiquette or the mechanics of conversation, such as how to initiate, sustain, or appropriately terminate a conversation. It is also remarkable how even very long and sophisticated segments of talk can be scripted word for word.

Nonverbal Language

Impaired nonverbal communication is another defining characteristic of the ASDs. Abnormalities of prosodic language (see Chap. 59), both during development and at outcome, parallel those of left-hemisphere language. Speaking individuals with ASD may sound robotic, flat, and pedantic or "professor-like." Volume may be inappropriately loud or quiet.

Abnormalities in the quantity of eye contact are well known, but qualitative abnormalities have recently been emphasized, given the increase in high-functioning children who develop eye contact and the amount of training that is directed at achieving eye contact in ASD children. This impairment is seen earliest in the lack of eye contact to coordinate and share attention (joint attention, social referencing) with others, a skill evident around age 9 months among typically developing children. Later, qualitative abnormalities vary from eye gaze that is intrusive and persistent to atypical timing. A recent pilot study found that adults with ASD failed to use gaze to demonstrate a "listening response" while a social partner spoke with them. In either case, eye gaze is not used in a fluid, natural manner to demonstrate attentiveness to and social relatedness with others.

Expression and comprehension of facial affect are also abnormal. These individuals are often sober-faced. Alternatively, they have one expression, typically smiling, regardless of the situation. Facial expression has a parkinsonian character in that there is little or no affect or animation during social communication; if emotion originates internally though, the individual's face becomes animated. Comprehension of facial affect may be nonexistent throughout life, or comprehension of basic expressions, if dramatic, may develop. Interestingly, these deficits in comprehension are apparent in the way that individuals with ASD visually examine faces, focusing on details of faces and processing them as if they were objects.[12,13] In addition, they focus on the mouth region of the face rather than the eyes to ascertain emotion.[14] Using only photographs of the eyes, participants with high-functioning autism and Asperger's disorder, compared with normal adults, were impaired at recognizing complex mental states.[15]

Normally developing children use many gestures as part of coordinating focus and attention with others, including pointing and nods during conversation to indicate agreement or interest. Individuals with ASD often do not "check in" with a communicative partner to acknowledge understanding, as with the nod of the head or the shrug of the shoulders. Hand gestures during conversation may be nonexistent, clumsy, or awkward. In the first year of life, the absence of pointing to indicate needs and later interests are among the early signs of autism.

Imaginative Play

Interest in and appropriate use of toys for play is another area of delay and disturbance in ASD. In its most severe manifestation, there is no interest in toys, or the interest is in the taste, smell, or texture of the toys or in one piece of the toy. A slightly higher level of function involves lining up of the toys or hoarding or collecting them. With developmental progress, isolated appropriate actions emerge at first, and, later, sequences of actions, but play remains repetitive and does not have the imaginative quality seen in normal children. At a less impaired level of functioning, PDD children play with toys by emulating cartoons or videos verbatim.

The ability to pretend that one object is, in fact, a certain other object, known as meta-representation, is notably diminished among individuals with ASD. Beginning at around age $2\frac{1}{2}$ years, typically developing children begin to engage in pretend play. A block becomes a telephone, two sticks become an airplane, and a toy action figure can speak. Pretend play requires the ability to hold in mind two representations, what it is and, at the same time, what one is pretending it to be. Despite an interest in toys, moderately impaired children with autism show notable deficits in pretend play. Higher-functioning children with autism can be taught play sequences, but when asked to make up something new, they lack the ability to see things in any way other than the way they are from one's current perspective.

The typical developmental sequence of play with peers is also disturbed among children with ASD. Severely impaired children with ASD often do not interact with or even maintain proximity to peers during play. Parallel play can be observed among moderately to mildly impaired children with autism. At a mild degree of autistic impairment, greater degrees of cooperative interaction can be expected. The child with high-functioning autism will often help build the sand castle but then fail to reference his peers when he decides it is time to "knock it down." In other words, he attempts to interact and join in the cooperative play, but then lacks the ability to monitor his behavior and the reactions of others to keep the play truly cooperative. Another occurrence is for the child with Asperger's disorder to become a "social dictator." Hence, even at the highest level of functioning, children with Asperger's disorder tend to become stuck in the process of cooperative play, failing to achieve true cooperation.

Restricted Range of Interests and Activities

The final symptom category includes a number of diverse behaviors, but the common theme is a focus on details and a failure to understand the whole. These behavioral abnormalities include preoccupation with the sensory aspects of objects or the pieces of an object rather than the whole object, resistance to change or rituals for coping with change, and a narrow range of interests (collections or topics) with a focus on details. In all cases, there is a common focus on details and failure to appreciate the whole. Recent research suggests that the major cognitive determinants of this behavior are the abstraction deficit[16] and resulting dependence on piecemeal processing. One important study has demonstrated a dissociation between concept formation and concept identification abilities in nonretarded individuals with autism. Essentially, these individuals do not develop strategy or novel problem-solving abilities, nor do they form prototypes; consequently they are rule-bound and detail-oriented. These individuals rely on slow verbally mediated reasoning and classification; they lack the rapid automatic processing that includes concept-, prototype-, and strategy-formation abilities. For these individuals, rituals and sameness become a way of coping with change that is unpredictable because of the lack of concepts that normally provide the capacity to cope with variability in details while preserving an appreciation that the overall outcome remains the same. Less able individuals do not even develop rules or categories and are preoccupied with the elementary properties of objects. The most impaired individuals are oblivious to any meaning.

Associated Features

Some signs and symptoms are common in autism but are not considered diagnostic features of the disorder. These include hyperactivity with or without attention deficit disorder, alterations in sensory sensitivity (hyper- or hyposensitivity), delayed motor development, and apraxia.

Neurologic Examination

The neurologic examination is generally unremarkable except for subtle hypotonia and hyperreflexia. Head circumference is increased in autism. In pooled samples, the mean is shifted up to the 60 or 70th percentile, with the majority of autistic individuals having head circumferences above the 50th percentile and about 20 percent having macrocephaly (>97th percentile).[17–19] Macrocephaly is also present at increased rates among relatives.[20]

Complications in Individuals with PDD and in Family Members

Seizure disorder and affective disorder are two well-known complications of the PDDs. Both should be considered in the differential diagnosis of a sustained deterioration of function. The onset of seizure disorders is cumulative across the life span but has a peak in early childhood and a smaller peak at puberty. New onset of seizures can occur at any age, however. In the absence of tuberous sclerosis, seizures are usually secondarily generalized or partial complex in type, with the latter being especially difficult to detect because of the aberrant social behavior and attentional focus of individuals with autism. The tricyclic antidepressants and the traditional neuroleptics all lower the seizure threshold and can exacerbate or precipitate seizures in individuals with PDD. Even the newer neuroleptics are not without risk of precipitating seizures. The occurrence of depression has been thought to be more a complication of high-functioning individuals, reflecting the stress of being required to function in settings that exceed their social and emotional capability. Frequently high-functioning and especially nonretarded children and adolescents with PDD excel academically but have social and emotional capabilities that may be as low as those of a 2- or 3-year-old and rarely higher than those of a 7- to 10-year-old. Their inability to cope socially and emotionally leads to maladaptive behavior and depression, sometimes to the point of suicidal ideation and attempted suicide, while persistent efforts are made to continue them in this setting because of their academic success. Mania may also occur in autism but is far less common. Anxiety is a nearly universal accompaniment of PDD in individuals who are sufficiently aware of their environment to experience change or teasing by peers or to be cognizant of expectations and their inability to fulfill them. The relief of anxiety is thought to be the basis for the success of the selective serotonin reuptake inhibitors in improving function in individuals with PDD. Attention deficit disorder with or without hyperactivity may also co-occur with autism and may respond to traditional pharmacologic management.

Family members of individuals with PDD have an increased incidence of affective disorder, anxiety disorder, obsessive-compulsive disorder, and the broader autism phenotype or traits of autism. These conditions often go unrecognized and untreated, so that, although effective pharmacologic intervention is readily available, they interfere with the treatment of the child and the functioning of the family.

NEUROPSYCHOLOGY

This section is not intended to provide comprehensive coverage of the neuropsychology of autism but to highlight areas of most relevance or new findings. In the past, 75 percent of autistic individuals were mentally retarded with IQ scores below 70 and 25 percent were not mentally retarded. Recent prevalence studies have reported that as many as 40 to 50 percent are not mentally retarded, and a growing proportion of preschoolers have IQ scores in the normal range at the time of diagnosis. The introduction of the Asperger's Syndrome diagnosis in ICD-10 and DSM-IV has contributed to improved recognition of verbal school-age children and to a lesser extent adults with autism spectrum disorder.

Mental Retardation

Mental retardation in autism is part and parcel of autism and not the result of the chance co-occurrence of two rare disorders, which could not, in any case, explain the high frequency of this association. The mental retardation in autism is the more severe expression of the pattern of cognitive deficits and intact abilities seen in individuals with autism who are not mentally retarded. As a result, the mental retardation retains the peculiarities typical of cognition in autism, which distinguish it from mental retardation resulting from other conditions. In essence the distinguishing features are the marked dissociation between IQ scores and adaptive behavior scores, reflecting the disproportionate loss in social, language, and abstract reasoning skills with declining IQ, and the peculiarities of behavior. These higher-order skills are the basis of adaptive and flexible behavior in society and are not accurately assessed by IQ tests. IQ tests assess simpler abilities, and predictions about real-life function based on IQ scores depend on the degree to which simpler skills predict these higher-order abilities and thus on normal brain development. Behaviorally, mentally retarded individuals with autism can be distinguished from nonautistic mentally retarded individuals with comparable IQ scores by their much poorer social, verbal, and nonverbal language and reasoning abilities, the inability to use the skills they do have in these areas in a functional manner, and their greater facility with trivial details. In essence, mentally retarded autistic individuals are functionally much more retarded than their nonautistic mentally retarded peers. This distinction between autistic and nonautistic individuals with comparable IQ scores holds true across the IQ spectrum.

IQ Score Profiles

At Full Scale and Verbal IQ scores below 70, Verbal IQ is often significantly below Performance IQ. When Full Scale and Verbal IQ scores are above 80, this "prototypic" pattern is not present and most do not have a significant disparity; when present, it can be in either direction.[21] Essentially, the IQ test ceases to be a sensitive indicator of the language deficit in nonretarded individuals with autism. In terms of subtests, Comprehension is typically the lowest and Block Design the highest subtest scores. The Comprehension subtest assesses social, not language comprehension, and Block Design assesses visuospatial ability. In higher-ability individuals, the deviations are often not marked. The above "prototypes" are based on group analyses, but individual scores vary widely and none of these patterns can be used for diagnosis. In addition, many factors besides PDD can affect these scores.

Profile of Neuropsychological Functioning

The profile of neuropsychological functioning in autism has been examined to identify a shared feature of the deficits to determine why they might be occurring together as a syndrome. The most comprehensive of the few studies done to date involved 33 individually matched pairs of adults and community volunteers and found intact attention, sensory perception, elementary motor movements, memory for simple information, formal language (spelling, reading decoding, fluency), the rule-learning aspects of abstract reasoning, and visuospatial processing.[22] Deficits were present in motor praxis, memory for complex information (organizational strategies that support memory), the interpretative aspects of language, and concept formation. The implications of this profile were several, the most obvious of which was that information acquisition and visuospatial processing were intact. Deficits involved information processing abilities and, within those domains, the abilities that made the highest demands on complex information processing. The deficits respected domains, and thus complexity was determined within domain rather than across domains. This profile, therefore, suggested that autism was a disorder of information processing that disproportionately impacted complex information processing. In applying this construct across the autism spectrum, the severity of autism is equivalent to the overall information processing capacity, while the autistic quality of the symptoms is preserved by the disproportionate impact on complex information processing at all levels of severity. The involvement of the motor domain, an area of relatively minor symptom involvement in today's society, suggests that the neuropathology involves a general architectural feature of the brain. This profile has now been replicated in a separate sample of adults and in a study of nonretarded children with autism. A similar neuropsychological profile has been observed in mildly mentally retarded autistic children.[23] Often, difficulties in function can be understood in terms of information processing demands, and reduction of these demands is effective in improving compliance and reducing behavior problems.

Part-Whole Processing

Another issue related to information processing that has been emphasized in autism is the performance advantage these individuals exhibit when piecemeal or local processing imparts an advantage. Thus, they are resistant to illusions and outperform controls on an embedded figures test.[24–26] However, for the same reason, they also have difficulty with face recognition and facial affect recognition, which require holistic processing. These issues are fascinating areas of research which involve the reciprocal cognitive and neural relationship between piecemeal or local processing and strategy or prototype formation. The failure of the latter cognitive abilities and neural substrate to develop leaves autistic individuals reliant on more elementary abilities and circuitry to perform tasks.[27]

Attention

Individuals with ASD may have attention deficit disorder, but it is not causative of their autistic symptoms. Purported deficits in shifting attention have been demonstrated to be deficits in executive function.[28,29]

Sensory Perception

Individuals with autism frequently complain of hypo- or hypersensitivity to sound, touch, and light, and nonverbal children have been reported to calm with sensory pressure or other input. These symptoms can be quite disabling, and yet there are no objective data regarding their neurologic basis. Evoked potential studies have demonstrated normal latencies and, in non-retarded individuals, normal perception of stimuli, so there is essentially no insight into the physiologic basis of this symptom. The only objective finding to date is that fingertip number writing is abnormal in a substantial percentage of nonretarded individuals with autism. These sensory perceptual distortions could be related to abnormal cortical integration or to abnormalities in thalamic gating.

Motor Function

A motor impairment is now widely accepted to be an integral part of the ASDs. The best-documented deficit involves motor praxis. Early in life, it may be apparent in the suboptimal formation of sign language. In higher-ability children, it is seen in their difficulty with scissors, crayons, tying shoes, handwriting, and motor coordination during walking and running. Gait is often visibly abnormal. A parkinsonian facies has also been described for decades, though its neurologic significance has been underappreciated.

Memory and Learning

Despite an early false analogy to amnesia, many studies have since demonstrated that basic memory processes are intact in autism. However, there is an inefficiency of memory and learning related to the failure to efficiently use organizational strategies to support memory. Thus, memory for simple material is intact but memory for larger amounts of material or material whose structure is inherently complex is deficient.[30] The particular test and material that will elicit deficits will depend on the general level of ability of the individual, as complexity or simplicity is relative to ability level. The implications of this deficit are that memory and learning can be improved by reducing the amount of material, preprocessing it, giving the bottom line, and increasing the processing time.

The impact of the memory deficit (which is actually a deficit in concept formation) on adaptive function has been demonstrated by Boucher[31] in a study of memory for a recently experienced event; she found that autistic children remembered less about a play activity than language-matched peers. Boucher proposed that autistic individuals would have difficulty with social situations because of the complexity of the information and the demands this would place on memory. In a recent study, Williams and colleagues[32] examined the memory of autistic individuals for common social scenes and found they remembered less about common daily activities than matched controls. The ability of normal individuals to rapidly process and make sense of information enables them to cope with voluminous amounts of information. Having to deal with information without such organizing and processing capacities results in loss of information and considerable reduction in function.

Language

Enormous amounts have been written about the language impairment in autism.[33] Perhaps the most important clinical issue to emphasize is that these individuals are hyperlexic regardless of language level. Their comprehension is always below their expressive level. This means that what they mean by what they say is always different from what normal individuals mean if they say the same thing. It also means that they may do what the rule says they should *not* do while they are saying the rule. Thus, it is critical to constantly monitor what their function demonstrates their comprehension to be. In addition, they do not understand the idioms, metaphors, irony, and satire that adults learning English as a second language typically do not understand. Finally, their acquisition of information is reduced across all language modalities and nonverbal input deficits are often underestimated in terms of their contribution to communication.

TREATMENT

Though not well appreciated, the first line of intervention in autism should be management of the environment: the physical environment, the people, and the events. Because of their deficits, individuals with autism are unable or slow to process information and are easily overwhelmed by the environment. They function best when the environment is highly structured and supervised, which means that the world is simplified, interactions are limited and superficial, known rules govern actions, events and people are predictable, and they are protected from scapegoating. This type of environment has the equivalent therapeutic effect to neuroleptics in schizophrenia. No medication will accomplish in autism what this type of environment will.

Behavioral intervention should be approached with a full understanding of the autistic quality of these people's deficits and behaviors, as approaches used in other disabilities are not suitable for autism. Early childhood intervention programs are a current major focus in autism. A number of programs have reported improvement in outcome in children participating in preschool programs that involve 15 to 40 h of school-based intervention. These programs report substantial gains in IQ by school age, with 50 percent participating in mainstream education classes; this does not, however, mean that the children did not have significant deficits at outcome.[34] Also, the only true replication study to date has failed to demonstrate improvement in outcome with early intensive intervention.[35] Most such programs have had selection criteria that identify those children with evidence of communicative intent at entry to the program, the absence of dysmorphic features, and the absence of high rates of stereotypic behavior. Some programs also exclude children who fail to make progress after a few months. These selection criteria capitalize on early signs of less severe autism. It is not clear whether such programs would be equally effective in lower ability autistic children, nor is it clear how many hours of intervention are needed to achieve an optimal response. The National Research Council has published a comprehensive report entitled *Educating Children with Autism,*[36] which is essential reading for all involved in making or implementing treatment recommendations. Dawson's chapter reviews a number of programs reporting success in autism. Each of the programs has a different approach, but all focus on training five basic skills.[37] The first is the ability to attend to people and to cooperate with teaching exercises. The second is the ability to imitate others, both verbal imitation and motor imitation. The third is the ability to comprehend and use language. Most teaching strategies provide immediate positive reward to the child's smallest attempt to communicate, such as a glance or slightest body movement. The fourth domain is the ability to play appropriately with toys, and the fifth is the ability to interact socially with others.

All of these programs involve Applied Behavior Analysis (ABA), a method in common parlance and essential knowledge to all dealing with autistic children. The principles of ABA involve manipulating the environment to effectively reduce maladaptive behaviors, such as self-injury and aggression, as well as to teach functional skills including speech, academic skills, ability to sustain attention, fine and gross motor skills, language comprehension, and daily living skills. Reinforcement, extinction, chaining, and shaping are four basic techniques of ABA frequently used as part of intervention programs for individuals with autism. When tasks are broken down into their component parts and skills are taught through massed rote trials, individuals with ASD eventually develop some of the abilities that typically developing individuals gain through incidental learning.

Behavior modification has provided empirically demonstrated treatment gains to individuals with autism through functional analysis and treatment of self-injurious and self-stimulatory behavior, teaching appropriate skills, and building language.[34,36] A number of programs have reported substantial improvement in outcome in children participating in preschool programs that involve 15 to 40 h of school-based intervention.[37] Methods of ABA have been used to teach functional communication skills through the Picture Exchange Communication System (PECS)[38]; functional speech, daily living, and play skills through video modeling[39]; and language, imitation, and academic skills through discrete trial procedures.[34] Visual strategies, such as photographic activity schedules, are helpful to enhance independent functioning through the sequencing of tasks into component parts.[40] Further, treatments are beginning to be developed that focus primarily on the social deficits of persons with ASD. For example, the Relationship Development Intervention[10,11] provides an intervention approach to teach joint attention and experience sharing by breaking down the skills needed for successful interpersonal relatedness into component parts, which are then reinforced primarily through enjoyable social encounters.

NEUROPATHOLOGY

Relatively few neuropathologic studies, involving approximately 24 whole-brain specimens, have been performed in autism.[41–43] The initial study of 19 cases reported several major findings. The first was an increase in brain weight in children and average brain weight in adults. The second was a substantial increase in neuronal cell-packing density in the hippocampus, areas of the amygdala, entorhinal cortex, septum, mammillary body, and anterior cingulate gyrus. The increase in cell-packing density was the result of a 60 to 90 percent increase in neuronal number, a reduction in neuronal size, and decreased number and length of dendritic branches—signs of developmental immaturity. A third finding involved a 50 to 60 percent reduction in Purkinje cells in the posteroinferior regions of the cerebellar hemispheres. This was accompanied by abnormalities in the emboliform, globose, fastigial, and dentate nuclei; in children, the neurons were enlarged and numerous, whereas in adults, they were reduced in size and number. The olivary nuclei likewise displayed small pale neurons in adults and enlarged plentiful neurons in children. The preservation of the olivary neurons in the face of marked reduction in the Purkinje cells was indicative of an onset of these disturbances in circuitry prior to 28 to 30 weeks of gestation. A more recent study reported additional findings of megalencephaly in four of six adult brains and a variety of developmental abnormalities of the cerebral cortex.[41] Most recently, Casanova and colleagues[43] have reported bilateral increase in the minicolumns or vertical columnar units of cerebral cortex in autism. In order for the increased number of minicolumns to maintain local and distant cortical connections, it would require an increase in connections that would result in an increase in white matter.[43]

NEUROIMAGING

Structural Imaging

The most common clinical neuroimaging finding in autism is that of normal neuroanatomy when cases of autism secondary to other disorders such as tuberous sclerosis, fetal rubella, or fetal cytomegalovirus are excluded. Mild to moderate enlargement of the lateral ventricles is occasionally seen but is not related to hydrocephalus or to the severity of autism; thus its significance is unknown. Because gross anatomic abnormalities are not an integral part of this syndrome, routine scanning is not recommended in children with autism spectrum disorders in the absence of other neurologic indicators of a need for further investigation.[9]

Reports of imaging abnormalities in autism are based on research protocols and quantitative measurements rather than clinically apparent imaging abnormalities. These abnormalities are not diagnostic and are based on group differences, not individual differences. The most significant neuroradiologic abnormality to be reported in the past 5 years has been an increase in total supratentorial brain volume in children with autism, which has been a consistent finding of several studies.[44–46] The increase in total brain volume appears to be present by 3 years of age, the youngest age for which imaging data are available, and appears to normalize at puberty as a result of brain growth in the normal population and a slight reduction in brain size in the autistic population.[44–46] Both gray and white matter volumes are increased. In the posterior fossa, the cerebellar hemispheres are also increased in volume.[44,45] The significance of this increase in white matter volume appears to be related to the abnormality in cerebral cortical minicolumns and the accompanying developmental abnormalities in neural connectivity. The early overgrowth concludes with the onset of symptoms in the second year of life, disrupting the development of the intricate circuitry that underlies the emergence of social language, and reasoning abilities.

Several studies have reported a reduction in the area of the corpus callosum, though the region involved has varied from anterior to posterior.[47–49] Such abnormalities suggest fewer myelinated fibers and reduced interhemispheric connectivity.

Functional Magnetic Resonance Imaging

Because of the invasiveness of methods used before the development of magnetic resonance imaging (MRI), there are limited functional imaging data with such methods. Two early studies are of interest because they presage fMRI findings that will appear in the literature in the next 2 to 3 years. A positron emission tomography study with 2,3 DPG[50] reported a reduction in the intra- and interhemispheric connectivity of frontal and parietal cortices with both cortical and subcortical regions. A second study[51] reported delayed maturation of the frontal lobes in 3- to 5-year-old autistic children using single photon emission computed tomography (SPECT) to study blood flow.

Only a few fMRI studies have been published so far, but many such studies are in progress and in various stages of the publication process. Functional MRI studies of individuals with high-functioning autism and Asperger's disorder demonstrated that they did not activate the amygdala when trying to discern emotional expression from eyes and faces.[52,53] Studies using theory-of-mind tasks have in one case shown failure to activate the left medial prefrontal gyrus[54] and in another the amygdala.[52]

Studies of face recognition have reported that autistic subjects did not activate fusiform gyrus but instead activated inferior temporal gyrus, a region that normal subjects activate when viewing objects.[13] Within the field of visual cognition, there is active debate as to whether the fusiform area is specialized for faces or is an area of expertise used for all difficult distinctions. Studies have shown that architects activate the fusiform or "face area" when making refined distinctions in their areas of expertise. In autism, the significant implication is that clinically they have difficulty processing complex information, in this case faces, and their neural circuitry lacks the specialization to process this information.

Two PET studies of serotonin receptors have been completed, but sample sizes have been small and results therefore preliminary. The most significant reported that the autistic children had a gradual increase in serotonin levels between 2 and 15 years of age, in contrast to the high levels of synthesis until 5 years of age in normal children, which decline thereafter.[55]

PATHOPHYSIOLOGY

Ideas about the pathophysiology of autism have continued to evolve with research findings. Up until a few years ago, autism was thought to be the result of a single primary cognitive deficit and an anatomic abnormality in a single brain structure. Autism is now generally thought to be a disorder of multiple primary deficits resulting from underdevelopment of selected neural systems.

The major cognitive deficits proposed in recent years to underlie autism involve executive function, shifting attention, theory of mind, central coherence, and complex information processing. The executive dysfunction model subsequently ceased to be a viable hypothesis because of the emergence of studies demonstrating this deficit was not universally present in autism.[56] The deficit in shifting attention also proposed to underlie much of the symptomatology in autism has been shown by several studies to be a deficit in executive function, not in attention.[28,58] The theory of mind deficit, though a major contribution to the neurobehavior of autism, was not sufficient to accommodate the nonsocial deficits in autism such as abstraction, nonverbal language, and motor abilities. The central coherence theory or lack of drive to make sense of the environment was derived from the same constellation of deficits in higher-order abilities that gave rise to the complex information processing theory, and the terms are essentially synonymous. However, the term *central coherence* is unknown outside the field of autism and substitutes a new term for traditional terms used to describe well-known neuropsychological deficits. The disadvantage of central coherence theory is that it does not readily accommodate deficits in motor skills or nonverbal language or expressive language. *Complex information processing* is a general term that is used in most disciplines and is broad enough to accommodate both cognitive and noncognitive deficits as well as expressive and receptive deficits. It also makes it relatively easy to relate these deficits to neurophysiologic abnormalities in autism and to classes of neural circuitry that might be relevant.

Autism is now generally viewed as a neural systems disorder rather than a disorder of one or more brain regions. These systems involve neocortex, limbic structures, and cerebellum, but the relative contributions of these structures to the function of the affected neural systems is debated.[41,42,57,58] Other brain structures are also likely to be involved. Abnormalities in face recognition suggest that specialization of regional circuitry may also be affected, in addition to distributed neural networks. The next decade promises to bring exciting revelations about the neurobiology of autism and this entire category of disorders.

REFERENCES

1. American Psychiatric Association: *Diagnostic and Statistic Manual of Mental Disorders,* 4th ed, Text Revision (DSM-IV-TR). Washington, DC: American Psychiatric Association, 2000.
2. Baird G, Charman T, Baron-Cohen S, et al: A screening instrument for autism at 18 months of age: a 6-year follow-up study. *J Am Acad Child Adolesc Psychiatry* 39(6):694–702, 2000.
3. Bertrand J, Mars A, Boyle C, et al: Prevalence of autism in a United States Population: The Brick Township, New Jersey Investigation. *Pediatrics* 108(5):1155–1161, 2001.
4. Chakrabarti S, Fombonne E: Pervasive developmental disorders in preschool children. *JAMA* 285:3093–3099, 2001.
5. Perisco AM, Agruma LD, Maiorano N, et al: Reelin gene alleles and haplotypes as a factor predisposing to autistic disorder. *Mol Psychiatry* 6:150–159, 2001.
6. Cook EH Jr, Courchesne RY, Cox NJ, et al: Linkage-disequilibrium mapping of autistic disorder with 15q11-13 markers. *Am J Hum Genet* 62:1077–1083, 1998.
7. Gillberg C: Chromosomal disorders and autism. *J Autism Dev Disord* 28:415–425, 1998.
8. International Molecular Genetic Study of Autism Consortium (IMGSAC): A genomewide screen for autism: Strong evidence for linkage to chromosomes 2q, 7q, and 16p. *Am J Hum Genet* 69:570–581, 2001.
9. Filipek PA, Accardo PJ, Baranek GT: The screening and diagnosis of autistic spectrum disorders. *J Autism Dev Disord* 29(6):439–484, 1999.
10. Mundy P, Sigman M: Specifying the nature of the social impairment in autism, in Dawson G (ed): *Autism: Nature, Diagnosis, and Treatment.* New York: Guilford Press, 1989.
11. Gutstein SE: *Autism and Asperger's: Solving the Relationship Puzzle.* Arlington, TX: Future Horizons, 2000.
12. Hobson RP, Ouston, J, Lee A: What's in a face? The case of autism. *Br J Psychol* 79:441–453, 1988.
13. Schultz RT, Gauthier I, Klin A, et al: Abnormal ventral temporal cortical activity among individuals with autism and Asperger syndrome during face discrimination. *Arch Gen Psychiatry* 57:331–340, 2000.
14. Klin A, Jones W, Schultz R, et al: Defining and quantifying the social phenotype in autism. *Am J Psychiatry* 159(6):895–908.
15. Baron-Cohen S, Wheelwright S, Jolliffe T: Is there a "language of the eyes"? Evidence from normal adults, adults with autism or Asperger syndrome. *Vis Cogn* 4(3):311–331, 1997.
16. Minshew NJ, Meyer J, Goldstein G: Abstract reasoning in autism: a dissociation between concept formation and concept identification. *Neuropsychology* 16(3):327–334.
17. Fombonne E, Roge B, Claverie J, et al: Microcephaly and macrocephaly in autism. *J Autism Dev Disord* 29(2):113–119, 1999.
18. Lainhart JE, Piven J, Wrozek M, et al: Macrocephaly in children and adults with autism. *J Am Acad Child Adolesc Psychiatry* 36:282–290, 1997.
19. Fidler DJ, Bailey JN, Smalley SL: Macrocephaly in autism and other pervasive developmental disorders. *Dev Med Child Neurol* 42(11):737–740, 2000.
20. Miles JH, Hadden LL, Takahashi TN, et al: Head circumference is an independent clinical finding associated with autism. *Am J Med Genet* 95(4):339–350, 2000.
21. Siegel DJ, Minshew NJ, Goldstein G: Wechsler IQ profiles in diagnosis of high functioning autism. *J Autism Dev Disord* 26(4):389–406, 1996.
22. Minshew NJ, Goldstein G, Siegel DJ: Neuropsychological functioning in autism: Profile of a complex information processing disorder. *J Int Neuropsychol Soc* 3:303–316, 1997.
23. Fein D, Dunn M, Allen DA, et al: Language and neuropsychological findings, in Rapin I (ed): *Preschool Children with Inadequate Communication: Developmental Language Disorder, Autism, Low IQ: Clinics in Development Medicine.* Cambridge, UK: Cambridge University Press, 1996, vol 139, pp 123–154.
24. Happe FG: Studying weak central coherence at low levels: children with autism do not succumb to visual illusions. A research note. *J Child Psychol Psychiatry Allied Disc* 37(7):873–877, 1996.
25. Jolliffe T, Baron-Cohen S: Are people with autism and Asperger syndrome faster than normal on the Embedded Figures Test? *J Child Psychol Psychiatry Allied Disc* 38(5):527–534, 1997.
26. Shah A, Frith U: Why do autistic individuals show superior performance on the block design task? *J Child Psychol Psychiatry* 34:1351–1363, 1993.
27. Luna B, Minshew NJ, Garver KE, et al: Neocortical system abnormalities in autism: an fMRI study of spatial working memory. *Neurology* 59(6):834–840.
28. Goldstein G, Johnson CR, Minshew NJ: Attentional processes in autism. *J Autism Dev Disord* 31(4):433–440.
29. Pascualvaca DM, Fantie BO, Papageorgiou, et al: Attentional capacities in children with autism: Is there a

general deficit in shifting focus? *J Autism Dev Disord* 28:467–478.

30. Minshew NJ, Goldstein G: The pattern of intact and impaired memory functions in autism. *J Child Psychiatry* 42(8):1095–1101, 2001.
31. Boucher J: Memory for recent events in autistic children. *J Autism Dev Disord* 11(3):293–301, 1981.
32. Williams DL, Minshew NJ, Goldstein G: Impaired memory for faces and social scenes in autism: clinical implications of the memory disorder. *Arch Clin Neuropsychol.* In press.
33. Tager-Flusberg H: Understand the language and communicative impairments in autism. *Int Rev Res Ment Retard* 23:185–205, 2001.
34. Lovaas OI, Schreibman L, Koegel RL: A behavior modification approach to the treatment of autistic children. *J Autism Child Schizophr* 4(2):111–129, 1974.
35. Smith T, Eikeseth S, Klevstrand M, et al: Intensive behavioral treatment for preschoolers with severe mental retardation and pervasive developmental disorder. *Am J Ment Retard* 102(3):238–249, 1997.
36. Committee on Education Interventions for Children with Autism, Division of Behavioral and Social Sciences and Education, and National Research Council: *Educating Children with Autism.* Washington, DC: National Academy Press, 2001.
37. Dawson G, Osterling J: Early intervention in autism, in Guralnick MJ (ed): *The Effectiveness of Early Intervention.* Baltimore, MD: Brookes, 1997, pp 307–325.
38. Bondy AS, Frost LA: The picture exchange communication system. *Semin Speech Lang* 19(4):373–388, 1998.
39. Charlop-Christy MH, Le L, Freeman KA: A comparison of video modeling with in vivo modeling for teaching children with autism. *J Autism Dev Disord* 30(6):537–552, 2000.
40. MacDuff GS, Krantz PJ, McClannahan LE: Teaching children with autism to use photographic activity schedules: maintenance and generalization of complex response chains. *J Appl Behav Anal* 26(1):89–97, 1993.
41. Bailey A, Luthert P, Dean A, et al: A clinicopathological study of autism. *Brain* 121(Pt 5):889–905, 1998.
42. Bauman ML, Kemper TL: Is autism a progressive process? *Neurology* 48:A285, 1997.
43. Casanova MF, Buxhoereden DP, Switala AE, et al: Minicolumnor pathology in autism. *Neurology* 58:428–432, 2002.
44. Courchesne E, Karns CM, Davis HR, et al: Unusual brain growth patterns in early life in patients with autistic disorder: an MRI study. *Neurology* 57(2):245–254, 2001.
45. Sparks BF, Friedman SD, Shaw DW, et al: Brain structural abnormalities in young children with autism spectrum disorder. *Neurology* 59(2):184–192.
46. Aylward EH, Minshew NJ, Field K, et al: Effects of age on brain volume and head circumference in autism. *Neurology* 59(2):175–183.
47. Egaas B, Courchesne E, Saitoh O: Reduced size of corpus callosum in autism. *Arch Neurol* 52(8):794–801, 1995.
48. Hardan AY, Minshew NJ, Keshavan MS: Corpus callosum size in autism. *Neurology* 55(7):1033–1036, 2000.
49. Piven J, Bailey J, Ranson BJ, et al: An MRI study of the corpus callosum in autism. *Am J Psychiatry* 154(8):1051–1056, 1997.
50. Horwitz B, Rapoport SI: Partial correlation coefficients approximate the real intrasubject correlation pattern in the analysis of interregional relations of cerebral metabolic activity. *J Nucl Med* 29:392–399, 1988.
51. Zilbovicius M, Garreau B, Samson Y, et al: Delayed maturation of the frontal cortex in childhood autism. *Am J Psychiatry* 152(2):248–252, 1995.
52. Baron-Cohen S, Ring HA, Wheelwright S, et al: Social intelligence in the normal and autistic brain: an fMRI study. *Eur J Neurosci* 11:1891–1898, 1999.
53. Critchley HD, Daly EM, Bullmore ET, et al: The functional neuroanatomy of social behavior: changes in cerebral blood flow when people with autistic disorder process facial expressions. *Brain* 123:2203–2212, 2000.
54. Happé F, Ehlers S, Fletcher P, et al: "Theory of mind" in the brain. Evidence from a PET scan study of Asperger syndrome. *Neuroreport* 8:197–201, 1996.
55. Chugani DC, Muzik O, Behen M, et al: Developmental changes in brain serotonin synthesis capacity in autistic and non-autistic children. *Ann Neurol* 45(3):287–295, 1999.
56. Minshew NJ, Goldstein G, Muenz LR, et al: Neuropsychological functioning in nonmentally retarded autistic individuals. *J Clin Exp Neuropsych* 14:749–761.
57. Carper RA, Courchesne E: Inverse correlation between frontal lobe and cerebellum sizes in children with autism. *Brain* 123(Pt 4):836–844, 2000.
58. Minshew NJ, Luna B, Sweeney JA: Oculomotor evidence for neocortical systems but not cerebellar dysfunction in autism. *Neurology* 52(5):917–922, 1999.

Chapter 69

MOLECULAR GENETICS OF COGNITIVE DEVELOPMENTAL DISORDERS

James Swanson
John Fossella
Deborah Grady
Robert Moyzis
Pam Flodman
Anne Spence
Michael Posner

Three disorders of childhood with important cognitive developmental components are addressed in this chapter: attention deficit hyperactivity disorder (ADHD), reading disorder (RD), and autistic spectrum disorder (ASD). The phenotypes (behavioral manifestations of these disorders) are discussed in Chaps. 66, 64, and 68, respectively. The cognitive neuroscience approach to understanding both phenotype and genotype (variations in DNA) to these disorders is discussed in a recent report by Posner et al.[1]

A first step in molecular genetic studies of ADHD, RD, and ASD is to find variations in DNA (genotypes) that may be associated with and linked to behavior of individuals with these psychopathologies (phenotypes). Two approaches are generally used to accomplish this: the genome scan approach and the candidate gene approach. The candidate gene approach starts with a hypothesis about a specific gene at a known chromosomal location, perhaps suggested by theories of the biological basis of etiology or treatment of the condition under investigation, and then tests whether a specific genotype is statistically associated with the disorder. The genome scan does not make such an assumption but instead starts with genetic markers spread across the entire genome and attempts to locate chromosomal regions by statistical methods (e.g., by finding markers that are shared at a greater-than-chance rate by affected relatives and thus are likely to be in chromosome regions harboring genes associated with and linked to the disorder). In general, the genome scan approach is most useful if the underlying genes are few, and their effect on predisposing risk is large. On the other hand, the candidate gene approach is more sensitive if the number of predisposing genes is large, and/or their individual effect on risk is small.

In this chapter, we present sections on some typical methods that are used to specify phenotypes of ADHD, RD, and ASD and some example methods used to specify genotypes used to investigate these disorders. Next we provide a brief review of quantitative statistical genetic methods that have been used to suggest a strong genetic basis for these three disorders. Then we will present a selective review of the literature of molecular genetic studies of ADHD, RD, and ASD, which fortunately provides excellent examples of candidate gene and genome scan approaches used to investigate genotype-phenotype relationships. Finally, we discuss the recent findings in each area that may point to important directions for future investigation of the genetics of cognitive developmental disorders.

PHENOTYPES OF ADHD, RD, AND ASD

One way in which phenotypes of ADHD, RD, and ASD have been specified is through clinical diagnosis of a psychiatric disorder. The criteria for clinical diagnoses are provided in the fourth edition of the American Psychiatric Association's *Diagnostic and Statistical Manual* (DSM-IV).[2] DSM-IV uses a categorical classification system that separates "mental" disorders into types based on consensus criteria (defining features) that are hierarchically organized. ADHD, RD, and ASD are classified as "Disorders Usually First Diagnosed in Infancy, Childhood, or Adolescence," which imposes a broad and overarching early age-of-onset criterion. This section of DSM-IV distinguishes 10 classes, each with multiple disorders having some common qualifying features: Mental Retardation, Learning Disorders (where RD is placed), Motor Skills Disorders, Communication Disorders, Pervasive Developmental Disorders (where ASD is placed), Attention-Deficit and Disruptive Behavior Disorders (where ADHD is placed), Feeding and Eating Disorders, Tic Disorders, Elimination Disorders, and Other Disorders. The DSM-IV criteria for ADHD, RD, and ASD are shown in Table 69-1.

The DSM-IV approach has an emphasis on phenomenology, not etiologies (which for psychiatric disorders are still treated as unknowns), and on reliability, not validity of diagnoses. DSM-IV is a categorical system, with diagnosis (classification) based on the presence of abnormal patterns of behavior assumed to be qualitatively different from the pattern of normal behavior in the population. This is appropriate when the boundaries between classes are clear, when the classes are mutually exclusive, and when within-class homogeneity is high. For ADHD, RD, and ASD, these conditions may not hold, so the use of the categorical system of DSM-IV and the qualitative psychiatric diagnoses that it generates may not be optimal for specifying phenotypes to be used in genetic investigations. Dimensional descriptions of phenotypes of these cognitive developmental disorders have been used, based on quantification of attributes that are distributed continuously and do not have clear boundaries to define separate categories of psychopathology.

Table 69-1
DSM-IV criteria for three cognitive developmental disorders

ADHD (DSM-IV, pp. 78–85):
- (a) age-inappropriate levels of inattention and/or impulsivity/hyperactivity (at least 6 of 9 symptoms present in one or both domains)
- (b) onset by the age of 7 years
- (c) impairment in two or more settings
- (d) interference with appropriate functioning
- (e) not better accounted for by other psychiatric disorders

RD (DSM-IV, pp. 48–50):
- (a) a discrepancy between ability and achievement
- (b) significant impairment in activities that require reading
- (c) difficulties not solely due to a sensory deficit

ASD (DSM-IV, pp. 66–71):
- (a) impaired social interaction
- (b) impaired language used in social communication
- (c) restricted patterns of behavior

A typical way to provide a quantitative description of a disorder is to use rating scales to obtain a subjective impression of the degree of behavior that defines or underlies the disorder. For example, in the assessment of ADHD, two rating scales are freely available on the Internet: the Swanson, Nolan, and Pelham (SNAP) scale of Swanson et al.[3] and the Strengths and Difficulties Questionnaire (SDQ) of Goodman et al.[4] The SNAP (*www.ADHD.net*) asks for ratings of the degree of psychopathology defined by the 18 DSM-IV symptoms of ADHD, using a scale of 0 to 3 (e.g., not at all = 0, just a little = 1, pretty much = 2, and very much = 3). The SDQ (*www.sdqinfo.com*) asks for ratings of the presence of 30 common behavioral and emotional difficulties of childhood, 5 of which are designated as ADHD items, using a scale of 0 to 2 (not present = 0, present = 1, or very much present = 2). For both the SNAP and SDQ, the sum of the ADHD items or the average rating per item assigns a severity score that can be used as a quantitative phenotype of ADHD. There are many commercial versions of ADHD rating scales available. Tharpar et al.[5] provide a recent review of the quantitative phenotype of ADHD.

For the assessment of ASD, the Autism Screening Questionnaire (ASQ), also known as the Social Communication Questionnaire (SCQ), is a 40-item screening instrument based on DSM-IV criteria and the Autism Diagnostic Interview-Revised.[6,7] The SCQ is not available on the Internet. The Checklist for Autism in Toddlers (CHAT) also provides a quantitative description of ASD for screening at 18 months of age,[6] based on five items about simple pretend play and joint attention that are assessed by parental report and direct testing. Baird et al.[7] provide a review of a variety of instruments that have been used to define the quantitative phenotypes of ASD.

In the assessment of RD, scores on psychometric tests (e.g., the discrepancy between IQ and achievement test scores) are part of the criteria for RD and provide a quantitative description of the disorder. In fact, IQ-achievement discrepancy cutoffs are specified in psychiatric manuals[2,8] and educational laws and regulations.[9] The current view is that the distribution of IQ-reading achievement discrepancies is smooth and normal, suggesting a quantitative, not qualitative, phenotype that places an individual on a continuum not in a category (see Ref. 10). However, the use of an IQ-achievement discrepancy has been questioned and the use of low achievement alone has been suggested as an alternative.[11] In some molecular genetic studies of RD, composite reading scores rather than discrepancy scores have been used.[12] Furthermore, multidimensional phenotypes of RD have been proposed that are not directly related to the DSM or IDEA criteria for diagnoses, based on auditory (phonologic awareness) and visual (orthographic decoding) processes, and these phenotypes have been used in molecular genetic studies of RD (e.g., Ref. 13). Schulte-Korne[14] provides a recent review that includes discussion of methods to define quantitative phenotypes of RD.

BEHAVIORAL (QUANTITATIVE) GENETICS

Family and twin studies of ADHD, ASD, and RD have been conducted and provide evidence of genetic bases of these disorders. These studies capitalize on the statistical properties of relatives, which can be used to evaluate whether individuals who are exposed to similar genetic factors have similar phenotypes. For example, the coefficient of relationship (R) shows the proportion of alleles shared identical-by-descent from one relative to another (or from a common ancestor). For monozygotic twins, R = 1 and for dizygotic twins R = 1/2. For first-degree relatives (parent-offspring, full siblings), R = 1/2; for second-degree relatives (uncles, aunts), R = 1/4; for third-degree relatives (first grandparents, cousins), R = 1/8 and so on (fourth degree, R = 1/16; fifth degree, R = 1/32; etc.). Thus, relatives of an individual with a disorder (e.g., ADHD, RD, or ASD) can be chosen who share genotypes to a different degree (100 percent, 50 percent, 25 percent, 12.5 percent, etc). Two important statistical terms are used to describe the results of family and twin studies of the genetics of ADHD, RD, and ASD: relative or recurrence risk (RR) and heritability (h^2).

To estimate RR, the population prevalence of the disorder and the prevalence of the disorder in different classes of relatives of the affected individual are obtained. Then, RR ratios (lambdas) are used to estimate the risks to relatives with different degrees of genetic relationship. Heritability (h^2) is defined as the ratio of genetic variance to phenotypic variance, but in a twin study it can be estimated from the observed correlation of phenotype and genotype in two types of twins (identical or monozygotic and fraternal or dizygotic). In a twin study, the genotypic correlation for monozygotic twins (1.0) and dizygotic twins (0.5) is known, and the correlations of phenotype across sets of the two types of twin pairs can be estimated. The difference in the correlations of the groups composed of monozygotic or dizygotic is used to estimate heritability: $h^2 = 2(r_{mz} - r_{dz})$. Even though heritabilty may change in different settings or for different measures of the phenotype, it is used as a way to estimate the percentage of total variation in the phenotype that may be due to genetic factors (whatever they might be).

Many family, twin, and adoption studies have been conducted to investigate the behavioral genetics of ADHD, RD, and ASD. For all three of these cognitive developmental disorders, estimates of lambda and h^2 are high and suggest that genetic factors play a large role in the etiologies of these disorders. Reviews of these studies are provides by Stevenson[15] and Faraone et al.[16] for ADHD, Pennington[17] and Schulte-Korne[14] for RD, and Smalley et al.[18] and Bailey et al.[19] for ASD.

These studies firmly establish that genetic factors play an important role in determining phenotype, but specific genetic factors are not uncovered by behavioral or quantitative genetic methods. Molecular genetic methods have this purpose, and some background on molecular genetics is provided in the next section.

Candidate gene studies are evaluated by simple statistical methods. For a population-based design, DNA is obtained from a group of affected probands and an unaffected (or randomly selected) control group. The prevalence of alleles (or a genotype) of the candidate gene are compared for the two groups, and a simple chi-square test is used to determine if the difference is statistically significant. In a family-based design, DNA is obtained from parents of the group of affected probands as well as from the affected probands. An initial step is to determine which two alleles (or genotype) were transmitted and which two were not transmitted to the child. For example, for four parental alleles (two for each parent), one allele from each parent (two of the four) are transmitted to the proband. The Transmission Disequilibrium Test (TDT) is used to determine whether the risk allele is "transmitted" more frequently than expected by chance in the group of affected probands. The alleles not transmitted represent a theoretical control group. A chi-square statistic is used to estimate if the candidate allele (or genotype) is prepresented at a greater-than-chance prevalence in the sample of affected probands. It is assumed that the actual transmission rate at meiosis is .5, but that the condition probability of having the disorder and being in the clinical group of affected probands is increased if the candidate allele increases risk for the disorder (or is close to a gene that does, and thus is in "linkage disequilibrium" with a risk allele).

Genome scan studies evaluate the marker alleles spread across the human genome. In an affected sibling design, families are recruited that have two children with the same disorder. DNA from the affected sib pair is used to determine the alleles present in markers spread across the genome. If the marker and the as-yet-unknown risk gene are far apart, then it is likely that recombination events over time would have separated them, but if they are close together, then recombination would be unlikely. The likehood of the observed data given linkage and nonlinkage are calculated, and the ratio is calculated. The logarithm of this ratio, labeled the "LOD" score, reflects the probability of linkage. A LOD score of 3.0 is typically required to confirm linkage. This represents 1000 to 1 odds of a chance occurrence, and it protects against false positive findings associated with the large number of markers and tests performed.

While genome scans are a useful tool for identifying DNA regions containing a major predisposing gene (for example the Huntington gene), they are less useful for complex genetic disorders, especially using reasonable sample sizes. In general, regions meeting the minimum acceptance for statistical significance (> LOD 3) have been difficult to find in studies of ADHD, ASD, and RD (Risch et al., 2000; Fisher et al., 2002).

MOLECULAR BIOLOGY

The starting point for the molecular genetic studies is the analysis of DNA, which is coiled up in long strings in the 46 chromosomes (23 pairs) in the nuclei of most cells. The basic building blocks of DNA are the four bases: adenine (A) and guanine (G) and cytosine (C) and thymine (T). When attached to a deoxyribose (sugar) and phosphate group, these bases form a nucleotide. Nucleotides have chemical properties that result in specific pairing of a "long" (A or G) and a "short" (C or T) base to a "base-pair" (bp). A long double string of bp forms Watson and Crick's famous double-helix structure. The length of a DNA string is measured in thousands of bp, or kilobases (kb). The 23 pairs of chromosomes are numbered based on length, from chromosome 1 (about 250,000 kp) to chromosome 22 (about 50,000 bp), plus the sex chromosomes X (about 100,000 kb) and Y (about 50,000 kb).

A gene is a segment of DNA that provides the code for a protein. A series of events occurs to build a protein from a gene. First, the double-stranded DNA unravels and the paired nucleotides separate into two complementary single strands. These single strands are translated into RNA. The specific order of the sequence in the single-stranded RNA provides a code for amino acids (the building block for proteins). Three nucleotides (triplets) are required to specify an amino acid. However, the four nucleotides taken three at a time can code for 64 different triplets, but there are only 20 amino acids incorporated into proteins. So, this is a redundant code, with 64 different triplets coding for one of 20 amino acids. The amino acids specified by the sequence of nucleotides are themselves chained together to form proteins.

Most of the 3 million kb of DNA in the human genome is "noncoding." The coding segments (genes) are spread out across each chromosome. Finding and counting genes was one of the primary purpose of the Human Genome Project (HGP), which identified far fewer (about 30,000 genes) than expected.[20,21] Even in a gene, not all of the DNA is used. The entire stretch is segregated into exons (which are used) and introns (which are not used). In the process of making a protein, the introns are cut out and the exons are joined to specify the final DNA sequence that provides the nucleotide code for a protein.

Although individuals have the same nucleotide sequence for 99 percent or more of the human genome, there are individual differences (polymorphisms) at many points in human DNA. Polymorphisms occur in the DNA segments comprising genes that build proteins (coding regions) as well as in the DNA segments that do not (noncoding regions). The polymorphisms in the noncoding regions of the human genome are used as markers in the genome scan studies (described below). The polymorphisms in the coding regions are used to specify genetic bases for structural differences in proteins of the body, and these are preferred (although not exclusively used) for specifying genotypes in candidate gene studies (also described below).

For particular locations on the human genome, DNA differences are called alleles. Some background is provided here about three methods for determining differences in DNA at a particular locus: SNPs, RFLPs, and VNTRs. At some loci, DNA varies across individuals at single points (nucleotides), and these differences are called single nucleotide polymorphisms (SNPs). Often, these single points can be detected by restriction enzymes that recognize and "cut" the DNA sequence into short or long fragments. These differences across individuals are called restriction fragment length polymorphisms (RFLPs). In some regions of chromosomes, a specific nucleotide sequence repeats, and the number of repeats varies across individuals. The length of the repeat sequence can be used to specify the number of repeats of the sequence in the variable number of tandem repeats (VNTRs).

MOLECULAR GENETICS OF ADHD, RD, AND ASD

ADHD and Candidate Gene Studies

The family and twin studies of ADHD (see above) stimulated molecular genetic studies to search for allelic variations of specific genes that are associated with this disorder. The initial investigations used the candidate gene approach (described above), and the following brief review of molecular genetic studies of ADHD provides excellent examples of the successful use of this approach. The candidate gene approach was based on two theories of ADHD: (1) the dopamine deficit theory of ADHD,[22,23] which suggests why the stimulant medications that are considered to be DA agonists (methylphenidate and amphetamine) are so effective for the treatment of this disorder, and (2) the neuroanatomic network theory of attention,[24] which suggests how DA is involved in the component processes of attention (alerting, orienting, and executive control). The candidate gene studies of ADHD have focused on two dopamine genes whose locations were known: the dopamine transporter (DAT) gene on chromosome 5 (5p15.3) and the dopamine receptor type 4 (DRD4) gene on chromosome 11 (11p15.5).

The DAT1 gene has a polymorphism (a 40-bp VNTR) in the 3′ noncoding region of the gene. In the human population, the primary allelic variants are defined by 3 repeats (in about 0.01 of alleles), 9 repeats (in about 0.25 of an alleles), or 10 repeats (in about 0.76 of alleles) repeats. Since a primary mechanism of action of methylphenidate is the inhibition of reuptake of DA,[25,26] an overactive DA transporter has been hypothesized as a factor in ADHD, and this suggests a plausible candidate gene based on the site of action of the primary treatment of this disorder.

In a family-based control association study, Cook et al.[27] investigated parent-to-child transmission rates of the DAT1 alleles. They reported an increased transmission of the most prevalent allele (10 repeat) in their ADHD sample. Subsequently, others have replicated this finding,[28,29] but some have not.[30–32] Nonreplication is expected for conditions with observed relative risk <1.5 when small sample sizes (<100) are used. Cook[33] performed a metanalysis that supported the statistical significance of this association.

The DRD4 gene has a polymorphism (a 48-bp VNTR) in a coding region (exon III). The polymorphism (from 2 to 11 repeats) produces differences across individuals in the size of an important region of the receptor (the third intracellular loop, which couples to G proteins and mediates postsynaptic effects). In humans, the allele frequencies of DRD4 vary across ethnic groups, but allele frequencies are well established within ethnic groups. For example, in a sample of 150 unrelated Caucasians (see Ref. 34), the allele frequencies were 0.10 (2R), 0.04 (3R), 0.67 (4R), 0.01 (5R), 0.02 (6R), 0.12 (7R), and 0.04 (8R).

We have described in detail elsewhere[35] why we chose the DRD4 as a candidate gene in our investigations of ADHD. Some contributing factors were that (1) the VNTR is in a coding region of the gene[36]; (2) the neuroanatomic foci of the gene product, D4 receptors, is in cortical areas including the anterior cingulate gyrus, a brain region that plays an important role in normal attention and motivation[24,37]; (3) the relatively less common 7R allele may code for a receptor that is subsensitive to DA,[38] although this is not just due to length[39]; and (4) the DRD4 7R allele is associated with higher-than-normal scores on the personality characteristic of novelty seeking (see Refs. 40 to 42).

Our initial candidate gene study,[43] using a case-control approach, reported that the percentage of DRD4 7R alleles was higher in a sample of ADHD subjects (29 percent) than in an ethnically matched control group (12 percent) (see Fig. 69-1, left). We noted that the percentage of subjects with at least one 7R allele (the 7-present genotype) in the ADHD sample was about 50 percent, which was greater than in the control group (about 20 percent), but that the presence of a 7R allele was not a necessary condition (since about 50 percent of the ADHD cases did not have this allele) or a sufficient condition (since about 20 percent of the non-ADHD cases did). Initial population-based candidate gene studies are always suspect, because for small sample sizes many positive findings turn out to be "false positives."[44] In a subsequent family-based association study of parent-child trios, we[45] replicated the percentage of 7R alleles in the probands (28 percent) and also reported that the transmission rate of the DRD4 7R allele from heterozygous parents to affected children was higher (64 percent) than expected (50 percent). This family-based design discounted the contention that the initial effect was a spurious association due to population stratification. Subsequently, many investigators replicated this finding,[46–49] but as expected for replications using a small sample size, some have not,[50–53] and others have only partially replicated the finding.[54,55]

Since there are so many genes expressed in the brain, it is typically assumed that an initial report of an association with any one gene will be a false positive.[44] However, when multiple replications of the same association are reported with family-based association methods, the assumption of a false-positive association is discounted. This is the case for the associations of the DRD4 and DAT1 genes and ADHD: at last count, over a dozen reports have confirmed these

Figure 69-1
Candidate gene studies of the DRD4 gene and ADHD.

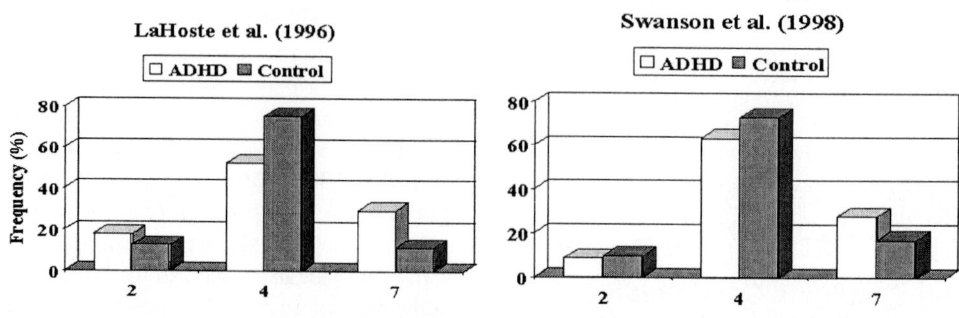

associations (see Refs. 33 and 56). In the literature, multiple replications of a candidate gene association for a psychiatric disorder is unusual if not unprecedented.[44] Thus, these initial molecular genetic studies of ADHD provide excellent examples of the successful use of the candidate gene approach.

RD and Quantitative Trait Linkage Studies

The biological descriptions of RD have also capitalized on advances in molecular biology. After twin and family studies documented a genetic influence on RD, several molecular genetic studies converged to identify a chromosome location of specific genes involved. These studies have used a variety of approaches, differing in the ways the study population was ascertained, how the phenotype was defined, and the type of statistical analysis.

Almost 20 years ago, Smith et al.[57] reported linkage to a site on chromosome 15. Others have confirmed and extended this linkage[13,58] based on a variety of phenotypes for RD.

Smith et al.[57] reported linkage to sites on chromosome 6 and Cardon et al.[12] confirmed this using quantitative trait analysis. Others have used somewhat different phenotypes of RD and have failed to document linkage to chromosome 6.[59–61] Nevertheless, others have confirmed and extended linkage to chromosome 6 for a variety of phenotypes of RD.[13,62,63] Thus, three research groups studying five independent populations have found evidence for linkage of reading disability to markers on 6p21.3.

Cardon et al.[12] used reading achievement to define a quantitative trait and selected a candidate region (the HLA region of chromosome 6) to investigate with a set of DNA. markers based on an autoimmune hypothesis of RD.[64] Strong evidence for linkage was reported. Grigorenko et. al.[13] investigating subtypes of RD found linkage in chromosome 6 just for phonological deficits. Gayan et al.[63] claim that 8 DNA markers on chromosome 6 are linked to word recognition, orthographic coding, phonological decoding, and phoneme awareness. Recently, analysis of multiple genome scans has identified another marker for RD on chromosome X.[65]

As reviewed by McGuffin and Martin[66] and by Schulte-Korne,[14] this degree of replication in the investigation of complex disorders is rare, so these studies provides a successful use of linkage analysis to narrow the search for genes involved in RD. The next steps will be to look in the regions on chromosome 6 and 15 to find the genes that may be involved. One approach is to look for candidate genes in these regions that may be related to biological pathways related to visual (orthographic) and auditory (phonologic) processes that are involved in reading.

ASD and Genome Scan Studies

There has been considerable investigation of the molecular genetics of ASD, but instead of the candidate gene approach, most of these studies have used the genome scan approach. Rutter[67] describes the background for molecular genetic studies of ASD and outlines why an affected-sib genome scan approach was favored (i.e., high heritability of ASD, relative small set of genes hypothesized, and reliable and standardized diagnostic methods were available). The widespread interest in ASD led to a multisite international study as well as multiple individual genome scan studies. Two of these are review here: IMGSAC[68] and Risch et al.[69]

The IMGSAC study used an affected sib-pair design with a broad phenotype of ASD. The genotypes used were based on markers spread across the chromosome about every 10 cM. This study[68] showed weak linkage of a marker in chromosome 7 as well as possible sites on five other chromosomes. Risch et al.[69] used affected sib pairs and discordant sib pairs and over 500 anonymous markers in a genome scan and showed only a slight increase in allele sharing in the affected sib pairs (51.6 percent) than discordant sib pairs (50.8 percent). However, only one marker was even moderate in size, and it was on chromosome 1, which was different than the finding of the Consortium study, which identified linkage in a broad region of chromosome 7. This is not unexpected for a condition (such as the broad phenotype of ASD) that may be associated with many genes.

The genetic bases of ASD continue to be the subject of intensive investigations. The lack of vertical transmission initially discounted the genetic basis of ASD, but family, twin, and adoption studies[18,70] revealed a high relative risk to siblings (60 to 100) and high heritability (about 0.9). The broad phenotype was more heritable than the narrow phenotype, suggesting that a categorical disorder of autism was not inherited but rather a range of social and cognitive anomalies. However, the application of the genome scan approach has not produced a clear direction for the next studies. Risch et al.[69] concluded that the next step in the genome scan approach (positional cloning of susceptibility loci) would be a formidable task because no specific region of the human genome was implicated by the genome scans.

NEXT STEPS IN MOLECULAR GENETICS OF ADHD, RD, AND AS

Some very recent studies have set the stage for the next round of molecular genetic studies of cognitive developmental disorders. Two of these are genome scan studies[71] and two are follow-up studies of the DRD4 candidate gene.[72,73]

First, Fisher et al.[71] reported the results of a genome scan for RD that combined prior samples from the United Kingdom[62] and the United States.[12,63] Based on the larger sample and refined statistical methods, this study identified a new region on chromosome 18 that was linked to RD phenotypes based on phonologic and orthographic processing. Second, Fisher et al.[71] reported the results for the first genome scan for ADHD. Based on a quantitative ADHD phenotype (number of ADHD symptoms on a structured psychiatric interview), no chromosome region was identified that exceeded the established significance thresholds, but four regions were identified with less rigorous criteria for linkage on chromosome 5 (5p12), chromosome 10 (10q26), chromosome 12 (12q23), and chromosome 16 (16p13). None of these regions contained the DAT or DRD4 genes that have been shown to be associated with ADHD in the candidate gene studies.

While the Fisher et al. (2002) study could not detect a gene with a lambda < 2–3, what magnitude of risk could one expect for disorders such as ADHD? The DRD4 7R/ADHD association can be used to answer this question, since it is one of the most reproduced in complex behavioral disorders (Swanson et al.[32,35]; Faraone et al.[56]). The approximately twofold risk associated with the DRD4 7R allele and ADHD has been described as "small" (Faraone et al.[56]; Fisher et al.[71]). While a twofold risk may be considered small in some contexts, this risk needs to be put in the perspective of observed DRD4 allele frequencies (Ding et al.[73]) and the predictions of the Common Variant-Common Disorder (CVCD) hypothesis (Zwick et al.[76]). In the CVCD hypothesis, disease-related alleles that are "common," usually defined as a frequency greater than 0.01 (Zwick et al., 2000) are proposed to be predisposing to common disorders, such as ADHD. Indeed, it is hypothesized that the reason these disorders are common is that their predisposing alleles are common (Zwick et al.[76]). The frequency of the DRD4 7R allele varies in different populations (Chang et al., 1996; Ding et al., 2002). In the populations of predominantly European origin used in most investigations of the DRD4/ADHD association (Swanson et al.[32,35]; Faraone et al.[56]), the allele frequency of DRD4 7R is approximately 12–15 percent (Ding et al.[73]). Therefore, even if the presence of a DRD4 7R allele was a necessary predisposing condition for ADHD (i.e., 100 percent of ADHD probands had at least one copy of this allele), and assuming Hardy-Weinberg equilibrium, the increase in observed frequency would be only 3.6-fold, barely detectable using current genome scan approaches. While more extensive genome scans are in the planning stages, involving many more individuals and orders of magnitude more markers (Risch and Merikangas[77]), it is unclear at present when the resources will be available (in terms of families, technologies, and money) to conduct such searches successfully.

Swanson et al.[72] evaluated a small sample of individuals with ADHD who had been genotyped for DRD4 and separated these subjects into subgroups defined by the presence (7R-present) and absence (7R-absent) of the presumed risk allele. The prior association studies were based on allele probabilities, either by contrasting the allele probabilities of the ADHD and control groups or by testing for distortion of the expected parent to proband allele transmission probability of 0.5, but these probabilities do not provide information about possible functional significance of the alleles (or of some linked alleles of other genes responsible for functional differences). Swanson et al.[72] followed up the positive associations with a test for functional differences between candidate genotypes. For the measures of function, a neuropsychological battery of reaction time tests (the Stroop color-word task, the Posner cue-detection task, and the Logan stop-change task) was used; for the candidate DRD4 genotype, subgroups based on the presence or absence of the hypothesized "high risk" 7R allele (7-present versus 7-absent) were used. Thus, genotype was used as an independent variable to evaluate the functional significance of the 7R allele on the quantitative traits of response speed (RT) and variability (SD). It was predicted that the 7-present subgroup (i.e., consisting of those ADHD subjects with at least one 7R allele) would have the greatest impairment, based on the simple hypothesis that the 7R form of the receptor when stimulated by DA would be less likely than other forms to transmit signals and activate brain areas important for attention and motivation.[74,75] However, the performance of 7-present subgroup was not different from that of the control group. Instead, only the 7-absent subgroup showed abnormal performance (longer RT and higher SD). This suggested that the hypothesized "risk" allele may not be associated with a cognitive impairment, even though it is associated with abnormal behavior documented by subjective impressions of symptoms of ADHD.

Finally, Ding et al.[73] showed by DNA resequencing/haplotyping of 600 DRD4 alleles, representing a worldwide population sample, that the origin of 2R through 6R alleles can be explained by simple one-step recombination/mutation events. In contrast, the 7R allele is not simply related to the other common alleles, differing by greater than 6 recombinations/mutations. Strong linkage disequilibrium (LD) was found between the 7R allele and surrounding DRD4 polymorphisms, suggesting this allele is at least 5–10-fold "younger" than the common 4R allele. Based on an observed bias towards nonsynonymous amino acid changes, the unusual DNA sequence organization, and the strong LD surrounding the DRD4 7R allele, Ding et al.[73] proposed that this allele originated as a rare mutational event, that nevertheless increased to high frequency in human populations by positive selection. Ding et al.[73] asked why an allele that appears to have undergone strong positive selection in human populations nevertheless is now disproportionately represented in individuals diagnosed with ADHD? The CVCD hypothesis, discussed above (Zwick et al., 2000) proposes that common genetic variation may be related to common disease, either because the disease is a product of a new environment (so that genotypes associated with the disorder were not eliminated in the past) or the disorder has a small effect on fitness (because it is late onset). For early onset disorders (such as ADHD) Ding et al.[73] suggested the possibility that predisposing alleles are in fact under positive selection, and only result in deleterious effects when combined with other environmental/genetic factors. Thus, it is possible that the very traits that may be selected for individuals possessing a DRD4 7R allele may predispose behaviors that are deemed inappropriate in a classroom setting in certain cultures today, and hence lead to diagnosis of ADHD.

SUMMARY

It is unlikely that RD, ASD, or ADHD are simple Mendelian conditions in which a single gene is the cause of a disorder in individual cases. Instead, it is likely that they are complex conditions for which a set of genes alters the probability of a disorder and individual genes are insufficient to cause a disorder outright.[76] When statistical methods for genome scans that were designed for the investigations of Mendelian diseases (e.g., affected sib-pair designs for detection of linkage) are applied to the study of complex diseases such as ADHD, RD, and ASD (which have low values of relative risk <2.0 and high population prevalence of the putative risk allele >10 percent), very large sample sizes (5000 to 65,000) are required for adequate statistical power.[77] This calls for different designs for molecular genetic investigations of complex disorders, such as candidate gene studies of association that are intended to detect linkage disequilibria. However, even these designs will require much larger sample sizes than usual nongenetic studies of these disorders (e.g., 250 to 1000).

Most alleles associated with complex genetic disorders will be neither necessary nor sufficient to predispose to the disease (as clearly observed for the DRD4 7R allele/ADHD association), since other alleles at an unknown number of genes will be involved as well. Further, we can only guess, based on heritability studies, what fraction of cases have a genetic origin, versus other environmental causes. Therefore, if the CVCD hypothesis is correct, one will never observe anything other than a small increase in risk for a single gene/allele. Indeed, the observed twofold increase in DRD4 7R allele frequency in ADHD probands is approximately 50 percent of the maximum possible (if all ADHD is genetic). It is simple to demonstrate that this allele, in combination with as few as one or two other alleles of a yet unidentified gene (at a comparable frequency), could account for the majority of ADHD cases. Yet neither of these hypothetical genes would be detected in current genome scans, because of their small individual effect on risk. In summary, common alleles associated with a particular disorder are expected to have only modest increase in allele frequency (λ) in affected individuals. This suggests that for the immediate future, candidate gene approaches may be the most sensitive way to identify alleles likely associated with cognitive developmental disorders.

The current plans for the identification of a large number of genetic markers (e.g., 100,000 SNPs—see Ref. 77) for use in molecular genetic studies do not take into consideration why statistical procedures for Mendelian genetics may not be applicable to the study of complex disorders. The power of an anonymous genome scan relying on linkage (i.e., an affected sib-pair study) or linkage disequilibrium (a TDT association study) relies on the ability of the observed phenotype to predict the underlying risk genotypes.[78] Since there are many genotypes that can produce the same phenotype (a many-to-one relationship), the conditional probability of genotype given phenotype would still be low, so mapping approaches may not work or at best have very low power. Instead, Weiss and Terwilliger[79] assert that if association studies use markers that are not causative, then they must be done with several preselected markers per gene that effectively represent the variation in chromosome regions of interest. An understanding of these problems and the use of statistical designs specifically tailored for studies of complex disorders seems essential in molecular genetics of developmental psychopathologies.[80]

REFERENCES

1. Posner MI, Rothbart MK, Farah M, Bruer J: Special issue: The developing human brain. *Develop Sci* 4:253–387, 2001.
2. American Psychiatric Association: *Diagnostic and Statistical Manual of Mental Disorders,* 4th ed (DSM-IV). Washington, DC: APA, 1994.
3. Swanson J: *School-Based Assessments and Interventions for ADD Students.* Irvine, CA: KC Publishing, 1994.
4. Goodman R, Ford T, Simons H, et al: Using the strengths and difficulties questionnaire (SDQ) to screen for child psychiatric disorders in a community sample. *Br J Psychiatry* 177:534–539, 2000.
   Goodman R, Ford T, Simons H, et al: Strengths and difficulties questionnaire (SDQ) (1995). (www.sdqinfo.com)
5. Tharpar A, Harrington R, Ross K, McGuffin P: *J Am Acad Child Adolesc Psychiatry* 39(12):1528–1536, 2000.
6. Robins DL, Fein D, Barton ML, Green JA: The modified checklist for autism in toddlers: An initial study investigating early detection of autism and pervasive developmental disorders. *J Autism Dev Disord* 31(2):131–144, 2001.
7. Baird G, Charman T, Cox A, et al: Screening and surveillance for autism and pervasive developmental disorders. *Arch Dis Child* 84:468–474, 2001.
8. World Health Organization: *International Classification of Diseases.* Geneva: WHO, 1993.
9. IDEA: *Seventeenth Annual Report to Congress on the Implementation of the Individuals with Disabilities Education Act.* Washington, DC: Office of Special Education Program, U.S. Department of Education, 1995.
10. Shaywitz SE, Escobar MD, Shawitz BA, et al: Evidence that dyslexia may represent the lower tail of a normal distribution of reading ability. *N Engl J Med* 326:145–150, 1992.
11. Fletcher JM, Shaywitz SE, Shaywitz BA: Comorbidity of learning and attention disorders: Separate but equal. *Pediatr Clin North Am* 46(5):885–897, 1999.
12. Cardon LR, Smith SD, Fulker DW, et al: Quantitative trait locus for reading disability on chromosome 6. *Science* 266:276–279, 1994.
13. Grigorenko EL, Wood FB, Meyer MS, et al: Susceptibility loci for distinct components of developmental dyslexia on chromosome 6 and 15. *Am J Hum Genet* 60:27–39, 1997.
14. Schulte-Korne G: Annotation: Genetics of reading and spelling disorder. *J Child Psychol Psychiatry* 42:985–997, 2001.

15. Stevenson J: Evidence for a genetic etiology in hyperactivity in children. *Behav Genet* 22:337–344, 1992.
16. Faraone SV, Doyle AE: The nature of heritability of attention-deficit hyperactivity disorder. *Child Adolesc Psychiatr Clin N Am* 10(2):299–316, 2001.
17. Pennington BF, Van Orden GC, Smith SD, et al: Phonological processing skills and deficits in adult dyslexics. *Child Dev* 61:1753–1778, 1990.
18. Smalley SL, Asarnow RF, Spence MA: Autism and genetics: A decade of research. *Arch Gen Psychiatry* 45:953–961, 1988.
19. Bailey A, Phillips W, Rutter M: Autism: Towards an integration of clinical, genetic, neuropsychological, and neurobiological perspectives. *J Child Psychol Psychiatry* 37:89–126, 1996.
20. Venter JC, Adams MD, Myers EW: The sequences of the attention genome. *Science* 291:1304–1351, 2001.
21. International Human Genome Sequencing Consortium. *Nature* 409:860–921, 2001.
22. Wender P: *Minimal Brain Dysfunction in Children.* New York: Wiley Liss, 1971.
23. Levy F: The dopamine theory of attention deficit hyperactivity disorder (ADHD). *Aust NZ J Psychiatry* 25:277–283, 1991.
24. Posner MI, Raichle ME: *Images of Mind.* New York: Scientific American Library, 1994.
25. Volkow ND, Ding YS, Fowler JS, et al: Is methylphenidate like cocaine? Studies on their pharmacokinetics and distribution in the human brain. *Arch Gen Psychiatry* 52:456–463, 1995.
26. Volkow ND, Wang G-J, Fowler JS, et al: Relationship between blockade of dopamine transporters by oral methylphenidate and increases in extracellular dopamine: Therapeutic implications. *Synapse* 43:181–187, 2002.
27. Cook EH, Stein MA, Krasowski MD, et al: Association of attention-deficit disorder and the dopamine transporter gene. *Am J Hum Genet* 56:993–998, 1995.
28. Gill M, Daly G, Heron S, et al: Confirmation of association between attention deficit hyperactivity disorder and a dopamine transporter polymorphism. *Mol Psychiatry* 2:311–313, 1997.
29. Waldman ID, Rowe DC, Abramowitz A, et al: Association and linkage of the dopamine transporter gene and attention-deficit hyperactivity disorder in children: Heterogeneity owing to diagnostic subtype and severity. *Am J Hum Genet* 63(6):1767–1776, 1998.
30. Sunohara G, Swanson JM, Larosa G: Association of dopamine receptor genes in attention deficit hyperactivity disorder. *Am J Hum Genet* 54(Suppl):A4–38, 1996.
31. Castellanos FX, Lau E, Tayebi N, et al: Lack of an association between a dopamine-4 receptor polymorphism and attention-deficit/hyperactivity disorder: Genetic and brain morphometric analysis. *Mol Psychiatry* 3:431–434, 1998.
32. Swanson J, Flodman P, Kennedy J, et al: Dopamine genes and ADHD. *Neurosci Biobehav Rev* 24:21–25, 2000.
33. Cook E: Website, University of Chicago, 2000.
34. Petronis A, Vantol HH, Lichter JB, et al. The D4 dopamine receptor gene maps on 11-p proximal to HRAS. *Genomics* 18(1):161–163, 1993.
35. Swanson JM, Posner M, Fosella J, et al: Genes and ADHD. *Curr Psychiatry Rep* 3:92–100, 2001.
36. Lichter JB, Barr DL, Kennedy JL, et al: A hypervariable segment in the human dopamine receptor D-4 gene. *Hum Mol Genet* 2(6):767–773, 1993.
37. Seeman P: Dopamine receptors and psychosis. *Sci Am Sci Med* 2(5):28–37, 1995.
38. Asghari V, Sanyal S, Buchwaldt S, et al: Modulation of intracellular cyclic AMP levels by different human dopamine D4 receptor variants. *J Neurochem* 65(3):1157–1165, 1995.
39. Jovanic V, Guan HC, Van Tol HH, et al: Comparative pharmacological and functional analysis of the human dopamine D4.2 and D4.10 receptor variants. *Pharmacogenetics* 9:561–568, 1999.
40. Benjamin J, Li L, Patterson C, et al: Population and familial association between the DRD4 gene and measures of novelty seeking. *Nat Genet* 12:81–84, 1996.
41. Ebstein RP, Novick O, et al: Dopamine D4 receptor (D4DR) exon III polymorphism associated with the human personality trait of novelty seeking. *Nat Genet* 12:78–80, 1996.
42. Cloninger CR, Adolfsson R, Svrakic NM: Mapping genes for human personality [news]. *Nat Genet* 12:3–4, 1996.
43. La Hoste GJ, Swanson JM, Wigal SB, et al: Dopamine D4 receptor gene polymorphism is associated with attention deficit hyperactivity disorder. *Mol Psychiatry* 1:121–124, 1996.
44. Crowe RR: Candidate genes in psychiatry: Epidemiological perspective. *Am J Med Genet* 48:74–77, 1993.
45. Swanson JM, Sunohara GA, Kennedy JL, et al: Association of the dopamine receptor D4 (DRD4) gene with a refined phenotype of attention deficit hyperactivity disorder (ADHD): A family-based approach. *Mol Psychiatry* 3:38–41, 1998.
46. Smalley SL, Bailey JN, Palmer CG, et al: Evidence that the dopamine D4 receptor is a susceptibility gene in attention deficit hyperactivity disorder. *Mol Psychiatry* 3:427–430, 1998.

47. Rowe DC, Stever C, Giedinghagen LN, et al: Dopamine DRD4 receptor polymorphism and attention deficit hyperactivity disorder. *Mol Psychiatry* 3:419–426, 1998.
48. Faraone SV, Biederman J, Weiffenbach B, et al: Dopamine D4 gene 7-repeat allele and attention deficit hyperactivity disorder. *Am J Psychiatry* 156:768–770, 1999.
49. Sunohara G, Roberts W, Malone M, et al: Linkage of the dopamine D4 receptor gene and ADHD. *J Am Acad Child Adolesc Psychiatry* 12:1537–1542, 2000.
50. Hawi Z, McCarron M, Kirley A, et al: No association of the dopamine DRD4 receptor (DRD4) gene polymorphism with attention deficit hyperactivity disorder (ADHD) in the Irish population. *Am J Med Genet (Neuropsychiatr Genet)* 96:268–272, 2000.
51. Eisenberg J, Zohar A, Mei-Tal G, et al: A haplotype relative risk study of the dopamine D4 receptor (DRD4) exon III repeat polymorphism and attention deficit hperactivity disorder (ADHD). *Am J Med Genet (Neuropsychiatr Genet)* 96:258–261, 2000.
52. Kotler M, Manor I, Sever Y, et al: Failure to replicate an excess of the long dopamine D4 exon III repeat polymorphism in ADHD in a family-based study. *Am J Med Genet (Neuropsychiatr Genet)* 96:278–281, 2000.
53. Todd RD, Neuman RJ, Lobos EA, et al: Lack of association of dopamine D4 receptor gene polymorphisms with ADHD subtypes in a population of twins. *Am J Med Genet (Neuropsychiatr Genet)* 105:432–438, 2001.
54. Holmes J, Payton A, Barrett J, et al: A family-based case-association study of the dopamine D4 receptor gene and dopamine transporter gene in attention deficit hyperactivity disorder. *Mol Psychiatry* 5:523–530, 2000.
55. Mills J, Curran S, Kent L, et al: ADHD and the DRD4 gene: Evidence of association but no linkage in a UK sample. *Mol Psychiatry* 6:440–444, 2001.
56. Faraone S, Doyle A, Mick E, Biederman J: Meta-analysis of the association between the dopamine D4 gene 7-repeate allele and ADHD. *Am J Psychiatry* 158:1052–1057, 2001.
57. Smith SD, Kimberling WJ, Pennington BF, Lubs HA: Specific reading disability: Identification of an inherited form through linkage analysis. *Science* 219:1345–1347, 1983.
58. Morris DW, Robinson L, Turic D, et al: Family-based association mapping provides evidence for a gene for reading disability on chromosome 15q. *Hum Mol Genet* 22:843–848, 2000.
59. Schulte-Korne G, Nothen MM, Muller-Myhsok B, et al: Evidence of linkage of spelling disability to chromosome 15. *Am J Hum Genet* 63:279–282, 1998.
60. Field LL, Kaplan BJ: Absence of linkage of phonological coding dyslexia to chromosome 6p23-p21.3 in a large family data set. *Am J Hum Genet* 63:1448–1456, 1998.
61. Petryshen TL, Kaplan BJ, Liu MF, Field LL: Absence of significant linkage between phonological coding dyslexia and chromosome 6p23-21.3, as determined by use of quantitative-trait methods: Confirmation of qualitative analyses. *Am J Hum Genet* 66:708–714, 2000.
62. Fisher SE, Marlow AJ, Lamb J, et al: A genome-wide search strategy for identifying quantitative trait loci involved in reading and spelling disability (developmental dyslexia). *Am J Hum Genet* 64:146–156, 1999.
63. Gayan J, Smith SD, Cherny SS, et al: Quantitative-trait locus for specific language and reading deficits on chromosome 6p. *Am J Hum Genet* 64:157–184, 1999.
64. Gilger JW, Pennington BF, DeFries JC: A twin study of the etiology of comorbidity: Attention deficit hyperactivity disorder and dyslexia. *J Am Acad Child Adolesc Psychiatry* 31:343–348, 1992.
65. Fisher SE, Francks C, Marlow AJ, et al: Independent genome scans identify a chromosome 18 quantitative locus influencing dyslexia. *Nat Genet* 30:86–91, 2002.
66. McGuffin P, Martin NS: Science, medicine and the future: Behaviour and genes. *Br Med J* 319:37–40, 1999.
67. Rutter M: Genetic studies of autism: From the 1970s into the millennium. *J Abnorm Child Psychol* 28:3–14, 2000.
68. International Molecular Genetic Study of Autism Consortium (IMGSAC): A full genome scan for autism with evidence for linkage on chromosome 7q. *Hum Mol Genet* 7:571–578, 1998.
69. Risch N, Spiker D, Lotspeich L, et al: A genome screen of autism: Evidence for a multilocus etiology. *Am J Hum Genet* 65:493–507, 1999.
70. Fostein S, Rutter M: Infantile autism: A genetic study of 21 twin pairs. *J Child Psychol Psychiatry* 18:297–321, 1977.
71. Fisher SE, Francks C, McCracken JT, et al: A genomewide scan for loci involved in ADHD. *Am J Hum Genet* 70:000-000, 2002.
72. Swanson J, Oosterlaan J, Murias M, et al: Attention deficit/hyperactivity disorder children with a 7-repeat allele of the dopamine receptor D4 gene have extreme behavior but normal performance on critical neurpsychological tests of attention. *Proc Natl Acad Sci U S A* 97:4754–4759, 2000.
73. Ding YC, Chi HC, Grady DL, et al: Evidence of positive selection acting at the human dopamine receptor D4 gene locus. *Proc Natl Acad Sci USA* 99(1):309–324, 2002.

74. Swanson JM, Sergeant JA, Taylor E, et al. *Lancet* 351: 429–433, 1998.
75. Swanson JM, Deutsch C, Cantwell D, et al: Genes and ADHD. *Clin Neurosci Res* 1:207–216, 2001.
76. Zwick M, Cutler DJ, Chakravarti A: *Annu Rev Genomics Hum Genet* 1:387–407, 2000.
77. Risch N, Merikangas K: The future of genetic studies of complex human diseases [see comments]. *Science* 273:1516–1517, 1996.
78. Terwilliger JD, Weiss KM: Linkage disequilibrium mapping of complex disease: Fantasy or reality? *Curr Opin Biotechnol* 9:578–594, 1998.
79. Weiss KM, Terwilliger JD. Commentary: How many diseases do you have to study to map one gene with SNPs? *Nat Genet* 26(2):151–157, 2000.
80. Terwilliger JD, Goring HH: Gene mapping in the 20th and 21st centuries: Statistical methods, data analysis, and experimental design. *Hum Biol* 72:63–132.

GLOSSARY OF LINGUISTIC TERMS*

Affix A MORPHEME that must be attached to another morpheme. Also known as a bound morpheme. Prefixes attach to the beginning of a morpheme (e.g., *re-* in *redefine*), and suffixes attach to the end of a morpheme (e.g., *-er* in *worker*).

Case A set of affixes or word forms that are used to distinguish the roles of nouns. For example, in English, *I, me,* and *my* have different cases.

Categorical perception The phenomenon whereby a continuous change in a physical characteristic of a speech signal is perceived discontinuously. For example, "ba" and "pa" differ in voice onset time (VOT). If one starts with a "ba" and gradually increases VOT, English speakers find it difficult to detect any change until a categorical boundary is reached. When the categorical boundary is crossed, subjects' perception of the sound suddenly switches from voiced (ba) to unvoiced (pa).

Closed class word See FUNCTION WORD.

Content word A word that has lexical meaning (SEMANTIC content). Examples include nouns, verbs, adjectives, and adverbs. Because new lexical words such as *modem* or *fax* can freely be invented (i.e., the number of possible lexical words is infinite), lexical words are sometimes referred to as OPEN CLASS WORDS.

Discourse The organization of continuous stretches of language larger than a sentence in a conversation or text.

Function word or functor A word or bound morpheme whose role is strictly or mostly to signal grammatical relationships. Examples include INFECTIONS, conjunctions, articles, auxiliary verbs, and pronouns. A given language has a limited and finite number of functors and, hence, function words are sometimes referred to as CLOSED CLASS WORDS or closed class morphemes.

Inflection Refers to affixes that signal grammatical relationships such as plural, past tense, progressive tense, and possession (in English, *-s, -ed, -ing,* and *'s,* respectively).

Lexical access The process of looking words up in one's lexicon (mental dictionary).

Lexical decision In psycholinguistic experiments, subjects are sometimes asked to decide whether a string or letters (or sounds) is a word in their language. For example, subjects might be presented English words such as "table" and nonwords such as "bivel." Because the only way to determine that "table" is a word and "bivel" is not a word is to determine whether they are in one's lexicon, lexical decision tasks are used to study LEXICAL ACCESS.

Morpheme The minimal distinctive unit of meaning that can be combined to form words. Morphemes can be bound (see AFFIX) or free (able to appear by themselves).

Morphology The branch of linguistics that investigates the form or structure of words and the processes and rules that govern the ways in which MORPHEMES are combined.

Open class word See CONTENT WORD.

Orthography The writing system of a language.

Phoneme The minimal unit of the sound system of a language that can be used to signal a potential

* Prepared by Karin Stromswold.

difference in meaning. For example, /b/ and /p/ are phonemes in English because there are minimal pairs of words such as /bat/ and /pat/ and /cab/ and /cap/ that differ only in whether a /b/ or a /p/ is present.

Phonemic awareness The awareness that words and morphemes are composed of PHONEMES. Specifically, phonemic awareness refers to the ability to break words into their component phonemes (e.g., /bat/ → /b/ + /a/ + /t/), report the number of syllables in a word, report whether a particular phoneme appears in a word, etc.

Phonology The branch of linguistics that studies the sound systems of languages, including the sounds that are used in a language and the way these sounds may be combined.

Pragmatics The branch of linguistics that investigates phenomena associated with the use of the language by individuals. Of particular interest is the constraints that people encounter when they use language in social settings and the effect their language has on the people with whom they are talking.

Prosody The overall sound pattern or contour of a word or sentence, including pitch, loudness, tempo, and rhythm.

Semantics The branch of linguistics that studies meaning in language.

Syntax The branch of linguistics that studies the grammar of language, particularly the rules that govern the way words combine to form sentences.

Thematic role A term used for semantic roles such as agent, patient, location, source, or goal. For example, in the sentence *John eats spaghetti, John* is the agent and *spaghetti* is the patient. In Government Binding Theory, every argument is given a particular thematic role by its predicate. Thematic roles are drawn from a universal set of thematic relations.

INDEX

Note: Page numbers followed by *f* indicate figures; those followed by *t* indicate tables.

A

Acalculia, parietal lobe and, 207–208
Acetylcholine (ACh)
  in Alzheimer's disease, 552*t*
  violence and, 758
Acetylcholinesterase (AChE) inhibitors, for Alzheimer's disease, 552–554, 553*t*
Achromatopsia
  central, 245–249
    clinical presentation of, 245
    definition of, 245
    neuroanatomic correlates of, 246–249, 248*f*
    neuro-ophthalmologic features of, 245
    neuropsychological features of, 245–246, 247*f*
  cerebral, 229
Activity limitation, definition of, 179–180
Activity restriction, in autism, 857
Acute confusional state (ACS), 495
Adaptive coding, prefrontal function and, 398
Aβ deposits, in Alzheimer's disease, 547–548
Affect. *See also* Depression; Emotion(s)
  mental status exam and, 24
Affective auditory agnosia, 263
Affective disorder. *See* Depression
Affective prosody, 744
  comprehension of, 747
  hemispheric lateralization of, 748–750, 749*f*
  repetition of, 746–747
  spontaneous, 746
Age. *See also* Children
  Alzheimer's disease and, 550
  childhood-acquired aphasia and, 793–794
Aggression. *See also* Violence
  ictal, 678
  interictal, 683
  postictal, 679
Aging, normal, 530–533
  atrophy and neuronal loss and, 531–533, 532*t*
  neuropathology and, 531
Agitation, treatment of, 759
  in Alzheimer's disease, 556–557
Agnosia
  apperceptive, 233–235
    behavior and anatomy of, 233–234, 234*f*
    interpretation of, 234
    relation to other disorders, 234–235
  associative, 235–237
    behavior and anatomy of, 235*f*, 235–236
    interpretation of, 236–237
    relation to other disorders, 237
  auditory. *See* Auditory agnosia
  color, 250–251
    case study of, 251
    definition of, 250
    neuroanatomic correlates of, 251
    neuropsychological correlates of, 250–251
  finger, 290
  landmark, 298–299
  orientation, 296
  tactile, 275–278
    anatomic considerations in, 277*f*, 277–278
    behavioral considerations in, 275–277
  visual, 246

Agrammatism, 148
  in aphasia, 171
  cognitive neuropsychological analysis of, 185*t*, 185–188, 186*f*
AIDS dementia complex (ADC), 629–631, 630*t*
AIT-082 (Neotrofin), for Alzheimer's disease, 560
Akinesia
  basal ganglia lesions and, 414–415
  limb, 303
Akinotopsia, cerebral, 229–230
Alcmaeon of Croton, 3
Alcohol
  prefrontal dysfunction due to, 391
  Wernicke-Korsakoff syndrome and, 639, 643
Alexia
  acquired, 246
  without agraphia (pure), 196–197
Alleles, 871
Allocortex, 46
Alzheimer's disease (AD), 501, 515–533, 545–562, 594*t*
  Aβ deposits in, 547–548
  anatomy in, 520*f*, 520–521
  aphasia due to, 159–160
  argyrophilic grains disease and, 528
  attention in, 577–578
  clinical picture in, 518
  cognitive neuropsychological issues in, 573–578
  diagnostic criteria for, 516–517, 517*t*
  differential diagnosis of, 505, 506*t*, 507
  emotional disturbances in relation to diffuse brain dysfunction in, 735–736
  focal cortical atrophies and, 528–530
  historical background of, 516, 516*f*
  laboratory tests in, 519–520
  Lewy bodies and, 527–528, 550
  main lesions and diagnosis of, 521*f*, 521–523
  neurofibrillary tangles in, 524*f*, 524–526, 525*f*, 532*t*, 532–533, 548–549
    biochemistry of, 548–549
    structure of, 548
  neuronal loss and atrophy in, 526–527, 549, 549*f*, 573–574
  neuropsychological tests in, 516
  normal aging and, 530–533
    atrophy and neuronal loss and, 531–533, 532*t*
    neuropathology and, 531
  normal-pressure hydrocephalus differentiated from, 664
  prefrontal dysfunction due to, 391
  risk factors for, 518–519, 550–551
  semantic memory in, 574–577
  senile plaques in, 521*f*, 521–523, 524–526, 545–546
    biochemistry of, 546–547, 547*f*
    cell biology of, 548
    structure of, 545–546, 546*f*
  storage in, 437
  synaptic loss in, 527, 549–550
  treatment and management of, 509, 551–562
    for behavioral manifestations, 555–557, 556*t*
    therapies aimed at slowing disease progression or delaying disease onset and, 557–562
    therapies aimed at symptomatic relief and, 551–555, 552*t*
  vascular dementia contrasted with, 615–616
Amino acids, excitatory, for Alzheimer's disease, 555
Amnesia, 431–441
  amnesic syndromes and, 432*f*, 432–433, 433*t*, 434*t*, 435
  anosognosia for, 354–355
  anterograde, 434*t*
    in Wernicke-Korsakoff syndrome, 641–642
  brain sites of memory processes and, 435*f*, 435–438, 436*f*, 437*t*, 439*f*
  classification of memory and, 431, 432*t*
  confabulation in
    in amnestic-dysexecutive syndrome, 364–366
    deficient strategic retrieval and, 367–368
    neuroanatomy of, 368–369, 369*f*
    neuropsychological mechanisms associated with, 364–368
    temporal/contextual displacement and, 366–367
  emotion and, 438, 440
  explicit memory and, 448–450
  functional, 434*t*
  global, transient, 434*t*
  implicit memory and, 448–449, 450–452
  in Korsakoff's syndrome, 433, 434*f*, 435
  mediotemporal lobe, 432–433
  posttraumatic
    assessment of, 465–466
    neurometabolism in, 466, 467*f*
    prognosis based on, 465, 465*f*
  psychogenic, 434*t*
  retrograde, 434*t*
    cognitive issues in, 445–446
    in Wernicke-Korsakoff syndrome, 642
  semantic memory in, 446–448
  somesthetic results of, 279
Amnestic-dysexecutive syndrome, confabulation in, 364–366
AMPAkines, for Alzheimer's disease, 555
Amusia, sensory/receptive, 257, 258*t*, 264–265

Amygdala
fear and, 713–714, 715*f*, 716
memory and, 438, 440
Anatomy, 45–54, 46*t*, 47*f*
in achromatopsia, central, 246–249, 248*f*
in agnosia
apperceptive, 239–240, 240*f*
associative, 241*f*, 241–242
color, 251
simultanagnosia, 331–332, 332*f*, 333*f*
tactile, 277*f*, 277–278
in Alzheimer's disease, 520*f*, 520–521
in amnesic confabulation, 368–369, 369*f*
in anomia, color, 252
in anosognosia for hemiplegia, 351
of ascending reticular activating system, 52–53
behavioral specialization and neural connectivity in cortex and, 48–50
cortical types and, 45–48
in delusional misidentification syndromes, 374
face recognition and, 240–241
functional, normal, 99–100
in memory impairment following anterior communicating artery aneurysms, 477, 478*f*
of neural networks, 53–54
from neuroimaging, 73
in pediatric neuropsychological assessment, focal versus neural substrates and, 774–775
plasticity and, 59
of subcortical structures, 50–52
globus pallidus, 50–51
striatum, 50
thalamus, 51*f*, 51–52
of thalamic lesions, in diencephalic amnesia, 425, 426*f*, 427
violence and, 756–757
Angelman's syndrome (AS), 847
Angiitis, of central nervous system, primary, 654*t*, 655
Anisometry, spatial, in neglect, 316
Anomia, 250–251
cognitive neuropsychological approach to, 183–185
analysis and, 183*f*, 183–184
treatment implications of, 184–185
color, 251–253
definition of, 251
neuroanatomic correlates of, 252
neuropsychological correlates of, 252
Anomic aphasia, 157
Anosodiaphoria, 350
Anosognosia, 345–358
for amnesia, 354–355
denial and, 355–357
for hemiplegia, 315, 349–354
anatomic considerations in, 351
confabulation and, 352–354, 353*t*
frequency and laterality of, 350–351
general intellectual functioning related to, 352
hemispatial neglect related to, 351–352, 352*t*
sensory loss and, 351
with neglect, 309–310
somesthetic results of, 279
types of unawareness and confabulation and, 357*t*, 357–358
for visual defects
for acquired scotoma and hemianopias, 345–347
for blindness, 348–349
for blind spot, 345
for divided visual fields in split-brain patients, 347–348
neuropathologic features of Anton's syndrome and, 349
Anoxia
childhood-acquired aphasia associated with, 792
emotional disturbances in relation to diffuse brain dysfunction in, 737
Anterior cerebral artery (ACA) aneurysms, prefrontal dysfunction due to, 387
Anterior choroidal artery region, infarctions due to thalamic lesions in, 424, 424*f*, 425*f*
Anterior communicating artery (ACoA) aneurysms
confabulation and, 364, 368, 369
memory impairment following, 477–482, 478*t*
anatomy and, 477, 478*f*
historical background of, 478–479, 479*f*
origin of amnestic symptoms and, 480–481, 481*f*
recovery and, 482
specific sequelae and, 481–482
Anterograde amnesia, 434*t*
in Wernicke-Korsakoff syndrome, 641–642
Anterograde disorientation, 299
Antiamyloid treatment, for Alzheimer's disease, 557–558
Anticholinergic drugs, for delirium, 500
Anticholinesterase-inhibitor agents, for dementia, 509
Anticonvulsants, for aggression, 760*t*
Antidepressants, for aggression, 760*t*
Antioxidants, for Alzheimer's disease, 560–561
Antiphospholipid (APL) syndrome, primary, 654*t*, 654–655
Antipsychotics, for aggression, 760*t*
Anton's syndrome, 348–349
neuropathologic features of, 349

Anxiety
in Alzheimer's disease, treatment of, 556
ictal, 677–678
interictal, 682–683
in Parkinson's disease, 737
Aβ peptide
in Alzheimer's disease, 522
normal aging and, 532
Aphasia, 147–160
anomic, 157
basal ganglia lesions and, 411–413, 413*f*
Broca's. *See* Broca's aphasia
childhood-acquired. *See* Childhood-acquired aphasia
clinical syndromes of, 147–148. *See also specific syndromes*
conduction, 152*f,* 152–153
crossed, 157–158
etiology of, 158–160
dementia and, 159–160
hemorrhage and, 159
herpes simplex encephalitis and, 159
infarction and, 158–159
traumatic, 159
tumors and, 159
global, 153–154
language processing and, 165–174
components of, 166
comprehension deficits and, 166–167, 167*f*
lexical processing disorders and, 168
new directions for, 173–174
phonologic processing disorders and, 167–168
production disorders and, 169–171
semantic processing disorders and, 168–169, 169*f*
sentence-level processing and, 171–173
in left-handers, 157
linguistic processing in, event-related potentials for study of, 123–124
optic, 237, 250–251
parallel distributed processing and, 141–143, 142*f*
primary progressive, 529, 584, 584*t*
rehabilitation of, 179–189
for agrammatism, 185*t,* 185–188, 186*f*
for anomia, 183*f,* 183–185
cognitive neuropsychology school of, 182–188, 183*f*
functional/pragmatic/social school of, 181–182, 182*f*
levels of analysis and, 179–180
modular-treatments approach to, 188–189
traditional language-oriented school of, 180–181, 181*f*
tactile, somesthetic results of, 279
transcortical
mixed, 157
motor, 154–156, 155*f*
sensory, 156, 156*f,* 168–169
Wernicke's. *See* Wernicke's aphasia
Aphasic mutism, 793
Apolipoprotein E, Alzheimer's disease and, 522, 551
Appearance, mental status exam and, 23
Apperceptive agnosia, 233–235
behavior and anatomy of, 233–234, 234*f*
interpretation of, 234
relation to other disorders, 234–235
Applied Behavior Analysis (ABA), for autism, 861
Apraxia
basal ganglia lesions and, 413–414
buccofacial, in global aphasia, 153
conceptual, 222–223
clinical findings in, 222–223
pathophysiology of, 223
conduction, 221–222
clinical findings in, 221
pathophysiology of, 222
constructional, 296–298, 297*f*
disassociation, 221
ideational, 221
ideomotor, 217
clinical findings in, 218–219
pathophysiology of, 219–221
limb. *See* Limb apraxia
oculomotor, 327
progressive, 530
in Wernicke's aphasia, 150
Apraxia-astereognosis syndrome, 278, 278*f*
Aprosodia, 745–750
crossed, developmental, 824
Aqueductal stenosis, association with idiopathic normal-pressure hydrocephalus, 670
Argyrophilic grains disease, 528
Ascending reticular activating system (ARAS)
anatomy of, 52–53
consciousness and, 338
Asomatognosia, 350
Asperger's syndrome, nonverbal, social, and emotional learning disabilities versus, 826
Assessment. *See* Mental status exam; Neuropsychological assessment; Psychometric tests
Association cortex, 46–48
heteromodal component of, 47–48
lesions of, visual perception and, 228–230
unimodal component of, 48, 49

Associative agnosia, 235–237
  behavior and anatomy of, 235*f,* 235–236
  interpretation of, 236–237
  relation to other disorders, 237
Associative visual agnosia, 237
Astereognosis, 275
  in apraxia-astereognosis syndrome, 278, 278*f*
Astrocytes
  in senile plaques, 523
  tufted, 530
Asymboly for pain, somesthetic results of, 279
Asyntactic comprehension, in aphasia, 171–172
Ataxia
  optic, 286, 325–327
  spinocerebellar, 601
Attention. *See also* Inattention; Sensory neglect
  in Alzheimer's disease, 577–578
  in autism, 859
  interhemispheric integration of perception and, 405–406
    sharing of attentional control and, 405–406
  mental status exam and, 26–27
  neglect right hemisphere damage and, event-related potentials for study of, 119–123, 122*f*
  processing without, in neglect, 318
  spatial, neglect and, 313–314
  visual, hemispheric sharing of control of, 405–406
Attentional dysfunction, in delirium, 496
Attentional dyslexia, 197
Attentional facilitation, prefrontal cortex and, event-related potentials for study of, 112–116, 114*f,* 115*f,* 117*f*
Attentional system, supervisory, prefrontal function and, 397
Attention deficit hyperactivity disorder (ADHD), 831–838
  brain mechanisms in, 834–835
    functional studies of, 834–835
    neurochemical studies of, 835
    structural studies of, 834
  definition of, 831–832
  epidemiology of, 832
  etiology of, 832–834
    environmental factors in, 833–834
    genetic, 832–833
  molecular genetics of, 867–873, 872*f,* 874–876
    behavioral genetics and, 869–870
    future directions for, 874–875
    molecular biology and, 870–871
    phenotype and, 867–869, 868*t*
  neuropsychology of, 835–837
  treatment of, 837–838
Attractors, parallel distributed processing networks and, 138
Aubertin, Ernest, 7, 7*f*
Auditory agnosia, 257–267, 258*t*
  affective, 263
  cortical auditory disorder, 257–259, 258*t*
  cortical deafness and, 257–259, 258*t*
  neuroimaging in, 265–266
  phonagnosia, 264
  pure word deafness, 257, 258*t*
  sensory/receptive amusia, 257, 258*t,* 264–265
  sound (for nonspeech sounds), 257, 258*t,* 262–263
  for speech (verbal). *See* Pure word deafness
Auras, in epilepsy, 676–677
Autism, 853–864
  attention in, 859
  complications in, 857–858
  features associated with, 857
  genetics of, 854
  imaginative pay in, 856–857
  interest and activity restriction in, 857
  IQ score profiles in, 858–859
  language in, 860
    nonverbal, 856
    verbal, 855–856
  learning in, 860
  memory in, 860
  mental retardation in, 858
  molecular genetics of, 867–871, 873–876
    behavioral genetics and, 869–870
    future directions for, 874–875
    molecular biology and, 870–871
    phenotype and, 867–869, 868*t*
  motor function in, 860
  neuroimaging in, 862–863
    functional, 862–863
    structural, 862
  neurologic examination in, 857
  neuropathology of, 861–862
  neuropsychological functioning profile in, 859
  nonverbal, social, and emotional learning disabilities versus, 826
  onset of, 854–855
  part-whole processing in, 859
  pathophysiology of, 863–864
  prevalence of, 853–854
  sensory perception in, 859–860
  social deficit in, 855
  treatment of, 860–861
Autism Screening Questionnaire (ASD), 868–869
Autotopagnosia, 289–290
Awareness
  of one's own body, 285, 289
  processing without, in neglect, 318–319

B

Backpropagation, parallel distributed processing and, 137
Bálint-Holmes syndrome, 329
Bálint's syndrome, 325, 333
Basal forebrain, 45–46
Basal forebrain amnesia, mediotemporal and diencephalic amnesia versus, 480–481, 481*f*
Basal ganglia lesions, 411–417, 412*f*
  aphasia and, 411–413, 413*f*
  apraxia and, 413–414
  emotional changes after, 415–416
  executive function after, 416
  frontal deficits after, 416
  ideomotor apraxia and, 220–221
  motor deficits after, 416
  neglect and, 414–415
Basolateral limbic circuit, 435, 436, 436*f*
Behavior, mental status exam and, 23–24
Behavior modification, for autism, 861
Bell, Charles, 4–5
Bell-Magendie law, 5
Bender-Gestalt Test, 37
Benzodiazepines
  for aggression, 760*t*
  for delirium, 500
Beta blockers, for aggression, 760*t*
Binswanger's disease, 613
  differential diagnosis of, 506*t*, 507–508
Blindness
  adaptation to, plasticity in, 63–68, 64*f*, 65*f*, 67*f*
  anosognosia for, 348–349
  cortical, unawareness of, 348–349
Blindsight, 228
Blind spot, anosognosia for, 345
Body-part phantoms, 286–288
  cerebral substrate of, 288
  in congenital absence of limbs, 287–288
  visual and somatosensory influences on, 287
Body perception, 285–292
  autotopagnosia and, 289–290
  awareness of one's own body and, 289
  body-part phantoms and, 286–288
    cerebral substrate of, 288
    in congenital absence of limbs, 287–288
    visual and somatosensory influences on, 287
  body-part specificity of knowledge about human body and, 291–292
  finger agnosia and, 290
  imitation of meaningless gestures and, 290–291, 291*f*
  levels of information about body and, 285–286
  neglect of one-half of body and, 288–289
  optic ataxia and, 286
BOLD fMRI, 86
  properties affecting experimental design, 93*f*, 93–94, 94*f*
  temporal structures of studies using, 94–96
  two-systems model of, 87*f*, 87–88, 88*t*
Bouillaud, Jean-Baptiste, 6–7, 7*f*
Braille, learning, plasticity in, 63–68, 64*f*, 65*f*, 67*f*
Brain at risk, 615
Brain damage
  event-related potentials and, 109–111, 111*f*
  with transcranial magnetic stimulation, 127
Brain injury, 463–472
  acute memory dysfunction following, 465–466
    assessment of, 465–466
    neurometabolism in, 466, 467*f*
    predicting outcome based on duration of, 465, 465*f*
  aphasia due to, 159
  childhood-acquired aphasia associated with, 785, 789*t*–790*t*
  chronic memory dysfunction following, 466–472
    frontal lobes and, 470–472, 471*f*
    nature of learning and memory deficits and, 468–470, 469*f*
    procedural and implicit memory and, 470
    prospective memory deficits and, 470
    semantic memory and, 470
    severity of brain injury and, 466–468
  emotional disturbances in relation to diffuse brain dysfunction in, 738–739
  memory processes in brain and, 463–464, 464*f*
  prefrontal dysfunction due to, 387, 388*f*
  violence associated with, 755
Brainstem auditory evoked potentials (BAEPs), 106
  signal averaging of, 108–109, 109*f*
Brain tumors
  aphasia due to, 159
  childhood-acquired aphasia associated with, 785, 790, 791*t*–792*t*
  prefrontal dysfunction due to, 388, 389*f*
BRAINVOX, 73–74, 75*f*, 76*f*
Broca, Paul, 7–8, 8*f*
Broca's aphasia, 148–150
  acute, 149, 149*f*
  chronic, 148–149, 149*f*
  cognitive neuropsychological analysis of, 185*t*, 185–188, 186*f*
  fractional syndromes of, 148
  frontal operculum damage and, 149
  improvement in, 150

linguistic processing in, event-related potentials for study of, 123–124
lower motor cortex lesions and, 149–150
Brodmann, Korbinian, 12
Brodmann's map, 45
Buccofacial apraxia, in global aphasia, 153
Building, impaired, 296–298, 297*f*
Buspirone, for aggression, 760*t*

C

Callosal disconnection. *See* Split-brain patients
Campbell, Alfred W., 12
Cancellation task, 304, 306*f*
Cancer treatments, childhood-acquired aphasia associated with, 790
Cannon-Bard theory of emotion, 711
Capgras' syndrome, 6, 373–374, 375, 376, 377*t*
Carbamazepine (CBZ), for aggression, 760*t*
Carbon monoxide poisoning, emotional disturbances in relation to diffuse brain dysfunction in, 738
Category fluency, prefrontal function and, 393
Category-specific impairment, of semantic memory, 458–459
Cerebral achromatopsia, 229
Cerebral akinotopsia, 229–230
Cerebral blood flow (CBF), regional, in normal-pressure hydrocephalus, 665
Cerebral commissurotomy, somesthetic results of, 278–279
Cerebral cortex, regions of, 45–48
Cerebral lesions, phantom sensations and, 288
Cerebritis, in systemic lupus erythematosus, 651
Cerebrospinal fluid (CSF) drainage procedures, in normal-pressure hydrocephalus, 666
Cerebrospinal fluid (CSF) infusion tests, in normal-pressure hydrocephalus, 666–667
Cerebrospinal fluid (CSF) pressure monitoring, in normal-pressure hydrocephalus, 667
Chemotherapy, childhood-acquired aphasia associated with, 790
Childhood-acquired aphasia, 783–795
adult-acquired aphasia versus, 785
age-related issues in, 793–794
brain bases of
nonfocal, 784
nonlateralized, 784–785
etiology of, 785–792
brain tumors and, 785, 790, 791*t*–792*t*
cancer treatments and, 790
hypoxic, 792
infectious, 790, 792
metabolic, 792
seizures and seizure-related disorders and, 785, 786*t*–787*t*
traumatic, 785, 789*t*–790*t*
vascular, 785, 788*t*
neuropathology of, 795
nonfluent characteristics of, 783–784
time-related issues in, 794–795
transient nature of, 784
Children
attention deficit hyperactivity disorder in. *See* Attention deficit hyperactivity disorder (ADHD)
autism in. *See* Autism
developmental reading disorders in. *See* Dyslexia, developmental
molecular genetics of cognitive developmental disorders in, 867–876, 872*f*
neurobehavioral examination in, 765–771, 766*t*, 768*t*, 769*t*, 770*f*
neuropsychological assessment of, 773–779
adult assessment contrasted with, 774–777
diagnostic method for, 777–778
focal versus neural substrates and, 774–775
intervention strategy formulation and, 778
modularity versus nonmodularity and, 775
neurobehavioral deficits versus environmental expectations and, 776–777
pathognomic signs versus developmental normality and, 776
predictions made on basis of, 778
reporting findings of, 778–779
stability versus developmental change and, 775–776
nonverbal, social, and emotional learning disabilities in. *See* Nonverbal, social, and emotional learning disabilities (NVLDs)
Pervasive Developmental Disorders in. *See* Asperger's syndrome; Autism; Pervasive Developmental Disorders (PDDs); Rett's syndrome (RS)
reading disorders in. *See* Dyslexia
Choline, for Alzheimer's disease, 554
Cholinergic agents, for Alzheimer's disease, 551–554
Chromosomal abnormalities, Alzheimer's disease and, 518–519
Chromosome 17 mutations, in frontotemporal lobar degeneration, 589
Chromosome 22q11.2-deletion syndrome, 848
Cisternography, in normal-pressure hydrocephalus, 665
Codman Hakim programmable valve, for normal-pressure hydrocephalus, 668
Cognitive conjunction design, for neuroimaging studies, 92

Cognitive decline, in systemic lupus erythematosus, 653–654
Cognitive defects, cognitive deficits and, 35
Cognitive deficits
  cognitive defects and, 35
  in delirium, 496
  identifying, 36
  measurement of, 36
Cognitive function, 685
  in attention deficit hyperactivity disorder, 835–837
  as computation, 135. *See also* Computational modeling
  ictal, 677
  interictal, 679–681
  in pediatric neuropsychological assessment, modularity versus nonmodularity and, 775
  screens of, mental status exam and, 25, 26*t*
Cognitive functions, 34
Cognitive models, constraints placed on, by functional neuroimaging, 98–99
Cognitive neuropsychology (CN), aphasia and. *See* Aphasia, language processing and
Cognitive neuropsychology (CN) school of aphasia therapy, 182–188, 183*f*
  for agrammatism, 185*t*, 185–188, 186*f*
  for anomia, 183*f*, 183–185
  modular-treatments approach to, 188–189
Cognitive psychology, marriage with experimental neuropsychology, 14–16
Cognitive subtraction, for neuroimaging studies, 91–92
Cohort effect, 531
Color agnosia, 250–251
  case study of, 251
  definition of, 250
  neuroanatomic correlates of, 251
  neuropsychological correlates of, 250–251
Color anomia, 251–253
  definition of, 251
  neuroanatomic correlates of, 252
  neuropsychological correlates of, 252
Color imagery, 243
  color perception related to, 249–250
  disorders of, 249–250
Color naming, 243
  disorders of, 251–253
  measurement of, 245
Color perception, 243
  color imagery related to, 249–250
  disorders of. *See* Achromatopsia, central
  measurement of, 243–244
  motor perception related to, 247–248
Color processing, 243–253, 244*f*. *See also* Color imagery; Color naming; Color perception; Color recognition
  terminology related to, 243
Color recognition, 243
  disorders of. *See* Color agnosia
  measurement of, 244
Coma, 338–339
  diagnostic criteria for, 338
  prognosis and outcome from, 338–339
Communication, elements of, 743–745
Compensatory cognitive strategies, recovery and, 102
Comprehension
  of affective prosody, 747
  in aphasia
    sentence-level, 171–173
    single words and, 166–167, 167*f*
  asyntactic, in aphasia, 171–172
  sentence-level, in aphasia, 171–173
  of single words, in aphasia, 166–167, 167*f*
Computational modeling, 135–143
  applications to behavioral neurology and neuropsychology, 138–143
  cognition as computation and, 135
  for covert face recognition, 140*f*, 140–141, 141*f*
  of dyslexia, 202–203
  of higher brain function, 17–18
  for neglect dyslexia, 139–140
  for optic aphasia, 141–143, 142*f*
  parallel distributed processing and, 135–138
    realism of PDP models and, 137
    spatial analogies for, 137–138
Computed tomography (CT)
  lesion identification using, 79
  in normal-pressure hydrocephalus, 661–662, 665
  timing of, for lesion method, 81–82
Conceptual apraxia, 222–223
  clinical findings in, 222–223
  pathophysiology of, 223
Conceptual functions, 34
Conceptual priming, in amnesia, 450–451
Conditioning, of fear, 713–718
  amygdala and, 713–714, 715*f*, 716
  background and definitions related to, 713, 714*f*
  hippocampus and, 716, 716*f*
  in humans, 716–718, 717*f*, 718*f*
  ventromedial prefrontal cortex and, 716
Conduction aphasia, 152*f*, 152–153
Conduction apraxia, 221–222
  clinical findings in, 221
  pathophysiology of, 222
Conduit d'approche, 152

Confabulation, 363–370
amnesic
in amnestic-dysexecutive syndrome, 364–366
deficient strategic retrieval and, 367–368
neuroanatomy of, 368–369, 369*f*
neuropsychological mechanisms associated with, 364–368
temporal/contextual displacement and, 366–367
anosognosia and, 357*t*, 357–358
for hemiplegia, 352–354, 353*t*
fantastic, 363
momentary, 363
neutral, 357*t*, 358, 363
personal, 357*t*, 358, 363
provoked, 363
simple, 363
spontaneous, 363
varieties of, 363–364
Confabulatory completion, in anosognosia, 348
Conflict-monitoring hypothesis, of prefrontal function, 397
Connectivity, parallel distributed processing and, 136
Consciousness, 337–342
arousal system and, 337
definition of, 337, 338*t*
disorders of, 338–342
gating system and, 337–338
Consolidation, 431, 432*t*, 464
brain sites of, 435*f*, 435–437, 436*f*, 437*t*
hippocampus in, 445–446
Consortium to Establish a Registry for AD (CERAD), criteria of, 517, 517*t*
Constructional apraxia, 296–298, 297*f*
Contextual displacement, amnesic confabulation and, 366–367
Contralateral neglect, 303
Contusions, aphasia due to, 159
Corpus callosum
disconnection of. *See* Split-brain patients
lesions of, ideomotor apraxia and, 219
specificity of callosal fibers and, 406
Cortical atrophies, focal, 528–530
Cortical auditory disorder, 257–259, 258*t*
Cortical blindness, unawareness of, 348–349
Cortical deafness, 257–259, 258*t*
Cortical lesions
in degenerative diseases, somatosensory disorders resulting from, 279, 279*f*
somatosensory disorders resulting from, 274–279
Cortical malformations, in dyslexia, 807–808
Cortical visual systems, dual, 230, 230*f*
Corticobasal degeneration, 530
Corticobasal ganglionic degeneration (CBGD)
cognitive characteristics of, 599–600
dementia in, 594*t*, 599–600
differential diagnosis of, 506*t*
epidemiology of, 599
pathology of, 600
COX-2 inhibitors, for Alzheimer's disease, 558
Cretinism, 845
Creutzfeldt-Jakob disease (CJD), dementia in, 631–632
Crossed aphasia, 157–158
Crossed aprosodia, developmental, 824
Cross-modal links, neglect and, 317–318
Crying, ictal, 678
Cytoarchitectonic maps, 45

D

Dax, Marc, 8–9
Deafferentation, differentiation from spatial neglect, 309
Deafness
cortical, 257–259, 258*t*
pure word, 257, 258*t*
in aphasia, 151–152, 167–168, 259–260
in Landau-Kleffner syndrome, 259, 260
mechanism of, 151–152
word-meaning, in aphasia, 168
Decision-making tasks, prefrontal lesions and, 395
Declarative memory, 463–464, 464*f*
following anterior communicating artery aneurysms, 481–482
Deep dyslexia, 197–199
Deep dysphasia, in aphasia, 168
Degenerative diseases. *See also specific diseases*
cortical sensory loss due to, 279, 279*f*
Déjerine, Joseph Jules, 10, 10*f*
Dejerine-Roussy syndrome, 419
Delayed response and span tasks, prefrontal lesions and, 394–395
Delirium, 495–500
attentional dysfunction in, 496
course and prognosis of, 497
definition of, 495–496, 496*t*
etiologies of, 498*t*, 498–499
laboratory features of, 497–498
management of, 499–500
movement disorders in, 497
neuropsychiatric features of, 496–497
nonattentional cognitive deficits in, 496
sleep-wake cycle disturbances in, 497
Delta Rule, parallel distributed processing and, 136–137

Delusion(s)
  in Alzheimer's disease, 735–736
  content-specific, secondary to brain damage, 729–730
  in Huntington's disease, 736
Delusional misidentification syndromes (DMSs), 373–378
  neuroanatomic correlates of, 374
  proposed framework for, 376–378, 377*t*
  representative theories of, 374–376
Dementia, 500–510
  aphasia due to, 159–160
  cortical, 503–505, 504*t*, 505*t*. *See also* Alzheimer's disease (AD)
    differential diagnosis of, 505, 506*t*, 507
  in corticobasal ganglionic degeneration, 594*t*, 599–600
  definition of, 500, 501*t*
  degenerative, 501
  of depression, differential diagnosis of, 506*t*, 507
  differential diagnosis of, 505, 506*t*, 507–509
    of cortical dementia, 505, 506*t*, 507
    of mixed cortical and subcortical dementia, 506*t*, 508–509
    of subcortical dementia, 506*t*, 507–508
  etiology of, 500–502
  frontotemporal
    aphasia due to, 160
    differential diagnosis of, 506*t*
    prefrontal dysfunction due to, 389–391, 390*f*
  future directions for, 510
  hereditary forms of, 501–502
  in Huntington's disease, 594*t*, 597–598
  infectious. *See* Infectious dementia
  with Lewy bodies, 527–528
    differential diagnosis of, 506*t*
  mixed cortical and subcortical dementia, differential diagnosis of, 506*t*, 508–509
  multi-infarct. *See* Vascular dementia
  neurochemistry in, 502–503
  neuroimaging in, 502
  in Parkinson's disease, 593, 594*t*, 595–596
  in progressive supranuclear palsy, 594*t*, 598–599
  semantic, 457, 584, 584*t*
  subcortical, 503–505, 504*t*, 505*t*
    differential diagnosis of, 506*t*, 507–508
  treatment and management of, 509–510
  violence in, 755
Dementia of frontal lobe type (DFT), 529–530
Denial, anosognosia and, 355–357
Depression
  in Alzheimer's disease, treatment of, 555–556
  in autism, 858
  dementia of, differential diagnosis of, 506*t*, 507
  in epilepsy
    ictal, 678
    interictal, 682
    treatment of, 684–685
  following brain injury, 739
  in Huntington's disease, 736
  in Parkinson's disease, 736–737
  poststroke, left frontal cortex lesions and, 728–729
Descartes, René, 4
Design fluency, prefrontal function and, 393
Developmental change, stability versus, in pediatric neuropsychological assessment, 775–776
Developmental crossed aprosodia, 824
Developmental dyscalculia, 210–211
Developmental normality, pathognomic signs versus, in pediatric neuropsychological assessment, 776
Developmental reading disorders. *See* Dyslexia, developmental
Diaschisis
  dynamic, 100
  reversal of, recovery and, 102
Diencephalic amnesia
  basal forebrain and mediotemporal amnesia versus, 480–481, 481*f*
  thalamic lesions and, 425–427
    anatomic basis of, 425, 426*f*, 427
    neuropsychological features of, 427
Diencephalic lesions, medial, in Korsakoff's syndrome, 433, 434*f*, 435
Diffuse axonal injury (DAI), emotional disturbances associated with, 738–739
Directional intentional neglect, 303
Disassociation apraxia, 221
Disorientation
  anterograde, 299
  egocentric, 298
  heading, 298
Dissociation(s)
  between number-processing operations, 209
  visual, 295–296
DNA, 870–871
Donepezil (Aricept), for Alzheimer's disease, 553, 553*t*
Dopamine (DA)
  in Alzheimer's disease, 552*t*
  in attention deficit hyperactivity disorder, 835
  violence and, 758
Dorsal left hemisphere systems, in dyslexia, 808–809
Dorsal simultagnosia, 329
Dorsomedial nucleus (DMN), in Wernicke-Korsakoff syndrome, 643

Dorsomedial somatosensory accessory cortex, 272, 273*t*
  apraxia-astereognosis syndrome and, 278, 278*f*
Down's syndrome (DS), 846
Drawing
  impaired, 296–298, 297*f*
  testing of, 304, 307*f*, 308*f*
Droperidol, for delirium, 500
Drugs. *See also specific drugs and drug types*
  violence induced by, 756
Dual cortical visual systems, 230, 230*f*
Dual-switch valve, for normal-pressure hydrocephalus, 668
Dynamic diaschisis, 100
Dyscalculia
  developmental, 210–211
  in Turner syndrome, 211
Dyslexia
  acquired, 195–203, 196*f*
    attentional, 197
    central, 197–201
    computation models of, 202–203
    deep, 197–199
    neglect, 139–140, 197
    peripheral, 196–197
    phonologic, 199
    right hemisphere and, 201–202
    surface, 199–200
  developmental, 801–813
    definitions related to, 801–802
    genetics of, 805–807
    historical background of, 801
    neurobiological foundations of, 807–809
    subtypes of, 803–804
    treatment of, 809–813
    visual and auditory temporal processes and, 804–805
    word recognition and phonological processes and, 802–803
Dysphasia, deep, in aphasia, 168
Dysprosody, 744
Dystonia, task-specific, plasticity and, 61

E

Education, Alzheimer's disease and, 519, 550–551
Egocentric disorientation, 298
Elaboration, 431, 432*t*, 464
  brain sites of, 435*f*, 435–437, 436*f*, 437*t*
  hippocampus in, 445–446
Electroencephalography (EEG)
  in delirium, 498
  event-related potentials and, 107–109, 109*f*
  plasticity studied using, 60
Electrophysiologic methods, 105–127. *See also* Brainstem auditory evoked potentials (BAEPs); Electroencephalography (EEG); Event-related potentials (ERPs); Somatosensory evoked responses (SERs); Transcranial magnetic stimulation (TMS); Visual evoked responses (VERs)
  endogenous, 106
Emotion(s), 711–719. *See also specific emotions*
  advances in understanding of, 713
  basal ganglia lesions and, 415–416
  hemispheric specialization and, 725–730
    autonomic components and experience of emotion and, 727–728
    comprehension and expression of emotions and, 726–727
    content-specific delusions secondary to brain damage and, 729–730
    first clinical studies and theoretical models of, 725–726
    poststroke depression and left frontal cortex lesions and, 728–729
  historical background of, 711–712, 712*f*
  ictal, 677–678
  integrated view of emotional brain and, 718–719
  limbic system concept of, 712, 712*f*
    contemporary challenges to, 712–713
  memory and, 438, 440
  neurology of, 750
Emotional behavior, 34–35
Emotional disorders, in relation to diffuse brain dysfunction, 735–739
  in Alzheimer's disease, 735–736
  in anoxia, 737
  in carbon monoxide poisoning, 738
  in closed head injury, 738–739
  in Huntington's chorea, 736
  in Parkinson's disease, 736–737
Emotional prosody, 744
Encephalitis, herpes simplex
  aphasia due to, 159
  childhood-acquired aphasia associated with, 790, 792
  lesion method for studying, 80
Encephalopathy
  anoxic, childhood-acquired aphasia associated with, 792
  in systemic lupus erythematosus, 653
Encoding, 431, 432*t*, 464
  brain sites of, 435*f*, 435–437, 436*f*, 437*t*
Energy, parallel distributed processing networks and, 138
Enumerative induction, 89
Environmental factors, in attention deficit hyperactivity disorder, 833–834

Environmental space, visuospatial disorders and, 298–299, 299*f*
Epilepsy, 675–686
  classification of, 675–676
  frontal lobe, 676
  ictal behavior in, 676–678
    cognitive phenomena, 677
    emotional phenomena, 677–678
    experiential phenomena, 677
  interictal behavior in, 679–684
    behavioral manifestations of, 681–684
    cognitive manifestations of, 679–681
  postictal behavior in, 678–679
  temporal lobe, surgery for, 695–701
    intellectual function and, 696
    language function and, 696–698
    memory and, 698–701
  temporolimbic, 676
  treatment of behavioral and cognitive symptoms in, 684–685
  violence in, 755
Episodic memory, 431, 432*t*
  semantic memory compared with, 446
Errorless learning, for memory rehabilitation, 490
Estrogens, for Alzheimer's disease, 559, 561–562
Event-related potentials (ERPs), 105, 106–124. *See also* Brainstem auditory evoked potentials (BAEPs); Somatosensory evoked responses (SERs); Visual evoked responses (VEPs)
  in brain-damaged patients, 109–111, 111*f*
  electroencephalogram and, 107–109, 109*f*
  exogenous, 106
  linguistic processing in aphasic patients and, 123–124
  with prefrontal damage, 111–119
    attentional facilitation and, 112–116, 114*f,* 115*f,* 117*f*
    inhibitory modulation and sensory gating and, 111–112, 113*f*
    novelty detection and, 116–119, 118*f,* 120*f,* 121*f*
  with right hemisphere damage, unilateral neglect and extinction after, 119–123, 122*f*
  technical aspects of, 106–109, 107*f*–109*f*
Evocation studies, neuroimaging for, 89
Evoked potentials. *See* Brainstem auditory evoked potentials (BAEPs); Event-related potentials (ERPs); Somatosensory evoked responses (SERs); Visual evoked responses (VEPs)
Excitatory amino acids, for Alzheimer's disease, 555
Executive control
  attentional facilitation and, 112–116, 114*f,* 115*f,* 117*f*
  following anterior communicating artery aneurysms, 481
  inhibitory modulation and sensory gating and, 111–112, 113*f*
  novelty detection and, 116–119, 118*f,* 120*f,* 121*f*
  prefrontal cortex and, 111. *See also* Prefrontal cortex (PFC)
Executive function (EF), 35
  in attention deficit hyperactivity disorder, 836–837
  basal ganglia lesions and, 416
  dysfunction of, confabulation and, 364–366
  interictal, 681
  mental status exam and, 29–30, 30*f*
  in nonverbal, social, and emotional learning disabilities, 822, 823*t,* 824
Experiential phenomena, ictal, 677
Experimental neuropsychology
  marriage with cognitive psychology, 14–16
  rise of, 13–14
Explicit memory, amnesia and, 448–450
External aids, for memory rehabilitation, 489
Extinction
  motor, 303
  testing for, 304
Extracellular matrix components, in senile plaques, 522
Extrapersonal neglect, 315

F

Face recognition
  anatomic bases of, 240–241
  covert, parallel distributed processing and, 140*f,* 140–141, 141*f*
  impairment of, 239–241, 246
    anatomic bases of face recognition and, 240–241
    functional deficit in, face-specificity of, 239–240
  in nonverbal, social, and emotional learning disabilities, 821–822
Family Intervention in Chronic Aphasia (FICA), 182
Fantastic confabulation, 363
Fatal familial insomnia (FFI), 631
Fear, ictal, 677–678
Fear conditioning, 713–718
  amygdala and, 713–714, 715*f,* 716
  background and definitions related to, 713, 714*f*
  hippocampus and, 716, 716*f*
  in humans, 716–718, 717*f,* 718*f*
  ventromedial prefrontal cortex and, 716
Feedforward networks, parallel distributed processing and, 136
Finger agnosia, 290
Flourens, Marie-Jean-Pierre, 6
Fluency tasks, prefrontal lesions and, 393–394

Fluent aphasia
  See Wernicke's aphasia
Fragile-X syndrome (FRAX), 846–847
Frégoli syndrome, 373, 375–376, 377*t*
Fritsch, Gustav, 9
Frontal deficits, basal ganglia lesions and, 416
Frontal lesions
  global aphasia and, 154
  transcortical motor aphasia and, 154–155, 155*f*
Frontal lobe(s), 385–391. *See also* Prefrontal cortex (PFC)
  injury to, memory and, 470–472, 471*f*
Frontal lobe degeneration (FLD), 529–530
Frontal lobe epilepsy (FLE), 676
Frontotemporal dementia (FTD), 582–589, 583*t*
  aphasia due to, 160
  clinical features of, 582–585, 583*t*
  differential diagnosis of, 506*t*, 585–586
  epidemiology of, 582
  FTLD variants and, 583–585, 584*t*
  neuroimaging in, 585*f*–587*f*, 586
  neuropathologic features of, 586, 587*f*, 588*f*, 588–589
  pathophysiology of, 589
  prefrontal dysfunction due to, 389–391, 390*f*
  treatment of, 589
Frontotemporal lobar degeneration (FTLD), 529–530, 582. *See also* Frontotemporal dementia (FTD)
  variants of, 583–585, 584*t*
Functional amnesia, 434*t*
Functional goals, for aphasia rehabilitation and, 180–181
Functional magnetic resonance imaging (fMRI), 17, 17*f*
  BOLD, 86
    properties affecting experimental design, 93*f*, 93–94, 94*f*
    temporal structures of studies using, 94–96
    two-systems model of, 87*f*, 87–88, 88*t*
  structural, 862–863
Functional neuroimaging, 85–96, 97–103. *See also specific imaging methods*
  advantages of, 97–98
  cognitive process manipulations and, 91–92
  constraints placed on cognitive models by, 98–99
  data provided by, properties of, 85–86
  inferences from, 88–90
  lesion studies related to, 90–91
  limitations of, 102–103
  normal functional anatomy on, 99–100
  properties affecting experimental design, 93*f*, 93–94, 94*f*
  recovery models and, 101–102
  two-systems model of, 87*f*, 87–88, 88*t*
Functional/pragmatic/social school of aphasia therapy, 181–182, 182*f*

G
Gabapentin, for aggression, 760*t*
Galactosemia, childhood-acquired aphasia associated with, 792
Galantamine (Reminyl), for Alzheimer's disease, 553*t*, 554
Galen of Pergamus, 3–4
Gall, Franz Josef, 5–6, 6*f*
Gamma-aminobutyric acid (GABA)
  in Alzheimer's disease, 552*t*
  violence and, 758
Gating system, consciousness and, 337–338
Gaze, paralysis of, psychic, 327
Gaze apraxia, 328
Gender, Alzheimer's disease and, 519, 551
Gene(s), 870
Generalized anxiety disorder (GAD), in Alzheimer's disease, 735
Generalized Delta Rule, parallel distributed processing and, 137
Genetic factors
  in Alzheimer's disease, 518–519, 551
  in attention deficit hyperactivity disorder, 832–833
  in autism, 854
  in dyslexia, 805–807
  in frontotemporal lobar degeneration, 589
  in nonverbal, social, and emotional learning disabilities, 825
Genetics, molecular, of cognitive developmental disorders, 867–876, 872*f*
  behavioral genetics and, 869–870
  future directions for, 874–875
  molecular biology and, 870–871
  phenotype and, 867–869, 868*t*
Geniculothalamic artery region, infarctions due to thalamic lesions in, 419–420, 421*f*
Geniculothalamic lacunae, 420, 421*f*
Gerstmann's syndrome, 208
Gerstmann-Straussler-Scheinker (GSS) syndrome, 631
Geschwind, Norman, 10
Gestures
  of affective prosody, 747–748, 748*f*
  meaningless, imitation of, 290–291, 291*f*
  spontaneous, 746
Giant cell arteritis, 654*t*
Ginkgo biloba, for Alzheimer's disease, 560–561, 562
Gliomas, lesion method for studying, 80
Global amnesia, transient, 434*t*
Global aphasia, 153–154
Globus pallidum, anatomy of, 50–51
Glutamate, in Alzheimer's disease, 552*t*
Goldman-Rakie, Patricia, 18

Goldstein, Kurt, 11, 12*f*
Grammatical class, lexical retrieval and, 170–171
Gratiolet, Pierre, 7

H

Hallucinations, in Huntington's disease, 736
Haloperidol, for delirium, 500
Halstead-Reitan Battery, 37
Handwriting, in pediatric motor examination, 768–769
Head, Henry, 11
Heading disorientation, 298
Head injury. *See* Brain injury
Hebb Rule, parallel distributed processing and, 136
Heilman, Kenneth, 18
Helm's Elicited Language Program for Syntax Stimulation (HELPSS), 180
Hemianopia, 227
  anosognosia for, 345–347
  right, in color anomia, 252
Hemiplegia
  anosognosia for. *See* Anosognosia, for hemiplegia
  after seizures, reversible, 679
Hemispatial neglect, 295
  anosognosia for hemiplegia related to, 351–352, 352*t*
Hemispheric dominance, 404–405
  evolution of, 404
  left hemisphere as interpreter and, 404
  visuospatial functions and, 404–405
Hemispheric lateralization. *See also* Left hemisphere; Right hemisphere
  of affective prosody, 748–750, 749*f*
  of praxis and visuospatial functions
    in crossed aphasia, 157
    in left-handers with aphasia, 158
Hemispheric specialization
  emotion and, 725–730
    autonomic components and experience of emotion and, 727–728
    comprehension and expression of emotions and, 726–727
    content-specific delusions secondary to brain damage and, 729–730
    first clinical studies and theoretical models of, 725–726
    poststroke depression and left frontal cortex lesions and, 728–729
  number processing and, 209–210
Hemodynamic response function (HRF), with BOLD fMRI, 93*f*, 93–94
Hemorrhage
  aphasia due to, 159
  intracerebral
    lesion method for studying, 81
    vascular dementia and, 614
  subarachnoid
    association with idiopathic normal-pressure hydrocephalus, 670
    vascular dementia and, 614
Herpes simplex encephalitis (HSE)
  aphasia due to, 159
  childhood-acquired aphasia associated with, 790, 792
  lesion method for studying, 80
Heteromodal cortex, 49
Hidden units, parallel distributed processing and, 136
Higher brain function, computational modeling of, 17–18
Hippocampus
  in consolidation, 445–446
  fear and, 716, 716*f*
  naming and, temporal lobe epilepsy surgery and, 698
Hippocrates, 3
History of behavioral neurology and neuropsychology, 3–18
  emergence of modern behavioral neurology and neuropsychology and, 9*f*–13*f*, 9–13
  localism/wholism debate and, 5–9, 6*f*–8*f*
  marriage of experimental neuropsychology and cognitive psychology and, 14–16
  new tools for study of mind and brain and, 16–18
  rise of experimental neuropsychology and, 13–14
  roots and, 3–5, 4*f*, 5*f*
Hitzig, Edward, 9
Homocystinuria, childhood-acquired aphasia associated with, 792
Homonymous hemianopia, 227. *See also* Hemianopia
Homovanillic acid (HVA), in attention deficit hyperactivity disorder, 835
Human immunodeficiency virus (HIV) infection, dementia due to, differential diagnosis of, 508
Huntington's disease (HD), 596–598
  cognitive characteristics of, 597
  dementia in, 594*t*, 597–598
  differential diagnosis of, 506*t*, 507, 508
  emotional disturbances in relation to diffuse brain dysfunction in, 736
  epidemiology of, 596–597
  pathology of, 597–598
Hydrocephalus
  differential diagnosis of, 506*t*, 507
  normal pressure. *See* Normal-pressure hydrocephalus (NPH)
  prefrontal dysfunction due to, 388–389, 389*f*

Hydroxychloroquine, for Alzheimer's disease, 558–559
Hyperactivity. *See* Attention deficit hyperactivity disorder (ADHD)
Hyperprosody, 744
Hypertension, systemic, association with idiopathic normal-pressure hydrocephalus, 670
Hypoarousal, in nonverbal, social, and emotional learning disabilities, 824
Hypokinesia, 303
Hypometria, 303
Hypothalamus, violence and, 756–757
Hypoxia, childhood-acquired aphasia associated with, 792

I

Ideational apraxia, 221
Idebenone, for Alzheimer's disease, 560
Ideomotor apraxia (IMA), 217
  clinical findings in, 218–219
  pathophysiology of, 219–221
Illusory limbs
  in anosognosia for hemiplegia, 353–354
  phantom limbs contrasted with, 353, 353*t*
Imageability, in deep dyslexia, 198
Imagery, mental, visual, 230–232
  image generation disorders and, 232
  image representation disorders and, 231*f*, 231–232
Imaginative play, in autism, 856–857
Imitation, of meaningless gestures, 290–291, 291*f*
Immunotherapy, for Alzheimer's disease, 557–558
Impairment, definition of, 179
Impersistence, 303
Implementation studies, neuroimaging for, 89
Implicit memory
  amnesia and, 448–449, 450–452
  following traumatic brain injury, 470
Impulsivity, in attention deficit hyperactivity disorder, 831
Inarticulate prosody, 744
Inattention. *See also* Sensory neglect
  in attention deficit hyperactivity disorder, 831
  in nonverbal, social, and emotional learning disabilities, 824
Inborn errors of metabolism, childhood-acquired aphasia associated with, 792
Infarctions
  aphasia due to, 158–159
  global aphasia due to, 154
  ischemic, prefrontal dysfunction due to, 386–387, 387*f*
  thalamic lesions due to, 419–424
    in anterior choroidal artery region, 424, 424*f*, 425*f*
    in geniculothalamic artery region, 419–420, 421*f*
    in interpeduncular profunda artery region, 422–424, 423*f*
    in tuberothalamic artery region, 420–422, 422*f*
Infections
  childhood-acquired aphasia associated with, 790, 792
  HIV, dementia due to, differential diagnosis of, 508
  prefrontal dysfunction due to, 389
Infectious dementia, 629–634
  AIDS dementia complex, 629–631, 630*t*
  differential diagnosis of, 508
  in Lyme disease, 633
  neurosyphilis, 632–633
  in postmeningitic syndromes, 634
  in prion diseases, 631–632
  progressive multifocal leukoencephalopathy, 631
  in progressive rubella panencephalitis, 634
  in subacute sclerosing panencephalitis, 633–634
  in Whipple's disease, 633
Inferior parietal lobe (IPL), neglect and, 306, 309
Inflammation, in senile plaques, 523
Inhibition, prefrontal cortex and, event-related potentials for study of, 111–112
Insight, mental status exam and, 25
Intellectual function. *See also* Mental retardation
  anosognosia for hemiplegia related to, 352
  in autism, 858–859
  interictal, 679–680
  temporal lobe epilepsy surgery and, 696
  in Wernicke-Korsakoff syndrome, 640, 640*t*
Intellectual prosody, 744
Intention, spatial, neglect and, 314
Intentional neglect, 303
  differentiating from representational neglect, 305
  testing for, 304
Interaction networks, parallel distributed processing and, 136
Interest restriction, in autism, 857
Interhemispheric integration of perception and attention, 405–406
  hemispheric isolation of visual and tactile information and, 405, 405*f*
  sharing of attentional control and, 405–406
Internal optic artery region, infarctions due to thalamic lesions in, 422–424, 423*f*
Interpeduncular profunda artery region, infarctions due to thalamic lesions in, 422–424, 423*f*
Intracerebral hemorrhage (ICH)
  lesion method for studying, 81
  vascular dementia and, 614
Intralaminar nuclei (ILN), consciousness and, 338

Intrinsic prosody, 744
Ipsilateral neglect, 303
Ischemic infarction, prefrontal dysfunction due to, 386–387, 387*f*
Isocortex, 46–48
  heteromodal component of, 47–48
  lesions of, visual perception and, 228–230
  unimodal component of, 48, 49

J

Jackson, John Hughlings, 11, 11*f*
James, William, 711
James-Lange theory of emotion, 711
Judgment, mental status exam and, 25

K

Kindling, violence and, 758
Kinesics, 743–744
  neurology of, 744–745
Klüver-Bucy syndrome, 438, 440, 711–712
Knowledge, about human body
  body-part specificity of, 291–292
  body perception and, 285–286
Koniocortex, 48
Korsakoff, Sergei S., 12, 13*f*
Korsakoff's syndrome, 433, 434*f*, 435
Kuru, 631

L

Lacunar strokes, multiple, differential diagnosis of, 506*t*, 507–508
Landau-Kleffner syndrome (LKS), 784, 785, 786*t*–787*t*
Landau-Kleffner syndrome, pure word deafness associated with, 259, 260
Landmark agnosia, 298–299
Language
  in autism, 860
  elements of, 743–745
  mental status exam and, 27–28
  in split-brain patients, 402–403
    right hemisphere control of speech and grammar and, 402–403
    right hemisphere reading and, 403
Language disorders
  neuropathology of, 795
  with thalamic lesions, 427–428
Language function
  in autism, 855–856
  interictal, 680–681
  temporal lobe epilepsy surgery and, 696–698
Language-oriented school of aphasia therapy, 180–181, 181*f*
Language processing
  aphasia and. *See* Aphasia, language processing and
  components of, 166
Lashley, Karl, 11, 12*f*
Lateralization. *See also* Left hemisphere; Right hemisphere
  of affective prosody, 748–750, 749*f*
  of praxis and visuospatial functions
    in crossed aphasia, 157
    in left-handers with aphasia, 158
Laughter, ictal, 678
Learning
  in autism, 860
  errorless, for memory rehabilitation, 490
Learning deficits, following traumatic brain injury, 468–470, 469*f*
Learning disabilities, nonverbal, social, and emotional. *See* Nonverbal, social, and emotional learning disabilities (NVLDs)
Learning rules, parallel distributed processing and, 136–137
Lecithin, for Alzheimer's disease, 554
Left-handedness, aphasia associated with, 157
Left hemisphere
  dominance of, 404–405
    evolution of, 404
    visuospatial functions and, 404–405
  as interpreter, 404
Leipmann, Hugo, 10
Lesion(s). *See also specific lesions*
  virtual, with transcranial magnetic stimulation, 126
Lesion method, 71–82
  BRAINVOX and, 73–74, 75*f*, 76*f*
  CT lesion identification and, 79
  for group analysis, 78–79
  limitations of, 82
  modern practice in humans, 73
  MRI lesion identification and, 79
  neuroanatomic resolution and, 79–80
  neuroanatomy from neuroimaging data and, 73
  neuroimaging studies related to, 90–91
  specimen choice for, 80–81
  template technique for, 74, 76–77
    improvement on, 77, 78*f*
  timing of imaging for, 81–82
Lesion studies, of achromatopsia, central, 246–248, 248*f*
Letter fluency, prefrontal function and, 393

Leukoaraiosis, 613
Lewy bodies
in Alzheimer's disease, 527–528, 550
dementia with, 527–528
differential diagnosis of, 506*t*
Lexical processing disorders, in aphasia, 168
Lexical retrieval, in aphasia, 170–171
Lichtheim, Ludwig, 10
Limb akinesia, 303
Limb apraxia, 217–224
conceptual, 222–223
conduction, 221–222
disassociation, 221
in global aphasia, 153
ideational, 217, 222
ideomotor, 217
clinical findings in, 218–219
pathophysiology of, 219–221
kinetic, 218
melokinetic, 217
testing for, 217–218
Limbic circuits, encoding and consolidation and, 435*f*, 435–437, 436*f*, 437*t*
Limbic structures, 49
Limbic system, violence and, 757
Limbic system theory of emotion, 712, 712*f*
contemporary challenges to, 712–713
Limb ideomotor apraxia, in conduction aphasia, 152
Linear activation functions, 136
Line bisection task, 304, 305*f*
Lingual gyrus, achromatopsia and, 249
Linguistic processing, in aphasia, event-related potentials for study of, 123–124
Lissencephaly, 844
Lithium, for aggression, 760*t*
Localism/wholism debate, 5–9, 6*f*–8*f*
Localization studies, neuroimaging for, 89
Location, impaired perception of, 295–296
Long-term depression (LTD), 59
Long-term potentiation (LTP), 59
Lorazepam, for delirium, 500
Luria, Aleksandr, 18
Lyme disease, dementia in, 633

M

MacQuarrie Test for Mechanical Ability, 37
Macropyramidal cortex, 48
Magendie, François, 4–5
Magnetic resonance imaging (MRI)
lesion identification using, 79
in normal-pressure hydrocephalus, 662, 664–665
timing of, for lesion method, 81–82
Magnetic resonance spectroscopy (MRS), plasticity studied using, 60
Magnetic source imaging (MSI), in dyslexia, 812–813
Magnetoencephalography (MEG), plasticity studied using, 60
Magnocellular system, in dyslexia, 804–805
Mania, ictal, 678
Marie, Pierre, 11
Meaning, reading without, 200–201
Medicare, aphasia rehabilitation and, 180–181
Medication effects, interictal, 681
Mediotemporal amnesia, basal forebrain and diencephalic amnesia versus, 480–481, 481*f*
Mediotemporal lobe lesions, amnesia and, 432–433
Memantine, for Alzheimer's disease, 555
Memory. *See also* Amnesia
acute dysfunction following brain injury
assessment of, 465–466
neurometabolism in, 466, 467*f*
predicting outcome based on duration of, 465, 465*f*
in autism, 860
chronic dysfunction following brain injury, 466–472
classification of, 431, 432*t*
declarative, 463–464, 464*f*
following anterior communicating artery aneurysms, 481–482
dysfunction following acute brain injury, 465–466
emotion and, 438, 440
episodic, 431, 432*t*
semantic memory compared with, 446
explicit, amnesia and, 448–450
following callosotomy, 403–404
impairment following anterior communicating artery aneurysm. *See* Anterior communicating artery (ACoA) aneurysms
implicit
amnesia and, 448–449, 450–452
following traumatic brain injury, 470
interictal, 680
mental status exam and, 28
procedural, 431, 432*t*, 463, 464*f*
following traumatic brain injury, 470
semantic. *See* Semantic dementia; Semantic memory
temporal lobe epilepsy surgery and, 698–701
working, 464
prefrontal function and, 397–398
Memory functions, 34
Memory processes, in brain, 463–464, 464*f*

Memory rehabilitation, 487–490
  approaches to, 487–488
  future directions for, 490
  methods of, 488–490
Meningiomas
  lesion method for studying, 80
  prefrontal dysfunction due to, 388, 389*f*
Meningitis
  childhood-acquired aphasia associated with, 790
  dementia following, 634
Mental imagery, visual, 230–232
  image generation disorders and, 232
  image representation disorders and, 231*f*, 231–232
Mental retardation, 843–849
  in Angelman's syndrome, 847
  in autism, 858
  in chromosome 22q11.2-deletion syndrome, 848
  in cretinism, 845
  in Down's syndrome, 846
  in fragile-X syndrome, 846–847
  in lissencephaly, 844
  neurobiological factors in, 843–844
  in Prader-Willi syndrome, 847
  in Rett's syndrome, 844–845
  in Rubenstein-Taybi syndrome, 845
  in Turner syndrome, 847–848
  violence associated with, 756
  in Williams' syndrome, 848–849
  X-linked, nonsyndromic, 845–846
Mental status exam, 23–31
  affect and, 24
  appearance and, 23
  attention and, 26–27
  behavior and, 23–24
  description of, 30–31
  executive function and, 29–30, 30*f*
  insight and, 25
  judgment and, 25
  language and, 27–28
  memory and, 28
  mood and, 24
  screens of cognitive function and, 25, 26*t*
  thought content and, 24–25
  thought processes and, 24
  visuospatial function and, 28–29, 29*f*
Mesulam, Marcel, 18
Metabolic disorders, childhood-acquired aphasia associated with, 792
Metachromatic leukodystrophy, prefrontal dysfunction due to, 391
Metal chelators, for Alzheimer's disease, 558
Mild cognitive impairment (MCI), progression to Alzheimer's disease, 561
Minimally conscious state (MCS), 340–342
  diagnostic criteria for, 340
  emergence from, criteria for, 340–341, 341*f*
  prognosis and outcome of, 341–342
Misidentification syndromes, 373–378
  neuroanatomic correlates of, 374
  proposed framework for, 376–378, 377*t*
  representative theories of, 374–376
Mismatch negativity (MMN), 116–118
  in neglect, 122, 122*f*
Misoplegia, 350
Mixed transcortical aphasia (MTA), 157
Mnemonic strategies, for memory rehabilitation, 489
Mnestic block syndrome, 440
Modality-specific impairment, of semantic memory, 459–460
Modular-treatments approach to aphasia, 188–189
Molecular genetics, of cognitive developmental disorders, 867–876, 872*f*
Molner, Brenda, 14
Momentary confabulation, 363
Montreal Neurological Institute, 13
Mood. *See also* Depression
  mental status exam and, 24
Motor actions, body-centered reference system for, 285
Motor aphasia, transcortical, 154–156, 155*f*
Motor cortex, 48
  lower, lesions of, Broca's aphasia and, 149–150
Motor deficits, basal ganglia lesions and, 416
Motor examination, in children, 768–770, 769*f*, 770*f*
Motor extinction, 303
Motor function, in autism, 860
Motor neglect, 303
  differentiating from representational neglect, 305
  testing for, 304
Motor pathways, speed of conduction in, transcranial magnetic stimulation for study of, 125–126
Motor perception, color perception related to, 247–248
Motor perseveration, 303
Movement disorders. *See also specific disorders*
  in delirium, 497
Multi-infarct dementia. *See* Vascular dementia
Multiple memory trace (MMT) theory, 446
Multiple system atrophy (MSA), 600–601
  cognitive characteristics of, 600–601
  epidemiology of, 600
  pathology of, 601
Munk, Hermann, 12
Mutism, aphasic, 793

N

Naming
  of colors, 243
    disorders of, 251–253
    measurement of, 245
  hippocampus and, temporal lobe epilepsy surgery and, 698
Neglect, 303–310, 313–319
  basal ganglia lesions and, 414–415
  contralateral, 303
  cross-modal and sensorimotor integration and, 317–318
  extrapersonal, 315
  hemispatial, 295
    anosognosia for hemiplegia related to, 351–352, 352*t*
  intentional (motor), 303
    differentiating from representational neglect, 305
    testing for, 304
  ipsilateral, 303
  levels of processing and, 318–319
    processing without attention and, 318
    processing without awareness and, 318–319
  of one-half of body, 288–289
  pathophysiology of, 306–309
  peripersonal, 315
  personal, 303, 315
  radial and vertical axes and, 315–316
  regions of space and, 315
  representational, 303
  representational instability and, 316–317
  after right hemisphere damage, event-related potentials for study of, 119–123, 122*f*
  sensory (inattention), 303
  spatial, 303
  spatial anisometry and, 316
  spatial reference frames and, 317
  testing for, 303–305, 305*f*–308*f*
    for extinction, 304
    for inattention (sensory neglect), 303–304
    for intentional (motor) neglect, 304
  theories of, 313–315
    attention and intention and, 314
    spatial attention and, 313–314
    spatial intention and, 314
    spatial representation and, 314–315
  treatment and management of, 309–310
Neglect dyslexia, 197
  parallel distributed processing and, 139–140
Neocortex, violence and, 757
Neural networks, anatomy of, 53–54
Neurites, of senile plaques, 523
Neurobehavioral examination
  in adults. *See* Mental status exam
  in children, 765–771, 766*t*, 768*t*, 769*t*, 770*f*
Neurofibrillary tangles (NFTs), in Alzheimer's disease, 524*f*, 524–526, 525*f*, 532*t*, 532–533, 548–549
  biochemistry of, 548–549
  structure of, 548
Neuroimaging. *See also specific methods*
  in achromatopsia, central, 248–249
  in auditory agnosia, 265–266
  in autism, 862–863
  in frontotemporal degeneration, 585*f*–587*f*, 586
  functional, 862–863
  neuroanatomy from, 73
  number processing and, 208–209
  structural, 862
Neuroleptics, for delirium, 500
Neurologic examination, in autism, 857
Neuronal configuration, event-related potentials and, 106–107, 107*f*
Neuronal loss/atrophy
  in Alzheimer's disease, 526–527, 549, 549*f*, 573–574
  with normal aging, 531–533
Neuronal membrane excitability, 59
Neuronal migration anomalies, in nonverbal, social, and emotional learning disabilities, 824
Neuropeptides, for Alzheimer's disease, 555
Neuropil threads, in Alzheimer's disease, 524
Neuropsychological assessment, 33–40
  in Alzheimer's disease, 516
  applications of, 33–34
  of children. *See* Children, neuropsychological assessment of
  evolution of, 33
  neuropsychological components of behavior and, 34–35
  of neuropsychological deficits, 35–36
  tests in, 36–37
Neuropsychological functioning, in autism, 859
Neurosyphilis, dementia in, 632–633
Neurotransmitters
  in Alzheimer's disease, 551, 552*t*
  violence and, 757–758
Neutral confabulation, 357*t*, 358, 363
NGF, for Alzheimer's disease, 559
Nicotinic acetylcholine receptor agonists, for Alzheimer's disease, 554
NINDS-AIREN criteria, 610, 612*t*
Noise, with BOLD fMRI, 94, 94*f*
Nonfluent aphasia. *See* Broca's aphasia
Nonhemorrhagic infarctions, for lesion method, 80
Nonspeech sounds, auditory agnosia for, 257, 258*t*, 262–263

Nonsteroidal anti-inflammatory drugs (NSAIDs), for Alzheimer's disease, 558, 562
Nonverbal, social, and emotional learning disabilities (NVLDs), 821–827
  differential diagnosis of, 826
  etiology of, 824–825
    acquired brain lesions in, 824
    genetic, 825
    prenatal neuromigrational anomalies and lesions in, 824–825
  hypoarousal in, 824
  inattention in, 824
  processing deficits at perceptual and motor level in, 821–822
  social cognition deficits in, 822, 823*t*, 824
  treatment of, 826–827
  workup and diagnostic evaluation of, 825–826
Norepinephrine (NE)
  in Alzheimer's disease, 552*t*
  violence and, 757
Normal-pressure hydrocephalus (NPH), 659–671, 660*f*, 661*f*
  Alzheimer's disease differentiated from, 664
  aphasia in, 661, 663*t*
  assessing patient improvement in, 667–668
  cisternography in, 665
  clinical evaluation of, 659–661, 663*t*
  computed tomography in, 661–662, 665
  congenital, detection of, 662
  CSF drainage procedures in, 666
  CSF infusion tests in, 666–667
  CSF pressure monitoring in, 667
  differential diagnosis of, 659, 662*t*
  idiopathic
    histopathology of, 669, 669*t*
    systemic hypertension related to, 670
  magnetic resonance imaging in, 662, 664–665
  regional cerebral blood flow in, 665
  shunt complications in, 668
  shunt outcome in, factors related to, 671, 671*t*
  shunt selection for, 668–669
  surgical outcome in, flow void on MRI as predictor of, 664–665
  white matter lesions in, 662, 664
Novel information, priming of, in amnesia, 451–452
Novelty detection, event-related potentials for study of, 116–119, 118*f*, 120*f*, 121*f*
Number processing, 207–212. *See also* Acalculia; Dyscalculia
  brain-imaging studies of, 208–209
  dissociations between operations and, 209
  hemispheric specialization and, 209–210
  isolation of number processing system and, 207
  parietal lobe and, 207–208

O

Occipital region lesions, achromatopsia and, 246–247
Occipitotemporal circuit, in dyslexia, 808, 809
Occipitotemporal junction lesions, achromatopsia and, 247
Occipitotemporal region
  color agnosia and, 251
  color anomia and, 252
Oculomotor apraxia, 327
Olanzapine
  for delirium, 500
  for dementia, 509
Optic aphasia, 237, 250–251
  parallel distributed processing and, 141–143, 142*f*
Optic ataxia, 286, 325–327
Optokinetic nystagmus, for reducing neglect, 310
Organic repression, 355
Orientation, impaired perception of, 295–296
Orientation agnosia, 296
Orton, Samuel, 801
Overt Aggression Scale (OAS), 758

P

Pain, asymboly for, somesthetic results of, 279
Paired helical filaments (PHFs), 524
Papez circuit, 435*f*, 435–436, 711–712
Paragrammatism, 148
Paralimbic zone, 46
Paralinguistic auditory agnosia, 257, 263–264
Parallel distributed processing (PDP), 135–138
  activation rule and, 136
  connectivity and, 136
  learning rules and, 136–137
Parallel distributed processing (PDP) models, 18
Paramedian thalamic artery region, infarctions due to thalamic lesions in, 422–424, 423*f*
Parametric designs, for neuroimaging studies, 92
Paramnesia, reduplicative, 355, 373, 434*t*. *See also* Misidentification syndromes
Parietal lobe
  lesions of
    conduction aphasia and, 153
    inferior, ideomotor apraxia and, 219–220
    tactile agnosia and, 277*f*, 277–278
  number processing and, 207–208

Parkinson's disease (PD)
cognitive characteristics of, 595–596
dementia in, 593, 594*t*, 595–596
differential diagnosis of, 506*t*, 507
emotional disturbances in relation to diffuse brain dysfunction in, 736–737
pathology of, 596
Participation restriction, definition of, 180
Part-of-speech effect, in deep dyslexia, 198
Part-whole processing, in autism, 859
Parvocellular pathway, 804
Patching, for reducing neglect, 310
Pencil grasp, in pediatric motor examination, 770, 770*f*
Perception
of body. *See* Body perception
color, 243
color imagery related to, 249–250
disorders of. *See* Achromatopsia, central
measurement of, 243–244
motor perception related to, 247–248
interhemispheric integration of attention and, 405–406
hemispheric isolation of visual and tactile information and, 405, 405*f*
sharing of attentional control and, 405–406
motor, color perception related to, 247–248
sensory, in autism, 859–860
tactile. *See* Tactile perception
visual, 227–230
association cortex lesions and, 228–230
organizing framework for higher-level disorders of, 230, 230*f*
phantom sensations and, 287
primary visual cortex and afferent lesions and, 227–228, 228*f*
Perceptual categorization deficit, 235
Perceptual functions, 34
Perceptual priming, in amnesia, 450–451
Periarteritis nodosa, 654*t*, 655
Perilesional activation, recovery and, 102
Peripersonal neglect, 315
Perisylvian lesions, global aphasia and, 153
Permanent vegetative state, 339–340
Persistent vegetative state, 339
Personal confabulation, 357*t*, 358, 363
Personality, in epilepsy, 683–684
Personal neglect, 303, 315
Pervasive Developmental Disorders (PDDs). *See also* Asperger's syndrome; Autism; Rett's syndrome (RS)
classification of, 853
prevalence of, 853–854
PHAB/DI (Phonological Analysis and Blending/Direct Instruction) Program, 810–811
Phantom(s), body-part, 286–288
cerebral substrate of, 288
in congenital absence of limbs, 287–288
visual and somatosensory influences on, 287
Phantom limbs, illusory limbs contrasted with, 353, 353*t*
PHAST (Phonological and Strategy Training) Track Reading Program, 811–812
Phenylketonuria, childhood-acquired aphasia associated with, 792
Phonagnosia, 264
Phonological processing
disorders of, in aphasia, 167–168
in dyslexia, 802–803
Phonologic dyslexia, 199
Physostigmine, for delirium, 500
Plasticity, 57–68
in adaptation to blindness, 63–68, 64*f*, 65*f*, 67*f*
on disease pathogenesis, 61–63
as intrinsic property of brain, 57–58
maladaptive, 60–61, 62*f*, 63*f*
mechanisms of, 58–59
methods for studying in humans, 59–60
Play, imaginative, in autism, 856–857
Polar artery region, infarctions due to thalamic lesions in, 420–422, 422*f*
Porteus's Mazes, 37
Positron emission tomography (PET), 16*f*, 16–17, 86
in auditory agnosia, 265–266
plasticity studied using, 60
Posner, Michael, 17
Posner paradigm, 123
Postmeningitic syndromes, dementia in, 634
Posttraumatic amnesia (PTA), 465–466
assessment of, 465–466
neurometabolism in, 466, 467*f*
prognosis based on, 465, 465*f*
Power spectrum, with BOLD fMRI, 94, 94*f*
Practice techniques, for memory rehabilitation, 488
Prader-Willi syndrome (PWS), 847
Prednisone, for Alzheimer's disease, 558
Prefrontal cortex (PFC), 385–391, 393–398
dysfunction and, etiology of, 386–391
degenerative dementias as, 389–391, 390*f*
hydrocephalus and, 388–389, 389*f*
infectious, 389
traumatic, 387, 388*f*
tumors and, 388, 389*f*
vascular, 386–387
event-related potentials for study of, 111–119

Prefrontal cortex (PFC) (*continued*)
attentional facilitation and, 112–116, 114*f*, 115*f*, 117*f*
inhibitory modulation and sensory gating and, 111–112, 113*f*
novelty detection and, 116–119, 118*f*, 120*f*, 121*f*
extrastriate neural activity regulation by, 113–116, 114*f*, 115*f*
function of, clinical aspects of, 385–386
lesions of, 393–395
decision-making tasks and, 395
delayed response and span tasks and, 394–395
diversity and commonality among patients and, 395
fluency tasks and, 393–394
response inhibition and, 394
sequencing tasks and, 393
theories of function of, 395–398, 396*f*, 397*t*
adaptive coding and, 398
supervisory attentional system and, 397
working memory and, 397–398
ventromedial, fear and, 716
Prerolandic gyrus lesions, Broca's aphasia and, 149–150
Primary progressive aphasia (PPA), 529, 584, 584*t*
Priming, 431, 432*t*
implicit memory and, 450–451
Prion diseases, dementia in, 631–632
Procedural memory, 431, 432*t*, 463, 464*f*
following traumatic brain injury, 470
Production
of sentences, in aphasia, 173
of single words, in aphasia, 169–171
Progressive apraxia, 530
Progressive multifocal leukoencephalopathy (PML), dementia in, 631
Progressive rubella panencephalitis, dementia in, 634
Progressive supranuclear palsy (PSP)
cognitive characteristics of, 598–599
dementia in, 594*t*, 598–599
differential diagnosis of, 506*t*, 507
epidemiology of, 598
pathology of, 599
prefrontal dysfunction due to, 391
Promoting Aphasics Communicative Effectiveness (PACE), 181
Propentofylline, for Alzheimer's disease, 559–560
Propranolol, for aggression, 760*t*
Prosody, 743
affective
comprehension of, 747
hemispheric lateralization of, 748–750, 749*f*
repetition of, 746–747
spontaneous, 746
neurology of, 744
Prosopagnosia, 239–241, 246
anatomic bases of face recognition and, 240–241
functional deficit in, face-specificity of, 239–240
Prospective memory deficits, following traumatic brain injury, 470
Provoked confabulation, 363
Psychiatric disorders, nonverbal, social, and emotional learning disabilities versus, 826
Psychic paralysis of gaze, 327
Psychogenic amnesia, 434*t*
Psychometric tests, 36–37
contributions to neuropsychological examination, 36–37
scores on
application and limitations of, 37–39
cutting, 39
double dissociation method and, 39
interpretation of, 39–40
pattern analysis and, 39
selection of, 37
Psychosis
in Alzheimer's disease, treatment of, 556–557
following brain injury, 739
interictal, 681–682
treatment of, 684
in Parkinson's disease, 737
postictal, 679
treatment of, 684
in systemic lupus erythematosus, 653
Purdue Pegboard Test, 37
Pure word deafness, 257, 258*t*
in aphasia, 167–168
Wernicke's aphasia and, 151–152, 259–260
in Landau-Kleffner syndrome, 259, 260
mechanism of, 151–152

Q

Quadrantanopsia, 228

R

Radiation therapy, childhood-acquired aphasia associated with, 790
Raichle, Marcus, 17
Rapid automatized naming (RAN) tasks, in dyslexia, 803
Raven's Progressive Matrices, 37

RAVE-O program, 812
Reaching, visually guided, impaired, 296, 296*f*
Reading. *See also* Alexia; Dyslexia
  right hemisphere and, 201–202, 403
  without meaning, 200–201
Reading disorder (RD), molecular genetics of, 867–871, 873, 874–876
  behavioral genetics and, 869–870
  future directions for, 874–875
  molecular biology and, 870–871
  phenotype and, 867–869, 868*t*
Recall, in split-brain patients, 403–404
Receptive amusia, 264–265
Recognition, in split-brain patients, 403–404
Recovery
  anatomic models of, 101–102
  cognitive models of, 101–102
Recurrent networks, parallel distributed processing and, 136
Redundancy
  recovery and, 101
  vicarious, recovery and, 101–102
Reduplicative paramnesia, 355, 373, 434*t*. *See also* Misidentification syndromes
Reference frames, spatial, neglect and, 317
Rehabilitation
  of aphasia. *See* Aphasia, rehabilitation of
  of memory dysfunction, 487–490
    approaches to, 487–488
    future directions for, 490
    methods of, 488–490
Rehearsal techniques, for memory rehabilitation, 488–489
Repetition, of affective prosody, 746–747
Representational instability, in neglect, 316–317
Representational neglect, 303
  testing for, 305
Repression, organic, 355
Resolution, in lesion method, 79–80
Response inhibition, prefrontal lesions and, 394
Rete mirabile, 3–4
Reticular formation (RF), consciousness and, 337
Retrieval
  brain sites of, 438, 439*f*
  lexical, in aphasia, 170–171
  strategic, deficient, confabulation and, 367–368
  of words, disorders of. *See* Anomia
Retrograde amnesia, 434*t*
  cognitive issues in, 445–446
  in Wernicke-Korsakoff syndrome, 642
Rett's syndrome (RS), 844–845
Rheumatoid arthritis, 654*t*
Ribot, Theodule, 12
Ribot's law, 12
Right hemisphere
  control of speech and grammar in, 402–403
  damage to, unilateral neglect after, 119–123, 122*f*
  in nonverbal, social, and emotional learning disabilities, 824
  reading and, 201–202, 403
Risperidone, for dementia, 509
Rivastigmine (Exelon)
  for Alzheimer's disease, 553*t*, 553–554
  for dementia, 509
Rubenstein-Taybi syndrome (RTS), 845

S

Scalp-current density (SCD), event-related potentials and, 107, 108*f*
Scleroderma, 654*t*
Scotoma, acquired, anosognosia for, 345–347
Scoville, William, 13
β-secretase inhibitors, for Alzheimer's disease, 557
τ-secretase inhibitors, for Alzheimer's disease, 557
Seizures. *See also* Epilepsy
  in autism, 857–858
  childhood-acquired aphasia associated with, 784, 785, 786*t*–787*t*
  complex, 675–676
  lesion method for studying, 80
  simple, 675
  in systemic lupus erythematosus, 652–653
Selection hypothesis, of prefrontal function, 397
Selective muscarinic receptor agonists, for Alzheimer's disease, 554
Selective serotonin reuptake inhibitors (SSRIs), for aggression, 760*t*
Selegiline, for Alzheimer's disease, 560
Semantic dementia, 457, 584, 584*t*
Semantic errors, in deep dyslexia, 198
Semantic memory, 431, 432*t*
  in Alzheimer's disease, 574–577
  in amnesia, 446–448
  deficits in, following traumatic brain injury, 470
  episodic memory compared with, 446–447
  impairment of, 237, 457–460
    category-specific, 458–459
    generalized, 457–458
    modality-specific, 459–460
Semantic processing disorders, in aphasia, 168–169, 169*f*

Senile plaques, in Alzheimer's disease, 521*f,* 521–523, 524–526, 545–546
  biochemistry of, 546–547, 547*f*
  cell biology of, 548
  structure of, 545–546, 546*f*
Sensorimotor links, neglect and, 318
Sensory amusia, 264–265
Sensory aphasia, transcortical, 156, 156*f*
Sensory cortex, 48
Sensory examination, in children, 767–768
Sensory function, in neglect, 121
Sensory gating, prefrontal cortex and, event-related potentials for study of, 112, 113*f*
Sensory loss, anosognosia for hemiplegia and, 351
Sensory neglect, 303
  testing for, 303–304
Sensory perception, in autism, 859–860
Sentence-level processing, 171–173
  comprehension and, 171–172
  production and, 173
  short-term memory and, 172–173
Sequencing tasks, prefrontal lesions and, 393
Serotonin (5-HT)
  in Alzheimer's disease, 552*t*
  violence and, 757–758
Short-term memory, sentence-level processing and, 172–173
Shunts, in normal-pressure hydrocephalus
  choice of, 668–669
  complications of, 668
Simple confabulation, 363
Simultanagnosia, 234, 327–328
  anatomic basis of, 326*f,* 331–332, 332*f,* 333*f*
  as disengage deficit, 329–330
  dorsal, 234, 329
  as spatial registration deficit, 330
  ventral, 329
  as visual feature integration deficit, 330
  visual impairments resembling, 332–333
  as what-where binding deficit, 330–331
Single-photon emission computed tomography (SPECT), 17
Sleep disturbances
  in Alzheimer's disease, treatment of, 557
  in Parkinson's disease, 737
Sleep-wake cycle disturbances, in delirium, 497
Social cognition, deficits in, in nonverbal, social, and emotional learning disabilities, 822, 823*t,* 824
Social deficit, in autism, 855
Somatic marker hypothesis, of prefrontal function, 397
Somatosensory cortex, 271–273
  association areas of, 272*f,* 272–273, 273*t*
  degenerative diseases and, 279, 279*f*
  primary, 271–272
Somatosensory evoked potentials (SEPs), 106
Somatosensory function
  clinical laboratory assessment of, 274
  phantom sensations and, 287
  tactile perception and. *See* Tactile perception
Somatostatins, for Alzheimer's disease, 552*t,* 555
Somatotopagnosia, 289
Somesthetic function
  amnesia and, 279
  anosognosia and, asymboly for pain and, 279
  asymboly for pain and, 279
  cerebral commissurotomy and, 278–279
  tactile aphasia and, 279
Sound, auditory agnosia for, 257, 258*t,* 262–263
Spatial analogies, for understanding parallel distributed processing network behavior, 137–138
Spatial anisometry, in neglect, 316
Spatial attention, neglect and, 313–314
Spatial function. *See* Visuospatial function
Spatial neglect, 303
  differentiation from deafferentation, 309
  intentional, 303, 314
Spatial representation, neglect and, 314–315
Specimen choice, for lesion method, 80–81
Speech, auditory agnosia for. *See* Pure word deafness
Speech disturbances, with thalamic lesions, 427–428
Sperry, Roger, 14
Spinocerebellar ataxia (SCA), 601
Split-brain patients, 401–407
  divided visual fields for, anosognosia for, 347–348
  hemispheric dominance in, 404–405
    evolution of, 404
    left hemisphere as interpreter and, 404
    visuospatial functions and, 404–405
  interhemispheric integration of perception and attention and, 405–406
    hemispheric isolation of visual and tactile information and, 405, 405*f*
    sharing of attentional control and, 405–406
  language in, 402–403
    right hemisphere control of speech and grammar and, 402–403
    right hemisphere reading and, 403
  recall and recognition in, 403–404
  specificity of callosal fibers and, 406
  techniques required to demonstrate disconnection phenomena and, 401

Spontaneous confabulation, 363
Stability, developmental change versus, in pediatric neuropsychological assessment, 775–776
State of California Alzheimer's Disease Diagnostic and Treatment Centers criteria, 610, 611*t*
Statins, for Alzheimer's disease, 561
Stimulation approach to aphasia therapy, 180
Stimulation language mapping, temporal lobe epilepsy surgery and, 697
Storage, 431, 432*t*
  brain sites of, 437–438
Strategic retrieval, deficient, confabulation and, 367–368
Strengths and Difficulties Questionnaire (SDQ), 868
Striatum, anatomy of, 50
Stroke
  depression following, left frontal cortex lesions and, 728–729
  in systemic lupus erythematosus, 651–652, 652*f*
  vascular dementia and. *See* Vascular dementia
Subacute sclerosing panencephalitis (SSPE), dementia in, 633–634
Subarachnoid hemorrhage
  association with idiopathic normal-pressure hydrocephalus, 670
  vascular dementia and, 614
Superior temporal sulcus (STS), neglect and, 306–309
Supervisory attentional system (SAS), prefrontal function and, 397
Supplementary motor area (SMA), 272, 273*t*
  lesions of, ideomotor apraxia and, 220, 220*f*
Supplementary sensory area (SSA), 272, 273*t*
Supramarginal gyrus lesions, conduction aphasia and, 152, 152*f*
Surface dyslexia, 199–200
Swanson, Nolan, and Pelham (SNAP) scale, 868
Synaptic loss, in Alzheimer's disease, 527, 549–550
Syphilis, dementia in, 632–633
Systemic lupus erythematosus (SLE), 651–654, 654*t*
  cognitive decline in, 653–654
  encephalopathy in, 653
  historical background of, 651
  psychosis in, 653
  seizures in, 652–653
  stroke in, 651–652, 652*f*
  vasculitis in, 654, 654*f*

T

Tacrine (Cognex), for Alzheimer's disease, 552–553, 553*t*
Tactile agnosia, 275–278
  anatomic considerations in, 277*f*, 277–278
  behavioral considerations in, 275–277
Tactile aphasia, somesthetic results of, 279
Tactile information, hemispheric isolation of, 405, 405*f*
Tactile perception, 271–279
  cortical lesions and
    clinical somatosensory disorders resulting from, 274–279
    in degenerative diseases, 279, 279*f*
  normal somatosensory function and, 273–274
  somatosensory cortices and, 271–273
    association, 272*f*, 272–273, 273*t*
    primary, 271–272
Takayasu arteritis, 654*t*
Tau, decreasing hyperphosphorylation of, for Alzheimer's disease, 561
Template technique, 74, 76–77
  improvement on, 77, 78*f*
Temporal arteritis, 654*t*
Temporal displacement, amnesic confabulation and, 366–367
Temporal lesions
  global aphasia and, 153, 154
  of gyrus
    superior, Wernicke's aphasia and, 150–151, 151*f*
    transcortical sensory aphasia and, 156, 156*f*
Temporal lobe epilepsy, surgery for, 695–701
  intellectual function and, 696
  language function and, 696–698
  memory and, 698–701
Temporal processing, in dyslexia, 805
Temporolimbic epilepsy (TLE), 676
Temporoparietal circuit, in dyslexia, 808–809
Tests. *See* Mental status exam; Neuropsychological assessment; Psychometric tests
Thalamic lesions, 419–428, 420*t*
  diencephalic amnesia and, 425–427
    anatomic basis of, 425, 426*f*, 427
    neuropsychological features of, 427
  ideomotor apraxia and, 221
  infarctions causing, 419–424
    in anterior choroidal artery region, 424, 424*f*, 425*f*
    in geniculothalamic artery region, 419–420, 421*f*
    in interpeduncular profunda artery region, 422–424, 423*f*
    in tuberothalamic artery region, 420–422, 422*f*
  speech and language disturbances associated with, 427–428
Thalamoperforating artery region, infarctions due to thalamic lesions in, 422–424, 423*f*
Thalamus, anatomy of, 51*f*, 51–52

Theory of Mind (ToM), in nonverbal, social, and emotional learning disabilities, 822, 823*t*, 824
Thiamine deficiency, Wernicke-Korsakoff syndrome and. *See* Wernicke-Korsakoff syndrome (WKS)
Third ventriculostomy, for normal-pressure hydrocephalus, 668–669
Thought content, mental status exam and, 24–25
Thought processes, mental status exam and, 24
Todd's paralysis, 679
Topographical disorientation, 246
Transcortical motor aphasia (TCMA), 154–156, 155*f*
Transcortical sensory aphasia (TCSA), 156, 156*f*, 168–169
Transcranial electrical stimulation (TES), 124
Transcranial magnetic stimulation (TMS), 105–106, 124–127
  application of, 125–127
  plasticity studied using, 60
  technical aspects of, 125, 125*f*
Transient global amnesia, 434*t*
Traumatic brain injury. *See* Brain injury
Trazodone, for aggression, 760*t*
Tuberothalamic artery region, infarctions due to thalamic lesions in, 420–422, 422*f*
Tufted astrocytes, 530
Tumors
  aphasia due to, 159
  childhood-acquired aphasia associated with, 785, 790, 791*t*–792*t*
  prefrontal dysfunction due to, 388, 389*f*
Turner syndrome, 847–848
  dyscalculia in, 211
Two cortical visual systems, 230, 230*f*

U

Uniparental disomy (UPD), 847
Unmasking, 59
  recovery and, 101

V

Valproic acid (VPA), for aggression, 760*t*
Vanishing cues, for memory rehabilitation, 489
Vascular cognitive impairment (VCI), 614–615
Vascular dementia, 609–620
  Alzheimer's disease contrasted with, 615–616
  aphasia due to, 159–160
  atrophy in, 613–614
  behavioral changes in, 616–617
  cognitive deficit pattern in, 610, 612
  criteria for, 609–615
    limitations of, 610, 612–614
    new concept for, 614–615
    NINDS-AIREN, 610, 612*t*
    of State of California Alzheimer's Disease Diagnostic and Treatment Centers, 610, 611*t*
  differential diagnosis of, 506*t*, 507, 618
  epidemiology of, 617
  infarct site in, 612
  infarct volume in, 612
  intracerebral hemorrhage and, 614
  investigation of, 618–619
  leukoaraiosis and, 613
  major stroke and, 614
  mechanism of cognitive impairment in, 615
  mixed dementia and, 614
  poststroke dementia and, 614
  prevention of, 619
  prognosis of, 620
  risk factors for, 617–618
  severity of, 612
  subarachnoid hemorrhage and, 614
  subcortical, 613
    differential diagnosis of, 506*t*, 507–508
  treatment of, 619
  types of, 612–613
Vascular disorders, childhood-acquired aphasia associated with, 785, 788*t*
Vasculitis, in systemic lupus erythematosus, 654, 654*f*
Vegetative state (VS), 339–340
  diagnostic criteria for, 339
  permanent, 339–340
  persistent, 339
  prognosis and outcome of, 339–340
Ventral left hemisphere systems, in dyslexia, 808, 809
Ventral simultanagnosia, 234–235, 329
Ventriculostomy, third, for normal-pressure hydrocephalus, 668–669
Ventrolateral somatosensory accessory cortex, 272, 273*t*
  tactile agnosia and, 272, 273*t*
    behavioral considerations in, 275–277
Ventroposterolateral (VPL) thalamic nucleus, damage to, 419
Ventroposteromedial (VPM) thalamic nucleus, damage to, 419
Veridical completion, in anosognosia, 348
Vicarious redundancy, recovery and, 101–102
Violence, 755–760. *See also* Aggression
  in dementia, 755
  differential diagnosis of, 756
  in epilepsy, 755
  evaluation of, 756

kindling and, 758
medication-related, 756
with mental retardation, 756
neuroanatomy of, 756–757
neurochemistry of, 757–758
psychosocial aspects of, 756
with traumatic brain injury, 755
treatment of, 758–759, 760*t*
Visible space, visuospatial disorders and, 295–298
impaired attention to space and, 295
impaired perception of location and orientation and, 295–296
impaired visually guided reaching and, 296, 296*f*
Visual agnosia, 246
Visual cortex
primary, lesions of, 227–228, 228*f*
with transcranial magnetic stimulation, 126–127
Visual defects, anosognosia for, 345–349
for acquired scotoma and hemianopias, 345–347
for blindness, 348–349
for blind spot, 345
for divided visual fields in split-brain patients, 347–348
neuropathologic features of Anton's syndrome and, 349
Visual disorientation, 295–296
Visual evoked responses (VERs), 106
in neglect, 121–122
Visual fields, divided, in split-brain patients, anosognosia for, 347–348
Visual impairments, simultanagnosia-like, 332–333
Visual information, hemispheric isolation of, 405, 405*f*
Visually guided reaching, impaired, 296, 296*f*
Visual mental imagery, 230–232
image generation disorders and, 232
image representation disorders and, 231*f*, 231–232
Visual object agnosia, 233–237, 246
apperceptive, 233–235
behavior and anatomy of, 233–234, 234*f*
interpretation of, 234
relation to other disorders, 234–235
associative, 235–237
behavior anorexia nervosa anatomy of, 235*f*, 235–236
interpretation of, 236–237
relation to other disorders, 237
Visual orientation, disturbances of, 328–332
Visual perception, 227–230
association cortex lesions and, 228–230
organizing framework for higher-level disorders of, 230, 230*f*
phantom sensations and, 287
primary visual cortex and afferent lesions and, 227–228, 228*f*
Visual processing
in dyslexia, 804–805
levels of, in neglect, 318–319
Visuospatial function, 295–299
environmental space and, 298–299, 299*f*
left hemispheric dominance and, 404–405
mental status exam and, 28–29, 29*f*
visible space and, 295–298
impaired attention to space and, 295
impaired construction and, 296–298, 297*f*
impaired perception of location and orientation and, 295–296
impaired visually guided reaching and, 296, 296*f*
Vitamin C, for Alzheimer's disease, 560
Vitamin E, for Alzheimer's disease, 509, 560
Vogt, Cécile, 12
Vogt, Oskar, 12
Von Haller, Albrecht, 4

W

Wada testing
of language function, temporal lobe epilepsy surgery and, 697–698
of memory, temporal lobe epilepsy surgery and, 700–701
Wandering, in Alzheimer's disease, treatment of, 557
Wechsler Intelligence Scales (WIS), 37
applications and limitations of, 38
Wegener's granulomatosis, 654*t*, 655
Weight space, parallel distributed processing networks and, 138
Wernicke, Carl, 9*f*, 9–10
Wernicke-Korsakoff syndrome (WKS), 639–644
anterograde amnesia in, 641–642
cognitive status in, 640*t*, 640–641
confabulation in. *See* Confabulation, amnesic
etiology of, 642–643
neuropathologic findings in, 643–644, 644*f*
retrograde amnesia in, 642
Wernicke's aphasia, 150–152, 151*f*
fractional syndromes of, 150
linguistic processing in, event-related potentials for study of, 123–124
pure word deafness in, 151–152, 259–260
Whipple's disease, dementia in, 633
White matter lesions, in normal-pressure hydrocephalus, 662, 664
Wholism/localism debate, 5–9, 6*f*–8*f*
Williams' syndrome (WS), 848–849
Wilson's disease, childhood-acquired aphasia associated with, 792

Wisconsin Card Sorting Test (WCST), of prefrontal function, 394
WIST (Word Identification Strategy Training) Program, 810–811
Word-meaning deafness, in aphasia, 168
Word recognition, in dyslexia, 802
Word retrieval disorders. *See* Anomia
Working memory (WM), 464
  prefrontal function and, 397–398

X

X-linked, nonsyndromic mental retardation (XMR), 845–846